ALL-IN-ONE

NURSING CARE PLANNING RESOURCE

Medical-Surgical, Pediatric, Maternity, and Psychiatric-Mental Health

ALL-IN-ONE

NURSING CARE PLANNING RESOURCE

Medical-Surgical, Pediatric, Maternity, and Psychiatric-Mental Health

4e

Pamela L. Swearingen, RN
Special Project Editor

ELSEVIER

ELSEVIER

3251 Riverport Lane
St. Louis, Missouri 63043

ALL-IN-ONE NURSING CARE PLANNING RESOURCE,   ISBN: 978-0-323-26286-6
FOURTH EDITION

Copyright © 2016 by Mosby, an imprint of Elsevier Inc.
Copyright © 2012, 2008, 2004 by Mosby, Inc., an affiliate of Elsevier Inc.

All rights reserved. No part of this publication may be reproduced or transmitted in any form or by any means, electronic or mechanical, including photocopying, recording, or any information storage and retrieval system, without permission in writing from the publisher. Details on how to seek permission, further information about the Publisher's permissions policies and our arrangements with organizations such as the Copyright Clearance Center and the Copyright Licensing Agency, can be found at our website: www.elsevier.com/permissions.

This book and the individual contributions contained in it are protected under copyright by the Publisher (other than as may be noted herein).

Notices

Knowledge and best practice in this field are constantly changing. As new research and experience broaden our understanding, changes in research methods, professional practices, or medical treatment may become necessary.

Practitioners and researchers must always rely on their own experience and knowledge in evaluating and using any information, methods, compounds, or experiments described herein. In using such information or methods they should be mindful of their own safety and the safety of others, including parties for whom they have a professional responsibility.

With respect to any drug or pharmaceutical products identified, readers are advised to check the most current information provided (i) on procedures featured or (ii) by the manufacturer of each product to be administered, to verify the recommended dose or formula, the method and duration of administration, and contraindications. It is the responsibility of practitioners, relying on their own experience and knowledge of their patients, to make diagnoses, to determine dosages and the best treatment for each individual patient, and to take all appropriate safety precautions.

To the fullest extent of the law, neither the Publisher nor the authors, contributors, or editors, assume any liability for any injury and/or damage to persons or property as a matter of products liability, negligence or otherwise, or from any use or operation of any methods, products, instructions, or ideas contained in the material herein.

Library of Congress Cataloging-in-Publication Data

All-in-one nursing care planning resource : medical-surgical, pediatric, maternity, psychiatric nursing care plans / Pamela L. Swearingen, special project editor. – 4th edition.
    p. ; cm.
  Includes bibliographical references and index.
  ISBN 978-0-323-26286-6
  I. Swearingen, Pamela L., editor.
  [DNLM: 1. Nursing Process–organization & administration.   2. Nursing Care–methods.
3. Patient Care Planning.   WY 100.1]
  RT49
  610.73–dc23
                                                         2014043475

Executive Content Strategist: Lee Henderson
Content Development Manager: Billie Sharp
Content Development Specialist: Charlene Ketchum
Publishing Services Manager: Hemamalini Rajendrababu
Project Manager: Maria Bernard
Design Direction: Ashley Miner

Printed in Canada

Last digit is the print number: 9 8 7 6 5 4 3 2 1

Working together to grow libraries in developing countries
www.elsevier.com • www.bookaid.org

Dedication

To the memory of Carol Monlux Swift, RN, BSN, CNRN,
whose integrity, talent, and dedication to
the nursing profession live on.

Contributors

MEDICAL-SURGICAL NURSING CARE PLANS

Lolita M. Adrien-Dunlap, RN, MS, CNS, CWON
Professor of Nursing, Retired
Contra Costa College
San Pablo, California
Contributed care plans for Crohn's Disease, Fecal Diversions, and Ulcerative Colitis.

Marianne Baird, RN, MN
Clinical Nurse Specialist
Magnet Program Director
Saint Joseph's Hospital of Atlanta
Atlanta, Georgia
Contributed Endocrine Care Plans.

Lynda K. Ball, RN, MSN, CNN
Quality Improvement Coordinator
Northwest Renal Network
Seattle, Washington
Contributed care plan for Care of the Renal Transplant Recipient.

Barbara S. Bishop, MS, ANP-BC, MSCN, CNRN
Nurse Practitioner, Adult Neurology and Multiple Sclerosis Specialist
Virginia Beach Neurology
Virginia Beach, Virginia
Contributed care plans for Neurologic Care Plans.

Maureen Bel Boardman, MSN, APRN-BC
Instructor
Dartmouth Medical School
Hanover, New Hampshire
Contributed care plans for Pneumonia and Respiratory Failure, Acute.

Jenny Bosley, RN, MS, CEN
Nursing Clinical Adjunct Faculty
Thomas Jefferson University
Philadelphia, Pennsylvania
Contributed care plans for Cholelithiasis, Cholecystitis and Cholangitis and Cirrhosis.

Michelle T. Bott, RN, MN
Senior Director, Patient Care Services
Guelph General Hospital
Guelph, Ontario, Canada
Contributed care plans for Acute Renal Failure, Chronic Kidney Disease, Care of the Patient Undergoing Hemodialysis, Care of the Patient Undergoing Peritoneal Dialysis, and Laboratory Tests: Reference Ranges for Adult Patients appendix.

Michael W. Day, RN, MSN CCRN
Trauma Care Coordinator
Providence Sacred Heart Medical Center & Children's Hospital
Spokane, Washington
Contributed care plan for COPD.

Vicki Good, MSN, RN, CENP, CPPS
Practitioner
System Director Clinical Safety
Cox Health
Springfield, Missouri
Contributed care plan for Pulmonary Tuberculosis.

R. Mark Hovis, CRNA
Nurse Anesthetist
Washington University School of Medicine
St. Louis, Missouri
Contributed care plan for Perioperative Care.

Patricia Jansen, RN, MSN, CNS, GCS-BC, OCN
Medical Surgical Clinical Nurse Specialist
Regional Medical Center of San Jose
San Jose, California
Contributed care plans for Benign Prostatic Hypertrophy, Older Adult Care, Ureteral Calculi, Urinary Diversions, and Urinary Tract Obstruction.

Suzanne Jed, MSN, FNP-BC
Instructor of Clinical Family Medicine
Pacific AIDS Education and Training Center
Keck School of Medicine
University of Southern California
Los Angeles, California
Contributed care plan for Caring for Individuals with Human Immunodeficiency Virus and Infection Prevention and Control appendix.

Kim Kuebler, DNP, APRN, ANP-BC
Associate Professor
South University
Savannah, Georgia
Contributed care plan for Palliative and End-of-Life Care.

Charlene Warren Myers
Associate Professor
University of South Alabama
Mobile, Alabama
Contributed care plans for Hepatitis, Pancreatitis, and Peritonitis

Misty Kirby-Nolan, MSN, APN-CNP
Nurse Practitioner
Northwestern Memorial Hospital
Adjunct Faculty
Saint Xavier University
Chicago, Illinois
Contributed care plan for Pain.

Ann Will Poteet, MS, RN, CCNS
Graduate Clinical Placements
Office of Academic Programs
University of Colorado, College of Nursing
Aurora, Colorado
Contributed care plans for Pneunothorax/Hemothorax and Pulmonary Embolus.

Barbara D. Powe, RN, PhD
Director, Underserved Populations Research
American Cancer Society
Atlanta, Georgia
Contributed care plan for Cancer Care, Psychosocial Support, and Psychosocial Support of the Patient's Family and Significant Other.

Dottie Roberts, RN, MSN, MACI, CMSRN, OCNS-C®
Nursing Instructor
South University
Clinical Nurse Specialist
Palmetto Health Baptist
Columbia, South Carolina
Contributed Musculoskeletal Care Plans.

Sandra Rome, RN, MN, AOCN
Hematology/Oncology Clinical Nurse Specialist
Cedars-Sinai Medical Center
Assistant Clinical Professor, UCLA School of Nursing
Los Angeles, California
Contributed Hematologic Care Plans.

Laura Steadman, EdD
Associate Professor of Nursing
University of Alabama
Birmingham, Alabama
Contributed care plan for Prolonged Bedrest.

Nancy A. Stotts, EdD, RN, FAAN
Professor Emeritus
University of California, San Francisco
San Francisco, California
Contributed care plan for Managing Wound Care.

Beth Taylor, RD, MS, CNSD, FCCM
Nutrition Support Specialist
Barnes-Jewish Hospital
St. Louis, Missouri
Contributed care plan for Providing Nutritional Support.

Mary E. Young, APRN, MSN, BC
Adult Nurse Practitioner
Assistant Dean and Director of Nursing and Allied Health
Hartnell College
Salinas, California
Contributed care plan for Abdominal Trauma and Cardiovascular Care Plans.

PEDIATRIC NURSING CARE PLANS

Sherry D. Ferki, RN, MSN
Adjunct Faculty
Old Dominion University, School of Nursing
Norfolk, Virginia
Contributed Pediatric Care Plans and Laboratory Tests: Reference Ranges for Pediatric Patients appendix.

MATERNITY NURSING CARE PLANS

Jacqueline Wright, RNC-OB, MSN, C-EFM, IBCLC
Professor of Nursing-Maternity
Contra Costa College
San Pablo, California

PSYCHIATRIC CARE PLANS

Donna Rolin-Kenny
Assistant Professor
Family Psychiatric Mental Health Nurse Practitioner Program
University of Texas at Austin School of Nursing
Austin, Texas
Contributed care plans for Dementia-Alzheimer's Type and Substance-Related and Addictive Disorders.

Anthony Steele, DNP, FNP-C, PMHNP-C
Director of Medical Services
Alcohol and Drug Services
Greensboro, North Carolina
Contributed care plans for Bipolar Disorder (Manic Component) and Schizophrenia.

Sylvia Rae Stevens, PhD APRN-BC
Professor
Montgomery College
Takoma Park/Silver Spring, Maryland
Contributed care plans for Anxiety Disorders and Major Depression.

Reviewers

Catherine Corrigan, APRN, MSN, BC
Assistant Professor
University of Detroit Mercy
Detroit, Michigan

Terry Delpier, RN, DNP, CPNP
Professor of Nursing
Northern Michigan University
Marquette, Michigan

Angela DiSabatino, RN, MS
Manager, Cardiovascular Clinical Trials
Center for Heart and Vascular Health
Christiana Care Health System
Newark, Delaware
Adjunct Nursing Faculty
Wilmington University
Wilmington, Delaware

Jennifer Duhon, RN, MS
Public Health Nurse
Peoria City/County Health Department
Peoria, Illinois

Jean Gash, APRN, PhD, BC
Assistant Professor
University of Detroit Mercy
Detroit, Michigan

Susan J. Grant, MSN, MS, APN, FNP-BC
Clinical Instructor
Family Nurse Practitioner
College of Nursing
University of Arkansas for Medical Sciences
Fayetteville, Arkansas

Leanna Kinney, RN
Director of Nursing
Pediatric Home Health Care
Epic MedStaff Services, Inc.
San Antonio, Texas

Margaret Malone, RN, MN, CCRN
Clinical Nurse Specialist
Critical Care and Cardiology
St. John Medical Center
Longview, Washington

Joyce Marrs, MS, FNP-BC, AOCNP
Nurse Practitioner
Hematology and Oncology
Dayton Physicians
Dayton, Ohio

Charles Preston Molsbee, MSN, RN, CNE
Assistant Professor
Nursing
University of Arkansas at Little Rock
Little Rock, Arkansas

Gina M. Newman, RN
Infection Preventionist
Infection Prevention and Clinical Epidemiology
Sharp Memorial Hospital
San Diego, California

Casey Norris, BSN, MSN, PCNS, BC
Pulmonary Clinical Specialist
East Tennessee Children's Hospital
Knoxville, Tennessee

Harriett Pitt, RN, MS, CIC
Infection Preventionist
President
EPIC Management Group, Inc.
Mount St. Mary School of Nursing
Adjunct Professor
Healthcare Epidemiology
Los Angeles, California

Mary Rodts, DNP, CNP, ONC, FAAN
Associate Professor
Rush College of Nursing
Chicago, Illinois

Richard J. Slote, RN, MS, ONC, RNC
Clinical Nurse II
Hospital for Special Surgery
New York, New York

Jessica Gaither Vandett, RN, MSN, ARNP, FNP-C
Assistant Professor
Department of Nursing
University of Arkansas at Little Rock
Little Rock, Arkansas

Kathleen S. Whalen, RN, PhD
Assistant Professor of Nursing
Loretto Heights School of Nursing
Regis University
Denver, Colorado

Alan H.B. Wu, PhD, DABCC
Professor
Laboratory Medicine
University of California San Francisco
San Francisco, California

Marge Zerbe, RN, BS
Consultant and Education
Noelle Project
Gaumard Scientific, Inc.
Miami, Florida
Adjunct Faculty
Lake Sumter Community College
Leesburg, Florida

All-in-One Nursing Care Planning Resource is a one-of-a-kind book featuring nursing care plans for all four core clinical areas. The inclusion of pediatric, maternity, and psychiatric-mental health nursing in addition to medical-surgical nursing care plans enables students to use one book throughout the entire nursing curriculum. This unique presentation—combined with solid content, an open and accessible format, and clinically relevant features—makes this a must-have care plans book for nursing students.

ORGANIZATION

This book is organized into four separate sections for medical-surgical, pediatric, maternal, and psychiatric-mental health care plans. Within each section, care plans are listed alphabetically by disorder or condition (the medical-surgical nursing care plans are organized alphabetically within each body system). General information that applies to more than one disorder can be found in the *General Care Plans* section, where nursing diagnoses and interventions for perioperative care, pain, prolonged bedrest, cancer care, psychosocial support for patients, psychosocial support for the patient's family and significant others, older adult care, and palliative/end-of-life care are discussed.

Each disorder uses the following consistent format:

- **Overview/Pathophysiology,** which includes a synopsis of the disorder and its pathophysiology, where appropriate
- **Health Care Setting,** such as hospital, primary, community, or long-term care
- **Assessment,** covering signs and symptoms and physical assessment
- **Diagnostic Tests**
- **Nursing Diagnoses with Desired Outcomes**
- **Assessment/Interventions and Rationales** in a clear, two-column format
- **Patient-Family Teaching and Discharge Planning**

This book is organized to provide the most important information related to various disorders. By providing a consistent format for each disorder, key information that a nurse needs to know is fully covered. For example, the rationales given for the interventions are supported by supplemental information provided in the "Overview/Pathophysiology" and "Assessment" sections.

FEATURES

The care plans in this book were written by clinical experts in each subject area to ensure the most current and accurate information. In addition to reliable content, the book offers the following special features:

- A **consistent, easy-to-use format** facilitates quick and easy retrieval of information.
- The **Health Care Setting** is specified for each care plan, because these conditions are treated in various settings such as hospital, primary care, long-term care facility, community, and home care.
- **Outcome criteria with specific timelines** assist in setting realistic goals for nursing outcomes and providing quality, cost-effective care.
- **Detailed, specific rationales** for each nursing intervention apply concepts to clinical practice.
- The **Patient-Family Teaching and Discharge Planning** section highlights key patient education topics, as well as resources for further information.
- The newest **NANDA-International** nursing diagnoses are included in each care plan.
- Separate care plans on **Pain** and **End-of-Life Care** focus on palliative care for patients with terminal illnesses, as well as relief of acute and chronic pain.
- **Current care and patient safety standards and clinical practice guidelines** in nursing and other health care disciplines are incorporated throughout the interventions and rationales.
- **Infection prevention and control guidelines** from the Centers for Disease Control and Prevention (CDC) are included in the appendix.
- **Normal laboratory values for adults** are listed in Appendix B, including separate tables for Complete Blood Count; Serum, Plasma, and Whole Blood Chemistry; and Urine Chemistry. **Normal laboratory values for pediatric patients** are included in Appendix C.

New to this edition are:

- A special index that lists all the nursing diagnoses used in this book along with their descriptive data and page numbers.
- **Safety alert icons** that alert nurses to interventions that necessitate special attention and care.
- **Complimentary and Alternative Therapies icons** that alert nurses to supplements that patients may be using and how they can interact with conventional medication.
- **Canadian Resources icons** that alert Canadian nurses to especially relevant references and journals.
- A new care plan for **Normal Labor and Birth**.

This book was carefully prepared to meet the needs of today's busy nursing student. We welcome comments on how we can enhance its usefulness in subsequent editions.

Pamela L. Swearingen

Contents

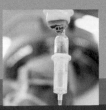

Cancer Care 1

OVERVIEW/PATHOPHYSIOLOGY

The term *cancer* refers to several disease entities, all of which have in common the proliferation of abnormal cells. To varying degrees, these cells have lost their ability to reproduce in an organized fashion, function normally, and die a natural death (apoptosis). As a result they may develop new functions not characteristic of their site of origin, spread and invade uncontrollably (metastasize), and cause dysfunction and death of other cells.

Cancer is the second leading cause of death in the United States after cardiac disease, accounting for nearly 1 of every 4 deaths (American Cancer Society, 2013b). It can cause damage and dysfunction at the site of origin, regionally, or metastasize and cause problems at more distant body sites. Eventually a malignancy may cause irreversible systemic damage and failure, resulting in death. Although the exact cause of many cancers remains unclear, cancers caused by cigarette smoking and heavy alcohol use could be prevented completely. The American Cancer Society (ACS) (American Cancer Society, 2013b) estimated that about 174,000 cancer deaths would be related to tobacco use and that about one fourth to one third of new cancer cases expected in the United States in 2013 would be related to overweight, obesity, physical inactivity, and poor nutrition, all of which are preventable (World Cancer Research Fund International, 2013). Certain cancers that are related to infectious agents such as human papillomavirus (HPV), hepatitis B virus (HBV), hepatitis C virus (HCV), human immunodeficiency virus (HIV), and *Helicobacter pylori (H. pylori)* could be prevented through behavioral changes, vaccines, or antibiotics. More than 2 million skin cancers are diagnosed annually. These could be prevented by protecting the skin from excessive sun exposure and avoiding indoor tanning (American Cancer Society, 2013b; World Cancer Research Fund International, 2013).

Early detection of cancer usually results in less extensive treatment and better outcomes. Regular screening has been shown to reduce mortality rate in cancers of the breast, colon, rectum, and cervix (American Cancer Society, 2013b). The 5-year relative survival rate for all cancers diagnosed between 2002 and 2008 is 68%, which is an increase from the 49% rate during the years 1975-1977 (American Cancer Society, 2013b). As of January 2012, there were an estimated 13.7 million cancer survivors in the United States with 59% of these being 65 years of age or older. Among survivors, the most common cancer sites include the female breast (22%), prostate (20%), colorectal (9%), and gynecologic (8%) (National Cancer Institute, 2013a).

HEALTH CARE SETTING

Medical or surgical floor in acute care; primary care, hospice, home care, long-term care

CARE OF PATIENTS WITH CANCER

Lung cancer

Lung cancer is the most common cause of cancer death among men and women in the United States, accounting for about 14% of all cancer diagnoses (American Cancer Society, 2013b). An estimated 159,480 deaths from lung cancer were expected in 2013, accounting for about 27% of all cancer deaths. Both incidence and death rates from lung cancer began declining for men over the past two decades, but these rates did not start declining for women until the mid-2000s (American Cancer Society, 2013b). The primary risk factor for lung cancer is cigarette smoking, and the risk increases with the amount and length of time someone smokes. Cigarette smoking is estimated to be responsible for 85% of all lung cancers (World Cancer Research Fund International, 2013). Despite treatment advances in surgery, chemotherapy, and radiation therapy, the cure rate remains low. Although exposure to known carcinogens such as second-hand smoke, radon, arsenic, asbestos, and air pollution (to name a few) may cause lung cancer, the single most important risk factor for lung cancer is smoking (National Cancer Institute, 2013).

Most cases of lung cancer are classified as small cell or non–small cell, but a small portion of lung cancer cases are mesotheliomas, bronchial gland tumors, or carcinoids. The cell type, diagnosed via biopsy and pathologic staging, determines the appropriate treatment. Because the disease has usually spread by the time it is diagnosed, chemotherapy and radiation are often used, sometimes in combination with surgery. The 1-year survival rate for lung cancer increased from 37% (1975-1979) to 44% (2005-2008); however, the 5-year survival rate for all stages of lung cancer combined is only 16% (American Cancer Society, 2013b). For patients with advanced disease for whom cure is not foreseen, palliative care (see p. 103) should be initiated concurrently with other treatment modalities but actually may be the only truly appropriate treatment course.

Screening: Annual screening with chest x-ray has not been shown to reduce lung cancer mortality. The National Lung Screening Trial (NLST), a clinical trial designed to determine the effectiveness of lung cancer screening in high-risk individuals, showed 20% fewer lung cancer deaths among current and former heavy smokers who were screened with spiral CT compared to standard chest x-ray (National Lung Screening Trial Research Team, 2011). Findings from this trial may not be applicable to everyone because these study participants had a history of smoking (about a pack of cigarettes per day for 30 years), so it is unclear whether those who have smoked less would show the same benefit (American Cancer Society, 2013b). Current lung cancer screening recommendations encourage shared decision making with the clinician in the use of spiral CT for patients who meet the same criteria as those in the NLST (American Cancer Society, 2013b).

See also: Chapter 3, "Perioperative Care," for appropriate nursing diagnoses, outcomes, and interventions, p. 45; and **Activity Intolerance**, p. 18, in this section.

Nervous system tumors

These tumors may be primary or secondary tumors of the central nervous system (CNS), which includes the brain and spinal cord. They are classified according to their cell of origin and graded according to their malignant behavior. Although histologically the tumor may be benign, the enclosed nature of the CNS may result in tumor effects causing significant damage or even death. The National Cancer Institute (NCI) estimated 22,910 new cases of primary malignant brain and central nervous system (CNS) tumors would be diagnosed in the United States in 2012. Among children, brain tumors are the most frequent cause of solid tumor cancer–related deaths. Incidence and mortality rates are highest among whites and men (National Cancer Institute, 2013f). Among children, there has been a slight rise in incidence and a decrease in mortality in the past 30 years (National Cancer Institute, 2013f).

There are relatively few known risk factors for brain and CNS cancers. Patients with exposure to radiation and vinyl chloride and those with certain genetic syndromes may be at higher risk. The primary CNS tumor may be diagnosed because of symptoms related to changes in functions of neurons, spinal cord or brain compression, or symptoms resulting from obstruction of the flow of cerebrospinal fluid (e.g., increased intracranial pressure). Surgery, radiation, and chemotherapy are commonly used treatments, while biologic therapy and hyperthermia therapy are being explored through clinical trials.

Screening: Currently there are no recommendations for screening for CNS tumors.

See also: Chapter 3, "Perioperative Care" for appropriate nursing diagnoses, outcomes, and interventions, p. 45, and Chapter 43, "Traumatic Brain Injury," **Deficient Knowledge: Craniotomy Procedure**, p. 346.

Gastrointestinal malignancies

Malignancies of the gastrointestinal (GI) system include carcinomas of the stomach, esophagus, bowel, anus, rectum, pancreas, liver, and gallbladder. Each disease site has its own staging criteria and prognostic factors. Most early stage tumors of all sites are surgically treated. Many treatment plans now begin with preoperative chemotherapy and/or concurrent radiation therapy in the weeks preceding surgery. This approach may eliminate the need for extensive surgeries, increase the chances for cure, or in the case of anorectal sparing approach, eliminate the necessity for a colostomy. Radiation therapy treatments are less common in gastric, colon, and liver tumors due to the toxicities associated with radiating these areas.

Screening: Currently the colon and rectum (colorectal) is the only GI site with recommended screening parameters. Colorectal cancer is the third most common cancer in men and women. It is estimated that 102,480 cases of colon and 40,340 cases of rectal cancer would be diagnosed in 2013 (American Cancer Society, 2013b). In 2008, ACS (American Cancer Society, 2013c) along with other organizations released update colorectal cancer screening guidelines. The guidelines make a clear distinction between screening tests that primarily detect cancer (stool tests) and those that are more likely to detect cancer and/or precancerous growths (i.e., flexible sigmoidoscopy, colonoscopy, double contrast barium enema, CT colonography). There is also emphasis on prevention of colorectal cancer. The ACS recommends routine screening for average risk individuals begin at age 50. Currently, there are several screening options. The nurse should explain the benefits and limitations of each these methods to the patient: (1) fecal occult blood test (FOBT) annually, (2) flexible sigmoidoscopy every 5 years, (3) colonoscopy every 10 years, (4) double-contrast barium enema every 5 years; (5) computed tomographic colonography (virtual colonoscopy) every 5 years; or (6) stool DNA test (recommended interval is unknown). When family history includes first-degree relatives with colorectal cancer or an individual has certain other medical conditions, screening should begin earlier than age 50.

See also: Chapter 3, "Perioperative Care," p. 45; Chapter 56, "Fecal Diversions," p. 429; and Chapter 73, "Managing Wound Care," p. 533; for appropriate nursing diagnoses, outcomes, and interventions.

RECOMMENDATIONS FOR COLORECTAL CANCER PREVENTION

- Have regular screening
- Maintain healthy weight
- Adopt a physically activity lifestyle
- Consume a healthy diet
- Limit alcohol

Neoplastic diseases of the hematopoietic system

Hematopoietic system cancers include lymphomas, leukemias, plasma cell disorders, and myeloproliferative disorders.

Lymphomas, including Hodgkin lymphoma and non-Hodgkin lymphoma (NHL) represent about 5% of all cancers in the United States. Lymphomas are characterized by abnormal proliferation of lymphocytes. In addition to characteristic lymph node enlargement, involvement of other lymphoid organs such as the liver, spleen, and bone marrow occurs. Due to improved treatments, the mortality rates associated with Hodgkin lymphoma have decreased by nearly 50% over the past 25 years. Incidence rates for NHL have increased over the past three decades but have remained stable since 2004; however, the mortality rate has declined since 1997 (National Cancer Institute, 2013h). Risk factors for both Hodgkin lymphoma and NHL include the presence of the HIV, Epstein-Barr virus, *H. pylori,* certain genetic immune disorders, or the human T-cell leukemia/lymphoma virus type 1 (HTLV-1) (National Cancer Institute, 2013h). The most common treatments are chemotherapy, targeted therapy, and watchful waiting.

Screening: Currently there is no routine screening recommended for the lymphomas.

Leukemia, the most common blood cancer, is the abnormal proliferation and accumulation of white blood cells (WBCs). Approximately 10 times more adults than children have leukemia, but leukemia is the most common cancer among children (National Cancer Institute, 2013g). Divided into two categories, leukemia presents as either acute or chronic, depending on cellular characteristics. In both types of leukemia, abnormal cells may interfere with normal production of other WBCs, red blood cells (RBCs), and platelets. Patients with chronic lymphocytic leukemia may have compromised immunity, resulting in frequent and possibly fatal infections. The four major types of leukemia include acute lymphocytic leukemia (also called *acute lymphoblastic leukemia, ALL*), chronic lymphocytic leukemia (CLL), acute myelogenous leukemia (AML), and chronic myelogenous leukemia (CML). Diagnosis usually occurs when the presenting symptoms include fever, malaise, bruising or bleeding, infections, adenopathy, hepatosplenomegaly, weight loss, or night sweats but may also be initially noted on routine complete blood count (CBC). Diagnosis is confirmed with a CBC and peripheral smear and by bone marrow biopsy. Depending on the type of leukemia, standard treatments include watchful waiting, chemotherapy, targeted therapy, biologic therapy, radiation therapy, donor lymphocyte infusion, and chemotherapy with stem cell transplant (National Cancer Institute, 2013g).

Screening: No screening recommendations currently exist for leukemia.

See also: Section 8, "Hematologic Care Plans," p. 468 for appropriate nursing diagnoses, outcomes, and interventions related to care of patients with abnormal blood cells.

Head and neck cancers

Head and neck cancers include tumors of the tonsils, larynx, pharynx, tongue, and oral cavity. Incidence is greatest in men older than age 50, and incidence rates are double in men compared to women. By far the greatest risk factors are tobacco consumption through smoking or smokeless tobacco and alcohol consumption. However, infection with cancer-causing HPV, especially HPV-16, is a risk factor for some types of head and neck cancers, particularly oropharyngeal cancers that involve the tonsils or the base of the tongue. In fact, the incidence of oropharyngeal cancers caused by HPV infection is increasing in the United States, while the incidence of oropharyngeal cancers related to other causes is decreasing (Adelstein et al., 2009; Chaturvedi et al., 2011; National Cancer Institute, 2013).

Screening: Although no formal recommendations regarding screening exist, routine dental examinations are one mechanism by which early detection occurs.

See also: Chapter 10, "Pneumonia," p. 119, **Ineffective Airway Clearance** for outcomes and interventions.

Breast cancer

With the exception of skin cancer, breast cancer is the most commonly occurring cancer in women, accounting for one in three cancer diagnoses (American Cancer Society, 2013a). Although Caucasian women have higher incidence rates, African American women have higher mortality rates associated with breast cancer (American Cancer Society, 2013a). Most women with breast cancer will have some type of surgery. Surgery is often combined with other treatments such as radiation therapy, chemotherapy, hormone therapy, and/or targeted therapy. The 5-year relative survival rate is lower among women diagnosed with breast cancer before age 40 (84%) compared to women diagnosed at 40 years of age or older (90%). This may be due to tumors diagnosed in younger women being more aggressive and/or less responsive to treatment (American Cancer Society, 2013a).

Screening: While there are clear similarities in screening recommendations across various agencies, there are also subtle differences. The United States Preventive Services Task Force (USPSTF) recommends biennial screening mammography for women ages 50 to 74 years and recommends against monthly breast self-examination (BSE) (U.S. Preventive Services Task Force, 2013). For women with average risk who are asymptomatic, the American Cancer Society (ACS) recommends clinical breast examinations (CBE) every 3 years for women ages 20 to 39. For women over age 40, ACS recommends annual mammogram and annual CBE. Women at higher risk for developing breast cancer may need to begin mammography before age 40. Women should be told about the benefits and limitations of BSE with the emphasis on breast self-awareness.

See also: Chapter 3, "Perioperative Care," p. 45, for appropriate nursing diagnoses, outcomes, and interventions; and **Risk for Disuse Syndrome**, p. 13, in this chapter.

Genitourinary cancers

For both men and women, genitourinary cancers include cancers of the bladder, kidney (renal cell), renal pelvis, ureter, and urethra and Wilms tumor and other childhood kidney tumors. Additional sites for men include the penis, prostate, and testicle. Sites of neoplasms of the female pelvis include the vulva, vagina, cervix, uterus, and ovaries. Selected cancers are briefly summarized in the following.

Bladder cancer: Incidence is much higher in Caucasians than in African Americans but mortality rates are only slightly higher due primarily to the later stage of diagnosis in African Americans. Smoking is the primary risk factor for bladder cancer. Standard treatment includes surgery, radiation, chemotherapy, and biologic therapy (National Cancer Institute, 2013e).

Screening: No standards currently exist for screening for bladder cancer; however, survival may depend on prompt evaluation of early symptoms.

Prostate cancer occurs most commonly in men older than age 50. More than 60% of all prostate cancer cases are diagnosed in men aged 65 and older, and 97% of all prostate cancers occur in men aged 50 and older (American Cancer Society, 2013b). African American men and Jamaican men of African descent have the highest documented prostate cancer incidence in the world (American Cancer Society, 2013b). Treatment varies depending on the man's age as well as the stage and grade (Gleason score) of the cancer along with his other medical conditions. Surgery (open, laparoscopic, or robotic-assisted), external beam radiation, or radioactive seed implants (brachytherapy) may be used to treat early stage disease (American Cancer Society, 2013b).

Screening: In recent years, there has been much discussion, debate, and controversy surrounding the use of Prostate Specific Antigen (PSA) to detect prostate cancer. Clinical trials aimed at testing the efficacy of PSA testing in reducing deaths for prostate cancer are inconclusive. Two European studies found a lower risk of death from prostate cancer among men receiving PSA screening while a study in the United States found no reduction (American Cancer Society, 2013b). Due to this level of insufficient evidence, ACS does not recommend for or against routine early prostate cancer testing with the PSA test. In contrast, the USPSTF (U.S. Preventive Services Task Force, 2012) recommends against the use of routine PSA to test for prostate cancer. The ACS (American Cancer Society, 2013b; National Cancer Institute, 2013c) recommends that beginning at age 50, men who are at average risk of prostate cancer and have a life expectancy of at least 10 years receive information about the potential benefits and known limitations associated with testing for early prostate cancer detection and have an opportunity to make an informed decision about testing. Men at higher risk (i.e., African Americans or men with a close relative diagnosed with prostate cancer) should have this discussion at age 45 or 40 (if a close relative was diagnosed at an early age).

Testicular cancer forms in tissues of one or both testicles and is most common in young or middle-aged men. Most testicular cancers begin in germ cells (cells that make sperm) and are called *testicular germ cell tumors* (National Cancer Institute, 2013d). Tumors are classified as seminomas and nonseminomas, depending on their cellular line of differentiation, with many consisting of a mixed cellular type. Nonseminomas tend to grow and metastasize more aggressively. Treatment options include surgery, radiation, and/or chemotherapy (PubMed Health, 2013).

Screening: Based on the low incidence of this condition and favorable outcomes of treatment, even in cases of advanced disease, there is adequate evidence that the benefits of screening for testicular cancer are small to none (U.S. Preventive Services Task Force, 2011). Any scrotal mass or changes identified by a man should be evaluated promptly.

Renal cell cancer, also called renal *adenocarcinoma,* or *hypernephroma,* can often be cured if it is diagnosed and treated when still localized to the kidney and the immediately surrounding tissue. Surgical resection is the standard treatment of this disease (National Cancer Institute, 2013b). Tobacco use is the primary risk factor, and early stage renal cancer usually has no symptoms. As the disease progresses, symptoms may include a pain or lump in the lower back or abdomen, fatigue, weight loss, fever, or swelling in the legs and ankles. Active surveillance may be an option for patients with small tumors while surgery is the primary treatment for most kidney cancers (American Cancer Society, 2013b). Kidney cancer tends to be resistant to traditional chemotherapy and radiation therapy.

Screening: No routine screening method exists to detect renal cell cancer.

See also: Chapter 3, "Perioperative Care," p. 45, Chapter 32, "Urinary Diversions," p. 230, and Chapter 26, "Benign Prostatic Hypertrophy" p. 197, for appropriate nursing diagnoses, outcomes, and interventions. Also see **Stress Urinary Incontinence** and **Sexual Dysfunction** in this chapter.

Cervical cancer incidence has decreased over the past several decades; however, these large declines have begun to taper off with rates becoming more stable (American Cancer Society, 2013b). Similarly, large declines in mortality rates have also begun to stabilize. The primary cause of cervical cancer is infection with certain types of HPV. Women who begin having sex at an early age or who have many sexual partners are at increased risk for HPV infection and cervical cancer (American Cancer Society, 2013b). However, a woman can become infected even if she has had only one sexual partner. Persistence of HPV infection and progression to cervical cancer may be influenced by many factors (e.g., immunosuppression, high parity, cigarette smoking). Preinvasisve lesions may be treated by electrocoagulation, cryotherapy, laser ablation, or local surgery. Invasive lesions are treated with surgery, radiation, and chemotherapy (in some cases) (American Cancer Society, 2013b).

Screening: The Pap test is the most widely used screening test for cervical cancer. For women ages 21 to 30, screening is recommended every 3 years using the Pap test. For women ages 30 to 65, screening is recommended every 5 years using HPV and PAP (called *co-testing*) (American Cancer Society, 2013b; U.S. Preventative Services Task Force, 2012). Women over age 65 who have had regular cervical cancer testing with normal results should *not* be tested for cervical cancer. At the time of this writing, two vaccines (Gardasil and Cervarix) have been approved for use in females 9 to 26 years of age for the prevention of the most common types of HPV infection that cause cervical cancer (American Cancer Society, 2013b). However, the overall effect of HPV vaccination on high-grade precancerous cervical lesions and cervical cancer is not yet known. Given these uncertainties, women who have been vaccinated should continue to be screened (U.S. Preventive Services Task Force, 2012).

Ovarian cancer accounts for about 3% of all cancers in women and usually has no obvious symptoms. The most common sign is swelling of the abdomen. The most important risk factor is a strong family history of breast or ovarian cancer. Treatment includes surgery and chemotherapy.

Screening: Currently, there is no screening test for the early detection of ovarian cancer.

Uterine Corpus (Endometrium) cancer usually occurs in the lining of the uterus. Abnormal uterine bleeding or spotting (especially in postmenopausal women) is a frequent early sign. Pain during urination, intercourse, or in the pelvic area is also a symptom (American Cancer Society, 2013b). Treatment usually includes surgery, radiation, hormones, and/or chemotherapy.

Screening: Currently, there is no screening test for the early detection of ovarian cancer.

See also: Chapter 3, "Perioperative Care," p. 45, for appropriate nursing diagnoses, outcomes, and interventions.

Nursing diagnoses and interventions for general cancer care

> **Note:** *The following nursing diagnoses, desired outcomes, and interventions relate to generalized cancer care. Those for care specific to chemotherapy, immunotherapy, and radiation therapy follow this section.*

Nursing Diagnosis:

Ineffective Breathing Pattern

related to hypoventilation occurring with pulmonary fibrosis, cellular damage, and decreased lung capacity (e.g., pneumonectomy or lobectomy)

> **Note:** *For desired outcome and interventions, see this nursing diagnosis in chemotherapeutic agents because some may cause pulmonary toxicity, an inflammatory reaction that results in fibrotic lung changes, cellular damage, and decreased lung capacity. Radiation therapy can also cause pulmonary damage and changes resulting in decreased lung capacity.*

Nursing Diagnosis:

Impaired Gas Exchange

related to altered oxygen supply occurring with anemia, pulmonary tumors, pneumonia, pulmonary emboli, pulmonary atelectasis, ascites, radiation, pericardial effusion, superior vena cava syndrome, hepatomegaly, and medication side effects

> **Note:** *For desired outcome and interventions, see this nursing diagnosis in Chapter 10, "Pneumonia," p. 118, and in Chapter 12, "Pulmonary Embolus," p. 129.*

Nursing Diagnosis:

Acute Pain

related to disease process, surgical intervention, or treatment effects

> **Note:** *For desired outcome and interventions, see Chapter 2, "Pain," p. 39.*

Nursing Diagnosis:

Chronic Pain

related to direct tumor involvement such as infiltration of tumor into nerves, bones, or hollow viscus; postchemotherapy pain syndromes (peripheral neuropathy, avascular necrosis of femoral or humeral heads, or plexopathy); or postradiation syndrome (plexopathy, radiation myelopathy, radiation-induced enteritis or proctitis, burning perineum syndrome, or osteoradionecrosis)

Desired Outcome: The patient participates in a prescribed pain regimen and reports that pain and side effects associated with the prescribed therapy are reduced to level of three or less within 1-2 hr of intervention, based on pain assessment tool (e.g., descriptive, numeric [on a scale of 0-10], or visual scale).

ASSESSMENT/INTERVENTIONS	RATIONALES
After the patient has undergone a complete medical evaluation for the causes of pain and the most effective strategies for pain relief, assess the patient's understanding of the evaluation and pain relief strategies.	This review helps determine the patient's level of understanding and reinforces findings, thereby promoting knowledge and adherence to pain relief strategies. It also empowers the patient as much as possible to participate in controlling his or her pain.
Assess the patient's cultural beliefs and attitudes about pain. *Never* ignore a patient's report of pain, taking into consideration that a patient's definition of pain may be different from that of the assessing nurse. Promptly report *any* change in pain pattern or new complaints of pain to the health care provider.	Cultural beliefs may influence how individuals describe their pain and its severity and their willingness to ask for pain medications. Pain is dynamic, and competent management requires frequent assessment at scheduled intervals.
Assess the patient's level of "discomfort" or abnormal sensations in addition to the usual pain queries.	Patients with *neuropathic pain* may not describe their discomfort as pain; therefore, be sure to use additional terms. *Nociceptive pain* refers to the body's perception of pain and its corresponding response. It begins when tissue is threatened or damaged by mechanical or thermal stimuli that activate the peripheral endings of sensory neurons known as *nociceptors*. In contrast, neuropathic pain is caused by damage to central or peripheral nervous system tissue or from altered processing of pain in the CNS. The resulting pain is chronic, may be difficult to manage, and is often described differently (burning, electric, tingling, numbness, pricking, shooting) from nociceptive pain.
Include the Following in Your Pain Assessments: - Characteristics (e.g., "burning" or "shooting" often describes nerve pain). - Location and sites of radiation.	Not all types of pain are managed solely by opioid therapy. Characterizing pain and documenting its location accurately will result in better pharmacologic intervention and help nurses develop a customized plan that incorporates nonpharmacologic measures as well.
- Onset and duration.	Determining precipitating factors (as with onset) may help prevent or alleviate pain.
- Severity: Use a pain scale that is comfortable for the patient (e.g., descriptive, numeric, or visual scale).	Severe pain can signal complications such as internal bleeding or leaking of visceral contents. Using a pain scale provides an objective measurement that enables the health care team to assess effectiveness of pain management strategies. Optimally, the patient's rated pain on a 0-10 scale is 4 or less. Be aware of literacy levels and/or cultural issues that may influence the patient's understanding of the pain scale.
- Aggravating and relieving factors.	This information may help prevent or alleviate pain.
- Previous use of strategies that have worked to relieve pain.	Strategies that have worked in the past may work for current pain.
Assess the patient's and caregiver's attitudes and knowledge about the pain medication regimen.	Many patients and their families have fears related to the patient's ultimate addiction to opioids. It is important to dispel any misperceptions about opioid-induced addiction when chronic pain therapy is necessary. Fears of addiction may result in ineffective pain management.

ASSESSMENT/INTERVENTIONS

Incorporate the Following Principles:

- Administer nonopioid and opioid analgesics in correct dose, at correct frequency, and via correct route.

- Recognize and report/treat side effects of opioid analgesia early.

- Use prescribed adjuvant medications.

- Assess for signs and symptoms of tolerance, and when it occurs discuss treatment with the health care provider.

[!] Never stop opioids abruptly in patients who have been taking them for a prolonged period.

- Use nonpharmacologic approaches, such as acupressure, biofeedback, relaxation therapy, application of heat or cold, and massage when appropriate. See Chapter 2, "Pain," p. 44, for details.

RATIONALES

Pharmacologic management of pain is often the mainstay of treatment of chronic cancer pain.

Chronic cancer analgesia is often administered orally. If pain is present most of the day, analgesia should be given around the clock (at scheduled intervals) rather than as needed because prolonged stimulation of the pain receptors increases the amount of drug required to relieve pain.

Side effects include respiratory depression, nausea and vomiting, constipation, sedation, and itching. The presence of these side effects does not necessarily preclude continued use of the drug. Consult with the care provider regarding prophylactic use of stool softeners to prevent constipation.

Adjuvant medications (see p. 40) help increase efficacy of opioids and may minimize their objectionable side effects as well.

Patients with chronic pain often require increasing doses of opioids to relieve their pain (tolerance). Respiratory depression occurs rarely in these individuals.

There is potential for physical dependence in patients taking opioids for a prolonged period; therefore, they should be tapered gradually to prevent withdrawal discomfort.

Nonpharmacologic approaches are often effective in enhancing effects of opioid therapy.

Nursing Diagnosis:

Ineffective Peripheral Tissue Perfusion

related to disease process (e.g,. interrupted blood flow occurring with lymphedema)

Desired Outcome: Following intervention/treatment, the patient exhibits adequate peripheral perfusion as evidenced by peripheral pulses greater than 2+ on a 0-4+ scale, normal skin color, decreasing or stable circumference of edematous site, equal sensation bilaterally, and ability to perform range of motion (ROM) in the involved extremity.

ASSESSMENT/INTERVENTIONS

Assess the involved extremity for degree of edema, quality of peripheral pulses, color, circumference, sensation, and ROM. Measure circumference of the affected and unaffected extremity for comparison.

Assess for tenderness, erythema, and warmth at edematous site.

Elevate and position the involved extremity on a pillow in slight abduction. If surgery has been performed, instruct the patient not to perform heavy activity with the affected limb during the recovery period.

RATIONALES

This assessment helps determine presence/degree of lymphedema and potential threat to the limb from hypoxia. Patients may be at risk based on a variety of disease processes, treatments, and medications.

These signs of infection need to be communicated to the health care provider for prompt intervention. A continuous supply of oxygen to the tissues through microcirculation is vital to the healing process and for resistance to infection.

As blood collects, waiting to get into the heart, pressure in the veins increases. The veins are permeable, and the increased pressure causes fluid to leak out of the veins and into the tissue. Elevating the extremity helps reduce venous pressure.

continued

ASSESSMENT/INTERVENTIONS	RATIONALES
Encourage the patient to wear loose-fitting clothing.	Tight-fitting clothing may cause areas of constriction, reducing lymph and blood flow, as well as creating potential areas for impaired skin integrity.
Avoid blood pressure (BP) readings, venipuncture, intravenous (IV) lines, and vaccinations in the affected arm. As indicated, advise the patient to get a medical alert bracelet that cautions against these actions.	BP cuffs can constrict lymphatic pathways, and injections or blood draws will cause an opening in the skin, providing an entrance for bacteria.
Consult physical therapist (PT) and health care provider about development of an exercise plan.	Exercise increases mobility, which promotes lymphatic flow. This in turn helps decrease edema.
As indicated, suggest use of elastic bandages, compression garments, or sequential compression devices. Ensure that compression garments are fitted properly and the patient understands when and how to use them.	Elastic bandages decrease edema in mild, chronic cases of lymphedema. The other devices decrease edema in more severe cases of lymphedema.

Nursing Diagnoses:

Ineffective Peripheral Tissue Perfusion
Risk for Decreased Cardiac Tissue Perfusion

related to interrupted venous flow occurring with deep venous thrombosis (DVT)/venous thromboembolism (VTE), lymphedema, and treatment side effects

Desired Outcome: Before hospital discharge, the patient and/or caregivers competently administer anticoagulant therapy as prescribed and describe reportable signs and symptoms suggestive of progressive coagulopathy.

ASSESSMENT/INTERVENTIONS	RATIONALES
Instruct the patient in the technique of self-administration of injectable low–molecular-weight heparin, if it is prescribed.	Individuals with certain malignancies (especially brain, breast, colon, renal, pancreatic, and lung) are at higher than average risk for DVT/VTE. Other possible contributing factors include recent surgery, presence of a venous access device, sepsis, obesity, concurrent cardiac disease, and underlying increased coagulability disorders.
If the patient is taking oral anticoagulants, teach dietary modifications with warfarin therapy.	Foods high in vitamin K (antidote to warfarin) may interfere with achievement of therapeutic anticoagulation. These include green leafy vegetables, avocados, and liver. However, some prescribers do not restrict dietary intake of vitamin K–containing foods. Instead, patients are instructed to maintain dietary consistency in moderation without large variations, and the warfarin dose is adjusted accordingly. If patients are consistent in their dietary intake, the prothrombin time (PT)/international normalized ratio (INR) should remain stable and therapeutic.
Teach reportable signs and symptoms, such as unilateral edema of a limb with possible associated warmth, erythema, and tenderness.	DVT/VTE may reoccur.
Caution that a sudden increase in shortness of breath with or without chest pain also should be reported immediately.	DVT/VTE may progress to pulmonary embolism.
For additional desired outcomes and interventions, see Chapter 24, "Venous Thrombosis/Thrombophlebitis," for **Ineffective Peripheral Tissue Perfusion/Risk for Decreased Cardiac Tissue Perfusion,** p. 186.	

Nursing Diagnosis:

Impaired Physical Mobility

related to musculoskeletal or neuromuscular impairment occurring with bone metastasis or spinal cord compression; pain and discomfort; intolerance to activity; or perceptual or cognitive impairment

> **Note:** *For desired outcome and interventions, see this nursing diagnosis in Chapter 69, "Osteo- arthritis," p. 507. Also see Chapter 73, "Managing Wound Care," p. 536 for discussions on care of patients at risk for pressure ulcers.*

Nursing Diagnoses:

Risk for Impaired Skin Integrity
Impaired Skin Integrity

related to disease state or related treatments

Desired Outcome: Following instruction, the patient verbalizes measures that promote comfort, preserve skin integrity, and promote competent management and infection prevention of open wounds.

ASSESSMENT/INTERVENTIONS	RATIONALES
Identify if your patient is at risk for skin lesions.	Individuals with breast, lung, colon, and renal cancers; T-cell lymphoma; melanoma; and extensions of head and neck cancers may be susceptible to skin lesions. These lesions often erode, providing challenges to wound care, patient dignity, body image, and odor control. Treatment may include radiation, systemic or local chemotherapy, cryotherapy, or excision.
Assess common sites of cutaneous lesions.	These sites include the anterior chest, abdomen, head (scalp), and neck and should be assessed in patients at risk.
Assess for local warmth, swelling, erythema, tenderness, and purulent drainage.	These are indicators of infection, which can occur as a result of nonintact skin.
Inspect skin lesions.	The presence of skin lesions necessitates being alert to and documenting general characteristics, location and distribution, configuration, size, morphologic structure (e.g., nodule, erosion, fissure), drainage (color, amount, character), and odor so that changes can be detected and reported promptly.
Perform the following skin care for nonulcerating lesions and teach these interventions to the patient and significant other, as indicated:	Maintaining skin integrity reduces risk of infection.
- Wash affected area with tepid water and pat dry.	Excessively warm temperatures damage healing tissue.
- Avoid pressure on the area.	Pressure would further damage friable tissue.
- Apply dry dressing.	This dressing will protect the skin from exposure to irritants and mechanical trauma (e.g., scratching, abrasion).
- Apply occlusive dressings, such as Telfa, using paper tape.	An occlusive dressing promotes penetration of topical medications.
Perform the following skin care for ulcerating lesions and teach these interventions to the patient and significant other, as indicated:	
For Cleansing and Débriding: Use ½-strength hydrogen peroxide and normal saline solution, followed by a normal saline rinse.	This solution will irrigate and débride the lesion. Rinsing removes peroxide and residual wound debris.

continued

ASSESSMENT/INTERVENTIONS	RATIONALES
Use cotton swabs or sponges to apply gentle pressure. As necessary, gently irrigate using a syringe.	Using gentle pressure with swabs or sponges débrides the ulcerated area and protects granulation tissue. If the ulcerated area is susceptible to bleeding, gentle pressure protects delicate granulation tissue.
Use soaks (wet dressings) of saline, water, Burrow's solution (aluminum acetate), or hydrogen peroxide on the involved skin.	These are methods of débridement, which will dislodge and remove bacteria and loosen necrotic tissue, foreign bodies, and exudate.
Thoroughly rinse hydrogen peroxide or aluminum acetate off the skin.	Failure to do so may cause further skin breakdown.
As necessary, use wet-to-dry dressings.	These dressings will provide gentle débridement.
For Prevention and Management of Local Infection: Irrigate and scrub with antibacterial agents, such as acetic acid solution or povidone-iodine.	These antibacterial agents prevent/manage local infection.
Collect wound cultures, as prescribed.	A culture will determine presence of infection and optimal antibiotic therapy.
Apply topical antibacterial agents (e.g., sulfadiazine cream, bacitracin ointment) to open areas, as prescribed.	These agents prevent infection in open areas that are susceptible.
Administer systemic antibiotics, as prescribed.	Systemic antibiotics are used for wounds that are more extensively infected.
To Maintain Hemostasis: Use silver nitrate sticks for cautery.	These sticks help maintain hemostasis in the presence of capillary oozing.
Use oxidized cellulose or pack the wound with Gelfoam or similar product.	These products are used for bleeding in larger surface areas.
Consult wound, ostomy, continence (WOC)/enterostomal therapy (ET) nurse as needed on wound-healing techniques.	When wounds fail to respond to more traditional interventions, a WOC/ET nurse may provide alternative suggestions.
Teach the patient to avoid wearing such fabrics as wool and corduroy.	These fabrics are irritating to the skin.
See also: Chapter 73, "Managing Wound Care," p. 533; Chapter 74, "Providing Nutritional Support," p. 539; and Appendix A, "Infection Prevention and Control," p. 747.	Wound healing depends on adequate intake of nutrients/protein for tissue synthesis.

Nursing Diagnosis:

Diarrhea

related to chemotherapeutic agents; radiation therapy; biologic agents; antacids containing magnesium; tube feedings; food intolerance; and bowel dysfunction such as Crohn's disease, ulcerative colitis, tumors, and fecal impaction

> **Note:** *For desired outcomes and interventions, see Chapter 61, "Ulcerative Colitis,"* **Diarrhea,** *p. 463 and* **Risk for Impaired Skin Integrity***: Perineal/Perianal, p. 464; Chapter 72, "Caring for Individuals with Human Immunodeficiency Virus,"* **Diarrhea,** *p. 525, and Chapter 74, "Providing Nutritional Support,"* **Diarrhea,** *p. 545.*
>
> *For patients receiving chemotherapy (e.g., 5-fluorouracil, irinotecan), teach the necessity of having appropriate antidiarrheal medications available and other methods used to combat effects of diarrhea (fluid replacement, addition of psyllium to the diet to provide bulk to stool, perineal hygiene). Instruct patients to notify their health care providers if experiencing more than six loose stools per day.*

Nursing Diagnosis:

Constipation

related to treatment with certain chemotherapy agents, opioids, tranquilizers, and antidepressants; less than adequate intake of food and fluids because of anorexia, nausea, or dysphagia; hypercalcemia; neurologic impairment (e.g., spinal cord compression); mental status changes; decreased mobility; or colonic disorders

> **Note:** *For desired outcomes and interventions, see Chapter 3, "Perioperative Care,"* **Constipation,** *p. 59; Chapter 4, "Prolonged Bedrest,"* **Constipation,** *p. 68; and Chapter 34, "General Care of Patients with Neurologic Disorders,"* **Constipation,** *p. 258. Patients with cancer should not go more than 2 days without having a bowel movement. Patients receiving Vinca alkaloids are at risk for ileus in addition to constipation. Preventive measures, such as use of senna products or docusate calcium with casanthranol, especially for patients taking opioids, are highly recommended. In addition, all individuals taking opioids should receive a prophylactic bowel regimen. The Oncology Nursing Society published a summary of evidence and recommended guidelines for the prevention and management of constipation, including a combination of a softener and stimulant. An algorithm for management includes first line treatment (oral combination of softener and stimulant), second line treatment (rectal suppositories, enemas, consideration of opioid antagonist), and third line treatment (manual evaluation), consideration of opioid antagonists if patient is taking opioids (Oncology Nursing Society, 2011).*

Nursing Diagnosis:

Stress Urinary Incontinence (or risk for same)

related to loss of muscle tone in the urethral sphincter after radical prostatectomy

Desired Outcome: Within the 24-hr period before hospital discharge, the patient relates understanding of incontinence cause and suggested regimen to promote bladder control.

ASSESSMENT/INTERVENTIONS	RATIONALES
Before surgery, explain that there is potential for permanent urinary incontinence after prostatectomy but that it may resolve within 6 months. Describe the reason for the incontinence.	A knowledgeable patient is not only less anxious but more likely to adhere to the treatment regimen. Aids such as anatomic illustrations will promote understanding.
Encourage the patient to maintain adequate fluid intake of at least 2-3 L/day (unless contraindicated).	Dilute urine is less irritating to the prostatic fossa, as well as less likely to result in incontinence. Paradoxically, patients with urinary incontinence often reduce their fluid intake to avoid incontinence.
Establish a bladder routine before hospital discharge.	Documenting time, amount voided, amount of fluid intake, timing of fluid intake followed by voiding, and related information such as degree of wetness experienced (e.g., number of incontinence pads used in a day, degree of underwear dampness) and exertion factor causing the wetness (e.g., laughing, sneezing, bending, lifting) may help patients manage incontinence. This helps estimate the amount of time patients can hold urine and avoid incontinence episodes.
	If successful, the patient can then attempt to lengthen time intervals between voidings. **Note:** Patients need to empty their bladders at least q4h to reduce risk of urinary tract infection (UTI) caused by urinary stasis.

continued

ASSESSMENT/INTERVENTIONS	RATIONALES
Teach the patient to avoid caffeine and alcoholic beverages.	Caffeine and alcoholic beverages are examples of irritants that may increase stress incontinence.
Teach Kegel exercises (see Chapter 26, "Benign Prostatic Hypertrophy," p. 204) to promote sphincter control. Begin teaching before surgery if possible.	Kegel exercises strengthen pelvic area muscles, which will help regain bladder control. Patients must first identify the correct muscle groups in order to perform Kegel exercises correctly. These exercises require diligent effort to reverse incontinence and in fact may need to be done for several months before any benefit is obtained.
Remind the patient to discuss any incontinence problems with health care provider during follow-up examinations.	Such a discussion will enable follow-up treatment for this problem.

Nursing Diagnosis:

Sexual Dysfunction

related to altered body function occurring with the disease process; psychosocial issues; radiation therapy to the lower abdomen, pelvis, and gonads; chemotherapeutic agents; or surgery

Desired Outcome: Following instruction, the patient identifies potential treatment side effects on sexual and reproductive function and acceptable methods of contraception during treatment if appropriate.

ASSESSMENT/INTERVENTIONS	RATIONALES
Assess the impact of diagnosis and treatment on the patient's sexual functioning and self-concept.	Sexual dysfunction affects every individual differently. It is important not to assume its meaning but rather explore it with the individual and allow him or her to give meaning to the changes.
Assess the patient's readiness to discuss sexual concerns.	Gentle, sensitive, open-ended questions allow patients to signal their readiness to discuss concerns.
Initiate discussion about effects of treatment on sexuality and reproduction, using, for example, the PLISSIT model.	The PLISSIT model provides an excellent framework for discussion. This four-step model includes the following: (1) **P**ermission—give the patient permission to discuss issues of concern; (2) **L**imited **I**nformation—provide patient with information about expected treatment effects on sexual and reproductive function, without going into complete detail; (3) **S**pecific **S**uggestions—provide suggestions for managing common problems that occur during treatment; and (4) **I**ntensive **T**herapy—although most individuals can be managed by nurses using the first three steps in this model, some patients may require referral to an expert counselor (Taylor & Davis, 2006).
If a female patient is of childbearing age, inquire if pregnancy is a possibility before treatment is initiated.	Pregnancy will cause a delay in treatment. The patient may be referred to a fertility specialist.
Discuss possibility of decreased sexual response or desire.	This may result from side effects of chemotherapy. Informing patient may allay unnecessary anxiety.
Encourage patients to maintain open communication with their partners about needs and concerns. Explore alternative methods of sexual fulfillment, such as hugging, kissing, talking quietly together, or massage.	Encouraging open dialogue promotes intimacy and helps prevent ill feelings or emotional withdrawal by either partner. In the presence of symptoms related to therapy, such interventions as taking a nap before sexual activity or use of pain or antiemetic medication may help decrease symptoms. Other suggestions include using a water-based lubricant for dyspareunia. If fatigue is a problem, partners might consider changing usual time of day for intimacy or using supine or side-lying positions, which require less energy expenditure.

ASSESSMENT/INTERVENTIONS	RATIONALES
Discuss the possibility of temporary or permanent sterility resulting from treatment.	This discussion could open the door to explaining possibility of sperm banking for men before chemotherapy treatment or oophoropexy (surgical displacement of ovaries outside the radiation field) for women undergoing abdominal radiation therapy. The patient may need referral to a fertility specialist.
Teach patients the importance of contraception during treatment if relevant. Discuss issues related to timing of pregnancy after treatment. Suggest that patients receive genetic counseling before attempting pregnancy, as indicated.	Healthy offspring have been born from parents who have received radiation therapy or chemotherapy, but long-term effects have not been clearly identified.
For patients undergoing lymphadenectomy for testicular cancer, explain that ejaculatory failure may occur if the sympathetic nerve is damaged, but erection and orgasm will be possible.	If ejaculatory failure does occur, the patient should know that artificial insemination is possible because the semen flows back into the urine, from which it can be extracted, enabling the ovum to become impregnated artificially.
If appropriate, explain that a silicone prosthesis may be placed after orchiectomy. Consult the health care provider about the potential for this procedure.	This will help the scrotum achieve a normal appearance.

Nursing Diagnosis:

Risk for Disuse Syndrome

related to upper extremity immobilization resulting from discomfort, lymphedema, treatment- or disease-related injury, or infection after breast surgery

Desired Outcomes: Before surgery, the patient verbalizes knowledge about importance of and rationale for upper extremity movements and exercises. Upon recovery, the patient has full or baseline level ROM of the upper extremity.

ASSESSMENT/INTERVENTIONS	RATIONALES
Consult the surgeon before breast surgery regarding such issues as wound healing, suture lines, and extent of the surgical procedure.	This consultation will determine the type of surgery anticipated and enable development of an individualized exercise plan in collaboration with physical and occupational therapists specific to the patient's needs.
Encourage finger, wrist, and elbow movement.	Such movements aid circulation, minimize edema, and maintain mobility in the involved extremity.
Elevate the extremity as tolerated.	Elevation decreases edema.
Encourage progressive exercise by having the patient use the affected arm for personal hygiene and activities of daily living (ADLs). Initiate other exercises (e.g., clasping hands behind the head and "walking" fingers up the wall) as soon as the patient is ready.	After drains and sutures have been removed (usually 7-10 days postoperatively), patients should begin exercises that will enhance external rotation and abduction of the shoulder. Ultimately they should be able to achieve maximum shoulder flexion by touching fingertips together behind the back if they were capable of this exercise before the surgery.
⚠ In patients who have had lymph node removal, avoid giving injections, measuring BP, or taking blood samples from affected arm. Remind the patient about lowered resistance to infection and importance of promptly treating any breaks in the skin. Advise the patient to treat minor injuries with soap and water after hospital discharge and to notify the health care provider if signs of infection occur.	Loss of lymph nodes alters lymph drainage, which may result in edema of the arm and hand and increases risk of infection as well.

continued

General Care Plans

ASSESSMENT/INTERVENTIONS — RATIONALES

ASSESSMENT/INTERVENTIONS	RATIONALES
Advise the patient to wear a medical alert bracelet that cautions against injections and tests in the involved arm.	Information on this bracelet optimally will help prevent infection caused by invasive procedures or ensure that the patient receives prompt treatment if an infection occurs.
Advise the patient to wear a thimble when sewing and a protective glove when gardening or doing chores that require exposure to harsh chemicals such as cleaning fluids.	This information promotes patient safety/infection prevention.
Explain that cutting cuticles should be avoided and lotion should be used to keep skin soft. An electric razor should be used for shaving the axilla.	This information promotes skin integrity and protects hand and arm from injury and subsequent infection.

Nursing Diagnosis:

Deficient Knowledge

related to unfamiliarity with the purpose, type, and management of venous access device (VAD)

Desired Outcome: Within the 24-hr period before hospital discharge, the patient and significant other/caregiver verbalize understanding regarding the VAD, including its purpose, appropriate management measures, and reportable complications.

ASSESSMENT/INTERVENTIONS	RATIONALES
Assess the patient's and caregiver's level of understanding of the VAD that will be or has been inserted and intervene accordingly.	A VAD can be used for venipunctures and administration of medications, fluids, and blood products. Determining the patient's and caregiver's current knowledge base helps the nurse devise an individualized teaching plan. Three types of VADs are generally used: tunneled catheters, nontunneled catheters, and implanted ports.
Nontunneled catheters (peripheral or central):	These catheters are inserted by venipuncture into the vessel of choice, usually basilic, cephalic, or medial cubital vein, near or at the antecubital area, or jugular or subclavian vein in the upper thorax. A peripherally inserted central catheter (PICC) is an example of a nontunneled catheter. Maintenance involves daily flushing after each use with normal saline and/or heparinized solution. Sterile dressing and cap changes are necessary. Refer to institutional policies for specific instructions.
Tunneled central venous catheters:	These catheters are inserted into a central vein with a portion of the catheter tunneled through subcutaneous tissue and exiting the body at a convenient area, usually the chest. A Dacron cuff encircles the catheter about 2 inches from the exiting end of the catheter. Tissue grows into this cuff, helping prevent catheter dislodgement and decreasing risk of microorganisms migrating along the catheter surface and entering the bloodstream. Single-lumen or multi-lumen catheters are available. Examples of tunneled central venous catheters include Broviac, Hickman, and Groshong. Maintenance involves flushing per institutional protocol and after each use with saline and/or heparinized saline solution. A sterile dressing change is performed 24 hr after insertion and then every 5-7 days until healed. Cap changes are performed using sterile technique. Refer to institutional policies for specific instructions.
Implanted venous access ports:	Implanted ports are commonly inserted when long-term therapy is anticipated or lack of venous access is expected to be a chronic issue. They consist of a catheter attached to a plastic or metal port inserted into a central or peripheral vein and then sutured in place in a surgically created subcutaneous pocket, most commonly on the chest. Venous access ports are completely embedded under the skin and may have single or dual access ports. Access to the port may be from the top or side, depending on port style.

ASSESSMENT/INTERVENTIONS

RATIONALES

Note: Noncoring needles must be used to access the port, which allows the system to reseal when the needle is removed.

This catheter must not be flushed with any syringe smaller than 10 mL due to excess pressures generated by smaller syringes. When removing the needle, pressure must be applied to sides of the port to promote ease of removal and patient comfort. Maintenance involves preparation of the site for access with an antibacterial preparation solution (e.g., povidone-iodine solution), optional local anesthetic, and flushing at least monthly or after each use with normal saline and/or heparinized solution. Refer to institutional policies for specific instructions. Dressings are not required after healing of the insertion site.

Teach patients to carry in their wallets the card provided by the manufacturer identifying type of catheter and recommended flushing solution.

There is a wide variety of catheter types, and the type of catheter determines the proper flushing solution. Refer to agency policy as indicated.

Provide a model of the device during patient teaching.

Visual aids augment understanding.

Explain where the device will be inserted.

Nontunneled catheters may be inserted at the bedside or in the clinic under local anesthesia. Tunneled central venous catheters and implanted ports are inserted in the operating room under local anesthesia.

Teach the patient that there may be mild discomfort, similar to a toothache, for 48 hr after the procedure but medication will ameliorate pain.

Explaining expected sensations and likely amelioration with analgesics reduces anxiety and provides the patient with guidelines for reportable symptoms.

If possible, introduce the patient and caregiver to another individual who has the device.

Conversing with someone who has already undergone a procedure may increase knowledge, decrease anxiety, and provide another avenue of support.

Teach VAD maintenance care. Provide both verbal and written instructions, including educational materials provided by the VAD manufacturer.

Maintenance care likely will be done while the patient is at home, where written materials will serve as a reference.

Have the patient or caregiver demonstrate dressing care, flushing technique, and cap-changing routine before hospital discharge. Provide 24-hr emergency number to call in case of problems.

This demonstration will reinforce previous teaching and, when done correctly, provides emotional support that this care can be done when at home.

Discuss potential complications associated with VADs, along with appropriate self-management measures.

Infection:

The patient should be taught how to assess the exit site for erythema, swelling, local increased temperature, discomfort, purulent drainage, and fever (temperature higher than 38° C [100.4° F]).

Bleeding:

The patient should be taught how to apply pressure to the site and to notify a health care team member if bleeding does not stop in 5 min.

Clot in the catheter:

The patient should be taught how to flush the catheter without using excessive pressure, which could damage or dislodge the catheter (particularly an implanted port). If flushing does not dislodge the clot, the patient or caregiver should notify a health care team member.

⚠ *Disconnected cap:*

The patient should be taught how to tape all connections and the importance of always carrying hemostats or alligator clamps with padded blades to prevent the catheter from tearing.

⚠ *Extravasation:*

Although this is a relatively rare complication, it can cause severe damage if a chemotherapy agent with vesicant properties is involved. The patient should be taught to report pain, burning, and stinging in the chest, clavicle, and port pocket or along the subcutaneous tunnel during medication administration.

Nursing Diagnosis:

Deficient Knowledge

related to unfamiliarity with side effects of antiandrogen therapy or bilateral orchiectomy

Desired Outcome: Within the 24-hr period before hospital discharge, the patient verbalizes knowledge about the extent and duration of body changes.

ASSESSMENT/INTERVENTIONS	RATIONALES
Assess the patient's health care literacy (language, reading, comprehension). Assess culture and culturally specific information needs.	This assessment helps ensure that information is selected and presented in a manner that is culturally and educationally appropriate. A knowledgeable patient likely will have less stress about his treatment, adhere to the treatment regimen accordingly, and report side effects promptly for timely treatment.
Inform the patient of side effects of estrogen therapy and orchiectomy.	Breast enlargement, breast tenderness, loss of sexual desire, and hot flashes can occur.
For patients undergoing estrogen therapy, provide instruction about symptoms related to complications of thromboembolic disorders and myocardial infarction, which should be reported promptly to the health care provider.	Shortness of breath; orthopnea; dyspnea; pedal edema; unilateral leg swelling or pain; and left arm, left jaw, or left-sided chest pain can occur with this therapy and should be reported promptly for timely intervention.
Explain that when therapy is discontinued, most side effects will resolve.	This knowledge may bring some reassurance to the patient.
If appropriate, explain that before initiating estrogen therapy, the health care provider may prescribe radiation therapy to areolae of the breasts.	Radiation therapy will minimize painful gynecomastia. However, this procedure will not decrease other side effects.

Nursing diagnoses and interventions specific to patients undergoing chemotherapy, immunotherapy, and radiation therapy

Nursing Diagnosis:

Risk for Infection

related to inadequate secondary defenses resulting from myelosuppression occurring with invasive procedures or cancer-related treatments

Desired Outcomes: The patient is free of infection as evidenced by oral temperature 38°C (100.4°F) or less, BP 90/60 mm Hg or higher, and heart rate (HR) 100 bpm or less. The patient identifies risk factors for infection, verbalizes early signs and symptoms of infection and reports them promptly to a health care professional if they occur, and demonstrates appropriate self-care measures to minimize risk of infection.

ASSESSMENT/INTERVENTIONS	RATIONALES
Assess each body system.	This assessment will help determine potential for and actual sources of infection. Patients with severe neutropenia have a significantly increased risk of infection because of invasion of surface bacteria in the mouth, intestinal tract, and skin. These patients frequently exhibit mucosal inflammation, particularly of the gingival and perirectal areas.
Assess vital signs (VS), temperature, and invasive sites q4h.	Temperature 38°C (100.4°F) or higher, increased HR, decreased BP, and the following clinical signs: tenderness, erythema, warmth, swelling, and drainage at invasive sites; chills; and malaise are signs of infection.

ASSESSMENT/INTERVENTIONS	RATIONALES
Before administering chemotherapy, ensure that blood counts and other related laboratory studies are within accepted parameters per institutional policy. See **Appendix B,** p. 754, for normal values.	Chemotherapy causes predictable drops in WBCs, RBCs, and platelet counts because it can damage normal, healthy blood cells forming in the bone marrow. Administering chemotherapy to individuals with counts below specified parameters may put them at risk for infection, bleeding, or worsening anemia.
Identify whether the patient is at risk for infection by reviewing the absolute neutrophil count (ANC). ANC = (% of segmented neutrophils + % of bands) × Total WBC count.	Neutropenia is a condition in which the number of neutrophils in the blood is too low. Because neutrophils are important in defending the body against bacterial and some viral infections, neutropenia places patients at increased risk for these infections. Severe neutropenia can lead to serious problems that require prompt care and attention inasmuch as the patient could develop bacterial, viral, fungal, or mixed infection at any time. ANC may be used to determine if patient is at unacceptable risk for infection when administering chemotherapy.
ANC of 1500-2000/mm^3 = No significant risk. ANC of 1000-1500/mm^3 = Minimal risk. ANC of 500-1000/mm^3 = Moderate risk. ANC of less than 500/mm^3 = Severe risk.	Neutropenic precautions need to be initiated based on agency policy.
Avoid invasive procedures when possible.	Invasive procedures increase risk of infection.
Note: Temperature of 38° C (100.4° F) or higher may be the only sign of infection in the neutropenic patient.	Other signs of infection may be absent in the presence of neutropenia.
Be alert to subtle changes in mental status: restlessness or irritability; warm and flushed skin; chills, fever, or hypothermia; increased urine output; bounding pulse; tachypnea; and glycosuria.	These are signs of impending sepsis, which often precede the classic signs of septic shock: cold, clammy skin; thready pulse; decreased BP; and oliguria. These signs should be reported promptly for timely intervention.
Place a sign on the patient's door indicating that neutropenic precautions are in effect for patients with ANC 1000/mm^3 or less.	These patients are vulnerable to infection.
Instruct all persons entering patient's room to wash hands thoroughly and to follow other appropriate Centers for Disease Control and Prevention (CDC) guidelines.	Hand hygiene is the most important form of infection prevention. Current CDC guidelines also state that individuals caring for patients at high risk for infection should not wear artificial nails and should consider keeping natural nails less than ¼ inch long.
Restrict individuals from entering who have transmissible illnesses.	Individuals with colds, influenza, chickenpox, or herpes zoster can transmit these illnesses to the patient.
Follow agency policy on restriction of fresh fruits or flowers.	More evidence is needed on the role of fresh fruits and flowers transmitting infection for patients with neutropenia.
Encourage the patient to practice good personal hygiene, including good perineal care after elimination.	Proper hygiene eliminates flora or bacteria that can easily lead to infection in an immunocompromised patient.
Notify the health care provider immediately if the patient's temperature is higher than 38° C (100.4° F).	This is a possible sign of infection and necessitates an emergent CBC.
Administer antibiotic therapy in a timely fashion (within 1 hr).	Inasmuch as the only sure sign of infection in a neutropenic patient is fever, initiation of antibiotic therapy in a timely fashion is imperative.
Implement routine oral care. Teach the patient to use a soft-bristle toothbrush after meals and before bed (bristles may be softened further by running them under hot water).	Gentle oral care helps prevent injury to oral mucosa that could result in infection.
Inspect the oral cavity daily, noting presence of lesions, erythema, or exudate on the tongue or mucous membranes.	Individuals with prolonged neutropenia are at risk for fungal, bacterial, and viral infections.
Encourage coughing, deep breathing, and turning.	These actions decrease risk of pneumonia and of skin breakdown, which could lead to infection.
Avoid use of rectal suppositories, rectal thermometer, or enemas. Caution the patient to avoid straining at stool.	These actions could traumatize the rectal mucosa, thereby increasing risk of infection because of infectious flora in the rectum.

continued

ASSESSMENT/INTERVENTIONS	RATIONALES
Suggest use of stool softener.	Patients with prolonged neutropenia are at increased risk for perirectal infection and should be monitored accordingly. Because the immune system is compromised, normal bacterial flora in the colon can be introduced to other parts of the body if perirectal abscesses are ruptured, leading to systemic infection.
Teach the patient to use electric shavers rather than razor blades, avoid vaginal douche and tampons, use emery board rather than clipper for nail care, check with the health care provider before dental care, and avoid invasive procedures.	These measures help maintain skin integrity, thereby minimizing risk for infection.
Use antimicrobial skin preparations before injections, and change IV sites q48-72h or per protocol.	These actions help prevent infection.
Instruct the patient to use water-soluble lubricant before sexual intercourse and avoid oral and anal manipulation during sexual activities. Caution the patient to abstain from sexual intercourse during periods of severe neutropenia.	These measures decrease risk of introducing infection because of nonintact skin.
If indicated, advise the patient to avoid foods with high bacterial count (raw eggs, raw fruits and vegetables, foods prepared in a blender that cannot adequately be cleaned); bird, cat, and dog excreta; plants, flowers, and sources of stagnant water. Follow institutional policy accordingly.	Empirical evidence for these strategies are underdeveloped. More research is needed in these areas.
As prescribed, administer colony-stimulating factors.	These agents minimize risk of myelosuppression associated with chemotherapy, especially for patients with a history of neutropenic fever.

See also: Appendix A, p. 747, "Infection Prevention and Control."

Nursing Diagnoses:

Activity Intolerance
Fatigue

related to decreased oxygen-carrying capacity of the blood occurring with anemia (caused by some chemotherapeutic drugs, radiation therapy, chronic disease such as renal failure, or surgery), or related to imbalance between oxygen supply and demand occurring with acute or chronic lung changes (e.g., due to lobectomy, pneumonectomy, pulmonary fibrosis)

Desired Outcome: After treatment, the patient reports that fatigue has decreased, rates perceived exertion at 3 or less on a 0-10 scale, and exhibits tolerance to activity as evidenced by respiratory rate (RR) 12-20 breaths/min with normal depth and pattern (eupnea), HR 100 bpm or less, and absence of dizziness and headaches.

ASSESSMENT/INTERVENTIONS	RATIONALES
Assess for fatigue and activity intolerance, and explain that they are manifestations of decreased oxygen-carrying capacity of the blood and can be tempered by various interventions mentioned below.	Fatigue and activity intolerance are temporary side effects of chemotherapy or radiation therapy and will abate gradually when therapy has been completed. Understanding this relationship likely will help the patient cope better with the treatment.
Stress the importance of good nutrition.	Vitamin and iron supplements and intake of foods high in iron such as liver and other organ meats, seafood, green vegetables, cereals, nuts, and legumes likely will help reverse the effects of anemia.
As prescribed, administer erythropoietin.	Epoetin alfa (Epogen, Procrit) is a synthetic form of erythropoietin that stimulates production of RBCs to treat anemia associated with cancer chemotherapy. (Erythropoietin will not be effective in patients who are iron deficient.)

ASSESSMENT/INTERVENTIONS	RATIONALES
[!] As the patient performs ADLs, be alert for dyspnea on exertion, dizziness, palpitations, headaches, and verbalization of increased exertion level.	These are signs of activity intolerance and decreased tissue oxygenation. If these signs are present, the patient may be at risk for falls, which necessitates implementation of safety measures.
Ask the patient to rate perceived exertion per Borg scale (see Chapter 4, "Prolonged Bedrest," **Risk for Activity Intolerance**, p. 61).	A rate of perceived exertion (RPE) greater than 3 is a sign of activity intolerance and usually necessitates stopping the activity.
Facilitate coordination of care providers to provide rest periods as needed between care activities.	Undisturbed rest periods of at least 90-min duration will help the patient regain energy stores. Frequent activity periods without associated rest periods may result in depleted energy stores and emotional exhaustion.
Assess oximetry and report significant findings.	Oxygen saturation at 92% or less indicates need for oxygen supplementation and may be necessary only during periods of activity.
Administer oxygen as prescribed, and encourage deep breathing.	Augmenting oxygen delivery to the tissues will help decrease fatigue.
Administer blood components as prescribed.	Infusing RBCs increases hemoglobin level and treats anemia.
[!] Double-check type and crossmatch with a colleague per institutional protocol; assess for and report signs of transfusion reaction.	These actions help prevent/assess for life-threatening transfusion reactions.
Encourage gradually increasing activities to tolerance as the patient's condition improves. Set mutually agreed-on goals with patient.	Mutually agreed-on goals promote adherence to increased activity levels, which will increase the patient's tolerance.

Nursing Diagnosis:

Risk for Bleeding

related to thrombocytopenia (for all patients receiving chemotherapy and radiation therapy, as well as those with cancers involving the bone marrow)

Desired Outcome: The patient is free of signs and symptoms of bleeding as evidenced by negative occult blood tests, HR 100 bpm or less, and systolic blood pressure (SBP) 90 mm Hg or greater.

ASSESSMENT/INTERVENTIONS	RATIONALES
[!] Monitor platelet counts; identify whether the patient is at risk for bleeding.	- Platelets 150,000-300,000/mm^3 = Normal risk for bleeding. - Platelets less than 50,000/mm^3 = Moderate risk for bleeding. Initiate thrombocytopenic precautions. - Platelets less than 10,000/mm^3 = Severe risk for bleeding. The patient may develop spontaneous hemorrhage.
Perform a baseline physical assessment; assess for evidence of bleeding.	Petechiae, ecchymosis, hematuria, hematemesis, tarry or bloody stools, hemoptysis, heavy menses, headaches, somnolence, mental status changes, confusion, and blurred vision signal bleeding and should be reported promptly for timely intervention.
[!] Assess VS at least every shift or with each appointment if the patient is not hospitalized. Report SBP higher than 140 mm Hg.	Hypotension and tachycardia are signs that signal bleeding and should be reported promptly for timely intervention. In the presence of thrombocytopenia, the patient is at risk for intracranial bleeding when SBP is elevated.
Perform a psychosocial assessment, including the patient's past experience with thrombocytopenia; the effect of thrombocytopenia on the patient's lifestyle; and changes in patient's work pattern, family relationships, and social activities.	This assessment identifies learning needs and necessity of skilled care after hospital discharge.
[!] Avoid invasive procedures when possible, including intramuscular (IM) injections.	IM injections and invasive procedures increase risk of bleeding. If punctures are necessary, use of smaller gauge needles and gentle pressure at the puncture site until bleeding stops will help prevent hemorrhage.

continued

ASSESSMENT/INTERVENTIONS	RATIONALES
Avoid use of rectal thermometer (use a tympanic thermometer when available).	A rectal thermometer can damage rectal mucosa and cause rectal bleeding.
Test all secretions and excretions.	These may contain occult blood.
For patients with platelet count less than 50,000/mm^3, place a sign on patient's door indicating that thrombocytopenia precautions are in effect.	Notifying all who enter the patient's room that the patient is at risk for bleeding optimally promotes the patient's safety.
In the presence of bleeding, begin pad count for heavy menses; measure quantity of vomiting and stool.	These actions quantify the amount of bleeding.
Discourage use of tampons.	Tampons may cause vaginal trauma during placement, resulting in bleeding.
Apply direct pressure and ice to site of bleeding (VAD, venipuncture).	Applying pressure and ice promote bleeding cessation.
Deliver platelet transfusions as prescribed and be alert to a transfusion reaction.	Patients may lose blood from surgery, or the cancer may cause internal bleeding. In addition, both radiation and chemotherapy affect cells in the bone marrow, leading to low blood cell counts. Transfusion reactions can occur when white cells or antigens were not removed properly.
Initiate oral care at frequent intervals.	Gentle oral care promotes integrity of gingiva and mucosa and helps prevent bleeding and infection.
Advise brushing with a soft-bristle toothbrush after meals and before bed (hot water run over bristles may soften them further).	Hard bristles may damage the gingival and oral mucosa.
Avoid oral irrigation tools. In the presence of gum bleeding, teach use of sponge-tipped applicator rather than toothbrush, avoiding dental floss, and avoiding mouthwash with alcohol content.	**Caution:** Dental care should not be performed until the platelet count approaches normal.
Suggest use of normal saline solution mouthwashes 4 times a day and water-based ointment for lubricating lips.	Alcohol-based products irritate impaired oral tissue and could promote bleeding.
Implement bowel program and check with the patient daily for bowel movement.	If the patient's platelet count is critically low, straining at stool must be avoided to prevent intraabdominal bleeding. Daily monitoring of bowel pattern promotes early intervention if it is needed.
Assess need for stool softeners or psyllium.	These agents help prevent constipation and straining, which could result in bleeding.
Encourage high-fiber foods and adequate hydration (at least 2500 mL/day) if not contraindicated due to co-morbid conditions.	Hydration and fiber promote stools that are soft with adequate bulk, both of which facilitate bowel movements without straining.
Avoid use of rectal suppositories, enemas, or harsh laxatives.	These products increase risk of bleeding/infection from inadvertent trauma to rectal mucosa.
Implement and teach measures that reduce risk of bleeding.	Patients should use electric shaver; apply direct pressure and elevation for 3-5 min after injections and venipuncture; and avoid vaginal douche and tampons and constrictive clothing. Alcohol is to be avoided as are medications that could induce bleeding, such as aspirin or aspirin-containing products, anticoagulants, and nonsteroidal antiinflammatory drugs (NSAIDs). Patients should perform gentle nose blowing and use emery board rather than clippers for nail care. Bladder catheterization should be avoided if possible.
Caution the patient to abstain from sexual intercourse when the platelet count is less than 50,000/mm^3. Otherwise, instruct the patient to use water-soluble lubrication during sexual intercourse. Caution the patient to avoid anal intercourse.	Sexual intercourse could traumatize vaginal, anal, and penile tissue, causing bleeding or introduction of bacteria.
Caution the patient to avoid activities that predispose to trauma or injury, and remove hazardous objects or furniture from the patient's environment. Assist with ambulating if physical mobility is impaired.	This information reduces the possibility of trauma that could result in bleeding.

PART I: Medical-Surgical Nursing

ASSESSMENT/INTERVENTIONS	RATIONALES
⚠ If the patient's platelet count is less than 20,000/mm³, teach the importance of avoiding activities such as moving up in bed, straining at stool, bending at the waist, and lifting heavy objects (more than 10 lb). Suggest bedrest if the platelet count is less than 10,000/mm³.	Valsalva's and other maneuvers that increase intracranial pressure put the patient at risk for intracerebral bleeding.

See also: Chapter 65, "Thrombocytopenia," p. 479.

Nursing Diagnoses:

Impaired Skin Integrity
Impaired Tissue Integrity

related to treatment with chemotherapy or biotherapy

Desired Outcome: Before chemotherapy, the patient identifies potential skin and tissue side effects of chemotherapy and measures that will maintain skin integrity and promote comfort.

ASSESSMENT/INTERVENTIONS	RATIONALES
Transient Erythema/Urticaria: Perform and document a pretreatment assessment of the patient's skin.	Pretreatment assessment enables a more accurate assessment of the posttreatment reaction. Alterations of skin or nails that occur in conjunction with chemotherapy are a result of destruction of the basal cells of the epidermis (general) or of cellular alterations at the site of chemotherapy administration (local). Transient erythema/urticaria may be generalized or localized at the site of chemotherapy administration.
⚠ If a skin reaction occurs and the chemotherapy is infusing, halt the chemotherapy temporarily.	This action may prevent further skin/tissue damage until the nature of the reaction can be ascertained.
Assess and document onset, pattern, severity, and duration of the reaction after treatment.	Reactions are specific to the agent used and vary in onset, severity, and duration. Usually they occur soon after chemotherapy is administered and disappear in several hours.
Hyperpigmentation: Inform the patient before treatment that this reaction is to be expected and may or may not disappear over the first few months when treatment is finished.	Hyperpigmentation is believed to be caused by increased levels of epidermal melanin-stimulating hormone. It can occur on the nail beds, on the oral mucosa, or along the veins used for chemotherapy administration, or it can be generalized. Hyperpigmentation is associated with many chemotherapeutic agents, but incidence is highest with alkylating agents and antitumor antibiotics. In addition, it can occur with tumors of the pituitary gland.
Caution the patient to wear sunscreen with a high sun protection factor (SPF) and cover exposed areas.	Sunlight may exacerbate hyperpigmentation.
Telangiectasis (Spider Veins): Inform the patient that this reaction is permanent but that the vein configuration will become less severe over time.	Telangiectasis is believed to be caused by destruction of the capillary bed and occurs as a result of applications of topical carmustine and mechlorethamine.
Photosensitivity: Assess onset, pattern, severity, and duration of the reaction.	Photosensitivity is enhanced when skin is exposed to ultraviolet light. Acute sunburn and residual tanning may occur with very short exposure to the sun when receiving certain chemotherapy drugs. Photosensitivity can occur during the time the agent is administered, or it can reactivate a skin reaction caused by recent sun exposure before chemotherapy.

continued

ASSESSMENT/INTERVENTIONS	RATIONALES
Teach the patient to avoid exposing skin to the sun. Advise wearing protective clothing and using an effective sun-screening agent (SPF of 15 or higher).	Photosensitivity is enhanced when skin is exposed to ultraviolet light. Acute sunburn and residual tanning can occur with short exposure to the sun.
Teach the patient to treat sunburns with comfort measures and to consult the health care provider accordingly.	Such measures as taking a tepid bath and using moisturizing cream and aloe are usually effective.

Hyperkeratosis:

For patients taking bleomycin, assess for the presence of skin thickening and loss of fine motor function of the hands.	Hyperkeratosis presents as a thickening of the skin, especially over hands, feet, face, and areas of trauma. It is disfiguring and causes loss of fine motor function of the hands.
In the presence of skin thickening, assess for fibrotic lung changes: dyspnea, cough, tachypnea, and crackles.	Hyperkeratosis may be an indicator of more severe fibrotic changes in the lungs that usually are not reversible.
Reassure the patient that skin thickening is usually reversible when bleomycin has been discontinued.	The patient will be less anxious knowing the condition is usually reversible.

Acne-Like Reaction:

Suggest use of commercial acne preparations, such as benzoyl peroxide lotion, gel, or cream, to treat blemishes.	An acne-like reaction presents as erythema, especially of the face, and progresses to papules and pustules, which are characteristic of acne and will disappear when the drug is discontinued.

Teach Proper Skin Care:

- Avoid hard scrubbing.	Scrubbing can cause skin breaks that enable bacterial entry.
- Avoid use of antibacterial soap. Use a mild plain soap.	Removal of nonpathogenic bacteria on the skin results in replacement by pathogens, which are implicated in the genesis of acne.
- Avoid use of oil-based cosmetics.	Oil can clog pores and trap bacteria.

Ulceration:

Assess for ulceration.	Ulceration presents as a generalized, shallow lesion of the epidermal layer and may be caused by several chemotherapeutic agents.
Treat ulcers with a solution of $\frac{1}{4}$-strength hydrogen peroxide and $\frac{3}{4}$-strength normal saline q4-6h.	This solution effectively cleanses the lesions.
Rinse with normal saline solution.	Normal saline rinses remove the cleansing solution from the skin.
Expose the ulcer to air, if possible.	A dark, moist, warm environment may promote bacterial growth and delay healing.
Be alert to signs of infection at the ulcerated site.	Local warmth, swelling, tenderness, erythema, and purulent drainage may be present at the site of ulceration and should be reported to the health care provider for treatment.

Radiation Recall Reaction:

Explain why radiation recall can occur and its signs and symptoms.	Radiation recall can occur when chemotherapy is given after treatment with radiation therapy. Radiation enhancement occurs when radiation and chemotherapy are given concurrently. Both present as erythema, followed by dry desquamation at the radiation site. More severe reactions can progress to vesicle formation and wet desquamation. After the skin heals, it may be permanently hyperpigmented.
Teach strategies to protect skin at the site of recall reaction. - Avoid sun exposure, which may precipitate a reaction similar to radiation recall. - Avoid wearing tight-fitting clothes and harsh fabrics. - Avoid excess heat or cold exposure to the area, salt water or chlorinated pools, deodorants, perfumed lotions, cosmetics, and shaving of the area. - Use mild detergents, such as Ivory Snow.	These are preventive strategies that may lessen severity of radiation recall reaction.

ASSESSMENT/INTERVENTIONS	RATIONALES
Dry, Pruritic Skin: Explain why dry, pruritic skin can occur and its signs and symptoms.	Dry, pruritic skin commonly occurs with biotherapy (e.g., Interferon, IL-2) or radiation recall reaction and should be treated aggressively. It may be accompanied by a rash and eventual desquamation.
Teach strategies for treating this condition. - Apply creams and water-based lotions several times a day, avoiding perfumed products. - Avoid hot bathing water and use only mild soaps. - Manage pruritus with antipruritic medications such as diphenhydramine or hydroxyzine hydrochloride. - Teach patients receiving IL-2 to check with their health care provider before using steroids because these may interfere with therapy.	These are strategies that may lessen severity of dry, pruritic skin.
See **Impaired Skin Integrity**, which follows, for more details about wound care.	

Nursing Diagnosis:

Impaired Skin Integrity

related to radiation therapy

Desired Outcome: Within 24 hr of instruction, the patient identifies skin reactions and management interventions that will promote comfort and skin integrity.

ASSESSMENT/INTERVENTIONS	RATIONALES
Assess the degree and extent of the skin reaction.	Severe skin reactions may necessitate a delay in radiation treatments. Skin reactions are graded as follows: *Grade 1:* Faint erythema or dry desquamation. *Grade 2:* Moderate to brisk erythema or patchy moist desquamation, moderate edema. *Grade 3:* Confluent moist desquamation, blisters, pitting edema. *Grade 4:* Skin ulceration or necrosis of full thickness dermis. (National Cancer Institute [NCI] Common Toxicity Criteria)
Teach the following skin care for the treatment field:	This information enables the patient to self-treat or obtain specialized help for the skin reaction stage.
- Cleanse skin gently and in a patting motion, using mild soap, tepid water, and soft cloth. Rinse the area and pat it dry.	Grade 1 reactions often do not require special interventions other than gentle, normal skin care.
- Apply cornstarch, A&D ointment, ointment containing aloe or lanolin, or mild topical steroids as prescribed.	This is the skin care protocol for a grade 2 reaction.
- Cleanse the area with ½-strength hydrogen peroxide and normal saline, using irrigation syringe. Rinse with saline or water and pat dry gently. - Use nonadhesive absorbent dressings for draining areas. Be alert to signs and symptoms of infection.	This is the skin care protocol for grade 3 skin reaction.
- Use moisture- and vapor-permeable dressings, such as hydrocolloids and hydrogels, on noninfected areas.	These dressings promote healing.
- Topical antibiotics (e.g., sulfadiazine cream) may be applied to open areas susceptible to infection.	This is the skin care protocol for grade 4 reaction.
Débride wound of eschar.	This measure is necessary before healing can occur.

continued

ASSESSMENT/INTERVENTIONS	RATIONALES
After removing eschar (results in yellow-colored wound), keep the wound clean. (Wet-to-moist dressings often are used to keep the wound clean.)	This measure prevents infection.
Collaborate with a Wound and Ostomy Care (WOC) nurse as needed.	This nurse is trained specifically and often certified in wound and ostomy care.
Teach about the potential for altered pigmentation, atrophy, fragility, or ulceration.	These long-term skin changes are associated with radiation.

Nursing Diagnoses:

Impaired Tissue Integrity (or risk for same)
Risk for Vascular Trauma

related to extravasation of vesicant or irritating chemotherapy agents

Desired Outcome: The patient's tissue remains intact without evidence of inflammation or tissue/vascular damage near the injection site.

ASSESSMENT/INTERVENTIONS	RATIONALES
⚠ Ensure that vesicant chemotherapy is administered by a nurse who is experienced in venipuncture and knowledgeable about chemotherapy.	Vesicant agents have the potential to produce tissue damage and therefore should be administered by a nurse skilled in venipuncture (Payne & Savarese, 2013). Vesicant agents include dactinomycin, daunomycin, doxorubicin, mitomycin C, epirubicin, estramustine, idarubicin, mechlorethamine, mitoxantrone, paclitaxel, vinblastine, vincristine, vindesine, and vinorelbine. The following irritants have the potential to produce pain along the injection site with or without inflammation: amsacrine, bleomycin, carmustine, dacarbazine, doxorubicin liposome, etoposide, ifosfamide, plicamycin, streptozocin, docetaxel, and teniposide.
Select the IV site carefully, using a new site if possible.	Ideally the IV site will be newly accessed for vesicant administration. A site older than 24 hr should be avoided because it will be difficult to ensure vessel integrity.
Avoid sites such as the antecubital fossa, wrist, or dorsal surface of the hand.	In these sites there is increased risk of damage to underlying tendons or nerves if extravasation occurs.
Assess patency of the venous site before and during administration of the drug. Instruct patient to report burning, itching, or pain immediately.	Extravasation of vesicants often causes immediate symptoms. Prompt reporting of these symptoms by the patient will enable early intervention to minimize tissue damage.
Assess venous access site at frequent intervals.	Pain, burning, and stinging are common with extravasation, as are erythema and swelling around the needle site. Blood return should not be used as the sole indicator to ascertain that extravasation has not occurred inasmuch as blood return is possible even in the presence of extravasation.
⚠ Keep an extravasation kit readily available, along with institutional guidelines for extravasation management.	Not all vesicants have antidotes. When administering vesicants with known antidotes, the antidote should be readily available in combination with the extravasation kit. Because time is of the essence to minimize tissue destruction when extravasation occurs, institutional guidelines or extravasation kit must be readily accessible before initiating drug delivery.
⚠ In the event of extravasation, follow these general guidelines:	Early intervention at the site of extravasation minimizes tissue damage.
- Stop the infusion immediately and aspirate any remaining drug from needle. To do this, first don latex gloves, then attach syringe to the tubing and aspirate the drug.	This action removes as much drug as possible from the extravasated site, thereby limiting tissue exposure.

ASSESSMENT/INTERVENTIONS	RATIONALES
- Consult chemotherapy infusion guidelines.	These guidelines provide specifics regarding management of extravasation of individual drugs.
- Leave the needle in place if using an antidote.	The needle enables access if an antidote is to be used with the extravasated drug.
- Do not apply pressure to the site. Apply a sterile occlusive dressing, elevate the site, and apply heat or cold as recommended by guidelines.	Pressure may cause added tissue damage.
- Document the incident, noting date, time, needle insertion site, venous access device type and size, drug, drug concentration, approximate amount of drug extravasated, patient symptoms, extravasation management, and appearance of the site. Review institutional guidelines regarding necessity of photo documentation. Assess the site at frequent intervals.	Documentation of actions taken ensures accuracy in case questions arise later about how the extravasation was managed. Photos provide a reference point for evaluation.
- Provide the patient with information about site care and follow-up appointments for evaluation of the extravasation. If appropriate, collaborate with health care provider regarding a plastic surgery consultation.	Tissue damaged by extravasation may take a long time to heal or may deteriorate so much that plastic surgery may be necessary. Patient needs to understand these possibilities to ensure optimal extravasation management.

Nursing Diagnosis:

Risk for Injury

(to staff, patients, and environment) *related to* improper preparation, handling, administration, and disposal of chemotherapeutic agents

Desired Outcome: There is minimal chemotherapy exposure of staff and environment by proper preparation, handling, administration, and disposal of waste by individuals familiar with these agents.

Note: *Pharmacists or specially trained and supervised personnel should prepare chemotherapy, and nurses familiar with these agents should administer them. Institutional guidelines should be readily available for safe preparation, handling, and potential complications such as spills or individual contact with these drugs. A chemotherapy administration certification course, which includes clinical mentoring, is highly recommended for nurses planning to administer chemotherapeutics.*

Although no information is available regarding reproductive risks of handling chemotherapy drugs in workers who use a biologic safety cabinet and wear protective clothing, employees who are pregnant, planning a pregnancy (male or female), breastfeeding, or have other medical reasons prohibiting exposure to chemotherapy drugs may elect to refrain from preparing or administering these agents or caring for patents during their treatment and up to 48 hr after completion of therapy. Both spontaneous abortion and congenital malformation excesses have been documented among workers handling some of these drugs without currently recommended engineering controls and precautions. The facility should have a policy regarding reproductive toxicity of hazardous drugs and worker exposure in male and female employees and should follow that policy (Centers for Disease Control and Prevention, 2013).

ASSESSMENT/INTERVENTIONS	RATIONALES
⚠ Implement the following measures when working with chemotherapy: use a biologic safety cabinet (laminar flow hood); an absorbent, plastic-backed pad placed on the work area; latex gloves (powder free and a minimum of 0.007 inch thick); full-length impervious (nonabsorbent) gown with cuffed sleeves and back closure; and goggles. Wear gloves and gowns during all handling and disposal of these agents.	These measures minimize the potential for aerosolization with resultant inhalation and direct skin contact with chemotherapeutic drugs during preparation.

continued

ASSESSMENT/INTERVENTIONS	RATIONALES
Prime the IV tubing with diluent rather than with fluid containing the chemotherapy agent.	This enables the nurse to challenge the vein before infusing potentially tissue-irritating or damaging agents.
Use syringes and IV administration sets with Luer-Lok fittings.	These fittings prevent accidental dislodgement of needles or tubing and thus an accidental chemotherapy spill.
When removing the IV administration set, wear latex gloves and wrap sterile gauze around the insertion port.	These actions prevent direct or aerosol contact with the drug.
Place all needles (that have not been crushed, clipped, or recapped), syringes, drugs, drug containers, and related material in a puncture-proof container that is clearly marked *Biohazardous Waste*. **Note:** Follow this procedure for disposal of immunotherapy waste as well.	Proper disposal of waste prevents accidental exposure to other workers and the environment.
Wear latex gloves (and impermeable gown and goggles if splashing is possible) when handling all body excretions for 48 hr after chemotherapy.	The drug is excreted through urine and feces and is present in blood and body fluids for approximately 48 hr after chemotherapy.
Ensure that only specially trained personnel clean a chemotherapy spill using a spill kit.	Chemotherapy spills could result in inadvertent exposure to other health care workers, the public, other patients, and the environment. Therefore, only staff properly trained in handling these agents should be allowed to manage a spill. Double-gloves, eye protection, and an appropriate, full-length gown is worn. Absorbent pads are used to absorb liquid; solid waste is picked up with moist absorbent gauze; glass fragments are collected with a small scoop—never with hands. These areas are cleansed three times with a detergent solution. All waste is put in a biohazardous waste container.
In the event of skin contact with the drug, wash the affected area with soap and water. Notify the health care provider for follow-up care. If eye contact occurs, irrigate the eye with water for 15 min and notify the health care provider for follow-up care.	Chemotherapeutic drugs may be absorbed through skin and mucous membranes.

Nursing Diagnosis:

Risk for Injury

(to staff, other patients, and visitors) *related to* potential for exposure to sealed sources of radiation, such as cesium-137 (^{137}Cs), iridium-192 (^{192}Ir), iodine-125 (^{125}I), palladium-103, strontium-90, or samarium-153 (^{153}Sm); or unsealed sources of radiation, such as iodine-131 (^{131}I) or phosphorus-32 (^{32}P)

Desired Outcome: Staff and visitors verbalize understanding about potential adverse effects of exposure to radiation and measures that must be taken to ensure personal safety.

ASSESSMENT/INTERVENTIONS	RATIONALES
Assign the patient a private room (with private bathroom), and place an appropriate radiation precaution sign on the patient's chart, door, and ID bracelet. Be aware of appropriate radiation precautions (listed on safety precaution sheet) before beginning care of the patient.	These measures minimize radiation exposure risk to employees, other patients, and visitors. Most institutions have a radiation safety committee that helps provide and enforce guidelines to minimize radiation risks to employees and the environment (committee guidelines should be kept readily available). The committee approves certain rooms that may be used for patients undergoing radioactive treatment to minimize exposure to employees and other patients.
Follow radiologist or agency protocol for visitor restrictions.	Visitors usually are restricted to 1 hr/day and should stand 6 ft from the bed for their own protection.
Ensure that pregnant women and children younger than age 18 do not enter the room.	Rapidly dividing cells (e.g., those of a fetus) are more susceptible to effects of radiation.

PART I: Medical-Surgical Nursing

ASSESSMENT/INTERVENTIONS	RATIONALES
⚠ Implement the two major principles involved in care of patients with radiation sources: *time* and *distance*.	These principles help ensure optimal care planning and staff and visitor safety by minimizing amount of time spent in room of patients with radiation sources, thus reducing exposure time and maximizing distance from implant (e.g., if the implant is in the patient's prostate, stand at the head of bed [HOB]). *Time:* Staff members should not spend more than 30 min/shift with the patient and should not care for more than two patients with implants at the same time. Staff should perform nondirect care activities in the hall (e.g., opening food containers, preparing food tray, opening medications). Linen should be changed only when it is soiled, rather than routinely, and complete bed baths should be avoided. *Distance:* Radiation exposure is greater the closer one is to the source.
⚠ Wear designated specialized gloves when in contact with secretions and excretions of all patients treated with unsealed radiation sources. Flush toilet at least three times after depositing urine or feces from commode.	Fluids from patients with unsealed radiation sources are a source of radiation exposure. **Note:** Urine from individuals with sealed radiation is not a source of radiation exposure and can be discarded in the usual manner. However, patients with implanted ^{125}I seeds should save all urine so that it may be assessed for presence of seeds.
⚠ Save all linen, dressings, and trash from patients with sealed sources of radiation.	The safety committee representative will analyze them before discard to ensure seeds have not been misplaced, which could result in accidental exposure to people or the environment.
⚠ Caution all staff members to use forceps, never the hands, to pick up seeds.	For protection against radiation exposure, long, disposable forceps and a sealed box should be kept in the room at all times in case displaced seeds are found.
⚠ Use disposable products for all patients with unsealed radiation. Cover all articles in the room with paper to prevent contamination.	These actions prevent inadvertent radiation exposure via body fluids, which will be radioactive for several days.
⚠ Attach a radiation badge (dosimeter) before entering the patient's room.	This badge monitors the amount of personal radiation exposure. According to federal regulations, radiation should not exceed 400 mrem/mo. Nurses who care for patients with radiation implants rarely receive this much exposure.

Nursing Diagnosis:

Imbalanced Nutrition: Less Than Body Requirements

related to nausea and vomiting or anorexia occurring with chemotherapy, radiation therapy, or disease; fatigue; or taste changes

Desired Outcome: At least 24 hr before hospital discharge, the patient and caregiver verbalize understanding of basic nutritional principles to prevent further weight loss.

ASSESSMENT/INTERVENTIONS	RATIONALES
For Anorexia: See Chapter 74, "Providing Nutritional Support," **Imbalanced Nutrition,** p. 542.	
Weigh the patient daily.	Nausea, vomiting, anorexia, and taste changes all may contribute to weight loss.
Assess food likes and dislikes, as well as cultural and religious preferences related to food choices.	Providing foods on the patient's "like" list as often as feasible and avoiding foods on "dislike" list optimally will promote sufficient intake. However, foods previously enjoyed may become undesirable, whereas previously disliked foods may appeal.

continued

ASSESSMENT/INTERVENTIONS	RATIONALES
Explain that anorexia may be caused by the pathophysiology of cancer and surgery or side effects of chemotherapy and radiation therapy.	Taste and olfactory receptors have a high rate of cell growth and may be sensitive to chemotherapy and radiation therapy.
Consult with a nutritionist and teach the importance of increasing caloric and protein intake.	Increasing calories augments energy, minimizes weight loss, and promotes tissue repair. Increasing protein facilitates repair and regeneration of cells.
Suggest that the patient eat several small meals at frequent intervals throughout the day.	Smaller, more frequent meals are usually better tolerated than larger meals.
Encourage use of nutritional supplements.	Adequate protein and calories are important for healing, fighting infection, and providing energy.
If indicated, consult the patient's health care provider regarding use of megestrol acetate and prednisone.	These agents have proved to have a positive influence on appetite stimulation and weight gain in individuals with cancer. Megestrol acetate is a progestogen similar to the hormone progesterone. It is used to treat breast cancer primarily, but because it is an appetite stimulant, it may be used for patients who have loss of appetite and weight loss in advanced cancer. Prednisone is a synthetic hormone called a "steroid" that is used in the treatment of many diseases and conditions, and it also has the effect of increasing appetite. These medications must be monitored closely for adverse effects.
For Nausea and Vomiting:	Nausea and vomiting may occur with advanced cancer, bowel obstruction, some medications, and metabolic abnormalities.
Assess the patient's pattern of nausea and vomiting: onset, frequency, duration, intensity, and amount and character of emesis.	Knowledge about the pattern of nausea and vomiting enables use of proper medication, route, and timing.
Explain that nausea and vomiting may be side effects of chemotherapy and radiation therapy.	The pathophysiology of nausea and vomiting is complex and involves transmission of impulses to receptors in the brain. Various antiemetics work at different points in the nausea/vomiting cycle. This action helps ensure coverage of the expected emetogenic period of the chemotherapy agent given.
Teach the patient to take the antiemetic, if prescribed, 1 hr before chemotherapy and to continue to take the drug as prescribed. Consider duration of previous nausea and vomiting episodes following chemotherapy when recommending antiemetic administration schedule.	Nausea is better controlled when the goal is prevention.
Explain that antiemetics are most effective if taken prophylactically or at nausea onset.	
Teach the patient to eat cold foods or foods served at room temperature.	The odor of hot food may aggravate nausea.
Suggest intake of clear liquids and bland foods.	Strong odors and tastes can stimulate nausea or suppress appetite.
Teach the patient to avoid sweet, fatty, highly salted, and spicy foods, as well as foods with strong odors, any of which may increase nausea.	Same as above.
Minimize stimuli such as smells, sounds, or sights, all of which may promote nausea.	Previous stimuli associated with nausea may provoke anticipatory nausea.
Encourage the patient to eat sour or mint candy during chemotherapy.	These candies decrease unpleasant, metallic taste.
If not contraindicated, teach the patient to take oral chemotherapy with antiemetics at bedtime.	This therapeutic combination and its timing help minimize incidence of nausea.
Encourage the patient to explore various dietary patterns. Suggest that the patient avoid eating or drinking for 1-2 hr before and after chemotherapy and to follow a clear liquid diet for 1-2 hr before and 1-24 hr after chemotherapy.	Some patients become nauseated in anticipation of chemotherapy. Reducing intake at this time may lessen this symptom.
Suggest that the patient avoid contact with food while it is being cooked and avoid being around people who are eating.	Prolonged exposure to smells can extinguish appetite or promote nausea.

ASSESSMENT/INTERVENTIONS	RATIONALES
Advise eating small, light meals at frequent intervals (5-6 times/day).	Presenting large volumes of food can be overwhelming, thereby extinguishing the appetite or causing nausea.
Suggest that the patient sit near an open window.	Breathing fresh air when feeling nauseated may relieve nausea.
Help the patient find an appropriate distraction technique (e.g., music, television, reading).	Helping focus on things other than nausea may be helpful in nausea management.
Teach the patient to use relaxation techniques.	These techniques may help prevent anticipatory nausea and vomiting.
Instruct the patient to slowly sip clear liquids such as broth, ginger ale, cola, tea, or gelatin; suck on ice chips; and avoid large volumes of water.	These actions help to increase oral moisture to relieve dry mouth.
For Fatigue:	
If easily fatigued, encourage the patient to eat frequent, small meals and document intake.	The energy required to consume and digest a large meal may exacerbate fatigue and discourage further nutritional intake.
Provide foods that are easy to eat.	"Finger foods" (e.g., crackers with cheese or peanut butter, nuts, chunks of fruit, smoothies) require less energy expenditure to eat and enable patient to eat in a position of comfort rather than sitting at a table, which requires more energy.
If the patient wears oxygen during exertion, encourage wearing it while eating.	Food consumption requires energy. A fatigued, hypoxic person likely will consume less food.
Avoid offering meals immediately after exertion.	A fatigued person will be less likely to want to eat and will tire quickly while eating, which also requires energy expenditure.
For Taste Changes:	
Suggest trying foods not previously enjoyed.	Previously enjoyed foods may no longer seem attractive, whereas foods that were once undesirable may now seem pleasant.
Encourage good mouth care; assess mucous membrane for thrush, lesions, or mucositis.	Thrush infections can cause taste alterations yet are easily treated. A coated tongue may interfere with ability to taste.
Suggest trying strongly flavored foods.	Patients often report that usual foods taste like sawdust.

Nursing Diagnosis:

Impaired Oral Mucous Membrane

related to side effects of chemotherapy or biotherapy; radiation therapy to the head and neck; ineffective oral hygiene; gingival diseases; poor nutritional status; tumors of the oral cavity and neck; and infection

Desired Outcomes: The patient complies with the therapeutic regimen within 1 hr of instruction. The patient's oral mucosal condition improves as evidenced by intact mucous membrane; moist, intact tongue and lips; and absence of pain and lesions.

ASSESSMENT/INTERVENTIONS	RATIONALES
Assess the oral mucosa for integrity, color, and signs of infection.	Patients receiving cancer treatments are at risk for problems of the oral cavity such as dryness, lesions, inflammation, infection, and discomfort.
For patients with myelosuppression, caution not to floss teeth or use oral irrigators or a stiff toothbrush.	The oral cavity is a prime site for infection in a myelosuppressed patient. Actions such as brushing with a stiff toothbrush and flossing could affect integrity of the oral mucous membrane and place patients at risk for infection. Patients should consult with a dentist as indicated.

continued

ASSESSMENT/INTERVENTIONS	RATIONALES
Be aware that some patients may require parenteral analgesics, such as morphine.	Parenteral analgesics may be necessary to relieve pain and promote adequate nutritional intake in patients with moderate to severe mucositis.
Suggest to patients with xerostomia (dryness of the mouth from a lack of normal salivary secretion) caused by radiation therapy that they may benefit from chewing sugarless gum; sucking on sugarless candy, frozen fruit juice pops, or sugar-free Popsicles; or taking frequent sips of water. Saliva substitutes are another option, although they are expensive and do not last long.	These products replenish oral hydration and promote mucous membrane integrity. A dry mouth also interferes with nutritional intake.
Advise frequent dental follow-ups.	Lack of or decrease in salivary fluid predisposes patients to dental caries. Fluoride treatment is recommended for these patients for this reason.

Nursing Diagnosis:

Impaired Swallowing

related to mucositis of the oral cavity or esophagus (esophagitis) occurring with radiation therapy to the neck, chest, and upper back; use of chemotherapy agents; obstruction (tumors); or thrush

Desired Outcomes: Before food or fluids are given, the patient exhibits the gag reflex and is free of symptoms of aspiration as evidenced by RR 12-20 breaths/min with normal depth and pattern (eupnea), normal skin color, and the ability to speak. Following instruction, the patient verbalizes early signs and symptoms of esophagitis, alerts the health care team as soon as they occur, and identifies measures for maintaining nutrition and comfort.

ASSESSMENT/INTERVENTIONS	RATIONALES
⚠ Assess for evidence of impaired swallowing with concomitant respiratory difficulties.	Esophagitis can occur with radiation therapy to the neck, chest, and upper back or be caused by chemotherapy agents, tumors, or thrush. Impaired swallowing places patients at risk for aspiration and necessitates aspiration precautions.
⚠ Teach the patient early signs and symptoms of esophagitis and of stomatitis and the importance of reporting symptoms promptly if they occur.	Sensation of a lump in the throat with swallowing, difficulty with swallowing solid foods, and discomfort or pain with swallowing occur early in esophagitis. Signs of stomatitis include generalized burning sensation of the oral cavity, white patches on oral mucosa, ulcerations, and pain. Patients should report these indicators promptly to the health care team if they occur so that timely interventions can be made.
Assess the patient's dietary intake and weight, teaching the following guidelines:	Impaired swallowing predisposes patients to nutritional deficits. Dietary intake should be monitored closely to evaluate early weight loss trends.
- Maintain a high-protein diet.	Protein promotes healing.
- Eat foods that are soft and bland.	These foods minimize pain while swallowing.
- Add milk or milk products to the diet (for individuals without excessive mucus production).	These products coat the esophageal lining to facilitate swallowing.
- Add sauces and creams to foods.	These foods may facilitate swallowing.
- Ensure adequate fluid intake of at least 2 L/day.	Patients with impaired swallowing are at risk for dehydration because they may avoid drinking and eating to prevent pain.
Implement the following measures that promote comfort, and discuss them with the patient accordingly:	Reducing pain associated with swallowing will assist in maintaining adequate nutritional intake.

PART I: Medical-Surgical Nursing

ASSESSMENT/INTERVENTIONS | RATIONALES

ASSESSMENT/INTERVENTIONS	RATIONALES
- Use a local anesthetic or solution as prescribed to minimize pain with meals.	Lidocaine 2% and diphenhydramine may be taken by the patient via swish and spit or swallow before eating. Some solutions such as Magic Mouthwash may be prescribed by the health care provider for oral mucositis symptom relief. Although the specific ingredients can be tailored by the provider, common ingredients include an antibiotic to kill bacteria around a sore, an antihistamine or local anesthetic such as lidocaine to reduce pain and discomfort, an antifungal, a corticosteroid, and an antacid to help coat the inside of the mouth (Mayo Clinic, 2013).
[!] Advise the patient to use the solution as directed and to be aware that his or her gag reflex may be decreased.	The patient should wait approximately 30 min before eating or drinking to allow the solution to work and to eat and drink carefully due to the potential decrease of the gag reflex.
- Suggest that the patient sit in an upright position during meals and for 15-30 min after eating.	Esophageal reflux may occur with obstructions and can be distressing.
- Obtain a prescription for analgesics and administer as prescribed. Teach the importance of taking analgesics before eating or drinking to promote proper nutrition and hydration.	Discomfort may prevent patients from maintaining adequate nutritional intake. If pain is unrelieved with mild analgesics, an opioid such as oxycodone or morphine may be necessary.
Encourage frequent oral care with normal saline and sodium bicarbonate solution (1 teaspoon of each to 1 quart of water).	Impaired mucous membranes are at risk for infection with bacteria, yeast, and viruses.
Teach the patient to avoid irritants, such as alcohol, tobacco, and alcohol-based commercial mouthwashes.	Irritants exacerbate discomfort and may prevent intake of adequate nutrients.
[!] Have suction equipment readily available in case the patient experiences aspiration. Educate the patient about ways to manage oral secretions.	Esophageal reflux may occur with obstructions and can be distressing and cause aspiration.
[!] Suction the mouth as needed, using low, continuous suction equipment.	Suction helps manage secretions and prevent aspiration.
Teach the patient to expectorate saliva into tissues, and dispose of it per institutional policy.	This intervention helps patient manage oral secretions using proper infection control measures.

See also: Chapter 74, "Providing Nutritional Support," **Impaired Swallowing,** p. 547, for desired outcomes and interventions.

Nursing Diagnosis:

Impaired Urinary Elimination

related to hemorrhagic cystitis occurring with cyclophosphamide/ifosfamide treatment; or renal toxicity caused by medications, disease process, or treatments

Desired Outcomes: Patients receiving cyclophosphamide/ifosfamide test negative for blood in their urine, and patients receiving cisplatin exhibit urinary output of 100 mL/hr or more 1 hr before treatment and 4-12 hr after treatment. Patients with leukemia and lymphomas and those taking methotrexate exhibit urine pH of 7.5 or higher.

ASSESSMENT/INTERVENTIONS | RATIONALES

ASSESSMENT/INTERVENTIONS	RATIONALES
[!] Assess for and ensure adequate hydration during treatment and for at least 24 hr after treatment for patients taking cyclophosphamide, ifosfamide, methotrexate, or cisplatin. Teach the importance of drinking at least 2-3 L/day. IV hydration also may be required, especially with high-dose chemotherapy.	Adequate hydration ensures sufficient dilution of the drug by urine in the urinary system and prevents exposure of renal cells to high drug concentrations and possible toxicity. Renal failure also may ensue when cellular breakdown products deposit in the renal tubules when patients have been inadequately hydrated before the chemotherapy given for leukemia or lymphoma.

continued

PART I: Medical-Surgical Nursing

ASSESSMENT/INTERVENTIONS	RATIONALES
Administer cyclophosphamide early in the day. Encourage the patient to urinate q2h during the day and before going to bed at night.	These actions help minimize retention of metabolites in the bladder, especially during the night.
Test urine for the presence of blood, and report positive results to the health care provider.	Hemorrhagic cystitis can occur in patients taking cyclophosphamide/ifosfamide and should be reported promptly to ensure timely intervention.
Assess input and output (I&O) at least q8h during high-dose treatment for 48 hr after treatment. Be alert to decreasing urinary output.	Most chemotherapy drugs are eliminated from the body within a 48-hr period. Maintaining adequate urine output for 48 hr prevents high drug metabolite concentrations in the kidneys and bladder.
Ensure that mesna is administered before or with ifosfamide but before high doses of cyclophosphamide. Then mesna is administered 4 and 8 hr after the infusion of Ifosfamide (or via a continuous infusion).	Mesna inhibits the hemorrhagic cystitis caused by ifosfamide/cyclophosphamide. The half-life of mesna is shorter than the half-life of ifosfamide/cyclophosphamide. Therefore, multiple doses or continuous infusion of mesna beyond the end of the ifosfamide/cyclophosphamide infusion is required to prevent urotoxicity.
Test all urine for the presence of blood.	Ifosfamide and cyclophosphamide can cause hemorrhagic cystitis.
Promote fluid intake to maintain urine output at approximately 100 mL/hr. Assess I&O during infusion and for 24 hr after therapy to ensure that this level of urinary output is attained.	Adequate fluid intake and resultant urinary output ensure that chemotherapy metabolites in high concentrations do not stay within the urinary system for prolonged periods.
For patients receiving cisplatin, prehydrate with IV fluid (150-200 mL/hr). Assess I&O hourly for 4-12 hr after therapy.	This amount of hydration helps ensure that urine output is maintained at 100-150 mL/hr or more, which decreases the potential for nephrotoxicity, a potential side effect of cisplatin. Patients may require diuretics to maintain this output. Cisplatin can be administered as soon as urine output is 100-150 mL/hr.
Promote fluid intake for at least 24 hr after treatment, especially for patients taking diuretics. Notify the health care provider promptly if urine output drops to less than 100 mL/hr.	Continual flushing of the urinary system prevents concentration of cisplatin metabolites in the kidneys and potential associated nephrotoxicity. Urine output should be kept at a relatively high level.
In patients with leukemia and lymphoma, assess I&O q8h, being alert to decreasing output. Test urine pH with each voiding to ensure that it is 7.5 or higher.	If cellular breakdown products that occur from the chemotherapy effect on tumor cells are allowed to concentrate in the renal tubules, renal failure can occur. Proper hydration prevents this potential cause of renal failure. Alkaline urine promotes excretion of uric acid that results from tumor lysis associated with treatment of leukemia and lymphoma.
Administer sodium bicarbonate or acetazolamide (Diamox) as prescribed.	These agents alkalinize the urine.
Administer allopurinol as prescribed.	Allopurinol prevents uric acid formation and is often administered before chemotherapy for patients with leukemia or lymphoma.
Assess patients with leukemia and lymphoma for the presence of urinary calculi. For more information, see Chapter 31, "Ureteral Calculi."	Hyperuricemia may be caused by chemotherapy treatment for leukemia and lymphoma. The rapid cell lysis and increased excretion of uric acid may result in renal calculi.
Teach signs of cystitis: fever, pain with urination, malodorous or cloudy urine, blood in the urine, and urinary frequency and urgency. Instruct the patient to notify the health care professional if these signs and symptoms occur.	Cystitis can occur secondary to cyclophosphamide and ifosfamide treatment and should be reported to the health care provider for timely intervention.

Nursing Diagnosis:

Deficient Knowledge

related to unfamiliarity with the type of, procedure for, and purpose of radiation implant (internal radiation) and measures for preventing and managing complications

Desired Outcome: Before the radiation implant is inserted, the patient and significant other/caregiver verbalize understanding of the implant type and procedure and identify measures for preventing and managing complications.

ASSESSMENT/INTERVENTIONS	RATIONALES
Assess the patient's health care literacy (language, reading, comprehension). Assess culture and culturally specific information needs.	This assessment helps ensure that materials are selected and presented in a manner that is culturally and educationally appropriate.
Determine the patient's and caregiver's level of understanding of the radiation implant. Explain the following, as Indicated.	Knowledge level will determine content of the individualized teaching plan.
- Afterloading	Implant carrier is inserted in the operating room, and radioactive source is inserted later.
- Preloading	Radioactive source is implanted with carrier.
Explain that the implant is used to provide high doses of radiation therapy to one area.	This method spares normal tissue from radiation.
Explain that radiation precautions (see **Risk for Injury**, p. 26) are required.	These precautions protect the patient, health care team, other patients, and visitors.
Teach the following assessment guidelines and management interventions for specific types of implants:	

Gynecologic Implants:

⚠ Explain that the following may occur: vaginal drainage, bleeding, or tenderness; impaired bowel or urinary elimination; and phlebitis. Instruct the patient to report any of these or any associated signs and symptoms.	An informed patient likely will report untoward signs and symptoms promptly to ensure timely treatment.
⚠ Explain that complete bedrest is required.	Bedrest helps prevent displacement of implants. HOB may be elevated to 30-45 degrees, and the patient may logroll from side to side. A urinary catheter is placed to facilitate urinary elimination.
Advise that a low-residue diet and medications to prevent bowel elimination may be prescribed.	These interventions help prevent bowel movements during the implant period. Generally a bowel clean-out (oral cathartics and/or enemas until clear) is prescribed.
⚠ Teach the patient to perform isometric exercises while on bedrest.	Isometric exercises minimize risk of contractures and muscle atrophy and promote venous return during bedrest.
Encourage the patient to take analgesics routinely for pain or to request analgesic before pain becomes severe.	These actions help keep pain at a minimal level. Prolonged stimulation of pain receptors results in increased sensitivity to painful stimuli and increase amount of drug required to relieve pain.
⚠ Explain the importance of and rationale for wearing antiembolism hose and performing calf-pumping and ankle-circling exercises while on bedrest. If prescribed, describe rationale for and use of sequential compression devices or pneumatic foot pumps.	These actions help prevent the lower extremity venostasis, thrombophlebitis, and emboli that can occur during enforced bedrest.
Explain that ambulation will be increased gradually when bedrest no longer is required (see Chapter 4, "Prolonged Bedrest," p. 61, for guidelines after prolonged immobility).	Gradual increments in ambulation will promote return to normal body function without undue stress on the body.
⚠ Explain that after the radiation source has been removed, the patient should dilate her vagina either through sexual intercourse or a vaginal dilator.	These actions help prevent vaginal fibrosis or stenosis.

Head and Neck Implants:

After a complete nutritional assessment, discuss measures for nutritional support during the implantation, such as a soft or liquid diet, a high-protein diet, and optimal hydration (more than 2500 mL/day).	Irradiated tissues may be swollen, irritated, and painful, which may interfere with nutritional intake. A high-protein diet promotes healing.
⚠ Teach signs and symptoms of infection at the site of implantation.	Fever, pain, swelling, local increased warmth, erythema, and purulent drainage at the implantation site may occur. Patients should report these indicators promptly to ensure timely treatment.

continued

PART I: Medical-Surgical Nursing

ASSESSMENT/INTERVENTIONS	RATIONALES
When appropriate, advise need for careful and thorough oral hygiene while the implant is in place.	Irradiated tissues are vulnerable to infection by bacteria, yeast, and viruses. **Note:** When implants are placed within the tongue, palate, or other structures of the buccal cavity, patients should not perform oral hygiene. Oral hygiene will be specifically prescribed by the health care provider and generally accomplished by the nurse. Improper mouth care could result in dislodgement of the device, pain, or improper cleansing.
Encourage the patient to take analgesics routinely for pain or to request analgesic before pain becomes severe.	These actions help ensure optimal pain management. Prolonged stimulation of pain receptors results in increased sensitivity to painful stimuli and increases amount of drug required to relieve pain.
Advise the patient to use a humidifier.	A humidifier will aid in maintaining moist mucous membranes and secretions. The patient should be instructed in procedures for cleaning the humidifier to avoid introduction of bacteria.
Identify alternative means for communication if the patient's speech deteriorates. Consult speech therapist as appropriate.	Patients should be aware that cards, Magic Slate, pencil and paper, and picture boards are potential communication measures. Preparing patients before impairment likely would reduce anxiety.

Breast Implants:

Teach signs of infection that may appear in the breast.	Pain, fever, swelling, erythema, warmth, and drainage at insertion site are indicators of infection and should be reported immediately for timely treatment.
Teach the importance of avoiding trauma at the implant site and keeping skin clean and dry.	These actions will help maintain skin integrity, prevent infection, and promote healing.
Encourage the patient to take analgesics routinely for pain or to request analgesic before pain becomes severe.	Pain is more efficiently managed when pain medications are administered promptly and before it becomes severe. Prolonged stimulation of pain receptors results in increased sensitivity to painful stimuli and will increase the amount of drug required to relieve pain.

Prostate Implants:

Explain need for the patient to use a urinal for voiding.	Use of a urinal will help ensure that urinary output is measured every shift and enable inspection of urine for the presence of radiation seeds.
Instruct the patient or caregiver to report dysuria, decreasing caliber of stream, difficulty urinating, voiding small amounts, feelings of bladder fullness, or hematuria.	Localized inflammation from radiation may cause urinary obstruction.
Inform the patient that linen, dressings, and trash need to be saved.	This information helps ensure that all radiation seeds will be accounted for.
Encourage the patient to take analgesics routinely for pain or to request analgesic before pain becomes severe.	Pain is more efficiently managed when pain medications are administered promptly and before it becomes severe. Prolonged stimulation of pain receptors results in increased sensitivity to painful stimuli and will increase amount of drug required to relieve pain.
Caution that the caregiver should limit amount of time spent close to implant site.	This precaution helps ensure the caregiver's protection from the radiation source.

Nursing Diagnosis:

Deficient Knowledge

related to unfamiliarity with the purpose and procedure for external beam radiation therapy, appropriate self-care measures after treatment, and available educational and community resources

Desired Outcome: Before external radiation beam therapy is initiated, the patient and significant other/caregiver identify its purpose and describe the procedure, appropriate self-care measures, and available educational and community resources.

ASSESSMENT/INTERVENTIONS | RATIONALES

ASSESSMENT/INTERVENTIONS	RATIONALES
See the first eight assessment/interventions under **Deficient Knowledge** related to chemotherapy, which follows.	
Provide information about the treatment schedule, duration of each treatment, and number of treatments planned.	Outlining the plan of care reduces anxiety and helps the patient and family plan their lives and activities accordingly. Radiation therapy usually is given 5 days/wk, Monday through Friday. The treatment itself lasts only a few minutes; the majority of the time is spent preparing patient for treatment. Immobilization devices and shields are positioned before treatment to ensure proper delivery of radiation and to minimize radiation to surrounding normal tissue.
Explain that the skin will be marked with pinpoint dots called *tattoos*.	Tattoos, which are permanent, assist technicians in positioning the radiation beam accurately and ensuring precise delivery of the radiation.
Caution that it is important not to use skin lotions, deodorants, or soaps unless approved by the radiation therapy provider.	Some products may interfere with radiation.
Discuss side effects that may occur with radiation treatment and appropriate self-care measures. See other nursing diagnoses and interventions in this section for more detail about local side effects.	Systemic side effects include fatigue and anorexia; however, the most commonly occurring side effects appear locally (e.g., side effects associated with head and neck radiation include mucositis, xerostomia, altered taste sensation, dental caries, sore throat, hoarseness, dysphagia, headache, and nausea and vomiting).
Teach strategies that help prevent skin breakdown.	These strategies include preventing local irritation by clothing, belts, or collars; avoiding chemical irritants such as alcohol, deodorants, or lotions; avoiding sun exposure of irradiated areas; and avoiding tape application to the radiation field.
Provide written materials that list radiation side effects and their management.	Supplemental written materials enhance knowledge and understanding.
Provide information about community resources for transportation to and from the radiation center and for skilled nursing care, as needed.	Stress associated with travel to a radiation center may interfere significantly with the lives of family members and may even give patients cause to terminate treatment. Home care nurses can assist the patient and family at home as treatment progresses and side effects become more pronounced.

Nursing Diagnosis:

Deficient Knowledge

related to unfamiliarity with chemotherapy and the purpose, expected side effects, and potential toxicities related to chemotherapy drugs; appropriate self-care measures for minimizing side effects; and available community and educational resources

Desired Outcome: Before the nurse administers specific chemotherapeutic agents, the patient and caregiver(s) verbalize knowledge about potential side effects and toxicities, appropriate self-care measures for minimizing side effects, and available community and educational resources.

ASSESSMENT/INTERVENTIONS | RATIONALES

ASSESSMENT/INTERVENTIONS	RATIONALES
Assess the patient's health care literacy (language, reading, comprehension). Assess culture and culturally specific information needs.	This assessment helps ensure that information is selected and presented in a manner that is culturally and educationally appropriate.
Establish the patient's and caregiver's current level of knowledge about the patient's health status, goals of therapy, and expected outcomes.	Understanding the knowledge level of the patient and caregiver will facilitate development of an individualized teaching plan.

continued

ASSESSMENT/INTERVENTIONS	RATIONALES
Assess the patient's and caregiver's cognitive and emotional readiness to learn.	To facilitate learning, teaching must be tailored to comprehensive abilities. The denial process may prevent comprehension of teaching content.
Assess barriers to learning. Define all terminology as needed. Correct any misconceptions about therapy and expected outcomes.	Barriers, including ineffective communication, inability to read, neurologic deficit, sensory alterations, fear, anxiety, or lack of motivation will affect learning and the teaching plan.
Provide written materials to reinforce information taught.	The ACS, NCI, pharmaceutical companies, and other organizations publish high-quality patient education materials the nurse may use to complement any verbal teaching.
Assess the patient's and caregiver's learning needs and establish short-term and long-term goals. Identify preferred methods of learning and amount of information they would like to receive.	Identifying preferred methods of learning and amount of information they would like to receive enables the nurse to develop a teaching plan based on this information.
Use individualized verbal and audiovisual strategies. Give simple, direct instructions; reinforce this information often.	These strategies promote learning and comprehension. Because anxiety may interfere with comprehension, repetition will help reinforce teaching.
Provide an environment free of distractions and conducive to teaching and learning.	A quiet setting free of distraction facilitates learning and retention.
Discuss medications the patient will receive. Provide both written and verbal information.	To help ensure that retention has occurred, the patients should be able to verbalize accurate knowledge about route of administration, duration of treatment, schedule, frequency of laboratory tests, most common side effects and toxicities, follow-up care, and appropriate self-care.
Provide emergency phone numbers.	These numbers should be used in case patient develops fever or side effects of chemotherapy that require emergent intervention.
Identify appropriate community resources to assist with transportation, costs of care, emotional support, and skilled care as appropriate.	Community resources may provide comfort for families under stress and prevent psychosocial issues from interfering with the plan of care.

Nursing Diagnosis:

Deficient Knowledge

related to unfamiliarity with immunotherapy and its purpose, potential side effects and toxicities; appropriate self-care measures to minimize side effects; and available community and education resources

Desired Outcome: Before immunotherapy is administered, the patient and significant other/caregiver verbalize understanding of its purpose, potential side effects and toxicities, appropriate self-care measures to minimize side effects, injection technique and site rotation (if appropriate), and available community and education resources.

ASSESSMENT/INTERVENTIONS	RATIONALES
See the first eight assessment/interventions under **Deficient Knowledge** related to chemotherapy, earlier.	
Teach proper injection technique and site rotation schedule. Teach the importance of recording the site of injection, time of administration, side effects, self-management of side effects, and any medications taken, as well as proper disposal of needles.	These patients often give their own injections of interferon. A diary or log will facilitate self-care.
Teach proper handling and storage of medication (e.g., refrigeration). As appropriate, arrange for community nursing follow-up for additional supervision and instruction.	Home care nursing support may reinforce teaching, assist with patient monitoring, and provide emotional support to patient and family.

ASSESSMENT/INTERVENTIONS	RATIONALES
Teach importance of being alert to the side effects of interferon.	Fever, chills, and flulike symptoms are expected side effects of interferon.
Suggest that the patient take acetaminophen, with health care provider's approval, to manage these symptoms, but avoid aspirin and NSAIDs.	Aspirin and NSAIDs may interrupt the action of interferon.
Assess I&O and weight closely for hospitalized patients and teach these assessments to patients.	Fluid shifts may occur with IL-2 treatment.
Teach the patient to monitor and record temperature twice daily and to drink 2000-3000 mL fluid/day.	These actions enable detection of fever, an expected interferon side effect, and replace fluid losses that can occur as a result.
Provide information regarding nutritional supplementation.	Dose-related anorexia and weight loss are other common side effects of interferon.

See also: Chapter 74, "Providing Nutritional Support," p. 539.

Nursing Diagnosis:

Disturbed Body Image

related to alopecia occurring with radiation therapy to the head and neck or administration of certain chemotherapeutic agents

Desired Outcome: The patient discusses the effects alopecia may have on self-concept, body image, and social interaction and identifies measures to cope satisfactorily with alopecia.

ASSESSMENT/INTERVENTIONS	RATIONALES
Discuss potential for hair loss before treatment.	Patients need to be informed about expected hair loss, depending on type of therapy, to develop strategies for coping and adaptation.
- Radiation therapy of 1500-3500 cGy to the head and neck will produce either partial or complete hair loss.	Hair loss is usually temporary and loss onset usually occurs 14-21 days from initiation of treatment. Regrowth begins as early as 2-3 months after final treatment but in some cases may take longer. This knowledge is likely to be reassuring to the patient.
- Radiation therapy of more than 4000 cGy usually results in permanent hair loss.	Patients may need to develop strategies for permanent hair loss.
- Hair loss associated with chemotherapy is temporary and related to specific agent, dose, and duration of administration.	Regrowth usually begins 1-2 mo after last treatment and hair often temporarily grows back a different texture. Common chemotherapeutic agents that cause alopecia include actinomycin D, amsacrine, bleomycin, cyclophosphamide, daunomycin, docetaxel, doxorubicin, epirubicin, etoposide (VP-16), topotecan (Hycamtin), idarubicin, ifosfamide, irinotecan (CPT-11), paclitaxel, teniposide, vinblastine, and vincristine.
Assess the impact hair loss has on the patient's self-concept, body image, and social interaction.	Alopecia is an extremely stressful side effect for most people. For some men, beard loss is disturbing as well.
Caution about the inadvisability of scalp hypothermia and tourniquet applications during IV chemotherapy.	These measures have not proved to be effective in minimizing hair loss and are contraindicated with some malignancies.
Suggest measures for women, such as cutting their hair short before treatment and selecting a wig before hair loss occurs that matches color and style of their own hair. Suggest wearing a hair net or turban during hair loss to help collect hair as it falls out.	These measures may help minimize the psychological impact of hair loss. Being prepared by having head coverings available when hair loss actually occurs may reduce anxiety surrounding the event. Wearing scarves, hats, caps, turbans, makeup, and accessories may enhance self-concept. **Note:** Wigs are tax deductible and often are reimbursed by insurance with appropriate prescriptions. Some centers and communities have wig banks that provide used and reconditioned wigs at no cost.

continued

ASSESSMENT/INTERVENTIONS	RATIONALES
Inform the patient that hair loss may occur on body parts other than the head.	Areas such as the axillae, groin, legs, eyes (eyelashes and eyebrows), and face also may lose hair. Loss of facial hair makes it difficult for makeup to stay on.
Instruct the patient to keep the head covered during summer and winter.	Covering the head minimizes sunburn during summer and prevents heat loss during winter. Certain chemotherapy agents and radiation therapy may sensitize skin to sun exposure.
Suggest resources that promote adaptation to alopecia.	For example, ACS hosts the "Look Good Feel Better" program, which provides women with encouragement and tips for managing body image changes during treatment.

Nursing Diagnosis:

Risk for Injury

related to changes in sensory perception (auditory, tactile, kinesthetic) and neuropathies associated with certain chemotherapeutic drugs

Desired Outcome: The patient reports early signs and symptoms of ototoxicity and peripheral neuropathy (functional disturbance of the peripheral nervous system), and measures are implemented promptly to minimize these side effects.

ASSESSMENT/INTERVENTIONS	RATIONALES
☒ Teach the patient and caregivers to report early symptoms of hearing loss the patient may experience.	Cumulative doses of cisplatin can result in irreversible loss of high-frequency range hearing or tinnitus.
Suggest that the patient face speakers and watch their lips during conversation while being aware that background noise may interfere with hearing ability.	This information promotes skills with which to cope with hearing loss.
Suggest a trial of a hearing aid before purchasing it.	A hearing aid may be helpful, or it may amplify background noise and worsen speech comprehension.
In instances of cisplatin-induced hearing loss, refer the patient to community resources for hearing-impaired persons.	Hearing loss from cisplatin is usually irreversible. A baseline audiogram may be done before cisplatin administration.
☒ Assess for development of peripheral neuropathy. Suggest consultation with PT or occupational therapist (OT) to assist with maintaining function. Explain that severity of symptoms may abate when treatment is halted; however, recovery may be slow and is usually incomplete.	Peripheral neuropathy can occur with several antineoplastic agents. Neurotoxicity is cumulative with some chemotherapy drugs, and therefore assessment of symptoms is done before delivery of each dose.
☒ Instruct the patient to report early signs and symptoms.	Numbness and tingling (paresthesias) of fingers and toes occur initially and can progress to difficulty with fine motor skills, such as buttoning shirts or picking up objects. The most severely affected individuals may lose sensation at hip level and have difficulty with balance and ambulation.
Assess for neuropathic pain. See **Chronic Pain**, p. 6, for desired outcomes and assessment/interventions.	Patients with neuropathies may experience neuropathic pain, which is often described and treated differently than nociceptive pain.
Assess bowel elimination daily in individuals at risk for paralytic ileus associated with neuropathy.	Patients receiving vinca alkaloids are at risk for paralytic ileus and require monitoring for this problem.
Administer stool softeners, psyllium, or laxatives daily if the patient does not have bowel movements at least every other day. Instruct the patient to increase dietary fiber and fluid intake.	If constipation is a problem, patients should be placed on a bowel regimen. Prevention of constipation is easier than treating constipation.

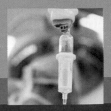

Pain 2

Nursing Diagnoses:

Acute Pain
Chronic Pain
Impaired Comfort

related to the disease process, injury, or surgical procedure

Desired Outcome: The patient's subjective report of pain using a pain scale, family's report, and behavioral and/or physiologic indicators reflect that pain is either reduced or at an acceptable level within 1-2 hr.

ASSESSMENT/INTERVENTIONS	RATIONALES
Obtain history about ongoing/previous pain experiences and previously used methods of pain control. Elicit what was/was not effective. Consider whether pain is acute, chronic, or acute with an underlying chronic component.	A pain history enables development of a systematic approach to pain management for each patient, using information gathered from pain history and the hierarchy of pain measurement (self-report, pathologic conditions or procedures that usually cause pain, behavioral indicators, report of family, and physiologic indicators). The Agency for Health Care Research and Quality (AHRQ, 2013) and the American Pain Society (APS, 2008) state that self-report of pain is the single most reliable indicator of pain.
Use a formal patient-specific method of assessing self-reported pain when possible, including description, location, intensity, and aggravating/alleviating factors.	The first step of effective pain management is accurate assessment of pain. Pain rating scales identify the intensity of pain over time and assist in evaluating the effectiveness of interventions. A numeric rating scale (NRS) of 0 (no pain) to 10 (worst possible pain), descriptive scales, and visual analog scale (VAS) are commonly used to assess intensity in adults who are cognitively intact. Pain intensity scales are available in many different languages when language barriers are present. The Wong-Baker FACES scale was developed for use in children. It is used in younger children and cognitively impaired adults. The Faces Pain Scale is appropriate for cognitively intact and cognitively impaired elders and appropriate for various cultures (Pasero & McCaffery, 2011). **Use the selected scale consistently.** **Note:** Although pain is multidimensional in nature, it is the subjective intensity of pain that is most often measured in clinical practice.
Assess for behavioral and physiologic indicators of pain at frequent intervals (e.g., during scheduled vital signs [VS] assessments). Document responses.	Behavioral and physiologic responses are potential indicators of pain in patients who are unable to self-report. This assessment optimizes reassessment and treatment intervals. **Note:** Not all patients demonstrate the same response to pain, nor does the lack of response negate the presence of pain.

continued

ASSESSMENT/INTERVENTIONS	RATIONALES
	Behavioral responses: Examples include facial expression (grimacing, facial tension, furrowed brow), vocalization (moaning, groaning, sighing, crying), verbalization (praying, counting), body action (rocking, rubbing, restlessness), and behaviors (massaging, guarding, short attention span, irritability, sleep disturbance). Behavioral examples may be seen in patients with impaired communication, including those who are cognitively impaired, unconscious, or conscious but unable to communicate.
	Physiologic responses: Examples include diaphoresis, vasoconstriction, increased or decreased blood pressure (15% or more from baseline), increased pulse rate (15% or more from baseline), pupillary dilation, change in respiratory rate (RR) (usually increased to greater than 20 breaths/min), muscle tension or spasm, and decreased intestinal motility (evidenced by nausea, vomiting). Physiologic indicators may reflect pain as a result of autonomic stimulation of the sympathetic and parasympathetic responses.
Teach patients that pain assessment and management are not only a part of their treatment but also their right.	Patients have the right to appropriate assessment and management of their pain (TJC, 2013).
Accept the patient's report of pain and plan interventions based on this report.	A patient's self-report should be the primary source of pain assessment when possible (AHRQ, 2013; APS, 2008).
Evaluate the patient's health history for alcohol and drug (prescribed and nonprescribed) use, which could affect effective doses of analgesics (i.e., patient may require more or less). Ensure that the surgeon, anesthesiologist, and other health care providers are aware of any significant findings. Consult a pain management team if available.	Other medication use could alter effective doses of analgesics or lead to undertreatment. All care providers must be consistent in setting limits while providing effective pain control through pharmacologic and nonpharmacologic methods. Psychiatric or clinical pharmacology consultation may be necessary.
Develop a systematic and collaborative approach to pain management for each patient, using information gathered from pain history and the hierarchy of pain measurement.	American Nurses Association & American Society for Pain Management in Nursing (2005) identifies importance of involvement of patient, family, and other health care providers in data collection, formulation of outcomes, and development of the pain management plan. The AHRQ (2013) and APS (2008) state self-report of pain is the single most reliable indicator of pain.
Use at least two identifiers (e.g., patient's name, medical record number) before administering medications.	Using two or more identifiers improves accuracy of patient identification in keeping with The Joint Commission (TJC, 2013) National Patient Safety Goals promoting the right patient receiving the right medication.
Use a preventive approach: administer prn pain medications before pain becomes severe as well as before painful procedures, ambulation, and bedtime.	Prolonged stimulation of pain receptors results in increased sensitivity to painful stimuli and the need to increase the amount of drug required to relieve pain.
Administer analgesics according to the World Health Organization (WHO) three-step analgesic ladder.	The WHO analgesic ladder focuses on selecting analgesics and adjuvants based on pain intensity. The WHO analgesic ladder has been endorsed by the APS (2008). **Note:** Not all patients start with the first step; the process is determined by the etiology and severity of the pain. The next level of analgesia builds on the previous analgesics. The three steps include: - Level one addresses mild pain: nonopioid, ± adjuvant. - Level two: opioid for mild to moderate pain, ± nonopioid, ± adjuvant. - Level three: opioid for moderate to severe pain, ± nonopioid, ± adjuvant.
Recognize that choice of analgesic agent is based on three general considerations: therapeutic goal, the patient's medical condition, and drug cost.	Individualized therapeutic goal and the stage of illness/disease process are important factors in agent selection to maximize pain relief and minimize potential of adverse side effects. The difference in cost of different agents used to accomplish the same goal may be large. Where there is no proven or expected benefit of using one medication in preference to another to accomplish a desired goal, the less costly medication should be considered. **The right medication is the one that works with the fewest side effects.**

ASSESSMENT/INTERVENTIONS

RATIONALES

ASSESSMENT/INTERVENTIONS	RATIONALES
Also consider convenience, anticipated analgesic requirements, side effects, and patient's previous experience with a specific agent or patient's recall of side effects experienced with a specific agent, including route.	The preferred route is the one that is least invasive while achieving adequate relief. Aversion to painful routes of delivery (e.g., subcutaneous, intramuscular [IM]) may lead to underreporting of pain by patients and to undermedication by nurses. - IM analgesia is inconsistent and has unreliable absorption; it is less titratable; and It can cause complications such as hematoma, granuloma, infection, aseptic tissue necrosis, and nerve injury. APS suggests that this route be used rarely, and that it be avoided when possible. - Oral route is least invasive, is convenient and flexible, and produces relatively steady analgesia. - Intravenous (IV) route is used for agents with quick time to onset of analgesia and for severe pain.
For relief of mild-moderate pain that may be associated with surgery, trauma, soft tissue and muscle injury, and inflammatory conditions, administer nonopioid agents, such as: - Salicylates (acetylsalicylic acid [aspirin]) - Para-aminophenol derivatives (acetaminophen) - Nonsteroidal antiinflammatory drugs (NSAIDs) (ibuprofen, ketorolac) - Indoleacetic acids (indomethacin) [!] Be certain that gastrointestinal (GI) function has returned (e.g., presence of bowel sounds, absence of vomiting) before administering oral agents.	**Note:** These agents also may be administered in conjunction with opioids. Ketorolac may be given IM or IV for patients unable to tolerate oral agents. NSAIDs have peripheral effects and a different mechanism of action and thus are very effective when combined or used with centrally acting opioid analgesics. They also have a dose-sparing effect and may contribute to the reduction of opioid side effects. Unless contraindicated, APS recommends use of nonopioid agents even if pain is severe enough to require addition of an opioid. Another advantage of NSAIDs is their dual antipyretic and antiinflammatory actions. Undesirable side effects such as GI disturbances (epigastric pain, nausea, dyspepsia), platelet dysfunction, bleeding, and renal compromise may occur.
[!] Use acetaminophen with caution. Be alert to the total amount of acetaminophen a patient is receiving through over-the-counter and other combined medications.	Dose adjustments are required for patients with impaired liver/renal function. For adults, the American Liver Foundation (2008) recommends acetaminophen not exceed 3 grams in 24 hr. Acetaminophen may cause serious skin reactions in some people, Stevens Johnson syndrome (see description in "Caring for Patients with Human Immunodeficiency Virus," p. 524), or toxic epidermal necrosis. Acetaminophen may be given IV for patients unable to tolerate oral agents.
[!] Use COX-2 selective NSAIDs and NSAIDs with caution.	NSAIDs and COX-2 selective NSAIDs should be used with caution in patients with a history of duodenal bleeding ulcer; preexisting renal impairment; advanced age; concomitant use of corticosteroids, anticoagulants, warfarin, heparin; or history of long-duration NSAID therapy. The Food and Drug Administration (FDA) alerts and manufacturers' withdrawals of rofecoxib (Vioxx) and valdecoxib (Bextra) mandate that all health care providers remain current and assess risks/benefits based on current information, safety data, and availability.
As prescribed, administer opioid analgesics (e.g., morphine) for pain of greater severity.	Morphine is the standard of comparison for opioid analgesics, and morphine or related "mu" (μ) receptor agonists are preferred when possible.
[!] Use meperidine and normeperidine, a metabolite of meperidine, with caution.	Normeperidine is a central nervous system (CNS) excitotoxin, which with repetitive dosing may produce anxiety, muscle twitching, and seizures. Patients with impaired renal function and those taking monoamine oxidase (MAO) inhibitors are particularly at risk. Recommended use is for less than 48 hr for acute pain in patients without renal or CNS dysfunction or dose less than 600 mg/24 hr (APS, 2008). In low doses meperidine has a role in alleviating shivering associated with general anesthesia and some biologic agents.
[!] Do not use naloxone (Narcan) to attempt to reverse normeperidine toxicity.	Naloxone does not reverse normeperidine and may potentiate hyperexcitability.

continued

PART I: Medical-Surgical Nursing

ASSESSMENT/INTERVENTIONS

RATIONALES

ASSESSMENT/INTERVENTIONS	RATIONALES
If use of naloxone is necessary, titrate with caution.	Too much too fast can precipitate severe pain, hypertension, tachycardia, and even cardiac arrest. More than one dose is sometimes necessary because naloxone has a shorter duration than most opioids.
Do not administer mixed agonist-antagonist analgesics concurrently with morphine or other pure agonists because reversal of analgesic effects may occur.	Mixed agonist-antagonist agents such as butorphanol (Stadol) and pentazocine (Talwin) produce analgesia by binding to opioid receptors, while blocking or remaining neutral to the μ receptors. To date, there is no convincing evidence that agonist-antagonists offer any advantage over morphine-like agonists in the treatment of acute pain. Mixed agonist-antagonist agents may be useful in patients who are unable to tolerate other opioids.
Assess patients receiving opioid analgesics for level of pain relief and potential side effects, including evidence of excessive sedation or respiratory depression (i.e., RR less than 10 breaths/min or SpO_2 less than 90%-92%). In the presence of respiratory depression, reduce amount or frequency of the dose as prescribed. Have naloxone readily available to reverse severe respiratory depression.	Sedative effects precede respiratory depression. Close monitoring of sedation level may prevent respiratory depression.
Monitor older adults and individuals with chronic obstructive pulmonary disease, obstructive sleep apnea, asthma, and other respiratory disorders closely for respiratory depression and excessive sedation when they are receiving opioid analgesics. Consider using reduced doses and titrate carefully.	Older adults who are opioid naive and patients with coexisting conditions are at higher risk of respiratory depression. The most critical time for monitoring for respiratory depression is the first 24 hr of opioid therapy in these populations (Pasero & McCaffery, 2011). Increased tolerance to respiratory depression occurs over days to weeks. Therefore, patients who are opioid naive (or have coexisting conditions) are at greater risk of respiratory depression than the patient who has been receiving an opioid for a week or more.
Wean patients as prescribed from opioid analgesics by decreasing dose or frequency.	In general, doses should be reduced by no more than 10%-20% per day with vigilant assessment for withdrawal signs and symptoms.
Convert to oral therapy as soon as possible. When changing route of administration or medication, be certain to use equianalgesic doses of the new medication.	**Note:** Changing the route of medication administration often results in inadequate pain relief because of ineffective equianalgesic conversion.
Reassess pain level and assess for side effects: - Routinely at scheduled intervals (e.g., q1h for the first 12 hr of opioid therapy, q2-4h with VS) - With each report of pain - Following administration of pain medication based on time to onset, time to peak effect, and duration of action	More opioid is required to produce respiratory depression than to produce sedation. Sedative effects precede respiratory depression. Close monitoring of the level of sedation and respiratory status may prevent respiratory depression.
Consult with the health care provider to discuss converting to scheduled dosing with supplemental prn analgesics when pain exists for 12 hr out of 24 hr.	Experts recommend around-the-clock (ATC) dosing for patients with continuous pain because it provides superior pain relief with fewer side effects (APS, 2008). Prolonged stimulation of pain receptors results in increased sensitivity to painful stimuli and the need to increase the amount of drug required to relieve pain. Addiction to opioids occurs infrequently in hospitalized patients.
Titrate the dose to achieve the desired effect.	The initial effect and duration of action of analgesics may differ vastly in acutely ill older adults who may require lower doses, whereas higher doses may be required for those with opioid tolerance or polysubstance use. It is important to consider factors such as these that can influence the initial effect and duration of action due to variations in the metabolism of analgesics. The goal is to develop a safe and effective pain management plan.

ASSESSMENT/INTERVENTIONS	RATIONALES
Provide patient-controlled analgesia (PCA) as prescribed.	PCA is a patient-activated system for pain control that uses an infusion pump to deliver specified doses of analgesics with options of continuous infusions, bolus dosing, or both. The PCA route can be IV, subcutaneous, epidural, wound infiltration, or perineural (around a nerve). Patient selection is important because patients must be capable of understanding and activating the device and be willing to participate in their own treatment. Morphine, fentanyl, and hydromorphone are examples of opioids available for PCA use. Examples of local anesthetics used in epidural, wound infiltration, or perineurally are Bupivacaine or Ropivacaine.
[!] Increase patient monitoring following initiation, during the initial 24 hr, and at night when the patient may hypoventilate. Do not assume pain is controlled; assess the patient to determine if relief has been obtained.	Monitoring involves pain, sedation, and respiratory assessments and may include Spo$_2$ and capnography. Safety issues with PCA have been described with suggested strategies to reduce risk in ISMP Medication Safety Alerts (2008, 2009, 2013).
Monitor patients in whom neuraxial analgesia is used based on drug(s) being administered, catheter placement, and drug concentration and volume.	Neuraxial analgesia (spinal, epidural, and caudal) is a widely used option for regional analgesia. It decreases many side effects associated with intravenous opioids, and there is evidence it can lead to increased mobility and postoperative recovery. Local anesthetics, opioids, steroids, and clonidine are examples of agents that may be used.
For *local anesthetics*, monitor motor examination/sensory level and pain intensity.	Assessments may include sensory level and motor examination evaluations, level of pain intensity, sedation level, VS, and side effects. Potential side effects/complications include catheter migration, occlusion, hematoma, respiratory depression, hypotension, nausea/vomiting, urinary retention, and pruritus. For local anesthetics sensory assessments are performed bilaterally along dermatomes.
For *opioids*, monitor respiratory rate, sedation level, and pain intensity.	Signs of local anesthetic systemic toxicity (LAST) are metallic taste, unusual sensations around and inside the mouth, ringing in the ears, muscle twitching, and confusion.
As prescribed, use analgesic adjuvants/co-analgesics.	These agents are used to prolong and enhance analgesia, not specifically to treat isolated incidents of anxiety or depression.
[!] Avoid substituting sedatives and tranquilizers for analgesics.	Sedatives and tranquilizers are not analgesics. Tricyclic antidepressant agents primarily used for neuropathic pain produce analgesia while improving mood and sleep. **Caution:** Concomitant use with opioids may lead to sedation and orthostatic hypotension. Amitriptyline has the best-documented analgesia but is the least tolerated because of anticholinergic effects, including dry mouth, blurred vision, and constipation. Benzodiazepines are anxiolytic/sedatives with little to no analgesic effect. They are useful for decreasing recall, treating acute anxiety, and decreasing muscle spasm associated with acute pain. They may decrease opioid requirement by decreasing pain perception. If administered without an analgesic, the patient's perception of pain may increase. Antiepileptics may be prescribed for pain associated with nerve injury from tumors or other destructive processes. Although the specific mechanism of action for pain reduction is unknown, it is believed to be the result of suppression of the paroxysmal discharges and reduction of neuronal hyperexcitability. Antihistamines potentiate the effect of opioid analgesics. **Note:** Phenergan may increase perceived pain intensity and increase restlessness.
Assess for and report analgesia side effects. For management of constipation, see **Constipation** in "Prolonged Bedrest," p. 68.	Other analgesia side effects can include sedation, respiratory depression, nausea/vomiting, pruritus, and hypotension.

continued

ASSESSMENT/INTERVENTIONS

RATIONALES

ASSESSMENT/INTERVENTIONS	RATIONALES
Augment action of the medication by advising nonpharmacologic methods of pain control, including weight reduction, physical therapy, cognitive behavioral therapies, acupuncture, massage, and biofeedback. Other methods include reflexology, acupressure, Reiki, thermotherapy, back and foot massage, range-of-motion exercises, transcutaneous electrical nerve stimulation, distraction, relaxation exercises, and guided imagery.	Patients in whom nonpharmacologic interventions may be most successful include those who express interest in the approach, express anxiety or fear, or those with inadequate relief with pharmacologic management (ASA, 2012). Many of these techniques may be taught to and implemented by the patient and significant other.
Maintain a quiet environment and plan nursing activities to enable long periods of uninterrupted rest at night.	Promoting rest and sleep may decrease level of pain.
Evaluate for and correct nonoperative sources of discomfort.	Such sources including uncomfortable positioning, full bladder, and infiltrated IV site can be corrected readily without resorting to drug use.
Carefully evaluate the patient if sudden or unexpected changes in pain intensity occur, and notify the health care provider immediately should this occur.	This may signal complications such as internal bleeding or leakage of visceral contents.
Document efficacy of analgesics and other pain control interventions using a pain scale or other formalized method.	This documentation communicates level of pain relief obtained, interventions, effectiveness of the interventions, and ongoing follow-up to meet the analgesic goal.

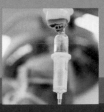

Perioperative Care 3

Nursing diagnoses for preoperative patients

Nursing Diagnosis:
Deficient Knowledge

related to unfamiliarity with the surgical procedure, preoperative routine, and postoperative care

Desired Outcome: The patient verbalizes knowledge about the surgical procedure, including preoperative preparations and sensations and postoperative care and sensations, and demonstrates postoperative exercises and use of devices before the surgical procedure or during the immediate postoperative period for emergency surgery.

ASSESSMENT/INTERVENTIONS	RATIONALES
Preoperatively: Evaluate the patient's desire for knowledge about the diagnosis and procedure.	Some individuals find detailed information helpful; others prefer very brief and simple explanations.
Assess the patient's understanding about the diagnosis, surgical procedure, preoperative routine, and postoperative regimen.	Assessment should include the patient's primary language and whether an interpreter is needed; the patient's readiness to learn; limitations on the patient's ability to learn such as blindness or decreased hearing; and the patient's self-assessment as to which modes of learning he or she finds most helpful, such as reading, listening, visual aids, or demonstration.
Determine past surgical experiences and their positive or negative effect on the patient. Assess the nature of any concerns or fears related to surgery. Document and communicate these assessment data to others involved in the patient's care.	Assessing the patient's knowledge, past experiences, and concerns about the surgical procedure will enable the nurse to focus on individual areas in need of the greatest intervention.
Based on your assessment, clarify and explain the diagnosis and surgical procedure accordingly. When possible, emphasize associated sensations (e.g., dry mouth, thirst, muscle weakness). Provide ample time for instruction and clarification and reinforce the health care provider's explanation of the procedure.	This information provides a knowledge base from which patients can make informed therapy choices and consent for procedures and presents an opportunity to clarify misconceptions.
Use anatomic models, diagrams, and other audiovisual aids when possible. Provide simply written information to reinforce learning. Provide written and verbal information in the patient's native language for non–English-speaking patients. **Note:** Evaluate the patient's reading comprehension before providing written materials.	Because individuals learn differently, using more than one teaching modality will provide teaching reinforcement of verbal information given.
Document if the patient provides an advance directive (see p. 104).	Laws about advance directives differ for each state.

continued

ASSESSMENT/INTERVENTIONS	RATIONALES
Explain the perioperative course of events. Review the following with the patient and significant other:	These measures increase the patient's knowledge of the surgical procedure, which optimally will promote adherence and minimize stress.
- Procedures for required preoperative assessment and testing and when and where they will be performed. Issue written directions, phone numbers, and maps as indicated. Discuss location and proper arrival time for the surgery.	Patients will need information regarding location of the preoperative testing center, parking arrangements, and expected length of time such testing will require.
- Where the patient will be before, during, and immediately after surgery.	Patients may be in postanesthesia care unit (PACU), intensive care unit (ICU), or specialty unit.
- Clarification of sounds and other sensations (e.g., sore throat, cool temperature, hard stretcher) the patient may experience during the immediate postoperative period. If possible, take the patient to the new unit and introduce him or her to the nursing staff.	Including sensory information in patient teaching is consistent with current nursing research that has determined patient outcomes are improved when expected sensations are explained.
- Preoperative medications and timing of surgery (scheduled time, expected duration).	
- If indicated, preoperative bowel preparation.	
- Pain management, including sensations to expect and methods of relief. If patient-controlled analgesia (PCA) or patient-controlled epidural anesthesia (PCEA) will be prescribed, have the patient give a return demonstration of use of the delivery device.	This information increases the likelihood of successful pain management. Some patients mistakenly expect to be pain free; others fear becoming addicted to narcotics (opioids).
- Use of pain assessment tools such as the numeric pain rating scale or the Wong-Baker FACES pain rating scale.	Pain assessment tools aid in the evaluation of pain and effectiveness of interventions.
- Placement of tubes, catheters, drains, cooling systems (Cryocuff), continuous passive motion (CPM) units, oxygen delivery devices, and similar devices routinely used for the patient's surgery. Show these devices to the patient when possible.	Patients may be unfamiliar with the use and purpose of these devices. Learning about them and seeing them in advance of surgery may help decrease fears and anxieties perioperatively.
- Use of antiembolism stockings, sequential compression devices (SCDs), pneumatic foot pumps, or similar devices.	These garments/devices prevent venous stasis and decrease risk of thrombus formation.
- Dietary alterations and progression, including nothing by mouth (NPO) status followed by clear liquids until return of full gastrointestinal (GI) function.	Traditionally, health care providers have progressed patients from clear liquids to a regular diet after surgery for a variety of reasons, including ease of swallowing and digestion and liquid diet being more readily tolerated in the presence of an ileus. However, practitioners are questioning the scientific basis of this diet advancement. Recent studies are indicating that a clear liquid diet may not always be indicated.
- Restrictions of activity and positions, as indicated by the specific surgical procedure.	For example, patients undergoing hip arthroplasty have specific positional limitations.
- Need to refrain from smoking during perioperative period.	Inhalation of toxic fumes/chemical irritants can damage lung tissue by decreasing ciliary function. Cilia line the respiratory tract and carry particles to the lower pharynx. Damaged lung tissue increases the likelihood of hypoxemia and lung infections, including pneumonia.
- Visiting hours and location of waiting room.	Families may feel less anxious when they are aware of a designated area where they can wait and receive updates on the progress of the surgery. Knowledge of visiting hours likely will reassure them they will have access to the patient after surgery.
Postoperatively: Explain postoperative activities, exercises, and precautions. Have the patient give a return demonstration of the following devices and exercises, as appropriate:	Adherence is enhanced when patients are knowledgeable about activities, exercises, and precautions. Patients gain confidence when they practice new skills before surgery and are provided feedback on their technique.
- Deep-breathing and coughing exercises (see **Ineffective Airway Clearance,** p. 49).	These actions help prevent atelectasis, pneumonia, and other respiratory disorders that can occur during the postoperative period.

ASSESSMENT/INTERVENTIONS	RATIONALES
Individuals for whom increased intracranial, intrathoracic, or intraabdominal pressure is contraindicated should not cough.	Coughing increases intracranial, intrathoracic, and intraabdominal pressure. Patients undergoing intracranial surgery, spinal fusion, eye and ear surgery, and similar procedures should avoid vigorous coughing because it raises intracranial pressure, which could cause harm. Coughing after a herniorrhaphy and some thoracic surgeries should be done in a controlled manner, with the incision supported carefully, to avoid raising intraabdominal and intrathoracic pressure dramatically.
- Use of incentive spirometry and other respiratory devices.	Incentive spirometry, when used with coughing and deep breathing, expands alveoli and mobilizes secretions, which helps prevent atelectasis, pneumonia, and other respiratory disorders.
- Calf-pumping, ankle-circling, and footboard-pressing exercises (see Chapter 24, "Venous Thrombosis/Thrombophlebitis," p. 188, for more information).	These exercises promote circulation and help prevent thrombophlebitis/venous thromboembolism (DVT/VTE) in the legs.
- Use of PCA/PCEA device.	Adequate pain management increases mobility, which decreases risk of nosocomial pneumonia and thrombosis formation and aids in the return of GI peristalsis.
- Movement in and out of bed.	Logrolling, raising self by using a trapeze device, and gradual movement are techniques that may be required.
Before the patient is discharged, teach prescribed activity precautions.	This teaching helps prevent excessive strain on the operative site. A patient who has a total hip replacement, for example, will need to follow activity precautions to prevent dislocation of the new joint. Increasing exercises gradually to tolerance, avoiding heavy lifting (more than 10 lb), and avoiding driving a car are precautions given to many surgical patients for safety because of the potential for decreased attention span and impaired reflexes resulting from opioid use. Lifting precautions may reduce stress on surgical incisions. Restrictions on sexual activity are indicated by the surgical procedure. Returning progressively to preoperative activity level promotes physical and psychosocial well-being.
Provide time for the patient to ask questions and express feelings of anxiety; be reassuring and supportive. Be certain to address the patient's main concerns.	Expressing feelings of anxiety and having questions answered are essential ways of reducing anxiety while learning new information.

Nursing Diagnosis:

Risk for Injury

related to exposure to pharmaceutical agents and other external factors during the perioperative period

Desired Outcome: Patient does not experience injury or untoward effects of pharmacotherapy or other external factors.

ASSESSMENT/INTERVENTIONS	RATIONALES
Assess need for holding, administering, or adjusting the patient's maintenance medications before or immediately after surgery.	Some medications, such as anticonvulsants, beta blockers, and other cardiac medications, should be continued throughout the perioperative period. Sometimes patients need to be weaned from medications such as baclofen for the perioperative period because stopping them suddenly could result in seizures or hallucinations. Other medications may require increased dosages during surgery (e.g., hydrocortisone in place of prednisone and with increased dosage for steroid-dependent patients) or alternative routes. Individuals with insulin-dependent diabetes need close monitoring of blood glucose levels and adjustments of insulin dosing based on testing.

continued

ASSESSMENT/INTERVENTIONS	RATIONALES
Reinforce the importance of NPO status.	Maintaining NPO status reduces risk of aspiration postoperatively. Clear liquids may be allowed up to 2 hr before surgery in patients with low risk of pulmonary aspiration. NPO policies vary widely from facility to facility.
Verify completion of preoperative activities and procedures, and document on the preoperative checklist or nursing documentation.	Documentation on the patient's preoperative checklist or inpatient's medical record helps ensure communication among health care team members, continuity, and optimal patient outcomes.
Be sure that consent has been signed and witnessed and the patient appears to understand what the procedure involves. Answer questions, or call the health care provider to answer patient's questions. Ensure that the patient's identification bracelet, blood transfusion bracelet, and allergy alert bracelet are in place.	These interventions help ensure that all appropriate documentation is present and that all steps have been taken to provide for the patient's safety and well-being.
Document allergies, any evidence of skin breakdown, bruises, rashes, or wounds; and presence of dressings, drains, or ostomy.	Documentation decreases risk of untoward outcomes. Noting the patient's preexisting wounds, dressings, and drains also helps ensure appropriate intraoperative positioning.
Assess for and document the patient's exposure to actual or potential abuse or neglect.	All states require health care providers to report suspected abuse and neglect of children and vulnerable adults who are in their care.
Document the patient's access to care and transportation upon discharge.	Surgery, pain, and analgesic medications may impede the patient's ability to care for self adequately after discharge.
Review the medical record to ensure that all appropriate documentation is present; report untoward findings to the health care provider.	The health care provider may not be aware of recent abnormal electrocardiogram (ECG), suspicious chest radiograph, or abnormal laboratory findings.
Prepare the surgical site and perform additional presurgical procedures as prescribed.	The AORN recommendations state that hair at the surgical site should be left in place whenever possible (AORN, 2011). When hair removal is indicated, the use of clippers or depilatory creams is preferable to shaving (Tanner, 2007). Additional presurgical procedures may involve showering with an antimicrobial agent, douching, enemas, or eye drops.
Administer preoperative antibiotics, sedation, or other medications as prescribed and on time.	This intervention helps ensure adequate serum levels of the prescribed medication. Giving antibiotics within 1 hour of the surgical incision may decrease risk of infection postoperatively (National Hospital Inpatient Quality Reporting Measures Specifications Manual, 2012).
[!] Make provisions for patient safety following sedative administration (e.g., bed in lowest position, side rails up, and reminding patient not to get out of bed without assistance).	Sedatives administered preoperatively may alter mental status and coordination, increasing the patient's risk for injury.
[!] Implement the preoperative verification and time out process as follows: 1. Confirm identification of the patient by all team members by verifying the patient's armband, patient speak back, or patient caregiver if the patient has been sedated.	This verification process should take place on admission to the facility, before the patient leaves the preoperative area, on entry to the surgical room, just prior to incision or start of procedure, and any time responsibility for patient care is transferred to another caregiver. If possible, the verification process should involve the patient while still awake and aware.
2. In the preoperative/holding area confirm that a mark has been made by the surgeon (who will have used a single-use surgical skin marker with a consistent mark type [e.g., surgeon's initials]) placed as close as anatomically possible to the incision site. 3. Perform a preoperative briefing in the operating room with patient involvement.	
4. Perform a standardized time-out process, which occurs after the prep and drape.	Prevention of the wrong site, wrong procedure, and wrong person surgery is accomplished by the use of a "time-out" procedure. A "time out" should include verification of the correct patient identity, the correct surgical site and side, and agreement on the procedure to be done.
5. Perform a pause between each surgical procedure that occurs within a single case to ensure that each procedure is performed accurately and according to the procedure, site, and laterality contained within the signed surgical consent.	

Nursing diagnoses for postoperative patients

Nursing Diagnosis:

Ineffective Airway Clearance

related to alterations in pulmonary physiology and function occurring with anesthetics, narcotics, mechanical ventilation, hypothermia, and surgery; increased tracheobronchial secretions occurring with effects of anesthesia combined with ineffective coughing; and decreased function of the mucociliary clearance mechanism

Desired Outcome: The patient's airway becomes clear as evidenced by normal breath sounds to auscultation, respiratory rate (RR) 12-20 breaths/min with normal depth and pattern (eupnea), normothermia, normal skin color, and O_2 saturation greater than 92% on room air.

ASSESSMENT/INTERVENTIONS	RATIONALES
Assess respiratory status, including breath sounds, q1-2h during immediate postoperative period and q8h during recovery.	This assessment will determine presence of rhonchi that do not clear with coughing, labored breathing, tachypnea (RR more than 20 breaths/min), mental status changes, restlessness, cyanosis, and presence of fever (38.3° C [101° F] or higher), which are all signs of respiratory system compromise.
Use pulse oximetry to assess oxygen saturation as indicated, and report saturation 92% or less to the health care provider.	Pulse oximetry is a noninvasive measure of arterial oxygen saturation. Values 92% or less are consistent with hypoxia and probably signal need for oxygen supplementation or workup to determine cause of desaturation. Pulse oximetry is especially indicated in patients with chronic obstructive pulmonary disease (COPD), respiratory or cardiovascular disease, morbid obesity, cardiothoracic surgery, major surgery, prolonged general anesthesia, and surgery for a fractured pelvis or long bone, as well as in debilitated patients and older adults, all of whom are at increased risk for desaturation.
Administer humidified oxygen as prescribed.	This intervention supplements oxygen and prevents further drying of respiratory passageways and secretions via added humidity.
⚠ Keep emergency airway equipment (e.g., Ambu bag and mask, intubation tray, endotracheal tubes, suctioning equipment, tracheostomy tray) readily available.	This ensures their availability in the event of sudden airway obstruction or ventilatory failure.
Encourage deep breathing and coughing q2h or more often for the first 72 hr postoperatively in nonambulatory patients. In the presence of fine crackles (rales) and if not contraindicated, have the patient cough to expectorate secretions. Facilitate deep breathing and coughing by demonstrating how to splint abdominal and thoracic incisions with hands or a pillow. If indicated, medicate ½ hr before deep breathing, coughing, or ambulation to promote adherence.	These actions expand alveoli and mobilize secretions. The effects of anesthesia and immobility may collapse alveoli and place patient at risk for nosocomial pneumonia and atelectasis. Proper positioning promotes chest expansion and ventilation of basilar lung fields. **Note:** Turning, coughing, and deep breathing (TCDB) are less effective than ambulation. Ambulation makes TCDB unnecessary in the vast majority of patients.
If the patient has a weak cough or poor reserve, try the "step-cough" technique. Coach the patient to cough in rapid succession.	A few weak coughs in a row may stimulate a larger, productive cough at the end of the cycle to clear the bronchial tree of secretions. **Caution:** Vigorous coughing may be contraindicated for some individuals (e.g., those undergoing intracranial surgery, spinal fusion, eye and ear surgery, and similar procedures). Coughing after a herniorrhaphy and some thoracic surgeries should be done in a controlled manner, with the incision supported carefully.
Consider whether the patient may be more motivated to perform pulmonary toilet with incentive spirometer or positive expiratory pressure (PEP) device.	Devices may be a motivating factor because the patient has a visual indicator of effectiveness of the breathing effort.

PART I: Medical-Surgical Nursing

Nursing Diagnosis:

Ineffective Breathing Pattern (or risk of same)

related to hypoventilation occurring with central nervous system (CNS) depression, pain, muscle splinting, recumbent position, obesity, narcotics, and effects of anesthesia

Desired Outcome: The patient exhibits effective ventilation as evidenced by relaxed breathing, RR 12-20 breaths/min with normal depth and pattern (eupnea), clear breath sounds, normal color, return to preoperative O_2 saturation on room air, PaO_2 80 mm Hg or greater, pH 7.35-7.45, $PaCO_2$ 35-45 mm Hg, and HCO_3^- 22-26 mEq/L.

ASSESSMENT/INTERVENTIONS	RATIONALES
See assessment/interventions under **Ineffective Airway Clearance**, p. 49.	
Review preoperative baseline assessment of the patient's respiratory system, noting rate, rhythm, degree of chest expansion, quality of breath sounds, cough, and sputum production, as well as smoking history and current respiratory medications. Note preoperative O_2 saturation and arterial blood gas (ABG) values if available.	Baseline assessment enables rapid detection of subsequent postoperative problems and timely intervention for same.
If appropriate, encourage the patient to refrain from smoking for at least 1 wk after surgery. Explain effects of smoking on the body.	Inhalation of toxic fumes/chemical irritants can damage lung tissue, increasing likelihood of hypoxemia and respiratory infection.
Monitor O_2 saturation continuously via oximetry in high-risk individuals (e.g., patients with obstructive sleep apnea [OSA] or who are heavily sedated, patients with preexisting lung disease, morbidly obese patients, patients having undergone upper airway surgery, or older patients) and at periodic intervals in other patients as indicated.	Pulse oximetry is a noninvasive method of measuring saturated hemoglobin in tissue capillaries. Factors that predispose the patient to OSA are: 1. History of snoring. 2. A history of feeling tired, fatigued, or sleepy during daytime. 3. History of stopping breathing during sleep. 4. History of hypertension. 5. BMI greater than 35. 6. Age greater than 50 yr. 7. Neck circumference greater than 40 cm. 8. Male gender.
Notify the health care provider of O_2 saturation 92% or less.	O_2 saturation of 92% or less may signal need for supplemental oxygen.
Evaluate ABG values, and notify the health care provider of low or decreasing PaO_2 and high or increasing $PaCO_2$.	Declining PaO_2 may signal hypoxemia and the need for supplemental oxygen.
Also assess for signs of hypoxia.	Early signs of hypoxia include restlessness, dyspnea, tachycardia, tachypnea, and confusion. Cyanosis, especially of the tongue and oral mucous membranes, and extreme lethargy or somnolence are late signs of hypoxia. Hypercapnia combined with acidosis and hypoxemia may result in pulmonary vasoconstriction that may be severe and life threatening.
Assist the patient with turning and deep-breathing/coughing exercises q2h until the patient is ambulatory.	These activities promote expansion of lung alveoli and prevent pooling of secretions, which could lead to nosocomial pneumonia.
If the patient has an incentive spirometer *or* PEP device, provide instructions and ensure adherence to its use q2h or as prescribed.	These devices promote expansion of the alveoli and help mobilize secretions in the airways; subsequent coughing further mobilizes and clears secretions.
Unless contraindicated, assist the patient with ambulation beginning on the day of surgery.	Ambulation promotes circulation and ventilation, which helps prevent formation of deep vein thrombosis and pulmonary embolus.

Nursing Diagnosis:

Risk for Aspiration

related to reduced level of consciousness, depressed cough and gag reflexes, decreased GI motility, abdominal distention, recumbent position, presence of gastric tube, gastroesophageal reflux disease (GERD), and impaired swallowing in individuals with oral, facial, or neck surgery

Desired Outcome: The patient's upper airway remains unobstructed as evidenced by clear breath sounds, RR 12-20 breaths/min with normal depth and pattern (eupnea), normal skin color, and a return to preoperative O_2 saturation.

ASSESSMENT/INTERVENTIONS	RATIONALES
If a sedated patient experiences nausea or vomiting, turn immediately into a side-lying position.	This position minimizes the potential for aspiration.
Encourage fully alert patients to remain in an upright position.	Maintaining a sitting position after meals decreases risk of aspiration by facilitating gravity drainage from the stomach to the small bowel. An upright position also helps prevent reflux.
As necessary, suction the oropharynx with Yankauer or similar suction device to remove vomitus.	Suctioning enables immediate removal of vomitus, which could be aspirated. Patients at high risk for aspiration should have suctioning apparatus immediately available for this life-saving intervention.
Administer antiemetics, histamine H_2-receptor blocking agents, omeprazole, metoclopramide, and similar agents as prescribed.	These agents decrease nausea, vomiting, and acidity of gastric contents and stimulate GI motility. H_2-receptor antagonists increase gastric pH, and nonparticulate antacids (e.g., Bicitra, Citra pH, and Alka Seltzer Gold) act as aspiration pneumonitis prophylaxis. Neutralizing gastric acidity may reduce severity of pneumonia if aspiration occurs.
Check placement and patency of gastric tubes q8h and before instillation of feedings and medications. Consult the health care provider before irrigating tubes for these individuals.	These actions prevent instillation of anything into the airway.
Use caution when irrigating and otherwise manipulating GI tubes of patients with recent esophageal, gastric, or duodenal surgery.	The tube may be displaced or the surgical incision disrupted by such activity.
Assess the patient's abdomen q4-8h by inspection, auscultation, palpation, and percussion for evidence of distention (increasing size, firmness, increased tympany, decreased bowel sounds).	A distended and rigid abdomen along with absent bowel sounds may indicate an ileus, which places patient at increased risk for vomiting and aspiration. Increased tympany or high-pitched or increased bowel sounds may signal mechanical obstruction, which also places patient at increased risk for vomiting and aspiration.
Notify the health care provider if distention is of rapid onset or if it is associated with pain.	Rapid abdominal distention postoperatively may indicate intraabdominal hemorrhage and can lead to a sometimes fatal condition called *abdominal compartment syndrome.*
Encourage early and frequent ambulation.	Ambulation improves GI motility and reduces abdominal distention caused by accumulated gases.
Introduce oral fluids cautiously, especially in patients with oral, facial, and neck surgery.	Swelling and irritation in the oropharynx may cause dysphagia and pain postoperatively. Nasal packing or intranasal splint aspiration also may cause airway obstruction.

For additional information, see Chapter 74, "Providing Nutritional Support," **Risk for Aspiration,** p. 544.

Nursing Diagnosis:

Risk for Infection

related to inadequate primary defenses (e.g., broken skin, traumatized tissue, decrease in ciliary action, stasis of body fluids), invasive procedures, or chronic disease

Desired outcome: The patient is free of infection as evidenced by normothermia; heart rate (HR) 100 bpm or less; RR 20 breaths/min or less with normal depth and pattern (eupnea); negative cultures; clear and normal-smelling urine; clear and thin sputum; no significant mental status changes; orientation to person, place, and time; and absence of unusual tenderness, erythema, swelling, warmth, or drainage at the surgical incision.

ASSESSMENT/INTERVENTIONS	RATIONALES
Monitor vital signs (VS) for evidence of infection, such as elevated HR and RR and increased body temperature.	With onset of infection, the immune system is activated, causing symptoms of infection to appear. Sustained temperature elevation after surgery may signal the presence of pulmonary complications, urinary tract infection, wound infection, or thrombophlebitis.
Notify the health care provider if these are new findings.	Presence of a fever affects treatment decisions.
Prevent transmission of infectious agents by washing your hands thoroughly before and after caring for the patient and by wearing gloves when contact with blood, drainage, or other body substance is likely.	Hand hygiene is an effective means of preventing microbial transmission. Wearing gloves protects the caregiver from the patient's body substances.
Encourage and assist the patient with coughing, deep breathing, incentive spirometry, and turning q2-4h, and note quality of breath sounds, cough, and sputum.	These activities expand alveoli in the lung and mobilize secretions, which will decrease the potential for respiratory infection/pneumonia. Optimally they will promote cough and improve quality of breath sounds.
Evaluate intravenous (IV) sites for erythema, warmth, swelling, tenderness, or drainage.	These are signs of infection. The body may be mounting a response to ward off offending pathogens.
Change the IV line and site if evidence of infection is present and according to agency protocol (q48-72h).	These are standard infection prevention guidelines.
Evaluate patency of all surgically placed tubes or drains. Irrigate, gently "milk," or attach to low-pressure suction as prescribed. Promptly report unrelieved loss of patency.	These actions prevent stasis and reflux of body fluids, which can result in infection. "Milking" the tube, however, may not be allowed in some facilities.
Assess stability of tubes/drains.	Movement of improperly secured tubes and drains enables access of pathogens at the insertion site.
Note color, character, and odor of all drainage. Report significant findings.	Foul-smelling, purulent, or abnormal drainage are indicators of infection.
Evaluate incisions and wound sites for unusual erythema, warmth, tenderness, induration, swelling, delayed healing, and purulent or excessive drainage.	These are indicators of localized infection.
Change dressings as prescribed, using "no touch" and sterile techniques. Prevent cross-contamination of wounds in the same patient by changing one dressing at a time and washing hands between dressing changes.	These are standard infection prevention guidelines.
Be alert to patient complaints of a feeling of "letting go" or to a sudden profusion of serous drainage on or a bulge in the dressing.	It is possible that a wound dehiscence or evisceration has occurred. Wound infection and poor wound healing put patients at risk for wound dehiscence.

ASSESSMENT/INTERVENTIONS

RATIONALES

ASSESSMENT/INTERVENTIONS	RATIONALES
! If the patient develops evisceration, do not reinsert tissue or organs. Place a sterile, saline-soaked gauze over eviscerated tissues and cover with a sterile towel until the wound can be evaluated by a health care provider.	Keeping viscera moist with a sterile towel increases viability of tissues and reduces risk of contamination and further infection.
Maintain the patient on bedrest, usually in semi-Fowler's position with knees slightly bent. Keep the patient NPO and anticipate need for IV therapy.	These actions provide comfort, prevent further evisceration, and prepare the patient for surgery.
! Ensure that the urinary catheter is removed on postoperative day 1 or day 2 whenever possible.	The risk of catheter-associated urinary tract infection (UTI) increases with prolonged duration of indwelling urinary catheterization.
When appropriate, encourage use of intermittent catheterization q4-6h instead of indwelling catheter.	Emptying the bladder routinely prevents stasis of urine and decreases presence of pathogens.
Keep the drainage collection container below bladder level, avoiding kinks or obstructions in drainage tubing.	This intervention prevents both reflux of urine (and potential pathogens) into bladder and urinary stasis, either of which could lead to infection.
Do not open the closed urinary drainage system unless absolutely necessary, and irrigate the catheter only with the health care provider's prescription and when obstruction is the known cause.	Keeping the system closed decreases risk of contamination and infection.
Assess the patient for chills; fever (temperature higher than 37.7° C [100° F]); dysuria; urgency; frequency; flank, low back, suprapubic, buttock, inner thigh, scrotal, or labial pain; and cloudy or foul-smelling urine.	These are indicators of UTI, which signal that the body is mounting a response to ward off offending pathogens.
Encourage intake of 2-3 L/day in nonrestricted patients.	Increasing hydration minimizes the potential for UTI by diluting the urine and maximizing urinary flow.
Ensure that the patient's perineum and meatus are cleansed during daily bath and the perianal area is cleansed after bowel movements. Do not hesitate to remind the patient of these hygiene measures.	Microorganisms can be introduced into the body via the catheter. Good hygiene decreases the number of microorganisms.
Be alert to meatal swelling, purulent drainage, and persistent meatal redness. Intervene if the patient is unable to perform self-care.	These are indicators of meatal infection and potential UTI.
Change the catheter according to established protocol or sooner if sandy particles are observed in its distal end or if the patient develops UTI. Change the drainage collection container according to established protocol or sooner if it becomes foul smelling or leaks.	Because the catheter can be a source of infection, changing the system per protocol (usually every month) is customary.
Obtain cultures of suspicious drainage or secretions (e.g., sputum, urine, wound) as prescribed. For urine specimens, be certain to use the sampling port, which is at the proximal end of the drainage tube.	Cultures determine if an infection is present and direct therapy with an appropriate antibiotic if it is.
Cleanse the sampling port with an antimicrobial wipe and use a sterile syringe with 25-gauge needle to aspirate urine.	Larger gauge needles form larger puncture holes that increase the risk of compromising the sterile system.
Evaluate mental status, orientation, and level of consciousness q8h.	Consider infection the likely cause if altered mental status or loss of consciousness is unexplained, especially in older adults.
Use precautions (see "Infection Prevention and Control," p. 747, for patients colonized with methicillin-resistant *Staphylococcus aureus* (MRSA), vancomycin-resistant *Enterococcus* (VRE), or other epidemiologically important organisms.	Such precautions prevent cross contaminating from infectious sources to uninfected patients.

Nursing Diagnosis:

Deficient Fluid Volume

related to active loss occurring with indwelling drainage tubes, wound drainage, or vomiting; inadequate intake of fluids occurring with nausea, NPO status, CNS depression, or lack of access to fluids; or failure of regulatory mechanisms with third spacing of body fluids due to the effects of anesthesia, endogenous catecholamines, blood loss during surgery, and prolonged recumbency

Desired Outcomes: The patient becomes normovolemic as evidenced by blood pressure (BP) 90/60 mm Hg or higher (or within the patient's preoperative baseline), HR 60-100 bpm, distal pulses greater than 2 on a 0-4 scale, urinary output 30 mL/hr or more, urine specific gravity 1.030 or less, stable or increasing weight, good skin turgor, warm skin, moist mucous membranes, and normothermia. The patient does not demonstrate significant mental status changes and verbalizes orientation to person, place, and time.

ASSESSMENT/INTERVENTIONS	RATIONALES
Monitor VS q4-8h during the recovery phase.	Decreasing BP, increasing HR, and slightly increased body temperature are indicators of dehydration.
Monitor urinary output q4-8h. Be alert for concentrated urine.	Concentrated urine (specific gravity more than 1.030) and low or decreasing output (average normal output is 60 mL/hr or 1400-1500 mL/day) are indicators of deficient fluid volume.
Administer and regulate IV fluids and electrolytes as prescribed until the patient is able to resume oral intake. When IV fluids are discontinued, encourage intake of oral fluids, at least 2-3 L/day in nonrestricted patients. As much as possible, respect the patient's preference in oral fluids, and keep them readily available in the patient's room.	Oral fluids usually are restricted until peristalsis returns and the nasogastric (NG) tube is removed. However, ice chips or small sips of clear liquids may be allowed.
Measure and record output from drains, ostomies, wounds, and other sources. Ensure patency of gastric and other drainage tubes. Record quality and quantity of output.	Both sensible and insensible losses need to be determined to ensure complete estimation of the patient's fluid volume status.
Measure, describe, and document any emesis. Be alert to and document excessive perspiration along with documentation of urinary, fecal, and other drainage.	Same as above.
Report excessive losses.	Replacement fluids likely will be indicated.
Monitor the patient's weight daily.	Daily weight measurement is an effective means of evaluating hydration and nutritional status.
Always weigh at the same time every day, using the same scale and same type and amount of bed clothing.	Weighing patients at the same time and under the same conditions avoids discrepancies that could reflect inaccurate losses or gains. **Note:** Weighing patients daily is not useful in detecting intravascular fluid loss due to third spacing. Movement of fluid from one area of the body to another will not change the total body weight.
If nausea and vomiting are present, assess for potential causes.	Potential causes include administration of opioid analgesics, loss of gastric tube patency, and environmental factors (e.g., unpleasant odors or sights).
Administer antiemetics (e.g., ondansetron, prochlorperazine, promethazine), metoclopramide, or similar agents as prescribed.	These agents combat nausea and vomiting, which could impair intake and add to fluid losses.
Instruct the patient to request medication *before* nausea becomes severe.	Postoperative vomiting is significantly less when patients receive nausea/vomiting prophylaxis.
Monitor for hypokalemia and hypocalcemia. See "Acute Renal Failure," p. 192, for **Acute Confusion/Ineffective Protection**.	A large fluid loss may cause electrolyte imbalances leading to life-threatening cardiac dysrhythmias.

PART I: Medical-Surgical Nursing

Nursing Diagnoses:

Risk for Bleeding

related to operative procedure

Risk for Shock

related to hypovolemia

Desired Outcomes: The patient is normovolemic as evidenced by BP 90/60 mm Hg or higher (or within the patient's preoperative baseline), HR 60-100 bpm, RR 12-20 breaths/min with normal depth and pattern (eupnea), brisk capillary refill (less than 2 sec), warm extremities, distal pulses greater than 2+ on a 0-4+ scale, urinary output 30 mL/hr or more, and urine specific gravity less than 1.030. The patient does not demonstrate significant mental status changes and verbalizes orientation to person, place, and time.

ASSESSMENT/INTERVENTIONS	RATIONALES
Assess VS and physical indicators at frequent intervals during the first 24 hr of the postoperative period for signs of internal hemorrhage and impending shock. See Chapter 17, "Cardiac and Noncardiac Shock (Circulatory Failure)," p. 145, for management.	There is greater potential for postoperative bleeding/hemorrhage during this period. Decreasing pulse pressure (difference between systolic blood pressure [SBP] and diastolic blood pressure [DBP]), decreasing BP, increasing HR, and increasing RR are indicators of internal hemorrhage and impending shock. Physical indicators include pallor, diaphoresis, cool extremities, delayed capillary refill, diminished intensity of distal pulses, restlessness, agitation, mental status changes, and disorientation, as well as subjective complaints of thirst, anxiety, or a sense of impending doom.
Inspect the surgical dressing; record saturated dressings and report significant findings to the health care provider.	Rapid saturation of the dressing with bright red blood is evidence of frank bleeding, which necessitates prompt intervention.
If the initial postoperative dressing becomes saturated, reinforce the dressing and notify the health care provider.	The health care provider may want to perform the initial dressing change.
Monitor wound drains and drainage systems, and report significant findings to the health care provider.	Excessive drainage (more than 50 mL/hr for 2-3 hr) should be reported promptly for timely intervention.
Note the amount and character of drainage from gastric and other tubes at least q8h. **Note:** After gastric and some other GI surgeries, patients will have small amounts of bloody or blood-tinged drainage for the first 12-24 hr. Be alert to large or increasing amounts of bloody drainage.	If drainage appears to contain blood (e.g., bright red, burgundy, or dark coffee ground appearance), it will be necessary to perform an occult blood test (may be performed in the laboratory). If the test is newly or unexpectedly positive, results should be reported to health care provider for timely intervention.
Monitor and measure urinary output q4-8h during the initial postoperative period. Report significant findings to the health care provider.	Average hourly output less than 30 mL/hr and specific gravity of 1.030 or more are indicators of deficient fluid volume, which can signal bleeding/hemorrhage.
Review complete blood count (CBC) values for evidence of bleeding; report significant decreases.	Evidence of bleeding may be indicated by decreases in hemoglobin (Hgb) from normal (male 14-18 g/dL; female 12-16 g/dL); and decreases in hematocrit (Hct) from normal (male 40%-54%; female 37%-47%). Significant decreases occur with active bleeding, an emergency situation.
Maintain a patent indwelling 18-gauge or larger IV catheter.	The gauge of this catheter will enable repeat infusions of blood products if hemorrhagic shock develops.

Nursing Diagnosis:

Excess Fluid Volume

related to compromised regulatory mechanisms after major surgery

Desired Outcome: Following intervention/treatment, the patient becomes normovolemic as evidenced by BP within normal range of the patient's preoperative baseline, distal pulses less than 4+ on a 0-4+ scale, presence of eupnea, clear breath sounds, absence of or barely detectable edema (1+ or less on a 0-4+ scale), urine specific gravity at least 1.010, and body weight near or at preoperative baseline.

ASSESSMENT/INTERVENTIONS	RATIONALES
Assess for and report any indicators of fluid overload, including elevated BP, bounding pulses, dyspnea, crackles (rales), and pretibial or sacral edema.	An increase in BP and an S3 galloping rhythm may indicate impending heart failure. Crackles and dyspnea may signal a shift of fluid from the vascular space to the pulmonary interstitial space and alveoli causing pulmonary edema.
Maintain a record of 8-hr and 24-hr input and output (I&O). Note and report a significant imbalance. Monitor urinary specific gravity and report consistently low (less than 1.010) findings.	Normal 24-hr output is 1400-1500 mL, and normal 1-hr output is 60 mL/hr or 480 mL per 8 hr. Decreased urinary output could be a sign of fluid volume excess.
Weigh the patient daily, using the same scale and same type and amount of bed clothing. Note significant weight gain.	Weight changes reflect changes in body fluid volume. One liter of fluid equals approximately 2.2 lb. Weighing the patient at the same time and under the same conditions avoids discrepancies that could reflect inaccurate losses or gains.
Administer diuretics as prescribed.	Diuretics mobilize interstitial fluid and decrease excess fluid volume.
Monitor patients carefully who are on diuretic therapy. See **Acute Confusion/Ineffective Protection** in "Acute Renal Failure," p. 192.	Diuretic therapy may cause dangerous K^+ depletion that could result in cardiac dysrhythmias. As well, diuretic therapy can lead to hyponatremia because of sodium losses.
Monitor older adults and individuals with cardiovascular disease especially carefully.	These individuals are especially at risk for developing postoperative fluid volume excess. Older adults have age-related changes of decreased glomerular filtration rate (GFR). Decreased kidney function and increased probability of chronic illness such as cardiac disease may signal higher risk of postoperative excessive fluid volume.
Anticipate postoperative diuresis approximately 48-72 hr after surgery.	This may occur because of mobilization of third-space (interstitial) fluid.

Nursing Diagnosis:

Risk for Trauma

related to weakness, balancing difficulties, and reduced muscle coordination due to anesthetics and postoperative opioid analgesics

Desired Outcome: The patient does not fall and remains free of trauma as evidenced by absence of bruises, wounds, and fractures.

ASSESSMENT/INTERVENTIONS	RATIONALES
Orient and reorient the patient to person, place, and time during the initial postoperative period. Inform the patient that the surgery is over. Repeat information until the patient is fully awake and oriented (usually several hours but may be days in heavily sedated or otherwise obtunded individuals).	Orientation and repeated explanations increase mental awareness and alertness, which decrease risk of trauma caused by disorientation. These measures also help the patient cope with unfamiliar surroundings.

ASSESSMENT/INTERVENTIONS	RATIONALES
! Maintain side rails on stretchers and beds in upright and locked positions.	Side rails help prevent trauma to the head and extremities. Some individuals experience agitation and thrash about as they emerge from anesthesia.
Secure all IV lines, drains, and tubing.	This action prevents their dislodgement.
! Maintain the bed in its lowest position when leaving the patient's room.	This action protects the patient from major trauma In case he or she falls out of bed.
Place the call mechanism within the patient's reach; instruct the patient in its use.	The patient can call for help when it is needed—for example, when needing to use the toilet. This will reduce risk of falls and injury.
! Identify patients at risk for falling. Correct or compensate for risk factors.	Risk factors include the following: - *Time of day:* Night shift, peak activity periods such as meals, bedtime. - *Medications:* Opioid analgesics, sedatives, hypnotics, and anesthetics. - *Impaired mobility:* Individuals requiring assistance with transfer and ambulation. - *Sensory deficits:* Diminished visual acuity caused by disease process or environmental factors; changes in kinesthetic sense because of disease or trauma.
Use restraints and protective devices if necessary and prescribed.	These devices provide protection during an emergent state. However, because they can cause agitation, their use should be infrequent and as a last resort. Behavioral intervention or a patient sitter Is preferred.

Nursing Diagnosis:

Risk for Impaired Skin Integrity

related to the presence of secretions/excretions around percutaneous drains and tubes

Desired Outcome: The patient's skin around percutaneous drains and tubes remains intact and nonerythematous.

ASSESSMENT/INTERVENTIONS	RATIONALES
Assess and change dressings as soon as they become wet. (The health care provider may prefer to perform the first dressing change at the surgical incision.) Use sterile technique for all dressing changes.	These interventions protect the wound from contamination and accumulation of fluids that may cause excoriation.
Keep areas around drains as clean as possible.	Intestinal secretions, bile, and similar drainage can lead quickly to skin excoriation (pepsin, conjugated bile acids, gastric acid, and lysolecithin all have a low [acidic] pH of 1-3). Sterile normal saline or a solution of saline and hydrogen peroxide or other prescribed solution may be used to clean around the drain site.
If some external drainage is present, position a pectin-wafer skin barrier around drain or tube. Ointments, such as zinc oxide, petrolatum, and aluminum paste, also may be used.	Skin barriers and ointments are used to protect the skin from drainage that could cause breakdown because of caustic enzymes, especially from the small bowel.
Consult a wound, ostomy, continence (WOC) or enterostomal therapy (ET) nurse as indicated.	These nurses provide specialized interventions if drainage is excessive, skin excoriation develops, or a collection bag needs to be placed over drains and incisions.
For additional information, see Chapter 73, "Managing Wound Care." p. 533.	

Nursing Diagnosis:

Disturbed Sleep Pattern

related to preoperative anxiety, stress, postoperative pain, noise, and altered environment

Desired Outcome: Following intervention/treatment, the patient relates minimal or no difficulty with falling asleep and describes a feeling of being well rested.

ASSESSMENT/INTERVENTIONS	RATIONALES
Use nonpharmacologic measures to promote sleep.	Behavioral interventions are the preferred method for insomnia because of their established efficacy and absence of drug side effects. Environmental stimulation should be reduced by use of minimum lighting and noise reduction. Pillows and bedding should be comfortable, and patients should be allowed to maintain their bedtime routine as close to normal as possible.
Administer analgesics and/or sedatives at bedtime when indicated.	This action reduces nighttime pain and augments effects of the hypnotic agent to promote sleep.
⚠ Use special care when administering sedative/hypnotic to patients with COPD. Monitor respiratory function, including oximetry, at frequent intervals in these patients.	Sedative/hypnotics could cause respiratory depression in patients who already have inadequate ventilation.
⚠ After administering the sedative/hypnotic, be certain to raise side rails, lower bed to its lowest position, and caution the patient not to smoke in bed.	The patient will become drowsy, which necessitates these safety measures.

Nursing Diagnosis:

Impaired Physical Mobility

related to postoperative pain, decreased strength and endurance occurring with CNS effects of anesthesia or blood loss, musculoskeletal or neuromuscular impairment occurring with the disease process or surgical procedure, sensoriperceptual impairment occurring with the disease process or surgical procedure (e.g., ocular surgery, neurosurgery), or cognitive impairment occurring with the disease process or effects of opioid analgesics and anesthetics

Desired Outcome: Optimally, by hospital discharge (depending on type of surgery), the patient returns to preoperative baseline physical mobility as evidenced by ability to move in bed, transfer, and ambulate independently or with minimal assistance.

ASSESSMENT/INTERVENTIONS	RATIONALES
Review the patient's preoperative physical mobility, including coordination and muscle strength, control, and mass.	Preoperative/baseline assessments enable accurate measurements of postoperative mobility problems.
Implement medically imposed restrictions against movement, especially with conditions or surgeries that are orthopedic, neurosurgical, or ocular.	Restricting movement and certain positions can prevent disruption of the surgical repair.
Evaluate and correct factors limiting physical mobility.	Factors such as oversedation with opioid analgesics, failure to achieve adequate pain control, and poorly arranged physical environment can be corrected.
Initiate movement from bed to chair and ambulation as soon as possible after surgery, depending on postoperative prescriptions, type of surgery, and the patient's recovery from anesthetics.	Patients usually can tolerate a graduated progression in activity and ambulation.

ASSESSMENT/INTERVENTIONS	RATIONALES
Assist with moving slowly to a sitting position in bed and then standing at the bedside before attempting ambulation. For more information, see **Risk for Ineffective Cerebral Tissue Perfusion**, p. 67	Many anesthetic agents depress normal vasoconstrictor mechanisms and can result in sudden hypotension with quick changes in position.
Encourage frequent movement and ambulation by postoperative patients. Provide assistance as indicated.	These actions reduce the potential for postoperative complications, including atelectasis, pneumonia, thrombophlebitis, skin breakdown, muscle weakness, and decreased GI motility.
Teach exercises that can be performed in bed and explain their purpose.	Exercises such as gluteal and quadriceps muscle sets (isometrics) and ankle circling and calf pumping promote muscle strength, increase venous return, and prevent stasis.
For additional information, see Chapter 4, "Prolonged Bedrest," **Risk for Activity Intolerance**, p. 61, and **Risk for Disuse Syndrome**, p. 63.	

Nursing Diagnosis:

Impaired Oral Mucous Membrane

related to NPO status and/or presence of NG or endotracheal tube

Desired Outcome: At the time of hospital discharge, the patient's oral mucosa is intact, without pain or evidence of bleeding.

ASSESSMENT/INTERVENTIONS	RATIONALES
Provide oral care and oral hygiene q4h and prn. Arrange for patients to gargle, brush teeth, and cleanse mouth with sponge-tipped applicators as necessary.	Oral care provides comfort and prevents excoriation and excessive dryness of oral mucous membrane.
Use a moistened cotton-tipped applicator to remove encrustations. Carefully lubricate lips and nares with antimicrobial ointment or emollient cream.	These interventions provide comfort and decrease risk of tissue breakdown caused by dry tissues.
If indicated, obtain a prescription for lidocaine gargling solution.	This solution provides comfort if the patient's throat tissue is irritated from the presence of an NG tube.

Nursing Diagnoses:

Risk for Dysfunctional Gastrointestinal Motility
Constipation

related to immobility, opioid analgesics and other medications, dehydration, lack of privacy, or disruption of abdominal musculature or manipulation of abdominal viscera during surgery

Desired Outcome: The patient returns to his or her normal bowel elimination pattern as evidenced by return of active bowel sounds within 48-72 hr after most surgeries, absence of abdominal distention or sensation of fullness, and elimination of soft, formed stools.

ASSESSMENT/INTERVENTIONS	RATIONALES
Assess for and document elimination of flatus or stool.	This signals return of intestinal motility.
Assess for abdominal distention, tenderness, absent or hypoactive bowel sounds, and sensation of fullness. Report gross distention, extreme tenderness, and prolonged absence of bowel sounds.	Gross distention, extreme tenderness, and prolonged absence of bowel sounds are signs of decreased GI motility and possible ileus. High-pitched bowel sounds may indicate impending bowel obstruction.

continued

PART I: Medical-Surgical Nursing

ASSESSMENT/INTERVENTIONS

RATIONALES

ASSESSMENT/INTERVENTIONS	RATIONALES
Encourage in-bed position changes, exercises, and ambulation to the patient's tolerance unless contraindicated.	These activities stimulate peristalsis, which promotes bowel elimination.
If an NG tube is in place, perform the following: - Check placement of the tube after insertion, before any instillation, and q8h. For a larger bore tube, aspirate gastric contents and assess for pH less than 5.0 for gastric tube placement. If the tube is in the trachea, the patient may exhibit signs of respiratory distress or consistently low O_2 saturation levels, or there may be absence of drainage. Reposition the tube immediately. Once assured of placement, mark tube to easily assess tube migration, and secure tubing in place. For smaller bore tubes, check recent x-ray film to confirm position before instilling anything.	A malpositioned NG tube will be ineffective in relieving gastric distention and pose a threat to the patient's well-being.
- For patients with gastric, esophageal, or duodenal surgery, notify the health care provider before manipulating the tube.	Manipulation of NG tubes in these patients could result in disruption of the surgical anastomosis.
- Keep the tube securely taped to the patient's nose, and reinforce placement by attaching the tube to the patient's gown with a safety pin or tape.	Securing the tube prevents its migration into the patient's airway.
- Measure and record quantity and quality of output, including color.	Typically the color will be green. For patients who have undergone gastric surgery, output may be brownish initially because of small amounts of bloody drainage but should change to green after about 12 hr.
- Test reddish, brown, or black output for the presence of blood. Reposition tube as necessary.	These colors may signal GI bleeding.
- Gently instill normal saline as prescribed.	This action helps maintain patency of the GI tube.
- Ensure low, intermittent suction of gastric sump tubes by maintaining patency of the sump port (usually blue).	When the port is open and air is entering the stomach, continuous suction is safe.
- If the sump port becomes occluded by gastric contents, flush the sump port with air until a *whoosh* sound is heard over the epigastric area.	If the port becomes occluded, the tube essentially becomes a single lumen tube and the continuous suction could damage the lining of the stomach.
- Never clamp or otherwise occlude the sump port. For patients with gastric, esophageal, or duodenal surgery, notify the health care provider before irrigating the tube.	Excessive pressure may accumulate and damage gastric mucosa or disrupt the surgical anastomosis.
- When the tube is removed, monitor for abdominal distention, nausea, and vomiting.	These are signs that GI motility is still decreased and requires further intervention.
Monitor and document the patient's response to diet advancement from clear liquids to a regular or other prescribed diet.	Poor response to diet advancement as evidenced by abdominal distention, nausea, and vomiting may signal continued decreased GI motility and should be reported for timely intervention. Postoperatively, decreased GI motility can result from stress (autonomic), surgical manipulation of the intestine, immobility, and effects of medications.
Encourage oral fluid intake (more than 2500 mL/day), especially intake of prune juice.	Increased hydration, including prune juice, helps promote soft stools that will minimize need to strain.
Administer stool softeners, mild laxatives, senna-based herbal teas, and enemas as prescribed. As appropriate, encourage a high-fiber diet (fresh vegetables and fruits). Monitor and record results.	These interventions promote bulk and softness in stools for easier evacuation.
Arrange periods of privacy during the patient's attempts at bowel elimination.	Privacy promotes relaxation and success with defecation.

ADDITIONAL NURSING DIAGNOSES/PROBLEMS:

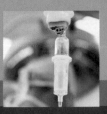

Prolonged Bedrest   4

OVERVIEW/PATHOPHYSIOLOGY

Patients on prolonged bedrest face many potential physiologic and psychosocial problems. Complications may include respiratory, cardiac, and musculoskeletal disorders as well as other problems resulting in permanent disabilities. This section reviews the most common physiologic and psychosocial problems that may occur. With patients being discharged from the hospital sooner, many health care problems are being treated in long-term care facilities or at home.

HEALTH CARE SETTING

Extended care, a̶c̶ ̶ ̶ ̶c̶are, home care

Nursing Diagnosis:

Risk for Activity Intolerance

related to deconditioned status

Desired Outcomes: Within 48 hr of discontinuing bedrest, the patient exhibits cardiac tolerance to activity or exercise as evidenced by heart rate (HR) 20 bpm or less over resting HR; systolic blood pressure (SBP) 20 mm Hg or less over or under resting SBP; respiratory rate (RR) 20 breaths/min or less with normal depth and pattern (eupnea); normal sinus rhythm; warm and dry skin; and absence of crackles (rales), new murmurs, new dysrhythmias, gallop, or chest pain. The patient rates perceived exertion (RPE) at 3 or less on a scale of 0 (none) to 10 (maximum) and maintains muscle strength and joint range of motion (ROM).

ASSESSMENT/INTERVENTIONS	RATIONALES
Assess for orthostatic hypotension: Prepare the patient for this change by increasing the amount of time spent in high Fowler's position and moving the patient slowly in stages.	Orthostatic hypotension can occur as a result of decreased plasma volume and difficulty in adjusting immediately to postural change. For more information about orthostatic hypotension, see **Risk for Ineffective Cerebral Tissue Perfusion,** p. 67.
Assess exercise tolerance: Be alert to signs and symptoms that the cardiovascular and respiratory systems are unable to meet the demands of the low-level ROM exercises.	Excessive shortness of breath may occur if (1) transient pulmonary congestion occurs secondary to ischemia or left ventricular dysfunction, (2) lung volumes are decreased, (3) oxygen-carrying capacity of the blood is reduced, or (4) there is shunting of blood from the right to the left side of the heart without adequate oxygenation. If cardiac output does not increase to meet the body's needs during modest levels of exercise, SBP may fall; the skin may become cool, cyanotic, and diaphoretic; dysrhythmias may be noted; crackles (rales) may be auscultated; or a systolic murmur of mitral regurgitation may occur.
Perform ROM exercises 2-4 times/day on each extremity. Individualize the exercise plan.	These exercises build stamina by increasing muscle strength and endurance

continued

ASSESSMENT/INTERVENTIONS	RATIONALES
Caution: Avoid isometric exercises in cardiac patients.	These exercises can increase systemic arterial blood pressure.
Mode or type of exercise: Begin with passive exercises, moving the joints through the motions of abduction, adduction, flexion, and extension. Progress to active-assisted exercises in which you support the joints while the patient initiates muscle contraction. When the patient is able, supervise him or her in active isotonic exercises, during which the patient contracts a selected muscle group, moves the extremity at a slow pace, and then relaxes the muscle group. Have the patient repeat each exercise 3-10 times.	Beginning with passive movement, progressing to active-assisted, and continuing with active isotonic takes patients from the least exerting to the most exerting exercises over a period of time, thus increasing gradual tolerance.
Caution: Stop the exercise if the patient becomes overly short of breath, has a rapid heart rate, passes out, or experiences severe pain, dizziness, or lightheadedness. Consult with the health care provider accordingly.	These exercises should be used with caution in any patient who has been recently ill or has unexplained weight gain or swelling of a joint because these may be signs of a serious health condition.
Caution: Stop any exercise that results in muscular or skeletal pain. Consult a physical therapist (PT) about necessary modifications.	This action prevents injury in a joint too inflamed or diseased to tolerate this type of exercise intensity.
Intensity: Begin with 3-5 repetitions as tolerated by the patient.	Starting with minimal intensity and progressing step-by-step to greater intensity enables gradual tolerance.
Measure HR and blood pressure (BP) at rest, peak exercise, and 5 min after exercise.	These assessments help determine tolerance to the exercise. If HR or SBP increases more than 20 bpm or more than 20 mm Hg over resting level, the number of repetitions should be decreased. If HR or SBP decreases more than 10 bpm or more than 10 mm Hg at peak exercise, this could be a sign of left ventricular failure, denoting that the heart cannot meet this workload. For other adverse signs and symptoms, see *Assess exercise tolerance.*
Duration: Begin with 5 min or less of exercise. Gradually increase the exercise to 15 min as tolerated.	Starting with minimal duration and progressing to greater duration enables gradual tolerance.
Frequency: Begin with exercises 2-4 times/day.	As duration increases, the frequency can be reduced.
Ask patient to rate perceived exertion experienced during exercise, basing it on the following scale developed by Borg (1982). 0 = Nothing at all 1 = Very weak effort 2 = Weak (light) effort 3 = Moderate effort 4 = Somewhat stronger effort 5 = Strong effort 7 = Very strong effort 9 = Very, very strong effort 10 = Maximum effort	Borg's Scale is a simple method of RPE that can be used to gauge a person's level of exertion in training. Exercises to prevent deconditioning should be performed at low levels of effort. Patients should not experience an RPE greater than 3 while performing ROM exercises.
If the patient tolerates the exercise, increase intensity or number of repetitions each day and increase activity as soon as possible to include sitting in a chair.	Tolerance is a sign that cardiovascular and respiratory systems are able to meet the demands of this low-level ROM exercise. To promote optimal conditioning, activity should be increased to correspond to the patient's increased tolerance.
Monitor CBC and report any abnormal value.	Disorders such as anemia can decrease the oxygen-carrying capacity of the blood and affect tolerance.
Progress activity in hospitalized patients as follows. **Level I: Bedrest** - Flexion and extension of extremities 4 times/day, 15 times each extremity - Deep breathing 4 times/day, 15 breaths - Position change from side to side q2h - Use of Vollman's prone positioners and kinetic therapy beds.	Signs of activity intolerance include decrease in BP more than 20 mm Hg, increase in HR to more than 120 bpm (or more than 20 bpm above resting HR in patients receiving beta-blocker therapy), and shortness of breath (discussed earlier). A strategy to promote lung expansion by the use of Vollman's prone positioner enables postural drainage. Kinetic therapy beds provide continual rotation of more than 200 times/day, which decreases the likelihood of pressure sores and pneumonia.

ASSESSMENT/INTERVENTIONS

Level II: Out of bed to chair
- As tolerated, 3 times/day for 20-30 min
- May perform ROM exercises 2 times/day while sitting in chair

Level III: Ambulate in room
- As tolerated, 3 times/day for 3-5 min in room

Level IV: Ambulate in hall

Initially, 50-200 ft 2 times/day, progressing to 600 ft 4 times/day
May incorporate slow stair climbing in preparation for hospital discharge
Monitor for signs of activity intolerance.

Have the patient perform self-care activities as tolerated.

Teach the patient's significant other interventions for preventing deconditioning and their purpose. Involve him or her in the patient's plan of care.

Pay attention to nonverbal behaviors and provide emotional support to the patient and significant other as the patient's activity level is increased.

RATIONALES

Gradually increasing activities by working up to 20- to 30-min sessions at least 3 to 4 times a week with the use of a walker or gait belt for support and providing nonskid footwear for ambulation not only promotes conditioning but patient safety as well.

Self-care activities such as eating, mouth care, and bathing may increase the patient's activity level.

Significant others can promote and participate in the patient's activity/exercises once they understand the rationale and are familiar with the interventions.

Emotional support helps allay fears of failure, pain, or medical setbacks.

Nursing Diagnosis:

Risk for Disuse Syndrome

related to paralysis, mechanical immobilization, prescribed immobilization, severe pain, or altered level of consciousness

Desired Outcomes: When bedrest is discontinued, the patient exhibits complete ROM of all joints without pain, and limb girth measurements are congruent with or increased over baseline measurements.

> **Note:** *ROM exercises should be performed at least 2 times/day for all immobilized patients with normal joints. Modification may be required for patients with spinal cord injuries.*

ASSESSMENT/INTERVENTIONS

Assess ROM of the patient's joints, paying special attention to the following areas: shoulder, wrist, fingers, hips, knees, and feet.

Assess for footdrop by inspecting the feet for plantar flexion and evaluating the patient's ability to pull the toes upward toward the head. Document the assessment daily.

Ensure that the patient changes position at least q2h. Post a turning schedule at the bedside.

RATIONALES

These areas are especially susceptible to joint contracture. Shoulders can become "frozen" to limit abduction and extension; wrists can "drop," prohibiting extension; fingers can develop flexion contractures that limit extension; hips can develop flexion contractures that affect the gait by shortening the limb or develop external rotation or adduction deformities that affect the gait; knees may have flexion contractures that can develop to limit extension and alter the gait; and feet can "drop" as a result of prolonged plantar flexion, which limits dorsiflexion and alters the gait.

Because feet lie naturally in plantar flexion, footdrop may occur when plantar flexion is prolonged. Inability to dorsiflex (pull the toes up toward the head) is a sign of footdrop, and it requires prompt intervention to prevent permanent damage. This may necessitate use of foot boards or high-top tennis shoes to facilitate normal dorsal flexion position.

Position changes not only maintain correct body alignment, thereby reducing strain on the joints, but also prevent contractures, minimize pressure on bony prominences, decrease venous stasis, and promote maximal chest expansion.

continued

ASSESSMENT/INTERVENTIONS	RATIONALES
Place the patient in a position that achieves proper standing. Maintain this position with pillows, towels, waffle boots, heel lift suspension boots, foam heal positioners, foot boards, PlexiPulse compression device, high-top tennis shoes, or other positioning aids.	A position in which the head is neutral or slightly flexed on the neck, hips are extended, knees are extended or minimally flexed, and feet are at right angles to the legs achieves proper standing alignment, which helps promote ambulation when the patient is ready to do so.
Ensure that the patient is prone or side lying, with hips extended, for the same amount of time spent in the supine position or, at a minimum, 3 times/day for 1 hr.	These positions prevent hip flexion contractures.
When the head of bed (HOB) must be elevated 30 degrees, extend the patient's shoulders and arms, using pillows to support the position.	This position maintains proper spinal posture.
Allow the patient's fingertips to extend over the pillow's edge.	This position maintains normal arching of the hands.
Place thin pads under the angles of the axillae and lateral aspects of the clavicles.	These pads help prevent internal rotation of the shoulders and maintain anatomic position of the shoulder girdle.
Ensure that the patient spends time with hips in extension (see preceding interventions).	This position helps prevent hip flexion contracture.
When the patient is in the side-lying position, extend the lower leg from the hip.	This position helps prevent hip flexion contracture.
When the patient can be placed in the prone position, move him or her to the end of the bed and allow the feet to rest between the mattress and footboard.	This prevents not only plantar flexion and hip rotation, but also injury to the heels and toes.
Use positioning devices liberally.	Using pillows, rolled towels, blankets, sandbags, antirotation boots, splints, knee abductors, drop seats, foot supports, back wedges, back support splints, wedges cushions, pommel cushions, and orthotics helps maintain joints in neutral position, which helps ensure that they remain functional when activity is increased.
When using adjunctive devices, monitor involved skin at least tid.	Assessing for alterations in skin integrity enables prompt interventions that prevent skin breakdown.
Teach the patient and significant other the rationale and procedure for ROM exercises, and have the patient give return demonstrations. Review **Risk for Activity Intolerance,** p. 61, to ensure that the patient does not exceed his or her tolerance. Provide passive exercises for patients unable to perform active or active-assisted exercises. In addition, incorporate movement patterns into care activities, such as position changes, bed baths, getting patient on and off the bedpan, or changing the patient's gown.	These actions facilitate adherence to the exercise regimen and help prevent contracture formation.
Provide the patient with a handout that reviews exercises and lists repetitions for each. Instruct the patient's significant other to encourage the patient to perform exercises as required.	These actions facilitate learning and adherence to the exercise program.
Perform and document limb girth measurements, dynamography, and ROM, and establish exercise baseline limits.	This assessment of existing muscle mass, strength, and joint motion enables subsequent evaluation and promotes exercise and ROM appropriate for the patient.
Explain to the patient how muscle atrophy occurs. Emphasize the importance of maintaining or increasing muscle strength and periarticular tissue elasticity through exercise. If there are complicating pathologic conditions, consult the health care provider about the appropriate form of exercise for the patient.	Muscle atrophy occurs because of disuse or failure to use the joint, often caused by immediate or anticipated pain. This explanation encourages patients to perform exercises inasmuch as disuse eventually may result in decreased muscle mass and blood supply and a loss of periarticular tissue elasticity, which in turn can lead to increased muscle fatigue and joint pain with use.
Explain the need to participate maximally in self-care as tolerated.	Self-care helps maintain muscle strength and promote a sense of participation and control.

ASSESSMENT/INTERVENTIONS

ASSESSMENT/INTERVENTIONS	RATIONALES
For noncardiac patients needing greater help with muscle strength, assist with resistive exercises (e.g., moderate weight lifting to increase size, endurance, and strength of the muscles). For patients in beds with Balkan frames or other types of over-bed frames, provide a means for resistive exercise by implementing a system of weights and pulleys.	Resistance increases the force needed to perform the exercise and promotes the maintenance or rebuilding of muscle strength.
Determine the patient's baseline level of performance on a given set of exercises, and then set realistic goals for repetitions.	Well-planned goals provide markers for assessing effectiveness of the exercise plan and progress made. For example, if the patient can do 5 repetitions of lifting a 5-lb weight with the biceps muscle, the goal may be to increase repetitions to 10 within 1 wk, to an ultimate goal of 20 within 3 wk, and then advance to 7.5-lb weights.
If the joints require rest, teach isometric exercises.	In these exercises, the patient contracts a muscle group and holds the contraction for a count of 5 or 10. The sequence is repeated for increasing counts or repetitions until an adequate level of endurance has been achieved. Thereafter, maintenance levels are performed. **Note:** These exercises do not build strength but, rather, help to maintain strength.
Provide a chart to show the patient's progress, and combine this with large amounts of positive reinforcement.	Attaining progress and having positive reinforcement promote continued adherence to the exercise plan.
Post the exercise regimen at the bedside. Instruct the patient's significant other in the exercise regimen, and elicit his or her support and encouragement of the patient's performance of the exercises.	These actions ensure consistency by all health care personnel and involvement and support of significant others.
As prescribed, teach transfer or crutch-walking techniques and use of a walker, wheelchair, or cane. Include the significant other in demonstrations, and stress the importance of proper body mechanics.	These interventions help ensure that patients can safely maintain the highest possible level of mobility while also improving circulation.
Employ gait belts, lifts, and bed assist devices.	These devices promote safety and help to improve movement.
Provide periods of uninterrupted rest between exercises/activities.	Rest enables patients to replenish energy stores.
Seek referral to PT or OT as appropriate.	Such a referral will help patients who have special needs or who are not in a care facility to attain the best ROM possible.

Nursing Diagnosis:

Ineffective Peripheral Tissue Perfusion

related to interrupted venous flow occurring with prolonged immobility

Desired Outcomes: At least 24 hr before hospital discharge, the patient has adequate peripheral perfusion as evidenced by normal skin color and temperature and adequate distal pulses (greater than 2+ on a 0-4+ scale) in peripheral extremities. The patient performs exercises independently, adheres to the prophylactic regimen, and maintains intake of 2-3 L/day of fluid unless contraindicated.

ASSESSMENT/INTERVENTIONS	RATIONALES
Assess for calf or groin tenderness, redness, unilateral swelling of a leg, warmth in the involved area, and coolness, unnatural color or pallor, and superficial venous dilation distal to the involved area.	Pain elicited with dorsiflexion along with these other indicators may be signs of deep vein thrombosis (DVT)/venous thromboembolism (VTE).
Measure the girth of the affected limb, comparing it to the opposite side.	If the girth of the affected limb is larger in comparison to the opposite limb, this is a sign of DVT/VTE.
Teach these indicators to the patient.	A knowledgeable patient is more likely to report these indicators promptly for timely intervention.

continued

ASSESSMENT/INTERVENTIONS	RATIONALES
In addition, assess vital signs and monitor erythrocyte sedimentation rate (ESR) results if they are available.	Additional signs of DVT/VTE may include fever, tachycardia, and elevated ESR. Normal ESR (Westergren method) in males younger than 50 yr is 0-15 mm/hr and older than 50 yr is 0-20 mm/hr; in females younger than 50 yr it is 0-20 mm/hr, and older than 50 yr it is 0-30 mm/hr.
Notify the patient's health care provider of significant findings.	If signs of DVT/VTE occur, further evaluation will be necessary to protect the patient from a pulmonary embolus or clot that could compromise the limb. For more information, see Chapter 24, "Venous Thrombosis/ Thrombophlebitis," p. 186.
Perform passive ROM or encourage active ROM exercises in the absence of signs of DVT.	These exercises increase circulation, which promotes peripheral tissue perfusion.
Teach patient calf-pumping (ankle dorsiflexion–plantar flexion) and ankle-circling exercises.	Same as above. The patient should repeat each movement 10 times, performing each exercise hourly during extended periods of immobility, as long as the patient is free of symptoms of DVT/VTE.
Encourage deep breathing.	Deep breathing increases negative pressure in the lungs and thorax to promote emptying of large veins and thus increase peripheral tissue perfusion.
When not contraindicated by peripheral vascular disease (PVD), ensure that the patient wears antiembolism hose, pneumatic foot pump devices, pneumatic sequential compression stockings, or thromboembolism-deterrent (TED) hose.	These garments/devices prevent venous stasis, the precursor to DVT/VTE. The pneumatic devices, which provide more compression than antiembolism hose, are especially useful in preventing DVT/VTE in patients who are mostly immobile. Patients with PVD may experience rest pain, which can be precipitated by TED hose, foot pump devices, and pneumatic sequential compression stockings.
Remove pneumatic sequential compress stockings for 10-20 min q8h. Reapply hose after elevating the patient's legs at least 10 degrees for 10 min.	Removing pneumatic sequential compress stockings enables inspection of underlying skin for evidence of irritation or breakdown. Elevating the legs before reapplying the pneumatic sequential compress stockings promotes venous return and decreases edema, which otherwise would remain and cause discomfort when the hose are reapplied.
Instruct the patient not to cross the feet at the ankles or knees while in bed.	These actions may cause venous stasis.
If the patient is at risk for DVT/VTE, elevate foot of the bed 10 degrees.	Elevating the foot of the bed increases venous return.
In nonrestricted patients, increase fluid intake to at least 2-3 L/day. Educate the patient about the need to drink large amounts of fluid (9-14 8-oz glasses) daily. Monitor intake and output (I&O) to ensure adherence.	Increased hydration reduces hemoconcentration, which can contribute to development of DVT/VTE.
Administer anticlotting medication as prescribed.	Patients at risk for DVT/VTE, including those with chronic infection and history of PVD and smoking, as well as patients who are older, obese, and anemic, may require anticoagulants to minimize the risk of clotting. Drugs such as aspirin, sodium warfarin, phenindione derivatives, heparin, or low-molecular-weight heparin (LMWH; e.g., enoxaparin sodium) may be given. Many patients are taught how to self-administer LMWH injections after hospital discharge.
Monitor appropriate laboratory values (e.g., prothrombin time [PT], international normalized ratio [INR], partial thromboplastin time [PTT]).	Optimal laboratory values for PTT are 60-70 sec or 1.5-2.5× control value if on anticoagulant therapy and INR 2.0-3.0 if on anticoagulant therapy. Values higher than these signify that the patient is at increased risk for bleeding.
Teach the patient to self-monitor for and report bleeding.	Anticoagulant drugs increase the risk of bleeding. It is important for the patient to know signs of bleeding so that he or she can report them as soon as they are noted to ensure timely intervention. Possible types of bleeding include epistaxis, bleeding gums, hematemesis, hemoptysis, melena, hematuria, hematochezia, menometrorrhagia, and ecchymoses.

ASSESSMENT/INTERVENTIONS	RATIONALES
Teach medication, food, and herbal interactions that can affect warfarin.	Many foods and over-the-counter herbals can prolong bleeding such as alfalfa/alfalfa sprouts, angelica (dong quai), borage, bromelain, celery, clove, Coenzyme Q-10, devils claw, echinacea, fenugreek, garlic, ginger, gingko biloba green tea, licorice, parsley, passion flower, quinine, red clover, and St. John's wort. Examples of medications and foods that decrease the effect of anticoagulation, thus increasing the chance of blood clots, are azathioprine, antithyroid medications, carbamazepine, dicloxacillin, glutethimide, griseofulvin, haloperidol, nafcillin, oral contraceptives, phenobarbital, rifampin, vitamin C, dark green leafy vegetables, spinach, kale, collards, broccoli, asparagus, cauliflower, and Brussels sprouts.

Nursing Diagnosis:

Risk for Ineffective Cerebral Tissue Perfusion

(orthostatic hypotension) *related to* interrupted arterial flow to the brain occurring with prolonged bedrest

Desired Outcome: When getting out of bed, the patient has adequate cerebral perfusion as evidenced by HR less than 120 bpm and BP 90/60 mm Hg or greater (or within 20 mm Hg of the patient's normal range) immediately after position change, dry skin, normal skin color, and absence of vertigo and syncope, with return of HR and BP to resting levels within 3 min of position change.

ASSESSMENT/INTERVENTIONS	RATIONALES
Assess for recent diuresis, diaphoresis, or change in vasodilator therapy.	These are factors that increase the risk of orthostatic hypotension because of fluid volume changes. For example, bedrest incurs a diuresis of about 600-800 mL during the first 3 days. Although this fluid decrease is not noticed when the patient is supine, the lost volume will be evident (i.e., with orthostatic hypotension) when the body tries to adapt to sitting and standing.
Be alert to diabetic cardiac neuropathy, denervation after heart transplantation, advanced age, or severe left ventricular dysfunction.	These are factors that increase risk of orthostatic hypotension because of altered autonomic control.
Assess BP in any high-risk patient for whom this will be the first time out of bed. Instruct the patient to report immediately symptoms of lightheadedness or dizziness.	Low BP, lightheadedness, and dizziness are signs of orthostatic hypotension and necessitate a return to the supine position.
Assess for a drop in SBP of 20 mm Hg or greater and an increased pulse rate, combined with symptoms of vertigo and impending syncope.	These are signs of orthostatic hypotension that signal the need for return to the supine position.
Explain cause of orthostatic hypotension and measures for preventing it.	Patients who are informed as to cause and ways of preventing orthostatic hypotension are more likely to avoid it. Measures to prevent orthostatic hypotension are discussed in subsequent interventions.
Apply antiembolism hose once the patient is mobilized.	Used to prevent DVT/VTE, antiembolism hose and sequential compression hose also may be useful in preventing orthostatic hypotension by promoting venous return once the patient is mobilized.
When the patient is in bed, provide instructions for leg exercises as described under **Ineffective Peripheral Tissue Perfusion,** p. 65. Encourage the patient to perform leg exercises immediately before mobilization.	Leg exercises promote venous return, which helps prevent orthostatic hypotension.

continued

ASSESSMENT/INTERVENTIONS	RATIONALES
Prepare the patient for getting out of bed by encouraging position changes within necessary restrictions.	Position changes help acclimate patients to the upright position. These changes may be accomplished with the assistance of an over-bed trapeze, hydraulic lift, and EZ lift.
Follow these guidelines for mobilization: - Have the patient dangle legs at the bedside. Be alert to indicators of orthostatic hypotension, including diaphoresis, pallor, tachycardia, hypotension, and syncope. Question patient about the presence of lightheadedness or dizziness. Again, encourage performance of leg exercises.	This action provides for a gradual adjustment to the possible effects of venous pooling and related hypotension in persons who have been supine or in Fowler's position for some time. Dangling of the legs may be necessary until intravascular fluid volume is restored. It also provides an opportunity for leg exercises that can reduce risk of venous stasis.
- If leg dangling is tolerated, have the patient stand at the bedside with two staff members in attendance. If no adverse signs or symptoms occur, have the patient progress to ambulation as tolerated.	This intervention helps ensure the patient's safety in the event of a fall.

Nursing Diagnosis:

Constipation

related to less than adequate fluid or dietary intake and bulk, immobility, lack of privacy, positional restrictions, and use of opioid analgesics

Desired Outcomes: Within 24 hr of this diagnosis, the patient verbalizes knowledge of measures that promote bowel elimination. The patient relates return of normal pattern and character of bowel elimination within 3-5 days of this diagnosis.

ASSESSMENT/INTERVENTIONS	RATIONALES
Assess the patient's bowel history.	This assessment elicits normal bowel habits and interventions that are used successfully at home.
Assess and document the patient's bowel movements, diet, and I&O.	This information tracks bowel movements and factors that promote or prevent constipation. Indications of constipation include the following: fewer than patient's usual number of bowel movements, abdominal discomfort or distention, straining at stool, and patient complaints of rectal pressure or fullness. Fecal impaction may be manifested by oozing of liquid stool and confirmed via digital examination.
If rectal impaction is suspected, use a gloved, lubricated finger to remove stool from the rectum.	Digital stimulation may be adequate to promote a bowel movement. Oil retention enemas may soften impacted stool.
Teach the importance of a high-fiber diet (20-35 grams/day) and a fluid intake of at least 2-3 L/day (unless this is contraindicated by a renal, hepatic, or cardiac disorder).	These measures increase peristalsis and the likelihood of normal bowel movements. High-fiber foods—including bran, nuts, raw and coarse vegetables, beans, and lentils—are rich in insoluble fiber. Good hydration softens the stool, making it easier to evacuate. Patients with renal, hepatic, and diverticular disease, cardiac disorders, or hemorrhoids may be on fluid restrictions.
Maintain the patient's normal bowel habits whenever possible by offering a bedpan; ensuring privacy; and timing medications, enemas, or suppositories so that they take effect at the time of day when the patient normally has a bowel movement.	These actions may facilitate regularity of bowel movements.
Provide warm fluids before breakfast, and encourage toileting.	These measures take advantage of the patient's gastrocolic and duodenocolic reflexes.
Maximize the patient's activity level within limitations of endurance, therapy, and pain.	Increased activity promotes peristalsis, which helps prevent constipation.

ASSESSMENT/INTERVENTIONS	RATIONALES
Request pharmacologic interventions from the health care provider when necessary. To help prevent rebound constipation, make a priority list of interventions.	Starting with the gentlest interventions helps prevent rebound constipation and ensures minimal disruption of patient's normal bowel habits. The following is a suggested hierarchy of interventions: - Bulk-building additives (psyllium), bran - Mild laxatives (apple or prune juice, milk of magnesia) - Stool softeners (docusate sodium, docusate calcium) - Potent laxatives and cathartics (bisacodyl, cascara sagrada) - Medicated suppositories - Enemas
Discuss the role that opioid agents and other medications play in causing constipation.	Opioids, antidepressants, anticholinergics, iron supplements, diuretics, and muscle relaxants are known to cause constipation. Methylnaltrexone, a μ-opioid receptor antagonist, is a medication that treats opioid-induced constipation.
Teach nonpharmacologic methods of pain control. See discussion in Chapter 2, "Pain," p. 44.	Nonpharmacologic methods that may decrease the need for opioid analgesics include transcutaneous electrical nerve stimulation (TENS), spinal cord stimulation (SCS), ice, massage therapy, guided imagery, music therapy, biofeedback, and acupuncture.

Nursing Diagnosis:

Ineffective Role Performance

related to necessity for dependence upon others during care vs. need/desire for independence/self-care as condition improves

Desired Outcome: Within 48 hr of this diagnosis, the patient collaborates with caregivers in planning realistic goals for independence and participates in self-care.

ASSESSMENT/INTERVENTIONS	RATIONALES
Assess the patient's response to the plan of care for recovery, which includes appropriate participation in self-care.	It is important to keep the patient gradually increasing activity and becoming more involved in self-care activities. Excessive activity may lead to fatigue and setbacks in recovery.
Encourage the patient to be as independent as possible within limitations of endurance, therapy, and pain.	Optimally, such encouragement will facilitate independence as much as feasible. Allow for temporary periods of dependence because they enable the individual to restore energy reserves needed for recovery.
Ensure that all health care providers are consistent in conveying expectations of eventual independence.	Consistency facilitates trusting relationships.
Alert the patient to areas of excessive dependence, and involve him or her in collaborative goal setting.	It is healthy to begin to foster a degree of independence as recovery progresses.
Do not minimize the patient's expressed feelings of depression. Allow expressions of emotions, but provide support, understanding, and realistic hope for a positive role change.	Minimizing a patient's expressed feelings of depression can add to anger and depression. Offering realistic goals and encouragement can provide needed emotional support in movement toward independence.
If indicated, provide self-help devices.	These devices, such as long-handled reachers or grabbers, canes, wheelchairs, and walkers, can increase the patient's independence with self-care.
Provide positive reinforcement when the patient meets or advances toward goals.	Positive reinforcement builds on the patient's strengths and promotes self-efficacy.

Nursing Diagnosis:

Deficient Diversional Activity

related to prolonged illness and hospitalization

Desired Outcome: Within 24 hr of intervention, the patient engages in diversional activities and relates absence of boredom.

ASSESSMENT/INTERVENTIONS	RATIONALES
Assess for evidence of the patient desiring something to read or do, daytime napping, and expressed inability to perform usual hobbies because of hospitalization.	These are indicators of boredom.
Assess the patient's activity tolerance as described on p. 61.	Activity tolerance will determine the amount of activity patients can engage in within limits of their diagnoses.
Collect a database by assessing the patient's normal support systems and relationship patterns with significant others. Question the patient and significant other about the patient's interests.	This enables the nurse to explore diversional activities that may be suitable for the health care setting and the patient's level of activity tolerance.
Personalize the patient's environment with favorite objects and photographs of significant others.	This intervention provides visual stimulation.
Provide low-level activities to the patient's tolerance.	These activities promote mental stimulation and reduce boredom. Examples include access to WiFi, laptop computers, Kindles, iPads, iPhones, iPods and Get Well Network. Providing books or magazines pertaining to the patient's recreational or other interests, computer games, television, and supplying writing implements for short intervals of activity are other possible actions.
Initiate activities that require little concentration, and proceed to more complicated tasks as the patient's condition allows (e.g., if reading requires more energy or concentration than the patient is capable of, suggest that the significant other read to patient or bring audiotapes of books).	Initially the patient may find difficult tasks frustrating. Physiologic problems such as anemia and pain may make concentration difficult.
Encourage discussion of past activities or reminiscence.	This could serve as a substitute for performing favorite activities during convalescence.
As the patient's endurance improves, obtain appropriate diversional activities such as puzzles, model kits, handicrafts, and computerized games and activities; encourage the patient to use them. Suggest that the patient's significant other bring hand-held devices, iPods, computers, DVD players, Kindles, phones, TV/tapes, computer, games, crafts, and grooming and beauty products from home.	Watching television, using the computer, listening to the radio or books on tape, and playing cards or board games often are good diversions.
Encourage significant others to visit within limits of the patient's endurance and to involve the patient in activities that are of interest to him or her.	Visiting and partaking in activities with loved ones likely reduce boredom.
As the patient's condition improves, assist him or her with sitting in a chair near a window so that outside activities can be viewed. When the patient is able, provide opportunities to sit in a solarium so that he or she can visit with other patients. If physical condition and weather permit, take the patient outside for brief periods.	New scenery, whether within the same room, such as looking out the window or into another area, can reduce boredom, as can meeting and speaking with other people. Being outdoors when it is possible changes the environment and optimally combats boredom.
Request consultation from OT, social services, pastoral services, and psychiatric nurse.	Such referrals may yield other diversional activities/interventions.
Increase the patient's involvement in self-care to provide a sense of purpose, accomplishment, and control.	Performing in-bed exercises (e.g., deep breathing, ankle circling, calf pumping), keeping track of I&O, and similar activities can and should be accomplished routinely by patients to provide a sense of purpose, accomplishment, and control, which likely will diminish boredom.

Nursing Diagnosis:

Ineffective Sexuality Patterns

related to actual or perceived physiologic limitations on sexual performance occurring with disease, therapy, or prolonged hospitalization

Desired Outcome: Within 72 hr of this diagnosis, the patient relates satisfaction with sexuality and/or understanding of the ability to resume sexual activity.

ASSESSMENT/INTERVENTIONS	RATIONALES
Assess the patient's normal sexual function, including importance placed on sex in the relationship, frequency of interaction, normal positions used, and the couple's ability to adapt or change to meet requirements of the patient's limitations.	This assessment helps determine the patient's normal sexual function and adaptations that will be necessary under current conditions.
Identify the patient's problem diplomatically, and clarify it with the patient.	This assessment helps determine if the patient suffers from sexual dysfunction resulting from lack of privacy, current illness, or perceived limitations. Indicators of sexual dysfunction can include regression, acting-out with inappropriate behavior such as grabbing or pinching, sexual overtures toward staff members, self-enforced isolation, and similar behaviors.
Encourage the patient and significant other to verbalize feelings and anxieties about sexual abstinence, having sexual relations in the hospital, hurting the patient, or having to use new or alternative methods for sexual gratification.	Open communication is the foundation for maintaining a strong intimate relationship.
Develop strategies in collaboration with the patient and significant other.	This information will promote understanding of ways to achieve sexual satisfaction.
Encourage acceptable expressions of sexuality by the patient.	Examples of positive and acceptable behaviors may eliminate inappropriate behaviors. Examples for a woman could include wearing makeup and jewelry and for a man, shaving and wearing his own shirts and shorts.
Inform the patient and significant other that it is possible to have time alone together for intimacy. Provide that time accordingly by putting a *Do not disturb* sign on the door, enforcing privacy by restricting staff and visitors to the room, or arranging for temporary private quarters.	These actions facilitate intimacy by ensuring privacy.
Encourage the patient and significant other to seek alternative methods of sexual expression when necessary.	Accustomed methods of sexual expression may not work under current circumstances. Alternative methods may include mutual masturbation, altered positions, vibrators, and identification of other erotic areas for each partner.
Refer the patient and significant other to professional sexual counseling as necessary.	Counseling may improve communication and acceptance of alternative therapies.

ADDITIONAL NURSING DIAGNOSES/PROBLEMS

General Care Plans

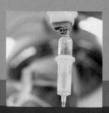

Psychosocial Support 5

Nursing Diagnosis:

Fatigue

related to disease process, treatment, medications, depression, or stress

Desired Outcome: Before hospital discharge, the patient and caregivers describe interventions that conserve energy resources.

ASSESSMENT/INTERVENTIONS	RATIONALES
Assess the patient's patterns of fatigue and times of maximum energy. (Use of a visual analog scale may be helpful in monitoring the fatigue level.)	This information helps identify areas for teaching energy conservation, relaxation, and diversional activities to reduce fatigue.
Assess how fatigue affects the patient's emotional status and ability to perform activities of daily living (ADLs). Suggest activity schedules to maximize energy expenditures (e.g., "After you eat lunch, take a 15-minute rest before you go to x-ray").	Developing an activity plan (e.g., rescheduling activities, allowing rest periods, asking for assistance, exercise) will help conserve energy, reduce fatigue, and maintain ADLs.
Assess for signs and symptoms of anemia.	Anemia can result from cancer or its treatments. Fatigue can occur because of decreased oxygen-carrying capacity of blood. Pharmacologic agents or transfusions may be needed to increase red blood cells.
Assess patterns of sleep.	Disturbance in sleep pattern may influence level of fatigue.
Help the patient maintain a regular sleep pattern by allowing for uninterrupted periods of sleep. Encourage rest when fatigued rather than attempting to continue activity. Encourage naps during the day.	Lack of effective sleep can lead to psychosocial distress (e.g., inability to concentrate, anxiety, uncertainty, and depression).
Reduce environmental stimulation overload (e.g., noise level, visitors for long periods of time, lack of personal quiet time).	This action helps promote uninterrupted sleep patterns.
Discuss how to delegate chores to family and friends who are offering to assist.	This action helps conserve energy and enables family and friends to feel a part of patient's care.
Encourage the patient to maintain a regular schedule once discharged, recognizing that attempting to continue previous activity levels may not be realistic.	This information helps patients engage in a realistic activity schedule to minimize fatigue and avoid frustration if physical functioning does not return to baseline levels.
Encourage mild exercise such as short walks and stretching, which may begin in the hospital if not contraindicated.	Such exercise will promote flexibility, muscle strength, and cardiac output and reduce stress.
⚠ Avoid exercise or use caution in patients with certain disease states.	Exercise should be used with caution and may be contraindicated in cases of - Bone metastases - Immunosuppression or neutropenia - Thrombocytopenia - Anemia - Fever or active infection - Limitations due to other illnesses (Oncology Nursing Society, 2011b)

Nursing Diagnosis:

Disturbed Sleep Pattern

related to environmental changes, illness, therapeutic regimen, pain, immobility, psychologic stress, altered mental status, or hypoxia

Desired Outcomes: After discussion, the patient identifies factors that promote sleep. Within 8 hr of intervention, the patient attains 90-min periods of uninterrupted sleep and verbalizes satisfaction with the ability to rest.

ASSESSMENT/INTERVENTIONS	RATIONALES
Assess the patient's usual (before and after diagnosis) sleeping patterns (e.g., bedtime routine, hours of sleep per night, sleeping position, use of pillows and blankets, napping during the day, nocturia).	Some or all of the patient's usual sleep pattern may be incorporated into the plan of care. A routine as similar to the patient's normal routine as possible will help promote sleep.
Assess causative factors and activities that contribute to the patient's insomnia, awaken the patient, or adversely affect sleep patterns.	Factors such as pain, anxiety, hypoxia, therapies, depression, hallucinations, medications, underlying illness, sleep apnea, respiratory disorder, caffeine, and fear may contribute to sleep pattern disturbance. Some may be ameliorated, and others may be modified.
Explore relaxation techniques that promote patient's rest/sleep.	Imagining relaxing scenes, listening to soothing music or taped stories, and using muscle relaxation exercises are relaxation techniques that are known to promote rest/sleep.
Administer sleep medicines at a time appropriate to induce sleep, taking into consideration time to onset and half-life.	Simulating the usual sleep/wake pattern aids in uninterrupted sleep.
As indicated, administer pain medications before sleep.	This intervention decreases the likelihood that pain will interfere with sleep.
Promote physical comfort via such measures as massage, back rubs, bathing, and fresh linens before sleep.	These measures may help relieve stress and promote relaxation. More research is needed to establish their effectiveness (Margaretta, 2006; Oncology Nursing Society, 2011c).
Organize procedures and activities to allow for 90-min periods of uninterrupted rest/sleep. Limit visiting during these periods.	Ninety minutes of sleep enables complete progression through the normal phases of sleep.
Whenever possible, maintain a quiet environment.	Excessive noise and light can cause sleep deprivation. Providing earplugs, reducing alarm volume, and using white noise (i.e., low-pitched, monotonous sounds: electric fan, soft music) may facilitate sleep. Dimming the lights for a period of time, drawing the drapes, and providing blindfolds are other ways of promoting sleep.
If appropriate, limit the patient's daytime sleeping. Attempt to establish regularly scheduled daytime activity (e.g., ambulation, sitting in chair, active range of motion), which may promote nighttime sleep.	Napping less during the day will promote a more normal nighttime pattern. Physical activity causes fatigue and may facilitate nighttime sleeping.
Promote nonpharmacologic comfort measures that are known to promote the patient's sleep.	Nonpharmacologic comfort measures such as earplugs, anxiety reduction, and use of the patient's own bed clothing and pillows may promote sleep.

Nursing Diagnosis:

Anxiety

related to actual or perceived threat of death, change in health status, threat to self-concept or role, unfamiliar people and environment, medications, preexisting anxiety disorder, the unknown, or uncertainty

Desired Outcome: Within 1-2 hr of intervention, the patient's anxiety has resolved or decreased as evidenced by the patient's verbalization of same, stabilization of vital signs (VS) if they were elevated due to anxiety (compared with the patient's normal levels), and absence of or decrease in irritability and restlessness.

ASSESSMENT/INTERVENTIONS	RATIONALES
Assess the patient's level of anxiety. Be alert to verbal and nonverbal cues. Assess for the following criteria that can contribute to anxiety: general medical condition, withdrawal from alcohol or narcotics, pain, generalized anxiety disorder, panic disorder, post-traumatic stress disorder, phobic disorder, or obsessive-compulsive disorder (Oncology Nursing Society, 2011a).	Being cognizant of a patient's level of anxiety enables the nurse to provide appropriate interventions, as well as modify the plan of care accordingly. Levels of anxiety include: - *Mild:* Restlessness, irritability, increased questions, focusing on the environment. - *Moderate:* Inattentiveness, expressions of concern, narrowed perceptions, insomnia, increased heart rate (HR). - *Severe:* Expressions of feelings of doom, rapid speech, tremors, poor eye contact. Patient may be preoccupied with the past; may be unable to understand the present; and may have tachycardia, nausea, and hyperventilation. - *Panic:* Inability to concentrate or communicate, distortion of reality, increased motor activity, vomiting, tachypnea.
Validate assessment of the anxiety with the patient.	Validating a patient's anxiety level provides confirmation of nursing assessment, as well as openly acknowledges their emotional state. In so doing, patients are given permission to share feelings. For example, "You seem distressed. Are you feeling uncomfortable now?"
Introduce self and other health care team members; explain each individual's role as it relates to the patient's care.	Familiarity with staff and their individual roles may increase the patient's comfort level and decrease anxiety.
Engage in honest communication with the patient, providing empathetic understanding. Listen closely.	These actions help establish an atmosphere that enables free expression.
For patients with severe anxiety or panic state, refer to psychiatric clinical nurse specialist, case manager, or other health care team members as appropriate.	Patients in severe anxiety or panic state may require more sophisticated interventions or pharmacologic management.
Approach the patient with a calm, reassuring demeanor. Show concern and focused attention while listening to the patient's concerns. Provide a safe environment and stay with the patient during periods of intense anxiety.	These actions reassure patients that you are concerned and will assist in meeting their needs.
Restrict the patient's intake of caffeine, nicotine, and alcohol.	Caffeine is a stimulant that may increase anxiety in persons who are sensitive to it. Cessation of caffeine, nicotine, and alcohol can lead to physiologic withdrawal symptoms including anxiety.
Avoid abrupt discontinuation of anxiolytics.	Abrupt withdrawal can cause headaches, tiredness, and irritability.
If the patient is hyperventilating, have him or her concentrate on a focal point and mimic your deliberately slow and deep-breathing pattern.	Modeling provides patients with a focal point for learning effective breathing technique.
After an episode of anxiety, review and discuss the thoughts and feelings that led to the episode.	This action validates the cause of the anxiety and explores interventions that may avert another episode.
Identify the patient's current coping behaviors. Review coping behaviors the patient has used in the past. Assist with using adaptive coping to manage anxiety.	Identifying maladaptive coping behaviors (e.g., denial, anger, repression, withdrawal, daydreaming, or dependence on narcotics, sedatives, or tranquilizers) helps establish a proactive plan of care to promote healthy coping skills. For example, "I understand that your wife reads to you to help you relax. Would you like to spend a part of each day alone with her?"
Encourage the patient to express fears, concerns, and questions.	Encouraging questions gives patients an avenue in which to share concerns. For example, "I know this room looks like a maze of wires and tubes; please let me know when you have any questions."
Provide an organized, quiet environment.	Such an environment reduces sensory overload that may contribute to anxiety.
Encourage social support network to be in attendance whenever possible.	Many people benefit from support of others and find that it reduces their stress level.
Teach relaxation and imagery techniques.	Relaxation and imagery skills empower individuals to manage anxiety-provoking episodes more skillfully and foster a sense of control.

Nursing Diagnosis:

Fear

related to recurrence of the disease, uncertainty, separation from support systems, unfamiliarity with environment or therapeutic regimen, or loss of sense of control

Desired Outcome: Following intervention, the patient expresses fears and concerns and reports feeling greater psychologic and physical comfort.

ASSESSMENT/INTERVENTIONS	RATIONALES
Assess the patient's fears and concerns and provide opportunities to express them. Also explore fear of recurrence of cancer or other complications.	These actions help determine factors contributing to feelings of fear. For example, "You seem very concerned about receiving more blood today."
Listen closely to the patient.	Reactions such as anger, denial, occasional withdrawal, and demanding behaviors may be coping responses.
Encourage the patient to ask questions and gather information about the unknown. Provide information about equipment, therapies, and routines according to the patient's ability to understand.	Increasing knowledge level about therapies and procedures reduces/eliminates fear of the unknown and affords a sense of control.
Acknowledge fears in an empathetic manner.	Acknowledging feelings encourages communication and hence reduces fear. For example, "I understand this equipment frightens you, but it is necessary to help you breathe." An empathic response promotes expression of fears and provides reassurance that concerns are acknowledged.
Encourage the patient to participate in and plan care whenever possible.	Participation promotes an increased sense of control, which helps decrease fears.
Provide continuity of care by establishing a routine and arranging for consistent caregivers whenever possible. Appoint a case manager or primary nurse.	Consistency in care providers promotes familiarity and trust.
Discuss with health care team members the appropriateness of medication therapy for patients with disabling fear or anxiety.	Pharmacologic interventions are sometimes necessary in assisting patients to cope with fears/anxieties about treatment, diagnosis, and prognosis.
Explore the patient's desire for spiritual or psychologic counseling.	Exploring spiritual/psychologic dimension of the current experience may assist patients to cope with fear and stress.
Explore the patient's desire to participate in support groups or meet with others with similar diagnoses.	Many people benefit from outside sources of support in decreasing fears. Interaction with another person who has had a similar experience provides hope and encouragement.

Nursing Diagnosis:

Ineffective Coping

related to the patient's health crisis, sense of vulnerability, or inadequate support systems

Desired Outcome: Before hospital discharge, the patient verbalizes feelings, identifies strengths and coping behaviors, and does not demonstrate ineffective coping behaviors.

ASSESSMENT/INTERVENTIONS	RATIONALES
Assess the patient's perceptions and ability to understand current health status. Discuss meaning of disease and current treatment with the patient, actively listening with a nonjudgmental attitude.	Evaluation of the patient's comprehension enables development of an individualized care plan.
Establish honest, empathetic communication with the patient.	This promotes effective therapeutic communication. For example, "Please tell me what I can do to help you."

continued

ASSESSMENT/INTERVENTIONS	RATIONALES
Support positive coping behaviors and explore effective coping behaviors used in the past.	These actions identify, reinforce, and facilitate positive coping behaviors, for example, "I see that reading that book seems to help you relax."
Identify factors that inhibit the patient's ability to cope.	This enables patients to identify areas such as unsatisfactory support system, deficient knowledge, grief, and fear that may contribute to anxiety and ineffective coping and to consider modification of these factors.
Help the patient identify previous methods of coping with life problems.	How individuals have handled problems in the past may be a reliable predictor of how they will cope with current problems.
Recognize maladaptive coping behaviors. If appropriate, discuss these behaviors with the patient.	Examples of maladaptive behaviors include severe depression; dependence on narcotics, sedatives, or tranquilizers; hostility; violence; and suicidal ideation. Patients may have used substances and other maladaptive behaviors in controlling anxiety. This pattern can interfere with the ability to cope with the current situation. If appropriate, nurses should discuss these behaviors with patients. For example, "You seem to be requiring more pain medication. Are you having more physical pain, or does it help you cope with your situation?"
Refer the patient to psychiatric liaison, clinical nurse specialist, case manager, or clergy, or recommend support groups or other programs as appropriate.	Professional intervention may assist with altering maladaptive behaviors.
Help the patient identify or develop a support system.	Many people benefit from outside support systems in helping them cope.
As the patient's condition allows, assist with reducing anxiety. See **Anxiety,** p. 73.	Anxiety makes effective coping more difficult to achieve.
Maintain an organized, quiet environment.	Such an environment helps reduce patient's sensory overload to aid with coping.
Encourage frequent visits by family and caregiver if visits appear to be supportive to patient. Encourage use of technology such as social media to stay in touch with family and friends.	Visitors and social media may help minimize a patient's emotional and social isolation, thereby promoting coping behaviors.
As appropriate, explain to the caregiver that increased dependency, anger, and denial may be adaptive coping behaviors used by the patient in early stages of crisis until effective coping behaviors are learned.	Lack of understanding about the patient's maladaptive coping can lead to unhealthy interaction patterns and contribute to anxiety within the family.
Arrange community referrals for discharge planning, as appropriate.	Support in the home environment promotes healthier adaptations and may avert crises.

Nursing Diagnosis:

Powerlessness

related to the absence of a sense of control over illness-related regimen and health care environment

Desired Outcome: Before hospital discharge, the patient begins to make decisions about care and therapies and reports onset of an attitude of realistic expectations and sense of self-control.

ASSESSMENT/INTERVENTIONS	RATIONALES
Assess the patient's personal preferences, needs, values, and attitudes. Before providing information, assess the patient's knowledge and understanding of condition and care.	This assessment helps develop a care plan individualized for the patient's needs, which optimally will decrease sense of powerlessness.
Assess for expressions of fear, lack of response to events, lack of interest in information, and lack of interest or participation in care.	These are signals of feelings of powerlessness.

ASSESSMENT/INTERVENTIONS	RATIONALES
Assess support systems; involve the significant other in patient care whenever possible. Refer to clergy and other support persons or systems as appropriate.	Many people feel empowered by outside support systems. Promoting family involvement reduces their feelings of powerlessness as well.
Evaluate caregiver practices, and adjust them to support the patient's sense of control.	For example, if a patient always bathes in the evening to promote relaxation before bedtime, modify the care plan to include an evening bath rather than follow the hospital routine of giving a morning bath.
Ask the patient to identify activities that may be performed independently.	Self-care activities likely will promote a sense of control.
Whenever possible, offer alternatives related to routine hygiene, diet, diversional activities, visiting hours, and treatment times.	Offering alternatives promotes a sense of control and power over daily routine.
When distant relatives and casual acquaintances request information about the patient's status, check with the patient for consent before sharing information.	This action ensures privacy and preserves the patient's territorial rights whenever possible.
Avoid overprotection and parenting behaviors toward the patient. Instead, act as an advocate for the patient and significant other.	Discouraging dependency on the staff will help promote independent behaviors.
Offer realistic hope for the future, realizing that within any situation there is always a reason to be hopeful, even if it is a "good" or peaceful death.	This likely will increase sense of control and power and promote hopefulness.
Determine the patient's wishes about end-of-life decisions, and document advance directives as appropriate. See Chapter 8, "Palliative and End-of-Life Care," for in-depth discussion.	These actions help promote a sense of control and power over these decisions.

Nursing Diagnosis:

Spiritual Distress

related to chronic illness, life change, or disturbances in belief and value systems that give meaning and a sense of hope

Desired Outcome: Before hospital discharge, the patient begins to verbalize religious or spiritual beliefs, continues previous practices, and expresses less distress and feelings of anxiety and fear.

ASSESSMENT/INTERVENTIONS	RATIONALES
Assess the patient's spiritual or religious beliefs, values, and practices.	This assessment will assist in development of an individualized care plan. For example, "Do you have a religious preference?" "How important is it to you?" "Are there any religious or spiritual practices in which you wish to participate while in the hospital?"
Inform the patient of availability of spiritual resources, such as a chapel or chaplain.	This information increases awareness of available spiritual resources and promotes a sense of acceptance of the patient's spirituality.
Display a nonjudgmental attitude toward the patient's religious or spiritual beliefs and values.	This action creates an environment that is conducive to free expression.
Identify available support persons or systems that may assist in meeting the patient's religious or spiritual needs (e.g., clergy, fellow church members, support groups).	Many people derive an increased sense of hope from religious and spiritual counselors.
Be alert to comments related to spiritual concerns or conflicts.	Comments such as "I don't know why God is doing this to me" and "I'm being punished for my sins" suggest that the patient is feeling some degree of spiritual distress.
Listen closely and ask questions.	These actions help the patient resolve conflicts related to spiritual issues and help the nurse plan how best to assist the patient. For example, "I understand that you want to be baptized. We can arrange to do that here."

continued

ASSESSMENT/INTERVENTIONS | RATIONALES

ASSESSMENT/INTERVENTIONS	RATIONALES
Provide privacy and opportunities for spiritual practices such as prayer and meditation.	Many people find prayer and meditation difficult in a nonprivate setting.
If spiritual beliefs and therapeutic regimens are in conflict, provide honest, substantiated information.	Such information promotes informed decision making. For example, "I understand your religion discourages receiving blood transfusions. We respect your position; however, it does not allow us to give you the best care possible."
Refer the patient for help with decision making if he or she is struggling with treatment-related decisions.	Such help assists in resolving care dilemmas, if appropriate. Many hospitals provide assistance in the form of educational materials and counseling in order to help resolve such dilemmas.

Nursing Diagnoses:

Grieving
Risk for Complicated Grieving

related to actual or anticipated loss of physiologic well-being (e.g., expected loss of body function or body part, changes in self-concept or body image, illness, death)

Desired Outcome: Following intervention, the patient expresses grief, participates in decisions about the future, and discusses concerns with health care team members.

ASSESSMENT/INTERVENTIONS | RATIONALES

ASSESSMENT/INTERVENTIONS	RATIONALES
Assess and accept the patient's behavioral response.	Reactions such as disbelief, denial, guilt, anger, and depression are normal reactions to grief.
Determine the patient's stage of grieving.	Comprehension of the stage of grief enables more effective therapeutic interventions. It is normal for a person to move from one stage to another and then revert to a previous stage. The time required to do so varies from individual to individual. If a patient is unable to move into the next stage, referral for professional intervention may be indicated. - *Protest stage:* denial, disbelief, anger, hostility, resentment, bargaining to postpone loss, appeal for help to recover loss, loud complaints, altered sleep and appetite. - *Disorganization stage:* depression, withdrawal, social isolation, psychomotor retardation, silence. - *Reorganization stage:* acceptance of loss, development of new interests and attachments, restructuring of lifestyle, return to preloss level of functioning.
Assess spiritual, religious, and sociocultural expectations related to loss.	Helping individuals find meaning in their experience may facilitate the grieving process. For example, "Is religion an important part of your life?" "How do you and your family deal with serious health problems?"
Assess the patient's grief reactions, and identify the potential for dysfunctional grieving reactions (e.g., absence of emotion, hostility, avoidance).	This assessment helps identify and reduce dysfunctional grieving, if present.
If dysfunctional grieving is present, refer the patient to a psychiatric clinical nurse specialist, case manager, clergy, or other source of counseling as appropriate.	Promoting normal progression through the grieving stages may allay unnecessary emotional suffering.
Refer to clergy or community support groups as appropriate.	Such a referral reinforces that there are support systems and resources to help work through grief.
Demonstrate empathy.	Empathetic communication (including respecting the desire not to communicate) promotes a trusting relationship and open dialogue. For example, "This must be a very difficult time for you and your family" or "Is there anything you'd like to talk about today?"

PART I: Medical-Surgical Nursing

ASSESSMENT/INTERVENTIONS   RATIONALES

ASSESSMENT/INTERVENTIONS	RATIONALES
In selected circumstances, explain the grieving process.	This approach may help the patient and family better understand and acknowledge their feelings and help family members better understand behaviors and verbalizations expressed by the patient.
When appropriate, provide referral for bereavement care.	Such a referral helps the patient and family grieve their loss.

Nursing Diagnosis:

Disturbed Body Image

related to physical trauma or loss or change in body parts or function

Desired Outcomes: Within the 24-hr period before hospital discharge, the patient begins to acknowledge bodily changes and demonstrates movement toward incorporating changes into self-concept. The patient does not demonstrate maladaptive response, such as severe depression.

ASSESSMENT/INTERVENTIONS   RATIONALES

ASSESSMENT/INTERVENTIONS	RATIONALES
Establish open, honest communication with the patient. Give the patient permission to grieve loss.	These actions promote an environment conducive to free expression in which the patient is comfortable talking about body image concerns. For example, "Please feel free to talk to me whenever you have any questions."
Assess for indicators of body image disturbance.	Patients may exhibit nonverbal indicators (avoidance of looking at or touching body part, hiding or exposing body part) or verbal indicators (expression of negative feeling about body, expression of feelings of helplessness, personalization or depersonalization of missing or mutilated part, or refusal to acknowledge change in structure or function of the body part).
Assess the patient's knowledge of the present health status and the pathophysiologic process that has occurred.	This assessment promotes understanding of health status and clarifies misconceptions that may be contributing to disturbed body image.
When planning the patient's care, be aware of therapies that may influence body image, and educate the patient accordingly before they are implemented.	Various drugs and surgical procedures can cause body changes. Monitoring equipment and invasive procedures can cause a diminished image of self and feelings of helplessness.
Discuss the loss or change with the patient. Practice nonjudgmental acceptance of the patient's reality.	Loss of any type has meaning of differing magnitudes for each individual. Talking about these issues may be a first step in accepting changes. What may seem to be a small change may be of great significance to the patient (e.g., arm immobilizer, catheter, hair loss, ecchymoses, facial abrasions).
Explore concerns, fears, and feelings of guilt.	Some body changes may reverse with time, and this information may lessen stress and concern. Assessing emotional reactions to the loss may help the nurse provide therapeutic support. For example, "I understand you are frightened. Your face looks different now, but you will see changes and it will improve. Gradually you will begin to look more like yourself."
Encourage the patient and family members to interact with one another. Help the family avoid reinforcement of their loved one's unhappiness over a changed body part or function.	Support and encouragement from loved ones help many people cope better with body changes. Guiding family members appropriately in their dealings with patients promotes healthy interactions that foster well-being. For example, "I know your son looks very different to you now, but it would help if you speak to him and touch him as you would normally."
Encourage the patient to participate gradually in self-care activities as he or she becomes physically and emotionally able.	Self-care activities and a sense of getting back to normal can contribute to a sense of wholeness and control. Assisting the patient with resuming a sense of normalcy promotes progression through the stages of grief.

continued

General Care Plans

ASSESSMENT/INTERVENTIONS	RATIONALES
Allow for some initial withdrawal and denial behaviors.	This is normal. For example, when changing dressings over a traumatized part, explain what you are doing but do not expect the patient to watch or participate initially.
Discuss opportunities for reconstruction or rehabilitation of the loss or change. Offer realistic hope for the future.	These actions promote a realistic sense of hope and help patients plan for the future. Examples include surgery, prosthesis, grafting, physical therapy, cosmetic therapies, modified clothing, and organ transplant.
Recognize manifestations of severe depression (e.g., sleep disturbances, change in affect, and change in communication pattern). As appropriate, refer to psychiatric clinical nurse specialist, case manager, clergy, or support group.	This knowledge enables referral of a patient who is at risk for self-harm, including suicide. See Chapter 98, "Major Depression," **Risk for Suicide,** p. 727.
Offer choices and alternatives whenever possible. Emphasize the patient's strengths, and encourage activities that interest the patient.	These actions help patients attain a sense of autonomy and control.
If possible, refer the patient to a support group, another patient who has had a similar experience, or on-line support resources.	Many people benefit from outside support systems and sharing experiences with another person who has had a similar experience.
Be aware that touch may enhance a patient's self-concept and reduce his or her sense of isolation.	Touch may mitigate a sense that patient is hideous or unattractive because of the body change.
See also: Chapter 56, "Fecal Diversions: Colostomy, Ileostomy, and Ileal Pouch Anal Anastomoses," **Disturbed Body Image,** p. 434.	

Nursing Diagnosis:

Impaired Verbal Communication

related to neurologic or anatomic deficit, psychologic or physical barriers (e.g., tracheostomy, intubation), or cultural or developmental differences

Desired Outcome: At the time of intervention, the patient communicates needs and feelings and reports decreased or absent feelings of frustration over communication barriers.

ASSESSMENT/INTERVENTIONS	RATIONALES
Assess the patient's health literacy level. Make sure materials are at an appropriate literacy level. Also assess digital literacy (ability to navigate websites or other technology) if they are used to provide information.	Although individuals may be able to read, their understanding of health-related materials may be low or they may have limited proficiency with computers.
Assess the cause of impaired communication (e.g., tracheostomy, stroke, cerebral tumor, Guillain-Barré syndrome).	Determining the cause of communication impairment will enable the nurse to develop a customized plan of care that incorporates communication skills patients can use, given their disability.
Involve the patient and/or caregiver in assessing the patient's ability to read, write, and understand English. If the patient speaks a language other than English, collaborate with an English-speaking family member or an interpreter to establish effective communication.	This assessment helps establish effective communication and ensure teaching materials provided are at a level appropriate for the patient.
When communicating, face the patient; make direct eye contact; and speak in a clear, normal tone of voice.	A visual or hearing-impaired person often develops compensatory methods—for example, lip reading for a person who is hearing-impaired.
When communicating with a deaf person about the treatment plan, arrange to have an interpreter present if possible.	An interpreter facilitates effective communication, promotes informed consent, and enables the patient to ask questions.
If the patient cannot speak because of a physical barrier (e.g., tracheostomy, wired mandibles), provide reassurance and acknowledge his or her frustration.	These actions will help decrease frustration caused by inability to communicate verbally. For example, "I know this is frustrating for you, but please do not give up. I want to understand you."

ASSESSMENT/INTERVENTIONS	RATIONALES
Provide slate, word cards, pencil and paper, alphabet board, pictures, computers, or other technology to assist with communication. Adapt call system to meet the patient's needs. Document meaning of signals used by the patient to communicate.	These actions will enable effective communication, promote continuity of care, and lessen the patient's anxiety.
Explain the source of the patient's communication impairment to the caregiver; teach the caregiver effective communication alternatives (see previous list).	Inability to communicate with ease may cause feelings of isolation that can be intensified if patients have difficulty communicating with caregivers.
Be alert to nonverbal messages. Validate their meaning with the patient.	Nonverbal response, such as facial expressions, hand movements, and nodding of the head, is a valid means of communication, and its meaning must be validated to facilitate understanding.
Encourage the patient to communicate needs; reinforce independent behaviors.	Inability to speak may foster maladaptive behaviors, and this reinforces the need for patients to be understood.
Be honest with the patient; do not pretend to understand if you are unable to interpret the patient's communication.	Pretending to understand patients will only add to their frustration and diminish trust.
If surgery is expected to create a physical condition that will interfere with communication, begin teaching preoperatively. Facilitate postoperative referrals for speech and swallowing.	These actions will help ensure that an effective method of communication will be in place postoperatively so that the patient's needs will be met.

Nursing Diagnosis:

Social Isolation

related to altered health status, inability to engage in satisfying personal relationships, altered mental status, body image change, or altered physical appearance

Desired Outcome: Before hospital discharge, the patient demonstrates movement toward interaction and communication with others.

ASSESSMENT/INTERVENTIONS	RATIONALES
Assess factors contributing to the patient's social isolation.	This assessment will help determine causes of social isolation and modify those factors. These may include: - Restricted visiting hours - Inability to access social media or use other technology - Absence of or inadequate support system - Inability to communicate (e.g., presence of intubation/ tracheostomy) - Physical changes that affect self-concept - Denial or withdrawal - Hospital environment
Identify patients at risk for social isolation.	Individuals most at risk for social isolation include older adults and disabled, chronically ill, and economically disadvantaged persons.
Help the patient identify feelings associated with loneliness and isolation.	This information facilitates interventions based on individual need. For example, "You seem very sad when your family leaves the room. Can you tell me more about your feelings?"
Determine the patient's need for socialization, and identify available and potential support person or systems. Explore methods for increasing social contact.	Assessing need for interaction and developing a care plan accordingly will reduce the sense of isolation surrounding the illness. Methods for increasing social contact include TV, radio, videos, use of computers and the Internet, social media, more frequent visitations, and scheduled interaction with nurse or support staff.

continued

ASSESSMENT/INTERVENTIONS	RATIONALES
Provide positive reinforcement for socialization that lessens the patient's feelings of isolation and loneliness.	Encouraging interaction gives patients permission to ask for social interaction from the nurse while decreasing sense of isolation. For example, "Please continue to call me when you need to talk to someone. Talking will help both of us better understand your feelings."
Facilitate patient's ability to communicate with others (see **Impaired Verbal Communication,** p. 80).	Impaired communication may be the cause of social isolation.

Nursing Diagnosis:

Deficient Knowledge

related to unfamiliarity with current health status and prescribed therapies

Desired Outcome: Before procedures or hospital discharge (as appropriate), the patient verbalizes understanding regarding current health status and therapies.

ASSESSMENT/INTERVENTIONS	RATIONALES
Assess the patient's health care literacy (language, reading, comprehension). Assess culture and culturally specific information needs as well as cognitive and emotional readiness to learn.	This assessment helps ensure that information is selected and presented in a manner that is culturally and educationally appropriate.
Assess other barriers to learning.	Barriers to learning include ineffective communication, educational deficit, neurologic deficit, sensory alterations, fear, anxiety, and lack of motivation.
Assess the patient's current level of knowledge regarding health status.	This assessment enables development of an individualized teaching plan, as well as correction of misperceptions and misinformation.
Assess learning needs and establish short-term and long-term goals. As appropriate, assess understanding of informed consent.	Well-planned goals provide markers for assessing effectiveness of the teaching plan and progress made. Patients will use information received to make informed decisions regarding care.
Use individualized verbal or written information to promote learning and enhance understanding. Give simple, direct instructions. As indicated, use audiovisual tools or technology assisted devices.	Because individuals learn differently, using more than one teaching modality will provide more opportunities to assimilate information.
Include the caregiver in all patient teaching, and encourage reinforcement of correct information regarding diagnosis and treatments.	Anxiety often filters the information given. Involving a spouse or other family member provides teaching reinforcement.
Encourage the patient's involvement in care information by planning care collaboratively. Explain rationale for care and therapies.	Involving patients in their own care planning promotes adherence to the treatment plan and engenders a sense of control and ownership.
Communicate often with the patient. Request feedback regarding what has been taught.	Anxiety may interfere with reception, comprehension, and retention. Individuals in crisis often need repeated explanations before information can be understood. Creating an environment of permission in which patients feel comfortable asking questions and revealing knowledge deficits facilitates learning.
Provide written information appropriate to the patient's comprehension and literacy levels. Also consider social media or other computer-assisted devices to provide verbal/visual information that can be replayed as needed.	Written and recorded material reinforces teaching and enables review at a later time.

ADDITIONAL NURSING DIAGNOSES/PROBLEMS:

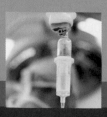

Psychosocial Support for the Patient's Family and Significant Others 6

Note: *The Health Insurance Portability and Accountability Act of 1996 (HIPAA) restricts who may request and receive health care–related information about a patient in order to protect confidentiality. Health care providers must be sensitive to and aware of expressed patient preferences before discussing the patient with others, including family. This includes divulging information regarding a patient's presence in the hospital.*

Nursing Diagnosis:

Fear

related to the patient's life-threatening condition and knowledge deficit

Desired Outcome: Following intervention, significant others/family members report that fear has lessened.

ASSESSMENT/INTERVENTIONS	RATIONALES
Assess the family's fears and their understanding of the patient's clinical situation.	Some fears may be realistic; others may not be and need clarification.
Evaluate verbal and nonverbal responses.	Some family members may not readily verbalize their fears but may give nonverbal cues such as withdrawing emotionally (evidenced by body position, facial expression, attitude of disinterest), refusing to be present during discussion, or disrupting discussion.
Acknowledge the family's fear.	Simple acknowledgment and giving more information can go a long way toward decreasing fear. For example, "I understand these tubes must frighten you, but they are necessary to help nourish your son."
Assess the family's history of coping behavior.	How a family has coped with fear in the past often is a reliable predictor of how they will cope in the current situation. For example, "How does your family react to difficult situations?" Awareness of maladaptive responses may assist the nurse in fostering more productive methods of coping.
Provide opportunities for family members to express fears and concerns.	Verbalizing feelings in a nonthreatening environment can help them deal with unresolved/unrecognized issues that may be contributing to the current stressor. Anger, denial, withdrawal, and demanding behavior may be adaptive coping responses during the initial period of crisis. Identifying fears also enables the nurse to dispel inaccuracies, which will help the family cope with the situation as it exists.

ASSESSMENT/INTERVENTIONS	RATIONALES
Provide information at frequent intervals about the patient's status, treatments, and equipment used.	This information increases the family's knowledge of the patient's health status, helping alleviate fear of the unknown.
Explain implications of HIPAA to the family and how this affects the type of information that can be given and how it can be given (e.g., no specific information can be given by phone or email).	Protection of patient privacy is critical. Helping families to understand what information can be provided and why will help alleviate anxiety.
Encourage the family to use positive coping behaviors by identifying fears, developing goals, identifying supportive resources, facilitating realistic perceptions, and promoting problem solving.	When under stress, the family may not recall sources of support without being reminded. For example, "Who usually helps your family during stressful times?"
Recognize anxiety, and encourage family members to describe their feelings.	Before family members can learn coping strategies, they must first clarify their feelings. For example, "You seem very uncomfortable tonight. Can you describe your feelings?"
Be alert to maladaptive responses to fear. Provide referrals to a psychiatric clinical nurse specialist or other staff member as appropriate.	Violence, withdrawal, severe depression, hostility, and unrealistic expectations for the staff or of the patient's recovery are maladaptive responses to fear, and they require expert guidance.
Offer *realistic* hope, even if it is hope for the patient's peaceful death.	Even though family members may have feelings of hopelessness, it sometimes helps to hear realistic expressions of hope.
Explore the family's desire for spiritual or other counseling.	People often derive hope and experience a decrease in fear and dread from spiritual counseling.
Assess your own feelings about the patient's life-threatening illness.	Without personal awareness of one's beliefs, a health care provider's attitude and fears may be reflected inadvertently to the family.
For other interventions, see **Interrupted Family Processes** and **Disabled Family Coping** listed later in this care plan.	

Nursing Diagnosis:

Interrupted Family Processes

related to the situational crisis (the patient's illness)

Desired Outcome: Following intervention, family members demonstrate effective adaptation to change/traumatic situation as evidenced by seeking external support when necessary and sharing concerns within the family unit.

ASSESSMENT/INTERVENTIONS	RATIONALES
Assess the family's character: social, environmental, ethnic, and cultural factors; relationships; and role patterns.	Having this detailed information will help the nurse develop an individualized care plan.
Identify the family's developmental stage.	The family may be dealing with other situational or maturational crises, such as managing an elderly parent or a teenager with a learning disability.
Assess previous adaptive behaviors.	How the family has dealt with problems in the past may be a reliable predictor of how they will adapt to current issues. For example, "How does your family react in stressful situations?"
Discuss observed conflicts and communications.	Awareness of this information will assist with development of an individualized plan of care, including referral for specialized care if appropriate. For example, "I noticed that your brother would not visit your mother today. Has there been a problem we should be aware of? Knowing about it may help us better care for your mother."
Acknowledge the family's involvement in patient care and promote strengths. Encourage the family to participate in patient care conferences. Promote frequent, regular patient visits by family members.	This reinforces positive ways of dealing with the crisis and promotes a sense of involvement and control for the family. For example, "You were able to encourage your wife to turn and cough. That is very important to her recovery."

continued

ASSESSMENT/INTERVENTIONS	RATIONALES
Provide the family with information and guidance related to the patient. Discuss the stresses of hospitalization, and encourage the family to discuss feelings of anger, guilt, hostility, depression, fear, or sorrow. Refer to clergy, clinical nurse specialist, or social services as appropriate.	Encouraging expressions of emotion helps family members begin the process of grieving. For example, "You seem to be upset since being told that your husband is not leaving the hospital today." Acknowledging their feelings promotes acceptance and facilitates therapeutic communication.
Evaluate patient and family responses to one another. Encourage the family to reorganize roles and establish priorities as appropriate.	These actions will help facilitate the family's adaptation to the situation regarding the patient and prevent unnecessary conflict. Helping family members redefine their roles may reduce confusion and provide direction. For example, "I know your husband is concerned about his insurance policy and seems to expect you to investigate it. I'll ask the financial counselor to talk with you."
Encourage the family to schedule periods of rest and activity outside the hospital and to seek support when necessary.	Persons undergoing stress sometimes require guidance of others to promote their own self-care. For example, "Your neighbor volunteered to stay in the waiting room this afternoon. Would you like to rest at home? I'll call you if anything changes."

Nursing Diagnoses:

Compromised Family Coping
Caregiver Role Strain

related to inadequate or incorrect information or misunderstanding, temporary family disorganization and role change, exhausted support persons or systems, unrealistic expectations, fear, anxiety, or financial burden

Desired Outcome: Following intervention, family members begin to verbalize feelings, identify ineffective coping patterns, identify strengths and positive coping behaviors, and seek information and support from the nurse or other support persons or systems outside the family.

ASSESSMENT/INTERVENTIONS	RATIONALES
Establish open, honest communication within the family. Help family members identify strengths, stressors, inappropriate behaviors, and personal needs.	These actions will help promote positive, effective communication among family members while enabling them to examine areas that contribute both to effective and ineffective coping in a nonthreatening environment. For example, "I understand your mother was very ill last year. How did you manage the situation?" "I know your loved one is very ill. How can I help you?"
Assess family members for ineffective coping and identify factors that inhibit effective coping.	Ineffective methods of coping (e.g., depression, chemical dependency, violence, withdrawal) can interfere with ability to deal with the current situation. Awareness of barriers to effective coping (e.g., inadequate support system, grief, fear of disapproval by others, and deficient knowledge) is the first step toward promoting changes and healthy adaptation. For example, "You seem to be unable to talk about your husband's illness. Is there anyone with whom you can talk about it?"
Assess the family's knowledge about the patient's current health status and treatment. Provide information often, and allow sufficient time for questions. Reassess the family's understanding at frequent intervals.	By providing information frequently and answering questions, stress, fear, and anxiety can be attenuated.
Provide opportunities in a private setting for family members to talk and share concerns with nurses. If appropriate, refer the family to a psychiatric clinical nurse specialist for therapy.	The family may need additional assistance in working through their issues.

ASSESSMENT/INTERVENTIONS	RATIONALES
Offer realistic hope. Help the family to develop realistic expectations for the future and to identify support persons or systems that will assist them.	These actions will foster realistic expectations about the patient's future health status and promote adaptation to impending changes.
Help the family to reduce anxiety and caregiver strain by encouraging diversional activities (e.g., time spent outside the hospital) and interaction with support persons or systems outside the family.	Promoting respites enhances coping and helps family members remain focused and supportive of the patient. For example, "I know you want to be near your son, but if you would like to go home to rest, I will call you if any changes occur."
For more information, see Chapter 8, "Palliative and End-of-Life Care," p. 104, for **Caregiver Role Strain.**	

Nursing Diagnosis:

Disabled Family Coping

related to unexpressed feelings, ambivalent family relationships, or disharmonious coping styles among family members

Desired Outcome: Within the 24-hr period before hospital discharge, family members begin to verbalize feelings; identify sources of support, as well as ineffective coping behaviors that create ambivalence and disharmony; and do not demonstrate destructive behaviors.

ASSESSMENT/INTERVENTIONS	RATIONALES
Establish open, honest communication and rapport with family members.	An atmosphere in which the family can express honest feelings and needs will help move them toward healthy coping and adaptation. For example, "I am here to care for your mother and to help your family as well."
Identify ineffective coping behaviors. Refer to a psychiatric clinical nurse specialist, case manager, clergy, or support group as appropriate.	Ineffective coping behaviors (e.g., violence, depression, substance misuse, withdrawal) can interfere with learning effective strategies. Awareness of ineffective or destructive coping behaviors is the first step toward promoting change. For example, "You seem to be angry. Would you like to talk to me about your feelings?"
Identify perceived or actual conflicts.	This information enables the family to examine areas that require change in a nonthreatening environment and identify potential sources of support. For example, "Are you able to talk freely with your family members?" "Are your brothers and sisters able to help and support you during this time?"
Assist in the quest for healthy functioning and adaptations within the family unit (e.g., facilitate open communication among family members and encourage behaviors that support family cohesiveness).	Facilitating open communication among family members and encouraging behaviors that support family cohesiveness promote skill acquisition in a nonthreatening environment and identify existing coping strengths. For example, "Your mother enjoyed your last visit. Would you like to see her now?"
Help family members develop realistic goals, plans, and actions. Refer them to clergy, psychiatric nurse, social services, financial counseling, and family therapy as appropriate.	These actions help provide direction in making necessary changes and adaptations.
Encourage family members to spend time outside the hospital and to interact with support individuals. Respect their need for occasional withdrawal.	A life out of balance adds to stress and promotes maladaptive coping.
Include family members in the patient's plan of care. Offer them opportunities to become involved in patient care.	Becoming involved in the patient's care (e.g., range-of-motion exercises, patient hygiene, and comfort measures such as back rubs) may decrease feelings of powerlessness, thereby increasing coping ability.

General Care Plans

Nursing Diagnosis:

Readiness for Enhanced Family Coping

related to use of support persons or systems, referrals, and choosing experiences that optimize wellness

Desired Outcomes: Family members express intent to use support persons, systems, and resources, and identify alternative behaviors that promote communication and strengths. Family members express realistic expectations and do not demonstrate ineffective coping behaviors.

ASSESSMENT/INTERVENTIONS	RATIONALES
Assess family relationships, interactions, support persons or systems, and individual coping behaviors.	This assessment facilitates development of an individualized care plan using existing family structure.
Permit movement through stages of adaptation. Encourage further positive coping.	Such an environment allows family members to process events surrounding the patient's illness in a healthy manner.
Acknowledge expressions of hope, plans, and growth among family members.	A sense of hopefulness is essential to process painful events in a healthy manner.
Provide opportunities in a private setting for family interactions, discussions, and questions.	Discussions and sharing of emotions in a nonpublic forum encourages development of open, honest communication within the family. For example, "I know the waiting room is very crowded. Would your family like some private time together?"
Refer the family to community or support groups (e.g., ostomy support group, head injury rehabilitation group).	Many people benefit from support of other people who have had similar experiences in learning new coping strategies.
Encourage the family to explore outlets that foster positive feelings.	Examples of outlets that foster positive feelings and thus promote effective coping include periods of time outside the hospital area, meaningful communication with the patient or support individuals, and relaxing activities such as showering, eating, exercising.

Nursing Diagnosis:

Deficient Knowledge

related to unfamiliarity with the patient's current health status or therapies

Desired Outcome: Following intervention, family members/significant others begin to verbalize knowledge and understanding about the patient's current health status and treatment.

ASSESSMENT/INTERVENTIONS	RATIONALES
Assess the family's health and digital literacy (language, reading, comprehension, ability to navigate and use computers/Internet for information seeking). Assess culture and culturally specific education needs.	This assessment helps ensure that information is selected and presented in a manner that is culturally and educationally appropriate.
At frequent intervals, inform the family about the patient's current health status, therapies, and prognosis. Use individualized verbal, written, and audiovisual strategies to promote their understanding.	Being informed frequently promotes accurate understanding of the patient's health status and allays unnecessary anxiety. In turn, this enables family members to process and plan.
At frequent intervals, evaluate the family's comprehension of information provided. Assess factors for misunderstanding, and adjust teaching as appropriate.	Some individuals in crisis need repeated explanations before comprehension can be ensured. For example, "I have explained many things to you today. Would you mind summarizing what I've told you so that I can be sure you understand your husband's status and what we are doing to care for him?"

ASSESSMENT/INTERVENTIONS	RATIONALES
Encourage the family to relay correct information to the patient.	This will reinforce comprehension for both the family and patient and promote open communication.
Inquire of family members if their information needs are being met.	This action reinforces understanding by family members and assures them that the information/support they desire will be met. For example, "Do you have any questions about the care your mother is receiving or about her condition?"
Help family members use the information they receive to make health care decisions about the patient.	Family members may require assistance in processing information and applying it appropriately (e.g., regarding surgery, resuscitation, organ donation).

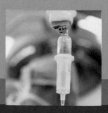

Older Adult Care 7

<u>Nursing Diagnoses:</u>

Acute Confusion
Risk for Injury

related to age-related decreased physiologic reserve, renal function, or cardiac function; altered sensory/perceptual reception occurring with poor vision or hearing; or decreased brain oxygenation occurring with illness state and decreased functional lung tissue

Desired Outcomes: The patient's mental status returns to normal for the patient within 3 days of treatment. The patient sustains no evidence of injury or harm as a result of mental status.

ASSESSMENT/INTERVENTIONS	RATIONALES
Assess the patient's baseline level of consciousness (LOC) and mental status on admission. Obtain preconfusion functional and mental status abilities from significant other or clinical caregiver. Ask the patient to perform a three-step task. For example, "Raise your right hand, place it on your left shoulder, and then place the right hand by your right side."	A component of the Mini-Mental Status Examination, this assessment of a three-step task provides a baseline for subsequent assessments of a patient's confusion. A three-step task is complex and is a gross indicator of brain function. Because it requires attention, it can also test for delirium.
Use the confusion assessment method (CAM) to help identify the presence or absence of confusion/delirium.	Delirium is a serious problem for hospitalized older adults and often goes unrecognized. The CAM tool (Waszynski, 2007) can be administered in a short period of time. CAM is a simple, standardized tool that can be used by bedside clinicians and has been validated in settings from medical-surgical areas to intensive care units. If your agency does not already employ this tool, there are several on-line sources that describe it in detail.
Test short-term memory by showing the patient how to use the call light, having the patient return the demonstration, and then waiting at least 5 min before having the patient demonstrate use of the call light again. Document the patient's actions in behavioral terms. Describe the "confused" behavior.	Inability to remember beyond 5 min indicates poor short-term memory.
Identify the cause of acute confusion.	Acute confusion is caused by physical and psychosocial conditions and not by age alone. For example, oximetry or arterial blood gas (ABG) values may reveal low oxygenation levels, serum glucose or fingerstick glucose may reveal high or low glucose level, and electrolytes and complete blood count (CBC) will ascertain imbalances and/or presence of elevated white blood cell (WBC) count as a determinant of infection. Hydration status may be determined by pinching skin over the sternum or forehead for turgor (tenting occurs with fluid volume deficit) and checking for dry mucous membranes and a furrowed tongue.

ASSESSMENT/INTERVENTIONS

RATIONALES

ASSESSMENT/INTERVENTIONS	RATIONALES
Assess for pain using a rating scale of 0-10. If the patient is unable to use a scale, assess for behavioral cues such as grimacing, clenched fists, frowning, and hitting. Ask the family or significant other to assist in identifying pain behaviors.	Acute confusion can be a sign of pain.
Treat the patient for pain, as indicated, and monitor behaviors.	If pain is the cause of the confusion, the patient's behavior should change accordingly.
Review cardiac status. Assess apical pulse and notify the health care provider of an irregular pulse that is new to the patient. If the patient is on a cardiac monitor or telemetry, watch for dysrhythmias; notify the health care provider accordingly.	Dysrhythmias and other cardiac dysfunctions may result in decreased oxygenation, which can lead to confusion.
Review current medications, including over-the-counter (OTC) drugs, with the pharmacist.	Toxic levels of certain medications, such as digoxin (rarely used), cause acute confusion. Medications that are anticholinergic also can cause confusion, as can drug interactions.
Monitor intake and output (I&O) at least q8h.	Optimally, output should match intake. Dehydration can result in acute confusion.
Review the patient's creatinine clearance test to assess renal function.	Renal function plays an important role in fluid balance and is the main mechanism of drug clearance. Blood urea nitrogen (BUN) and serum creatinine are affected by hydration status and in older patients reveal only part of the picture. Therefore, to fully understand and assess renal function in older patients, creatinine clearance must be tested.
Have the patient wear glasses and hearing aid, or keep them close to the bedside and within easy reach for patient use.	Glasses and hearing aids are likely to help decrease sensory confusion.
Keep the patient's urinal and other routinely used items within easy reach for the patient.	A confused patient may wait until it is too late to seek assistance with toileting.
If the patient has short-term memory problems, toilet or offer the urinal or bedpan q2h while awake and q4h during the night. Establish a toileting schedule and post it on the patient care plan and, inconspicuously, at the bedside.	A patient with a short-term memory problem cannot be expected to use the call light.
Check on the patient at least q30min and every time you pass the room. Place the patient close to the nurses' station if possible. Provide an environment that is nonstimulating and safe.	A confused patient requires extra safety precautions.
Provide music but not TV.	Patients who are confused regarding place and time often think the action on TV is happening in the room.
Attempt to reorient the patient to his or her surroundings as needed. Keep a clock with large numerals and a large print calendar at the bedside; verbally remind the patient of the date and day as needed.	Reorientation may decrease confusion
Tell the patient in simple terms what is occurring. For example, "It's time to eat breakfast," "This medicine is for your heart," "I'm going to help you get out of bed."	Sentences that are more complex may not be understood.
Encourage the patient's significant other to bring items familiar to the patient, including blanket, bedspread, and pictures of family and pets.	Familiar items may promote orientation while also providing comfort.
If the patient becomes belligerent, angry, or argumentative while you are attempting to reorient, *stop this approach.* Do not argue with the patient or the patient's interpretation of the environment. State, "I can understand why you may [hear, think, see] that."	This approach prevents escalation of anger in a confused person.
If the patient displays hostile behavior or misperceives your role (e.g., nurse becomes thief, jailer), leave the room. Return in 15 min. Introduce yourself to the patient as though you had never met. Begin dialogue anew.	Patients who are acutely confused have poor short-term memory and may not remember the previous encounter or that you were involved in that encounter.

continued

ASSESSMENT/INTERVENTIONS	RATIONALES
If the patient attempts to leave the hospital, walk with him or her and attempt distraction. Ask the patient to tell you about the destination. For example, "That sounds like a wonderful place! Tell me about it." Keep your tone pleasant and conversational. Continue walking with the patient away from exits and doors around the unit. After a few minutes, attempt to guide the patient back to the room. Offer refreshments and a rest. For example, "We've been walking for a while and I'm a little tired. Why don't we sit and have some juice while we talk?"	Distraction is an effective means of reversing a behavior in a patient who is confused.
If the patient has a permanent or severe cognitive impairment, check on her or him at least q30min and reorient to baseline mental status as indicated; however, do not argue with the patient about his or her perception of reality.	Arguing can cause a cognitively impaired person to become aggressive and combative. **Note:** Individuals with severe cognitive impairment (e.g., Alzheimer's disease or dementia) also can experience acute confusional states (i.e., delirium) and can be returned to their baseline mental state.
If the patient tries to climb out of bed, offer a urinal or bedpan or assist to the commode.	The patient may need to use the toilet.
Alternatively, if the patient is not on bedrest, place him or her in chair or wheelchair at the nurses' station.	This action provides added supervision to promote a patient's safety while also promoting stimulation and preventing isolation.
Bargain with the patient. Try to establish an agreement to stay for a defined period, such as until the health care provider, meal, or significant other arrives.	This is a delaying strategy to defuse anger. Because of poor memory and attention span, the patient may forget he or she wanted to leave.
Have the patient's significant other talk with the patient by phone or come in and sit with the patient if the patient's behavior requires checking more often than q30min.	These actions by the significant other may help promote the patient's safety.
If the patient is attempting to pull out tubes, hide them (e.g., under blankets). Put a stockinette mesh dressing over intravenous (IV) lines. Tape feeding tubes to the side of the patient's face using paper tape, and drape the tube behind the patient's ear.	Remember: Out of sight, out of mind.
Evaluate the continued need for certain therapies.	Such therapies may become irritating stimuli. For example, if the patient is now drinking, discontinue the IV line; if the patient is eating, discontinue the feeding tube; if the patient has an indwelling urethral catheter, discontinue the catheter and begin a toileting routine.
Use restraints with caution and according to agency policy.	Patients can become more agitated when wrist and arm restraints are used.
Use medications cautiously for controlling behavior.	Follow the maxim "start low and go slow" with medications because older patients can respond to small amounts of drugs. Neuroleptics, such as haloperidol, can be used successfully in calming patients with dementia or psychiatric illness (contraindicated for individuals with parkinsonism). However, if the patient is experiencing acute confusion or delirium, short-acting benzodiazepines (e.g., lorazepam) are more effective in reducing anxiety and fear. Anxiety or fear usually triggers destructive or dangerous behaviors in acutely confused older patients. **Note:** Neuroleptics can cause akathisia, an adverse drug reaction evidenced by increased restlessness.
Also see Chapter 97, "Dementia—Alzheimer's Type," p. 716, as appropriate.	

Nursing Diagnosis:

Impaired Gas Exchange (or risk for same)

related to decreased oxygenation occurring with decreased functional lung tissue

Desired Outcomes: The patient's respiratory pattern and mental status are normal for the patient. The patient's ABG or pulse oximetry values are within the patient's normal limits.

ASSESSMENT/INTERVENTIONS	RATIONALES
Assess and document the following on admission and routinely thereafter: respiratory rate (RR), pattern, and depth; breath sounds; cough; sputum; and sensorium.	This assessment establishes a baseline for subsequent assessments of the patient's respiratory system.
Assess the patient for subtle changes in mentation or behavior such as increased restlessness, anxiety, disorientation, and hostility. If available, monitor oxygenation status via ABG findings (optimally Pao_2 80%-95% or greater) or pulse oximetry (optimally greater than 92%).	Mentation changes such as increased restlessness, anxiety, disorientation, and hostility can signal decreased oxygenation. To adequately evaluate pulse oximetry, the hemoglobin (Hgb) must be known. Patients with low Hgb can have a higher pulse oximeter reading and yet display restlessness or acute confusion. This is due to the lack of Hgb to circulate oxygen.
Assess the lungs for adventitious sounds.	The aging lung has decreased elasticity. The lower part of the lung is no longer adequately aerated. As a result, crackles commonly are heard in individuals 75 years of age and older. This sign alone does not mean that a pathologic condition is present. Crackles (rales) that do not clear with coughing in an individual with no other clinical signs (e.g., fever, increasing anxiety, changes in mental status, increasing respiratory depth) are considered benign.
Encourage the patient to cough and breathe deeply. When appropriate, instruct the patient in use of incentive spirometry.	These actions promote alveolar expansion and clear the secretions from the bronchial tree, thereby helping ensure better gas exchange.
Unless contraindicated by a cardiac or renal condition, encourage fluid intake to greater than 2.5 L/day.	Hydration helps ensure less viscous pulmonary secretions, which are more easily mobilized.
Treat fevers promptly, decrease pain, minimize pacing activity, and lessen anxiety.	These interventions reduce the potential for increased oxygen consumption.
Instruct the patient in use of support equipment such as oxygen masks or cannulas.	Knowledge helps promote adherence to therapy.

Nursing Diagnosis:

Risk for Aspiration

related to depressed cough and gag reflexes or ineffective esophageal sphincter

Desired Outcomes: The patient swallows independently without choking. The patient's airway is patent and lungs are clear to auscultation both before and after meals.

ASSESSMENT/INTERVENTIONS	RATIONALES
Perform a baseline assessment of the patient's ability to swallow by asking if he or she has any difficulty swallowing or if any foods or fluids are difficult to swallow or cause gagging. If the patient is unable to answer, consult the patient's caregiver or significant other. Document findings.	This assessment helps determine a patient's ability to swallow without choking and should be compared with subsequent assessments to document improvements or deficits.

continued

ASSESSMENT/INTERVENTIONS	RATIONALES
Assess the patient's ability to swallow by placing your thumb and index finger on both sides of the laryngeal prominence and asking the patient to swallow. Check for the gag reflex by gently touching one side and then the other of the posterior pharyngeal wall using a tongue blade. Document both findings.	Ability to swallow and an intact gag reflex are necessary to prevent aspiration and choking before the patient takes foods or fluids orally.
Place the patient in an upright position with the chin tilting down slightly while eating or drinking, and support the upright position with pillows on the patient's sides.	This position minimizes risk of choking and aspirating by closing off the airway and facilitating gravitational flow of foods and fluids into the stomach and through the pylorus.
Monitor the patient when he or she is swallowing.	This assessment will help determine the patient's ability to swallow without choking. Deficits may necessitate aspiration precautions.
Watch for drooling of saliva or food or inability to close the lips around a straw.	These are signs of limited lip, tongue, or jaw movement.
Check for retention of food in sides of the mouth.	This is an indication of poor tongue movement.
Monitor intake of food. Document consistencies and amounts of food the patient eats, where the patient places food in the mouth, how the patient manipulates or chews before swallowing, and the length of time before the patient swallows the food bolus.	Other caregivers will find this information useful during subsequent feedings.
Monitor the patient for coughing or choking before, during, or after swallowing.	Coughing or choking may occur up to several minutes following placement of food or fluid in the mouth and signals aspiration of material into the airway.
Monitor the patient for changes in lung auscultation (e.g., crackles [rales], wheezes, rhonchi), shortness of breath, dyspnea, decreasing LOC, increasing temperature, and cyanosis.	These are signs of silent aspiration. For example, some older patients, especially those in declining health, have increased risk for silent aspiration when the esophageal sphincter fails to close completely between swallows.
Monitor the patient for a wet or gurgling sound when talking after a swallow.	This sound indicates aspiration into the airway and signals delayed or absent swallow and gag reflexes.
For a patient with poor swallowing reflex, tilt the head forward 45 degrees during swallowing. **Note:** For patients with hemiplegia, tilt the head toward the unaffected side.	This head position will help prevent inadvertent aspiration by closing off the airway.
As indicated, request evaluation by a speech therapist.	This evaluation will enable specialized assessment of gag and swallow reflexes.
Anticipate swallowing video fluoroscopy in evaluation of the patient's gag and swallow reflexes.	This procedure is used to determine whether patients are aspirating, consistency of materials most likely to be aspirated, and aspiration cause. Using four consistencies of barium, the radiologist and speech therapist watch for the presence of reduced or ineffective tongue function, reduced peristalsis in the pharynx, delayed or absent swallow reflex, and poor or limited ability to close the epiglottis that protects the airway.
Based on results of the swallowing video, fluoroscopy, thickened fluids may be prescribed.	Agents are added to the fluid to make it more viscous and easier for patients to swallow. Similarly, mechanical soft, pureed, or liquid diets may be prescribed to enable patients to ingest food with less potential for aspiration.
Provide adequate rest periods before meals.	Fatigue increases risk for aspiration.
Remind patients with dementia to chew and swallow with each bite. Check for retained food in sides of the mouth.	Patients with dementia might forget to chew and swallow.
Ensure that the patient has dentures in place, if appropriate, and that they fit correctly.	Chewing well minimizes risk of choking.
Ensure that someone stays with the patient during meals or fluid intake.	This ensures added safety in the event of choking or aspiration.
Provide adequate time for the patient to eat and drink.	Generally, patients with swallowing deficits require twice as much time for eating and drinking as those whose swallowing is adequate.

ASSESSMENT/INTERVENTIONS	RATIONALES
! Be aware of the location of suction equipment to be used in the event of aspiration.	If the patient is at increased risk for aspiration, suction equipment should be available at the bedside.
! If the patient aspirates, implement the following:	
- Follow American Heart Association (AHA) standards if the patient displays characteristics of complete airway obstruction (i.e., choking).	This is an emergency situation.
- For partial airway obstruction, encourage the patient to cough as needed.	This action will clear the airway.
- For partial airway obstruction in an unconscious or nonresponsive individual who is not coughing, suction the airway with a large-bore catheter such as Yankauer or tonsil suction tip.	Suctioning clears the airway.
- For either a complete or partial aspiration, inform the health care provider and obtain a prescription for chest x-ray examination.	X-ray will determine if food/fluid remains in the airway.
- Implement nothing by mouth (NPO) status until a diagnosis is confirmed.	NPO prevents further risk to patient.
- Monitor breathing pattern and RR q1-2h after a suspected aspiration for alterations (i.e., increased RR).	This assessment helps determine that a change in the patient's condition has occurred.
- Anticipate use of antibiotics.	There is risk for infection/pneumonia after aspiration.
Encourage the patient to cough and deep breathe q2h while awake and q4h during the night.	These measures promote expansion of available lung tissue and help prevent infection.

Nursing Diagnosis:

Risk for Deficient Fluid Volume

related to inability to obtain fluids because of illness or placement of fluids or *related to* use of osmotic agents during radiologic tests

Desired Outcomes: The patient's mental status; vital signs (VS); and urine specific gravity, color, consistency, and concentration remain within normal limits for the patient. The patient's mucous membranes remain moist, and there is no "tenting" of skin. The patient's intake equals output.

ASSESSMENT/INTERVENTIONS	RATIONALES
Assess fluid intake. In nonrestricted individuals, encourage fluid intake of 2-3 L/day. Specify intake goals for day, evening, and night shifts.	These actions help ensure that the patient's hydration status is adequate. Restrictions may apply to patients with cardiopulmonary and renal disorders.
Assess and document skin turgor. Check hydration status by pinching skin over the sternum or forehead.	Skin that remains in the lifted position (tenting) and returns slowly to its original position indicates dehydration. A furrowed tongue signals severe dehydration.
Assess and document color, amount, and frequency of any fluid output, including emesis, urine, diarrhea, or other drainage.	This assessment enables comparison of intake to output amounts. Urine that is dark in color signals concentration and thus dehydration.
Monitor the patient's orientation, ability to follow commands, and behavior.	Loss of the ability to follow commands, decrease in orientation, and confused behavior can signal a dehydrated state.
Weigh the patient daily at the same time of day (preferably before breakfast) using the same scale and bed clothing.	Using comparable measurements ensures more accurate comparisons. Wide variations in weight (e.g., 2.5 kg [5 lb] or greater) can signal increased or decreased hydration status.
In patients who are dehydrated, anticipate elevations in serum Na^+, BUN, and serum creatinine levels.	These elevations often occur with dehydration.

continued

ASSESSMENT/INTERVENTIONS	RATIONALES
If the patient is receiving IV therapy, assess cardiac and respiratory systems for signs of overload. Assess the apical pulse and listen to lung fields during every VS assessment.	Overload could precipitate heart failure or pulmonary edema. Rising heart rate (HR), crackles, and bronchial wheezes can be signals of heart failure or pulmonary edema.
Carefully monitor I&O when the patient is receiving tube feedings or dyes for contrast. Watch for evidence of third spacing of fluids, including increasing peripheral edema, especially sacral; output significantly less than intake (1:2); and urine output less than 30 mL/hr.	These agents act osmotically to pull fluid into the interstitial tissue.
Whenever in the room, offer the patient fluids. Offer a variety of drinks the patient likes, but limit caffeine because it acts as a diuretic.	Older persons have a decreased sense of thirst and need encouragement to drink.
Assess the patient's ability to obtain and drink fluids by himself or herself. Place fluids within easy reach. Use cups with tops to minimize concern over spilling.	These actions remove barriers to adequate fluid intake.
Ensure access to the toilet, urinal, commode, or bedpan at least q2h when the patient is awake and q4h at night. Answer the call light quickly.	The time between recognition of the need to void and urination decreases with age.

Nursing Diagnosis:

Risk for Infection

related to age-related changes in immune and integumentary systems and/or suppressed inflammatory response occurring with long-term medication use (e.g., antiinflammatory agents, steroids, analgesics), slowed ciliary response, or poor nutrition

Desired Outcome: The patient remains free of infection as evidenced by orientation to person, place, and time and behavior within the patient's normal limits; RR and pattern within the patient's normal limits; urine that is straw colored, clear, and of characteristic odor; core temperature and HR within the patient's normal limits; sputum that is clear to whitish in color; and skin that is intact and of normal color and temperature for the patient.

ASSESSMENT/INTERVENTIONS	RATIONALES
Assess baseline VS, including LOC and orientation. Also be alert to HR greater than 100 bpm and RR greater than 24 breaths/min. Auscultate lung fields for adventitious sounds. Be aware, however, that crackles (rales) may be a normal finding when heard in the lung bases.	A change in mentation is a leading sign of infection in older patients. Other signs of infection include tachycardia and tachypnea. Adventitious breath sounds may or may not be seen until late in the course of illness.
Assess the patient's temperature, using a low-range thermometer if possible.	Older adults may run lower temperatures because of decreasing metabolism in individuals who are inactive and sedentary. They also tend to lose heat readily to the environment and may not be kept at the right temperature. A temperature of 35.5° C (96° F) may be normal, whereas a temperature of 36.67°-37.22° C (98°-99° F) may be considered febrile.
Obtain temperature readings rectally if the oral reading does not match the clinical picture (i.e., skin is very warm, the patient is restless, mentation is depressed) or if the temperature reads 36.11° C (97° F) or higher.	If the oral reading seems unreliable, rectal readings may help ensure the patient's core temperature is accurately determined.
If possible, avoid use of a tympanic thermometer.	Reliability of the electronic tympanic thermometer may be inconsistent because of improper use.

ASSESSMENT/INTERVENTIONS	RATIONALES
Assess the patient's skin for tears, breaks, redness, or ulcers. Document condition of the patient's skin on admission and as an ongoing assessment (refer to **Risk for Impaired Skin Integrity**).	Skin that is not intact is susceptible to infection.
Assess quality and color of the patient's urine. Document changes when noted, and report findings to the health care provider. Also be alert to urinary incontinence, which can signal urinary tract infection (UTI).	UTI, as manifested by cloudy, foul-smelling urine without painful urination and urinary incontinence, is the most common infection in older adults.
Avoid insertion of urinary catheters when possible.	Urinary catheter use increases risk of infection.
Obtain drug history in reference to use of antiinflammatory or immunosuppressive drugs or long-term use of analgesics or steroids.	These drugs mask fever, a sign of infection.
If infection is suspected, anticipate initiation of IV fluid therapy.	Fluid therapy will help maintain optimal hydration as well as replace losses caused by fever and thin the secretions for easier expectoration.
Anticipate blood cultures, urinalysis, and urine culture.	Cultures will isolate the bacteria type.
Anticipate WBC count.	WBC count 11,000/mm^3 or higher can be a late sign of infection in older patients because the immune system is slow to respond to insult.
Expect a chest x-ray examination if the patient's chest sounds are not clear.	This will be performed to rule out pneumonia.
If infection is present, prepare for initiation of broad-spectrum antibiotic therapy, oxygen therapy, and use of an antipyretic.	These interventions will eliminate infection, promote oxygenation to the brain, and decrease fever. Fever increases cardiac workload (i.e., HR rises) as the body responds to infection. Because of decreased physiologic reserve, older patients may have increased risk of heart failure or pulmonary edema from prolonged tachycardia.

Nursing Diagnosis:

Hypothermia

related to age-related changes in thermoregulation and/or environmental exposure

Desired Outcome: The patient's temperature and mental status remain within the patient's normal limits, or they return to the patient's normal limits at a rate of 1° F/hr, after interventions.

ASSESSMENT/INTERVENTIONS	RATIONALES
Assess the patient's temperature, using a low-range thermometer if possible.	This assessment will determine if the patient has hypothermia. Older adults can have a normal temperature of 35.5° C (96° F).
Assess the temperature orally by placing a thermometer far back in the patient's mouth.	This method provides the most accurate assessment of a patient's core temperature.
Note: Do not take axillary temperature in the older adult. If unable to measure the temperature orally, measure tympanic or temporal temperature but note that reliability of these thermometers may be inconsistent because of improper use.	Older persons have decreased peripheral circulation and loss of subcutaneous fat in the axillary area, resulting in formation of a pocket of air that may make readings inaccurate.
Assess and document the patient's mental status.	Increasing disorientation, mental status changes, or atypical behavior can signal hypothermia.
Be alert to use of sedatives, hypnotics (including anesthetics), and muscle relaxants.	These medications decrease shivering and therefore place patients at risk for environmental hypothermia. In addition, all older adults are at risk for environmental hypothermia at ambient temperatures of 22.22°-23.89° C (72°-75° F).

continued

PART I: Medical-Surgical Nursing

ASSESSMENT/INTERVENTIONS	RATIONALES
Ensure that patients going for testing or x-ray examination are sent with enough blankets to keep warm.	This intervention will help prevent hypothermia.
If the patient is mildly hypothermic, initiate slow rewarming.	To reverse mild hypothermia, one method of slow rewarming is raising the room temperature to at least 23.89° C (75° F). Other methods of external warming include use of warm blankets, head covers, and warm circulating air blankets.
If the patient's temperature falls below 35° C (95° F), warm the patient internally by administering warm oral or IV fluids.	To reverse moderate to severe hypothermia, patients are warmed internally by administering warm oral or IV fluids. Warmed saline gastric or rectal irrigations or introduction of warmed humidified air into the airway are other methods of internal warming.
Be alert to signs of too rapid rewarming.	Signs of too rapid rewarming include irregular HR, dysrhythmias, and very warm extremities caused by vasodilation in the periphery, which causes heat loss from the core.
If the patient's temperature fails to rise 1° F/hr using these techniques, anticipate laboratory tests, including WBC count for possible sepsis, thyroid test for hypothyroidism, and glucose level for hypoglycemia.	Causes other than environmental ones may be responsible for the hypothermia.
As prescribed, administer antibiotics for sepsis, thyroid therapy, or glucose for hypoglycemia.	The patient's temperature will not return to normal unless the underlying condition has been treated.

Nursing Diagnosis:

Risk for Impaired Skin Integrity

related to decreased subcutaneous fat and decreased peripheral capillary networks in the integumentary system

Desired Outcome: The patient's skin remains nonerythremic and intact.

ASSESSMENT/INTERVENTIONS	RATIONALES
Assess the patient's skin on admission and routinely thereafter.	This assessment provides a baseline for subsequent assessments of skin integrity.
Note any areas of redness or any breaks in the skin surface.	Redness or breaks in skin integrity necessitate aggressive skin care interventions to prevent further breakdown and infection.
Ensure that the patient turns frequently (at least q2h).	Turning alternates sites of pressure and pressure relief.
Lift or roll the patient across sheets when repositioning.	Pulling, dragging, or sliding across sheets can lead to shear (cutaneous or subcutaneous tissue) injury.
Monitor skin over bony prominences for erythema.	Skin that lies over the sacrum, scapulae, heels, spine, hips, pelvis, greater trochanter, knees, ankles, costal margins, occiput, and ischial tuberosities is at increased risk for breakdown because of excessive external pressure.
Use pillows or pads around bony prominences, even when the patient is up in a wheelchair or sits for long periods.	This intervention maintains alternative positions and pads the bony prominences, thereby protecting overlying skin. The ischial tuberosities are susceptible to breakdown when a patient is in the seated position. Gel pads for the chair or wheelchair seats aid in distributing pressure.
Use lotions liberally on dry skin.	Lotions promote moisture and suppleness. Lanolin-containing lotions are especially useful.
Use alternating-pressure mattress, air-fluidized mattress, waterbed, air bed, or other pressure-sensitive mattress for older patients who are on bedrest or unable to get out of bed.	These mattresses protect skin from injury caused by prolonged pressure.

ASSESSMENT/INTERVENTIONS	RATIONALES
Avoid placing tubes under the patient's limbs or head. Place a pillow or pad between the patient and tube for cushioning.	Excess pressure from tubes can create a pressure ulcer.
Get the patient out of bed as often as possible. Liberally use mechanical lifting devices to aid in safe patient transfers. If the patient is unable to get out of bed, assist with position changes q2h.	These actions promote blood flow, which helps prevent skin breakdown.
Establish and post a turning schedule on the patient care plan and at the bedside.	Schedules increase awareness of the staff and patient/family of turning schedule.
Ensure that the patient's face, axillae, and genital areas are cleansed daily.	Complete baths dry out older adults' skin and should be given every other day instead.
Use tepid water (32.2°-40.5° C [90°-105° F]) and super-fatted, nonperfumed soaps.	Hot water can burn older adults, who have decreased pain sensitivity and decreased sensation to temperature. Super-fatted soaps help decrease dryness of skin.
Minimize use of plastic protective pads under the patient. When used, place at least one layer of cloth (drawsheet) between the patient and the plastic pad to absorb moisture. For incontinent patients, check the pad at least q2h. Discourage use of adult diapers unless the patient is ambulatory, going for tests, or is up in a chair.	Pads and diapers trap moisture and heat and can lead to skin breakdown (macerated associated skin damage).
Document the percentage of food intake with meals. Encourage the significant other to provide the patient's favorite foods. Suggest nutritious snacks if the patient's diet is not restricted. Obtain nutritional consultation with a dietitian as needed.	Food/snacks high in protein and vitamin C help prevent skin breakdown.
For more information, see Chapter 73, "Wound Care," Pressure Ulcers," p. 536, and Chapter 74, "Providing Nutritional Support," p. 539.	

Nursing Diagnosis:

Disturbed Sleep Pattern

related to unfamiliar surroundings and hospital routines/interruptions

Desired Outcomes: Within 24 hr of interventions, the patient reports attainment of adequate rest. Mental status remains normal for the patient.

ASSESSMENT/INTERVENTIONS	RATIONALES
Assess and document the patient's sleeping pattern, obtaining information from the patient, the patient's caregiver, or significant others.	Older adults typically sleep less than they did when they were younger and often awaken more frequently during the night.
Ask questions about naps and activity levels.	Individuals who take naps and have a low level of activity frequently sleep only 4-5 hr/night.
Determine the patient's usual nighttime routine and attempt to emulate it.	Following the usual nighttime rituals may facilitate sleep.
Attempt to group together activities such as medications, VS, and toileting.	This reduces the number of interruptions and facilitates rest and sleep.
Provide pain medications, back rub, and pleasant conversation at sleep time.	These comfort measures may facilitate sleep.
Monitor the patient's activity level.	If the patient complains of being tired after activities or displays behaviors such as irritability, yelling, or shouting, encourage napping after lunch or early in the afternoon. Otherwise, discourage daytime napping, especially in the late afternoon, because it can interfere with nighttime sleep.

continued

ASSESSMENT/INTERVENTIONS	RATIONALES
Discourage caffeinated coffee, cola, and tea after 6 PM.	Stimulants can make it difficult to fall asleep and stay asleep as well as increase nighttime awakenings to urinate.
Provide a quiet environment and minimize interruptions during sleep hours.	Excessive noises, bright overhead lights, noisy roommates, and loud talking can cause sleep deprivation. Use of sound generators (e.g., of ocean waves) or white noise (e.g., fan) may promote sleep.

Nursing Diagnosis:

Constipation

related to changes in diet, decreased activity, and psychosocial factors

Desired Outcomes: The patient states that his or her bowel habit has returned to normal within 3-4 days of this diagnosis. Stool appears soft, and the patient does not strain in passing stools.

ASSESSMENT/INTERVENTIONS	RATIONALES
On admission, assess and document the patient's normal bowel elimination pattern. Include frequency, time of day, associated habits, and successful methods used to correct constipation in the past. Consult the patient's caregiver or significant other if the patient is unable to provide this information.	This assessment establishes a baseline and determines a patient's normal bowel elimination pattern.
Inform the patient that changes occurring with hospitalization may increase the potential for constipation. Urge the patient to institute successful nonpharmacologic methods used at home as soon as this problem is noticed or prophylactically as needed.	Constipation is easier to treat preventively than it is when present and/or prolonged.
Teach the relationship between fluid intake and constipation. Unless otherwise contraindicated, encourage fluid intake that exceeds 2500 mL/day. Monitor and record bowel movements (date, time, consistency, amount).	A high fluid intake promotes soft stool and decreases risk/degree of constipation. A high fluid volume may be contraindicated in patients with renal, cardiac, or hepatic disorders who may have fluid restrictions.
Encourage the patient to include roughage (e.g., raw fruits and vegetables, whole grains, nuts, fruits with skins) as a part of each meal when possible. For patients unable to tolerate raw foods, encourage intake of bran via cereals, muffins, and breads.	Eating roughage reduces the potential for constipation by promoting bulk in the stool.
Titrate the amount of roughage to the degree of constipation.	Too much roughage taken too quickly can cause diarrhea, gas, and distention.
Teach the patient the relationship between constipation and activity level. Encourage optimal activity for all patients. Establish and post an activity program to enhance participation; include devices necessary to enable independence.	Exercise can prevent or decrease constipation by promoting peristalsis.
If the patient's usual bowel movement occurs in the early morning, use the patient's gastrocolic or duodenocolic reflex to promote colonic emptying. If the patient's bowel movement occurs in the evening, ambulate the patient just before the appropriate time.	Scheduling interventions that coincide with a patient's bowel habit are more likely to promote bowel movements. Drinking hot liquids in the morning, for example, also promotes peristalsis. Digital stimulation of the inner anal sphincter may facilitate a bowel movement.
Attempt to use methods the patient has used successfully in the past. Follow the maxim "go low, go slow" (i.e., use the lowest level of nonnatural intervention and advance to more powerful interventions slowly).	Aggressive interventions may result in rebound constipation and interfere with subsequent bowel movements.
When requesting a pharmacologic intervention, use the more benign, oral methods first.	Older persons tend to focus on the loss of habit as an indicator of constipation rather than on the number of stools. Do not intervene pharmacologically until the older adult has not had a stool for 3 days.

ASSESSMENT/INTERVENTIONS

RATIONALES

	The following hierarchy is suggested: - Bulk-building additives such as psyllium or bran. - Mild laxatives (apple or prune juice, Milk of Magnesia). - Stool softeners (docusate sodium, docusate calcium). - Potent laxatives or cathartics (bisacodyl, cascara sagrada). - Medicated suppositories (glycerin, bisacodyl). - Enema (tap water, saline, sodium biphosphate/phosphate).
After diagnostic imaging of the gastrointestinal tract with barium, ensure that the patient receives a postexamination laxative.	The laxative facilitates removal of the barium. After any procedure involving a bowel clean-out, there may be rebound constipation from the severe disruption of bowel habit.
Monitor hydration status for signs of dehydration. Emphasize diet, fluid, activity, and resumption of routines. If no bowel movement occurs in 3 days, begin with mild laxatives to try to regain the normal pattern.	Dehydration can occur as a result of the osmotic agents used. Deficient fluid volume can result in hard stools, which are more difficult to evacuate.

See also: Chapter 4, "Prolonged Bedrest," **Constipation,** p. 68.

Nursing Diagnosis:

Adult Failure to Thrive

related to loss of independence, loss of functional ability, malnutrition, depression, cognitive impairment, impaired immune function, and the impact of chronic disease

Desired Outcome: The patient exhibits or verbalizes improvement in at least one of the following: weight gain, increased appetite, increased functional ability, sense of hopefulness, peaceful death.

ASSESSMENT/INTERVENTIONS

RATIONALE

Perform a thorough physical assessment. Assess status of a chronic disease.	A complete system assessment provides a baseline for subsequent comparison.
Review laboratory and other studies such as CBC with differential, basic metabolic panel, thyroid-stimulating hormone (TSH), albumin, and pre-albumin levels.	A review of laboratory information identifies issues in nutrients and electrolytes essential for basic body function, status of protein and thyroid function, and presence/absence of infection.
Perform a thorough patient history; engage caretakers as needed. Analyze critical factors such as the death of a spouse or family member.	A thorough history focusing on timing of the change in behaviors and appetite, medications, and decline in activities of daily living (ADLs) and instrumental activities of daily living (IADLs) will help identify contributing factors to the decline in function. Examples of contributing factors include hypothyroidism, dementia, decreased sense of taste or smell, and depression.
Encourage the patient to verbalize feelings of despair, frustration, fear, anger, and concerns about hospitalization and health.	Verbalization of feelings and the knowledge that they are normal often help minimize feelings of despair.
Discuss normal age changes with the patient and family.	As people age, their physiologic reserve decreases and affects multiple systems. Failure to thrive can occur from interaction of three components: physical frailty, disability or decline in functional ability, and impaired neuropsychiatric function. Frailty is defined by decreased physiologic reserve affecting many systems. Disability is defined as difficulty or decline in completing ADLs. Neuropsychiatric impairment is a complex phenomenon that can occur from life circumstances leading to depression, physiologic disruption leading to delirium, or neurologic changes resulting in cognitive impairment.

continued

ASSESSMENT/INTERVENTIONS

As indicated, consult with other health care professionals.

RATIONALE

A multidisciplinary approach is necessary for this complex condition. Speech therapists and dietitians can help assess unexplained decline in eating. Physical and occupational therapists can help analyze physical limitations/strengths and the potential for improvement with a program or assistive device. Social Services can help assess support networks and readiness for end-of-life possibility.

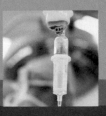

Palliative and End-of-Life Care 8

OVERVIEW

The concept of palliative care is undergoing significant change in the United States in the face of an increasingly aging society. The 80 million baby boomers who began to turn 65 in 2010 and entered into the Medicare system have prompted significant changes in approaches to health care delivery. Currently 70% of the U.S. population is diagnosed with a chronic disease and four out of six patients live with more than one chronic symptomatic condition—or multiple chronic conditions (MCCs) (Institutes of Medicine [IOM], 2012). To address these issues the Affordable Care Act (ACA) has provided extensive funding to almost every agency under the U.S. Department of Health and Human Services to focus on initiatives that address symptomatic MCCs in order to provide better care, improve health, and reduce the cost of care to support the needs of this fastest growing patient population.

The premise of palliative care is to provide optimal symptom management. The symptom burden that accompanies MCCs and malignancies requires the skilled use of palliative interventions. Optimally managing symptoms reduces disease exacerbations, promotes physical activity, reduces hospital use, and improves patients' quality of life.

As the trajectory of the disease progresses toward the end of life, palliative interventions increase in use, complexity, and intensity. At the end of life, patients become more symptomatic, require full assistance with activities of daily living, and are profoundly weaker and often bedbound. Physical, emotional, and spiritual symptoms may become more pronounced during this time and will require skilled and knowledgeable interventions by an interdisciplinary team of professionals (e.g., medicine, nursing, social work, clergy, ancillary support). The use of a team-based approach is essential to address and meet the multiple needs of the patient and family.

HEALTH CARE SETTING

Primary care, outpatient clinic, rehabilitation center, surgical center, acute care, home care, long-term care, skilled hospital, and hospice

Nursing Diagnosis:

Decisional Conflict

related to uncertainly about the course of action as the patient moves from an acute curative medical model into a palliative care/symptom management plan of care

Desired Outcome: The patient and family will effectively transition from the acute medical management of advanced disease into palliative care with minimal conflict and confusion.

ASSESSMENT/INTERVENTION	RATIONALE
Assess understanding of the underlying disease pathophysiology and concomitant symptoms that interfere with the patient's perceived quality of life.	Individuals who gain an understanding of the disease that is nonresponsive to acute medical interventions will be better prepared to understand the transition from acute medical management to palliative care.

continued

ASSESSMENT/INTERVENTION	RATIONALE
Assess the preparation and previous discussions on advance care planning. If the patient has a Durable Power of Attorney (DPA), document this information in the patient's health record.	Discussing the patient's advance care planning helps to avoid a crisis-like approach to advanced disease management. These discussions promote a realistic approach to disease and disability. The DPA identifies the person who will serve as an advocate for the patient. The DPA and the patient's health care wishes are documented in the event that patients are unable to speak for themselves. Refer the patient and family to credible resources and interdisciplinary support if the patient needs to complete his or her advance directive. Examples of advance directives can be found from: Caring Connections, which provides free advance directives and instructions for state-specific advance directives: http://www.caringinfo.org/i4a/pages/index.cfm?pageid=3289 Aging with Dignity has developed the *Five Wishes* document, which meets the legal requirements in 42 states and is useful in all 50 states. http://www.agingwithdignity.org/five-wishes.php
Determine if there are conflicts associated with the transition of care from acute to palliative.	Individuals who understand the rationale for moving from being acutely managed to symptom management or to less invasive medical management will be more likely to move with greater ease along the trajectory of their disease. Certain physiologic indicators can be used to determine the progressive nature of a chronic condition. These indicators, which include ejection fraction, pulmonary and renal function, and metastatic disease, show when a disease can no longer be reversed or improved through aggressive medical intervention.
As needed, facilitate added support for the patient and family members.	The patient and family may require support from multiple disciplines such as advanced practice nurses, medical social workers, dietitians, nursing assistants, physical therapists, and spiritual advisors.
Promote physical activity and social engagement and active participation in life for as long as possible.	Physical activity helps to reduce disease exacerbations, minimize depression, reduce discomfort, promote socialization, reduce isolation, and prevent complications associated with immobility.
Help the patient and family differentiate palliative care from hospice care.	Not all individuals are comfortable with or want to be referred to hospice care. Palliative care interventions do not depend on a 6-month or less prognosis nor are they mandated by reimbursement criteria.
Explain that palliative care can be provided concomitantly with advanced disease management by the patient's primary care provider and is reimbursed as routine medical management.	Palliative care is integrated into the management of advanced disease with a primary focus on symptom management and is not contingent on the treatment being provided during the last months, days, or weeks of life. This enables coordinated and continuous medical management by the patient's familiar primary care provider.

Nursing Diagnosis:
Caregiver Role Strain

related to the demands associated with the patient's physical care needs as the patient's disease progresses and contributes to physical limitations and disability

Desired Outcome: Caregivers are assisted with providing care and offered frequent respite opportunities.

ASSESSMENT/INTERVENTIONS	RATIONALES
Assess the specific support systems used to provide the patient with advanced disease care management.	This assessment will help determine if an appropriate support system is in place to address the physical, emotional, and spiritual demands associated with advanced disease, illness, and disability.

ASSESSMENT/INTERVENTIONS	RATIONALES
Determine the specific roles of the patient's family or support system. Identify the primary caregiver and any additional caregivers who can support the patient and primary caregiver.	In addition to a primary caregiver, a secondary caregiver should be identified and mobilized to reduce the potential for burn-out. Burn-out occurs when only one person provides all the caregiving.
Evaluate community-based services or supportive programs that can be used to provide caregiver respite.	Services for the aging, adult daycare, and church-specific services, as well as help provided by volunteers, friends, and neighbors, may be considered to provide respite for the primary caregiver.
Encourage communication between the patient and caregiver.	Communication will provide an opportunity to identify and verbalize fears and concerns regarding the demands of meeting the patient's activities of daily living. This communication will provide earlier identification of problems that require prompt attention and problem-solving in order to reduce caregiver burn-out.
Elicit interdisciplinary support to assist the caregiver in problem-solving and seeking additional supportive resources.	Social workers, spiritual advisors, and advanced practice nurses will have additional ideas and be familiar with community resources that can be facilitated to support the primary caregiver, thereby reducing the potential for burn-out.
If caregiving demands are increased out of proportion to the caretaker's abilities and physical reserves, reevaluate the plan of care and the expectations of both the patient and caregiver.	Progressive symptomatic disease may increase the physical demands on the caregiver. For example, a dementia patient who becomes combative and is not sleeping may require admission into a long-term care facility or nursing home. Reevaluation should occur when it is no longer safe for the patient or the caregiver to continue to meet the many needs of the patient.

Nursing Diagnosis:

Impaired Comfort

related to the pathophysiologic and psychological consequences associated with advanced symptomatic disease and illness

Desired Outcome: The patient's discomfort level decreases as evidenced by a self-rated symptom intensity score of less than a 5 on a 1-10 numerical multisymptom rating scale.

ASSESSMENT/INTERVENTION	RATIONALE
Identify and recognize the multiple symptoms associated with progressive advanced disease, using a multisymptom, numerical self-rating scale of 1-10 (e.g., Edmonton Symptom Assessment Scale).	Significant evidence suggests that any symptom rated at 5 or higher interferes with the patient's perceived quality of life (Foley & Abernathy, 2008). Multiple symptoms that accompany advanced disease can include pain, dyspnea, fatigue, edema, weakness, anxiety, depression, and insomnia.
Assess the multidimensional aspects of specific symptoms: modifying or aggravating factors, location, quality, character, timing, intensity, and/or relieving factors.	Use of a numerical scale captures the intensity of the symptom but does not help to determine the full impact of the symptom's influence on the patient's perceived quality of life. Obtaining a full description of the symptom helps to identify specific physiologic aspects and guide appropriate interventions. In addition, emotional and spiritual aspects can interface with and intensify symptom complaints.
Assess for and report the use of all medications that are used to manage specific symptoms.	The use of polypharmacy may reduce or exacerbate the efficacy of specific medications prescribed to reduce symptoms. Multiple providers may have prescribed specific medications that alter the effects of other medications. It is important to report all of the medications used by the patient to the managing provider to ensure their use does not interfere with the efficacy of necessary medications.

continued

ASSESSMENT/INTERVENTION	RATIONALE
Promote and recognize the use and implementation of evidence-based pharmacologic interventions that are used to generate optimal patient quality of life.	Evidence-based interventions have been studied and evaluated to promote patient well-being and improved quality of life. Using off-label or compounded medications that have not undergone rigorous evaluation or approval from the Food and Drug Administration (FDA) places patients at risk for complications and unknown drug-drug interactions.
Document the patient's symptom intensity rating before an intervention and again following the intervention.	Evaluating the pre- and postsymptom intensity score and reporting these findings in the patient health record promote standardized communication among the interdisciplinary team and help identify the efficacy of the intervention.
Provide early and prompt identification and assessment of pain and other problems—physical, psychologic, and spiritual.	Approaching the patient from a multidimensional perspective will promote a holistic approach to pain and symptom management, thereby preventing or reducing the incidence of somatization and poorly managed symptoms.
Recognize common symptoms associated with specific diseases and preemptively prepare the patient and family regarding what to look for and how to be proactive in seeking symptom management.	Two systematic reviews (Cherny & Radbruch, 2009; Doorenbos et al., 2006) have identified the most common symptoms in advanced disease and end-of-life care as pain, fatigue, dyspnea, and depression.
Assess and differentiate among acute, chronic, neuropathic, and somatic (nociceptive) pain syndromes.	Specific analgesic interventions are based on the type of pain. Acute pain is a normal response to injury or a warning of potential injury and resolves with healing (e.g., surgical incision). Chronic pain persists and may last for months or years (e.g., arthritis). Patients can have an acute exacerbation of chronic pain. Neuropathic pain involves nerves, while somatic pain comes from bone, muscle, joints, and hollow organs. The patient's verbal descriptors will help to identify neuropathic pain (sharp, shooting, hot, radiating) from somatic (nociceptive) pain (dull, constant, gnawing, deep, constant).
Explain to the patient and significant others how pain may be treated in the palliative and end-of-life care settings.	Mild to moderate pain may be managed with nonopioid analgesics. Opioids are appropriate for moderate to severe pain or persistent mild to moderate pain.
Apply the World Health Organization's three-step approach to the management of chronic malignant and non-malignant pain.	See Figure 8-1.
Recognize the four general principles when initiation, titration, and/or discontinuation of opioid analgesics are considered.	1. Establish the pain relief goal (e.g., 30% reduction in numerical pain score) 2. Initiate analgesia with a short-acting, low-dose upload 3. Use a titration schedule based on the opioid's pharmacologic properties 4. Frequently monitor for analgesia and adverse effects These activities are carried out by the prescribing provider.

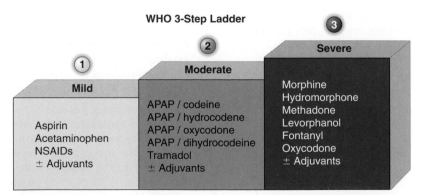

WHO 3-Step Ladder

FIGURE 8-1 The World Health Organization's three-step approach to the management of chronic malignant and nonmalignant pain. APAP, abbreviation for acetaminophen.

ASSESSMENT/INTERVENTION	RATIONALE
Explain the common side effects of opioid analgesics and the therapeutics than can help mitigate these symptoms.	Common side effects include nausea, vomiting, itchiness (pruritus), and drowsiness, all of which resolve or decrease with continued use. Opioids may slow breathing when therapy is initiated, but if the dose is titrated, this symptom should be limited. Constipation is predictable, and a stool softener or stimulant should accompany the use of opioid therapy.
Explain the value of adjuvant analgesics in promoting optimal management of neuropathic and somatic (nociceptive) pain syndromes.	Adjuvant analgesics are medications that, when combined with opioid analgesics, help to reduce neuropathic and nociceptive pain. No amount of opioid alone will effectively manage these two pain syndromes. Neuropathic pain syndromes benefit from the adjuvant use of antidepressants, anticonvulsants, muscle relaxants, and corticosteroids. Somatic or nociceptive pain syndromes respond to nonsteroidal antiinflammatory agents, corticosteroids, and bisphosphonates (e.g., Boniva, Fosamax).
Assess the need for around-the-clock analgesic dosing versus as-needed dosing.	Patients who self-rate their pain intensity at a 5 or greater and are using short-acting analgesics (q4h) and remain without optimal pain relief should be considered for longer-acting opioid analgesics. Long-acting opioids are administered q12h, once daily, or every 3 days (q36h such as Duragesic). Short-acting opioids are used for breakthrough pain and to increase therapeutic systemic opioid levels. Frequent or excessive use of rescue dosing signifies the need for a reassessment of the patient's pain and its management.
Assess for barriers that may affect the optimal and effective management of the patient's pain.	Barriers to optimal pain management can occur through providers, patients themselves, and the health care system. Provider barriers include concerns about medication risks, lack of appropriate assessment skills, limited knowledge of treatment options, or cultural or social barriers. Patient barriers include cognitive communication issues, fear of side effects or influence on mentation, and cultural or social barriers. Barriers associated with the health care system include limited specialists or access to care, formulary limitations, or inventory system restrictions.
[!] Provide the patient and caregiver with tips for safe opioid use.	1. Patients should not combine opioids with other central stimulating medications, including alcohol. 2. Patients should consult with their health care provider before stopping or changing an opioid dose. Abrupt withdrawal can precipitate excessive symptoms. 3. Store medication in a locked or secure cabinet to prevent wrongful use or theft. 4. Because opioids can cause drowsiness, impair concentration, and slow reflexes, patients should avoid driving or performing complex tasks when initiating therapy.
Offer the patient and caregiver resources to promote effective pain management education.	Chronic pain resources include Pain Action: www.painaction.com American Chronic Pain Association: www.theacpa.org American Pain Foundation: www.painfoundation.org American Pain Society: www.ampainsoc.org/people The Neuropathy Association: www.neuropathy.org American Cancer Society: www.cancer.org

Nursing Diagnoses:

Adult Failure to Thrive
Deficient Fluid Volume
Decreased Cardiac Output
Anxiety
Fatigue
Acute Confusion
Impaired Swallowing
Impaired Gas Exchange

related to the normal process of death and dying and its effects on the human body

Desired Outcome: The patient and family acknowledge their acceptance of the normal process of death and dying and understanding of the effects on the human body.

ASSESSMENTS/INTERVENTIONS	RATIONALES
Be proactive in assessing for and preventing or controlling distressing symptoms with the goal of the patient's peaceful death.	Patients who are in the final stages of disease and illness tolerate symptoms poorly, largely because of weakness and generalized debility. Uncontrolled symptoms, especially at this stage of the disease trajectory, can easily escalate into a crisis for both the patient and family.
Assess for a decrease in cardiac function as death nears, including a decreased blood pressure (BP).	The BP decreases due to a combination of the heart's ineffective pumping ability, dehydration, and renal insufficiency.
Assess for increased heart rate (HR), even though the pulse is weak, thready, and irregular.	This is a compensatory mechanism of the heart as death approaches.
Monitor for cyanosis and coolness and a mottling appearance to the skin.	Cyanosis is often present and becomes progressive as death nears, resulting from ineffective delivery of blood, nutrients, and oxygen to the body's tissues. This causes the patient's skin to become cool and appear mottled. Circulatory blood is shunted to essential organs and is no longer adequately perfusing the kidneys and the peripheral structure.
Monitor for changes in the patient's breathing.	Compensatory mechanisms of the pulmonary system used to regulate normal homeostasis are often seen as changes in the patient's breathing. Respirations may become increasingly shallow or labored as the dying process nears. Patients experience and families observe more frequent periods of apnea. Pulmonary secretions increase and the patient may have difficulty managing a cough, swallowing, or clearing the airway.
Help prevent uncontrolled respiratory secretions.	Early use of anticholinergic interventions (e.g., scopolamine) can help to reduce respiratory secretions. Anticholinergics are not effective when secretions are already present.
If the patient experiences dyspnea, facilitate simple environmental comfort (e.g., use a fan, elevate head of bed, and reposition the patient from side to side).	Dyspnea is one of the most distressing symptoms for dying patients and their families and can be difficult to manage. Measures other than providing environmental comfort include bronchodilators, cough suppressants, diuretics (use cautiously in patients with established dehydration), anticholinergics, opiates, corticosteroids, and oxygen.

ASSESSMENTS/INTERVENTIONS	RATIONALES
Assess for dyspnea, tachypnea, Cheyne-Stokes, apnea, labored breathing, and/or noisy respirations.	Dyspnea is difficulty in breathing; tachypnea is a rapid respiratory rate; and Cheyne-Stokes is an abnormal pattern of breathing characterized by progressively deeper and sometimes faster breathing, which can also be identified as labored or apneic or irregular. Noisy respirations occur close to death and are often termed "death rattle." To effectively manage these symptoms, providers may prescribe specific medications such as opiates, bronchodilators, anxiolytics, and oxygen. The nurse can help to position the patient (high Fowler's, 45-degree angle, moving the patient from side to side), minimize the patient's energy expenditure, and provide reassurance.
Teach the family how to provide good oral hygiene for the patient.	Patients who are mouth breathing and prescribed anticholinergic medications will have a dry oral mucosa. Keeping the mouth moist with water and ice chips will promote patient comfort.
Monitor for decreased or absent urine output on each daily assessment.	Absent or diminished urine output is often an expected reaction to dying, a result of decreased cardiac perfusion, decreased oral intake of fluids, medications, or decreased renal function. Renal insufficiency is more pronounced in patients with renal disease, chronic diabetes, unmanaged hypertension, and heart failure (HF).
	Urinary retention can result from an enlarged prostate, anticholinergic or opioid medications, weakness, disinterest due to depression, lack of cognitive awareness, or a full rectal vault. It is important to recognize the underlying cause and consider indwelling catheterization. While incontinence may be manageable at the end of life, it may require frequent linen and position changes, which may be uncomfortable for the patient.
Base your decisions regarding the need for hydration on the patient's comfort level, symptom burden, use of opioid medications, and proximity to death.	Dehydration is a result of various etiologies, and at the end stage of disease, patients are further debilitated and have diminished oral intake, which increases the risk for dehydration. Opioid metabolite accumulation as a result of dehydration can create nausea, confusion, restlessness, myoclonus, delirium, nightmares, hallucinations, and hyperalgesia. Light hydration can help to relieve these symptoms. Patients who are not given hydration and who are taking opioids should have the dose titrated down from their original opiate dose to lessen the accumulation of toxic metabolites.
	There remains a debate whether actively dying patients can benefit from intravenous or subcutaneous fluid administration. Instead of thinking that hydration is either good or bad, hydration can be thought of as a comfort intervention.
Assess changes in cognition that often occur close to death, with the most common being somnolence, delirium, difficulty communicating, labile mood, hallucinations, agitation, or restlessness.	Delirium is frequently seen near the end of life, but it is important to evaluate for a reversible etiology and provide treatment when warranted. Several studies have identified the presence of delirium in as many as 88% of cancer patients in their final weeks. Delirium is generally multifactorial and can be reversible—e.g., in opiate and benzodiazepine toxicities, metabolic disorders, or dehydration.
Differentiate delirium from dementia.	Determinant factors in delirium are sudden onset, inattention, scattered thought process, and altered consciousness; in dementia the onset is gradual and consciousness is unimpaired. Delirium can occur concurrently with dementia or other cognitive impairments.
Assess and evaluate reversible causes of delirium that require prompt attention and intervention.	All medications require a thorough investigation to determine if they are contributing to delirium (e.g., opioids, benzodiazepines, antidepressants, antihistamines, anticonvulsants, nonsteroidal antiinflammatory agents, corticosteroids, metoclopramide, ranitidine, ACE inhibitors, and digoxin). Other causes include hypoxia, visual and hearing deficits, hypertension, infection, trauma, surgery, hepatic or renal failure, and metabolic abnormalities (e.g., hypercalcemia, hypernatremia, uremia, hypercapnia, hyponatremia, and hypoglycemia).

continued

ASSESSMENTS/INTERVENTIONS	RATIONALES
Differentiate agitation and restlessness from delirium and dementia and intervene accordingly. Educate the family that the patient may "act out" toward them during these episodes because they are "safe" targets.	Uncontrolled pain, full bladder, constipation, or emotional issues can be misinterpreted as restlessness. Adding more opiates can aggravate agitation. If pain is suspected as the cause of restlessness, administer a breakthrough dose of pain medication. If this is ineffective, the underlying cause requires further evaluation. Haloperidol is the drug of choice (titrated to effect) should the restlessness not be reversible.
Monitor for dysphagia and impaired cognition. As indicated, administer medications by sublingual, rectal, transdermal, or subcutaneous routes.	Patients at the end of life can have impaired cognition and develop dysphagia resulting from progressive weakness and be unable to swallow oral medications.
Prepare the family for the patient's expected death awareness.	Death awareness is not confusion or hallucinations but important work for the patient. The family should listen to what the patient may be trying to communicate, address any unresolved issues, and prepare to finalize their time with the patient.
Identify the patient's withdrawal from close and social relationships and activities. Educate the family to expect withdrawal and not to take it personally as the patient turns inward.	The dying process is unique for each individual. The patient may shift focus and disengage from loved ones. The patient does not have the energy for relationships.

Nursing Diagnosis:

Grieving

related to the anticipatory loss of one's own life or that of a loved one

Desired Outcome: The patient and family acknowledge and eventually reach a state of acceptance of the impending loss.

ASSESSMENT/INTERVENTIONS	RATIONALES
Assess for signs of grieving and encourage expressions of feelings by the patient, family, and interdisciplinary health care team.	Signs of grieving include tearfulness and feelings of sadness or disbelief in the ending of life. Expressions of grief can be cathartic. Anger is often substituted for grief and is considered normal.
Teach the family how to differentiate normal grieving from complicated grieving.	Complicated grief may be present when an individual's ability to resume normal activities and responsibilities is continually disrupted beyond 6 months of the time of death.
Help the patient and family identify successful past coping strategies that have worked in stressful situations.	Building from past strategies that have worked can be encouraged for use in the current situation.
Respect the patient's and family's need to use denial occasionally.	Denial can be an effective coping mechanism for grief.
Give the family permission to express culturally specific concerns and issues about the patient's impending death.	Many cultures handle death and dying differently.
Encourage family members to engage in conversations that involve sensitive issues or unfinished business. Honor their wishes, for example, by contacting the spiritual advisor or people with whom the patient desires to have closure.	Verbalizing unfinished or sensitive issues might require the integration of interdisciplinary support (social worker, spiritual advisor) to help resolve difficult or sensitive issues between the patient and family.

ADDITIONAL NURSING DIAGNOSES/PROBLEMS:

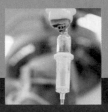

Chronic Obstructive Pulmonary Disease (COPD)

9

OVERVIEW/PATHOPHYSIOLOGY

Chronic obstructive pulmonary disease (COPD) is the third leading cause of death and 12th leading cause of morbidity in the United States. It is a disease state characterized by airflow limitation that is not fully reversible. Airflow limitation is progressive and associated with an abnormal inflammatory response of the lungs to noxious particles or gases and characterized by chronic inflammation throughout the airways, parenchyma, and pulmonary vasculature.

The chronic airflow limitation characteristic of COPD is caused by a mixture of small airway inflammation (bronchitis) and parenchymal destruction (emphysema), the relative contributions of each varying from person to person.

HEALTH CARE SETTING

COPD may be found in any health care setting, such as the home, primary care, hospitalized patients (medical, surgical floors or critical care units) and long-term care facilities.

ASSESSMENT

Signs and symptoms, acute and chronic: Common symptoms associated with chronic COPD include dyspnea, chronic cough, and chronic sputum production. Dyspnea that interferes with daily activities is the main reason patients seek medical attention. Increased sputum production may be prominent. As lung function deteriorates and dyspnea worsens, arterial hypoxemia and hypercarbia become more pronounced and additional complications such as weight loss, right heart failure (cor pulmonale), and respiratory failure occur.

Key health history: Environmental exposure is the most common cause of COPD. Cigarette smoking, or passive exposure to cigarette smoke, is the most commonly encountered risk factor. Chronic occupational exposure to dust or volatile gases is an important risk factor. Indoor air pollutants, especially from burning biomass fuels in confined spaces, is associated with increased risk for COPD in developing countries, especially among women who are primarily responsible for meal preparation. Genetic factors (e.g., hereditary deficiency of alpha-1 antitrypsin) may be responsible for disease development and progression. Any process that affects lung development and growth (such as low birth weight or recurrent respiratory infections) may increase the potential for developing COPD later in life. Multiple risk factors magnify the possibility of developing COPD.

Significant comorbidities include cardiovascular disease, osteoporosis, anxiety/depression, lung cancer, respiratory infections and diabetes. All of the above may have significant impact on the COPD patient. The comorbidities are treated in the usual manner in the COPD patient.

Physical assessment: Prolonged expiratory phase, decreased thoracic expansion, adventitious breath sounds (especially wheezing), use of accessory muscles of respiration, development of a barrel chest, digital clubbing, dullness on percussion over areas of consolidation, ankle edema, distended neck veins.

DIAGNOSTIC TESTS

Spirometry: When the common symptoms associated with chronic COPD are present, spirometry confirms the diagnosis of COPD. It is expressed as a ratio of the forced expiratory volume (FEV_1), or the volume of air that is forcefully exhaled in the first second, divided by the forced vital capacity (FVC), or the maximum volume of air that can be forcefully exhaled post–bronchodilator use. The ratio is expressed as FEV_1/FVC but sometimes simply abbreviated to FEV_1. Clinical symptoms and a post–bronchodilator use FEV_1 of less than 0.70 are used to diagnose and classify the severity and prognosis of COPD.

Pulse Oximetry (SpO_2): A useful tool for both screening and monitoring disease progression, with the normal for COPD patients being between 88%-92%.

Chest x-ray examination: Rarely diagnostic unless bullous disease is present. Radiologic changes in COPD include signs of hyperinflation (i.e., flattened diaphragm on lateral chest film and increase in volume of the retrosternal airspace).

Arterial blood gas (ABG) values: Important in monitoring COPD during exacerbations or respiratory failure (PaO_2 less than 60 mm/Hg with or without $PaCO_2$ greater than 50 mm/Hg).

Alpha-1 antitrypsin deficiency screen: Performed in patients who develop COPD at a young age (younger than 45 yr) or who have a strong family history of the disease.

Differential diagnosis: COPD may mimic many other diseases.

PART I: Medical-Surgical Nursing

Nursing Diagnosis:

Ineffective Breathing Pattern

related to ineffective inspiration and expiration occurring with chronic airflow limitations

Desired Outcome: Following treatment/intervention, the patient's breathing pattern improves as evidenced by reduction in or absence of reported dyspnea and related symptoms.

ASSESSMENTS/INTERVENTIONS	RATIONALES
Assess respiratory status q2-4h and as indicated by the patient's condition. Report significant findings.	Restlessness, anxiety, mental status changes, shortness of breath, tachypnea, and use of accessory muscles of respiration are signs of respiratory distress, which should be reported promptly for immediate intervention.
Auscultate breath sounds q2-4h and as indicated by the patient's condition.	A decrease in breath sounds or an increase in adventitious breath sounds (crackles, wheezes, rhonchi) may indicate respiratory status change and necessitate prompt intervention.
Administer bronchodilator therapy as prescribed.	Bronchodilators increase FEV_1 by altering airway smooth muscle tone, with long acting formulations being preferred. If symptoms do not improve with a single agent, combined short- and long-acting agents are used.
Administer inhaled corticosteroids as prescribed.	This treatment is used for patients with FEV_1 at less than 30%, whose frequent exacerbations are not well controlled with long acting bronchodilators.
Administer oral corticosteroids as prescribed.	Short-term corticosteroids shorten recovery time, improve lung function and arterial hyoxemia, and decrease hospital length of stay. A typical course is 10-14 days. Long- term oral corticosteroid monotherapy is not recommended because the side effects outweigh the minimal advantage oral corticosteroids provide over inhaled corticosteroids.
Administer combination inhaled corticosteroids and bronchodilator therapy as prescribed. Advise the patient about the increased risk for pneumonia.	Corticosteroids combined with a long-acting beta-2 agonist are more effective than any one individual treatment in reducing exacerbations and overall improvement of lung function. However, its use also carries an increased risk for pneumonia.
Monitor for tachycardia and dysrhythmias.	These are side effects of bronchodilator therapy.
Deliver humidified oxygen as prescribed and monitor the patient's response..	Long-term oxygenation for chronic hypoxemia has been shown to reduce mortality. Delivering O_2 with humidity will help minimize convective losses of moisture, decreasing dry mucous membranes and enhancing lung compliance.
Monitor pulse oximetry readings and titrate oxygen to keep SpO_2 between 88%-92%.	SpO_2 saturation at 87% or less can indicate need for initiating or increasing O_2 therapy. SpO_2 saturation at 93% or more can indicate need for decreasing O_2 therapy to prevent the complications of oxygen toxicity in the patient with COPD, including oxygen-free radicals and capillary leakage (Collopy KT, et al, 2012).

Nursing Diagnosis:

Impaired Gas Exchange

related to altered oxygen supply occurring with small airway inflammation and parenchymal destruction or alveolar edema

Desired Outcomes: Optimally within 1-2 hr following treatment/intervention or by discharge, the patient has adequate gas exchange as evidenced by respiratory rate (RR) of 12-20 breaths/min (or values consistent with patient's baseline). Before discharge from the care facility, the patient's arterial blood gas (ABG) values are as follows: PaO_2 60 mm Hg or higher, $PaCO_2$ 35-45 mm Hg, and pH 7.35-7.45, or SpO_2 88%-92% or values consistent with the patient's baseline.

ASSESSMENTS/INTERVENTIONS | RATIONALES

ASSESSMENTS/INTERVENTIONS	RATIONALES
[!] Assess for signs and symptoms of hypoxia and report significant findings.	Hypoxia (evidenced by agitation, anxiety, restlessness, changes in mental status or level of consciousness [LOC]) indicates oxygen deficiency and necessitates prompt treatment.
[!] Auscultate breath sounds q2-4h and as indicated by the patient's condition and report significant findings.	A decrease in breath sounds or an increase in adventitious breath sounds (crackles, wheezes, rhonchi) may indicate respiratory status change and necessitate prompt intervention.
Deliver humidified oxygen as prescribed, and monitor the patient's response.	Long-term oxygenation for chronic hypoxemia has been shown to reduce mortality. Delivering O_2 with humidity will help minimize convective losses of moisture, decreasing dry mucous membranes and enhancing compliance.
[!] Monitor pulse oximetry readings and titrate oxygen to keep SpO_2 between 88%-92%.	SpO_2 at 87% or less can indicate need for O_2 therapy. SpO_2 at 93% or more can indicate need for decreasing O_2 therapy. See this rationale with **Ineffective Breathing Pattern,** earlier.
Position the patient in high Fowler's position, with the patient leaning forward and elbows propped on the over-the-bed table. Pad the over-the-bed table with pillows or blankets. Record the patient's response to positioning.	This position promotes comfort and optimal gas exchange by enabling maximal chest expansion, using activation of accessory muscles during inspiration and gravity during expiration.
Administer noninvasive positive pressure ventilation (NIPPV) as prescribed.	NIPPV has been shown to increase blood pH, reduce $Paco_2$, and reduce severity of dyspnea in the first 4 hr of treatment, possibly eliminating the need for mechanical ventilation in some patients. If the patient is able to tolerate PO intake, switch the NIPPV to nasal cannula oxygen during meals to facilitate eating and prevent aspiration while using NIPPV.
Explain, as indicated, that intubation, mechanical ventilation, pressure support, and minimal positive end expiratory pressure may be necessary and this would necessitate intensive care support.	Exacerbations of COPD or complications (e.g., pneumonia, surgery, trauma) may require endotracheal intubation and short-term mechanical ventilation. Goals and possible outcomes should be discussed with the patient and/or significant others BEFORE intubation and mechanical ventilation are instituted, if possible. Pressure support provides inspiration assistance to overcome the resistance of the endotracheal tube and ventilator circuit. PEEP is limited to exert the least internal pressure on the fragile lungs.
Monitor serial ABG values as indicated by the patient's condition.	PaO_2 likely will continue to decrease as the patient's disease progresses. Patients with chronic CO_2 retention may have chronically compensated respiratory acidosis with a low normal pH (7.35-7.38) and a $Paco_2$ greater than 50 mm Hg.

Nursing Diagnosis:

Activity Intolerance

related to imbalance between oxygen supply and demand due to inefficient work of breathing

Desired Outcome: The patient reports decreasing dyspnea during activity or exercise and rates perceived exertion at 3 or less on a 0-10 scale. See Chapter 4, "Prolonged Bedrest," **Risk for Activity Intolerance,** p. 62 for a description of the Borg scale.

ASSESSMENTS/INTERVENTIONS	RATIONALES
Monitor the patient's respiratory response to activity, including assessment of oxygen saturations.	Activity intolerance is indicated by excessively increased RR (e.g., more than 10 breaths/min above baseline) and depth, and use of accessory muscles of respiration. Ask the patient to rate perceived exertion. If activity intolerance is noted, instruct the patient to stop the activity and rest. Individuals with COPD may become hypoxic during increased activity and require oxygen therapy to prevent hypoxemia, which increases the risk for exacerbations of the COPD.
Maintain prescribed activity levels, and explain rationale to the patient.	Prescribed activity levels will increase the patient's stamina while minimizing dyspnea. COPD is a progressive disease, and affected individuals can gradually become totally disabled because they must use all available energy for breathing.
Allow at least 90 min between activities for undisturbed rest. Facilitate coordination across health care providers.	Ninety minutes of undisturbed rest decreases oxygen demand and enables adequate physiologic recovery.
Assist with active range-of-motion (ROM) exercises. For more information, see **Risk for Activity Intolerance** in "Prolonged Bedrest," p. 61.	ROM exercises help build stamina and prevent complications of decreased mobility.
Request consultation from pulmonary rehabilitation.	A comprehensive program includes exercise training, nutrition counseling, and education and provides benefits to patients with all stages of COPD. Pulmonary rehabilitation is strongly recommended for any patient with an FEV_1 less than 50%. Patients who have completed a pulmonary rehabilitation program have been shown to experience improved quality of life and slowed progression of the disease (American College of Physicians, American College of Chest Physicians, American Thoracic Society, and European Respiratory Society, 2011).

Nursing Diagnosis:

Imbalanced Nutrition: Less Than Body Requirements

related to decreased intake occurring with fatigue and anorexia

Desired Outcome: For a minimum of 24 hr before hospital discharge, the patient has adequate nutrition as evidenced by intake of at least 50% of prescribed calories/meals.

ASSESSMENTS/INTERVENTIONS	RATIONALES
Assess food and fluid intake.	This assessment provides data that will determine need for dietary consultation.
Provide the diet in small, frequent, high caloric meals that are nutritious and easy to consume.	Small meals are easier to consume in individuals who are fatigued. Patients with COPD expend an extraordinary amount of energy simply on breathing and require high caloric meals to maintain body weight and muscle mass. Cachexia (loss of muscle and fat despite adequate nutrition) is associated with higher mortality in individuals with COPD. Although a common belief is that carbohydrates increase CO_2 production, there are no conclusive data to support high fat, low carbohydrates diets for COPD patients.
Request consultation with a dietitian as indicated.	Such a consultation enables a comprehensive nutritional assessment and possible additional therapies, including nutritional counseling related to the disease process. The dietitian also may facilitate establishment of enteral or parental nutrition in the cachectic or intubated patient or those who are not able to consume adequate nutrition orally.

ASSESSMENTS/INTERVENTIONS

RATIONALES

ASSESSMENTS/INTERVENTIONS	RATIONALES
For patients who require an oxygen mask or NIPPV and are able to eat, consult with respiratory therapy for the most appropriate device to allow the patient to eat.	Attempting oral intake while using NIPPV may result in aspiration. Changing devices for short periods to enable the patient to eat may avoid the need for enteral or parental nutrition support.
When not otherwise indicated, encourage fluid intake (2.5 L/day or more).	Adequate hydration helps decrease sputum viscosity for patients with chronic increased sputum production.
Discuss with the patient and significant others the importance of good nutrition in the treatment of COPD.	This information optimally will promote adequate nutrition and stable body weight. A knowledgeable patient is more likely to adhere to the treatment plan.

✓ PATIENT-FAMILY TEACHING AND DISCHARGE PLANNING

When providing patient-family teaching, focus on sensory information, avoid giving excessive information, and initiate a visiting nurse referral for necessary follow-up teaching and/or pulmonary rehabilitation program. Include verbal and written information about the following:

✓ Use of home O_2, including instructions for when to use it, importance of not increasing prescribed flow rate, precautions, community resources for O_2 replacement when necessary, and an absolute restriction of smoking near O_2.

✓ Importance of respiratory therapy consultation to assist with teaching related to O_2 therapy, if indicated.

✓ Medications, including drug name, route, purpose, dosage, schedule, precautions, and potential side effects. Also discuss drug-drug, herb-drug, and food-drug interactions. If patient will take corticosteroids while at home, provide instructions accordingly to ensure patient takes the prescribed amount. The patient should return demonstration of the correct use of inhalers, including spacers and rinsing of the mouth after steroid inhalation.

✓ Smoking cessation: Single most effective way of reducing risk of development and progression of COPD. Nicotine replacement therapy reliably decreases smoking rates.

✓ Staying alert to public health announcements about air quality alerts. If significant COPD is present, the patient should avoid outdoor exercise or stay indoors during these alerts.

✓ Signs and symptoms that necessitate medical attention to such conditions as COPD exacerbation, pneumonia/infections, or heart failure:

- increased dyspnea, fatigue, and coughing
- changes in amount, color, or consistency of sputum
- fever
- increased swelling of ankles and legs or sudden weight gain. Patients with COPD often have right-sided heart failure and fluid retention related to the cardiac effects of the disease. For more information, see Chapter 21, "Heart Failure," p. 168.
- Early treatment of COPD exacerbations decreases mortality and health care costs and shortens recovery.

✓ Importance of avoiding contact with infectious individuals, especially those with respiratory infections, and limiting exposure in general during seasonal outbreaks.

✓ Recommendation that patient receives a pneumococcal vaccination and annual influenza vaccination.

✓ Review of sodium-restricted diet and other dietary considerations as indicated.

✓ The need to remain active and the importance of pacing activity level and taking frequent rest periods to conserve energy.

✓ Follow-up appointment with the health care provider; confirm date and time of next appointment.

✓ Introduction to pulmonary rehabilitation programs. Physical training programs may improve ventilation and cardiac muscle function, which may compensate for nonreversible lung disease.

✓ Additional resources and patient education materials may be found at:
- The American Lung Association at *www.lung.org*
- The Lung Association at *www.lung.ca*
- The Canadian Cancer Society at *www.cancer.ca* for educational tools to support smoking cessation

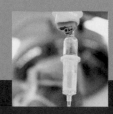

Pneumonia 10

OVERVIEW/PATHOPHYSIOLOGY

Pneumonia is an acute bacterial or viral infection that causes inflammation of the lung parenchyma (alveolar spaces and interstitial tissue). As a result of the inflammation involved, lung tissue becomes edematous and air spaces fill with exudate (consolidation), gas exchange cannot occur, and nonoxygenated blood is shunted into the vascular system, causing hypoxemia. Bacterial pneumonias involve all or part of a lobe, whereas viral pneumonias appear diffusely throughout the lungs.

Influenza, which can cause pneumonia, is the most serious viral airway infection for adults. Patients older than 50 yr, residents of extended care facilities, and individuals with chronic health conditions have the highest mortality rate from influenza.

Pneumonias generally are classified into two types: community acquired and hospital associated (nosocomial). A third type is pneumonia in the immunocompromised individual.

Community acquired: The most common. Individuals with community-acquired pneumonia generally do not require hospitalization unless an underlying medical condition, such as chronic obstructive pulmonary disease (COPD), cardiac disease, or diabetes mellitus, or an immunocompromised state complicates the illness.

Hospital associated (nosocomial): Nosocomial pneumonias usually occur following aspiration of oropharyngeal flora or stomach contents in an individual whose resistance is altered or whose coughing mechanisms are impaired (e.g., a patient who has decreased level of consciousness [LOC], dysphagia, diminished gag reflex, or a nasogastric tube or who has undergone thoracoabdominal surgery or is on mechanical ventilation). Bacteria invade the lower respiratory tract via three routes: (1) gastric acid aspiration (the most common route), causing toxic injury to the lung, (2) obstructions (foreign body or fluids), and (3) infections (rare). Gram-negative pneumonias are associated with a high mortality rate, even with appropriate antibiotic therapy. Aspiration pneumonia is a nonbacterial (anaerobic) cause of hospital-associated pneumonia that occurs when gastric contents are aspirated. Pneumonia is the second most common nosocomial infection in critically ill patients and is a leading cause of death in hospital-acquired infection.

Ventilator-associated pneumonia (VAP) is defined as pneumonia occurring more than 48 hr after patients have been intubated and receive mechanical ventilation. Eighty-six percent of nosocomial pneumonias are classified as VAP. The risk of pneumonia increases 3- to 10-fold in patients receiving mechanical ventilation. VAP is associated with increases in morbidity and mortality, hospital length of stay, length of stay in the ICU, and in significant incremental cost estimated to be in the billions of dollars annually (Augustyn, 2007).

Pneumonia in the immunocompromised individual: Immunosuppression and neutropenia are predisposing factors in the development of nosocomial pneumonias from both common and unusual pathogens. Severely immunocompromised patients are affected not only by bacteria but also by viruses (cytomegalovirus) and fungi (*Candida, Aspergillus, Pneumocystis jirovecii*). Most commonly, *P. jirovecii* is seen in persons with human immunodeficiency virus infection or in persons who are immunosuppressed therapeutically following organ transplantation.

HEALTH CARE SETTING

Primary care, with acute or intensive care hospitalization resulting from complications

ASSESSMENT

Findings are influenced by patient's age, extent of the disease process, underlying medical condition, and pathogen involved. Generally, any factor that alters integrity of the lower airways, thereby inhibiting ciliary activity, increases the likelihood of developing pneumonia.

General signs and symptoms: Cough (productive and nonproductive), increased sputum (rust colored, discolored, purulent, bloody, or mucoid) production, fever, pleuritic chest pain (more common in community-acquired bacterial pneumonias), dyspnea, chills, headache, and myalgia. Older adults may be confused or disoriented and run low-grade fevers but may present with few other signs and symptoms.

General physical assessment findings: Restlessness, anxiety, decreased skin turgor and dry mucous membranes secondary to dehydration, presence of nasal flaring and expiratory grunt, use of accessory muscles of respiration (scalene, sternocleidomastoid, external intercostals), decreased chest expansion caused by pleuritic pain, dullness on percussion over affected (consolidated) areas, tachypnea (respiratory rate [RR] more than 20 breaths/min), tachycardia (resting heart rate [HR] more than 100 bpm), increased vocal fremitus, egophony ("e" to "a" change) over area of consolidation, decreased breath sounds, high-pitched and inspiratory crackles (rales) increased by or heard only after coughing, low-pitched inspiratory crackles (rales) caused by airway secretions, and circumoral cyanosis (a late finding).

DIAGNOSTIC TESTS

Chest x-ray examination: To confirm presence of pneumonia (i.e., infiltrate appearing on the film).

Sputum for Gram stain and culture and sensitivity tests: Sputum is obtained from the lower respiratory tract before initiation of antibiotic therapy to identify causative organism. It can be obtained via expectoration, suctioning, transtracheal aspiration, bronchoscopy, or open-lung biopsy.

White blood cell (WBC) count: Will be increased (more than 12,000/mm^3) in the presence of bacterial pneumonias. Normal or low WBC count (less than 4000/mm^3) may be seen with viral or mycoplasma pneumonias.

Chemistry panel: To detect presence of hypernatremia, hyperglycemia, and/or dehydration.

Blood culture and sensitivity: To determine presence of bacteremia and help identify causative organism. To attain the best yield, blood cultures should be drawn before administration of antibiotics.

Urinary antigen test: To detect *Legionella pneumophila* and *Streptococcus pneumoniae*.

Oximetry: May reveal decreased O$_2$ saturation (92% or less).

Arterial blood gas (ABG) values: May vary, depending on degree of lung involvement or other coexisting disease. Findings may demonstrate hypoxemia (PaO$_2$ less than 80 mm Hg) and hypocarbia (PaCO$_2$ less than 32-35 mm Hg), with a resultant respiratory alkalosis (pH more than 7.45) in the absence of an underlying pulmonary disease. However, with increasing respiratory difficulty, respiratory acidosis may occur.

Serologic studies: Acute and convalescent antibody titers drawn to diagnose viral pneumonia. A relative rise in antibody titers suggests viral infection.

Acid-fast stains and cultures: To rule out tuberculosis.

Nursing diagnosis for patients *at risk* for developing pneumonia

Nursing Diagnosis:

Risk for Infection (nosocomial pneumonia)

related to inadequate primary defenses (e.g., decreased ciliary action), invasive procedures (e.g., intubation), and/or chronic disease

Desired Outcome: Patient is free of infection as evidenced by normothermia, WBC count 12,000/mm^3 or less, and sputum clear to whitish in color.

ASSESSMENT/INTERVENTIONS	RATIONALES
Identify presurgical candidates who are at increased risk for nosocomial pneumonia.	This assessment helps ensure that surgical patients remain free of infection because nosocomial pneumonia has a high morbidity and mortality rate. Factors that increase risk for nosocomial pneumonia in surgical patients include the following: older adult (older than 70 yr), obesity, COPD, other chronic pulmonary conditions (e.g., asthma), history of smoking, abnormal pulmonary function tests (especially decreased forced expiratory flow rate), intubation, and upper abdominal/thoracic surgery.
Perform thorough hand hygiene before and after contact with the patient (even when gloves have been worn).	This intervention helps prevent spread of infection by removing pathogens from the hands. Hand hygiene involves using alcohol-based waterless antiseptic agent if hands are not visibly soiled or using soap and water if hands are dirty or contaminated with proteinaceous material.
Provide preoperative teaching, explaining and demonstrating pulmonary activities that will be used postoperatively to prevent respiratory infection.	Pulmonary activities that help to prevent infection/pneumonia include deep breathing, coughing, turning in bed, splinting wounds before breathing exercises, ambulation, maintaining adequate oral fluid intake, and use of a hyperinflation device.
Make sure the patient verbalizes knowledge of these activities and their rationales and returns demonstrations appropriately.	These actions help ensure the patient is knowledgeable and capable of performing these activities. Learning how to apply information via a return demonstration is more helpful than receiving verbal instruction alone. A knowledgeable patient is more likely to adhere to therapy.

continued

ASSESSMENT/INTERVENTIONS	RATIONALES
Advise individuals who smoke to discontinue smoking, especially during preoperative and postoperative periods. Refer to a community-based smoking cessation program as needed or provide nicotine replacement therapy.	Inhalation of toxic fumes/chemical irritants can damage cilia and lung tissue and is a factor that increases the likelihood of developing pneumonia.
Administer analgesics ½ hr before deep-breathing exercises. Support (splint) the surgical wound with hands, pillows, or folded blanket placed firmly across the site of incision.	These interventions help control pain, which otherwise would interfere with lung expansion.
Identify patients who are at increased risk for aspiration.	Individuals with depressed LOC, advanced age, dysphagia, or a nasogastric (NG) or enteral tube in place are at risk for aspiration, which predisposes them to pneumonia.
Maintain the head of bed (HOB) at 30- to 45-degree elevation, and turn the patient into a side-lying position. When the patient receives enteral alimentation, recommend continuous rather than bolus feedings. Hold feedings when the patient is lying flat.	Aspiration is one of the two leading causes of nosocomial pneumonia. Aspiration precautions include maintaining the HOB at 30-degree elevation, turning the patient onto the side rather than the back, and using continuous rather than bolus feedings when the patient receives enteral alimentation.
Recognize risk factors for infection in patients with tracheostomy and intervene as follows:	Risk factors include the presence of underlying lung disease or other serious illness, increased colonization of oropharynx or trachea by aerobic gram-negative bacteria, greater access of bacteria to the lower respiratory tract, and cross-contamination caused by manipulation of the tracheostomy tube.
- Wear gloves on both hands when handling the tube or when handling mechanical ventilation tubing.	Loss of skin integrity or space around the tube would enable ingress of pathogens via the wound or tube.
- Suction as needed rather than on a routine basis.	Frequent suctioning increases risk of trauma and cross-contamination.
- Always wear gloves on both hands to suction. Use a sterile catheter for each suctioning procedure. Consider use of closed suction system; replace closed suction system per agency policy. Always replace the suction system between patients. Use only sterile fluids and dispense them using sterile technique. Change breathing circuits according to agency policy. Fill fluid reservoirs immediately before use (not far in advance).	These practices further decrease risk of contamination.
- Avoid saline instillation during suctioning. If the patient has tenacious secretions, increase heat and humidity.	Saline instillation can cause dislodgement of bacteria into the lower lung fields, increasing the risk of inflammation and invasion of sterile tissue. It can also stimulate coughing.
- Avoid the following when working with nebulizer reservoirs: introduction of nonsterile fluids or air, manipulation of the nebulizer cup, or backflow of condensate from delivery tubing into the reservoir or into the patient when tubing is manipulated. - Discard any fluid that has condensed in tubing; do not allow it to drain back into the reservoir or into the patient.	These are ways in which nebulizer reservoirs can contaminate patients.

Nursing diagnoses for patients *with* pneumonia

Nursing Diagnosis:

Impaired Gas Exchange

related to altered oxygen supply and alveolar-capillary membrane changes occurring with the inflammatory process and exudate in the lungs

Desired Outcome: Hospital discharge is anticipated when the patient exhibits at least five of the following indicators: temperature 37.7°C or less, HR 100 bpm or less, RR 24 breaths/min or less, systolic blood pressure (SBP) 90 mm Hg or more, oxygen saturation more than 92%, and ability to maintain oral intake.

ASSESSMENT/INTERVENTIONS	RATIONALES
[!] Monitor for and promptly report signs and symptoms of respiratory distress.	Signs and symptoms of respiratory distress include restlessness, anxiety, mental status changes, shortness of breath, tachypnea, and use of accessory muscles of respiration. Respiratory distress necessitates prompt medical intervention.
[!] Auscultate breath sounds at least q2-4h or as indicated by the patient's condition. Report significant findings.	Decreased or adventitious sounds (e.g., crackles, wheezes) can signal potential respiratory failure that would further aggravate hypoxia and necessitate prompt intervention.
[!] Monitor and document vital signs (VS) q2-4h or as indicated by the patient's condition. Report significant findings.	A rising temperature and other changes in VS (e.g., increased HR and RR) may signal presence of worsening inflammatory response in the lungs. This could cause further hypoxia, contributing to adult respiratory distress syndrome and need for mechanical ventilation.
Administer antibiotics within 6 hr of hospital admission and ongoing as prescribed.	Early administration of antibiotics decreases inflammatory response in the lung, promoting healing and reducing risk of mortality. Typical antibiotic therapy for community-acquired pneumonia includes use of a B-lactam (high-dose amoxicillin or amoxicillin-clavulanate) and cephalosporins (ceftriaxone, cefotaxime, and cefpodoxime) along with macrolides (azithromycin, clarithromycin, and erythromycin). Cephalosporins alone will not provide coverage against atypical bacteria without the addition of a macrolide. Fluoroquinolones (gatifloxacin, levofloxacin, moxifloxacin, and gemifloxacin) may be used solely because of their broad-spectrum coverage. However, they are not routinely the first drug of choice because of concerns about increasing resistance. Proper identification of the organism and determination of sensitivity to specific antibiotics are critical for appropriate therapy.
Monitor oximetry readings; report O_2 saturation of 92% or less.	O_2 saturation of 92% or less is a sign of a significant oxygenation problem and can indicate need for O_2 therapy.
Administer oxygen as prescribed.	Oxygen is administered when O_2 saturation or ABG results demonstrate hypoxemia. Initially, oxygen is delivered in low concentrations, and oxygen saturation is watched closely. If O_2 saturation does not rise to an acceptable level (more than 92%), FiO_2 is increased in small increments, with concomitant checks of O_2 saturations or obtaining ABG values. Significant increases in oxygen requirements to maintain O_2 saturations greater than 92% should be reported promptly.
Monitor ABG results.	Acute hypoxemia (PaO_2 less than 80 mm Hg) often indicates need for oxygen therapy. Hypocarbia ($PaCO_2$ less than 35 mm Hg), with a resultant respiratory alkalosis (pH greater than 7.45) in the absence of an underlying pulmonary disease, is consistent with pneumonia. However, if pneumonia progresses to acute respiratory distress, respiratory acidosis will result.
Position the patient for comfort (usually semi-Fowler's position).	This position provides comfort, promotes diaphragmatic descent, maximizes inhalations, and decreases work of breathing. Gravity and hydrostatic pressure when the patient is in this position promote perfusion and ventilation-perfusion matching. In patients with unilateral pneumonia, positioning on the unaffected side (i.e., "good side down") promotes ventilation-perfusion matching.
Facilitate coordination across the health care team to provide rest periods between care activities. Allow 90 min for undisturbed rest.	Rest decreases oxygen demand in a patient whose reserves are likely limited.

Nursing Diagnosis:

Ineffective Airway Clearance

related to the presence of tracheobronchial secretions occurring with infection

Desired Outcomes: The patient demonstrates effective cough. Following intervention, the patient's airway is free of adventitious breath sounds.

ASSESSMENT/INTERVENTIONS	RATIONALES
Auscultate breath sounds q2-4h (or as indicated by the patient's condition), and report changes in the patient's ability to clear pulmonary secretions.	This assessment determines the presence of adventitious breath sounds (e.g., crackles, wheezes). Coarse crackles are a sign the patient needs to cough. Fine crackles at lung bases likely will clear with deep breathing. Wheezing is a sign of airway obstruction, which necessitates prompt intervention to ensure effective gas exchange.
Inspect sputum for quantity, odor, color, and consistency; document findings.	As the patient's condition worsens, sputum can become more copious and change in color from clear/white to yellow and/or green, or it may show other discoloration characteristic of underlying bacterial infection (e.g., rust colored; "currant jelly").
Ensure that the patient performs deep breathing with coughing exercises at least q2h.	These exercises help clear airways of secretions. Controlled coughing (tightening upper abdominal muscles while coughing 2 to 3 times) ensures a more effective cough because it uses the diaphragmatic muscles, which increases forcefulness of the effort.
Assist the patient into a position of comfort, usually semi-Fowler's position.	This position provides comfort and facilitates ease and effectiveness of these exercises by promoting better lung expansion (there is less lung compression by abdominal organs) and gas exchange.
Assess need for hyperinflation therapy.	The patient's inability to take deep breaths is a sign of the need for this therapy. Deep inhalation with a hyperinflation device expands alveoli and helps mobilize secretions to the airways, and coughing further mobilizes and clears the secretions. Emphasis of this therapy is on inhalation to expand the lungs maximally. The patient inhales slowly and deeply 2× normal tidal volume and holds the breath at least 5 sec at the end of inspiration. To maintain adequate alveolar inflation, 10 such breaths/hr are recommended.
Report complications of hyperinflation therapy to the health care provider.	Complications include hyperventilation, gastric distention, headache, hypotension, and signs and symptoms of pneumothorax (shortness of breath, sharp chest pain, unilateral diminished breath sounds, dyspnea, cough).
Teach the patient to splint the chest with pillow, folded blanket, or crossed arms.	This action reduces pain while coughing, thereby promoting a more effective cough.
Instruct patients who are unable to cough effectively in a cascade cough.	A cascade cough removes secretions and improves ventilation via a succession of shorter and more forceful exhalations than are done with the usual coughing exercise.
Deliver oxygen with humidity as prescribed.	This intervention provides oxygenation while decreasing convective losses of moisture and helping mobilize secretions.
Assist the patient with position changes q2h. If the patient is ambulatory, encourage ambulation to the patient's tolerance.	Movement and activity help mobilize secretions to facilitate airway clearance.
Suction as prescribed and indicated.	Suctioning maintains a patent airway by removing secretions.
When not contraindicated, encourage fluid intake (2.5 L/day or more).	Increasing hydration decreases viscosity of the sputum, which will make it easier to raise and expectorate.

Nursing Diagnosis:

Deficient Fluid Volume

related to increased insensible loss occurring with tachypnea, fever, or diaphoresis

Desired Outcome: At least 24 hr before hospital discharge, the patient is normovolemic as evidenced by urine output 30 mL/hr or more, stable weight, HR less than 100 bpm, SBP greater than 90 mm Hg, fluid intake approximating fluid output, moist mucous membranes, and normal skin turgor.

ASSESSMENT/INTERVENTIONS

RATIONALES

ASSESSMENT/INTERVENTIONS	RATIONALES
Assess intake and output (I&O). Be alert to and report urinary output less than 30 mL/hr or 0.5 mL/kg/hr.	This assessment monitors the trend of fluid volume. An indicator of deficient fluid volume is urinary output less than 30 mL/hr for 2 consecutive hours. Consider insensible losses if the patient is diaphoretic and tachypneic.
Weigh the patient daily at the same time of day and on the same scale; record weight. Report weight changes of 1-1.5 kg/day.	These actions ensure consistency and accuracy of weight measurements. Weight changes of 1-1.5 kg/day can occur with fluid volume excess or deficit.
Encourage fluid intake (at least 2.5 L/day in unrestricted patients). Maintain intravenous (IV) fluid therapy as prescribed.	These actions help ensure adequate hydration.
Promote oral hygiene, including lip and tongue care.	Oral hygiene moistens dried tissues and mucous membranes in patients with fluid volume deficit.
Provide humidity for oxygen therapy.	Humidity helps minimize convective losses of moisture during oxygen therapy.

ADDITIONAL NURSING DIAGNOSIS FOR PATIENTS ON MECHANICAL VENTILATION

"General Care of Patients with Neurologic Disorders" for **Risk for Infection** related to inadequate primary defenses occurring with intubation.   p. 246

 PATIENT-FAMILY TEACHING AND DISCHARGE PLANNING

When providing patient-family teaching, focus on sensory information, avoid giving excessive information, and initiate a visiting nurse referral for necessary follow-up teaching. Include verbal and written information about the following:

- ✓ Techniques that promote gas exchange and minimize stasis of secretions (e.g., deep breathing, coughing, use of hyperinflation device, increasing activity level as appropriate for patient's medical condition, percussion, and postural drainage as necessary).
- ✓ Medications, including drug name, purpose, dosage, frequency or schedule, precautions, and potential side effects, particularly of antibiotics. Also discuss drug-drug, herb-drug, and food-drug interactions. Instruct patient to complete full dose of antibiotics to prevent reinfection and subsequent readmission.
- ✓ Signs and symptoms of pneumonia and importance of reporting them promptly to the health care professional should they recur. Teach the patient's significant others that changes in mental status may be the only indicator of pneumonia if the patient is elderly.
- ✓ Importance of preventing fatigue by pacing activities and allowing frequent rest periods.
- ✓ Importance of avoiding exposure to individuals known to have flu and colds and reducing exposure in general during seasonal outbreaks.
- ✓ Vaccinations: The Centers for Disease Control now recommends two different pneumococcal vaccines for adults.
  - One dose of pneumococcal conjugate vaccine (PCV 13) is recommended for adults ages 19 yrs and older with asplenia, sickle cell disease, cerebrospinal leaks,

cochlear implants, or any other conditions that cause immunocompromise.

- Adults ages 19-64 yr with medical conditions such as certain kidney diseases, cigarette smoking, chronic heart or lung disease, asplenia, or any other conditions that cause immunocompromise should receive one or two doses of pneumococcal polysaccharide vaccine (PPSV 23).
- All adults 65 yr and older should receive one dose of PPSV 23.
- If patients have a diagnosis that requires both PPSV 23 and PCV13 vaccines, they should be administered the PCV 13 vaccine first, followed by the PPSV 23 8 weeks later.
- ✓ Recommendation that the following individuals receive an influenza vaccination annually: all persons 6 mo and older with rare exception (e.g., allergy, history of Guillain-Barré). Influenza vaccines are routinely administered from the months of October through March, but ideally should be given in October.
- ✓ Minimizing factors that can cause reinfection, including close living conditions, poor nutrition, and poorly ventilated living quarters or work environment.
- ✓ Importance of smoking cessation education and community resources to assist in cessation.
- ✓ Phone numbers to call in case questions or concerns arise about therapy or disease after discharge. Additional general information can be obtained by visiting *www.lungusa.org*.
- ✓ Information in the following free brochures that outline ways to help patients stop smoking:
  - "How to Help Your Patients Stop Using Tobacco: A National Cancer Institute Manual for the Oral Health Team," from the Smoking and Tobacco Control Program of the National Cancer Institute; call (800) 4-CANCER.
  - "Clinical Practice Guideline: A Quick Reference Guide for Smoking Cessation Specialists," from the Agency for Health Care Policy and Research (AHCPR); call (800) 358-9295.
  - The American Lung Association at *www.lung.org*.
  - The Canadian Lung Association at *www.lung.ca*.

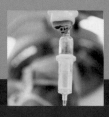

Pneumothorax/Hemothorax 11

PNEUMOTHORAX

OVERVIEW/PATHOPHYSIOLOGY

Pneumothorax is an accumulation of air in the pleural space that leads to increased intrapleural pressure. Risk factors include blunt or penetrating chest injury, chronic obstructive pulmonary disease (COPD), previous pneumothorax, and positive pressure ventilation. The three types of pneumothorax are as follows.

Spontaneous: Also referred to as *closed pneumothorax* because the chest wall remains intact with no leak to the atmosphere. It results from rupture of a bleb or bulla on the visceral pleural surface, usually near the apex. Generally, the cause of the rupture is unknown, although it may result from a weakness related to a respiratory infection or from an underlying pulmonary disease (e.g., COPD, tuberculosis, malignant neoplasm). Smoking also increases the risk of spontaneous pneumothorax. The affected individual is usually young (20-40 yr), previously healthy, and male. Generally, onset of symptoms occurs at rest rather than with vigorous exercise or coughing. Potential for recurrence is great, with the second pneumothorax occurring an average of 1-3 yr after the first.

Traumatic: Can be open or closed. An *open pneumothorax* occurs when air enters the pleural space from the atmosphere through an opening in the chest wall, such as with a gunshot wound, stab wound, or invasive medical procedure (e.g., lung biopsy, thoracentesis, or placement of a central line into a subclavian vein). A sucking sound may be heard over the area of penetration during inspiration, accounting for the classic wound description as a "sucking chest wound." A closed pneumothorax occurs when the visceral pleura is penetrated but the chest wall remains intact with no atmospheric leak. This usually occurs following blunt trauma that results in rib fracture and dislocation. It also may occur from use of positive end-expiratory pressure (PEEP) or after cardiopulmonary resuscitation.

Tension: Generally occurs with closed pneumothorax; also can occur with open pneumothorax when a flap of tissue acts as a one-way valve. Air enters the pleural space through the pleural tear when the individual inhales, and it continues to accumulate but cannot escape during expiration because the tissue flap closes. With tension pneumothorax, as pressure in the thorax and mediastinum increases, it produces a shift in the affected lung and mediastinum toward the unaffected side, which further impairs ventilatory efforts. The increase in pressure also compresses the vena cava, which impedes venous return, leading to a decrease in cardiac output and, ultimately, to circulatory collapse if the condition is not diagnosed and treated quickly. Tension pneumothorax is a life-threatening medical emergency.

HEMOTHORAX

OVERVIEW/PATHOPHYSIOLOGY

Hemothorax is an accumulation of blood in the pleural space. Hemothorax generally results from blunt trauma to the chest wall, but it can also occur following thoracic surgery, after penetrating gunshot or stab wounds, as a result of anticoagulant therapy, after insertion of a central venous catheter, or following various thoracoabdominal organ biopsies. Mediastinal shift, ventilatory compromise, and lung collapse can occur, depending on the amount of blood accumulated.

HEALTH CARE SETTING

Acute care, primary care

ASSESSMENT

Clinical presentation will vary, depending on the type and size of the pneumothorax or hemothorax.

DIAGNOSTIC TESTS

Chest x-ray: Will reveal presence of air or blood in the pleural space on the affected side, pneumothorax/hemothorax size, and any shift in the mediastinum.

Computed tomography (CT) scanning: Used when a chest x-ray cannot confirm or exclude the presence of a pneumothorax or hemothorax or for evaluation of recurrent spontaneous pneumothorax.

Oximetry: Will reveal decreased O_2 saturation (90% or less).

Arterial blood gas (ABG) values: Hypoxemia (PaO_2 less than 80 mm Hg) may be accompanied by hypercarbia ($PaCO_2$ greater than 45 mm Hg) with resultant respiratory acidosis (pH less than 7.35). Arterial oxygen saturation may be decreased initially but usually returns to normal within 24 hr.

Complete blood count (CBC): May reveal decreased hemoglobin proportionate to amount of blood lost in a hemothorax.

Assessment

Spontaneous or Traumatic Pneumothorax		Tension Pneumothorax	Hemothorax
Closed	**Open**		
Signs and Symptoms			
Shortness of breath, cough, chest tightness, chest pain	Shortness of breath, sharp chest pain	Dyspnea, chest pain	Dyspnea, chest pain
Physical Assessment			
Tachypnea, decreased thoracic movement, cyanosis, subcutaneous emphysema, hyperresonance over affected area, diminished breath sounds, paradoxical movement of chest wall (may signal flail chest), change in mental status	Agitation, restlessness, tachypnea, cyanosis, presence of chest wound, hyperresonance over affected area, sucking sound on inspiration, diminished breath sounds, change in mental status	Anxiety, tachycardia, cyanosis, jugular vein distention, tracheal deviation toward the unaffected side, absent breath sounds on affected side, distant heart sounds, hypotension, change in mental status	Tachypnea, pallor, cyanosis, dullness over affected side, tachycardia, hypotension, diminished or absent breath sounds, change in mental status

Nursing Diagnosis:

Ineffective Breathing Pattern

related to decreased lung expansion occurring with pneumothorax/hemothorax, pain, or malfunction of the chest drainage system

Desired Outcome: Following intervention, the patient becomes eupneic; lung expansion is noted on chest x-ray.

ASSESSMENT/INTERVENTIONS	RATIONALES
! Assess the patient's mental, respiratory, and cardiac status at frequent intervals (q2-4h, as appropriate).	This assessment monitors the patient's status while the chest drainage system is in place. The purpose of a chest drainage system is to drain air or fluid and reexpand the lung. Diminished breath sounds, along with tachycardia, restlessness, anxiety, and changes in mental status, are signs of respiratory distress that may occur as a result of chest drainage system malfunction. If these signs are present, prompt intervention is necessary to prevent further hypoxia and distress.
! Assess and maintain the closed chest drainage system as follows: - Tape all connections and secure the chest tube to the thorax with tape or other securement device.	These actions help ensure maintenance of the closed chest drainage system and facilitate drainage.
- Avoid all tubing kinks, and ensure that the bed and equipment are not compressing any component of the system. Eliminate all dependent loops in tubing.	These actions help ensure maintenance of the chest drainage system and facilitate drainage.
- Many closed systems come prefilled with water. Otherwise, maintain fluid in the water-seal chamber and suction chamber at appropriate levels.	The suction apparatus does not regulate the amount of suction applied to the closed chest drainage system. The amount of suction is determined by the water level in the suction control chamber.
- Monitor bubbling in the water-seal chamber.	Intermittent bubbling in this chamber is normal and signals that air is leaving the pleural space. Intermittent bubbling with coughing and exhalation is also normal. Absence of bubbling indicates the system is malfunctioning and suction is not being maintained.
- Locate and seal any leak in the system if possible.	Continuous bubbling in the water-seal chamber may be a signal that air is leaking into the drainage system.
- Dial the level of dry suction per the health care provider's recommendation.	This action maintains air and fluid removal from the pleural space. **Note:** Suction aids in lung reexpansion, but removing suction for short periods, such as for transporting, will not be detrimental or disrupt the closed chest drainage system.

continued

ASSESSMENT/INTERVENTIONS	RATIONALES
- Monitor fluctuations in the water-seal chamber.	These fluctuations are characteristic of a patent chest tube, and the water level may rise and fall with respirations. Fluctuations stop when either the lung has reexpanded or there is a kink or obstruction in the chest tube.
- Avoid stripping of the chest tubes.	This mechanism for maintaining chest tube patency is not recommended and has been associated with creating high negative pressures in the pleural space, which can damage fragile lung tissue.
[!] Keep the following necessary emergency supplies at the bedside.	
- Petrolatum gauze pad.	This gauze pad is applied over the insertion site if the chest tube becomes dislodged. Use of this dressing provides an airtight seal to prevent recurrent pneumothorax.
- A bottle of sterile water.	Submerging the chest tube in a bottle of sterile water if it becomes disconnected from the water-seal system provides for a temporary closed-chest drainage system.
[!] Never clamp a chest tube without a specific directive from the health care provider.	Clamping may lead to tension pneumothorax because air in the pleural space no longer can escape.

Nursing Diagnosis:

Impaired Gas Exchange

related to ventilation-perfusion mismatch

Desired Outcomes: Following treatment/intervention, the patient exhibits adequate gas exchange and ventilatory function as evidenced by respiratory rate (RR) 20 breaths/min or less with normal depth and pattern (eupnea); no significant mental status changes; and orientation to person, place, and time. At a minimum of 24 hr before hospital discharge, the patient's ABG values are as follows: PaO_2 80 mm Hg or more and $PaCO_2$ 35-45 mm Hg (or values within patient's acceptable baseline parameters), or O_2 saturation greater than 92%.

ASSESSMENT/INTERVENTIONS	RATIONALES
[!] Monitor serial ABG results or oximetry readings. Report significant findings to the health care provider.	These assessments detect decreasing PaO_2 or O_2 saturation and increasing $PaCO_2$, which can signal impending respiratory compromise and necessitate prompt intervention.
[!] Assess for indicators of hypoxia. Report significant findings.	Increased restlessness, anxiety, tachycardia, and changes in mental status are early indicators of hypoxia and can signal impending respiratory compromise, which would necessitate prompt intervention.
[!] Assess vital signs and breath sounds q2h or as indicated by the patient's condition. Report significant findings.	These assessments monitor patient trends. Significant changes such as increased heart rate (HR), increased RR, and unilateral decreased breath sounds signal a worsening or unresolved condition.
[!] Following chest tube placement or exploratory thoracotomy, assess the patient q15min until stable. Report significant findings.	These assessments enable prompt detection of respiratory distress for timely intervention, including increased RR, diminished or absent movement of the chest wall on the affected side, paradoxical movement of the chest wall, increased work of breathing, use of accessory muscles of respiration, complaints of increased dyspnea, unilateral diminished breath sounds, and cyanosis.
	Chest tubes may be placed in any patients who are symptomatic to remove air or fluid from the pleural space and enable reexpansion of the lung. A thoracotomy may be indicated if the patient has had two or more spontaneous pneumothoraces or if the current pneumothorax does not resolve within 7 days. In the presence of a hemothorax, a thoracotomy may be indicated to locate the source and control the bleeding if loss exceeds 200 mL/hr for 2 hr.

ASSESSMENT/INTERVENTIONS	RATIONALES
Evaluate HR and blood pressure for tachycardia and hypotension. Report significant findings.	Tachycardia, along with tachypnea, is a compensatory mechanism that occurs due to hypoxia/hypoxemia. Tachycardia and hypotension are indicators of shock.
Support the patient in an optimal position (e.g., semi-Fowler's).	This position provides comfort and enables full expansion of the unaffected lung, adequate expansion of the chest wall, and descent of the diaphragm.
Change the patient's position q2h.	This intervention promotes drainage and lung reexpansion and facilitates alveolar perfusion.
Encourage the patient to take deep breaths, providing necessary analgesia to decrease discomfort during deep-breathing exercises. Instruct the patient in splinting the thoracotomy site with arms, a pillow, or folded blanket.	Deep breathing promotes full lung expansion and decreases risk of atelectasis. Analgesia and splinting decrease discomfort during deep-breathing exercises. Coughing facilitates mobilization of tracheobronchial secretions, if present.
Deliver and monitor oxygen and humidity as indicated for patients with oxygen saturations of 92% or less.	This intervention ensures adequate oxygen levels if the patient has hypoxemia, which is likely to be present if the pneumothorax/hemothorax is large. Humidity minimizes convective losses of moisture.

Nursing Diagnosis:

Acute Pain

related to impaired pleural integrity, inflammation, presence of a chest tube, or surgical intervention

Desired Outcome: Within 1 hr of intervention, the patient's subjective perception of pain decreases, as documented by a patient-reported pain scale.

ASSESSMENT/INTERVENTIONS	RATIONALES
At frequent intervals, assess the patient's degree of discomfort, using the patient's verbal and nonverbal cues. Use a self-report pain scale with the patient, rating pain from 0 (no pain) to 10 (worst pain).	These assessments monitor the patient's trend of pain and help determine the success of subsequent pain interventions. Because of rich innervation of the pleura, chest tube placement is painful; significant analgesia is usually required.
Medicate with analgesics as prescribed, using a pain scale to evaluate and document medication effectiveness.	These actions provide pain relief and determine effectiveness of the analgesia.
Encourage the patient to request analgesics before the pain becomes severe or, alternatively, administer analgesics at scheduled intervals.	Prolonged stimulation of pain receptors results in increased sensitivity to painful stimuli and increases the amount of analgesia required to relieve pain.
Premedicate the patient 30 min before initiating coughing, exercising, or repositioning and 30 min before, during, and after chemical pleurodesis.	This intervention provides comfort during painful exercises and repositioning and facilitates compliance. Chemical pleurodesis is extremely painful and requires diligent pain management.
Teach the patient to splint the affected side when coughing, moving, or repositioning.	This action reduces discomfort and promotes adherence to the treatment plan.
Facilitate coordination among health care providers to provide rest periods between care activities. Allow 90 min for undisturbed rest.	Relaxation and rest decrease oxygen demand and may decrease the level of pain.
Stabilize the chest tube with tape or a securement device securely to the thorax, positioning the tube to ensure there are no dependent loops.	These actions reduce pull or drag on latex connector tubing, prevent discomfort, and facilitate drainage and appropriate functioning.
For additional interventions, see Chapter 2, "Pain," p. 39.	

ADDITIONAL NURSING DIAGNOSES/PROBLEMS:

✓ PATIENT-FAMILY TEACHING AND DISCHARGE PLANNING

When providing patient-family teaching, focus on sensory information, avoid giving excessive information, and initiate a visiting nurse referral for necessary follow-up teaching.

Include verbal and written information about the following:

✓ Purpose for chest tube placement and maintenance.

✓ Pain management.

✓ Purpose for surgical intervention, if required, including risks/benefits and recovery.

✓ Potential for recurrence of spontaneous pneumothorax. Average time between occurrences is 1-3 yr. Explain the importance of seeking medical care immediately if symptoms recur (see Assessment).

✓ Medications, including drug name, purpose, dosage, schedule, precautions, and potential side effects. Also discuss drug-drug, herb-drug, and food-drug interactions.

✓ Importance of smoking cessation to prevent further pulmonary injury.

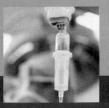

Pulmonary Embolus 12

OVERVIEW/PATHOPHYSIOLOGY

Pulmonary embolus (PE) is an obstruction of the pulmonary artery or one of its branches by substances (i.e., blood clot, fat, air, amniotic fluid) that originated elsewhere in the body. The most common source is a dislodged blood clot from the systemic circulation, typically the deep veins of the legs or pelvis. Thrombus formation is the result of the following factors: blood stasis, alterations in clotting factors, and injury to vessel walls. PE is classified as acute or chronic. In *acute PE*, patients develop signs and symptoms immediately after obstruction to the pulmonary vessels. In *chronic PE*, patients develop slow and progressive dyspnea over years as a result of pulmonary hypertension. Massive acute PE causes hypotension (systolic blood pressure [SBP] less than 90 mm Hg or a greater than or equal to 40-mm Hg decrease from baseline in a 15-min period), with accompanying right heart failure unexplained by a cardiac cause. Early diagnosis and intervention can reduce mortality as well as hospital length of stay (Smith et al., 2010). With treatment, most pulmonary emboli resolve and leave no residual deficits; however, some patients may be left with chronic pulmonary hypertension. A fat embolus is the most common nonthrombotic cause of pulmonary perfusion disorders. It is the result of release of free fatty acids causing a toxic vasculitis, followed by thrombosis and obstruction of small pulmonary arteries by fat.

Total obstruction leading to pulmonary infarction is rare because the pulmonary circulation has multiple sources of blood supply.

HEALTH CARE SETTING

Acute care

ASSESSMENT

Signs and symptoms often are nonspecific and variable, depending on extent of obstruction and whether the patient has an infarction as a result of the obstruction.

Pulmonary embolus: Sudden onset of dyspnea and sharp chest pain, restlessness, anxiety, nonproductive cough or hemoptysis, palpitations, nausea, and syncope. With a large embolism, oppressive substernal chest discomfort and signs of diastolic (right-sided) heart failure will be present. See Chapter 21, "Heart Failure," p. 168, for signs and symptoms.

Pulmonary infarction: Fever, pleuritic chest pain, and hemoptysis.

Physical assessment: Tachypnea, tachycardia, hypotension, crackles (rales), decreased chest wall excursion secondary to splinting, S_3 and S_4 gallop rhythms, transient pleural friction rub, jugular venous distention, diaphoresis, edema, and cyanosis. Temperature may be elevated if infarction has occurred.

Specific findings for fat embolus: Typically, the patient is asymptomatic for 12-24 hr following embolization. This period ends with sudden cardiopulmonary and neurologic deterioration: apprehension, restlessness, mental status changes, confusion, delirium, coma, and dyspnea.

Physical assessment for fat embolus: Tachypnea, tachycardia, and hypertension; fever; petechiae, especially of conjunctivae, neck, upper torso, axillae, and proximal arms; inspiratory crowing; pulmonary edema; profuse tracheobronchial secretions; fat globules in sputum; and expiratory wheezes.

HISTORY AND RISK FACTORS

Immobility: Especially significant when it coexists with surgical or nonsurgical trauma, carcinoma, or cardiopulmonary disease. Risk increases as the duration of immobility increases.

Cardiac disorders: Atrial fibrillation, heart failure, myocardial infarction, rheumatic heart disease.

Surgical intervention: Risk increases in prolonged surgeries of more than 30-min duration or during the postoperative period, especially for patients with orthopedic, pelvic, thoracic, or abdominal surgery and for those with extensive burns or musculoskeletal injuries of the hip or knee. This risk is present for 3 mo postoperatively.

Pregnancy: Especially during the postpartum period.

Chronic pulmonary and infectious diseases

Trauma: Especially lower extremity fractures and burns. The degree of risk is related to severity, site, and extent of trauma.

Mechanical ventilation: Risk increases because of immobility and inflammatory processes.

Carcinoma: Particularly neoplasms involving the breast, lung, pancreas, and genitourinary and alimentary tracts.

Obesity: A body mass index greater than 29 is associated with an increased incidence of PE, especially in women.
Varicose veins or prior thromboembolic disease
Age: Risk of thromboembolism is greatest for patients older than 55 yr.

History and risk factors for fat embolus

Multiple long bone fractures, especially fractures of the femur and pelvis; trauma to adipose tissue or liver; burns; osteomyelitis; sickle cell crisis.

DIAGNOSTIC TESTS
General findings for pulmonary emboli

Arterial blood gas (ABG) values: Hypoxemia (PaO_2 less than 80 mm Hg), hypocarbia ($PaCO_2$ less than 35 mm Hg), and respiratory alkalosis (pH more than 7.45) usually are present. A normal PaO_2 does not rule out the presence of pulmonary emboli.

Brain natriuretic peptide (BNP): Levels are typically greater in patients with PE compared to patients without PE; however, the test is insensitive since there are multiple causes for an elevated BNP. BNP does correlate the risk of subsequent complications and prolonged hospitalization.

D-dimer: A degradation product produced by plasmin-mediated proteolysis of cross-linked fibrin, D-dimer is measured by an enzyme-linked immunosorbent assay. The higher the result (with more than 500 ng/mL usually considered abnormal), the more likely it is the patient has a PE. This test is not sensitive or specific enough to diagnose PE, but it may be used in conjunction with other diagnostic tests.

Chest x-ray examination: Initially findings are normal, or an elevated hemidiaphragm may be present. After 24 hr, x-ray examination may reveal small infiltrates secondary to atelectasis that result from the decrease in surfactant. If pulmonary infarction is present, infiltrates and pleural effusions may be seen within 12-36 hr.

Electrocardiogram (ECG) results: If PEs are extensive, signs of acute pulmonary hypertension may be present: right-shift QRS axes, tall and peaked P waves, ST-segment changes, and T-wave inversion in leads V_1-V_4.

Spiral or helical computed tomography (CT): Enables image acquisition of pulmonary arteries during a single breath hold and with optimal contrast enhancement. Spiral CT is rapidly becoming the test of choice in diagnosing PE because of its higher specificity and sensitivity.

Pulmonary ventilation-perfusion scan: Used to detect abnormalities of ventilation or perfusion in the pulmonary system. Radiopaque agents are inhaled and injected peripherally. Images of distribution of both agents throughout the lung are scanned. If the scan shows a mismatch of ventilation and perfusion (i.e., pattern of normal ventilation with decreased perfusion), vascular obstruction is suggested.

Pulmonary angiography: The definitive study for PE, this is an invasive procedure that involves right heart catheterization and injection of dye into the pulmonary artery (PA) to visualize pulmonary vessels. An abrupt vessel "cutoff" may be seen at the site of embolization. Usually, filling defects are seen. More specific findings are abnormal blood vessel diameters (e.g., obstruction of the right PA would cause dilation of the left PA) and shapes (e.g., the affected blood vessel may taper to a sharp point and disappear).

Findings specific for fat emboli

ABG values: Should be drawn on patients at risk for fat embolus for the first 48 hr following injury because early hypoxemia indicative of fat embolus is apparent only with laboratory assessment. Hypoxemia (PaO_2 less than 80 mm Hg) and hypercarbia ($PaCO_2$ more than 45 mm Hg) will be present with a respiratory acidosis (pH less than 7.35).

Chest x-ray examination: A pattern similar to adult respiratory distress syndrome is seen: diffuse, extensive bilateral interstitial and alveolar infiltrates.

Complete blood count (CBC): May reveal decreased hemoglobin (Hgb) and hematocrit (Hct) secondary to hemorrhage into the lung. In addition, thrombocytopenia (platelets 150,000/mm^3 or less) is indicative of fat embolism.

Serum lipase: Will rise with fat embolism.

Urinalysis: May reveal fat globules following fat embolus.

Nursing Diagnosis:
Risk for Injury

related to venous stasis, hypercoagulable state, and/or vessel injury contributing to venous thromboembolism (VTE)

Desired Outcome: Following intervention/treatment, the patient exhibits no venous thromboembolic events (see descriptions under Assessment, earlier).

ASSESSMENT/INTERVENTIONS

RATIONALES

ASSESSMENT/INTERVENTIONS	RATIONALES
Assess for risk factors relating to VTE.	Risk factors alone or in combination increase the risk for developing VTE. Examples include advanced age, surgery, and immobility.
Collaborate with the health care provider regarding appropriate treatment with prophylaxis.	Prophylaxis may include unfractionated heparin or low-molecular-weight heparin (LMWH) and/or pneumatic compression devices. *Low dose unfractionated heparin:* Started immediately in patients without bleeding; typically given in 2-3 doses. *LMWH:* An alternative to low-dose heparin and given as a one-time dose. Most of the LMWH is excreted by the kidneys, and therefore the dose must be adjusted for individuals with renal impairment (creatinine clearance less than 30 mL/min). LMWH has been shown to be safe if given during pregnancy. *Pneumatic compression devices:* Prevent VTE via arterial compression. These devices are used in patients who cannot have heparin because of high risk of bleeding; once the risk of bleeding subsides, recommendations change to heparin. (Guyatt, et al, 2012).
Encourage ambulation and monitor activity.	Increased ambulation prevents venous stasis, a major risk factor for development of VTE.

Nursing Diagnosis:

Impaired Gas Exchange

related to ventilation-perfusion mismatch

Desired Outcomes: Following intervention/treatment, the patient exhibits adequate gas exchange and ventilatory function as evidenced by respiratory rate (RR) 12-20 breaths/min with normal pattern and depth (eupnea); no significant changes in mental status; and orientation to person, place, and time. At a minimum of 24 hr before hospital discharge, the patient has O_2 saturation greater than 92% or PaO_2 80 mm Hg or higher, $PaCO_2$ 35-45 mm Hg, and pH 7.35-7.45 (or values consistent with the patient's acceptable baseline parameters, or PaO_2 adjusted for altitude).

ASSESSMENT/INTERVENTIONS

RATIONALES

ASSESSMENT/INTERVENTIONS	RATIONALES
[!] Assess the patient for RR increased from baseline and increasing dyspnea, anxiety, restlessness, confusion, and cyanosis. Report significant findings.	These signs and symptoms of increasing respiratory distress and indicators of PE necessitate prompt intervention.
[!] As indicated, monitor oximetry readings. Report O_2 saturation of 92% or less.	A low O_2 saturation may indicate need for O_2 therapy. A poor response to treatment or worsening O_2 saturation necessitates prompt reporting for timely evaluation and further treatment. Hypoxia is common with PE, although its absence does not mean that patient does not have a PE.
Instruct the patient not to cross legs when lying in bed or sitting in a chair.	Legs that are crossed impede venous return from the legs and can increase risk of PE.
Pace the patient's activities and procedures.	Pacing activities and procedures decreases metabolic demands for oxygen and prevents further complications related to immobility. **Note:** It is safe for patient to ambulate once anticoagulation has been started.
Ensure that the patient performs deep breathing and coughing exercises 3-5 times q2h.	These exercises mobilize secretions and improve ventilation.
Ensure delivery of prescribed concentrations and humidity of oxygen.	Supplemental oxygen helps maintain a PaO_2 greater than 60 mm Hg and optimally 80 mm Hg or greater. Humidifying the oxygen minimizes convective losses of moisture.

Nursing Diagnosis:

Risk for Bleeding

related to anticoagulation therapy

Desired Outcome: The patient is free of frank or occult bleeding and exhibits the following signs of hemodynamic stability: heart rate (HR) less than 120 bpm, SBP greater than 90 mm Hg or returned to baseline, and RR 20 breaths/min or less.

ASSESSMENT/INTERVENTIONS	RATIONALES
Assess vital signs for indicators of profuse bleeding or hemorrhage. Report significant findings.	Hypotension, tachycardia, and tachypnea are signs of bleeding/hemorrhage, which can occur with anticoagulant therapy and necessitate prompt intervention.
At least once each shift inspect wounds, oral mucous membranes, any entry site of an invasive procedure, and nares.	This assessment helps determine if blood is present at any of these sites.
At least once each shift inspect the torso and extremities.	The presence of petechiae or ecchymoses signals bleeding within the tissues.
Apply pressure to all venipuncture or arterial puncture sites until bleeding stops completely.	To ensure that all bleeding stops completely, it is necessary to apply pressure for longer than the usual amount of time.
Ensure easy access to the following antidotes for the prescribed treatment: - Fresh frozen plasma - Vitamin K (vitamin K₁ [phytonadione] or K₃ [menadione]) - Four factor prothrombin complex concentrate	This product may be required in cases of serious bleeding or given to maintain coagulation for expected emergent procedure. 20 mg is given subcutaneously to counteract effects of oral anticoagulants. This agent is administered for warfarin reversal in cases of acute significant bleeding, usually 5-10 mg IV (Guyatt, et al, 2012). **Note:** Reversal agents should not be the first line of therapy unless a patient is actively bleeding.
If the patient is receiving heparin therapy, monitor serial partial thromboplastin time (PTT).	This will confirm that PTT is in the desired range (1.5-2.5× control).
If the patient is receiving warfarin therapy, monitor serial prothrombin time (PT).	This will confirm that PT is in the desired range (1.25-1.5× control, or international normalized ratio value of 2.0-3.0).
Report values outside the desired range.	This will enable prompt intervention.
Consult the pharmacist about compatibility before infusing other intravenous (IV) drugs through heparin IV line. For patients on warfarin therapy, consult the pharmacist to obtain specific information about the patient's medication profile.	For patients on heparin therapy, the following agents decrease the effect of heparin therapy: digitalis, tetracycline, nicotine, and antihistamines. Numerous drugs result in a decrease or increase in response to treatment with warfarin.
Discuss with the patient and significant others the effects of anticoagulant therapy and importance of reporting promptly the presence of bleeding.	Hematuria, melena, frank bleeding from the mouth, epistaxis, hemoptysis, and excessive vaginal bleeding (menometrorrhagia) are potential effects of anticoagulant therapy and necessitate timely intervention to prevent further blood loss.
Teach the necessity of using a soft toothbrush and mouthwash for oral care. Instruct the patient to shave with electric rather than straight or safety razor.	These measures minimize risk of bleeding.
If the patient is restless and combative, provide a safe environment. Use extreme care when moving the patient.	These actions help prevent falls and avoid bumping extremities into side rails, which could result in severe bleeding.
Assess for and teach the patient about herbal, food or over-the-counter medications that could affect coagulation and/or have an affect on anti-coagulant medications.	Herbal remedies, such as Ginko biloba, garlic, and ginseng have been shown to adversely affect clotting (Cordier, et al., 2012). Over-the-counter medications, such as aspirin, acetaminophen, non-steroidal anti-inflammatories (e.g., ibuprofen, naproxen), and cough and cold medications, as well as foods with high levels of vitamin K, such as dark green leafy vegetables, broccoli, and cabbage can adversely affect anti-coagulant medications.

Nursing Diagnosis:

Deficient Knowledge

related to unfamiliarity with oral anticoagulant therapy, potential side effects, and foods and medications to consider during therapy

Desired Outcome: Before hospital discharge, the patient verbalizes knowledge of the prescribed anticoagulant, potential side effects, and foods and medications to consider while receiving oral anticoagulant therapy.

ASSESSMENT/INTERVENTIONS	RATIONALES
Assess the patient's health care literacy (language, reading, comprehension). Assess culture and culturally specific learning needs.	This assessment helps ensure that information is selected and presented in a manner that is culturally and educationally appropriate.
Determine the patient's knowledge of oral anticoagulant therapy. As appropriate, discuss the medication name; purpose; dose; schedule; precautions; food-drug, herb-drug, and drug-drug interactions; and potential side effects.	Knowledgeable patients are more likely to adhere to the therapeutic regimen.
⚠ Teach the potential side effects/complications of anticoagulant therapy: easy bruising, prolonged bleeding from cuts, spontaneous nosebleeds, bleeding gums, black and tarry or bloody stools, vaginal bleeding, and blood in urine and sputum.	This information increases patients' awareness of side effects and complications to report to their health care providers for timely intervention.
⚠ Discuss the importance of laboratory testing and follow-up visits with the health care provider.	Laboratory testing helps ensure that the blood clotting time stays within therapeutic range. To promote safety, patients need close management by health care providers while undergoing anticoagulant therapy.
Explain the importance of informing all health care providers (including dentist) that the patient is taking an anticoagulant. Suggest the patient wear a medical alert tag or otherwise carry identification informing health care providers about the anticoagulant therapy.	These actions help ensure that patients are not given drugs or therapies that will have adverse effects on anticoagulant therapy, causing greater risk for hemorrhaging or clotting.
Teach the patient to notify the health care provider when ingesting large amounts of foods high in vitamin K or a subsequent change in the usual dietary pattern.	Foods high in vitamin K (e.g., asparagus, avocados, beef liver, broccoli, cabbage, soybeans, lettuce, olive oil, and canola oil) can interfere with anticoagulation.
Caution the patient that a soft-bristle rather than hard-bristle toothbrush and electric rather than straight or safety razor should be used during anticoagulant therapy.	These devices minimize risk of injury that could cause severe bleeding.
⚠ Instruct the patient to consult the health care provider before taking over-the-counter or prescribed medications that were used before initiating anticoagulant therapy.	Aspirin, cimetidine, trimethaphan, and macrolides are among the many medications that enhance response to warfarin. Medications that decrease response include antacids, diuretics, oral contraceptives, and barbiturates, among others.

ADDITIONAL NURSING DIAGNOSES/PROBLEMS:

"Perioperative Care"	p. 45
"Prolonged Bedrest"	p. 61
"Venous Thrombosis/Thrombophlebitis"	p. 186

 PATIENT-FAMILY TEACHING AND DISCHARGE PLANNING

When providing patient-family teaching, focus on sensory information, avoid giving excessive information, and initiate a visiting nurse referral for necessary follow-up teaching. Include verbal and written information about the following.

Note: Rehabilitation and family teaching concepts for fat emboli are nonspecific.

✓ Risk factors related to development of thrombi and embolization and preventive measures to reduce the risk.

✓ Signs and symptoms of thrombophlebitis: calf swelling; tenderness or warmth in the involved area; slight fever; and distention of distal veins, coolness, edema, and pale color in the distal affected leg.

✓ Signs and symptoms of pulmonary embolism: sudden onset of dyspnea and anxiety, nonproductive cough or hemoptysis, palpitations, nausea, syncope.

✓ Importance of preventing impairment of venous return from the lower extremities by avoiding prolonged sitting, crossing legs, and constrictive clothing.

✓ Medications, including drug name, dosage, purpose, schedule, precautions, and potential side effects. Also discuss drug-drug, herb-drug, and food-drug interactions.

Pulmonary Tuberculosis 13

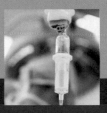

OVERVIEW/PATHOPHYSIOLOGY

Tuberculosis (TB) is an infectious disease caused primarily by *Mycobacterium tuberculosis*. In 2011, nearly 9 million persons around the world became sick with TB, the majority of whom have latent tuberculosis infection (LTBI), in which the bacteria are in the body (usually the lungs) in a dormant form that neither causes disease nor is communicable to other persons. A small proportion of persons (about 10%) with LTBI will develop active TB in their lifetimes.

For many years (from 1953 to 1984), reported cases of TB in the United States decreased almost 6% each year, and there was a general perception that TB was no longer a problem. This decline was due to many factors, including improved living conditions (less crowding and better ventilation), better nutrition, and antituberculosis drugs. As a result, the public health infrastructure to support TB control weakened as other diseases, for example, human immunodeficiency virus (HIV)/acquired immunodeficiency syndrome (AIDS), became more prominent. It was not until the late 1980s that the link between TB and HIV/AIDS became apparent as was manifested partially by multidrug-resistant (MDR) TB outbreaks occurring in seven hospitals between 1990 and 1992, resulting in many cases of LTBI, TB disease, and death. In addition, reported cases of TB increased 20% between 1985 and 1992. After the hospital outbreaks and subsequent administrative and legislative support to control TB, cases have steadily declined again in most areas of the country. In 2011, there were fewer than 11,000 reported cases of TB in the United States, more than half of which were among foreign-born persons. Worldwide, however, TB remains a leading cause of death in undeveloped countries and in persons who are HIV infected, with the World Health Organization estimating that approximately one third of the world's population is infected with M. *tuberculosis*.

M. *tuberculosis* is transmitted by the airborne route via minute, invisible particles called *droplet nuclei*. When individuals with TB disease of the lungs or throat cough, sneeze, speak, or sing, their respiratory secretions harbor TB organisms that are expelled into the air and transform quickly into tiny droplet nuclei that can remain suspended in air for several hours, depending on the environment (especially ventilation). In order to become infected, another person must breathe the air containing the droplet nuclei. A person's natural defenses of the nose and upper airway and immune system will often prevent sufficient numbers of organisms from reaching the alveoli to cause infection. In fact, it generally takes 5 to 200 organisms implanted in the alveoli to cause LTBI. When organisms reach the alveoli, they are ingested by macrophages. Some of the bacilli spread through the bloodstream when the macrophages die; however, the immune system response usually prevents the individual from developing TB disease. Although the majority of TB cases are pulmonary (85%), TB can occur in almost any part of the body or as disseminated disease. About half of people with LTBI who develop active TB (5%) will do so within the first year or two after infection. The remainder (5%) will develop active TB within their lifetimes.

HEALTH CARE SETTING

Primary care or long-term care, with possible hospitalization (acute care) resulting from complications

ASSESSMENT

For an accurate diagnosis of TB, a complete medical and psychosocial history should be taken along with a physical examination that includes a tuberculin skin test or an interferon gamma release assay (IGRA) blood test (there are currently two Food and Drug Administration [FDA]–approved IGRA tests available: the QuantiFERON®-TB Gold (QFT-G) and T-SPOT®), chest x-ray and CT scan examinations, and sputum examination (including acid-fast bacilli [AFB] smears, cultures, and drug sensitivity studies).

Signs and symptoms: TB is often suspected based on a group of symptoms that may include productive prolonged cough, fever, and night sweats, as well as chest pain, hemoptysis, chills, loss of appetite, unintended weight loss over a short period of time, and tiredness.

> **Note:** *Close contacts of the patient require identification so that they can undergo evaluation for the presence of LTBI. TB is reportable to the Public Health Department.*

History/risk factors for developing active TB: Immunocompromised state, especially HIV infection; injection drug use; radiographic evidence of prior, healed TB; weight loss of 10% or more of ideal body weight; and other medical conditions, including diabetes mellitus, silicosis, end-stage renal disease, some types of cancers, elders, infants, and certain immunosuppressive therapies. Persons who have emigrated from areas of the world with high rates of TB are also more likely to have LTBI than persons born in the United States.

DIAGNOSTIC TESTS

Tuberculin skin test or intradermal injection of antigen (purified protein derivative [PPD]): This test uses a PPD of mycobacterial organisms that is administered intradermally and interpreted as positive or negative using measured millimeters of induration. The test is considered positive when an area of induration 10 mm or greater is present within 48-72 hr after injection. High-risk categories such as persons with HIV infection and recent exposure are considered positive with 5 mm or greater induration. Those who are immunocompromised and some patients with active TB may have a negative PPD test, even in the presence of active TB disease. A positive PPD test indicates LTBI and is not diagnostic for active disease.

Interferon gamma release assays (IGRAs): Until recently, the only way to diagnose LTBI was with the tuberculin skin test (TST). Since 2001 an alternative to the TST, the IGRA blood test, has been approved by the FDA. This whole-blood interferon gamma assay requires only one patient visit for a blood specimen to assess for LTBI (rather than for active disease) and will become more widely used as laboratories implement the requirements for specimen evaluation. Two IGRA blood tests are currently available: the QuantiFERON®-TB Gold (QFT-G) test and the T-SPOT® test. These tests have high specificity (greater than 95%) and are not affected by prior vaccination with Bacille Calmette-Guérin (BCG).

Acid-fast stain: Detection of AFB in stained smears examined under a microscope usually provides the first bacteriologic clue of TB. Smear results should be available within 24 hr of specimen collection. AFB in the smear may be mycobacteria other than M. *tuberculosis*; many patients can have TB and have a negative smear. Specimens are generally collected by asking the patient to expectorate sputum into a cup; however, tracheal washing, bronchoscopy, thoracentesis of pleural fluid, and lung biopsy are other options.

Chest x-ray examination: Involvement is most characteristically evident in the apex and posterior segments of the upper lobes. Although not diagnostically definitive, it will reveal calcification at the original site, enlargement of hilar lymph nodes, parenchymal infiltrate, pleural effusion, and cavitation. Patients with HIV infection may have an atypical radiographic presentation of TB. Any abnormality on an AIDS patient's chest x-ray film should be considered possible TB until ruled out.

Gastric washings: May reveal presence of tubercle bacilli secondary to swallowed sputum. Gastric washings are usually used for children who cannot expectorate sputum.

Nursing Diagnosis:

Deficient Knowledge

related to unfamiliarity with the spread of TB and the procedure for Airborne Infection Isolation (AII)

Desired Outcome: Following instruction, the patient and significant others verbalize how TB is spread and measures necessary to prevent the spread.

ASSESSMENT/INTERVENTIONS	RATIONALES
Assess the patient's health care literacy (language, reading, comprehension). Assess culture and culturally specific information needs. Then teach the patient about TB and the mechanism by which it is spread (respiratory droplet nuclei).	This assessment helps ensure that information is selected and presented in a manner that is culturally and educationally appropriate. A well-informed patient is more likely to adhere to precautions against spreading the disease.
Post a notice of isolation/airborne precautions on the patient's room door.	Until antimicrobial therapy is successful as indicated by AFB smears, AII (or "airborne precautions" in the nomenclature of Standard Precautions) requires a private room with special ventilation that dilutes and removes airborne contaminants and controls the direction of airflow. The negative pressure is monitored continuously or checked and recorded daily while the patient is isolated in this room. Patients should wear a regular surgical mask if it is necessary to leave the room.

ASSESSMENT/INTERVENTIONS	RATIONALES
Explain to the patient and significant others. Remind staff and visitors of the need to keep the patient's door closed.	A closed door enables effective function of the ventilation system.
[!] Explain to the staff and visitors the importance of wearing N-95 or other high-efficiency respirators, including proper fit and use. Provide appropriate respirators at the doorway or other convenient place.	N-95 respirators, designed to provide a tight face seal and filter particles in the 1- to 5-micron range, are worn by all individuals entering the patient's room to reduce the possibility of infection.
[!] Teach the patient the importance of covering mouth and nose with tissues when sneezing or coughing and of disposing used tissues in the appropriate waste container.	These actions reduce the possibility of spreading infection.

✓ PATIENT-FAMILY TEACHING AND DISCHARGE PLANNING

When providing patient-family teaching about TB, focus on sensory information, avoid giving excessive information, and initiate a referral to the public health department for investigation and follow-up of household members and other contacts exposed to the patient with TB. Include verbal and written information about the following:

✓ Antituberculosis medications, including drug name, purpose, dosage, schedule, precautions, and potential side effects. Also discuss drug-drug, herb-drug, and food-drug interactions. Remind patients that medications are to be taken without interruption for the prescribed period. Remind patients of the need for continued laboratory monitoring for complications of pharmacotherapy. Describe directly observed therapy (DOT) if that is the medication administration method selected.

✓ Importance of periodic reculturing of sputum.

✓ Importance of basic hygiene measures, including hand hygiene practices, covering cough with tissues, and proper disposal of contaminated items.

✓ Phone numbers to call in case questions or concerns arise about therapy or disease after discharge. Additional general information can be obtained by contacting the following:
- *www.cdc.gov/tb* (Centers for Disease Control and Prevention)
- *www.lung.org* (American Lung Association)
- *www.lung.ca* (Canadian Lung Association and the Canadian Thoracic Society)
- *www.thoracic.org* (American Thoracic Society)
- *http:globaltb.njms.rutgers.edu* (Rutgers: Global Tuberculosis Institute)
- *http://ntcc.ucsd.edu* (National Tuberculosis Curriculum Consortium at the University of California San Diego)

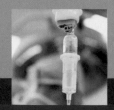

Respiratory Failure, Acute 14

OVERVIEW/PATHOPHYSIOLOGY

Acute respiratory failure (ARF) develops when the lungs are unable to exchange O_2 and CO_2 adequately. Clinically, respiratory failure exists when PaO_2 is less than 60 mm Hg with the patient at rest and breathing room air. $PaCO_2$ of 50 mm Hg or more or pH less than 7.35 is significant for respiratory acidosis, which is the common precursor to ARF.

Although a variety of disease processes can lead to the development of respiratory failure, four basic mechanisms are involved.

Alveolar hypoventilation: Occurs secondary to reduction in alveolar minute ventilation. Because differential indicators (cyanosis, somnolence) occur late in the process, the condition may go unnoticed until tissue hypoxia is severe.

Ventilation-perfusion mismatch: Considered the most common cause of hypoxemia. Normal alveolar ventilation occurs at a rate of 4 L/min, with normal pulmonary vascular blood flow occurring at a rate of 5 L/min. Normal ventilation/perfusion ratio is 0.8:1. Any disease process that interferes with either side of the equation upsets physiologic balance and can lead to respiratory failure as a result of reduction in arterial O_2 levels.

Diffusion disturbances: Processes that physically impair gas exchange across the alveolar-capillary membrane. Diffusion is impaired because of the increase in anatomic distance the gas must travel from alveoli to capillary and capillary to alveoli.

Right-to-left shunt: Occurs when the previously mentioned processes go untreated. Large amounts of blood pass from the right side of the heart to the left and out into the general circulation without adequate ventilation; therefore, blood is poorly oxygenated. This mechanism occurs when alveoli are atelectatic or fluid filled, inasmuch as these conditions interfere with gas exchange. Unlike the first three responses, hypoxemia secondary to right-to-left shunting does not improve with O_2 administration because the additional FiO_2 is unable to cross the alveolar-capillary membrane.

HEALTH CARE SETTING

Primary care; acute care resulting from complications

ASSESSMENT

Clinical indicators of ARF vary according to the underlying disease process and severity of the failure. ARF is one of the most common causes of impaired level of consciousness. Often it is misdiagnosed as heart failure, pneumonia, or stroke.

Early indicators: Restlessness, changes in mental status, anxiety, headache, fatigue, cool and dry skin, increased blood pressure, tachycardia, cardiac dysrhythmias.

Intermediate indicators: Confusion, increased agitation, and increased oxygen requirements with decreased oxygen saturations. Patients who have hypoventilation respiratory failure often exhibit lethargy and bradypnea. Patients with ventilation-perfusion mismatch often exhibit tachypnea.

Late indicators: Cyanosis, diaphoresis, coma, respiratory arrest.

DIAGNOSTIC TESTS

Arterial blood gas (ABG) analysis: Assesses adequacy of oxygenation and effectiveness of ventilation and is the most important diagnostic tool. Typical results are PaO_2 60 mm Hg or less, $PaCO_2$ 50 mm Hg or more, and pH less than 7.35, which are consistent with severe respiratory acidosis.

Chest x-ray examination: Ascertains the presence of underlying pathophysiology or disease process that may be contributing to the failure.

NURSING DIAGNOSES/PROBLEMS: (THE LISTED DISORDERS MAY BE PRECURSORS TO ARF)	
"Psychosocial Support"	p. 72
"Chronic Obstructive Pulmonary Disease"	p. 111
"Pneumonia" for **Impaired Gas Exchange**	p. 118
Deficient Fluid Volume	p. 120
"Pneumothorax/Hemothorax"	p. 122
"Pulmonary Embolus"	p. 127
"Guillain-Barré Syndrome"	p. 267
"Multiple Sclerosis"	p. 286

✓ **PATIENT-FAMILY TEACHING AND DISCHARGE PLANNING**

ARF is an acute condition that is symptomatically treated during the patient's hospitalization. Discharge planning and teaching should be directed at educating the patient and significant others about the underlying pathophysiology and treatment specific for that process. See chapters in this Respiratory section, shown above, as precursors that relate specifically to the underlying pathophysiology contributing to development of ARF.

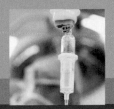

Aneurysms 15

OVERVIEW/PATHOPHYSIOLOGY

An aneurysm is a pathologic expansion in a section of an arterial wall. The most common cause is atherosclerosis, which alters the vessel pathology, weakens the vessel wall, and allows expansion. Additional causes include vessel wall trauma, congenital connective tissue disorders (e.g., Marfan's syndrome), and infection, particularly syphilis or acquired immunodeficiency syndrome (AIDS). Primary risk factors are heredity, age, and smoking. Because undiagnosed and untreated aneurysms are at risk for rupture and embolization, early diagnosis is imperative. Although aneurysms can develop in any artery, the abdominal aorta is the most common site. Abdominal aortic aneurysms (AAAs) occur more often in men and represent approximately 80% of all aneurysms. As the aneurysm enlarges, the risk of rupture increases. Aneurysms larger than 5.5 cm have the highest risk of rupture and require frequent monitoring and intervention.

Aneurysms in the thoracic aorta are most often attributed to the modifiable risk factors of hypertension and cigarette smoking. Thoracic aneurysms are more susceptible to dissection. The atherosclerotic lesions present in *dissecting aneurysms* develop intimal tears, which allow bleeding into the layers of the vessel, causing false lumens to form that obstruct or limit blood flow in the true lumen of the vessel. This pathology is distinctly different from that of AAAs.

Early diagnosis and periodic evaluation of aneurysms are essential to protect the patient from emergent life-threatening rupture. Physical assessment combined with ultrasound and radiologic screening of patients with risk factors leads to diagnosis.

HEALTH CARE SETTING

Chronic aneurysms may be monitored in primary care, with periodic radiographic or ultrasound assessment. Surgical intervention requires hospitalization and acute or intensive care during the perioperative period. Rehabilitation and home care services may be necessary during recovery.

ASSESSMENT

Abdominal aortic aneurysm: A pulsatile, nontender mass may be palpated on both sides of the abdominal midline.

Assessment is more difficult in obese patients. Severe acute abdominal pain, of sudden onset with radiation to the back, may be indicative of aneurysm rupture and is a surgical emergency. Rupture carries a high mortality of up to 75% (Radvany & Seguritan, 2008).

Thoracic aneurysm: Patients may be asymptomatic for years; however, pressure from the aneurysm on adjacent structures can result in dull pain in the upper back, dyspnea, cough, dysphasia, hemoptysis, tracheal deviation, and hoarseness. If there is pain associated with these aneurysms, it is more likely to be nonradiating central chest pain.

Femoral aneurysm: Leg or groin pain, decreased pulses, and swelling of the affected leg may occur. Femoral aneurysms may rupture or thrombose. See indicators discussed in Chapter 16, "Atherosclerotic Arterial Occlusive Disease," p. 140.

Acute indicators (rupture or dissection): Sudden onset of severe pain in the area of aneurysm with radiation, pallor, diaphoresis, and sudden loss of consciousness.

Physical assessment with acute rupture: Sudden drop of blood pressure (BP), weak and thready peripheral pulses, tachycardia, cyanosis, cool and clammy skin, and altered level of consciousness. Hypovolemic shock and death may occur, depending on severity of the bleeding.

DIAGNOSTIC TESTS

CT scan: Imaging standard with 100% accuracy, depicting exact location and size. It must be used in urgent situations in which suspicion for rupture is high and the patient is stable.

Ultrasound: Sound waves evaluate aneurysm size, shape, and location. This is a noninvasive and efficient examination, used for initial and emergent screening, especially when the patient is unstable.

Abdominal x-ray examination: May detect calcifications in the vessel wall but is not used for aneurysm evaluation.

Contrast arteriography: Determines size of the aneurysm, leaking, and origin of blood vessels arising from the aorta.

Nursing Diagnoses:

Risk for Decreased Cardiac Tissue Perfusion
Risk for Ineffective Renal Perfusion
Risk for Ineffective Gastrointestinal Perfusion

related to interrupted arterial flow occurring with rupture, bleeding, or embolization following the invasive procedure

Desired Outcome: The patient has adequate perfusion as evidenced by peripheral pulse amplitude greater than 2+ on a 0-4+ scale, brisk capillary refill (less than 2 sec), and exhibits baseline extremity sensation, motor function, color, and temperature.

ASSESSMENT/INTERVENTIONS	RATIONALES
Assess vital signs (VS) and peripheral pulses frequently in the perioperative period. Use a Doppler if necessary.	This provides ongoing assessment of perfusion. Pulse amplitude 2 or less (or other than "N") could signal embolization. Some health care centers use A (absent), D (requires Doppler), W (weak), N (normal), and B (bounding) to describe peripheral pulses. A Doppler is necessary for detection of a pulse that cannot be palpated.
If indicated, mark the location of peripheral pulses with a pen.	Location marking enables rapid identification of the pulses by all members of the health care team.
Assess peripheral sensation with VS. Instruct the patient to report impaired sensation promptly.	Impaired sensation could signal impaired perfusion secondary to embolization or bleeding. The patient is the first to notice changes in sensation.
Assess urine output frequently, recording intake and output measurements.	Severe hypotension or renal artery occlusion can decrease renal perfusion. Optimally urine output is 30 mL/hr or greater.
⚠ Report to the health care provider immediately any changes in vital signs, extremity color, capillary refill, temperature, motor function, sensation, or increasing pain.	These are assessments of peripheral perfusion; changes from baseline (e.g., VS variance of 20% or greater, capillary refill 3 sec or greater, coolness, pallor, or mottling, decreased motor function or sensation, and pain) may signal embolization or bleeding. Arterial obstruction and bleeding must be treated emergently to prevent hemorrhage, ischemia, and potential loss of the extremity.
Maintain the patient in neutral position and on bedrest until otherwise directed.	Bedrest helps maintain BP and perfusion. The neutral position maintains integrity of the graft and minimizes risk of postprocedure embolization.
⚠ Report any bloody diarrhea to the health care provider.	This may be a sign of bowel ischemia.
As prescribed, administer beta-blockers (i.e., metoprolol, atenolol, propanolol) to decrease myocardial irritability and contractility.	These agents slow the heart rate and decrease BP, which aids in preventing dissection.

✔ PATIENT-FAMILY TEACHING AND DISCHARGE PLANNING

When providing patient-family teaching, focus on sensory information, avoid giving excessive information, and initiate a visiting nurse referral for necessary follow-up teaching. Include verbal and written information about the following:

✔ Importance of regular medical follow-up to ensure graft patency, arterial integrity, and adequate perfusion.

✔ Reduction and/or management of risk factors (i.e., cigarette smoking, hypertension, obesity, diabetes) to prevent postoperative complications and slow the progression of atherosclerosis.

✔ Necessity of a regularly scheduled exercise program that may progress as the patient recovers.

✔ Indicators of wound infection and thrombus or embolus formation, and the need to report them promptly to the health care provider should they occur.

✔ Medications, including drug name, purpose, dosage, schedule, precautions, and potential side effects. Also discuss drug-drug, herb-drug, and food-drug interactions.

✓ Phone number of nurse or health care provider available to discuss concerns and questions.
✓ Importance of follow-up visits with health care provider; confirm date and time of next appointment.
✓ Potential need for assessment of other family members to rule out aneurysm, if heredity is a factor.

Additional resources and patient educational materials may be found at:

✓ The Heart and Stroke Foundation at *www.heartandstroke.com*
✓ The Canadian Lung Association at *www.lung.ca* or the Canadian Cancer Society at *www.cancer.ca* for educational tools to support smoking cessation
✓ American Heart Association at *www.americanheart.org*.

Atherosclerotic Arterial Occlusive Disease 16

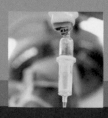

OVERVIEW/PATHOPHYSIOLOGY

Atherosclerosis is the primary etiology of peripheral artery disease. Damage to the intima of the artery occurs by the pathogenesis of atherosclerosis, which includes inflammation, plaque formation, lipid deposits, and hemorrhage. This process leads to vessel narrowing and hardening, decreasing lumen size and blood flow. Risk factors for atherosclerosis include smoking, heredity, advancing age, hyperlipidemia, hypertension, diabetes, metabolic syndrome, and a sedentary lifestyle.

Arterial occlusive disease is systemic and progressive and is of grave concern when 75% or more of a cross section of an artery becomes blocked. This disease is often associated with other comorbidities, such as coronary artery disease, hypertension, chronic obstructive pulmonary disease, and diabetes. The complexity of these comorbidities may lead to loss of limb or life in affected patients.

HEALTH CARE SETTING

Acute care or primary care

ASSESSMENT

Signs and symptoms: Severe, cramping pain (intermittent claudication) with exercise that is relieved by rest is the classic symptom of ischemia secondary to decreased blood flow. Additionally, decreased sensory or motor function, thin shiny legs, leg or foot ulcers, pallor or dependent rubor, pain, delayed wound healing, and gangrene all may be present.

Physical assessment: Decreased pulse amplitude, decreased hair distribution, muscle atrophy, and cool, pale or bluish discoloration of the extremities may be present. Skin often appears shiny, and the nails may be thick. Audible bruits may be assessed with a stethoscope over partially occluded vessels. Capillary filling may be 2 or more sec (with normal circulation, capillary filling occurs in less than 2 sec); pulses may be diminished and detected only by Doppler examination.

Risk factors: Cigarette smoking, hypertension, diabetes mellitus, family history of atherosclerotic disease, metabolic syndrome, and hyperlipidemia.

DIAGNOSTIC TESTS

Ankle-brachial index (ABI): Determines the degree of arterial occlusion and subsequent ischemia. Blood pressure (BP) is measured at the ankle (using either posterior tibial or dorsalis pedis pulse) and at the brachial artery. The pressure obtained at the ankle is divided by that at the brachial artery. Normally ABI is greater than 1.0; resting pain occurs with an ABI 0.3 or less.

Doppler flow studies: Uses a transducer that emits sound waves through a probe to determine the amount of blood flow through arteries in which palpable pulses are difficult to obtain. Waveforms also can be assessed similar to those on an electrocardiogram. The more normal or triphasic waveform looks like a regular heart rhythm. A flatter line with lengthening, called *monophasic*, indicates more severe disease. Pressures also can be obtained for ABIs.

Duplex imaging: Uses ultrasound and Doppler to assess arterial flow and velocity.

Pulse-volume recording: BP cuffs are placed over the thighs, calves, or feet to obtain pulse-volume recordings and pulse waveforms.

Exercise testing: Determines the amount of exercise that precipitates claudication.

Angiography of peripheral vasculature: Locates obstruction(s) and reveals the extent of vascular lesions by injecting dye into arteries and taking pictures of the arteries in a timed sequence. This imaging study is most used when angioplasty or stenting is planned.

Digital subtraction angiography: Arteriogram in which the computer subtracts early images from late images, deleting bone and soft tissue, so that only contrast-filled arteries appear.

Magnetic resonance imaging: Demonstrates vessels in multiple projections and can be used with or without contrast. It is used widely but is more expensive and not suitable for all patients. Implanted metal (e.g., pacemakers, automatic defibrillators) and prosthetic joint replacements preclude this study from being performed.

Nursing Diagnosis:

Impaired Tissue Integrity

related to altered arterial circulation occurring with atherosclerotic process

Desired Outcome: Over a period of days or weeks, the patient's lower extremity circulation improves and perfusion is maximized as evidenced by palpable pulses, decreased leg pain, and improvement in mobility and sensation.

ASSESSMENT/INTERVENTIONS	RATIONALES
Assess legs, feet, and between the toes for ulcerations.	Ulcerations can occur with decreased arterial circulation. A decrease in circulation significantly decreases oxygen delivery to the tissues and subsequently impairs healing of even the most minor break in the skin. A baseline assessment enables timely interventions.
Teach the importance of walking and range-of-motion (ROM) exercises for the hip, knee, and ankle.	Walking is the best activity and patients can be instructed to walk until they have pain, rest until recovery, and then resume walking. Walking and exercise improve collateral circulation. This is especially useful for patients who claudicate, along with other risk factor modifications. Activity may be contraindicated for some patients with severe disease.
Determine the allowed activity and exercise with the health care team, and discuss this with the patient.	Exercise promotes circulation. **Note:** Bedrest without exercise may be prescribed in acute, severe cases to decrease oxygen demand to the tissues, which optimally will decrease pain.
⚠ Teach the patient how to assess peripheral pulses, warmth, sensation, and color of the lower extremities (LE). Encourage daily foot inspections by the patient or family members if the patient's vision or assessment ability is compromised.	Monitoring status of the LE is essential for early identification of breaks in skin integrity, because early identification and care may prevent serious problems.
⚠ Encourage cessation of smoking and other tobacco use. Provide smoking and tobacco cessation literature. Discuss with the health care provider use of medication for smoking cessation.	Stopping tobacco use helps prevent increased vasoconstriction and severity of the circulation deficit, as well as the effects of nicotine on the lungs and other body organs.
Discuss the importance of keeping the feet warm and protected by wearing socks when walking or in bed.	Decreased circulation because of vasoconstriction results in decreased blood flow to the LE, which promotes hypothermia. Keeping warm promotes vasodilatation and a more optimal blood supply.
⚠ Caution the patient about using heating pads.	Heating pads increase metabolism and may promote ischemia if circulation is limited. Also, the patient's sensitivity to temperature is often decreased and burns may result.
Discuss the importance of nightlights being placed in bedrooms and bathrooms.	Nightlights promote visibility and may help avoid tissue trauma at night when getting up.
Caution the patient to avoid pressure over areas of bony prominence.	Pressure increases the risk of skin breakdown; areas over bony prominence are particularly susceptible.
Caution the patient to cover all exposed areas when going outside in cooler weather.	This action helps prevent hypothermia, to which patients with decreased circulation may be susceptible. Cold temperatures cause vasoconstriction, which further results in decreased tissue perfusion.

Nursing Diagnosis:

Chronic Pain

related to reduced circulation and ischemia

Desired Outcome: Over several days or weeks, following nonsurgical interventions to improve perfusion, the patient's pain decreases as documented by pain scale.

ASSESSMENT/INTERVENTIONS	RATIONALES
Assess for the presence of pain on initial contact and periodically throughout care, using a pain scale from 0 (no pain) to 10 (worst pain).	This assessment helps determine the degree and trend of pain.
Administer pain medications as prescribed.	Usually mild analgesics are given to reduce pain. Opioids may be given for perioperative pain. Opioids may not be effective in some patients for rest pain, and must be used cautiously in older adults.
Document pain relief obtained using the pain scale.	This documentation helps determine effectiveness of the medication.
Teach the patient to rest when claudication (severe, cramping pain) occurs. If claudication occurs at rest, encourage the patient to position legs so that they are dependent, and ensure warmth with socks and blankets, as appropriate.	Intermittent claudication from activity is relieved by rest. Claudication at rest implies severe circulatory compromise; measures such as leg dependency and warmth may reduce pain.
Explore alternative methods of pain relief, such as visualization, guided imagery, biofeedback, meditation, relaxation exercises, or music.	Because the pain may be chronic and continuous, pain relief should be augmented with nonpharmacologic methods, which do not have side effects.
Institute measures to improve circulation, such as dependence of extremities, ensuring warmth, walking, and use of medications (see **Impaired Tissue Integrity,** p. 141) as directed by the health care provider.	These measures increase circulation to ischemic extremities, which optimally will increase the patient's comfort level.

Nursing Diagnosis:

Deficient Knowledge

related to unfamiliarity with the potential for infection and impaired tissue integrity caused by decreased arterial circulation

Desired Outcome: Following teaching, the patient verbalizes knowledge about the potential for infection and impaired tissue integrity, as well as measures to prevent these problems.

ASSESSMENT/INTERVENTIONS	RATIONALES
Assess the patient's health care literacy (language, reading, comprehension). Assess culture and culturally specific information needs.	This assessment helps ensure that information is selected and presented in a manner that is culturally and educationally appropriate.
Teach how to assess for signs of infection or breaks in skin integrity, and to report significant findings to the health care provider.	This information facilitates understanding of symptoms that occur with infection or impaired skin integrity and describes symptoms that should be reported for timely intervention. This includes any new or enlarging wound or ulceration, redness, swelling, increased pain, or drainage.
Caution about the increased potential for easily traumatizing skin (e.g., from bumping lower extremities).	Decreased circulation in the legs diminishes the healing process after tissue trauma.
Instruct the patient to inspect both feet each day for any open wounds or bruises. If necessary, suggest the use of a long-handled mirror to see bottoms of the feet. Advise the patient to report any open areas to the health care provider.	Decreased circulation in the legs diminishes sensation, and therefore careful inspection is important to identify breaks in skin integrity. Open wounds can lead to infection, which should be reported promptly for timely intervention.
Stress the importance of wearing shoes or slippers that fit properly without areas of stress or friction.	Improper fit can lead to traumatized tissues. Bare feet in an individual with decreased sensation can lead to trauma.
Instruct the patient to cut toenails straight across or have them cut by a podiatrist.	Ingrown toenails can lead to infection.
Advise the patient to cover corns or calluses with pads.	Protection helps prevent further injury.

ASSESSMENT/INTERVENTIONS	RATIONALES
Encourage the patient to keep feet clean and dry, using mild soap and warm water for cleansing, and apply a mild lotion.	This promotes hygiene and prevents dryness, which could result in skin breakdown that could lead to infection.
Advise the patient not to scratch the feet.	Abrasions can easily become infected.
Advise keeping the feet warm with warm soaks and loose-fitting socks.	Decreased circulation leaves patients vulnerable to hypothermia. Keeping warm promotes vasodilatation and increased blood supply to the area.
Caution the patient to check temperature of warm soaks and bath water carefully with an elbow prior to stepping into the water.	Water temperature exceeding comfort can cause burns in an individual whose temperature sensitivity is decreased. Bath water should feel lukewarm to the elbow (a sensitive way to test water temperature).

Nursing Diagnosis:

Ineffective Peripheral Tissue Perfusion (or risk for same)

related to decreased arterial flow occurring with atherosclerosis or to acute occlusion occurring with a postsurgical graft embolus

Desired Outcome: Optimally, following interventions, the patient has adequate peripheral perfusion as evidenced by BP within 15-20 mm Hg of baseline BP and absence of the six Ps in the involved extremities: pain, pallor, pulselessness, paresthesia, poikilothermia (coolness), and paralysis.

ASSESSMENT/INTERVENTIONS	RATIONALES
Assess peripheral pulses and the involved extremity for the six Ps. Report significant findings.	Sensory changes usually precede other symptoms of ischemia, (i.e., pain, loss of two-point discrimination, and paresthesia). Such findings should be reported promptly for timely intervention. **Note:** Some health care centers document pulses as A (absent), D (requires Doppler), W (weak), N (normal), or B (bounding).
Administer the following medications as prescribed:	Use these medications for the following reasons:
- Antiplatelet agents (e.g., aspirin, clopidogrel, or ticlopidine)	- Help prevent platelet adherence and thromboembolism.
- Anticoagulants (e.g., heparin, low–molecular weight heparin, or warfarin)	- May be used in the postoperative period to prevent thrombus formation.
- Thrombolytics (e.g., urokinase or tissue plasminogen activator)	- May be used to lyse clot formation if an embolus or thrombus is present.
- Blood viscosity–reducing/antiplatelet agent (e.g., pentoxifylline or cilostazol)	- May increase flexibility of erythrocytes, thereby enhancing their movement through the microcirculation and preventing aggregation of red blood cells and platelets. This therapy has the potential to increase circulation at the capillary level and reduce or alleviate symptoms caused by lack of blood flow.
- Lipid-lowering agents (e.g., lovastatin, atorvastatin, simvastatin, and pravastatin)	- Reduce serum cholesterol levels and decrease inflammation in vessel walls.
- Antihypertensive agents (e.g., angiotensin-converting enzyme inhibitors, beta-blockers, diuretics, or calcium channel blockers)	- Decrease systolic and diastolic blood pressures, which is important in patients with peripheral arterial disease. Increased BP promotes further arterial wall damage, plaque formation, and rupture.

continued

PART I: Medical-Surgical Nursing

ASSESSMENT/INTERVENTIONS	RATIONALES
Explain the surgical intervention if one is planned.	For patients who have tissue loss, rest pain, or disabling claudication, surgical intervention may be necessary to open the occluded vessel or bypass the vessel to improve distal circulation.
- Endarterectomy	Endarterectomy involves removal of the atheromatous obstruction via arterial incision.
- Distal revascularization	Revascularization bypasses the obstructed segment by suturing an autogenous vein or graft proximally and distally to the obstruction.
- Percutaneous transluminal angioplasty (PTA or PTLA)	A balloon-tipped catheter is inserted through the artery to the area of occlusion. The balloon is gradually inflated to ablate the obstruction.
- Stent	During an arteriogram, a hollow tube is positioned and deployed within a stenosed vessel to stretch and improve blood flow. Combined with angioplasty, a stent may provide longer patency of the vessel.
If necessary, use a Doppler ultrasonic probe to check pulses, holding the probe to the skin at a 45-degree angle to the blood vessel. Record the presence or absence of pulsations, as well as rate, character, frequency, and intensity of sounds.	Doppler probes are capable of evaluating the amount of blood flow in arteries in which pulses are difficult to palpate. Optimally, pulsatile blood flow will be heard. In the presence of normal blood flow, wavelike, whooshing sounds will be heard.
[!] Protect legs and feet from pressure or damage.	Decreased LE sensation increases risk of injury. Foam protectors, special mattresses, cotton socks, and blankets are useful.
Monitor BP. Report to the health care provider any significant increase or decrease greater than 15-20 mm Hg, or as directed.	BP is another indicator of peripheral perfusion pressure. An increase in BP may interrupt the surgical site; decreased BP may cause graft occlusion.
[!] For the first 48-72 hr after surgery (or as directed), prevent acute joint flexion in the presence of a graft.	Joint flexion can impede blood flow and perfusion. Mild foot elevation or light Ace-wrapping may help ease hyperemia of the extremity.
In the absence of acute cardiac or renal failure, encourage adequate fluid intake.	Adequate fluid intake enhances perfusion; inadequate fluid intake can lead to dehydration and poor perfusion.

ADDITIONAL NURSING DIAGNOSES/PROBLEMS:

"Perioperative Care"   p. 45

PATIENT-FAMILY TEACHING AND DISCHARGE PLANNING

When providing patient-family teaching, focus on sensory information, avoid giving excessive information, and initiate a visiting nurse referral for necessary follow-up teaching. Include verbal and written information about the following:

✓ Progressive exercise program as prescribed by the health care team; importance of rest periods if claudication occurs.

✓ Meticulous, routine skin and foot care.

✓ Medications, including drug name, purpose, dosage, schedule, precautions, and potential side effects. Also discuss drug-drug, food-drug, and herb-drug interactions.

✓ Referral to a smoking/tobacco cessation program if appropriate.

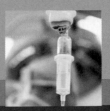

Cardiac and Noncardiac Shock (Circulatory Failure) 17

OVERVIEW/PATHOPHYSIOLOGY

Shock occurs when tissue perfusion is severely decreased, causing cellular metabolic dysfunction. Shock is classified according to the causative event.

Hypovolemic shock: Occurs when volume in the intravascular space is severely decreased and the metabolic needs of tissues cannot be met, as with severe hemorrhage or dehydration.

Cardiogenic shock: Occurs when cardiac pump failure results in decreased cardiac output, resulting in decreased systemic perfusion, as with severe myocardial infarction.

Distributive shock conditions: Characterized by a significant decrease in vascular volume. The three types are neurogenic shock, anaphylactic shock, and septic shock.

Neurogenic shock occurs when a neurologic event (e.g., spinal cord injury) causes loss of sympathetic tone, resulting in massive vasodilation and decreased perfusion pressures.

Anaphylactic shock is caused by a severe systemic response to an allergen (foreign protein), resulting in massive vasodilation, increased capillary permeability, decreased perfusion, decreased venous return, and subsequent decreased cardiac output.

Septic shock occurs when bacterial toxins cause an overwhelming systemic infection, resulting in severe hypotension and decreased cardiac output.

Regardless of the cause, shock results in cellular hypoxia secondary to decreased perfusion and ultimately in cellular, tissue, and organ dysfunction. A prolonged shock state can result in death; therefore early recognition and intervention are essential.

HEALTH CARE SETTING

Critical care unit (e.g., cardiogenic shock in coronary care unit; distributive shock in medical intensive care unit [ICU])

ASSESSMENT

Early signs and symptoms: Cool, pale, and clammy skin; decreased pulse strength; dry and pale mucous membranes; restlessness; change in level of consciousness; hyperventilation; anxiety; nausea; thirst; weakness.

Physical assessment: Rapid heart rate (HR); decreased systolic blood pressure (SBP) and increased diastolic blood pressure (DBP) secondary to catecholamine (sympathetic nervous system [SNS]) response.

Late signs and symptoms: Decreased urinary output, hypothermia, drowsiness, diaphoresis, confusion, and lethargy, all of which can progress to a comatose state.

Physical assessment: Thready, rapid HR; low or decreasing blood pressure (BP), usually with SBP less than 90 mm Hg; rapid and possibly irregular respiratory rate (RR).

DIAGNOSTIC TESTS

Diagnosis is usually based on presenting symptoms and clinical signs.

Arterial blood gas (ABG) values: May reveal metabolic acidosis or respiratory alkalosis (bicarbonate [HCO_3^-] less than 22 mEq/L and pH less than 7.40) caused by anaerobic metabolism.

Serial measurement of urinary output: Less than 30 mL/hr (0.5 mL/kg/hr) indicates decreased perfusion and decreased renal function.

Blood urea nitrogen (BUN) and creatinine: Increase with decreased renal perfusion.

Serum electrolyte levels: Identify renal complications and metabolic dysfunction as evidenced by hyperlactatemia and elevated levels of electrolytes.

Cultures of blood, sputum, wound, and urine: To identify the causative organism in septic shock.

White blood cell (WBC) count: Extremely elevated in septic shock due to infection. Increased eosinophils may be present in anaphylactic shock.

Complete blood count (CBC): Hematocrit (Hct) and hemoglobin (Hgb) may be increased in severe dehydration or decreased in the presence of hemorrhage.

Nursing Diagnoses:

Risk for Ineffective Peripheral Tissue Perfusion
Risk for Decreased Cardiac Tissue Perfusion
Risk for Ineffective Cerebral Tissue Perfusion
Risk for Ineffective Renal Perfusion
Risk for Electrolyte Imbalance

related to decreased circulating blood volume occurring with shock

Desired Outcome: Within 1-2 hr of treatment, the patient has adequate perfusion as evidenced by peripheral pulse amplitude more than 2+ on a 0-4+ scale; brisk capillary refill (less than 2 sec); SBP greater than 90 mm Hg; SaO_2 greater than 92%; mean arterial pressure (MAP) 70-100 mm Hg; HR regular and 100 bpm or less; no significant change in mental status; orientation to person, place, and time; normalized electrolytes; and urine output at least 30 mL/hr (0.5 mL/kg/hr).

ASSESSMENT/INTERVENTIONS	RATIONALES
Assess and document peripheral perfusion status. Report significant findings.	Significant findings include coolness and pallor of the extremities, decreased amplitude of pulses, and delayed capillary refill. Ineffective peripheral perfusion is an early sign of decreased cardiac output and shock and necessitates prompt intervention.
Assess BP and indicators of hypotension at frequent intervals. Notify the health provider promptly of significant findings.	Indicators of hypotension include decreased SBP of greater than 20 mm Hg below the patient's normal range, dizziness, altered mentation, and decreased urinary output. Immediate intervention is necessary to avoid irreversible organ damage due to poor perfusion.
If severe hypotension is present, place the patient in a supine position.	This position promotes venous return. BP must be at least 80/60 mm Hg for adequate coronary and renal artery perfusion.
Assess for restlessness, confusion, mental status changes, and decreased level of consciousness (LOC). If these indicators occur, intervene to keep the patient safe from harm; reorient as indicated.	These are indicators of ineffective cerebral perfusion/cerebral hypoxia. Patients with mental status changes due to poor cerebral perfusion are at risk of falling or making inappropriate decisions regarding mobility (e.g., getting out of bed without assistance).
Monitor for the presence of chest pain and an irregular HR. Report significant findings.	These are indicators of decreased coronary artery perfusion. Decreased coronary artery perfusion necessitates prompt intervention to prevent ischemia.
Monitor urinary output hourly and check weight daily; notify the health care provider of significant findings, including urine output less than 30 mL/hr (0.5 mL/kg/hr) in the presence of adequate intake and/or weight gain.	Decreased urinary output is a sign of decreased cardiac output and ineffective renal perfusion. Weight gain may be a sign of fluid retention, which can occur with ineffective renal perfusion.
Monitor laboratory results for elevated BUN and creatinine levels; report increases.	BUN more than 20 mg/dL and creatinine more than 1.5 mg/dL are signals of ineffective renal perfusion.
Monitor serum electrolyte values for evidence of imbalances, particularly of lactate, Na^+, and K^+. Assess for clinical signs of hyperkalemia, such as muscle weakness, hyporeflexia, and irregular HR, and for clinical signs of hypernatremia, such as fluid retention and edema. Notify the health care provider of significant findings.	Hyperlactatemia (more than 2-4 mmol/L), hypernatremia (Na^+ more than 147 mEq/L), and hyperkalemia (K^+ more than 5.0 mEq/L) may be signs of renal and metabolic complications of shock as a result of ineffective renal perfusion and the kidneys' inability to regulate lactate and electrolytes. Electrolyte imbalances and acidosis are life threatening and need immediate correction. Correction likely will include oxygen therapy, fluid resuscitation, and replacement or excretion of electrolytes.
Avoid use of sedatives or tranquilizers.	LOC can be altered by these medications, and tissue hypoperfusion makes absorption unpredictable.

ASSESSMENT/INTERVENTIONS	RATIONALES
Administer fluids and medications as prescribed and according to the type of shock, the patient's clinical situation, and hemodynamic interventions. See the following table.	Interventions are determined by the clinical presentation and severity of the shock state. Patients are transferred to ICU for invasive hemodynamic monitoring with pulmonary artery catheter and use of vasoactive intravenous (IV) drips to improve tissue perfusion.
⚠ Avoid rapid delivery of colloidal fluids in the treatment of hypovolemic shock.	Very rapid infusion of colloidal fluids may precipitate pulmonary edema.

Cardiogenic Shock

- Vascular support	To reduce cardiac workload.
- Intraaortic balloon counterpulsation	To augment perfusion pressures.
- Ventricular assist devices	To bypass or assist the ventricles, lowering myocardial oxygen requirements, reducing cardiac stress, and permitting cardiac muscle rest.
- Fluid administration or diuretics	To optimize blood volume. Fluids may be limited to prevent overload (the heart is not able to handle the volume already in the intravascular space), yet dehydration must be avoided. Decreasing preload (fluids) may be the treatment of choice to take the workload off the heart. An indwelling urinary catheter should be inserted for accurate output measurement.
- Inotropes (e.g., dopamine)	To increase cardiac contractility.
- Antidysrhythmics	To control rapid, irregular heart rate.
- Morphine	To reduce severe chest pain and reduce preload and afterload.
- Vasodilators (e.g., nitroprusside, nitroglycerin)	To increase peripheral perfusion and reduce afterload vasoconstriction caused by vasopressors.
- Osmotic diuretics	To increase renal blood flow.
- O_2 support	To increase oxygen availability to the tissues.

Anaphylactic Shock

- Epinephrine (0.5 mL, 1:1000 in 10 mL saline):	To promote vasoconstriction and decrease the allergic response by counteracting vasodilation caused by histamine release.
- Bronchodilators	To relieve bronchospasm.
- Antihistamines	To prevent relapse and relieve urticaria.
- Hydrocortisone	For its antiinflammatory effects.
- Vasopressors	May be necessary for reversing shock state.
- O_2 and airway support	To increase oxygen availability to the tissues.
- Albumin	Colloidal infusion to increase vascular volume.
- Ringer's solution	Isotonic solution to replace intravascular fluid, electrolytes, and ions. In shock states, fluid leaves the intravascular spaces.

Septic Shock

- Antibiotic therapy	Initial therapy is broad spectrum. Once the causative organism is identified, specific antibiotic therapy can be initiated.
- Fluid administration	To maintain adequate vascular volume.
- Vasoactive agents (e.g., norepinephrine, dopamine)	To reverse vasodilation and maintain perfusion.
- Positive inotropic medications (e.g., dopamine)	To augment cardiac contractility.

continued

PART I: Medical-Surgical Nursing

ASSESSMENT/INTERVENTIONS	RATIONALES
Hypovolemic Shock	
- Control of volume loss	Essential to decrease life-threatening complications and mortality.
- Blood transfusion	To increase O_2 delivery at the tissue level when more than 2 L of blood has been lost. Often a combination of packed red blood cells (RBCs) and a crystalloid solution is administered.
- Albumin	Colloidal infusion to increase vascular volume.
- Ringer's solution	Isotonic solution to replace fluids, electrolytes, and ions lost with bleeding.

Nursing Diagnosis:

Impaired Gas Exchange

related to altered oxygen supply occurring with decreased respiratory muscle function

Desired Outcome: Within 1-2 hr of intervention, the patient has adequate gas exchange as evidenced by SaO_2 greater than 92%; PaO_2 at least 80 mm Hg; $PaCO_2$ 45 mm Hg or less; pH at or near 7.35; presence of eupnea; and orientation to person, place, and time.

ASSESSMENT/INTERVENTIONS	RATIONALES
Monitor ABG results. Report significant findings.	The presence of hypoxemia (decreased PaO_2), hypercapnia (increased $PaCO_2$), acidosis (decreased pH, increased $PaCO_2$, and increased lactate levels) are signs of decreased gas exchange.
Monitor SaO_2. Report significant findings.	Readings of 92% or less are indicators of decreased oxygenation, and oxygen therapy likely will be required.
Assess respirations q30min; note and report presence of tachypnea or dyspnea.	Fast or labored breaths may signal respiratory distress and possibly respiratory failure. Tachypnea and dyspnea also may be signs of pain, anxiety, or infection and should be evaluated accordingly.
Assess for mental status changes, restlessness, irritability, and confusion.	Often these are symptoms of hypoxia.
Report significant findings.	Supplemental oxygen or other respiratory interventions likely will be required.
Teach the patient to breathe slowly and deeply in through the nose and out through the mouth.	These actions slow the respiratory cycle for better alveolar gas exchange.
Ensure the patient has a patent airway; suction secretions as needed.	This intervention promotes gas exchange.
Administer O_2 as prescribed; deliver O_2 with humidity.	These interventions increase oxygen supply and help prevent its convective drying effects on oral and nasal mucosa.

ADDITIONAL NURSING DIAGNOSES/PROBLEMS:

"Psychosocial Support"	p. 72
"Psychosocial Support for the Patient's Family and Significant Other"	p. 84

✓ PATIENT-FAMILY TEACHING AND DISCHARGE PLANNING

For interventions, see discussion of the patient's primary diagnosis.

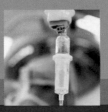

Cardiac Surgery 18

OVERVIEW/PATHOPHYSIOLOGY

Surgical intervention may be necessary to treat acquired or congenital heart disease. *Coronary artery bypass grafting (CABG)* is performed to treat blocked coronary arteries. A portion of the saphenous vein, internal mammary artery, gastroepiploic artery, or radial artery is excised and anastomosed to coronary arteries, revascularizing the affected myocardium. *Valve repair* or *replacement* is performed for patients with valvular stenosis or valvular incompetence of the mitral, tricuspid, pulmonary, or aortic valve. *Aortic surgery* may be done to remove or repair an aortic aneurysm. Other types of cardiac surgeries are performed to correct heart defects that are either acquired or congenital, such as ventricular aneurysm, ventricular or atrial septal defects, transposition of the great vessels, and tetralogy of Fallot. *Heart transplantation* may be considered for some patients diagnosed with end-stage cardiac disease; however, the national shortage of acceptable donor organs remains an obstacle. Some patients waiting for heart transplants may have a ventricular assist device placed to serve as a bridge until transplant. *Combined heart-lung transplantation* is performed for patients with end-stage disease affecting both organs.

Many patients undergoing cardiac surgery may have temporary epicardial pacing wires placed. These wires are placed on the heart at the time of surgery and pulled through the chest wall where they can be attached to a temporary pacemaker. They are used for temporary pacing postoperatively if needed. When no longer needed, they may be removed by nurses or other health care providers who have demonstrated technical proficiency.

HEALTH CARE SETTING

When the surgery is elective, patients are often admitted to the hospital on the day of surgery. However, many patients undergoing cardiac surgery may be in an emergent or urgent situation and may be directly admitted from an emergency room, clinic, or medical office.

During the perioperative period, many patients may need to be in a cardiac or intensive care unit (CCU/ICU) for monitoring and stabilization. When stable they may be transferred to a cardiac unit.

Nursing Diagnosis for Preoperative Patients:

Deficient Knowledge

related to unfamiliarity with the diagnosis, surgical procedure, preoperative routine, and postoperative course

Desired Outcome: Before surgery, the patient verbalizes knowledge about the diagnosis, surgical procedure, and preoperative and postoperative regimens.

ASSESSMENT/INTERVENTIONS	RATIONALES
Assess the patient's health care literacy (language, reading, comprehension). Assess culture and culturally specific information needs.	This assessment helps ensure that information is selected and presented in a manner that is culturally and educationally appropriate.
Assess the patient's level of knowledge about the diagnosis and surgical procedure, and provide information as necessary. Encourage questions, and allow time for verbalization of concerns and fears.	Knowledge level will vary from patient to patient. Some patients find detailed explanations helpful; others prefer brief and simple explanations. The amount of information given depends on learning needs and should be individualized.
When appropriate, provide orientation to the ICU and equipment that will be used postoperatively.	Familiarity with the unit and equipment optimally will promote understanding and minimize stress.

ASSESSMENT/INTERVENTIONS	RATIONALES
Provide instructions for and demonstrate deep breathing and coughing techniques; ask the patient to give a return demonstration.	Deep breathing and coughing are essential postoperative techniques that reinflate the lungs after heart-lung bypass and help prevent atelectasis and pneumonia.
Reassure the patient that postoperative pain will be managed with medication. Explain the types of medication administration available—i.e., epidural, patient-controlled analgesia (PCA), intermittent intravenous (IV), and by mouth (PO).	This information may aid in reducing anxiety about postoperative pain and increase understanding of the types of pain medications.
Advise the patient that in the immediate postoperative period, speaking will be impossible but that other means of communication (e.g., nodding, writing) will be available.	An endotracheal tube that will assist with breathing will prevent speech. Knowledge that alternative methods will be employed will reassure and help prepare patients.
Review and demonstrate sternal precautions.	Sternal precautions include how to get in and out of the bed and chair without using upper extremities; not lifting, pushing, or pulling more than 5-10 lb with each upper extremity for a period of 4-6 wk; and not driving a car for the same period of time.

Nursing Diagnosis:

Activity Intolerance

related to generalized weakness and bedrest following cardiac surgery

Desired Outcome: By a minimum of 24 hr before hospital discharge, the patient rates perceived exertion at 3 or less on a 0-10 scale and exhibits cardiac tolerance to activity after cardiac surgery as evidenced by heart rate (HR) 110 bpm or less, systolic blood pressure (SBP) within 20 mm Hg of resting SBP, and respiratory rate (RR) 20 breaths/min or less with normal depth and pattern (eupnea).

ASSESSMENT/INTERVENTIONS	RATIONALES
Assess vital signs at frequent intervals, and be alert to any changes. Notify the health care provider of significant findings, including a blood pressure (BP) change greater than 20 mm Hg.	Hypotension, tachycardia, crackles (rales), tachypnea, and diminished amplitude of peripheral pulses are signs of cardiac complications and should be reported promptly for timely intervention.
Ask the patient to rate perceived exertion (RPE) during activity, and monitor for evidence of activity intolerance. Notify the health care provider of significant findings.	An RPE greater than 3, along with cool, diaphoretic skin, is a signal to stop the activity and notify the health care provider. See Chapter 4, "Prolonged Bedrest," **Risk for Activity Intolerance,** p. 62, for a discussion of RPE.
Facilitate coordination of health care providers to provide rest periods between care activities and thus decrease cardiac workload.	Uninterrupted rest of at least 90 min helps decrease cardiac workload. An increased cardiac workload is likely if too many activities are performed without concomitant rest.
Assist with exercises, depending on tolerance and prescribed activity limitations. As prescribed, initiate physical therapy (PT) and/or cardiac rehabilitation.	Monitored exercise increases activity tolerance.
See Chapter 4, "Prolonged Bedrest," **Risk for Activity Intolerance,** p. 61, and **Risk for Disuse Syndrome,** p. 63, for a discussion of in-bed exercises.	

ADDITIONAL NURSING DIAGNOSES/PROBLEMS:

PATIENT-FAMILY TEACHING AND DISCHARGE PLANNING

When providing patient-family teaching, focus on sensory information, avoid giving excessive information, and initiate a visiting nurse referral for follow-up teaching. Include written information with verbal reinforcement and allow time for questions.

✓ Medications, including drug name, dosage, schedule, purpose, precautions, and potential side effects. Also discuss drug-drug, herb-drug, and food-drug interactions.

✓ Technique for assessing radial pulse, temperature, and weight, if these indicators require monitoring at home, and the importance of reporting significant changes to the health care provider.

✓ Signs and symptoms that necessitate immediate medical attention: chest pain, dyspnea, shortness of breath, weight gain, edema, inability to urinate, nausea, vomiting, and decrease in exercise tolerance.

✓ Care of incision site; importance of assessing for signs of infection, such as increased incisional pain, drainage, swelling, fever, persistent redness, and local warmth and tenderness.

✓ Symptoms requiring medical attention for patients taking warfarin, such as bleeding from the nose (epistaxis) or gums, hemoptysis, hematemesis, hematuria, melena, hematochezia, menometrorrhagia, and excessive bruising. In addition, stress the following: take warfarin at the same time every day, notify the health care provider if any signs of bleeding occur, avoid over-the-counter and herbal medications (e.g., aminosalicylates [ASAs], nonsteroidal antiinflammatory drugs [NSAIDs], garlic supplements, feverfew, ginkgo, sweet clover) unless approved by the health care provider, carry a medical alert bracelet or card, avoid constrictive or restrictive clothing, and use a soft-bristled toothbrush and electric razor.

✓ Importance of pacing activities at home and allowing frequent rest periods.

✓ Referral to a cardiac rehabilitation program.

✓ Activity restrictions (e.g., no heavy lifting, pushing, or pulling anything heavier than 5-10 lb with upper extremities for at least 4-6 wk); prescribed exercise program; and resumption of sexual activity, work, and driving a car, as directed.

✓ Maintenance of a low-sodium and low-cholesterol diet. Encourage patients to use food labels to determine sodium, fat, and cholesterol content of foods.

✓ Telephone number of the nurse and health care provider to discuss concerns and questions or clarify instructions.

✓ Importance of follow-up visits the with health care provider; confirm date and time of next appointment.

✓ Discussion of the patient's home environment and potential need for changes or adaptations (e.g., too many steps to climb, activities of daily living that are too strenuous).

✓ Introduction to local Heart Association activities. Provide the address or telephone number for the local chapter or encourage the patient to contact the following:

• American Heart Association at *www.americanheart.org*.

• For patients awaiting heart transplantation, as appropriate: The United Network for Organ Sharing at *www.unos.org*.

• The Heart and Stroke Foundation at *www.heartandstroke.com*.

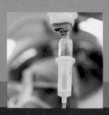

Coronary Artery Disease 19

OVERVIEW/PATHOPHYSIOLOGY

Coronary artery disease (CAD) is the leading cause of death in the United States, affecting more than 17 million Americans. The coronary arteries supply the myocardial muscle with oxygen and the nutrients necessary for optimal function. In CAD, the arteries are narrowed or obstructed, potentially resulting in cardiac muscle death. Atherosclerotic lesions, arterial spasm, platelet aggregation, and thrombus formation all may cause obstruction. The most common symptom of CAD is angina, affecting 50% of patients with this disease. Angina results from the decreased blood flow and insufficient oxygen supply to the heart muscle.

Acute coronary syndrome (ACS) refers to an imbalance between myocardial oxygen supply and demand secondary to an acute plaque disruption or erosion. ACS is an umbrella term that includes stable coronary artery disease (SCAD), unstable angina (USA), non–ST-elevation myocardial infarction (NSTEMI), and ST-segment elevation myocardial infarction (STEMI).

USA is defined as an increase in severity, frequency, or intensity of anginal pain or a new onset of rest angina, lasting more than 20 min. NSTEMI is defined by clinical presentation of chest pain with an elevation in cardiac biomarkers and electrocardiograph (ECG) changes that may include T-wave inversion or ST-segment depression but no ST-segment elevation. Diagnosis of STEMI is based on elevated cardiac biomarkers plus ST-segment elevation on ECG signifying ischemia. Of the three, STEMI is the most serious and life threatening.

Time is essential in diagnosing and treating patients with ACS. Patients presenting with a STEMI are high priority for intervention. An ECG is the primary assessment tool that guides the intervention strategy. Primary angioplasty is the therapy of choice for reperfusion in acute myocardial infarction (AMI). However, not all acute care hospitals in the United States can provide percutaneous coronary intervention (PCI). Because time is so critical in patients presenting with STEMI, a decision must be made by the health care provider to proceed with either fibrinolytic therapy or primary PCI within 10 min of presentation. The goal for door-to-needle time is within 30 min and door-to-balloon time within 60-90 min. Initiating thrombolysis within 70 min of symptom onset is key to reducing mortality and morbidity. If catheterization laboratory facilities for primary intervention are not available within this "golden hour," fibrinolytics are administered until transport can be arranged.

HEALTH CARE SETTING

Primary care, acute care, intensive/coronary care unit

ASSESSMENT

Signs and symptoms: Chest pain, substernal pressure and burning, and pain that radiates to the jaw, shoulder, or arm are the most common symptoms of ischemia. Weakness, diaphoresis, nausea, vomiting, shortness of breath, and acute anxiety also may occur. Heart rate (HR) may be abnormally slow (bradycardia), especially in right coronary artery (RCA) infarct, or it may be rapid (tachycardia). Stable or progressively worsening angina occurs when myocardial demand for O_2 is more than the supply, such as during exercise. Pain is often described as a feeling of pressure or as a crushing or burning substernal pain that radiates down one or both arms. It can be felt also in the neck, cheeks, and teeth. Usually anginal pain is relieved by discontinuation of exercise, rest, or administration of nitroglycerin (NTG).

Physical assessment: Anxiety, hypertension, tachycardia, tachypnea, and dynamic ECG changes are the most common symptoms of acute ischemia. Severe hypotension may occur in shock states. Temperature elevations can occur secondary to the inflammatory process. Intensity of S_1 and S_2 heart sounds may be decreased. Pulmonary congestion may occur if ventricular failure is present, and S_3 and S_4 sounds may be auscultated.

History and risk factors: Family history, increasing age, male gender, smoking, low high-density lipoprotein (HDL) values, hypercholesterolemia, diabetes mellitus, hypertension, and metabolic syndrome. Obesity, glucose intolerance, and a sedentary, stressful lifestyle also contribute to increased risk. Chest pain occurring with exertion is a warning sign of CAD.

DIAGNOSTIC TESTS

ECG: Reveals dynamic changes in the presence of ischemia. When the ECG is performed during chest pain, characteristic changes may include ST-segment elevation or depression greater than 0.05 mV in leads over the area of ischemia. The presence of a bundle branch block also can be determined on ECG as well as dysrhythmias. Serial ECGs are often done on patients with acute syndromes. As ischemia advances, the muscle does not transmit electrical impulses, and the ECG helps determine the area and extent of the infarct.

Cardiac biomarkers: Creatinine phosphokinase (CPK), CK-MB, and troponin I and T are proteins released in response to ischemia or MI. Elevations of these biomarkers usually occur 4-6 hr after ischemic damage. Serial tests q8h for 24 hr are recommended and help determine the extent of myocardial damage.

C-reactive protein: If elevated from the normal range of 0.03-1.1 mg/dL, this signals that coronary artery plaques are inflammatory and the patient is at higher risk of an acute coronary event.

Echocardiogram: Assesses ventricular function, chamber size, valvular function, ejection fraction, wall motion, and hemodynamic measurements. Heart muscle damage may alter ventricular function, wall motion, and hemodynamic pressures. A heart muscle that moves weakly may have been damaged during an acute ischemic attack, or it may be receiving too little oxygen.

Chest x-ray examination: Usually normal unless heart failure is present.

Total lipid panel: Obtained during the patient's evaluation and treatment to assess for hyperlipidemia, a risk factor in CAD. Low HDL (value less than 40 mg/dL) and high low-density lipoprotein (LDL) (value greater than 100 mg/dL) are linked to atherosclerotic heart disease. (Values may change in the presence of acute ischemia, and therefore are considered more valid when they are obtained before hospital discharge.)

Stress tests: Stress testing with concurrent imaging of the heart is the standard means of noninvasive cardiac evaluation. Stress tests are prescribed to assess coronary artery flow, valvular function, and wall motion abnormalities.

Exercise treadmill test: To determine the amount of exercise-induced ischemia, hemodynamic response, and ECG changes with exercise. Significant findings include 1 mm or more ST-segment depression or elevation, dysrhythmias, or a sudden decrease in blood pressure (BP).

Stress echocardiogram: Typically performed using either a treadmill or bicycle. Echocardiograms are obtained before and immediately after exercise. A stress-induced imbalance in the myocardial supply/demand ratio will produce myocardial ischemia and regional wall motion abnormality (the area of ischemia affects muscle contraction). Stress echocardiography is particularly useful for identifying CAD in patients with multivessel disease.

Stress echocardiogram: Dobutamine, adenosine, or dipyridamole is used as a stress agent with echocardiogram imaging for patients who cannot exercise.

Cardiac nuclear imaging modalities:
Myocardial perfusion imaging:
- Detection of CAD is found by differential blood flow through the left ventricular myocardium. Normal blood flow and normal tracer uptake are seen with unobstructed coronary arteries; diminished flow and diminished tracer uptake are found with coronary stenosis. An abnormality will be present in an area of myocardial infarction (MI) resulting from lack of blood flow.
- Commonly used radiopharmaceutical agents are thallium-201 and technetium-99m sestamibi. Dobutamine, adenosine, and dipyridamole are pharmacologic stress agents used in combination with a radiopharmaceutical agent if patients are unable to exercise or fail to reach 85% of age-predicted maximum HR.
- Single-photon emission computed tomography (SPECT) is used to develop three-dimensional views of cardiac processes and cellular level metabolism by viewing the heart from several different angles and using tomography methods to reconstruct the image. SPECT enables clearer resolution of myocardial ischemia and better quantification of cardiac damage.

Radionuclide angiography: Used to evaluate left and right ventricular ejection fraction (EF), left ventricular volume, and regional wall motion. The first-pass technique is a fast acquisition of myocardial images. Gated pool ejection or multiple-gated acquisition (MUGA) scan permits calculation of the amount of blood ejected with ventricular contraction and is used for risk stratification of patients after MI or with CAD.

CT: May be helpful in differentiating AMI from aortic dissection in patients with severe, tearing back pain and associated dyspnea and/or syncope.

Ambulatory monitoring: 24-hr ECG monitoring (Holter monitor) can show activity-induced ST-segment changes or ischemia-induced dysrhythmias.

Coronary arteriography via cardiac catheterization: The gold standard of diagnostic testing for CAD. Arterial lesions (plaque) are located and the amount of occlusion determined. During this test, feasibility for coronary artery bypass grafting (CABG) or percutaneous coronary intervention (PCI) is determined. For details, see **Chapter 18,** "Cardiac Surgery," p. 149.

Intravascular ultrasound: A flexible catheter with a miniature transducer at the tip is threaded to the coronary arteries to provide information on the interior of the coronary arteries. Ultrasound is used to create a cross-sectional image of the three layers of the arterial wall and its lumen to assess the degree of atherosclerosis.

Nursing Diagnosis:

Acute Pain (Angina)

related to decreased oxygen supply to the myocardium

Desired Outcomes: Within 30 min of onset of pain, the patient's subjective perception of angina decreases, as documented by a pain scale. Objective indicators, such as grimacing and diaphoresis, are absent or decreased.

ASSESSMENT/INTERVENTIONS	RATIONALES
Assess location, character, and severity of the pain. Record severity on a subjective 0 (no pain) to 10 (worst pain) scale.	This assessment monitors degree, character, precipitator, and trend of pain for the initial check and subsequent comparisons.
Assess HR and BP during episodes of chest pain. Be alert to and report significant findings.	Increases in HR and changes in systolic blood pressure (SBP) greater than 20 mm Hg from baseline signal increased myocardial O_2 demands and necessitate prompt medical intervention.
Administer O_2 as prescribed.	Hypoxia is common because of the decreased perfusion and adds stress to the compromised myocardium.
Deliver O_2 with humidity.	Humidity helps prevent oxygen's convective drying effects on oral and nasal mucosa.
Administer sublingual NTG at the onset of pain (if not on an IV NTG drip), and explain to the patient that it is to be administered as soon as angina begins, repeating q5min ×3 if necessary.	NTG increases microcirculation, perfusion to the myocardium, and venous dilation. Venous dilation causes pooling in the periphery so that less blood comes back to the right side of the heart, which in turn lowers O_2 demand.
Notify the health care provider of unrelieved pain.	If pain is unrelieved or returns very quickly, emergency medical treatment is advised.
As prescribed, increase intravenous (IV) NTG drip in increments of 10 mcg if pain persists, and continue to monitor SBP. Notify the health care provider if SBP is below 90 mm Hg, HR is less than 60, or RR is less than 10.	SBP should be maintained at 90 mm Hg or higher until pain is relieved to avoid worsening ischemia secondary to hypotension. NTG lowers BP.
As prescribed, add IV morphine sulfate in small increments (2 mg). Monitor HR, RR, and BP.	IV morphine sulfate is added in small increments to titrate for adequate pain relief. Morphine also decreases heart rate, BP, RR, and anxiety.
Obtain ECG as prescribed.	ECG patterns may reveal ischemia, as evidenced by dynamic ST- or T-wave changes, evidence of new Q waves, or left bundle branch block.
Stay with the patient and provide reassurance during periods of angina.	These measures reduce anxiety, which might otherwise worsen the angina.
Monitor for the presence of headache and hypotension after administering NTG.	These are side effects of NTG as a result of vasodilation.
Maintain the patient in a recumbent position with the head of bed (HOB) elevated no higher than 30 degrees during angina and NTG administration.	This position minimizes the potential for headache/hypotension by enabling better blood return to the heart and head.
Emphasize to the patient the importance of immediately reporting angina to the health care team.	Early treatment decreases morbidity and mortality.
Instruct the patient to avoid activities and factors known to cause stress.	Stress may precipitate angina.
Discuss the value of relaxation techniques, including tapes, soothing music, biofeedback, meditation, or yoga. See **Deficient Knowledge** (relaxation techniques) later.	Relaxation helps reduce stress and anxiety, which otherwise may precipitate angina.
Administer beta-blockers (e.g., metoprolol, atenolol, carvedilol) as prescribed.	These medications block beta stimulation to the sinoatrial (S-A) node and myocardium. HR, BP, and contractility are decreased, subsequently reducing workload of the heart and myocardial oxygen demand, ultimately improving myocardial oxygenation. Metoprolol may be administered IV as the initial treatment.

ASSESSMENT/INTERVENTIONS	RATIONALES
Administer long-acting nitrates (isosorbide preparations) and/or topical nitrates as prescribed.	Nitrates are given for anginal prophylaxis via vasodilation, lowering of BP, and decreasing O_2 demand.
Administer angiotensin-converting enzyme (ACE) inhibitor (e.g., enalapril, captopril, quinapril, ramipril) as prescribed.	ACE inhibitors reduce BP, down-regulate the renin-angiotensin-aldosterone system (RAAS), and improve long-term survival.
Administer calcium channel blockers (e.g., nifedipine, diltiazem) as prescribed.	Calcium channel blockers decrease coronary artery vasospasm, a potential cause of ischemia and subsequent angina. They also cause the vessels to dilate, increasing blood flow to the heart.
Administer aspirin as prescribed.	Aspirin reduces platelet aggregation, which helps prevent obstruction of the coronary arteries.
Administer antihyperlipidemic agents (e.g., atorvastatin, rosuvastatin) as prescribed.	These agents, also known as "statin" drugs, are used to reduce hyperlipidemia and can stabilize plaque.
Administer stool softeners as prescribed.	Straining at stool or constipation can increase myocardial work.

Nursing Diagnosis:

Activity Intolerance

related to generalized weakness and imbalance between oxygen supply and demand occurring with tissue ischemia secondary to MI.

Desired Outcome: During activity, the patient rates perceived exertion at 3 or less on a 0-10 scale and exhibits cardiac tolerance to activity as evidenced by respiratory rate (RR) 20 breaths/min or less, HR 120 bpm or less (or within 20 bpm of resting HR), SBP within 20 mm Hg of resting SBP, and absence of chest pain and new dysrhythmias.

ASSESSMENT/INTERVENTIONS	RATIONALES
Assess the frequency of angina, noting alleviating and precipitating factors. Observe whether angina occurs at rest and is relieved or unrelieved by NTG. Document accordingly.	This assessment detects evidence of imbalance between oxygen supply and demand and hence potential activity intolerance. The four classifications of angina are as follows: *Class I:* Angina occurs only with strenuous activity. *Class II:* Angina occurs with moderate activity such as walking quickly or climbing stairs, walking uphill, or walking at a normal pace more than two blocks or one flight of stairs. *Class III:* Angina occurs with mild activity such as climbing one flight of stairs or walking level for one to two blocks. *Class IV:* Angina occurs with any physical activity and may be present at rest.
Assess the patient's response to activity and report significant findings.	Chest pain, increase in HR (greater than 20 bpm), change in SBP (20 mm Hg over or under resting BP), excessive fatigue, and shortness of breath are signs of activity intolerance that should be reported promptly for timely intervention.
Ask the patient to rate perceived exertion (RPE). See "Prolonged Bedrest," Risk for Activity Intolerance, p. 62, for details.	RPE higher than 3 is a signal to stop the activity.
Help the patient recognize and limit activities that increase O_2 demands, such as exercise and anxiety.	This information helps patients recognize and attempt to control factors that increase ischemia.
Administer O_2 as prescribed for angina episodes.	This measure increases oxygen supply to the myocardium.
Deliver O_2 with humidity.	Humidity helps prevent oxygen's convective drying effects on oral and nasal mucosa.
Have the patient perform range-of-motion (ROM) exercises, depending on tolerance and prescribed activity limitations.	Cardiac intolerance to activity can be further aggravated by prolonged bedrest.

continued

ASSESSMENT/INTERVENTIONS	RATIONALES
Consult the health care provider about in-bed exercises and activities that can be performed by the patient as the condition improves.	This intervention enables progressive pacing toward the patient's optimal activity potential. In addition, the cardiac rehabilitation department should be consulted for early and progressive activity.
For further interventions, see "Prolonged Bedrest," **Risk for Activity Intolerance,** p. 61, and **Risk for Disuse Syndrome,** p. 63.	

Nursing Diagnosis:

Imbalanced Nutrition: More Than Body Requirements

related to excessive intake of calories, sodium, or fats

Desired Outcome: Within the 24-hr period before hospital discharge, the patient demonstrates knowledge of the dietary regimen by planning a 3-day menu that includes and excludes appropriate foods.

ASSESSMENT/INTERVENTIONS	RATIONALES
Assess body weight and body mass index (BMI). If the patient is over ideal body weight, discuss benefits of weight loss.	Being overweight is a risk factor for CAD and puts more workload on the heart.
Discuss ways to decrease dietary intake of saturated (animal) fats and increase intake of polyunsaturated (vegetable oil) fats.	Reducing dietary saturated fat is effective in lowering the risk of heart and blood vessel disease in many individuals.
Teach the patient to limit dietary intake of cholesterol to less than 300 mg/day. Encourage use of food labels to determine cholesterol content of foods.	Reducing cholesterol intake is effective in lowering the risk of heart and blood vessel disease in many individuals.
Teach the patient to limit dietary intake of refined/processed sugar.	Refined sugars are empty calories that can convert to fat stores.
Teach the patient to limit dietary intake of sodium chloride (NaCl) to less than 4 g/day (mild restriction). Encourage reading food labels to determine sodium content of foods.	Increased sodium intake can lead to water retention, which increases vascular volume and cardiac workload.
Instruct the patient and significant other in use of "Nutrition Facts" (federally mandated public information on all food product labels).	This information reveals the amount of calories, total fat, saturated fat, cholesterol, and sodium in foods. Patients should be especially aware of the serving size listed for respective nutrients. (A serving size listed as 4 oz on a package containing 12 oz would mean patients would get 3 times the amount of each ingredient if they eat the entire contents of the container!)
Encourage intake of fresh fruits, natural (unrefined or unprocessed) carbohydrates, fish, poultry, legumes, fresh vegetables, and grains.	These food groups ensure a healthy, balanced diet.

Nursing Diagnosis:

Deficient Knowledge

related to unfamiliarity with the purpose, precautions, and side effects of nitrates

Desired Outcome: Within the 24-hr period before hospital discharge, the patient verbalizes understanding of the purpose, precautions, and side effects of nitrates.

PART I: Medical-Surgical Nursing

ASSESSMENT/INTERVENTIONS	RATIONALES
Assess the patient's health care literacy (language, reading, comprehension). Assess culture and culturally specific information needs.	This assessment helps ensure that information is selected and presented in a manner that is culturally and educationally appropriate.
Teach the purpose of the prescribed nitrate (isosorbide, NTG).	These medications are given during angina to increase microcirculation, venous dilation, and blood to the myocardium, which should decrease angina. A patient who is knowledgeable about the purpose of this drug will be more likely to adhere to the therapeutic regimen.
Instruct the patient to report to the health care provider or staff the presence of a headache associated with nitrates.	The vasodilation effect of nitrates can result in transient headaches, in which case the health care provider may alter the dose of the isosorbide. Tylenol may be recommended for treatment of headaches if not contraindicated.
Teach the patient to assume a recumbent position with HOB slightly elevated if a headache occurs.	This position may reduce pain by enabling better blood return to the heart and head.
Instruct the patient to rise slowly from a sitting or lying position and to remain by the chair or bed for 1 min after standing to ensure he or she is not going to experience orthostatic changes.	Vasodilation from nitrates also may decrease BP, which can result in orthostatic hypotension and injury to the patient.

Nursing Diagnosis:

Deficient Knowledge

related to unfamiliarity with the purpose, precautions, and side effects of beta-blockers

Desired Outcome: Within the 24-hr period before hospital discharge, the patient verbalizes understanding of the purpose, precautions, and side effects of beta-blockers.

ASSESSMENT/INTERVENTIONS	RATIONALES
Assess the patient's readiness and ability to learn.	This assessment helps ensure that information is selected and presented at a time and in a manner that is appropriate for the patient.
Teach the purpose of beta-blockers.	Patients who are knowledgeable about the purpose of this medication will be more likely to adhere to therapy. These medications block beta stimulation to the S-A node and myocardium. HR and contractility are decreased, subsequently decreasing workload of the heart. As well, they decrease myocardial oxygen demand, thereby improving myocardial oxygenation.
Instruct the patient to be alert to depression, fatigue, dizziness, erythematous rash, respiratory distress, and sexual dysfunction. Explain the importance of notifying the health care provider promptly if these side effects occur.	Side effects may discourage patients from continuing taking the medication.
Explain that BP and HR are assessed before administration of beta-blockers.	These medications can cause hypotension and excessive slowing of the heart.
Caution the patient not to omit or abruptly stop taking beta-blockers.	Stopping this medication abruptly may result in rebound tachycardia, potentially causing angina or MI.

Nursing Diagnosis:

Deficient Knowledge

related to unfamiliarity with drug-drug and herb-drug precautions and adverse effects

Desired Outcome: Within the 24-hr period before hospital discharge, the patient verbalizes understanding of the potential drug-drug and herb-drug precautions and adverse effects.

ASSESSMENT/INTERVENTIONS	RATIONALES
Ascertain any herbs currently being taken.	Determining current herb usage will guide the teaching plan.
Plan a teaching strategy to include precautions and adverse effects of potential drug-drug and herb-drug interactions.	Patients who are knowledgeable about the precautions and adverse effects of herb to drug interactions may avoid adverse effects.
Instruct the patient to be alert to adverse signs such as bleeding with excessive garlic intake or garlic supplements when taking anticoagulant or antiplatelet drugs.	Because risk of bleeding in persons using anticoagulant or antiplatelet agents increases, concomitant use with garlic should be avoided. Garlic supplements should be discontinued about 10 days before elective surgical procedures, especially by patients taking aspirin or warfarin.
Caution the patient to avoid use of ginseng.	Ginseng can cause hypertension.
Caution the patient to avoid taking St. John's wort while taking cardiac medications.	Coadministration of this herb with antiarrhythmics, beta blockers, and calcium channel blockers may result in reduced medication bioavailability and effectiveness with subsequent recurrence of dysrhythmias, hypertension, or other undesirable effects.
Caution the patient to avoid grapefruit when taking statin medications.	Grapefruit contains a compound that interacts with enzymes needed to metabolize statins, resulting in their accumulation. Accumulation of statins can cause liver or kidney failure.

Nursing Diagnosis:

Deficient Knowledge

related to unfamiliarity with the disease process and lifestyle implications of CAD

Desired Outcome: Within the 24-hr period before hospital discharge, the patient verbalizes knowledge about the disease process of CAD and concomitant lifestyle implications.

ASSESSMENT/INTERVENTIONS	RATIONALES
Teach the patient about CAD, including pathophysiologic processes of cardiac ischemia, angina, and infarction.	Increasing patients' knowledge of their health status optimally will promote adherence to the treatment regimen.
Assist with identifying risk factors for CAD and risk factor modification.	Risk factor identification optimally will result in risk factor modification, including: - Diet low in cholesterol and saturated fat - Smoking cessation - Regular activity/exercise program - Weight loss (if appropriate)
Discuss symptoms that necessitate medical attention.	Progression to unstable angina, loss of consciousness, decreased exercise tolerance, angina unrelieved by NTG, increasing frequency of angina, and need to increase the number of NTG tablets to relieve angina are symptoms that necessitate medical attention to prevent MI.
Discuss guidelines for sexual activity.	Drugs for erectile dysfunction (e.g., Viagra, Cialis, Levitra) cannot be taken simultaneously with NTG because this may cause a sudden drop in BP. Resting before intercourse, finding a comfortable position, taking prophylactic NTG, and postponing intercourse for 1-1½ hr after a heavy meal are valid guidelines that help minimize oxygen demand on the heart.
Discuss the rationale for antihyperlipidemic therapy, which may include the following:	
- HMG-CoA reductase inhibitors (e.g., lovastatin, simvastatin, fluvastatin, pravastatin, atorvastatin)	These agents inhibit the enzyme involved in early cholesterol formation, thereby reducing total cholesterol levels, including LDL and triglycerides, while increasing HDL.
- Nicotinic acid (niacin)	This vitamin lowers triglyceride and LDL levels while raising HDL levels.

ASSESSMENT/INTERVENTIONS	RATIONALES
- Fibric acid derivatives (e.g., gemfibrozil, fenofibrate)	These agents lower triglycerides and raise HDL.
- Bile acid sequestrant resins (e.g., cholestyramine, colestipol)	These agents bind with bile acids in the intestine and remove LDL and cholesterol from the blood.
Discuss procedures such as cardiac catheterization, PCI, and CABG, if appropriate.	PCI is a procedure that improves coronary blood flow by using a balloon inflation catheter to rupture plaque and dilate the artery. It is performed in the cardiac catheterization laboratory under local anesthesia and with mild sedation, enabling patients to be awake and interact with the health care team. PCI is a common alternative to bypass surgery for individuals with discrete lesions. Balloon angioplasty traditionally is followed by stent placement. Following the procedure, patients routinely are placed on antiplatelet agents (e.g., ASA and Plavix) to reduce risk of in-stent restenosis post PCI. Additionally, drug-eluting stents further reduce risk of restenosis. An antirestenotic medication contained within the polymer of these stents is released over a period of time to modify the healing response that would result in restenosis. Complications of PCI include bleeding, acute in-stent thrombosis, vascular injury, infection, MI, stroke, contrast-induced nephropathy, allergic reaction to medications or contrast, and death. Cardiac catheterization is discussed later in this section, and CABG is discussed in Chapter 18, "Cardiac Surgery," p. 149.

Nursing Diagnosis:

Deficient Knowledge

related to unfamiliarity with relaxation techniques effective for stress reduction

Desired Outcome: The patient reports subjective relief of stress after using a relaxation technique.

ASSESSMENT/INTERVENTIONS	RATIONALES
Assess the patient's stress level. Discuss the importance of relaxation for patients with CAD if appropriate.	Relaxation decreases nervous system tone (sympathetic), energy requirements, and O₂ consumption. Knowledgeable patients are more likely to adhere to techniques that promote relaxation.
Introduce methods of relaxation, such as music, imagery, massage, art therapy, biofeedback.	Relaxation methods may decrease energy requirements.
Encourage the patient to practice relaxation techniques whenever feeling stressed or tense.	These techniques can become part of the patient's lifestyle, reducing stress on a daily level.

Nursing diagnoses for patients undergoing cardiac catheterization procedure:

Nursing Diagnosis:

Deficient Knowledge

related to unfamiliarity with the catheterization procedure and postcatheterization regimen

Desired Outcome: Before the procedure, the patient verbalizes knowledge about cardiac catheterization and the postcatheterization plan of care.

ASSESSMENT/INTERVENTIONS	RATIONALES
Assess the patient's health care literacy (language, reading, comprehension). Assess culture and culturally specific information needs.	This assessment helps ensure that information is selected and presented in a manner that is culturally and educationally appropriate.
Assess the patient's knowledge about the catheterization procedure. As appropriate, reinforce the health care provider's explanation, and answer any questions or concerns. Describe the catheterization lab and sensations the patient may experience.	Knowledge about the procedure and what to expect may help reduce anxiety.
Before cardiac catheterization, have the patient practice techniques that will be used during the procedure.	Valsalva's maneuver, coughing, and deep breathing may be required during the cardiac catheterization, and many people are unfamiliar with the proper technique.
Explain that a "flushing" feeling may occur when dye in initially injected.	Dye injection causes vasodilation, which often induces flushing.
Explain the postcatheterization regimen and caution that flexing the insertion site is contraindicated, often for 4-6 hr postprocedure.	After the procedure bedrest will be required and vital signs, circulation, and the insertion site will be checked at frequent intervals to ensure integrity. Flexing the insertion site (arm or groin) is contraindicated to prevent bleeding.
⚠ Stress the importance of promptly reporting signs and symptoms of concern.	Groin, leg, or back pain; dizziness; chest pain; or shortness of breath may signal hemorrhage or embolization of the stent. Prompt reporting enables rapid intervention.

Nursing Diagnosis:

Risk for Decreased Cardiac Tissue Perfusion

related to interrupted arterial flow occurring with the cardiac catheterization procedure

Desired Outcome: Within 1 hr after the procedure, the patient has adequate perfusion as evidenced by HR regular and within 20 bpm of baseline HR; apical/radial pulse equality; BP within 20 mm Hg of baseline BP; peripheral pulse amplitude greater than 2+ on a 0-4+ scale; warmth and normal color in the extremities; no significant change in mental status; and orientation to person, place, and time.

ASSESSMENT/INTERVENTIONS	RATIONALES
Assess BP q15min until stable on 3 successive checks, q2h for the next 12 hr, and q4h for 24 hr unless otherwise indicated.	These assessments monitor BP trend.
Note: If the insertion site was the antecubital space, measure BP in the unaffected arm.	This measure prevents bleeding or blood vessel injury.
If the femoral artery was the insertion site, maintain HOB at no greater than a 30-degree elevation.	This measure prevents acute hip joint flexion, which could compromise arterial flow.
⚠ If the SBP drops 20 mm Hg or more below previous recordings, lower the HOB and notify the health care provider.	A drop in BP could signify acute bleeding or shock. Lowering the HOB aids perfusion to the heart and brain.
⚠ Assess HR, and notify the health care provider if dysrhythmias occur. If the patient is not on a cardiac monitor, auscultate apical and radial pulses with every BP check, and report irregularities or apical/radial discrepancies.	Dysrhythmias and apical/radial discrepancies may be signs of cardiac ischemia.
⚠ Be alert to and report cool extremities, decreased amplitude of peripheral pulses, cyanosis, changes in mental status, decreased level of consciousness, and shortness of breath.	These are indicators of decreased perfusion.

Nursing Diagnoses:

Risk for Bleeding
Risk for Deficient Fluid Volume

related to the potential for hemorrhage caused by arterial puncture and/or osmotic diuresis caused by the contrast dye

Desired Outcomes: The patient remains normovolemic as evidenced by HR 100 bpm or less; BP 90/60 mm Hg or greater (or within 20 mm Hg of baseline range); no significant change in mental status; and orientation to person, place, and time. The dressing is dry, and there is no swelling at the puncture site.

ASSESSMENT/INTERVENTIONS	RATIONALES
⚠ Assess vital signs and promptly report a decrease in BP, increase in HR, and decreasing level of consciousness (LOC).	These are indicators of hemorrhage and/or shock. Rapid reporting enables prompt intervention.
⚠ Inspect the dressing on the groin or antecubital space at frequent intervals, and report significant findings.	This measure detects presence of frank bleeding or hematoma formation (fluctuating swelling), which would necessitate prompt intervention.
⚠ Assess for and report diminished amplitude or absence of distal pulses, delayed capillary refill, coolness of the extremities, and pallor.	These signs of decreased peripheral perfusion may signal embolization or hemorrhagic shock.
Caution the patient about flexing the elbow or hip more than 30 degrees for 6-8 hr, or as prescribed.	These restrictions minimize risk of bleeding and circulation compromise.
If bleeding occurs, maintain pressure at the insertion site as prescribed, usually 1 inch proximal to the puncture site or introducer insertion site.	Pressure stabilizes bleeding. Typically this is done with a pressure dressing or a 2- to 5-lb sandbag.

Nursing Diagnosis:

Risk for Ineffective Peripheral Tissue Perfusion

related to interrupted arterial flow in the involved limb occurring with embolization

Desired Outcome: Within 1-2 hr following intervention, the patient has adequate perfusion in the involved limb as evidenced by peripheral pulse amplitude greater than 2+ on a 0-4+ scale; normal color, sensation, and temperature; and brisk capillary refill (less than 2 sec).

ASSESSMENT/INTERVENTIONS	RATIONALES
⚠ Assess peripheral perfusion by palpating peripheral pulses q15min for 30 min, then q30min for 1 hr, then hourly for 2 hr, or per protocol.	Prompt recognition of a diminished or absent pulse is essential to prevent limb damage.
⚠ Be alert to and report faintness or absence of pulse; coolness of the extremity; mottling; decreased capillary refill; cyanosis; and complaints of numbness, tingling, and pain at the insertion site. Instruct the patient to report any of these indicators promptly.	These are signs of embolization in the involved limb. Prompt recognition will result in rapid intervention.
If there is no evidence of an embolus or thrombus formation, instruct the patient to move the fingers or toes and rotate the wrist or ankle.	These measures promote circulation in the involved limbs.
Ensure that the patient maintains bedrest for 4-6 hr or as prescribed.	Bedrest or immobility enables the puncture site to stabilize, thereby avoiding bleeding.

PART I: Medical-Surgical Nursing

Nursing Diagnosis:

Risk for Ineffective Renal Perfusion

related to interrupted blood flow occurring with decreased cardiac output or reaction to contrast dye

Desired Outcome: The patient has adequate renal perfusion as evidenced by a stable blood urea nitrogen (BUN)/creatinine, urinary output of at least 30 mL/hr (0.5 mL/kg/hr), specific gravity less than 1.030, good skin turgor, and moist mucous membranes.

ASSESSMENT/INTERVENTIONS	RATIONALES
Assess for indicators of dehydration, such as poor skin turgor, dry mucous membranes, and high urine specific gravity (1.030 or more).	Contrast dye for cardiac catheterization may cause osmotic diuresis.
Assess intake and output.	This assessment determines if urine output is sufficient.
⚠ Notify the health care provider if urinary output is less than 30 mL/hr (0.5 mL/kg/hr) in the presence of adequate intake.	A fall in urinary output is a sign of dehydration or renal insufficiency.
⚠ Monitor BUN and creatinine daily.	A rise in these renal markers may signify renal insufficiency or acute renal failure. See Appendix B, "Laboratory Tests Discussed in This Manual: Normal Values," p. 754, for optimal values.
If urinary output is insufficient despite adequate intake, restrict fluids.	This measure helps prevent fluid overload.
⚠ Be alert to and report crackles (rales) on auscultation of lung fields, distended neck veins, and shortness of breath; notify the health care provider about significant findings.	These signs are other indicators of fluid overload. Prompt detection and reporting enable rapid intervention.
If the patient does not exhibit signs of cardiac or renal failure, encourage daily intake of 2-3 L of fluids or as prescribed.	Increasing hydration helps flush contrast dye out of the system more quickly.

ADDITIONAL NURSING DIAGNOSES/PROBLEMS:

PATIENT-FAMILY TEACHING AND DISCHARGE PLANNING

When providing patient-family teaching, focus on sensory information, avoid giving excessive information, and initiate a visiting nurse referral for necessary follow-up teaching. Include verbal and written information about the following:

✓ Signs and symptoms necessitating immediate medical attention, including chest pain unrelieved by NTG, decreased exercise tolerance, increasing shortness of breath, increased leg edema or pain (postcatheterization), and loss of consciousness.

✓ Importance of reporting to the health care provider any change in pattern or frequency of angina.

✓ Importance of follow-up with the health care provider; confirm date and time of next appointment.

✓ Importance of getting BP checked at regular intervals (at least monthly if the patient is hypertensive).

✓ Pulse monitoring: how to self-measure pulse, including parameters for target heart rates and limits.

✓ Avoiding strenuous activity for at least 1 hr after meals to help prevent excessive O₂ demands.

✓ Medications, including drug name, dosage, purpose, schedule, precautions, and potential side effects. Also discuss drug-drug, food-drug, and herb-drug interactions (see appropriate Deficient Knowledge). Explain the potential for headache and dizziness after NTG administration. Caution the patient about using NTG more frequently than prescribed and notifying the health care provider if three tablets do not relieve angina.

✓ Importance of reducing or eliminating intake of caffeine, which causes vasoconstriction and increases HR.

✓ Dietary changes: low saturated fat, low sodium, low cholesterol, and need for weight loss if appropriate. Encourage use of food labels to determine caloric, cholesterol, fat, and sodium content of foods.

✓ Prescribed exercise program and importance of maintaining a regular exercise schedule, with referral to a cardiac rehabilitation program, in which individualized exercise programs are outlined for the patient.

✓ Practice of stress reduction techniques.

✓ Elimination of smoking and tobacco use. Refer patient to a "stop smoking" program as appropriate. The following Internet resources support and describe methods and reasons to advise patients to stop smoking:

- *http://smokefree.gov/*
- *http://www.cancer.gov/cancertopics/tobacco/smoking*
- Importance of involvement and support of significant others in patient's lifestyle changes.
- Availability of community and medical support, such as American Heart Association at *www.americanheart .org.*
- The Heart and Stroke Foundation at *www .heartandstroke.com.*

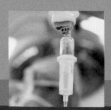

Dysrhythmias and Conduction Disturbances 20

OVERVIEW/PATHOPHYSIOLOGY

Dysrhythmias are abnormal rhythms of the heart caused by conditions that alter electrical conduction. Dysrhythmias originate in different areas of the conduction system, such as the sinus node, atrium, atrioventricular (A-V) node, His-Purkinje system, bundle branches, and ventricular tissue. Many conditions and diseases may cause dysrhythmias; the most common are coronary artery disease (CAD) and myocardial infarction (MI). Other causes include fluid and electrolyte imbalance, hormonal imbalance, changes in oxygenation, medications, and drug toxicity. Cardiac dysrhythmias may result from the following mechanisms:

Disturbances in automaticity: May involve an increase or decrease in automaticity in the sinus node (e.g., sinus tachycardia or sinus bradycardia). Premature beats may arise from the atria, A-V junction, or ventricles. Abnormal rhythms, such as atrial or ventricular tachycardia, also may occur.

Disturbances in conductivity: Conduction may be too rapid, as in conditions caused by an accessory pathway (e.g., Wolff-Parkinson-White syndrome), or too slow (e.g., A-V block). Reentry occurs when a stimulus reexcites a conduction pathway through which it already has passed. Once started, this impulse may circulate repeatedly. For reentry to occur, there must be two different pathways for conduction: one with slowed conduction and one with unidirectional block.

Combinations of altered automaticity and conductivity: Several dysrhythmias occur together, for example, a first-degree A-V block (disturbance in conductivity) and premature atrial contractions (disturbance in automaticity).

HEALTH CARE SETTING

Primary care, acute care, and intensive/coronary care unit (ICU/CCU)

ASSESSMENT

Signs and symptoms: Can vary from absence of symptoms to complete cardiopulmonary collapse. General indicators include alterations in level of consciousness (LOC), vertigo, syncope, seizures, weakness, fatigue, activity intolerance, shortness of breath, dyspnea on exertion, chest pain, palpitations, sensation of "skipped beats," anxiety, and restlessness.

Physical assessment: Increases or decreases in heart rate (HR), blood pressure (BP), and respiration rate (RR); changes in heart rhythm; dusky color or pallor; crackles (rales); cool skin; decreased urine output; weakened and paradoxical pulse; and abnormal heart sounds (e.g., paradoxical splitting of S_1 and S_2).

Electrocardiogram (ECG) results: Changes with dysrhythmias include abnormalities in rate, such as sinus bradycardia or sinus tachycardia, irregular rhythm such as atrial fibrillation, extra beats such as premature atrial contractions (PACs) and premature junctional contractions (PJCs), wide and bizarre-looking beats such as premature ventricular contractions (PVCs) and ventricular tachycardia (VT), a fibrillating baseline such as ventricular fibrillation (VF), and a straight line as with asystole.

History and risk factors: CAD, recent MI, electrolyte disturbances, substance abuse, drug toxicity, obesity, diabetes mellitus, obstructive sleep apnea, advanced age, genetic factors, thyroid problems, certain medications and supplements, and hypertension.

DIAGNOSTIC TESTS

12-lead ECG: To detect dysrhythmias and identify possible origin.

Serum electrolyte levels: To identify electrolyte abnormalities that can precipitate dysrhythmias. The most common are potassium and magnesium abnormalities.

Drug levels: To identify toxicities (e.g., of digoxin, quinidine, procainamide, aminophylline) that can precipitate dysrhythmias, or to determine substance abuse that can affect heart rate and rhythm, such as cocaine.

Ambulatory monitoring (e.g., Holter monitor or cardiac event recorder): To identify subtle dysrhythmias, associate abnormal rhythms by means of patient's symptoms, and assess response to exercise.

Electrophysiology study: Invasive test in which two to three catheters are placed into the heart, giving it a pacing stimulus at varying sites and of varying voltages. The test determines origin of dysrhythmia, inducibility, and effectiveness of drug therapy in dysrhythmia suppression.

Exercise stress testing: Used in conjunction with Holter monitoring to detect advanced grades of PVCs (those caused by ischemia) and to guide therapy. During the test, ECG and BP readings are taken while the patient walks on a treadmill or pedals a stationary bicycle; response to a constant or increasing workload is observed. The test continues until the patient reaches target heart rate or symptoms such as chest pain, severe fatigue, dysrhythmias, or abnormal BP occur.

Oximetry or ABG values: To document trend of hypoxemia.

Nursing Diagnosis:

Decreased Cardiac Output

related to altered rate, rhythm, or conduction or to negative inotropic changes

Desired Outcome: Within 1 hr of treatment/intervention, the patient has improved cardiac output as evidenced by BP 90/60 mm Hg or higher, HR 60-100 bpm, and normal sinus rhythm on ECG.

ASSESSMENT/INTERVENTIONS	RATIONALES
Assess the patient's heart rhythm continuously on a monitor.	This assessment will reveal whether dysrhythmias occur or increase in occurrence.
Assess BP and symptoms when dysrhythmias occur.	Signs of decreased cardiac output include decreased BP and symptoms such as unrelieved and prolonged palpitations, chest pain, shortness of breath, weakened and rapid pulse (more than 150 bpm), sensation of skipped beats, dizziness, and syncope.
Report significant findings to the health care provider.	Decreased cardiac output should be reported promptly for timely intervention, because it may be life threatening.
If symptoms of decreased cardiac output occur, prepare to transfer the patient to intensive care.	Transfer to a specialized intensive care unit for continual monitoring is essential.
Document dysrhythmias with a rhythm strip, using a 12-lead ECG as necessary.	This assessment will identify dysrhythmias and their general trend.
Monitor the patient's laboratory data, particularly electrolyte and digoxin levels.	Serum potassium levels less than 3.5 mEq/L or more than 5.0 mEq/L can cause dysrhythmias. Digoxin toxicity may cause heart block or dysrhythmias.
Administer antidysrhythmic agents as prescribed; note patient's response to therapy based on action of the following classifications:	
Class IA: sodium channel blockers: quinidine, procainamide, disopyramide	Decrease depolarization moderately and prolong repolarization.
Class IB: sodium channel blockers: phenytoin, mexiletine, tocainide	Decrease depolarization and shorten repolarization.
Class IC: sodium channel blockers: encainide, flecainide, propafenone	Significantly decrease depolarization with minimal effect on repolarization.
Class II: beta-blockers: propranolol, metoprolol, atenolol, acebutolol	Slow sinus automaticity, slow conduction via A-V node, control ventricular response to supraventricular tachycardias, and shorten the action potential of Purkinje fibers.
Class III: potassium channel blockers: amiodarone, sotalol, ibutilide, dofetilide	Increase the action potential and refractory period of Purkinje fibers, increase ventricular fibrillation threshold, restore injured myocardial cell electrophysiology toward normal, and suppress reentrant dysrhythmias.
Class IV: calcium channel blockers: verapamil, diltiazem, nifedipine	Depress automaticity in the sinoatrial (S-A) and A-V nodes, block the slow calcium current in the A-V junctional tissue, reduce conduction via the A-V node, and are useful in treating tachydysrhythmias because of A-V junction reentry. This class of drugs also vasodilates.
Monitor corrected QT interval (QTc) when initiating drugs known to cause QT prolongation (e.g., sotalol, propafenone, dofetilide, flecainide).	When QTc is prolonged, it can increase risk of dysrhythmias. QTc equals QT (in seconds) divided by the square root of the R-to-R interval (in seconds).
Provide humidified O_2 as prescribed.	O_2 may be beneficial if dysrhythmias are related to ischemia or are causing hypoxia. Humidity helps prevent oxygen's drying effects on oral and nasal mucosa.
Maintain a quiet environment, and administer pain medications promptly.	Both stress and pain can increase sympathetic tone and cause dysrhythmias.

continued

PART I: Medical-Surgical Nursing

ASSESSMENT/INTERVENTIONS	RATIONALES
If life-threatening dysrhythmias occur, initiate emergency procedures and cardiopulmonary resuscitation (as indicated by advanced cardiac life support [ACLS] protocol).	This action provides circulation to vital organs and restores the heart to normal or viable rhythm.
When dysrhythmias occur, stay with the patient; provide support and reassurance while performing assessments and administering treatment.	This action reduces stress and provides comfort, which optimally will decrease dysrhythmias.

Nursing Diagnosis:

Deficient Knowledge

related to unfamiliarity with the mechanism by which dysrhythmias occur and lifestyle implications

Desired Outcome: Within the 24-hr period before hospital discharge, the patient and significant other verbalize knowledge about causes of dysrhythmias and implications for the patient's lifestyle modifications.

ASSESSMENT/INTERVENTIONS	RATIONALES
Assess the patient's health care literacy (language, reading, comprehension). Assess culture and culturally specific information needs.	This assessment helps ensure that information is selected and presented in a manner that is culturally and educationally appropriate.
Discuss causal mechanisms for dysrhythmias, including resulting symptoms. Use a heart model or diagrams as necessary.	This information increases the patient's knowledge about health status. Visual aids augment understanding of verbal information. A knowledgeable patient is more likely to adhere to the therapeutic regimen.
Teach signs and symptoms of dysrhythmias that necessitate medical attention.	Indicators such as unrelieved and prolonged palpitations, chest pain, shortness of breath, rapid pulse (more than 120 bpm), dizziness, and syncope are serious and should be reported promptly for timely intervention.
Teach the patient and significant other how to check pulse rate for a full minute.	Checking the pulse rate for a full minute ensures a better average of rate and rhythm than if it were measured for 15 seconds and multiplied by 4.
Teach about medications that will be taken after hospital discharge, including drug name, purpose, dosage, schedule, precautions, and potential side effects. Also discuss drug-drug, food-drug, and herb-drug interactions. See **Decreased Cardiac Output,** earlier, for a description of these medications and their actions.	The more knowledgeable the patient is, the more likely he or she is to adhere to therapy and report side effects and complications promptly for timely intervention.
Stress that the patient will be taking long-term antidysrhythmic therapy and that it could be life threatening to stop or skip these medications without health care provider involvement.	Stopping or skipping these drugs may decrease blood levels effective for dysrhythmia suppression.
Advise about the availability of support groups and counseling; provide appropriate community referrals. Explain that anxiety and fear, along with periodic feelings of denial, depression, anger, and confusion, are normal following this experience.	Patients who survive sudden cardiac arrest may experience nightmares or other sleep disturbances at home.
Stress the importance of leading a normal and productive life. If the patient is going on vacation, advise taking along sufficient medication and investigating health care facilities in the vacation area.	This concept may be difficult to implement for patients who fear breakthrough of life-threatening dysrhythmias and alter their lives accordingly.
Advise the patient and significant other to take cardiopulmonary resuscitation classes; provide addresses for community programs.	Emergency life-saving procedures may be necessary in the future.

ASSESSMENT/INTERVENTIONS	RATIONALES
Teach the importance of follow-up care; confirm date and time of the next appointment if known. Explain that outpatient Holter monitoring is performed periodically.	Medical follow-up is important for ongoing assessment and management of cardiac dysrhythmias.
Explain dietary restrictions that individuals with recurrent dysrhythmias should follow. Discuss need for reduced intake of products containing caffeine, including coffee, tea, chocolate, and colas.	Caffeine is a stimulant that can cause abnormal heart rhythms.
Provide instruction for a general low-cholesterol diet. Encourage reading of food labels to determine cholesterol content of foods.	There is an overlap between dysrhythmias and CAD, often necessitating a low-cholesterol diet that decreases hyperlipidemia.
As indicated, teach relaxation techniques.	Such techniques enable patients to reduce stress and decrease sympathetic tone. In some types of dysrhythmias, stress can increase incidence of occurrence.

If the Patient Has Had an Implantable Cardioverter-Defibrillator (ICD) Inserted or Is Wearing a Defibrillator Life Vest, Teach the Following:

- The device is programmed to deliver the electrical stimulus at a predetermined rate and/or after assessing morphology of the ECG. (First- and second-generation ICDs provide for only cardioversion or defibrillation; third-generation ICDs also provide overdrive pacing and backup ventricular pacing).	Implantable or portable defibrillators are recommended for patients who have survived an episode of sudden cardiac death (cardiac arrest), patients with CAD who have had a cardiac arrest, and those in whom conventional antidysrhythmic therapy has failed.
- The ICD will have a pulse generator.	The pulse generator is powered by lithium batteries and surgically inserted (in the operating room [OR] or catheterization laboratory) into a "pocket" formed in the pectoral area. Leads are tunneled beneath the skin from the pocket to the subclavian vein through which they are advanced to the right ventricle.
[!] - Postoperative complications include atelectasis, pneumonia, seroma at the generator "pocket," pneumothorax, and thrombosis. Lead migration and lead fracture are the two most common structural problems. Interference from unipolar pacemakers and "myopotentials" (electrical interference) are common mechanical complications.	Patients should be informed of these complications and structural problems in order to report them promptly for timely intervention.
[!] - Some procedures interfere with and may change programming of the device. In addition, the ICD may "see" these procedures as a dysrhythmia and shock the patient.	ICDs may need to be deactivated during surgical procedures, use of electrocautery, and magnetic resonance imaging.
- Patients should keep a pocket card on hand with all relevant ICD data on it.	This card ensures that medical information is available at all times in case a medical event occurs.
Explain the importance of follow-up care; confirm date and time of the next appointment if known.	Follow-up care helps ensure proper functioning of the device.
Explain that home monitoring using the telephone also may be indicated and will need further instruction.	Home monitoring is an efficient and easy method of monitoring the device for many patients.
If indicated, teach about left ventricular aneurysmectomy and infarctectomy.	Surgical excision of possible focal spots of ventricular dysrhythmias may be indicated, depending on etiology and severity of the disease.

✓ **PATIENT-FAMILY TEACHING AND DISCHARGE PLANNING**

See the patient's primary diagnosis.

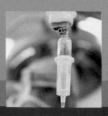

Heart Failure 21

OVERVIEW/PATHOPHYSIOLOGY

Heart failure (HF) is a complex clinical syndrome in which the heart is unable to pump sufficient blood to meet the body's metabolic demands. It is caused by structural or functional cardiac disorders that impair the ventricle's ability to fill with or eject blood. HF is a chronic condition that is prone to acute exacerbations (termed *acute decompensated heart failure* [ADHF]). In most cases of ADHF, severe volume overload and pulmonary edema are present. HF usually results from either systolic or diastolic cardiac dysfunction or a combination of both.

Systolic dysfunction: Ventricular dilation and impaired ventricular contraction are caused by myocardial muscle injury or abnormality (see dilated cardiomyopathy, below). The initial injury or stressor to the heart muscle results in impaired cardiac output. This triggers a cascade of compensatory mechanisms, which together contribute to the development and progression of HF.

Increased neurohormonal activation: Activation of the sympathetic nervous system (SNS) and renin-angiotensin system (RAS) stimulates catecholamines and other neurohormones, causing increases in heart rate (HR) and blood pressure (BP), systemic vasoconstriction, decreased renal perfusion, and sodium and fluid retention in an effort to increase cardiac output.

Hemodynamic alterations: Increase in left ventricular end-diastolic volume/pressure (preload) and thickening and elongation of the myofibrils (stretch) initially result in increased force of contraction (Frank-Starling law). The rise in myocardial oxygen demand further stimulates the neurohormonal response. Increases in preload and afterload (because of increased systemic resistance) add to left ventricular workload and cause excessive "stretch" of the myofibrils, thereby impairing ventricular contraction.

Remodeling: The neurohormonal and hemodynamic responses eventually cause hypertrophy (enlargement and thickening of the left ventricular [LV] wall). The heart becomes more spherical (dilated) because of lengthening of the myofibrils, cell slippage, fibrosis, and myocyte death. These progressive changes in size, shape, and structure of the heart muscle are termed *remodeling*.

The structural, hemodynamic, and neurohormonal alterations cause progressive deterioration in systolic function associated with decreased left ventricular ejection fraction (LVEF), increased intracardiac pressures, impaired valvular function, decreased forward flow to vital organs and tissues, and increased pulmonary pressures. This results in pulmonary (left-sided failure) and hepatic (right-sided failure) congestion, edema, renal impairment, and impaired oxygenation and metabolism. Ventricular and atrial dysrhythmias are common because of structural changes to the myocytes and increased myocardial oxygen demand, contributing to a major cause of mortality for persons with heart failure.

Diastolic dysfunction: The ventricle becomes noncompliant and unable to accommodate increased preload and afterload (or decreased preload). Symptoms of HF may occur because of volume overload without a reduction in systolic function as seen in individuals with long-standing hypertension, coronary artery disease (CAD), and hypertrophic and restrictive cardiomyopathies (see below).

Cardiomyopathies: HF commonly occurs in the presence of an underlying cardiomyopathy (disorder of the heart muscle). Cardiomyopathies are classified according to the cause and abnormality in structure and function.

- *Dilated cardiomyopathy (DCM):* The most prevalent type characterized by enlargement of one (usually left) or both ventricles and impaired contraction (systolic dysfunction). The most common form is ischemic cardiomyopathy caused by severe coronary (ischemic) heart disease and/or myocardial infarction. DCM also occurs secondary to hypertension, valvular heart disease, diabetes mellitus (DM), cardiotoxins, genetic causes, and metabolic, infectious, or systemic diseases. DCM is termed *idiopathic* when the cause cannot be identified. See "Systolic dysfunction," earlier, for additional information.

- *Hypertrophic cardiomyopathy:* Characterized by an abnormally enlarged left ventricle but without a concomitant increase in cavity size. Filling is restricted and may be associated with left ventricular outflow tract obstruction. Cardiac function can remain normal for varying periods before decompensation occurs. Symptoms include HF symptoms, chest pain, palpitations, dizziness, near-syncope, or syncope. Ventricular dysrhythmias may occur. Hypertrophic cardiomyopathy may have a hereditary link. Often etiology is not known.

- *Restrictive cardiomyopathy:* Least common in Western countries, it is characterized by inadequate compliance causing restriction of diastolic filling.

Other causes of heart failure

Acute HF and pulmonary edema can occur secondary to other conditions that place excessive demands on cardiac output, such as hypertensive crisis, tachycardia due to hyperthyroidism, severe anemia, valvular insufficiency, congenital heart defects, dysrhythmias, cardiomyopathy, myocarditis, trauma, infection, volume overload (i.e., caused by intravenous [IV] fluids, postoperative fluid shifts), pregnancy, and conditions that affect capillary permeability. In these cases, treatment of the underlying cause is essential and may result in normalization or improvement of cardiac function.

Severe pulmonary diseases, including chronic obstructive pulmonary disease (COPD), pulmonary hypertension, and obstructive sleep apnea (OSA), can lead to diastolic HF (cor pulmonale). This is less likely to be reversible. Poorly compensated pulmonary disease, upper respiratory infection, and pneumonia can exacerbate all types of HF and need to be treated aggressively.

HEALTH CARE SETTING

Primary care with possible hospitalization, including intensive care unit (ICU), resulting from complications

ASSESSMENT

General

Signs and symptoms: Dyspnea on exertion (DOE) or at rest, fatigue, decreased exercise tolerance, weakness, orthopnea (unable to lie flat; may need to sleep on pillows or sitting in a chair), paroxysmal nocturnal dyspnea, wheezing, cough, cyanosis, irregular or rapid HR, sudden weight gain from fluid retention, lower extremity edema, abdominal distention, nausea, early satiety, and nocturia. Associated indicators include chest/anginal pains, palpitations, near-syncope, and syncope. *Low-output symptoms* include positional lightheadedness, weakness, mental status changes, and decreased urine output.

Physical assessment: Decreased or elevated blood pressure (BP), dysrhythmias, tachycardia, tachypnea, increased venous pulsations, pulsus alternans (alternating strong and weak heartbeats), increased central venous pressure (CVP), jugular venous distention, crackles (rales), wheezes, decreased breath sounds, cardiac gallop and/or murmur, hepatomegaly, ascites, and pitting edema in dependent areas (lower extremities, sacrum).

History/risk factors: CAD, hypertension, DM, OSA or other pulmonary disease, recent IV fluid infusions, surgery, pregnancy, recent/current infectious illness, pneumonia, nonadherence to medication or diet regimen, obesity, hypercholesterolemia, and recent nonsteroidal antiinflammatory drug or COX-2 inhibitor use. In addition, see "Other causes of heart failure," earlier.

Acute decompensated heart failure

Signs and symptoms: Typified by marked severity of HF symptoms and deterioration of one or more New York Heart Association (NYHA) functional classes. Pulmonary edema and cardiogenic shock (see p. 145) may be present and, in more severe cases, renal dysfunction.

Acute pulmonary edema

Signs and symptoms: Extreme dyspnea, anxiety, restlessness, frothy and blood-tinged sputum, severe orthopnea, and paroxysmal nocturnal dyspnea. Patient exhibits "air hunger" and may thrash about and describe a sensation of drowning.

Physical assessment: Crackles (rales), wheezing, decreased breath sounds, increased BP, tachycardia, tachypnea, engorged neck veins, cool and clammy skin, and cardiac gallop/murmur.

DIAGNOSTIC TESTS

Chest x-ray examination: May show cardiomegaly, engorged pulmonary vasculature, "Kerley-B lines" suggestive of HF, and pleural or pericardial effusions.

Electrocardiogram (ECG): Changes may indicate CAD, acute myocardial ischemia, left ventricular hypertrophy (widened QRS), conduction defects, and dysrhythmias.

Left ventricular ejection fraction: The percentage of blood ejected from the left ventricle during systole. Normal LVEF is 50%-70%. In systolic dysfunction, it is reduced. LVEF less than 35% is associated with increased risk for mortality-related HF and dysrhythmias. In hypertrophic cardiomyopathy, LVEF may be greater than 70%. LVEF assessment can be measured during echocardiogram, magnetic resonance imaging (MRI), or radionuclide studies (multiple-gated acquisition scan, nuclear stress test [see below]).

Echocardiography: The most commonly used method of evaluating ventricular function. It assesses left- and right-sided systolic function, LVEF, degree of ventricular dilation, wall thickness, abnormal wall and septal motion, valvular function, estimated pulmonary pressure, presence of thrombus, restrictive outflow, and pericardial effusion. Diastolic dysfunction may be evident. Tissue Doppler/three-dimensional echocardiography may reveal the degree of ventricular synchrony and utility of cardiac resynchronization therapy.

Cardiac catheterization: Determines ischemic heart disease and assesses hemodynamics (left- and right-sided filling pressures, cardiac output, and systemic and pulmonary vascular resistance).

Left ventriculography: Evaluates LV function and LVEF.

Endomyocardial biopsy: Performed during right heart catheterization. It is usually done for severe, refractory HF in nonelderly patients to help identify pathologic agent and reversible causes, or in posttransplant patients.

Radionuclide stress test, stress echocardiogram: To assess for underlying ischemic heart disease and reversible or fixed ischemic defects.

Pulmonary function tests: Useful in differentiating causes of shortness of breath and other HF symptoms. Pulmonary function tests (PFTs) may reveal underlying COPD or reactive airways disease (asthma).

Oximetry/arterial blood gas (ABG) values: Measure oxygen levels in the blood. ABGs assess oxygen, carbon dioxide, bicarbonate, and pH levels. Hypoxemia and metabolic/respiratory acidosis often occur in acute myocardial ischemia, cardiac arrest, and severe HF. Overnight (sleep) oximetry evaluates obstructive sleep apnea.

Serum blood urea nitrogen (BUN), creatinine: Elevated in renal insufficiency and chronic kidney disease. It may be elevated in poor renal perfusion associated with low cardiac output and hypotension. Treatment with diuretics, angiotensin-converting enzyme (ACE) inhibitors, angiotensin receptor blockers (ARBs), or aldosterone antagonists also affects these renal markers.

Serum electrolytes: Altered in multiple cardiac and renal conditions/diseases. Careful monitoring is essential to avoid cardiac arrest due to dysrhythmias caused by alterations in potassium, magnesium, calcium, sodium, and phosphorous.

Cardiac enzymes: Mild elevation in cardiac troponins (with normal creatinine kinase [CK]) is common in patients with chronic HF or chronic kidney disease. Cardiac troponin and enzyme elevation indicate myocardial ischemia.

Liver function tests, including serum aspartate aminotransferase and serum bilirubin: May be elevated in patients with hepatic congestion.

Brain natriuretic peptide (BNP): Released from the ventricles in response to wall stress. This test is useful in differentiating HF from other causes of dyspnea, including pulmonary disease. Negative BNP (less than 100 pg/mL) suggests non-HF etiology. When used in conjunction with standard clinical assessment, elevated BNP may support diagnosis of HF and evaluate the patient's response to treatment.

Digoxin level: The goal in patients with HF is a level less than 1.0 ng/mL. Hypokalemia and impaired renal function can predispose patients to digoxin toxicity.

Complete blood count (CBC): May reveal decreased hemoglobin (Hgb) and hematocrit (Hct) in the presence of anemia.

Thyroid-stimulating hormone level: To rule out hyperthyroidism or hypothyroidism, either of which may contribute to HF and dysrhythmias.

Nursing Diagnosis

Impaired Gas Exchange

related to alveolar-capillary membrane changes (fluid accumulation in the alveoli)

Desired Outcome: Within 30 min of treatment/intervention, the patient has adequate gas exchange as evidenced by normal breath sounds and skin color, presence of eupnea, HR 100 bpm or less, PaO_2 80 mm Hg or higher, and $PaCO_2$ 45 mm Hg or less.

ASSESSMENT/INTERVENTIONS	RATIONALES
Assess all lung fields for breath sounds.	The presence of crackles (rales) may signal alveolar fluid congestion and systolic dysfunctional (left-sided) HF. Decreased breath sounds signify fluid overload or decreased ventilation. Wheezing may signify associated bronchitis or asthma.
Monitor oximetry and ABG values and report significant findings.	Oximetry of 92% or less and the presence of hypoxemia (decreased PaO_2) and hypercapnia (increased $PaCO_2$) signify decreased oxygenation.
Assess respiratory rate (RR), lung excursion, use of accessory muscles, air hunger, mental status changes, cyanosis, and changes in HR or BP. Report significant changes.	These are signs of increasing respiratory distress that require prompt intervention.
Assist the patient into high Fowler's position with the head of bed (HOB) up 90 degrees.	This position decreases work of breathing, reduces cardiac workload, and promotes gas exchange.
Teach the patient to take slow, deep breaths.	Taking deep breaths increases oxygenation to the myocardium and improves prognosis. Hypoxia adds stress to the already distressed myocardium.
Administer oxygen as prescribed. Deliver oxygen with humidity.	In ADHF/pulmonary edema, high-flow O_2 may be given either by non-rebreathing mask, positive airway pressure devices, or endotracheal intubation and mechanical ventilation. Once stabilized, O_2 is titrated to keep pulse oximetry readings higher than 92%. Humidity helps prevent oxygen's convective drying effects on oral and nasal mucosa.

ASSESSMENT/INTERVENTIONS	RATIONALES
Administer diuretics as prescribed.	Diuretics promote normovolemia by reducing fluid accumulation and blood volume. Fluid overload decreases perfusion in the lungs, causing hypoxemia.
Monitor K⁺ levels.	There is potential for hypokalemia (K⁺ less than 3.5 mEq/L) in patients taking some diuretics, such as furosemide and metolazone.
Administer vasodilators as prescribed.	Vasodilators increase venous capacitance (dilation) and decrease pulmonary congestion, which will improve gas exchange. *Hydralazine* is an oral vasodilator and afterload reducer. It is used in combination with nitrates in patients who are ACE inhibitor/ARB intolerant because of renal dysfunction. It improves mortality and HF symptoms to a lesser degree than ACE inhibitors and can cause reflex tachycardia. *Nitrates* are coronary vasodilators used in conjunction with hydralazine (see above). They are also used in ischemic heart disease as antianginal drugs. *ACE inhibitors* (enalapril, lisinopril, benazepril, captopril, quinapril, ramipril) suppress effects of the renin-angiotensin system by reducing angiotensin II and causing decreased aldosterone secretion. These drugs lower BP and reduce preload and afterload, decreasing work of the left ventricle. *Angiotensin II receptor antagonists* (ARBs—losartan, valsartan, candesartan) are used for patients who do not tolerate ACE inhibitors because of cough caused by bradykinin release.
⚠ As indicated, have emergency equipment (e.g., airway, manual resuscitation bag) available and functional.	Patients with severely decompensated HF may suffer cardiac arrest.
As indicated, prepare to transfer the patient to ICU.	The patient may require invasive and/or closer monitoring.

Nursing Diagnosis

Excess Fluid Volume

related to compromised regulatory mechanisms occurring with decreased cardiac output

Desired Outcomes: Within 1 hr of intervention/treatment, the patient demonstrates less shortness of breath and has output greater than intake on intake and output (I&O) monitoring. Within 1 day of treatment/intervention, edema is 1+ or less on a 0-4+ scale. Weight becomes stable within 2-3 days.

ASSESSMENT/INTERVENTIONS	RATIONALES
At frequent intervals assess I&O, including insensible losses from diaphoresis and respirations.	Decreasing urinary output can signal decreased cardiac output, which decreases renal blood flow.
Assess daily morning weight; record and report steady losses or gains.	This assessment helps identify fluid retention and fluid loss, enabling titration of diuretics.
Assess for edema (interstitial fluids), especially in dependent areas such as the ankles and sacrum.	The presence of weight gain and edema is a key determinant of fluid retention. If diligent assessment is maintained and early intervention is practiced, the occurrence of rehospitalization can be decreased dramatically.
Assess the respiratory system for indicators of fluid extravasation, such as crackles (rales) or pink-tinged, frothy sputum.	These are signs of fluid volume excess and systolic dysfunction (left-sided) HF.
Monitor for jugular vein distention, peripheral edema, and ascites.	These are other indicators of fluid overload.
Monitor laboratory results for increased urinary specific gravity, decreased Hct, increased urine osmolality, hyponatremia, hypokalemia, and hypochloremia.	These findings are indicators of fluid imbalance.

continued

PART I: Medical-Surgical Nursing

ASSESSMENT/INTERVENTIONS	RATIONALES
Monitor IV rate of flow. Use an infusion control device.	These measures are essential to prevent volume overload during IV infusion.
Unless contraindicated, provide ice chips or ice pops. Record amount on the I&O record. Provide frequent mouth care to reduce dry mucous membranes.	These measures help the patient control thirst while providing minimal amounts of fluid. **Note:** Some care centers advocate small amounts of room-temperature water instead because it may relieve thirst better.
Administer diuretics as prescribed, and record the patient's response.	Diuretics promote normovolemia by reducing fluid accumulation and blood volume.
Loop diuretics (furosemide, bumetanide, torsemide): These agents promote excretion of water and sodium, reduce preload, and prevent fluid retention. In ADHF, these diuretics are administered via IV bolus or in drip form until stabilization occurs. These drugs can cause neurohormonal activation and aggravate preexisting renal dysfunction or hypokalemia.
Thiazide diuretics (hydrochlorothiazide, metolazone): Hydrochlorothiazide may be used for mild fluid retention. Metolazone is a potent drug that, when given $\frac{1}{2}$ hr before loop diuretics, markedly potentiates diuresis and therefore is reserved for more severe volume overload in ADHF or late-stage HF. Hyponatremia, hypokalemia, and worsening of renal function may occur and necessitate careful assessment.
Administer morphine sulfate if prescribed.	Morphine induces vasodilation and decreases venous return to the heart.
Teach patients and families about the importance of adhering to a low-sodium diet.	Hypernatremia can promote excess fluid retention. A 2-g-per-day sodium diet is recommended for most patients.

Nursing Diagnosis

Risk for Decreased Cardiac Tissue Perfusion

related to interrupted blood flow occurring with decreased cardiac output

Desired Outcome: By at least the 24-hr period before hospital discharge, the patient has adequate tissue perfusion as evidenced by BP within 20 mm Hg of baseline BP; HR 100 bpm or less with regular rhythm; RR 20 breaths/min or less with normal depth and pattern (eupnea); brisk capillary refill (less than 2 sec); and significant improvement in mental status or orientation to person, place, and time.

ASSESSMENT/INTERVENTIONS	RATIONALES
Assess BP q15min or more frequently if unstable. Be alert to decreases greater than 20 mm Hg over patient's baseline or associated changes such as dizziness and altered mentation.	Hypotension is a side effect of many HF medications, as well as a consequence of aggressive diuresis. Careful monitoring is essential to avoid decreased perfusion to vital organs.
Assess HR q15-30min. Monitor for irregularities, increased HR, or skipped beats.	These signs may signal decompensation and decreased function of the heart.
Assess the extremities for pulse presence and amplitude, capillary refill, edema, color, and temperature.	Decreased pulse amplitude, delayed capillary refill (more than 2 sec), pallor, and coolness are indicators of peripheral vasoconstriction (from SNS compensation). Edema is evidence of fluid overload.
Report any assessment changes immediately to the health care provider.	Significant alterations may be life threatening.
Assess for restlessness, anxiety, mental status changes, confusion, lethargy, stupor, and coma. Institute safety precautions accordingly.	These are indicators of decreased cerebral perfusion and hypoxia and should be addressed promptly for rapid intervention.

ASSESSMENT/INTERVENTIONS

RATIONALES

⚠ Administer inotropic medications and vasodilators as prescribed. Monitor effects closely. Be alert to problems such as hypotension and irregular heartbeats.

IV inotropic medications (dobutamine, dopamine, milrinone) increase strength of contractions and are reserved for use in ADHF-associated low-cardiac output and cardiogenic shock until the patient is stabilized. They may be used longer term in advanced-stage HF as a bridge to transplantation or for palliation of symptoms. Use may be associated with increased mortality and ventricular dysrhythmias. Administration of inotropic medications may require transfer to the coronary care unit (CCU) to monitor for hemodynamic effects and dysrhythmias.

IV vasodilators (nitroglycerin [NTG], nitroprusside, nesiritide) are used in ADHF to decrease cardiac workload by reducing ventricular filling pressures and systemic vascular resistance (SVR, afterload). These medications are avoided in low-output HF, cardiogenic shock, and systolic blood pressure (SBP) less than 90 mm Hg.

- *Nesiritide:* Balanced arterial and venous vasodilator. This medication can alleviate acute dyspnea and reduce pulmonary capillary wedge pressure (PCWP) within the first 30 min of therapy. It promotes diuresis and natriuresis but does not replace need for diuretic therapy. It improves cardiac output by off-loading the heart and decreases neurohormonal activation. It does not require CCU monitoring.
- *NTG:* Arterial and venous vasodilator. It also reduces PCWP and may require ICU/CCU monitoring. Because of tachyphylaxis (tolerance), patients may need escalating doses to achieve the desired effect.
- *Nitroprusside:* Potent arterial and venous vasodilator and afterload reducer. It must be administered in intensive care due to the need for continual hemodynamic monitoring.
- *Morphine sulfate:* A coronary vasodilator that may be given in ADHF or acute pulmonary edema to decrease anxiety and work of breathing and to relieve angina if ischemic heart disease is present.

Nursing Diagnosis

Decreased Cardiac Output

related to negative inotropic changes in the heart (decreased cardiac contractility)

Desired Outcomes: By at least the 24-hr period before hospital discharge, the patient exhibits adequate cardiac output as evidenced by SBP at least 90 mm Hg, HR 100 bpm or less, urinary output at least 30 mL/hr (0.5 mL/kg/hr), stable weight, eupnea, normal breath sounds, and edema 1+ or less on a 0-4+ scale. By at least 48 hr before hospital discharge, the patient is free of new dysrhythmias, does not exhibit significant changes in mental status, and remains oriented to person, place, and time.

ASSESSMENT/INTERVENTIONS

RATIONALES

⚠ Assess for jugular venous distention, extra heart sounds such as S_3, changes in mental status or level of consciousness, cool extremities, hypotension, tachycardia, and tachypnea.

These are indicators of decreased cardiac output, which should be reported promptly for timely intervention.

⚠ Assess lungs for adventitious breath sounds and shortness of breath.

Dyspnea, crackles, and shortness of breath signal fluid accumulation in the lungs and may be a direct indicator of ventricular failure and decreased cardiac output. Cardiac output decreases as HF progresses.

⚠ Monitor I&O; weigh the patient daily.

Decreasing urine output and weight gain can occur as a result of decreased cardiac contractility, which can cause decreased renal perfusion and fluid retention.

continued

ASSESSMENT/INTERVENTIONS	RATIONALES
Assess for peripheral (sacral, pedal) edema.	Edema can occur with diastolic dysfunction (right-sided) HF/myocardial infarction.
Assist with activities of daily living and facilitate coordination of health care providers, allowing 90 min for undisturbed rest. If necessary, limit visitors.	Rest decreases cardiac workload.
Administer medications as prescribed, such as beta-blockers, calcium channel blockers, and antidysrhythmic agents.	*Beta-blockers* (metoprolol XL) and *alpha/beta-adrenergic blockers* (carvedilol): Block effects of SNS and toxic effects of neurohormones on the myocardium. These medications decrease HR and BP, thereby decreasing cardiac workload. *Calcium channel blockers:* May be used in diastolic HF to assist with relaxation and filling and reduce outflow tract obstruction (hypertrophic cardiomyopathy). Except for amlodipine or felodipine, calcium channel blockers are avoided in LV systolic dysfunction because they decrease cardiac contractility. Amiodarone is an example of an *antidysrhythmic* given for patients with HF.
Explain the potential for dysrhythmia management under the guidance of an electrophysiologist/cardiologist.	Dysrhythmias have become a major factor in quality-of-life issues and rehospitalization in patients with HF. Many of these patients require an implantable cardioverter-defibrillator (ICD) because of repeated life-threatening episodes of ventricular tachycardia from an irritable myocardium. Patients with ventricular asynchrony, as seen in bundle branch blocks, may benefit from a biventricular pacer. Pacing each ventricle in synchrony may result in better cardiac output.
Assist the patient into a position of comfort, usually semi-Fowler's position (HOB up 30-45 degrees).	This position decreases work of breathing and reduces cardiac workload.

Nursing Diagnosis

Activity Intolerance

related to imbalance between oxygen supply and demand occurring with a decrease in cardiac muscle contractility

Desired Outcome: During activity, the patient rates perceived exertion at 3 or less on a 0-10 scale and exhibits cardiac tolerance to activity as evidenced by RR 20 breaths/min or less, SBP within 20 mm Hg of resting range, HR within 20 bpm of resting HR, and absence of chest pain and new dysrhythmias.

ASSESSMENT/INTERVENTIONS	RATIONALES
Assess the patient's physiologic response to activity and report significant findings.	Chest pain, new dysrhythmias, increased shortness of breath, HR increased greater than 20 bpm over resting HR, and SBP greater than 20 mm Hg over resting SBP are significant findings of decreased cardiac output or cardiac failure that can manifest during activity.
Ask the patient to rate perceived exertion (RPE) (see p. 62 for a description).	Optimally, patients should not experience RPE of more than 3. If this happens, intensity of the activity should be decreased and its frequency increased until RPE of 3 or less is achieved.
Assess vital signs q4h, and report significant findings.	Findings such as irregular HR, HR greater than 100 bpm, or decreasing BP may be signs of cardiac ischemia.
Before hospital discharge teach the patient self-measurement of HR for gauging exercise tolerance.	An HR that is too high increases myocardial O_2 demand; an HR that is too low may cause more ischemia. Patients should use an exertion scale and a pain scale to gauge exercise tolerance and ensure that HR is less than 20 bpm over baseline or as prescribed by the health care provider.

PART I: Medical-Surgical Nursing

ASSESSMENT/INTERVENTIONS	RATIONALES
! Assess for and report oliguria, decreasing BP, decreased mentation, and dizziness.	These are signs of acute decreased cardiac output.
! Assess peripheral pulses, distal extremity skin color, and urinary output. Report significant findings.	These assessments reveal the integrity of peripheral perfusion. Changes such as decreased amplitude of pulses, pallor or cyanosis, and decreased urinary output are significant findings that should be reported for timely intervention.
Ensure that the patient's needs are met (e.g., by keeping water at the bedside and urinal or commode nearby, maintaining a quiet environment, and limiting visitors as necessary).	These measures promote adequate rest, prevent activity intolerance, and decrease cardiac workload.
Facilitate coordination of health care providers to provide rest periods between care activities. Allow 90 min for undisturbed rest.	Rest helps decrease cardiac workload.
Administer O_2 as prescribed.	Increasing oxygen supply to the myocardium promotes activity tolerance.
Assist with passive and some active or assistive range-of-motion and other exercises, depending on the patient's tolerance and prescribed limitations.	Exercise prevents complications to joints and tissue caused by prolonged immobility.
Also discuss with the health care provider the patient's potential participation in an exercise program after hospital discharge.	Progressive monitored exercise for patients with HF can improve quality of life, activity tolerance, heart function, and disease outcomes.

Nursing Diagnosis

Fear

related to a potentially life-threatening situation

Desired Outcome: Within 24 hr of this diagnosis, the patient communicates fears and concerns and relates attainment of increasing physical and psychological comfort.

ASSESSMENT/INTERVENTIONS	RATIONALES
Assess for and acknowledge the patient's fears and provide opportunities for the patient and significant other to express their feelings. Be reassuring and supportive.	Identifying and acknowledging feelings encourages communication and hence reduces fear. Empathy lessens a sense of isolation and fear.
Assist the patient in being as comfortable as possible, with prompt pain relief and positioning, typically high Fowler's position (HOB up 90 degrees).	Comfort measures may decrease the intensity of the physiologic event that is contributing to the fear.
Create and maintain a calm and quiet environment.	These measures prevent or reduce the sensory overload that may contribute to fear.
Explain all treatment modalities, especially those that may be uncomfortable (e.g., O_2 face mask and rotating tourniquets).	Increasing a patient's knowledge level about therapies and procedures reduces/eliminates fear of the unknown and affords a sense of control.
Remain with the patient if possible, providing emotional support for both the patient and significant other.	Many individuals benefit from the support of others and find that it reduces their stress/fear level.
For further interventions, see "Psychosocial Support," **Fear,** p. 75.	

Nursing Diagnosis

Deficient Knowledge

related to unfamiliarity with the purpose, precautions, and side effects of diuretic therapy

Desired Outcome: Within the 24-hr period before hospital discharge, the patient verbalizes knowledge of the precautions and side effects of diuretic therapy.

ASSESSMENT/INTERVENTIONS	RATIONALES
Assess the patient's health care literacy (language, reading, comprehension). Assess culture and culturally specific information needs.	This assessment helps ensure that information is selected and presented in a manner that is culturally and educationally appropriate.
Teach the purpose of the prescribed diuretic.	These medications control fluid accumulation and reduce blood volume. Patients who are knowledgeable about their medication's purpose are more likely to adhere to the therapeutic regimen.
Depending on the type of diuretic used, teach the patient to report signs and symptoms of the following:	A knowledgeable patient will know how to monitor for and report symptoms that necessitate medical attention.
Hypokalemia: Anorexia, irregular pulse, nausea, apathy, and muscle cramps.	Use of furosemide and metolazone, which are potassium-wasting diuretics, can cause these symptoms.
Hyperkalemia: Muscle weakness, hyporeflexia, and irregular HR.	Use of amiloride and spironolactone, which are potassium-sparing diuretics, can cause these symptoms.
Hyponatremia: Fatigue, weakness, and edema (caused by fluid extravasation).	Use of bumetanide, a diuretic that promotes excretion of NaCl, may cause these symptoms.
For patients on long-term diuretic therapy, explain the importance of follow-up monitoring of blood levels of potassium and sodium.	Although the most common electrolyte problem with diuretic use is hypokalemia, the potential for hyperkalemia and electrolyte imbalance of sodium continues with long-term therapy.
For patients receiving potassium-wasting diuretics (e.g., furosemide), teach the need to consume supplemental high-potassium foods.	Foods high in potassium content, such as apricots, bananas, oranges, and raisins, will help replenish potassium lost via diuretics.
As appropriate, instruct the patient to use care when rising from a sitting or recumbent position.	There is potential for injury from orthostatic hypotension, which can occur with diuretic use because of diuresis.

Nursing Diagnosis

Deficient Knowledge

related to unfamiliarity with the purpose, precautions, and side effects of digoxin therapy

Desired Outcome: Within the 24-hr period before hospital discharge, the patient verbalizes understanding of the purpose, precautions, and side effects associated with digoxin therapy.

ASSESSMENT/INTERVENTIONS	RATIONALES
Assess the patient's health care literacy (language, reading, comprehension). Assess culture and culturally specific information needs.	This assessment helps ensure that information is selected and presented in a manner that is culturally and educationally appropriate.
Teach the purpose of digoxin therapy.	Digoxin slows conduction through the atrioventricular (A-V) node and increases strength of contractility. Although not a first-line drug as originally believed for HF patients, it is used for dysrhythmia management when atrial fibrillation coexists or to improve symptoms in class III-IV HF patients. A patient who is knowledgeable about the purpose of digoxin will be more likely to adhere to the therapy.
Teach the technique and importance of assessing HR before taking digoxin.	Although patients should obtain HR parameters from their health care providers, digoxin is usually withheld when the HR is less than 60 bpm (unless the patient's usual HR is less than 60 bpm).

ASSESSMENT/INTERVENTIONS	RATIONALES
Teach the patient to hold the dose if there is a 20-bpm or greater change from his or her normal rate and to notify the health care provider if he or she has omitted a dose because of a slow or significantly changed HR.	Such a change may signal that the patient is receiving too much medication and a dose adjustment may be necessary if slowing of the HR persists.
Explain that serum potassium levels are monitored routinely.	Low levels of potassium can potentiate digoxin toxicity.
Explain that apical HR and peripheral pulses are assessed for irregularity.	Irregularity may signal the presence of dysrhythmias (e.g., heart block), which is associated with digoxin toxicity.
[!] Teach the patient to be alert to nausea, vomiting, anorexia, headache, diarrhea, blurred vision, yellow-haze vision, and mental confusion. Explain the importance of reporting signs and symptoms promptly to the health care provider or staff if they occur.	These are other indicators of digoxin toxicity that necessitate prompt medical attention for timely intervention.

Nursing Diagnosis

Deficient Knowledge

related to unfamiliarity with the purpose, precautions, and side effects of vasodilators

Desired Outcome: Within the 24-hr period before hospital discharge, the patient verbalizes knowledge of the purpose, precautions, and side effects of vasodilators.

ASSESSMENT/INTERVENTIONS	RATIONALES
Assess the patient's health care literacy (language, reading, comprehension). Assess culture and culturally specific information needs.	This assessment helps ensure that information is selected and presented in a manner that is culturally and educationally appropriate.
Teach the purpose of vasodilators.	See discussion in **Impaired Gas Exchange**, p. 170.
Explain that a headache can occur after administration of a vasodilator.	Headache can occur because of dilation of the cranial vessels or from orthostatic hypotension.
Suggest that lying down will help alleviate pain.	A supine position may help alleviate the pain by increasing blood flow to the heart and head, although blood flow to the head may worsen the headache. Pain medication and decreased dosage of the vasodilator may be necessary.
Teach the importance of assessment for weight gain and signs of peripheral or sacral edema.	A possible side effect of vasodilator therapy is a decrease in venous return to the right side of the heart with subsequent accumulation in the periphery.
[!] For patients on long-term ACE inhibitor therapy, explain the importance of follow-up monitoring of blood levels of serum creatinine.	ACE inhibitors may cause kidney damage, resulting in decreased creatinine clearance. If this occurs, the patient may need to be taken off the medication.
[!] For patients receiving ACE inhibitors, teach the importance of using care when rising from a sitting or recumbent position.	There is potential for injury caused by orthostatic hypotension, a potential side effect of ACE inhibitors.
Teach the patient receiving ACE inhibitors the technique for and importance of assessing BP before taking the medication. Explain that it is possible to purchase automatic BP machines from local pharmacies and if necessary to seek reimbursement or funding information from a social worker.	Vasodilators can cause an excessive reduction in BP. Although patients should obtain BP parameters from their health care providers, ACE inhibitors are usually withheld when BP is less than 110/60 mm Hg.
Teach the patient to notify the health care provider if he or she has omitted a dose because of a low or significantly changed BP.	It may be necessary to lower the dose or change the medication.

ADDITIONAL NURSING DIAGNOSES/PROBLEMS:

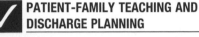

PATIENT-FAMILY TEACHING AND DISCHARGE PLANNING

When providing patient-family teaching, focus on sensory information, avoid giving excessive information, and initiate a visiting nurse referral for necessary follow-up teaching. Include verbal and written information about the following:

✓ Medications, including drug name, purpose, dosage, schedule, precautions, and potential side effects. Also discuss drug-drug, food-drug, and herb-drug interactions.

✓ Signs and symptoms that necessitate immediate medical attention: dyspnea, decreased exercise tolerance, alterations in pulse rate/rhythm, alterations in or loss of consciousness (caused by dysrhythmias or decreased cardiac output), oliguria, and weight gain of greater than 2-3 lb in 24 hr or 3-5 lb in 48 hr.

✓ Reinforcement that heart failure/cardiomyopathy is a chronic disease requiring lifetime treatment.

✓ Importance of abstaining from alcohol, which increases cardiac muscle deterioration.

✓ Importance of a low-sodium diet (less than 1000 mg/day) to prevent fluid retention.

✓ Need for physical support from family and outside agencies as the disease progresses.

✓ Availability of community and medical support, such as:
  • The American Heart Association at *www.americanheart.org*
  • The Heart and Stroke Foundation at *www.heartandstroke.com*

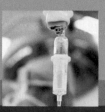

OVERVIEW/PATHOPHYSIOLOGY

Hypertension affects more than one of three adults in the United States, with more than 60% of individuals older than 65 years diagnosed with hypertension (AHA, 2013). Hypertension occurs when cardiac output and peripheral vascular resistance are altered. Most commonly, endothelial changes of peripheral arterioles cause restriction of blood flow, raising arterial pressure.

Risk factors include age, heredity, ethnicity (incidence is higher in African Americans), renal disease, obesity, hyperlipidemia, smoking, and some endocrine disorders (e.g., Cushing's disease, thyroid disease, primary aldosteronism, pheochromocytoma).

Complications of hypertension include increased incidence of transient ischemic attack/stroke, retinopathy, cardiovascular disease, heart failure, aortic aneurysm, and renal failure.

Hypertension is defined by the Joint National Committee on Prevention, Detection, Evaluation and Treatment of Hypertension (JNC 7) (based on the average of two or more properly measured readings at each of two or more visits after an initial screen) as:

- Normal blood pressure: systolic blood pressure (SBP) less than 120 mm Hg and diastolic blood pressure (DBP) less than 80 mm Hg
- Prehypertension: SBP 120-139 mm Hg or DBP 80-89 mm Hg
- Hypertension
  - Stage 1: SBP 140-159 mm Hg or DBP 90-99 mm Hg
  - Stage 2: SBP 160 mm Hg or greater or DBP 100 mm Hg or greater
  - Treatment goals of hypertension in persons 60 yr of age and older is to achieve blood pressure of less than 150/90 (JNC 8). In persons less than 60 yr of age, or those with chronic kidney disease or diabetes, the treatment goal is less than 140/90 (JNC 8).

HEALTH CARE SETTING

Primary care or cardiology clinic setting most commonly; patients with severe hypertension may require acute hospitalization.

Nursing Diagnosis:

Deficient Knowledge

related to unfamiliarity with the need for frequent blood pressure (BP) checks, adherence to antihypertensive therapy, and lifestyle changes

Desired Outcome: Following teaching, the patient verbalizes knowledge of the importance of frequent BP checks and adhering to antihypertensive therapy and lifestyle changes.

ASSESSMENT/INTERVENTIONS	RATIONALES
Assess the patient's health care literacy (language, reading, comprehension). Assess culture and culturally specific information needs.	This assessment helps ensure that information is selected and presented in a manner that is culturally and educationally appropriate.
Teach the importance of assessing BP at frequent intervals and adhering to the prescribed medication therapy.	Frequent assessment provides feedback on response to therapy and may help improve adherence to therapy. Self-assessment is also helpful for evaluating "white coat hypertension," the phenomenon of increased BP when assessed by a health care provider.

continued

ASSESSMENT/INTERVENTIONS

ASSESSMENT/INTERVENTIONS	RATIONALES
Provide teaching guidelines on the importance of exercise, stress reduction, weight loss (if appropriate), decreased alcohol intake, and a less than 2 g/day sodium diet. Review how to read food labels and choose low sodium foods. Refer to a nutritionist and exercise program, if appropriate.	Primary treatment for this disease includes promotion of lifestyle modification, which can lower BP significantly when adhered to.
Teach medication actions, administration times, side effects, adverse effects, and the importance of taking as prescribed. Include drug-drug, food-drug, and herb-drug interactions.	Knowledge about and adherence to the prescribed regimen can lower morbidity and mortality risk and improve patient outcomes.
Teach the importance of seeking medical evaluation if BP reading is greater than 200/100 mm Hg or less than 90/60 mm Hg, or if headache, dizziness, lightheadedness, or blurred vision occurs.	Severe hypertension or hypotension can be life threatening, compromising perfusion to vital organs.

ADDITIONAL NURSING DIAGNOSES/PROBLEMS:

✔ PATIENT-FAMILY TEACHING AND DISCHARGE PLANNING

When providing patient-family teaching, focus on sensory information, avoid giving excessive information, and initiate a visiting nurse referral for necessary follow-up teaching. Include verbal and written information about the following:

- ✓ Signs and symptoms that necessitate immediate medical attention: elevated or decreased BP readings (greater than 200/100 mm Hg or less than 90/60 mm Hg), headache, dizziness, lightheadedness, blurred vision, chest pain, dyspnea, or syncope.

- ✓ Self blood pressure evaluation when indicated. Monitoring machines are available in local stores and pharmacies and on-line. Remind the patient that evaluation of BP should be done while seated, after resting for 5 min, and recorded. Taking 3 readings 1 min apart in the morning and evening is recommended by the American Society for Hypertension (ASH). Appropriate cuff size must be selected (AHA guidelines). Measurement of standing BP can be obtained when indicated, i.e., in diabetic autonomic neuropathy, when orthostatic symptoms are present, or when a dose increase in antihypertensive therapy has been made (ASH).

- ✓ Medications, including name, purpose, dosage, schedule, precautions, and potential side effects. Discuss drug-drug, food-drug, and herb-drug interactions.

- ✓ Importance of abstaining from smoking and excessive salt and alcohol intake, which increase blood pressure.

- ✓ Reinforcement that hypertension is a chronic disease requiring lifetime treatment.

- ✓ Need for physical support from the family and outside agencies.

- ✓ Availability of community and medical support such as the American Heart Association at *www.americanheart.org*

- ✓ The Heart and Stroke Foundation at *www.heartandstroke.com*

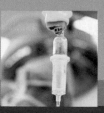

Pulmonary Arterial Hypertension 23

OVERVIEW/PATHOPHYSIOLOGY

Pulmonary blood vessels exchange the primary gases CO_2 and O_2 at the arteriole level. In healthy individuals, this exchange occurs with each respiration. However, the pulmonary vasculature's ability to provide adequate gas exchange may be altered in the presence of lung and heart disease. When pulmonary pressures rise, pulmonary arterial hypertension (PAH) results.

PAH may be idiopathic (rare), which has a poor prognosis and affects primarily young and middle-age women; or it can be secondary (most common), which often responds to therapy and may be present in a variety of medical conditions. The cause of idiopathic pulmonary arterial hypertension (IPAH) is unknown. It may be familial and has been linked to the bone morphogenetic protein receptor 2 (BMPR2). Often the etiology of secondary PAH is chronic hypoxia, which can result from increased pulmonary blood flow from a ventricular or atrial shunt, left ventricular failure, chronic obstructive pulmonary disease (COPD) or obstructive sleep apnea (OSA), pulmonary embolus, interstitial lung disease, human immunodeficiency virus (HIV) infection, collagen vascular disorders such as scleroderma or lupus, portal hypertension due to liver disease, or any physiologic occurrence that increases pulmonary vascular resistance or constriction of the vessels in the pulmonary tree.

HEALTH CARE SETTING

Primary care with possible hospitalization in a cardiac or medical-surgical unit resulting from complications or in a special center for heart-lung transplantation

ASSESSMENT

Acute indicators: Exertional dyspnea and fatigue (the most common presenting symptoms), eventually progressing to dyspnea at rest. Syncope, precordial chest pain, and palpitations can occur because of low cardiac output or hypoxia.

Chronic indicators: Signs of right or left ventricular failure as a result of right ventricular enlargement and eventual fluid overload.

Right (diastolic) ventricular failure: Peripheral edema, increased venous pressure and pulsations, liver engorgement, distended neck veins.

Left (systolic) ventricular failure: Dyspnea; shortness of breath, particularly on exertion; decreased blood pressure (BP); oliguria; orthopnea; anorexia.

Physical assessment: Pale, cool skin with peripheral cyanosis due to decreased cardiac output, systemic vasoconstriction and ventilation-perfusion mismatch, systolic murmur caused by tricuspid regurgitation or pulmonary stenosis, diastolic murmur caused by pulmonary valvular incompetence, accentuated S_2 heart sound, possible S_3 or S_4 heart sound, distended neck veins, and a parasternal heave caused by right ventricular enlargement.

DIAGNOSTIC TESTS

Chest x-ray examination: Demonstrates enlargement of the pulmonary artery and right atrium and ventricle. Pulmonary vasculature may appear engorged.

Echocardiography: Valuable for showing increased right ventricular dimension, thickened right ventricular wall, and possible tricuspid or pulmonary valve dysfunction. This test indirectly measures pulmonary artery systolic pressure.

Radionuclide imaging: Equilibrium-gated blood pool imaging and thallium imaging assess function of the right ventricle.

Computerized tomography (CT) scan: Evaluates diameter of the main pulmonary arteries, which is helpful in evaluating severity of disease. High-resolution CT can confirm the presence of interstitial lung disease. Spiral CT is more specific in evaluating pulmonary embolus.

Right heart catheterization: Gold standard for diagnosing PAH. It also provides helpful information regarding severity of the disease and establishing prognosis. Pulmonary vascular resistance will be very high, and pulmonary artery and right ventricular pressures can approach or equal systemic arterial pressures. Vasodilator challenge is often performed to assess reactivity and guide treatment. Adenosine, epoprostenol, and nitric oxide typically are used.

Pulmonary perfusion scintigraphy (perfusion scan): A noninvasive way to assess pulmonary blood flow. This study involves intravenous (IV) injection of serum albumin tagged with trace amounts of a radioisotope, most often technetium. The particles pass through the circulation and lodge in the pulmonary vascular bed. Subsequent scanning reveals concentrations of particles in areas of adequate pulmonary blood flow.

The scan is normal in PAH. An abnormal scan suggests presence of thromboembolic pulmonary hypertension.

Electrocardiogram (ECG) results: Will show evidence of right atrial enlargement and right ventricular enlargement (evidenced by right axis deviation, right bundle branch block, tall and peaked P waves, and large R waves in V_1) secondary to the increased pressure needed to force blood through the hypertensive pulmonary vascular bed.

Pulmonary function test: Results are usually normal, although some individuals will have increased residual volume, reduced maximum voluntary ventilation, and decreased vital capacity.

Sleep study: Confirms diagnosis of obstructive sleep apnea as etiology for associated PAH.

Exercise testing: Symptom-limited stress test or 6-min walk test can help assess severity of symptoms and guide response to treatment.

Arterial blood gas (ABG) analysis: May show low $PaCO_2$ and high pH, which occur with hyperventilation, or increased $PaCO_2$ with decreased gas exchange.

Oximetry: May show decreased O_2 saturation (92% or less).

Blood tests to rule out secondary causes of PAH: Anti-nuclear antibody, rheumatoid arthritis, erythrocyte sedimentation rate (tests for collagen vascular disorders), HIV, and thyroid-stimulating hormone (thyroid abnormalities commonly coexist with PAH).

Complete blood count (CBC): Polycythemia can occur in the presence of chronic hypoxemia as a result of compensation.

Liver function tests: May be abnormal if venous congestion is significant. Examples include increased aspartate aminotransferase (AST), alanine aminotransferase (ALT), and bilirubin.

Nursing Diagnosis:

Impaired Gas Exchange

related to altered blood flow occurring with pulmonary capillary constriction

Desired Outcome: The patient has improved gas exchange by at least 24 hr before hospital discharge, as evidenced by O_2 saturation greater than 92% (90% or greater for patients with COPD) and PaO_2 80 mm Hg or higher.

ASSESSMENT/INTERVENTIONS	RATIONALES
Assess O_2 saturation; report O_2 saturation 92% or less to the health care provider.	Low O_2 saturation may signal the need for oxygen supplementation.
Monitor ABG results. Report significant findings to the health care provider.	ABG results can reveal signs of hypoventilation (decreased PaO_2, increased $PaCO_2$, and decreased pH), which can signal respiratory failure, or hyperventilation (low $PaCO_2$ and high pH), which can occur with anxiety or respiratory distress. Hypoxemia is the key gas deficit seen with pulmonary vascular vasoconstriction. Blood flow through the lungs is impaired, making it difficult to exchange O_2 for CO_2. O_2 becomes low (hypoxemia) and CO_2 becomes high (hypercarbia). Hypercarbia causes a change in pH to the acid side. Although initially respiratory in origin, hypoxemia eventually results in metabolic acidosis because of lactic acid production. Values outside of normal or acceptable range should be reported promptly for timely intervention.
Assess all lung fields for breath sounds q4-8h or more frequently as indicated.	Adventitious sounds (especially rales) can occur with fluid overload; diminished breath sounds are congruent with disease severity.
Assess respiratory rate (RR), pattern, and depth; chest excursion; and use of accessory muscles of respiration q4h.	Increased RR, abdominal breathing, use of accessory muscles, and nasal flaring are signals of hypoxia and respiratory distress.
Inspect skin and mucous membranes for cyanosis or skin color change.	These color changes are significant and later signs of decreased gas exchange.
Assess mental status and report significant changes.	Changes in mental acuity or level of consciousness (LOC) may be indications of hypoxemia or acid-base imbalance.
Assist the patient into high Fowler's position (head of bed [HOB] up 90 degrees), if possible.	This position reduces work of breathing and maximizes chest excursion.

ASSESSMENT/INTERVENTIONS	RATIONALES
Teach the patient to take slow, deep breaths.	This promotes gas exchange.
Administer prescribed O_2 as indicated.	Oxygen treats hypoxia. It can be administered continuously or only at bedtime or with exercise when oxygen desaturation is most likely to occur. If hypoxia is severe, O_2 is administered by mask.
[!] Use care when administering O_2 to patients with a history of COPD.	High concentrations of O_2 can depress the respiratory drive in individuals with chronic CO_2 retention.
Deliver O_2 with humidity.	Humidity helps prevent oxygen's drying effects on oral and nasal mucosa.

Nursing Diagnosis:

Activity Intolerance

related to generalized weakness and imbalance between oxygen supply and demand occurring with right and left ventricular failure

Desired Outcome: By at least 24 hr before hospital discharge, the patient rates perceived exertion at 3 or less on a 0-10 scale and exhibit cardiac tolerance to activity as evidenced by RR 20 breaths/min or less, heart rate (HR) 20 bpm or less over resting HR, and systolic blood pressure (SBP) within 20 mm Hg of resting range.

ASSESSMENT/INTERVENTIONS	RATIONALES
[!] Assess vital signs at least q4h and before and after activity and report significant findings.	A drop in BP greater than 10-20 mm Hg signals decompensation of the cardiac muscle, which must be reported for prompt intervention.
Ask the patient to rate perceived exertion (RPE) during activity, and monitor for evidence of activity intolerance. For details, see, "Prolonged Bedrest," p. 61, for **Risk for Activity Intolerance**. Notify the health care provider of significant findings.	This assessment helps determine if activity intolerance is present (RPE higher than 3).
Assess for dyspnea, shortness of breath, crackles (rales), and decreased O_2 saturation (92% or less) as determined by oximetry.	These are signs of left (systolic) ventricular failure.
Measure and document intake and output and weight, reporting any steady gains or losses. Assess for peripheral edema (pedal and sacral), ascites, distended neck veins, and increased central venous pressure (more than 12 cm H_2O).	These are signs of right (diastolic) ventricular failure.
Administer diuretics, vasodilators, and calcium channel blockers as prescribed.	*Diuretics:* These medications are used in the presence of right-sided (diastolic dysfunction) or left-sided (systolic dysfunction) heart failure and fluid overload.
	Vasodilators: The goal of medical therapy is to decrease pulmonary artery pressure by vasodilation. Epoprostenol is a prostanoid, a potent IV vasodilator that also inhibits platelet aggregation. It is continuously infused through a long-term venous access device. Drawbacks to this medication include significant cost and severe side effects, including rebound pulmonary hypertension if stopped abruptly. Treprostinil is a prostacyclin analogue that is a potent vasodilator, administered continuously via subcutaneous infusion, intravenously, or inhaled. Like epoprostenol, it is expensive, must be initiated in the hospital, and cannot be discontinued abruptly. Bosentan and ambrisentan are oral endothelin receptor antagonists, which are oral vasodilators approved for use in pulmonary hypertension. Sildenafil is a phosphodiesterase-5 inhibitor approved for use as a vasodilator in pulmonary hypertension.
	Calcium channel blockers: These are helpful in patients who demonstrate response to vasodilator challenge and are administered in higher doses than when they are used to treat hypertension.

continued

ASSESSMENT/INTERVENTIONS	RATIONALES
Facilitate coordination of health care providers. Allow time for undisturbed rest. If necessary, limit visitors.	Rest helps decrease oxygen demand.
Place frequently used items within the patient's reach.	This measure conserves energy, reducing oxygen demand.
Assist with maintaining prescribed activity level and progress as tolerated. If activity intolerance is observed, stop the activity and have the patient rest.	These measures increase activity tolerance while preventing overexertion.
Assist with range-of-motion exercises at frequent intervals. Plan progressive ambulation and exercise based on the patient's tolerance and prescribed activity restrictions.	These measures help prevent complications caused by immobility while avoiding overexertion.

Nursing Diagnosis:

Deficient Knowledge

related to unfamiliarity with the disease process and treatment

Desired Outcome: Within the 24-hr period before hospital discharge, the patient and significant other verbalize knowledge of the disease, its treatment, and measures that promote wellness.

ASSESSMENT/INTERVENTIONS	RATIONALES
Assess the patient's health care literacy (language, comprehension, reading). Assess culture and culturally specific information needs.	This assessment helps ensure that information is selected and presented in a manner that is culturally and educationally appropriate.
Assess the patient's level of knowledge of the disease process and its treatment.	This information enables development of an individualized teaching plan. A knowledgeable patient is more likely to adhere to the treatment.
Discuss purposes of the medications:	
- Vasodilators	Vasodilators ease workload of the heart by decreasing systemic resistance.
- Calcium channel blockers	Calcium channel blockers "relax" the heart by decreasing coronary artery spasm.
- Diuretics	Diuretics enhance renal output, reducing fluid accumulation.
- Anticoagulants (warfarin sodium)	Anticoagulants promote improved long-term survival by preventing thromboembolic complications.
Provide emotional support to the patient adapting to living with a chronic disease.	This action reinforces the need to adhere to lifetime therapy while also expressing empathy.
Reinforce explanations of the disease process and treatment.	A knowledgeable patient is more likely to adhere to the treatment regimen.
Discuss lifestyle changes that may be necessary.	Changes may be necessary to maintain quality of life and prevent complications of the disease.
Explain the value of relaxation techniques, including soothing music, meditation, and biofeedback.	Relaxation can promote decreased myocardial demand, lowering HR, BP, and RR.
If the patient smokes, provide materials that explain benefits of smoking cessation, such as pamphlets prepared by the American Heart Association *(www.americanheart.org)*. Provide telephone numbers for local smoking cessation programs.	Smoking increases workload of the heart by causing vasoconstriction.
Confer with the health care provider about an exercise program that will benefit the patient; provide patient teaching as indicated.	Exercise improves vascular tone and strengthens skeletal muscles. In collaboration with the health care provider and physical therapist, the nurse can assist the patient in maximizing the benefits of exercise.

ASSESSMENT/INTERVENTIONS	RATIONALES
If appropriate, involve the dietitian to assist the patient with planning low-sodium meals.	A diet low in sodium may be necessary if signs of heart failure are present.
Discuss treatment of causative factors if they are known.	Examples include surgical closure of arteriovenous shunts; replacement of defective valves; or treatment of obstructive sleep apnea, pulmonary embolism, or COPD.
As directed by the health care provider, explain the possibility of a heart-lung transplantation and refer to appropriate team members.	Transplantation may be considered for advanced (end-stage) pulmonary vascular disease that is not responsive to medical therapy. Early referral is necessary to begin the planning stages.

ADDITIONAL NURSING DIAGNOSES/PROBLEMS:

✓ PATIENT-FAMILY TEACHING AND DISCHARGE PLANNING

When providing patient-family teaching, focus on sensory information, avoid giving too much information, and initiate a visiting nurse referral for necessary follow-up teaching. Include verbal and written information about the following:

✓ Indicators that necessitate medical attention: decreased exercise tolerance, increasing shortness of breath or dyspnea, swelling of ankles and legs, steady weight gain.

✓ Medications, including drug name, purpose, dosage, schedule, precautions, and potential side effects.

Also discuss drug-drug, food-drug, and herb-drug interactions.

✓ Support and information sites available on the Internet, which include:
  - Pulmonary Hypertension Association at *http://www.phassociation.org/*.
  - American Lung Association at *http://www.lung.org/lung-disease/pulmonary-arterial-hypertension/*.
  - Canadian Lung Association at *www.lung.ca.*
  - National Heart, Lung, and Blood Institute at *http://www.nhlbi.nih.gov/health/health-topics/topics/pah/*.

✓ Elimination of smoking; refer patient to a local smoking cessation program as appropriate. The following web sites describe programs, provide printed materials, and explain multiple ways to help patients stop smoking:
  - Smoking and Tobacco Control Program of the National Cancer Institute at *http://www.cancer.gov/cancertopics/tobacco/smoking*.
  - *www.smokefree.gov.*
  - Centers for Disease Control and Prevention: smoking and tobacco use at *http://www.cdc.gov/tobacco/tobacco_control_programs/*.
  - The Canadian Cancer Society at *www.cancer.ca.*

For additional information, see **Deficient Knowledge** in this chapter.

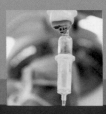

Venous Thrombosis/ 24 Thrombophlebitis

OVERVIEW/PATHOPHYSIOLOGY

Venous thromboembolism (VTE) describes the conditions of deep vein thrombophlebitis (DVT) and pulmonary embolism. Predisposing conditions that affect coagulation or stasis of the blood contribute to the incidence of VTE. Hemoconcentration, vessel trauma or inflammation, hypercoagulability, and immobility are the most common risk factors for VTE.

Hemoconcentration is caused by dehydration, including inadequate fluid resuscitation in the perioperative period. Vessel trauma or inflammation may result from chemical irritation caused by intravenous (IV) solutions, direct trauma, including venipuncture, and improper prolonged positioning. Hypercoagulability is often due to malignancies, hereditary factors, or estrogen therapy.

Immobility resulting from prolonged bedrest, inability to move due to paralysis or stroke, or extended operating room table positioning contributes to venous stasis. Additionally, venous stasis may occur with chronic heart failure, shock states, structural disorders of the veins, and following abdominal, pelvic, or orthopedic operative procedures, and extended air travel.

DVT describes thrombosis and inflammation in the deep venous system, most commonly of the lower extremities. The most serious complication of DVT is embolization, causing a pulmonary embolus (PE).

HEALTH CARE SETTING

Acute care or primary care

ASSESSMENT

Signs and symptoms: At the site of the thrombus signs and symptoms often include pain, tenderness, erythema, local warmth, and swelling. Distal to the thrombus, the extremity may be cool, pale or cyanotic, and edematous with prominent superficial veins. Sometimes the condition is clinically "silent," and the late presenting sign may be a PE (see "Pulmonary Embolus," p. 127).

Physical assessment: Assessment at the site of the thrombus (associated with inflammation) and distal to the clot (associated with venous congestion) is important. A knot or bump at the site of the thrombus may be palpated, along with pain, increased warmth, redness, and edema. Distal to the site, assess pulses, limb circumference, and skin temperature. Calf pain elicited with foot dorsiflexion (Homans' sign) may be a sign of DVT. Additional findings include unilateral limb swelling, fever, and tachycardia.

Risk factors: Prolonged bedrest and immobility, leg trauma, recent surgery, malignancy, hormonal therapy, hypercoagulability, obesity, varicose veins.

DIAGNOSTIC TESTS

Doppler ultrasound: Identifies changes in blood flow secondary to the presence of a thrombus. Doppler venous sounds may be absent if a thrombus is present, occluding blood flow.

Duplex imaging: Use of ultrasound to assess veins for changes in flow and increased velocity when a clot is obstructing flow. Accuracy and sensitivity of this imaging technique are helpful diagnostic measures for DVT.

Impedance plethysmography: Estimates blood flow using measures of resistance and normal changes that occur during pulsatile blood flow. It is highly accurate above the knee.

Plasma markers (D-dimer test): A positive plasma D-dimer test is indicative of fibrin breakdown, and further evaluation is warranted. A negative D-dimer test is helpful in excluding DVT if noninvasive testing also is negative.

Nursing Diagnoses:

Ineffective Peripheral Tissue Perfusion
Risk for Decreased Cardiac Tissue Perfusion

related to thrombus formation or embolization

Desired Outcome: Following emergency interventions, the patient has adequate peripheral and cardiac perfusion as evidenced by normal extremity color, temperature, and sensation;

respiratory rate (RR) 12-20 breaths/min with normal depth and pattern (eupnea); heart rate (HR) 100 bpm or less; blood pressure (BP) within 20 mm Hg of baseline BP; O_2 saturation greater than 92%; and normal breath sounds.

ASSESSMENT/INTERVENTIONS	RATIONALES
⚠ Assess for lower extremity pain, erythema, increased limb circumference, local warmth, distal pale skin, edema, and venous dilation. If indicators appear, maintain the patient on bedrest and notify the health care provider promptly.	These are early indicators of peripheral thrombus formation (DVT), which necessitate bedrest and prompt medical attention to prevent embolization.
⚠ Assess for and immediately report sudden onset of chest pain, dyspnea, tachypnea, tachycardia, hypotension, hemoptysis, shallow respirations, crackles (rales), O_2 saturation 92% or less, decreased breath sounds, and diaphoresis.	These are signs of PE, a life-threatening situation. If they occur, prompt medical attention is required.
Administer anticoagulants as prescribed.	Anticoagulants prevent propagation of a clot. Heparin is used during the acute phase, and long-term warfarin therapy is used after the acute phase. Six months of anticoagulation is recommended for a first occurrence of DVT. Low-molecular-weight heparin may be prescribed, enabling outpatient management of DVT until warfarin levels are therapeutic. **Note:** A vena caval filter may be surgically implanted transvenously, which filters blood from distal sites to prevent PE. This is most often used when patients cannot be anticoagulated or have had PEs while being therapeutically anticoagulated.
⚠ Double-check anticoagulant doses with a colleague. Always use a pump for heparin administration.	Correct dosing is essential to avoid bleeding while preventing clot formation.
Maintain the patient on bedrest, provide passive range-of-motion (ROM) exercises, and apply support hose, sequential compression device, or pneumatic foot compression device as prescribed to the alternate extremity.	These measures decrease lower extremity edema and minimize risk of or prevent further DVTs in the alternate extremity.
Maintain elevation of the affected limb.	This measure promotes venous drainage.

Nursing Diagnosis:

Acute Pain

related to the inflammatory process caused by thrombus formation

Desired Outcomes: Within 1 hr of intervention, the patient's subjective perception of pain decreases, as documented by a pain scale. Objective indicators, such as grimacing, are absent.

ASSESSMENT/INTERVENTIONS	RATIONALES
Assess for the presence of pain, using a pain scale from 0 (no pain) to 10 (worst pain). Administer analgesics as prescribed, and document medication and relief obtained using the pain scale.	This assessment and interventions evaluate the patient's perception of pain and determine the most effective analgesic and dosing required to relieve the pain.
⚠ Ensure that the patient maintains bedrest and limb elevation during the acute phase.	These measures minimize painful engorgement, promote venous drainage, and decrease the potential for embolization.
If prescribed, apply warm, moist packs. Be sure packs are warm (but not extremely so) and not allowed to cool.	Continuous moist heat may be beneficial in reducing discomfort and pain by promoting vasodilation and blood supply to the area.
Avoid flexion of hips or knees.	Flexion contributes to venous stasis and discomfort.

Nursing Diagnosis:

Ineffective Peripheral Tissue Perfusion

related to interrupted venous flow occurring with venous engorgement or edema

Desired Outcome: Following interventions, the patient has adequate peripheral perfusion as evidenced by absence of discomfort and presence of normal extremity temperature, color, sensation, and motor function.

ASSESSMENT/INTERVENTIONS	RATIONALES
Assess for pain and changes in skin temperature, color, and motor or sensory function. Be alert to venous engorgement (prominence) in the lower extremities.	These are signs of inadequate peripheral perfusion.
Elevate the patient's legs.	Elevation promotes venous drainage.
As prescribed for patients without evidence of thrombus formation, apply antiembolic hose.	These hose compress superficial veins to increase blood flow to the deeper veins.
Remove stockings for approximately 15 min q8h.	This measure enables skin inspection for evidence of irritation and decreased circulation.
In the absence of known DVT, apply a sequential compression device or pneumatic foot compression device as prescribed.	These devices increase blood flow in the deep and superficial veins to prevent DVT and are often indicated for patients who are mostly immobile.
Remove these devices for 15 min q8h.	Removal enables skin inspection for evidence of irritation and decreased circulation.
Place a cloth sleeve (stockinette) beneath the plastic device.	This measure prevents trapping of heat and moisture, which could irritate or harm skin.
Encourage the patient to perform ankle circling and active or assisted ROM exercises of the lower extremities. Perform passive ROM exercises if the patient cannot.	These exercises prevent venous stasis, which is a known cause of venous disorders.
If there are any signs of acute thrombus formation, such as calf hardness or tenderness, exercises are contraindicated. Notify the health care provider accordingly.	This restriction minimizes risk of embolization.
Encourage deep breathing.	Deep breathing creates increased negative pressure in the lungs and thorax to assist in emptying of the large veins.
Assess peripheral pulses regularly.	Although arterial circulation usually will not be impaired unless there is arterial disease or severe edema compressing arterial flow, regular pulse assessment will confirm presence of good arterial flow.

Nursing Diagnosis:

Deficient Knowledge

related to unfamiliarity with the disease process of VTE and the necessary at-home treatment/management measures after hospital discharge

Desired Outcome: Before hospital discharge, the patient verbalizes knowledge of the disease process and treatment/management measures that are to occur after hospital discharge.

ASSESSMENT/INTERVENTIONS	RATIONALES
Assess the patient's health care literacy (language, reading, comprehension). Assess culture and culturally specific education needs.	This assessment helps ensure that information is selected and presented in a manner that is culturally and educationally appropriate.

ASSESSMENT/INTERVENTIONS   RATIONALES

ASSESSMENT/INTERVENTIONS	RATIONALES
Discuss the process of VTE and ways to prevent thrombosis and discomfort.	Avoiding restrictive clothing and prolonged periods of standing and elevating legs above heart level when sitting promote venous return and help prevent DVT while promoting comfort. In addition, regular walking and active ankle and leg ROM exercises promote venous return, strengthen leg muscles, and facilitate development of collateral vessels.
Discuss the prescribed anticoagulant therapy. (Refer to "Patient-Family Teaching," below, and to "Pulmonary Embolus," p. 131.)	Most patients will be maintained on anticoagulation therapy for several months or longer.
Teach signs of venous stasis ulcers, and advise the patient to report any breaks in skin to the health care provider.	Such indicators as redness and skin breakdown are signals of venous stasis ulcers, which necessitate medical attention before they lead to complications such as infection or even gangrene.
Stress the importance of avoiding trauma to the extremities and keeping the skin clean and dry.	Avoiding trauma decreases risk of skin breakdown; clean and dry skin helps prevent infection that could develop in broken skin.
Instruct the patient to inspect both feet each day. If necessary, suggest use of a long-handled mirror to see bottoms of the feet. Advise the patient to report any open areas to the health care provider.	Foot inspection will detect bruises or open wounds, because tissues of the lower extremities may be susceptible to injury.
Discuss the prescribed exercise program.	Walking usually is considered the best exercise, although other exercises involving the lower extremities also prevent venous stasis, strengthen lower leg muscles, and help develop collateral vessels where circulation may be routed.
Teach the patient how to apply antiembolic hose if prescribed.	Decreasing venous distention with these hose optimally will increase blood flow back to the heart. These hose should be applied after the legs have been elevated above heart level for at least a minute to prevent entrapment of the edema in the feet and ankles.
Describe indicators that necessitate medical attention.	Persistent redness, swelling, tenderness, weak or absent pulses, and ulcerations in the extremities may be signs of infection and worsening venous congestion. This must be reported to the health care provider promptly to avoid systemic infection and further compromise to the circulation.
Encourage long-term management of venous stasis with elastic stockings.	This measure will help prevent sequelae associated with postphlebitic syndrome and chronic venous insufficiency.

ADDITIONAL NURSING DIAGNOSES/PROBLEMS:

"Pulmonary Embolus" for **Risk for bleeding** related to   p. 130
    anticoagulation therapy

✓ PATIENT-FAMILY TEACHING AND DISCHARGE PLANNING

When providing patient-family teaching, focus on sensory information, avoid giving excessive information, and initiate a visiting nurse referral for necessary follow-up teaching. Include verbal and written information about the following:

  ✓ See **Deficient Knowledge** for topics to discuss, both verbally and through written information, with the patient and significant other.

  ✓ If the patient is discharged from the hospital on warfarin therapy, provide information about the following:

- As directed, see the health care provider for scheduled international normalized ratio (INR) evaluation.
- Take warfarin at the same time each day; do not skip days unless directed to by the health care provider.
- Wear a medical alert bracelet.
- Avoid alcohol consumption and changes in diet (e.g., changing to a vegetarian diet), both of which can alter the body's response to warfarin.
- When making appointments with other health care providers and dentists, inform them that warfarin is being taken.
- Be alert to indicators that necessitate immediate medical attention: hematuria, hematemesis, meno-metrorrhagia, hematochezia, melena, epistaxis, bleeding gums, ecchymosis, hemoptysis, dizziness, and weakness.
- Avoid taking over-the-counter medications (e.g., aspirin, which also prolongs coagulation time) without consulting the health care provider or nurse.
- Avoid trauma to extremities.

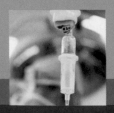

Acute Renal Failure 25

OVERVIEW/PATHOPHYSIOLOGY

Acute renal failure (ARF) is a sudden loss of renal function as a result of reduced blood flow or glomerular injury, which may or may not be accompanied by oliguria. The kidneys lose their ability to maintain biochemical homeostasis, causing retention of metabolic wastes and dramatic alterations in fluid, electrolyte, and acid-base balance. Although alteration in renal function usually is reversible, ARF may be associated with a mortality rate of 40%-80%. Mortality varies greatly with the cause of ARF, patient's age, and comorbid conditions.

Causes of ARF are classified according to development as prerenal, intrarenal, and postrenal. A decrease in renal function secondary to decreased renal perfusion but without renal parenchymal damage is called *prerenal failure*. Causes of prerenal failure include fluid volume deficit, shock and decreased cardiac function. If hypoperfusion has not been prolonged, restoration of renal perfusion will restore normal renal function. A reduction in urine output because of mechanical obstruction to urine flow is called *postrenal failure*. Conditions causing postrenal failure include neurogenic bladder, tumors, and urethral strictures. Early detection of prerenal and postrenal failure is essential because, if prolonged, they can lead to parenchymal damage. Restoration of renal function in cases of postrenal failure is directly related to removal of the obstruction.

The most common cause of *intrinsic* or *intrarenal failure*, or renal failure that develops secondary to renal parenchymal damage, is acute tubular necrosis (ATN). Although typically associated with prolonged ischemia (prerenal failure) or exposure to nephrotoxins (aminoglycoside antibiotics, heavy metals, radiographic contrast media), ATN also can occur after transfusion reactions, septic abortions, or crushing injuries. Additional medications associated with the development of ARF include nonsteroidal antiinflammatory drugs (NSAIDs), angiotensin-converting enzyme (ACE) inhibitors, immunosuppressants (e.g., cyclosporine), antineoplastics (e.g., cisplatin), and antifungals (e.g., amphotericin B). The clinical course of ATN can be divided into the following three phases: oliguric (urine output of greater than 100 mL and less than 400 mL/day, lasting approximately 7-21 days), diuretic (7-14 days), and recovery (3-12 mo). Causes of intrinsic renal failure other than ATN include acute glomerulonephritis (GN), malignant hypertension, hepatorenal syndrome, and autoimmune syndromes.

HEALTH CARE SETTING

Acute medical-surgical care unit

ASSESSMENT

Physical assessment: Pallor, edema (peripheral, periorbital, sacral), jugular vein distention, crackles (rales), and elevated blood pressure (BP) in a patient who has fluid overload.

Excess fluid volume: Oliguria, pitting edema, hypertension, pulmonary edema.

Metabolic acidosis: Kussmaul respirations (hyperventilation), lethargy, headache.

Electrolyte disturbance: Muscle weakness and dysrhythmias.

Infection: Urinary tract infection, septicemia, pulmonary infections, peritonitis.

Uremia (retention of metabolic wastes): Altered mental state, anorexia, nausea, diarrhea, pale and sallow skin, purpura, decreased resistance to infection, anemia, fatigue. **Note:** Uremia adversely affects all body systems.

GI system: Nausea, vomiting, diarrhea, constipation, gastrointestinal (GI) bleeding, anorexia, abdominal distention.

History of: Exposure to nephrotoxic substances, recent blood transfusion, prolonged hypotensive episodes or decreased renal perfusion, sepsis, administration of radiolucent contrast media, or prostatic hypertrophy.

DIAGNOSTIC TESTS

Creatinine clearance: Measures the kidney's ability to clear the blood of creatinine and approximates the glomerular filtration rate. It will decrease as renal function decreases. Creatinine clearance is normally decreased in older persons.

Note: *Failure to collect all urine during the period of study can invalidate the test.*

Blood urea nitrogen (BUN) and serum creatinine: Assess progression and management of ARF. Although both BUN and creatinine will increase as renal function decreases, creatinine is a better indicator of renal function because it is not affected by diet, hydration, or tissue catabolism.

Urinalysis: Can provide information about the cause and location of renal disease as reflected by abnormal urinary sediment (renal tubular cells and cell casts).

Urinary osmolality and urinary sodium levels: To rule out renal perfusion problems (prerenal). In ATN, the kidney loses its ability to adjust urine concentration and conserve sodium, producing urine Na$^+$ level greater than 40 mEq/L (in prerenal azotemia the urine Na$^+$ is less than 20 mEq/L).

Note: *All urine samples should be sent to the laboratory immediately after collection or should be refrigerated if this is not possible. Urine left at room temperature has greater potential for bacterial growth, turbidity, and alkalinity, any of which can distort the reading.*

Renal ultrasound: Provides information about renal anatomy and pelvic structures, evaluates renal masses, and detects obstruction and hydronephrosis. Because no intravenous (IV) contrast agent is used, this procedure limits risk of further compromise to renal function.

Renal scan: Provides information about perfusion and function of the kidneys.

Computed tomography (CT) scan: Identifies dilation of renal calices in obstructive processes.

Retrograde urography: Assesses for postrenal causes (i.e., obstruction).

Nursing Diagnosis:

Risk for Infection

related to the presence of uremia

Desired Outcome: The patient is free of infection as evidenced by normothermia; white blood cell (WBC) count 11,000/mm^3 or less; urine that is clear and of normal odor; normal breath sounds; eupnea; and absence of erythema, warmth, tenderness, swelling, and drainage at the catheter or IV access sites.

Note: *One of the primary causes of death in ARF is sepsis.*

ASSESSMENT/INTERVENTIONS	RATIONALES
Assess temperature and secretions for indicators of infection.	Even minor increases in temperature can be significant because uremia masks the febrile response and inhibits the body's ability to fight infection.
Use meticulous sterile technique when changing dressings or manipulating venous catheters, IV lines, or indwelling catheters.	These measures prevent infection via spread of pathogens.
Avoid long-term use of indwelling urinary catheters. Whenever possible, use intermittent catheterization instead.	Indwelling urinary catheters are a common source of infection.
Provide oral hygiene and skin care at frequent intervals.	Intact skin and oral mucous membranes are barriers to infection.
Use emollients and gentle soap.	These measures prevent drying and cracking of the skin, which could lead to breakdown and infection.
Rinse off all soap when bathing the patient.	Soap residue may further irritate the skin and affects its integrity.

Nursing Diagnoses:

Acute Confusion
Ineffective Protection

related to neurosensory, musculoskeletal, and cardiac changes occurring with uremia, electrolyte imbalance, and metabolic acidosis

Desired Outcomes: After treatment, the patient verbalizes orientation to person, place, and time and is free of injury caused by neurosensory, musculoskeletal, or cardiac disturbances. Within the 24-hr period before hospital discharge, the patient verbalizes signs and symptoms of electrolyte imbalance and metabolic acidosis and the importance of reporting them promptly should they occur.

ASSESSMENT/INTERVENTIONS	RATIONALES
Assess for and alert the patient to indicators of alterations in fluid, electrolyte, and acid-base balance.	In ARF, the kidneys lose their ability to maintain biochemical homeostasis, causing retention of metabolic wastes and dramatic alterations in fluid, electrolyte, and acid-base balance. The following may occur:
	Hypokalemia: Muscle weakness, lethargy, dysrhythmias, abdominal distention, and nausea and vomiting (secondary to ileus). It may occur during the diuretic phase because of urinary potassium losses.
	Hyperkalemia: Muscle cramps, dysrhythmias, muscle weakness, increased QRS duration, and peaked T waves on electrocardiogram. Hyperkalemia is a common and potentially fatal complication of ARF during the oliguric phase. It may occur if the kidney is unable to excrete potassium ions into the urine.
	Caution: A normal serum K^+ level is necessary for normal cardiac function.
	Hypocalcemia: Neuromuscular irritability, for example, positive Trousseau's sign (carpopedal spasm) and Chvostek's sign (facial muscle spasm), and paresthesias. Hypocalcemia may occur because of increased serum phosphate (there is a reciprocal relationship between calcium and phosphorus—as one rises, the other decreases).
	Hyperphosphatemia: Although usually asymptomatic, it may cause bone or joint pain and painful/itchy skin lesions. Serum phosphorus may increase because of a decreased ability of the kidneys to excrete this ion.
	Uremia: Anorexia, nausea, metallic taste in the mouth, irritability, confusion, lethargy, restlessness, and itching. Uremic symptoms result from increased BUN as the kidney loses its ability to excrete nitrogenous wastes.
	Metabolic acidosis: Rapid, deep respirations; confusion. A buildup of hydrogen ions occurs in the serum because of the kidneys' inability to buffer and secrete this ion.
Avoid giving foods high in potassium content.	This restriction helps potassium levels return to more normal levels. Salt substitutes also contain potassium and should be avoided along with apricots, avocados, bananas, cantaloupe, carrots, cauliflower, chocolate, dried beans and peas, dried fruit, mushrooms, nuts, oranges, peanuts, potatoes, prune juice, pumpkins, spinach, sweet potatoes, Swiss chard, tomatoes, and watermelon.
Maintain adequate nutritional intake (especially calories).	If caloric intake is inadequate, body protein will be used for energy, resulting in increased end products of protein metabolism (i.e., nitrogenous wastes). A high-carbohydrate diet helps minimize tissue catabolism and production of nitrogenous wastes.

ASSESSMENT/INTERVENTIONS	RATIONALES
Prevent infections.	This measure minimizes tissue catabolism by controlling fevers. See **Risk for Infection**, earlier.
⚠ Avoid or use with caution the following medications: NSAIDs, ACE inhibitors, and potassium-sparing diuretics.	NSAIDs may further damage kidney function and/or cause electrolyte imbalances including hyperkalemia or hyponatremia. ACE inhibitors and potassium sparing diuretics may cause an increase in serum potassium. **Note:** Soon after renal disease is initially diagnosed, ACE inhibitors may be prescribed for their renal protective effects. However, after chronic kidney disease has developed, ACE inhibitors may require dose adjustment or may be contraindicated because of hyperkalemia.risk.
Prepare the patient for the possibility of altered taste and smell.	Alterations in taste and smell may occur with uremia as a result of toxin buildup due to inability of the kidneys to excrete nitrogenous waste.
Avoid use of magnesium-containing medications.	Patients with renal failure are at risk for increased magnesium levels because of decreased urinary excretion of dietary magnesium. Patients using magnesium-containing antacids such as Maalox typically are switched to aluminum hydroxide preparations such as ALternaGEL or Amphojel. Milk of Magnesia should be substituted with another, non–magnesium-containing laxative such as casanthranol.
Administer aluminum hydroxide or calcium antacids as prescribed. Experiment with different brands, or try capsules for patients who refuse certain liquid antacids.	These agents are administered to control hyperphosphatemia. Phosphate binders vary in their aluminum or calcium content, however, and one may not be exchanged for another without first ensuring that the patient is receiving the same amount of elemental aluminum or calcium. These medications must be administered with meals. **Note:** Aluminum-containing phosphate binders should not be used long term because of their potential to cause bone damage.
Administer other medications as prescribed:	
- Diuretics	These medications are used in nonoliguric ARF for fluid removal. For example, furosemide (Lasix) (100-200 mg) or mannitol (12.5 g) may be given early in ARF to limit or prevent development of oliguria.
- Antihypertensives	These medications are used to control BP in the presence of underlying illness, fluid overload, sodium retention, or stimulation of the renin-angiotensin system in patients with renal ischemia.
- Cation exchange resins (Kayexalate)	These resins are used to control hyperkalemia. Kayexalate is most effectively administered orally, but it may be administered as an enema. The resin acts in the intestinal tract via exchange of sodium ions (from the Kayexalate) for potassium ions. Kayexalate is usually administered with sorbitol to prevent constipation and fecal impaction. **Note:** Severe hyperkalemia may be treated also with *IV sodium bicarbonate*, which shifts potassium into the cells temporarily, or *glucose and insulin*. Insulin also helps move potassium into the cells, and glucose helps prevent dangerous hypoglycemia, which could result from the insulin. *IV calcium* is given to reverse the cardiac effects of life-threatening hyperkalemia.
- Calcium or vitamin D supplements	These supplements are given to patients with hypocalcemia.
- Sodium bicarbonate	This is given to treat metabolic acidosis when the serum bicarbonate level is less than 15 mmol/L.
Avoid or use cautiously in patients with hypocalcemia, edema, or sodium retention.	Rapidly rising serum pH may result in muscle spasms in patients with hypocalcemia.
- Vitamins B and C	These vitamins replace losses if the patient is on dialysis.

continued

ASSESSMENT/INTERVENTIONS	RATIONALES
Reassure the patient and significant other that irritability, restlessness, and altered thinking are temporary and will improve with treatment.	Reassurance may help allay added anxiety.
Display calendars and request that significant others bring radios and familiar objects.	These measures will help orient the patient to person, place, and time.
Ensure safety measures (e.g., padded side rails, airway) for patients who are confused or severely hypocalcemic. For patients who exhibit signs of hyperkalemia, have emergency supplies (e.g., manual resuscitator bag, crash cart, emergency drug tray) available.	These measures are for the patient's protection until electrolyte disturbance is reversed.

Nursing Diagnosis:

Excess Fluid Volume

related to compromised regulatory mechanisms occurring with renal dysfunction: *Oliguric phase*

Desired Outcome: The patient adheres to prescribed fluid restrictions and becomes normovolemic as evidenced by decreasing or stable weight, normal breath sounds, edema 1+ or less on a 0-4+ scale, central venous pressure (CVP) 10 mm Hg or less, and BP and heart rate (HR) within the patient's normal range.

ASSESSMENT/INTERVENTIONS	RATIONALES
Closely assess and document intake and output (I&O).	This assessment detects trend of fluid volume, particularly decreasing urinary output when compared to intake. Patients with ARF may/may not develop oliguria. Urine volume does not necessarily reflect renal function in patients with ARF. For example, in postrenal failure, large volumes of urine may be associated with relief of obstruction. In ARF, the kidneys lose their ability to maintain biochemical homeostasis. This causes retention of metabolic wastes and dramatic alterations in fluid, electrolyte, and acid-base balance. For details about likely electrolyte imbalances and metabolic acidosis, see **Acute Confusion/Ineffective Protection**, earlier.
Monitor weight daily. Weigh the patient at the same time each day, using the same scale and with the patient wearing the same amount of clothing.	The patient likely will lose 0.5 kg/day if not eating; a sudden weight gain suggests excessive fluid volume. This ensures that weight measurements are performed under the same conditions with each assessment, thereby facilitating more precise measurements of fluid volume.
Assess for edema, hypertension, crackles (rales), tachycardia, distended neck veins, shortness of breath, and increased CVP.	These signs are indicators of fluid volume excess. In ARF, dependent edema likely will be detected in the legs or feet of patients who are ambulatory, and in the sacral area of patients who are on bedrest. Periorbital edema may also result from excessive fluid overload. Jugular veins are likely to be distended with the head of bed elevated 45 degrees due to increased intravascular volume. Crackles and shortness of breath can occur as a result of pulmonary fluid volume overload. Low serum albumin decreases colloid osmotic pressure, allowing fluid to leak into the extravascular space. Low serum albumin also may contribute to generalized edema and pulmonary edema. Hypertension, tachycardia, and increased CVP may result from sodium and fluid retention. Decreased renal perfusion also may activate the renin-angiotensin system, exacerbating these symptoms.
Carefully adhere to the prescribed fluid restriction.	This measure helps patients return to normovolemia. Fluids usually are restricted on the basis of "replace losses 400 mL/24 hr." Insensible fluid losses are only partially replaced to offset water formed during the metabolism of proteins, carbohydrates, and fats.

ASSESSMENT/INTERVENTIONS	RATIONALES
Provide oral hygiene at frequent intervals, and offer fluids in the form of ice chips or ice pops. Spread allotted fluids evenly over a 24-hr period, and record the amount given. Instruct the patient and significant others about the need for fluid restriction.	These interventions minimize thirst during fluid restriction. Hard candies also may be given to decrease thirst. **Note:** Patients nourished via total parenteral nutrition are at increased risk for fluid overload because of the necessary fluid volume involved and its hypertonicity.
Monitor results of BUN, serum creatinine, and creatinine clearance tests.	Although both BUN and creatinine will increase as renal function and renal excretion decrease, creatinine is a better indicator of renal function because it is not affected by diet, hydration, or tissue catabolism. Creatinine clearance measures the ability of the kidney to clear the blood of creatinine and approximates the glomerular filtration rate. It will decrease as renal function decreases. **Note:** Creatinine clearance is normally decreased in older persons.
Administer medications that promote diuresis as prescribed.	Control of fluid overload in ARF may include use of large doses of furosemide in nonoliguric patients to induce diuresis.
Arrange for or administer renal dialysis as prescribed. For more information, see "Care of the Patient Undergoing Hemodialysis," p. 212, or, "Care of the Patient Undergoing Peritoneal Dialysis," p. 216, as indicated.	Hemodialysis treatments remove excess fluid through the process of ultrafiltration (removal of fluids using pressure). Peritoneal dialysis removes fluid via osmotic pressures across the peritoneal membrane. The present trend is to use dialysis early in ARF. It is done q1-3days (but may be done continuously in critical care). Prophylactic use of dialysis has reduced the incidence of complications and rate of death in patients with ARF.

Nursing Diagnosis:
Deficient Fluid Volume

related to active loss occurring with excessive urinary output: *Diuretic phase*

Desired Outcome: The patient becomes normovolemic as evidenced by stable weight, balanced I&O, good skin turgor, CVP 4 mm Hg or greater, and BP and HR within the patient's normal range.

ASSESSMENT/INTERVENTIONS	RATIONALES
Closely assess and document I&O.	This assessment detects the trend of fluid volume. Following relief of the obstruction in patients with postrenal failure, postobstructive diuresis may occur if the kidney is unable to concentrate the urine. Consequently, large volumes of solute and fluid may be lost (8-20 L/day of urinary losses), resulting in volume depletion.
Monitor weight daily. Weigh the patient at the same time each day, using the same scale and with the patient wearing the same amount of clothing.	A weight loss of 0.5 kg/day or more may reflect excessive volume loss. When weight is measured under the same conditions, more precise measurements of fluid volume can be anticipated.
Monitor the patient for complaints of lightheadedness, poor skin turgor, hypotension, postural hypotension, tachycardia, and decreased CVP.	These are indicators of volume depletion, which may result from loss of intravascular volume caused by urinary fluid losses and could lead to falls and other injuries.
As prescribed, encourage fluids in the dehydrated patient.	This intervention promotes rehydration and prevents life-threatening electrolyte abnormalities caused by the large-volume urinary and solute losses.
Report significant findings to the health care provider.	Although renal function usually can be reversed, there is a mortality rate of 40%-80% associated with ARF, depending on cause and the patient's age and comorbid conditions.

Nursing Diagnosis:

Imbalanced Nutrition: Less Than Body Requirements

related to nausea, vomiting, anorexia, and dietary restrictions

Desired Outcome: Within 2 days of admission, the patient has stable weight and demonstrates normal intake of food within restrictions, as indicated.

ASSESSMENT/INTERVENTIONS	RATIONALES
Assess for and alert the health care provider to untoward GI symptoms, and monitor BUN levels.	The presence of nausea, vomiting, and anorexia may signal increased uremia. BUN levels 80-100 mg/dL usually require dialytic therapy.
Provide frequent, small meals in a pleasant atmosphere, especially controlling unpleasant odors.	Smaller, more frequent meals are usually better tolerated than larger meals.
Administer prescribed antiemetics as necessary. Instruct the patient to request medication before discomfort becomes severe.	Antiemetics are given to reduce nausea, which is better controlled when it is treated early.
Coordinate meal planning and dietary teaching with the patient, significant others, and renal dietitian.	Dietary restriction may include reduced protein, sodium, potassium, phosphorus, and fluid intake.
Provide fact sheets that list foods to restrict.	Protein is limited to minimize retention of nitrogenous wastes. Sodium is limited to prevent thirst and fluid retention. Potassium and phosphorus are limited because of the kidney's decreased ability to excrete them.
Demonstrate with sample menus examples of how dietary restrictions may be incorporated into daily meals.	Sample menus show the patient how to apply this new knowledge.
Provide oral hygiene at frequent intervals.	Oral hygiene decreases metallic taste in the mouth associated with uremia.

ADDITIONAL NURSING DIAGNOSES/PROBLEMS:

PATIENT-FAMILY TEACHING AND DISCHARGE PLANNING

When providing patient-family teaching, focus on sensory information, avoid giving excessive information, and initiate a visiting nurse referral for necessary follow-up teaching. Include verbal and written information about the following:

✓ Medications: Include drug name, purpose, dosage, schedule, precautions, and potential side effects. Also discuss drug-drug, herb-drug, and food-drug interactions.

✓ Diet: Include fact sheets that list foods to restrict. Provide sample menus with examples of how dietary restrictions may be incorporated into daily meals.

✓ Care and observation of dialysis access if the patient is being discharged with one. If the patient requires dialysis after discharge, coordinate discharge planning with the dialysis unit staff.

✓ Importance of continued medical follow-up of renal function.

✓ Signs and symptoms of potential complications. These should include electrolyte imbalance (see **Acute Confusion/Ineffective Protection** in this chapter); indicators of infection (see **Risk for Infection** in this chapter); **Excess Fluid Volume** in this chapter; and bleeding (especially from the GI tract for patients who are uremic).

✓ Telephone numbers to call in case questions or concerns arise about therapy or disease after discharge. Additional general information can be obtained by contacting the following:

✓ National Kidney and Urologic Diseases Information Clearinghouse at *www.kidney.niddk.nih.gov*

✓ National Kidney Foundation at *www.kidney.org*

✓ The Kidney Foundation of Canada at *www.kidney.ca*

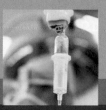

Benign Prostatic Hypertrophy 26

OVERVIEW/PATHOPHYSIOLOGY

The prostate is an encapsulated gland that surrounds the male urethra below the bladder neck and produces a thin, milky fluid during ejaculation. As a man ages, the prostate gland grows larger. Although the exact cause of enlargement is unknown, one theory is that hormonal changes affect the estrogen-androgen balance. This noncancerous enlargement is common in men older than 50 yr, and as many as 80% of men older than 65 yr are thought to have symptoms of prostatic enlargement. Treatment options include two classes of medications, alpha-adrenergic antagonists and 5 alpha-reductase inhibitors, and surgical treatment. Medical management may reduce the need for surgery. Treatment is given when symptoms of bladder outlet obstruction appear.

HEALTH CARE SETTING

Primary care; outpatient acute (surgical) care

ASSESSMENT

Chronic indicators: Urinary frequency, hesitancy, urgency, and dribbling or postvoid dribbling; decreased force and caliber of stream; nocturia (several times each night); hematuria. Scores on American Urological Association (AUA) questionnaire are 0-7 (mild), 8-19 (moderate), and 20-35 (severe).

Acute indicators/bladder outlet obstruction: Anuria, nausea, vomiting, severe suprapubic pain, severe and constant urgency, flank pain during micturition.

Physical assessment: Bladder distention, kettledrum sound with percussion over the distended bladder. Rectal examination reveals a smooth, firm, symmetric, and elastic enlargement of the prostate.

DIAGNOSTIC TESTS

Urinalysis: Checks for the presence of white blood cells (WBCs), leukocyte esterase, WBC casts, bacteria, and microscopic hematuria.

Urine culture and sensitivity: Verifies presence of an infecting organism, identifies type of organism, and determines the organism's antibiotic sensitivities. **Note:** All urine specimens should be sent to the laboratory immediately after they are obtained, or they should be refrigerated if this is not possible (specimens for urine culture should not be refrigerated). Urine left at room temperature has a greater potential for bacterial growth, turbidity, and alkaline pH, any of which can distort test results.

Hematocrit (Hct) and hemoglobin (Hgb): Decreased Hct and Hb values may signal mild anemia from local bleeding.

Blood urea nitrogen (BUN) and creatinine: To evaluate renal and urinary function. **Note:** BUN can be affected by the patient's hydration status, and results must be evaluated accordingly: fluid volume excess reduces BUN levels, whereas fluid volume deficit increases them. Serum creatinine may not be a reliable indicator of renal function in older adults because of decreased muscle mass and decreased glomerular filtration rate; results of this test must be evaluated along with those of urine creatinine clearance, other renal function studies, and the patient's age.

Prostate-specific antigen: Elevated above normal (0-4.0 ng/mL; normal range may increase with age); correlates well with positive digital examination findings. This glycoprotein is produced only by the prostate and reflects prostate size.

Cystoscopy: Visualizes the prostate gland, estimates its size, and ascertains presence of any damage to the bladder wall secondary to an enlarged prostate. **Note:** Because patients undergoing cystoscopy are susceptible to septic shock, this procedure is contraindicated in patients with acute urinary tract infection (UTI) because of the possible danger of hematogenous spread of gram-negative bacteria.

Transrectal ultrasound: Assesses prostate size and shape via a probe inserted into the rectum.

Maximal urinary flow rate: Rate less than 15 mL/sec indicates significant obstruction to flow.

Postvoid residual volume: Normal volume is less than 12 mL; higher volumes signal obstructive process.

Nursing Diagnosis:

Acute Confusion

related to fluid volume excess occurring with absorption of irrigating fluid during surgery; or cerebral hypoxia occurring with sepsis

Desired Outcome: The patient's mental status returns to normal for the patient within 3 days of treatment.

ASSESSMENT/INTERVENTIONS	RATIONALES
Assess the patient's baseline level of consciousness (LOC) and mental status on admission. Ask the patient to perform a three-step task.	Asking patients to perform a three-step task (e.g., "Raise your right hand, place it on your left shoulder, and then place the right hand by your side") is an effective way to evaluate baseline mental status because patients may be admitted with chronic confusion.
Assess short-term memory.	Short-term memory can be tested by showing the patient how to use the call light, having him return the demonstration, and then waiting 5 min before having him demonstrate use of the call light again. Inability to remember beyond 5 min indicates poor short-term memory.
Document the patient's response.	A patient's baseline status can then be compared with postsurgical status for evaluation, which will help determine the presence of acute confusion.
Document the patient's actions in behavioral terms. Describe the "confused" behavior.	This ensures that the patient's current/postsurgical status is compared with his normal status.
Obtain a description of prehospital functional and mental status from sources familiar with the patient (e.g., family, friends, personnel at the nursing home or residential care facility).	The cause may be reversible.
Identify the cause of acute confusion as follows:	
- Assess oximetry or request arterial blood gas values.	Low levels of oxygen can contribute to diminished mental status.
- Check serum sodium.	Dilutional hyponatremia can be caused by absorption of irrigating fluid.
- Request current serum electrolytes and WBC count.	Imbalances in electrolytes and the presence of infection (reflected by elevated WBC count) can affect mental status.
- Assess hydration status by reviewing intake and output (I&O) records after surgery. Output should match intake.	Both excess and deficient fluid volumes can affect mental status.
- Assess the legs for dependent edema.	Dependent edema can signal overhydration with poor venous return, which can affect mental status.
- Assess cardiac and lung status.	Abnormal heart sounds or rhythms and the presence of crackles (rales) in lung bases can signal fluid excess, which could affect mental status.
- Assess the mouth for a furrowed tongue and dry mucous membranes.	These signs signal fluid deficit, which can affect mental status.
- For oximetry readings 92% or less, anticipate initiation of oxygen therapy to increase oxygenation.	Patients usually require supplementary oxygen at these levels. Decreased levels of oxygen can adversely affect mental status.
- As appropriate, anticipate initiation of antibiotics in the presence of sepsis, diuretics to increase diuresis, and increased fluid intake by mouth or intravenous (IV) to rehydrate the patient.	These interventions may help reverse acute confusion.
As appropriate, have the patient wear glasses and hearing aid, or keep them close to the bedside and within easy reach.	Disturbed sensory perception can contribute to confusion.
Keep the urinal and other commonly used items within easy reach.	Patients with short-term memory problems cannot be expected to use a call light.
As indicated by mental status, check on the patient frequently or every time you pass by the room.	This intervention helps ensure the patient's safety.
If indicated, place the patient close to the nurses' station if possible. Provide an environment that is nonstimulating and safe.	These measures provide a safer and less confusing environment for patients.

ASSESSMENT/INTERVENTIONS

ASSESSMENT/INTERVENTIONS	RATIONALES
Provide music, but avoid use of television.	Individuals who are acutely confused regarding place and time often think the action on television is happening in the room.
Attempt to reorient the patient to his surroundings as needed. Keep a clock and calendar at the bedside, and remind him verbally of the date and place.	These orientation measures help reduce confusion.
Encourage the patient or significant other to bring items familiar to the patient.	Familiar items provide a foundation for orientation and can include blankets, bedspreads, and pictures of family or pets.
If the patient becomes belligerent, angry, or argumentative while you are attempting to reorient him, *stop this approach.* Do not argue with him or his interpretation of the environment.	Arguing with confused patients likely will increase their belligerence. State, "I can understand why you may (hear, think, see) that."
If the patient displays hostile behavior or misperceives your role (e.g., nurse becomes thief, jailer), leave the room. Return in 15 min. Introduce yourself to him as though you have never met. Begin dialogue anew.	Patients who are acutely confused have poor short-term memory and may not remember the previous encounter or that you were involved in that encounter.
If the patient attempts to leave the hospital, walk with him and attempt distraction. Ask him to tell you about his destination. For example, "That sounds like a wonderful place! Tell me about it." Keep your tone pleasant and conversational. Continue walking with him away from exits and doors around the unit. After a few minutes, attempt to guide him back to his room.	Distraction is an effective technique with individuals who are confused.
If the patient has permanent or severe cognitive impairment, check on him frequently and reorient to baseline mental status as indicated; however, do not argue with him about his perception of reality.	Arguing can cause a cognitively impaired person to become aggressive and combative. Patients with severe cognitive impairments (e.g., Alzheimer's disease, dementia) also can experience acute confusional states (i.e., delirium) and can be returned to their baseline mental state.

Nursing Diagnosis:

Risk for Bleeding

related to invasive procedure or actions that put pressure on the prostatic capsule

Desired Outcomes: The patient is normovolemic as evidenced by a balanced I&O; heart rate (HR) 100 bpm or less (or within the patient's normal range); blood pressure (BP) 90/60 mm Hg or more (or within the patient's normal range); respiratory rate (RR) 20 breaths/min or less; and skin that is warm, dry, and of normal color. Following instruction, the patient relates actions that may result in hemorrhage of the prostatic capsule and participates in interventions to prevent them.

ASSESSMENT/INTERVENTIONS	RATIONALES
On the patient's return from the recovery room, assess vital signs (VS) as his condition warrants or per agency protocol.	These assessments evaluate trend of the patient's recovery. Increasing pulse, decreasing BP, diaphoresis, pallor, and increasing respirations can occur with hemorrhage and impending shock.
Monitor and document I&O q8h. Subtract the amount of fluid used with continuous bladder irrigation (CBI) from the total output.	This assessment evaluates trend of the patient's hydration status and assesses for postsurgical bleeding.
Assess catheter drainage closely for the first 24 hr. Watch for dark red drainage that does not lighten to reddish pink or drainage that remains thick in consistency after irrigation.	Drainage should lighten to pink or blood tinged within 24 hr after surgery. Dark red drainage that does not lighten to reddish pink or drainage that remains thick in consistency after irrigation can signal bleeding within the operative site.
Be alert to bright red, thick drainage at any time.	This drainage can occur with arterial bleeding within the operative site.

continued

ASSESSMENT/INTERVENTIONS	RATIONALES
Do not measure temperature rectally or insert tubes or enemas into the rectum. Instruct the patient not to strain with bowel movements or sit for long periods.	These actions can result in pressure on the prostatic capsule and may lead to hemorrhage.
Obtain prescription for and provide stool softeners or cathartics as necessary. Encourage a diet high in fiber and increased fluid intake.	These measures aid in producing soft stool and preventing straining.
Maintain traction on the indwelling urethral catheter for 4-8 hr after surgery or as directed.	The surgeon may establish traction on the indwelling urethral catheter in the operating room to help prevent bleeding. **Note:** Urethral catheters used after prostatic surgery commonly have a large retention balloon (30 mL).
Monitor for signs of disseminated intravascular coagulation (DIC). Report significant findings promptly if they occur. For more information, see p. 471, "Disseminated Intravascular Coagulation."	DIC can result from release of large amounts of tissue thromboplastins during a transurethral prostatectomy (TURP). Indicators of DIC include active bleeding (dark red) without clots and unusual oozing from all puncture sites.

Nursing Diagnoses:

Excess Fluid Volume (or risk for same)
Risk for Electrolyte Imbalance

related to absorption of irrigating fluid during surgery (TURP syndrome)

Desired Outcomes: Following surgery, the patient is normovolemic as evidenced by balanced I&O (after subtraction of irrigant from total output); orientation to person, place, and time with no significant changes in mental status; BP and HR within the patient's normal range; absence of dysrhythmias; and electrolyte values within normal range. Urinary output is 30 mL/hr or more.

ASSESSMENT/INTERVENTIONS	RATIONALES
Assess and record VS.	This assessment evaluates hydration status. Sudden increases in BP with corresponding decrease in HR can occur with fluid volume excess.
Assess pulse for dysrhythmias, including irregular rate and skipped beats.	Dysrhythmias, including irregular HR and skipped beats, can signal electrolyte imbalance, which can occur as a result of the high volumes of fluid used during irritation.
Monitor and record I&O. To determine true amount of urinary output, subtract the amount of irrigant (CBI) from the total output.	Large amounts of fluid, commonly plain sterile water, are used to irrigate the bladder during the operative cystoscopy to remove blood and tissue, thereby enabling visualization of the surgical field. Over time, this fluid may be absorbed through the bladder wall into the systemic circulation.
Report discrepancies between I&O.	Differences may signal either fluid retention or fluid loss.
Monitor the patient's mental and motor status. Assess for muscle twitching, seizures, and changes in mentation.	These are signs of water intoxication and electrolyte imbalance, which can occur within 24 hr after surgery because of the high volumes of fluid used in irrigation.
Monitor electrolyte values, in particular those of Na^+.	Normal range for Na^+ is 137-147 mEq/L. Values less than that signal hyponatremia, which can occur with absorption of the extra fluids and its dilutional effect.
Promptly report indications of fluid overload and electrolyte imbalance to the health care provider.	This intervention ensures prompt treatment, which may include diuretics.

Nursing Diagnosis:

Acute Pain

related to bladder spasms

Desired Outcomes: Within 1 hr of intervention, the patient's subjective perception of pain decreases, as documented by pain scale. Objective indicators, such as grimacing, are absent or diminished.

ASSESSMENT/INTERVENTIONS	RATIONALES
Assess and document quality, location, and duration of pain. Devise a pain scale with the patient, rating pain from 0 (no pain) to 10 (worst pain).	This assessment establishes a baseline, monitors the trend of pain, and determines subsequent response to medication.
Medicate the patient with prescribed analgesics, narcotics, and antispasmodics as appropriate; evaluate and document the patient's response, using the pain scale.	Suppositories (e.g., belladonna and opium [B&O] suppositories) are contraindicated because of the potential for disrupting the incision, which is close to the rectum. Oral anticholinergics, such as oxybutynin, are used as antispasmodics instead.
Instruct the patient to request analgesic before pain becomes severe.	Prolonged stimulation of the pain receptors results in increased sensitivity to painful stimuli and will increase the amount of drug required to relieve pain.
Provide warm blankets or heating pad to the affected area.	These measures increase regional circulation and relax tense muscles.
Monitor for leakage around the catheter.	Leakage can signal the presence of bladder spasms.
If the patient has spasms, assure him that they are normal.	Spasms can occur from irritation of the bladder mucosa or from a clot that results in backup of urine into the bladder with concomitant mucosal irritation.
Encourage fluid intake.	Adequate hydration helps prevent spasms.
If the health care provider has prescribed catheter irrigation for the removal of clots, follow instructions carefully.	Gentle irrigation will avoid discomfort and injury to the patient.
Monitor for the presence of clots in the tubing. If clots are present for a patient with CBI, adjust the rate of bladder irrigation to maintain light red urine (with clots). If clots inhibit the flow of urine, irrigate the catheter by hand according to agency or health care provider's directive.	Total output should be greater than the amount of irrigant instilled. If output equals the amount of irrigant or the patient complains that his bladder is full, the catheter may be clogged with clots.

Nursing Diagnosis:

Risk for Impaired Skin Integrity

related to wound drainage from suprapubic or retropubic prostatectomy

Desired Outcome: The patient's skin remains nonerythremic and intact.

ASSESSMENT/INTERVENTIONS	RATIONALES
Assess the skin and incisional dressings frequently during the first 24 hr; change or reinforce dressings as needed.	If an incision has been made into the bladder, irritation can result from prolonged contact of urine with the skin.
Use Montgomery straps or gauze net (Surginet) rather than tape to secure the dressing.	These measures ensure that the dressing is secure without the damage that tape can cause to the skin.
If drainage is copious after drain removal, apply a wound drainage or ostomy pouch with a skin barrier over the incision.	This measure provides a barrier between the skin and drainage.
Use a pouch with an antireflux valve.	This valve prevents contamination from reflux.

Nursing Diagnosis:

Deficient Knowledge

related to unfamiliarity with postsurgical sexual function

Desired Outcome: Following intervention/patient teaching, the patient discusses concerns about sexuality and relates accurate information about sexual function.

ASSESSMENT/INTERVENTIONS	RATIONALES
Assess the patient's level of readiness to discuss sexual function; provide opportunities for the patient to discuss fears and anxieties.	This assessment enables the appropriate time to provide patient teaching and optimally will reveal the patient's specific fears and anxieties.
Assure patients who have had a simple prostatectomy that the ability to attain and maintain an erection is unaltered.	Retrograde ejaculation (backward flow of seminal fluid into the bladder, which is eliminated with the next urination) or "dry" ejaculation will occur in most patients, but this probably will end after a few months. However, it will not affect the ability to achieve orgasm.
Be aware of your own feelings about sexuality.	If you are uncomfortable discussing sexuality, request that another staff member take responsibility for discussing concerns with the patient.
As indicated, encourage continuation of counseling after hospital discharge. Confer with the health care provider and social services to identify appropriate referrals.	Conferring with the health care provider and social services will help identify appropriate referrals.

Nursing Diagnosis:

Constipation

related to postsurgical discomfort or fear of exerting excess pressure on the prostatic capsule

Desired Outcome: By the third to fourth postoperative day, the patient relates the presence of a bowel pattern that is normal for him with minimal pain or straining.

ASSESSMENT/INTERVENTIONS	RATIONALES
Assess and document the presence or absence and quality of bowel sounds in all four abdominal quadrants.	A patient whose bowel sounds have not yet returned but who states that he needs to have a bowel movement during the first 24 hr after surgery may have clots in his bladder that are creating pressure on the rectum. Assess for the presence of clots (see **Acute Pain,** earlier) and irrigate the catheter as indicated.
Gather baseline information on the patient's normal bowel pattern and document findings.	Each patient has a bowel pattern that is normal for him.
Caution the patient to avoid straining when defecating.	Straining puts excess pressure on the prostatic capsule.
Unless contraindicated, encourage the patient to drink 2-3 L of fluids on the day after surgery.	Adequate hydration helps ensure a softer stool with less of a tendency to strain.
Consult the health care provider and dietitian about the need for increased fiber in the patient's diet.	Adding bulk to stools will minimize the risk of damaging the prostatic capsule by straining.
Encourage the patient to ambulate and be as active as possible.	Increased activity helps promote bowel movements by increasing peristalsis.
Consult the health care provider about use of stool softeners for the patient during the postoperative period.	Soft stool will be less painful to evacuate following surgery and will cause less straining.
See "Prolonged Bedrest," p. 68, **Constipation**, for more information.	

Nursing Diagnosis:

Urge Urinary Incontinence

related to urethral irritation after removal of the urethral catheter

Desired Outcome: The patient reports increasing periods of time between voidings by the second postoperative day and regains a normal pattern of micturition within 4-6 wk after surgery.

ASSESSMENT/INTERVENTIONS	RATIONALES
Before removing the urethral catheter, explain to the patient that he may void in small amounts for the first 12 hr after catheter removal.	Irritation from the catheter may cause the patient to void in small amounts. Initially the patient may void q15-30min, but the interval between voidings should increase toward a more normal pattern.
Instruct the patient to save urine in a urinal for the first 24 hr after surgery. Inspect each voiding for color and consistency.	First urine specimens can be dark red from passage of old blood. Each successive specimen should be lighter in color.
Note and document the time and amount of each voiding.	Initially patients may void q15-30min, but the time interval between voidings should increase toward a more normal pattern.
Encourage the patient to drink 2.5-3.0 L/day if not contraindicated.	Low intake leads to highly concentrated urine, which irritates the bladder and can lead to incontinence.
Before hospital discharge, inform the patient that dribbling may occur for the first 4-6 wk after surgery.	Dribbling occurs because of disturbance of the bladder neck and urethra during prostate removal. As muscles strengthen and healing occurs (the urethra reaches normal size and function), dribbling stops.
Teach Kegel exercises (see **Deficient Knowledge** later in this chapter.)	These exercises improve sphincter control.

Nursing Diagnosis:

Stress Urinary Incontinence

related to temporary loss of muscle tone in the urethral sphincter after radical prostatectomy

Desired Outcome: Within the 24-hr period before hospital discharge, the patient relates understanding of the cause of the temporary incontinence and the regimen that must be observed to promote bladder control.

ASSESSMENT/INTERVENTIONS	RATIONALES
Explain that there is a potential for urinary incontinence after prostatectomy but that it should resolve within 6 mo. Describe the reason for the incontinence, using aids such as anatomic illustrations.	A knowledgeable patient likely will adhere to the therapeutic regimen. Understanding that incontinence is a possibility but that it usually resolves should be encouraging.
Encourage the patient to maintain adequate fluid intake of at least 2-3 L/day (unless contraindicated by an underlying cardiac dysfunction or other disorder).	Dilute urine is less irritating to the prostatic fossa and less likely to result in incontinence.
Instruct the patient to avoid caffeine-containing drinks.	These fluids irritate the bladder and have a mild diuretic effect, which would make bladder control even more difficult.
Establish a bladder routine with the patient before hospital discharge.	The goal of bladder training is to reduce the number of small voidings and thereby return the patient to a more normal bladder function. The amount of time between voidings is determined to estimate how long the patient can hold his urine. The patient schedules times for emptying his bladder and has a copy of the written schedule. An example initially would be q1-2h when awake and q4h at night. Then, if this is successful, the patient lengthens the intervals between voidings.

continued

ASSESSMENT/INTERVENTIONS	RATIONALES
Teach Kegel exercises (see next nursing diagnosis).	These exercises promote sphincter control, thereby decreasing incontinence episodes.
Remind the patient to discuss any incontinence problems with the health care provider during follow-up examinations.	This information helps ensure that the patient's needs are addressed and treated.

Nursing Diagnosis:

Deficient Knowledge

related to unfamiliarity with the pelvic muscle (Kegel) exercise program to strengthen perineal muscles (effective for individuals with mild to moderate stress incontinence)

Desired Outcome: Within the 24-hr period following teaching, the patient verbalizes and demonstrates accurate knowledge about the pelvic muscle (Kegel) exercise program.

ASSESSMENT/INTERVENTIONS	RATIONALES
Explain the purpose of Kegel exercises.	Kegel exercises strengthen pelvic area muscles, which will help regain bladder control.
Assist the patient with identifying the correct muscle group.	A common error when attempting to perform this exercise is contracting the buttocks, quadriceps, and abdominal muscles.
Teach the exercise as follows:	
- Attempt to shut off urinary flow after beginning urination, hold for a few seconds, and then start the stream again.	This strengthens the proximal muscle. If it can be accomplished, the correct muscle group is being used.
- Contract the muscle around the anus as though to stop a bowel movement.	This strengthens the distal muscle.
- Repeat these exercises 10-20 times, qid.	These exercises must be done frequently throughout the day and for 2-9 mo before benefits are obtained.

ADDITIONAL NURSING DIAGNOSES/PROBLEMS:

"Perioperative Care" p. 45

✓ PATIENT-FAMILY TEACHING AND DISCHARGE PLANNING

When providing patient-family teaching, focus on sensory information, avoid giving excessive information, and initiate a visiting nurse referral for necessary follow-up teaching. Include verbal and written information about the following:
- ✓ Medications, including drug name, purpose, dosage, schedule, precautions, and potential side effects. Also discuss drug-drug, herb-drug, and food-drug interactions.
- ✓ Necessity of reporting the following indicators of UTI to the health care provider: chills; fever; hematuria; flank, costovertebral angle, suprapubic, low back, buttock, or scrotal pain; cloudy and foul-smelling urine; frequency; urgency; dysuria; and increasing or recurring incontinence.
- ✓ Care of incision, if appropriate, including cleansing, dressing changes, and bathing. Advise the patient to be aware of indicators of infection: persistent redness, increasing pain, edema, increased warmth along the incision, or purulent or increased drainage.
- ✓ Care of catheters or drains if the patient is discharged with them.
- ✓ Daily fluid requirement of at least 2-3 L/day in nonrestricted patients.
- ✓ Importance of increasing dietary fiber or taking stool softeners to soften stools. This will minimize the risk of damage to the prostatic capsule by preventing straining with bowel movements. Caution the patient to avoid using suppositories or enemas for the treatment of constipation.
- ✓ Use of a sofa, reclining chair, or footstool to promote venous drainage from legs and to distribute weight on the perineum, not the rectum.
- ✓ Avoiding the following activities for the period prescribed by the health care provider: sitting for long periods, heavy lifting (more than 10 lb), and sexual intercourse.
- ✓ Kegel exercises to help regain urinary sphincter control for postoperative dribbling. See **Deficient Knowledge**, above.

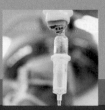

Chronic Kidney Disease 27

OVERVIEW/PATHOPHYSIOLOGY

Chronic kidney disease (CKD) is a progressive, irreversible loss of kidney function that develops over days to years. Aggressive management of hypertension and diabetes mellitus (DM) and avoidance of nephrotoxic agents may slow progression of CKD; however, loss of glomerular filtration is irreversible, and eventually CKD can progress to end-stage renal disease (ESRD), at which time renal replacement therapy (dialysis or transplantation) is required to sustain life. Before ESRD, the individual with CKD can lead a relatively normal life managed by diet and medications. The length of this period varies, depending on the cause of renal disease and the patient's level of renal function at the time of diagnosis.

Of the many causes of CKD, some of the most common are DM, hypertension, glomerulonephritis (GN), long-term exposure to certain classes of medications (e.g., nonsteroidal antiinflammatories) or metals (e.g., gold therapy, lead), and polycystic kidney disease. Regardless of the cause, clinical presentation of CKD, particularly as the individual approaches ESRD, is similar. Retention of metabolic end products and accompanying fluid and electrolyte imbalances adversely affect all body systems. Alterations in neuromuscular, cardiovascular, and gastrointestinal (GI) function are common. Renal osteodystrophy and anemia are early and common complications, with alterations being seen when the glomerular filtration rate (GFR) decreases to 60 mL/min. The collective manifestations of CKD are termed *uremia*.

HEALTH CARE SETTING

Primary care with possible hospitalization resulting from complications or during ESRD

ASSESSMENT

Anemia: Pallor, shortness of breath on exertion, headache, persistent fatigue, dizziness.

Fluid volume abnormalities: Crackles (rales), hypertension, edema, oliguria, anuria.

Electrolyte disturbances: Muscle weakness, dysrhythmias, pruritus, neuromuscular irritability, tetany.

Metabolic acidosis: Deep respirations, lethargy, headache.

Uremia—retention of metabolic wastes: Weakness, malaise, anorexia, dry and discolored skin, peripheral neuropathy, irri-

tability, clouded thinking, ammonia odor to breath, metallic taste in mouth, nausea, vomiting. **Note:** Uremia adversely affects all body systems.

POTENTIAL ACUTE COMPLICATIONS

Heart failure: Crackles (rales), dyspnea, orthopnea.

Pericarditis: Heart pain, elevated temperature, presence of pericardial friction or rub on auscultation.

Cardiac tamponade: Hypotension, distant heart sounds, pulsus paradoxus (exaggerated inspiratory drop in systolic blood pressure [SBP]).

Dysrhythmias: Increased QRS duration and/or peaked T waves on electrocardiogram.

Physical assessment: Pallor, dry and discolored skin, edema (peripheral, periorbital, sacral); fluid overload, crackles, and elevated blood pressure (BP) may be present.

History: GN; DM; polycystic kidney disease; hypertension; systemic lupus erythematosus; chronic pyelonephritis; and analgesic abuse, especially the combination of phenacetin and aspirin.

DIAGNOSTIC TESTS

GFR: May be calculated using a mathematical formula. The simplified Modification of Diet in Renal Failure equation to calculate GFR is:

$$GFR = 175 \times (\text{plasma creatinine in mg/dL})^{-1.154} \times (\text{age})^{-0.203}$$
$$\times (0.742 \text{ if female}) \times (1.212 \text{ if the patient is black})$$

Creatinine clearance: Measures the kidney's ability to clear the blood of creatinine and approximates the GFR. Creatinine clearance decreases as renal function decreases. Dialysis is usually begun when the GFR is 12 mL/min if the patient is symptomatic or the GFR is less than 6 mL/min. Creatinine clearance normally is decreased in older adults. Creatinine clearance may be measured through collection of a 24-hr urine sample or calculated using the Cockcroft-Gault equation:

$$\text{For men: } CrCl = (140 - \text{age}) \times \text{weight (in kg)}/$$
$$\text{plasma creatinine (in mg/dL)} \times 72$$
$$\text{For women: } CrCl = (140 - \text{age}) \times \text{weight (in kg)}/$$
$$\text{plasma creatinine (in mg/dL)} \times 85$$

Note: *Failure to collect all urine specimens during the period of study will invalidate test results.*

Blood urea nitrogen (BUN) and serum creatinine: Both will be elevated. **Note:** Nonrenal problems, such as dehydration or gastrointestinal (GI) bleeding, also can cause the BUN to increase, but there will not be a corresponding increase in creatinine.

Serum chemistries and serum hematology (electrolytes, phosphate, CBC); and chest and hand x-ray examinations: To assess for development and progression of uremia and its complications.

Kidney-ureter-bladder (KUB) x-ray examination: Documents the presence of two kidneys, changes in size or shape, and some forms of obstruction.

Intravenous pyelogram, renal ultrasound, renal biopsy, renal scan (using radionuclides), and computed tomography (CT) scan: Additional tests for determining the cause of renal insufficiency. Once the patient has reached ESRD, these tests are not performed. **Note:** Acetylcysteine (Mucomyst) may be prescribed as a prophylactic therapy before, during, and/or after administration of intravenous (IV) contrast in order to reduce the risk of further insult to the kidneys or dye-mediated acute renal failure.

Nursing Diagnosis:

Imbalanced Nutrition: Less Than Body Requirements

related to nausea, vomiting, anorexia, and dietary restrictions

Desired Outcome: Within 2 days of admission, the patient has stable weight and demonstrates normal intake of food within restrictions, as indicated.

ASSESSMENT/INTERVENTIONS	RATIONALES
See also Chapter 25, "Acute Renal Failure," p. 196, Imbalanced Nutrition: Less Than Body Requirements.	
In addition:	
Administer multivitamins and folic acid, if prescribed.	Anorexia and nausea and vomiting may occur with increased anorexia. Vitamin supplementation assists with ensuring that patients maintain adequate nutrition. Multivitamins for patients on dialysis are specially formulated (e.g., Nephro-Vite, Dialyvite).
Caution against the use of over-the-counter (OTC) vitamins.	Use of OTC multivitamins is contraindicated in CKD patients because some vitamin levels (e.g., of vitamin A) may be toxic.
Monitor for proteinuria, and refer to the dietitian if excessive protein losses and/or low serum albumin is noted.	Proteinuria results in malnutrition. Patients with poor nutritional status at the start of dialysis have increased risk of mortality.

Nursing Diagnosis:

Impaired Skin Integrity

related to uremia, hyperphosphatemia (if severe), and edema

Desired Outcome: The patient's skin is intact and free of erythema and abrasions.

ASSESSMENT/INTERVENTIONS	RATIONALES
Assess for the presence/degree of pruritus.	Pruritus is common in patients with uremia and occurs when accumulating nitrogenous wastes begin to be excreted through the skin, causing frequent and intense itching with scratching. Pruritus also may result from prolonged hyperphosphatemia.

ASSESSMENT/INTERVENTIONS

RATIONALES

ASSESSMENT/INTERVENTIONS	RATIONALES
Encourage use of phosphate binders and reduction of dietary phosphorus if elevated phosphorus level is a problem.	Pruritus often decreases with a reduction in BUN and improved phosphorus control. Phosphate binders are medications that, when taken with food, bind dietary phosphorus and prevent GI absorption. Calcium carbonate, sevelamer hydrochloride, aluminum hydroxide, and calcium acetate are common phosphate binders.
Note: Administer phosphate binders while food is present in the stomach.	Prolonged elevation of serum phosphorus and/or calcium absorption from ingestion of phosphate binders on an empty stomach results in an increased calcium-phosphorus product (serum calcium × serum phosphorus). When this product exceeds a level of 55 (normal product is approximately 40), phosphorus binds with calcium, and the resulting calcium-phosphate complex is deposited in soft tissues of the body. Deposition of these complexes in the skin produces necrotic patches. In addition, elevation in calcium-phosphate product is associated with increased risk of death, aortic calcification, mitral valve calcification, and coronary artery calcification.
If necessary, administer prescribed antihistamines.	Antihistamines help control itching.
Keep the patient's fingernails short.	If the patient is unable to control scratching, short fingernails will cause less damage.
Instruct the patient to monitor scratches for evidence of infection and to seek early medical attention if signs and symptoms of infection appear.	Uremia retards wound healing; nonintact skin can lead to infection.
Encourage use of skin emollients and soaps with high fat content. Advise bathing every other day and to apply skin lotion immediately upon exiting the bath/shower.	Uremic skin is often dry and scaly because of reduction in oil gland activity. Patients should avoid harsh soaps, soaps or skin products containing alcohol, and excessive bathing.
Advise the patient and significant others that easy bruising can occur.	Patients with uremia are at increased risk for bruising because of clotting abnormalities and capillary fragility.
Provide scheduled skin care and position changes for patients with edema.	These measures decrease risk of skin/tissue damage resulting from decreased perfusion and increased pressure.

Nursing Diagnosis:

Activity Intolerance

related to generalized weakness occurring with anemia and uremia

Desired Outcome: Following treatment, the patient rates perceived exertion at 3 or less on a 0-10 scale and exhibits improving endurance to activity as evidenced by heart rate (HR) 20 bpm or less over resting HR, SBP 20 mm Hg or less over or under resting SBP, and respiratory rate (RR) 20 breaths/min or less with normal depth and pattern (eupnea).

Note: *Anemia is better tolerated in the uremic than in the nonuremic patient.*

ASSESSMENT/INTERVENTIONS

RATIONALES

ASSESSMENT/INTERVENTIONS	RATIONALES
Assess the patient during activity, and ask the patient to rate perceived exertion (RPE) (see "Prolonged Bedrest," p. 61, for **Risk for Activity Intolerance**).	This assessment evaluates the degree of activity intolerance. Optimally RPE should be at 3 or less on a 0-10 scale.

continued

ASSESSMENT/INTERVENTIONS

RATIONALES

ASSESSMENT/INTERVENTIONS	RATIONALES
Notify the health care provider of increased weakness, fatigue, dyspnea, chest pain, or further decreases in hematocrit (Hct).	This action enables rapid treatment of anemia and dose adjustment of epoetin alfa, which induces erythrocyte production and reticulocyte production in the bone marrow. Low levels of hemoglobin (Hgb) and Hct may result in angina. Shortness of breath and shortness of breath on exertion in the long term contribute to the development of ventricular hypertrophy, increasing the risk of morbidity from cardiovascular disease (CVD), the most significant cause of death in CKD patients. Conversely, high levels of Hgb may result in hypertension and increased thrombosis.
Administer epoetin alfa, if prescribed.	Current clinical practice guidelines recommend that epoetin alfa (Epogen) be started when Hgb decreases below 10 g/dL. Target Hgb for patients receiving epoetin alfa is 11.5 g/dL (or a range of 11.0-12.0 g/dL). Epoetin alfa may be contraindicated in patients with uncontrolled hypertension or sensitivity to human albumin.
Gently mix the container; use only one dose per vial (do not reenter used vials; discard unused portions).	Shaking may denature the glycoprotein.
Assess for increasing hypertension, dyspnea, chest pain, seizures, calf pain, erythema, swelling, severe headache, and seizures.	These are potential untoward effects of epoetin alfa (Epogen) therapy. Dose adjustment or discontinuation may be necessary. Hypertension may occur as a side effect of Epogen therapy during the period in which Hct levels are rapidly rising. Headaches may accompany the rise in blood pressure. Epogen has also been associated with increased thrombosis. Patients should be monitored for evidence of thrombotic events (i.e., symptoms of myocardial infarction [MI], deep vein thrombosis [DVT]/venous thromboembolism [VTE], stroke, transient ischemic attack [TIA], or clotting of the vascular access in hemodialysis patients), and those symptoms should be reported immediately to the health care provider. Epogen should be used with caution in patients with a known seizure history as there is an increased risk of seizures within the first 3 mo of Epogen therapy.
Assess for and report evidence of occult blood and blood loss.	Blood loss can cause anemia.
Administer oral or parenteral iron if prescribed.	Iron deficiency anemia is common in CKD patients. In addition, iron is required for epoetin alfa to make new red blood cells. Thus, effectiveness of epoetin alfa requires that patients maintain their iron stores. **Note:** Anaphylaxis is a possible complication of intravenous (IV) iron administration, most commonly during the first dose.
For patients receiving oral iron, assess for signs and symptoms of constipation.	Constipation is a common side effect of oral iron. See Chapter 4, "Prolonged Bedrest," **Constipation,** p. 68.
Coordinate laboratory studies.	This intervention minimizes blood drawing. CKD patients are already at risk for anemia.
Provide and encourage optimal nutrition and consider referral to a renal dietitian.	Protein and phosphorus are initially restricted to slow progression of CKD and prevent early development of renal osteodystrophy. (*Renal osteodystrophy* is a collective term for changes in the bone structure of patients with CKD, resulting most often in rapid bone turnover. These changes result from a combination of hyperphosphatemia, hypocalcemia, stimulation of parathyroid hormone, and alterations in the kidney's ability to convert vitamin D to its active form.) Carbohydrates are increased for patients on protein-restricted diets to ensure adequate caloric intake, thereby preventing tissue catabolism, which would contribute to buildup of nitrogenous wastes. As the patient approaches ESRD, sodium intake is limited to reduce thirst and fluid retention, K⁺ intake is limited because of the kidneys' decreased ability to excrete this ion, and protein may be further restricted to limit production of nitrogenous wastes. For patients on protein-restricted diets, protein intake should be restricted to sources primarily of high biologic value. Over-restriction of protein may lead to malnutrition; therefore, referral to a renal dietitian is recommended to ensure adequate intake.

PART I: Medical-Surgical Nursing

ASSESSMENT/INTERVENTIONS	RATIONALES
Do not administer ferrous sulfate at the same time as antacids.	To maximize absorption of ferrous sulfate, antacids or calcium carbonate medications are given at least 1 hr before or after ferrous sulfate.
Assist with identifying activities that increase fatigue and adjusting those activities accordingly.	It is important to minimize fatigue while attempting to promote tolerance to activity.
Assist with activities of daily living (ADLs) while encouraging maximum independence to tolerance. Establish realistic, progressive exercises and activity goals that are designed to increase endurance. Ensure that they are within the patient's prescribed limitations. Examples are found Chapter 4, "Prolonged Bedrest," **Risk for Activity Intolerance,** p. 61, and **Risk for Disuse Syndrome,** p. 63.	Same as above.
Administer packed red blood cells as prescribed.	This measure treats severe or symptomatic anemia.

Nursing Diagnosis:

Deficient Knowledge

related to unfamiliarity with the need for frequent BP checks and adherence to antihypertensive therapy and the potential for change in insulin requirements for individuals who have DM

Desired Outcomes: Within the 24-hr period before hospital discharge, the patient verbalizes knowledge about the importance of frequent BP checks and adherence to antihypertensive therapy. Patients with DM verbalize knowledge about the potential for a change in insulin requirements.

ASSESSMENT/INTERVENTIONS	RATIONALES
Assess the patient's current level of knowledge about his or her therapy and health care literacy (language, reading, comprehension). Assess culture and culturally specific information needs.	This assessment helps ensure that information is selected and presented in a manner that is culturally and educationally appropriate.
Teach the importance of getting BP checked at frequent intervals and adhering to prescribed antihypertensive therapy.	Patients with CKD may experience hypertension because of fluid overload, excess renin secretion, or arteriosclerotic disease. Control of hypertension may slow progression of chronic renal insufficiency and decrease risk of CVD.
Teach about antihypertensive medications, including drug name, purpose, dosage, schedule precautions, and potential side effects. Also discuss drug-drug, herb-drug, and food-drug interactions.	These medications control BP, slow progression of CKD, and/or reduce proteinria/microalbuminuria. Angiotensin-converting enzyme (ACE) inhibitors and angiotensin receptor blockers (ARBs) are considered first-line medications for management of patients with CKD and coexisting diabetes, proteinuria, and/or microalbuminuria. Additional antihypertensives are often added in the following order to achieve a target BP of less than 130/80 mm Hg: diuretic, then beta-blocker or calcium channel blocker. Patients may require up to four antihypertensives to control BP adequately. Because increased release of angiotensin may occur with renal pathology, some patients require bilateral nephrectomies to control excessive hypertension.
Teach the importance of a target BP of less than 130/80 mm Hg.	This knowledge will help the patient keep BP within optimal levels by following the antihypertensive medication regimen.
Teach patients with DM that insulin requirements often decrease as renal function decreases. Instruct these patients to be alert to weakness, blurred vision, and headache.	Anorexia or nausea/vomiting, which occur with uremia, may decrease dietary consumption and thereby decrease insulin requirements. These symptoms are indicators of hypoglycemia, which can occur as insulin requirements decrease.

continued

ASSESSMENT/INTERVENTIONS	RATIONALES
Teach patients on ACE inhibitors or ARBs the importance of medical follow-up.	Follow-up is important for monitoring GFR, potassium levels, and hypotension. Hypotension and cough are common side effects. ACE inhibitors and ARBs may increase serum potassium and decrease GFR. Angioedema is a potential side effect.
Teach patients receiving diuretics the importance of medical follow-up.	Follow-up enables monitoring for volume depletion, decreased GFR, and electrolyte abnormalities. Use of diuretics can result in dehydration and hypokalemia and may hasten loss of renal function.
Explain that restriction of sodium to less than 2.4 g/day is recommended. Consider referral to a dietitian.	These measures help manage hypertension and slow the progression of CKD.
Teach that weight loss should be considered if body mass index is greater than 25 kg/m². Refer to a dietitian as indicated.	Obesity increases hypertension, resulting in progression of CKD and increased mortality rates due to CVD.
Teach the importance of limiting alcohol intake to less than 2 drinks/day for men, and less than 1 drink/day for women.	Excessive alcohol intake may increase the risk of malnutrition, hypertension, and CVD resulting in progression of CKD and increased mortality.
Counsel patient on smoking cessation if applicable.	CVD is the leading cause of death in CKD patients. Smoking increases the risk of CVD and arteriosclerosis.
Teach the benefits of exercise and physical activity.	Thirty minutes of physical activity of moderate intensity most days of the week is recommended for hypertension management in patients with CKD. Management of hypertension may slow the progression of CKD.

ADDITIONAL NURSING DIAGNOSES/PROBLEMS:

"Prolonged Bedrest" for **Constipation** related to   p. 68
changes in dietary intake and immobility. In
addition, the patient may experience constipation
because of oral iron supplementation.

"Psychosocial Support" for **Disturbed Body Image**   p. 79
related to changes in body parts or function. In
addition, the patient may experience body image
disturbance because of the presence of dialysis
catheters.

"Care of the Patient Undergoing Hemodialysis"   p. 212

"Care of the Patient Undergoing Peritoneal Dialysis"   p. 216

✓ PATIENT-FAMILY TEACHING AND DISCHARGE PLANNING

When providing patient-family teaching, focus on sensory information, avoid giving excessive information, and initiate a visiting nurse referral for necessary follow-up teaching. Include verbal and written information about the following:
   ✓ Medications, including drug name, purpose, dosage, schedule, precautions, and potential side effects. Also discuss drug-drug, herb-drug, and food-drug interactions.
   ✓ For patients not on dialysis but requiring epoetin alfa, teach the patient and/or significant other preparation of the medication and subcutaneous injections. Demonstrate how to gently mix the container (shaking may denature the glycoprotein); use only one dose per vial (do not reenter used vials, discard unused portions). Instruct the patient and/or significant other to store epoetin alfa in the refrigerator but not to allow it to freeze. Teach importance of monitoring for and rapidly reporting to the health care provider any of the following: dyspnea, chest pain, seizures, and severe headache.
   ✓ Diet, including fact sheet listing foods that are to be restricted or limited. Inform the patient that diet and fluid restrictions may be altered as renal function decreases. Provide sample menus, and have the patient demonstrate understanding by preparing 3-day menus that incorporate dietary restrictions.
   ✓ Care and observation of the dialysis access if the patient has one (see next two care plans).
   ✓ Signs and symptoms that necessitate medical attention: irregular pulse, fever, unusual shortness of breath or edema, sudden change in urine output, and unusual muscle weakness.
   ✓ Need for continued medical follow-up; confirm date and time of next health care provider appointment.
   ✓ Importance of avoiding infections and seeking treatment promptly should one develop. Teach indicators of frequently encountered infections, including upper respiratory infection (URI), urinary tract infection (UTI), impetigo, and otitis media. For details, see "Care of the Renal Transplant Recipient," **Risk for Infection**, p. 220.
   ✓ Telephone numbers to call in case questions or concerns arise about the therapy or disease after discharge.

Additional general information and patient education resources can be obtained by contacting the following:

✓ National Kidney and Urologic Diseases Information Clearinghouse at *www.kidney.niddk.nih.gov*

✓ National Kidney Foundation at *www.kidney.org*

✓ The Kidney Foundation of Canada at *www.kidney.ca*

✓ For patients with or approaching ESRD, provide data concerning various treatment options and support groups. The local chapter of the National Kidney Foundation can be helpful in identifying support groups and organizations in the area. The patient and significant others should meet with the renal dietitian and social worker before discharge.

✓ Coordinate discharge planning and teaching with the dialysis unit or facility. If possible, have the patient visit the dialysis unit before discharge.

✓ For individuals with ESRD, teach the importance of coordinating all medical care through their nephrologist and alerting all medical and dental personnel to ESRD status because of increased risk of infection and the need to adjust medication dosages. In addition, dentists may want to premedicate ESRD patients with antibiotics before dental work and avoid scheduling dental work on the day of dialysis because of the heparinization that is used with dialytic therapy.

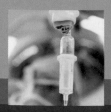

Care of the Patient Undergoing Hemodialysis 28

OVERVIEW/PATHOPHYSIOLOGY

During hemodialysis, blood is removed via a special vascular access, heparinized, pumped through an artificial kidney (dialyzer), and then returned to the patient's circulation. Hemodialysis is a temporary, acute procedure performed as needed, or it is performed long term 2-4 times/wk for 3-5 hr each treatment.

Indications for hemodialysis: Acute renal failure or acute episodes of renal insufficiency that cannot be managed by diet, medications, and fluid restriction; end-stage renal disease (ESRD) with low glomerular filtration rate (GFR); uremia; drug overdose; hyperkalemia; fluid overload; and metabolic acidosis.

Continuous venovenous hemodiafiltration (CVVHD): A double-lumen catheter is placed in a large vein and blood is pumped from the vein, through the dialysis circuit, passing through the hemofilter and returning to the patient's circulation via a venous access. Ultrafiltrate (fluid, metabolic wastes, and electrolytes) drains from the hemofilter into a collection device.

HEALTH CARE SETTING

Dialysis center or in an acute care hospital outpatient or inpatient setting

Use of CVVHD is currently limited to patients in critical care settings because it requires continuous monitoring.

Components of hemodialysis

Artificial kidney (dialyzer): Composed of a blood compartment and dialysate compartment, separated by a semipermeable membrane that allows diffusion of solutes and filtration of water. Protein and bacteria do not cross the artificial membrane.

Dialysate: Electrolyte solution similar in composition to normal plasma. Each of the constituents may be varied according to patient need. The most commonly altered components are K^+ and bicarbonate. Glucose may be added to prevent sudden drops in serum osmolality and serum glucose during dialysis.

Vascular access: Necessary to provide a blood flow rate of 300-500 mL/min for an effective dialysis. Vascular access sites may include an arteriovenous fistula, arteriovenous graft, internal jugular catheters (right side preferred), femoral vein catheters, or subclavian catheters.

Nursing Diagnosis:

Risk for Imbalanced Fluid Volume

related to excessive fluid removal from dialysis resulting in hypovolemia or fluid volume depletion; or *related to* compromised regulatory mechanism resulting in fluid retention due to renal failure

Desired Outcomes: After dialysis the patient is normovolemic as evidenced by stable weight, respiratory rate (RR) 12-20 breaths/min with normal depth and pattern (eupnea), central venous pressure (CVP) 4-10 mm Hg, heart rate (HR), and blood pressure (BP) within the patient's normal range, and absence of abnormal breath sounds and abnormal bleeding. After instruction, the patient relates signs and symptoms of fluid volume excess and deficit.

ASSESSMENT/INTERVENTIONS	RATIONALES
⚠ Assess for and instruct the patient/family to assess for and report edema, hypertension, crackles (rales), tachycardia, distended neck veins, shortness of breath, and increased central venous pressure (CVP).	These are indicators of fluid volume excess. Dependent edema likely will be detected in the legs or feet of patients who are ambulatory, whereas the sacral area will be edematous in those who are on bedrest. Periorbital edema also may result from excessive fluid overload. Jugular veins are likely to be distended with the head of bed (HOB) elevated 45 degrees owing to increased intravascular volume. Crackles and shortness of breath can occur as a result of fluid volume overload. Low serum albumin decreases colloid osmotic pressure, allowing fluid to leak into the extravascular space. Low serum albumin also may contribute to generalized edema and pulmonary edema. Hypertension, tachycardia, and increased CVP may result from sodium and fluid retention.
⚠ After dialysis, assess for and report hypotension, decreased CVP, tachycardia, and complaints of dizziness or lightheadedness. Describe signs and symptoms to the patient, and explain importance of reporting them promptly if they occur.	These are indicators of fluid volume deficit, which may result from rapid or excessive fluid losses during dialysis. It should be noted that patients with uremia may not develop compensatory tachycardia owing to autonomic neuropathy, which can occur with uremia. **Note:** Antihypertensive medications usually are held before and during dialysis to help prevent hypotension during dialysis. Clarify medication prescriptions with the health care provider.
Assess intake and output (I&O) and daily weight as indicators of fluid status.	Intake greater than output and steady weight gain indicate retained fluid. Weight is an important guideline for determining the quantity of fluid to be removed during dialysis.
Weigh the patient at the same time each day, using the same scale and with the patient wearing same amount of clothing (or with same items on the bed if using a bed scale).	Weighing patients under the same conditions helps ensure accurate measurement of fluid status.
Weigh the patient before and after dialysis treatment.	Weighing the patient before and after dialysis therapy assesses the effectiveness of treatment in removing fluid volume.
⚠ Monitor for postdialysis bleeding (needle sites, incisions). Alert the patient to the potential for bleeding from these areas.	This bleeding can occur because of use of heparin during dialysis. If these signs and symptoms occur, the patient will be able to report them promptly to the staff or health care provider for timely intervention.
⚠ Do not give intramuscular (IM) injection for at least 1 hr after dialysis.	Avoiding IM injections for this amount of time prevents hematoma formation.
Test all stools for the presence of blood. Report significant findings.	Gastrointestinal (GI) bleeding is common in patients with renal failure, especially after heparinization.

Nursing Diagnoses:
Risk for Bleeding
related to vascular access puncture or its disconnection

Ineffective Peripheral Tissue Perfusion (or risk for same)
related to interrupted blood flow that can occur with clotting in the vascular access

Risk for Infection
related to invasive procedure (creation of vascular access for hemodialysis and frequency of site access)

Desired Outcomes: The patient's vascular access remains intact and connected, and the patient is normovolemic (see description in **Risk for Imbalanced Fluid Volume**). The patient has adequate tissue perfusion as evidenced by normal skin temperature and color and brisk capillary refill (less than 2 sec) distal to the vascular access. The patient's access is patent as evidenced by presence of thrill with palpation and bruit with auscultation of fistula or graft. The patient is free of infection as evidenced by normothermia and absence of erythema, local warmth, exudate, swelling, and tenderness at access site.

ASSESSMENT/INTERVENTIONS	RATIONALES
After surgical creation of the vascular access, assess for patency, auscultate for bruit, and palpate for thrill.	These assessments reveal whether the patient's vascular access is patent. A bruit is a hissing sound that is made when blood moves through the access. A thrill is a vibration felt when placing a hand over the access, denoting blood flow.
Report complaints of severe or unrelieved pain, numbness, and tingling of the area of vascular access or extremity distal to the access.	These indicators can signal impaired tissue perfusion caused by occlusion of the vascular access.
Assess for postoperative swelling along the graft or fistula or area around the shunt; elevate the extremity accordingly.	Postoperative swelling along the graft or fistula or area around the shunt is expected and will diminish with extremity elevation.
Notify the health care provider if the extremity distal to the vascular access becomes cool or swollen, has decreased capillary refill, or has decreased pulse or is discolored.	These problems can indicate hypoxia as a result of reduced blood supply to the extremity (called *steal syndrome*).
Follow the three principles of nursing care common to all types of vascular access: (1) prevent bleeding, (2) prevent clotting, and (3) prevent infection. Never use the vascular access for instillation of intravenous (IV) medications or phlebotomy. Monitor it closely, and handle it with care.	The vascular access is the patient's lifeline, and it must be monitored closely to ensure maintenance of patency and prevention of infection.
Explain monitoring and care procedures to the patient.	A knowledgeable patient is more likely to adhere to these principles.
Vascular accesses include the following:	
Subclavian or femoral lines	External, temporary catheters inserted into a large vein.
1. Anchor the catheter securely because it might not be sutured in. Tape all connections. Keep clamps at the bedside in case the line becomes disconnected. If the line is removed or accidentally pulled out, apply firm pressure to site for at least 10 min. **Caution:** If an air embolus occurs: a. Immediately clamp the line.	These measures prevent bleeding. An air embolus can occur if a subclavian line accidentally becomes pulled out or disconnected.
b. Turn the patient onto a left-side-lying position.	This position helps prevent air from blocking the pulmonary artery.
c. Lower the HOB into Trendelenburg position. Administer 100% oxygen by mask, and obtain vital signs. Notify the health care provider *stat!*	This position increases intrathoracic pressure, which will decrease the flow of inspiratory air into the vein.
2. Allow only the dialysis staff to access the line.	Improper heparin flushing increases the risk of clotting. Accessing the line for nondialysis treatments increases risk of infection.
3. Monitor for and report the presence of erythema, local warmth, exudate, swelling, and tenderness at exit site.	These are indicators of infection. Dressing changes and cultures of any drainage should be performed only by the dialysis staff. If a dressing loosens, it needs to be reinforced and the dialysis unit contacted to perform the dressing change.
Fistula or graft	Internal, permanent connection between an artery and a vein, or the insertion of an internal graft that is joined to an artery and vein. Grafts can be straight or U-shaped. Grafts and fistulas are most commonly located in the arm but may be placed in the thigh.
1. Inspect needle puncture sites. If bleeding occurs, apply just enough pressure over the site to stop it. Release the pressure and check for bleeding q5-10min.	These measures assess for and intervene in the event of postdialysis bleeding.
2. Place a sign above HOB indicating extremity in which the fistula or graft has been placed, and stating not to take BP, start an IV, or draw blood from the affected limb. Ensure that this information is clearly documented on the patient's medical record and care plan. Caution the patient to avoid tight clothing, jewelry, name bands, or restraint on affected extremity.	These procedures and precautions help prevent blood clotting in the vascular access.
3. Palpate for thrill and auscultate for bruit at least every shift and after hypotensive episodes. Notify the health care provider *stat* if bruit or thrill has changed significantly or is absent.	These assessments determine whether the vascular access is patent and enable rapid intervention if changes occur.
4. Observe for and report the presence of erythema, local warmth, swelling, exudate, and unusual tenderness at graft, fistula, or shunt site.	These are indicators of infection. Dressing changes and cultures of any drainage should only be performed by dialysis staff. If a dressing loosens, it needs to be reinforced and the dialysis unit contacted to perform the dressing change.

✓ PATIENT-FAMILY TEACHING AND DISCHARGE PLANNING

When providing patient-family teaching, focus on sensory information, avoid giving excessive information, and initiate a visiting nurse referral if indicated for follow-up teaching. Include verbal and written information about the following:

- ✓ Medications, including drug name; purpose; dosage; schedule; drug-drug, herb-drug, and food-drug interactions; precautions; and potential side effects.
- ✓ Diet and fluid restrictions: Include fact sheets that list foods to limit or restrict. Review fluid restrictions. Provide sample menus with examples of how dietary restrictions may be incorporated into daily meals. Have the patient demonstrate understanding of dietary restrictions by preparing 3-day menus.
- ✓ Care of fistula or graft to prevent/detect bleeding, clotting, and infection.
- ✓ Need for and importance of monitoring daily weights, I&O, and monitoring of BP at home, if necessary.

- ✓ Importance of continued medical follow-up; confirm date and time of next health care provider and hemodialysis appointments.
- ✓ Signs and symptoms that necessitate medical attention: increased weight gain, unusual shortness of breath, edema, dizziness or fainting, fever, increased hypertension, redness around access site, decrease in bruit or thrill (fistulas, graft), prolonged bleeding from fistula or graft, discoloration or coldness distal to fistula or graft, accidental pulling on the subclavian line.
- ✓ Telephone numbers to call in case questions or concerns arise about therapy or disease after discharge. Additional general information and patient educational materials can be obtained by contacting:
  - National Kidney and Urologic Diseases Information Clearinghouse at *www.kidney.niddk.nih.gov*
  - National Kidney Foundation at *www.kidney.org*
  - The Kidney Foundation of Canada at *www.kidney.ca*

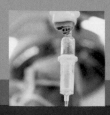

Care of the Patient Undergoing Peritoneal Dialysis 29

OVERVIEW/PATHOPHYSIOLOGY

Peritoneal dialysis uses the peritoneum as the dialysis membrane. Dialysate is instilled into the peritoneal cavity via a catheter surgically placed in the abdominal wall. Once the dialysate is within the abdominal cavity, movement of solutes and fluid occurs between the patient's capillary blood and the dialysate. At set intervals, the peritoneal cavity is drained and new dialysate is instilled.

Indications for peritoneal dialysis: Episodes of renal insufficiency that cannot be managed by diet, medications, and fluid restriction; end-stage renal disease (ESRD); drug overdose; hyperkalemia; fluid overload; and metabolic acidosis.

Components of dialysis

Catheter: Silastic tube that is either implanted using general anesthesia as a surgical procedure for patients who will have long-term treatment or is inserted using local anesthetic at the bedside for short-term dialysis.

Dialysate: Sterile electrolyte solution similar in composition to normal plasma. The electrolyte composition of the dialysate can be adjusted according to individual need. Glucose is added to the dialysate in varying concentrations to remove excess body fluid via osmosis.

Note: Some glucose crosses the peritoneal membrane and enters the patient's bloodstream. Patients with diabetes mellitus may require additional insulin. Observe for and report indicators of hyperglycemia (e.g., complaints of thirst, changes in sensorium). Insulin and other medications may be added directly to the dialysate by dialysis nurses or a pharmacist.

Types of dialysis

Continuous ambulatory peritoneal dialysis (CAPD): Using sterile technique, the patient attaches a new bag of dialysate to the peritoneal catheter, allows the dialysate to drain out, and then allows new dialysate to drain in. The patient then clamps the catheter and places a new cap on the tubing using sterile technique. This process is repeated q4-6h (8 hr at night), 7 days/wk. CAPD is used primarily for ESRD.

Continuous cycling peritoneal dialysis (CCPD): This is a combination of intermittent peritoneal dialysis (IPD) and CAPD. A cycler performs three dialysate exchanges at night. In the morning, a fourth exchange is instilled and left in the peritoneal cavity for the entire day. At the end of the day, the fourth exchange is allowed to drain out and the process is repeated. The patient is ambulatory by day and restricted to bed at night. CCPD is commonly done every night.

HEALTH CARE SETTING

Home setting; acute care setting if the patient has complications or has been hospitalized for other medical reasons

Nursing Diagnosis:

Risk for Infection

related to invasive procedure (direct access of the catheter to the peritoneum)

Desired Outcomes: The patient is free of infection as evidenced by normothermia and absence of the following: abdominal pain, cloudy outflow, nausea, malaise, erythema, edema, increased local warmth, drainage, and tenderness at the exit site. Before hospital discharge, the patient verbalizes signs and symptoms of infection and the need for sterile technique for bag, tubing, and dressing changes.

ASSESSMENT/INTERVENTIONS	RATIONALES
Assess for and report indications of peritonitis (see "Peritonitis," p. 454).	The most common complication of peritoneal dialysis is peritonitis. Indicators include fever, abdominal pain, distention, abdominal wall rigidity, rebound tenderness, cloudy outflow, nausea, and malaise. Recurrent/relapsing peritonitis is one of the most common reasons that peritoneal dialysis treatment must be discontinued.
Assess color and clarity of dialysate following outflow.	Bloody and cloudy outflow or the presence of fibrin in the outflow may be an initial sign of peritonitis. Note that bloody outflow may occur in female patients during menstruation.
Assess for and report redness, local warmth, edema, drainage, or tenderness at the exit site. Culture any exudate, and report results to the health care provider.	These are signs of infection at the exit site.
Maintain sterile technique when making systems connections, disconnecting, and capping the system, or adding medications to the dialysate.	To minimize the risk of peritonitis and other infections, the dialysate must remain sterile because it is instilled directly into the body.
Follow agency policy for care of the catheter exit site.	Exit site infections may lead to development of peritonitis.
Report to the health care provider if dialysate leaks around the catheter exit site.	This leakage can signal an obstruction or need for another purse-string suture around the catheter site. Leakage around the exit site has been associated with increased risk of tunnel infections, exit site infections, and peritonitis. Organisms may track through subcutaneous tissue into the peritoneum, causing infection.
Instruct the patient in the preceding interventions and observations if peritoneal dialysis will be performed after hospital discharge.	An informed patient likely will adhere to infection prevention interventions and know when to report untoward signs to the health care provider.

Nursing Diagnosis:

Risk for Imbalanced Fluid Volume

related to hypertonicity of the dialysate or inadequate exchange

Desired Outcomes: Postdialysis the patient is normovolemic as evidenced by balanced intake and output (I&O), stable weight, good skin turgor, central venous pressure (CVP) 4-10 mm Hg, respiratory rate (RR) 12-20 breaths/min with normal depth and pattern (eupnea), and blood pressure (BP) and heart rate (HR) within the patient's normal range. The volume of dialysate outflow equals or exceeds inflow.

ASSESSMENT/INTERVENTIONS	RATIONALES
Assess for and report hypertension, dyspnea, tachycardia, distended neck veins, or increased CVP.	These are indicators of fluid overload and should be reported promptly for timely intervention.
Assess the patient for respiratory distress.	Respiratory distress can occur because of compression of the diaphragm by the dialysate, especially when the patient is supine.
If respiratory distress occurs, elevate the head of bed (HOB), and notify the health care provider.	Raising the HOB may help alleviate this problem because the diaphragm will be less compressed by the dialysis solution. If respiratory distress continues, the dialysis nurse should be notified because drainage of the solution may alleviate diaphragmatic pressure.
Assess I&O and weight daily, using the same scale and with the patient wearing the same amount of clothing (or with same items on the bed if using a bed scale).	The patient's weight is one of the key indicators in choosing dialysis solutions. For example, a steady weight gain indicates fluid retention and may indicate a need for increased dialysis. Weighing the patient under the same conditions helps ensure accurate measurements of fluid status.
Assess for and report indicators of volume depletion.	Volume depletion (e.g., poor skin turgor, hypotension, tachycardia, and decreased CVP) can occur with excessive use of hypertonic dialysate and should be reported promptly for timely intervention.

continued

ASSESSMENT/INTERVENTIONS	RATIONALES
Assess for the presence of incomplete dialysate returns.	Fluid retention can occur because of catheter complications that prevent adequate outflow, a severely scarred peritoneum that prevents adequate exchange, or inadequate dialysis prescriptions. Accurate measurement and recording of outflow are critical to detect these problems promptly.
In the presence of outflow problems, monitor for the following: *Full colon:* Use stool softeners, high-fiber diet, laxatives, or enemas if necessary. *Catheter occlusion by fibrin* (usually occurs soon after insertion): Obtain prescription to irrigate with heparinized saline. *Catheter obstruction by omentum:* Turn the patient from side to side, elevate HOB or foot of bed, or apply firm pressure to the abdomen. Notify the health care provider for unresolved outflow problems.	These factors are potential causes of outflow problems, and they necessitate intervention to reverse the problem.

Nursing Diagnosis:

Imbalanced Nutrition: Less Than Body Requirements

related to protein loss in the dialysate

Desired Outcomes: At a minimum of 24 hr before hospital discharge, the patient exhibits adequate nutrition as evidenced by stable weight. The patient's protein intake is 1.2-1.5 g/kg/day.

ASSESSMENT/INTERVENTIONS	RATIONALES
Assess the patient's dietary intake of protein to ensure it is 1.2-1.5 g/kg/day.	Protein crosses the peritoneum, and a significant amount is lost in the dialysate. An increased intake of protein is necessary to prevent excessive tissue catabolism. Protein loss increases with peritonitis.
Ensure that a dietary evaluation and teaching program are performed when the patient changes from one type of dialysis to the other.	Patients undergoing peritoneal dialysis typically have fewer dietary restrictions than those on hemodialysis. Usually sodium and potassium restrictions are less for a patient receiving peritoneal dialysis than for one on hemodialysis. This is due, in part, to the fact that dialysis is provided continuously to peritoneal dialysis patients versus only 3 times/wk for those receiving hemodialysis.
Provide lists of restricted and encouraged foods with menus that illustrate their integration into the daily diet.	This information helps ensure the patient's understanding of the dietary regimen.
Request that the patient plan a 3-day menu that incorporates appropriate foods and restrictions.	Asking the patient to apply newly learned information via menu planning is a valid way of teaching and evaluating the patient's understanding.

ADDITIONAL NURSING DIAGNOSES/PROBLEMS:

"Prolonged Bedrest" for **Constipation** related to changes in dietary intake and immobility. Constipation also can occur as a result of oral iron supplementation.   p. 68

"Psychosocial Support" for **Disturbed Body Image** related to changes in body parts or function. Disturbed body image also can occur as a result of the presence of the dialysis catheter.   p. 79

 PATIENT-FAMILY TEACHING AND DISCHARGE PLANNING

When providing patient-family teaching, focus on sensory information, avoid giving excessive information, and initiate a visiting nurse referral if indicated for follow-up teaching. Include verbal and written information about the following:

✓ Medications, including drug name, purpose, dosage, schedule, drug-drug and food-drug interactions, precautions, and potential side effects.

✓ Diet and fluid restrictions: Include fact sheets that list foods to limit or restrict. Review fluid restrictions.

Provide sample menus with examples of how dietary restrictions may be incorporated into daily meals. Have the patient demonstrate understanding of dietary restrictions by preparing 3-day menus.

✓ Care and observation of exit site as per agency protocol.

✓ Need for and importance of monitoring daily weights, intake and output, and monitoring of BP at home, if necessary.

✓ Importance of continued medical follow-up; confirm date and time of next health care provider appointment.

✓ Signs and symptoms that necessitate medical attention. For example, symptoms that may indicate need for alteration in dialysis prescription: increased weight gain, unusual shortness of breath, edema, dizziness or fainting; symptoms that may indicate infection: fever, abdominal pain, redness or discharge from exit site, cloudy or decreased outflow, or nausea.

✓ Telephone numbers to call in case questions or concerns arise about therapy or disease after discharge. Additional general information and patient education materials can be obtained by contacting:
- National Kidney and Urologic Diseases Information Clearinghouse at *www.kidney.niddk.nih.gov*
- National Kidney Foundation at *www.kidney.org*
- The Kidney Foundation of Canada at *www.kidney.ca*

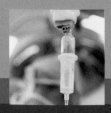

Care of the Renal Transplant Recipient 30

OVERVIEW/PATHOPHYSIOLOGY

Individuals with end-stage renal disease (ESRD) have several treatment modalities from which to choose—hemodialysis, peritoneal dialysis, no treatment, and renal transplantation. Renal transplantation is the only modality that restores kidney function to normal. The caveat is that patients need to take immunosuppressive medications for the life of the graft. The literature reports that non-compliance occurs in approximately 20% of renal recipients, making it a major cause of graft loss. Renal transplantation is not a cure for renal failure. There are several types of donors for renal transplant patients: deceased (formerly cadaveric), living related, living unrelated, voluntary nondirected (anonymous), directed, paired kidney exchange, domino, and expanded-criteria donors. Postoperatively, patients are sent to specialized units where nephrology nurses monitor them on an hourly basis for the first 24-36 hr. Subsequent admissions may occur at any hospital for treatment of a rejection episode, infection, medication complication, or unrelated illness. Rejection is the major complication of renal transplantation. Long-term complications occur secondary to use of immunosuppressive agents and include hyperglycemia, electrolyte imbalance, infection, hypertension, hyperlipidemia, cardiovascular disease, chronic liver disease, bone demineralization, cataracts, gastrointestinal (GI) hemorrhage, and cancer.

HEALTH CARE SETTING

Transplant center; acute care surgical unit or critical care unit; medical/surgical unit for complications or rejection

Immunosuppression

With the exception of identical twin donors, all transplant recipients must take drugs that suppress their immune system to prevent graft rejection. Each transplant center has a drug protocol outlining which combination of medications will be given to each patient. **Note:** A complete list of the patient's medications, including herbal remedies, should be included on the patient's chart. Some herbs interfere with absorption of immunosuppressive medications, causing patients to have lower levels of medications in their systems and potentially resulting in episodes of graft rejection and/or loss of the graft. The National Kidney Foundation has a list of the most common herbal supplements that would be harmful for patients with chronic kidney disease (www.kidney.org/atoz/content/herbalsupp.cfm). For more indepth information regarding herbal supplements, check Micromedex if unsure about interactions.

Rejection

Acute: Usually occurs days to weeks post transplant; potentially reversible; treated with increased immunosuppression.

Chronic: Usually classified as starting 1 year after transplant; irreversible; managed conservatively with diet and antihypertensive agents until dialysis is required.

Indicators of rejection: Oliguria, tenderness over graft site (located in iliac fossa), sudden weight gain (2-3 lb/day), fever, malaise, hypertension, and increased blood urea nitrogen (BUN) and serum creatinine. In addition, hyperglycemia will develop with combined kidney-pancreas transplants.

Nursing Diagnosis:

Risk for Infection

related to invasive procedures, exposure to infected individuals, and immunosuppression

Desired Outcomes: The patient is free of infection as evidenced by normothermia; heart rate (HR) 100 bpm or less (or within the patient's normal range); respiratory rate (RR) 12-20 bpm with normal depth and pattern; and absence of erythema, edema, increased local warmth, tenderness, or purulent drainage at wounds or catheter exit sites. The patient is free of signs and symptoms of oral, esophageal, respiratory, gastrointestinal (GI), genitourinary, and cutaneous infections. The patient verbalizes indicators of infection and the importance of reporting them promptly to the health care provider or staff.

ASSESSMENT/INTERVENTIONS	RATIONALES
! When caring for the patient, increase your sensitivity to *any* indicator of infection as a cue to increase depth and frequency of assessments for infection.	Transplant recipients are taking large doses of immunosuppressive agents, and their immune response and thus response to infectious agents will be muted. Infections therefore are potentially life threatening in an individual who is immunosuppressed.
- Assess for low-grade temperature elevation, fever, and unexplained tachycardia.	These are indicators that might signal infection in a transplant recipient.
- Assess for indicators of cytomegalovirus (CMV), including fever, malaise, fatigue, and muscle aches.	CMV is a common infectious agent among these patients. Other infectious complications include *Legionella pneumophila*; cutaneous herpes zoster (shingles); varicella (chickenpox); Epstein-Barr virus (EBV); oral, esophageal, deep fungal, or mycotic pseudoaneurysm caused by *Candida*; and *Pneumocystis jiroveci* (formerly called *Pneumocystis carinii*).
! Use sterile technique with all invasive procedures and dressing changes.	Following sterile technique reduces the possibility of infection, which is increased with invasive procedures into the body and involving nonintact skin.
! Instruct the patient to be alert to signs and symptoms of commonly encountered infections and caution about the following:	Infections and their indicators include *urinary tract infection* (UTI)—cloudy and malodorous urine; dysuria, frequency, and urgency; pain in the suprapubic area, buttock, thighs, labia, or scrotum; *upper respiratory tract infection* (URI)—productive cough, malodorous, purulent, colored, and copious secretions, chest pain or heaviness; *pharyngitis*—painful swallowing; *otitis media*—malaise, earache; *impetigo*—inflamed or draining areas on the skin.
- Importance of reporting these indicators to the health care provider promptly.	Prompt reporting of these indicators is essential because infections can be life threatening in a patient undergoing immunosuppression.
- Avoiding exposure to individuals known to have infections and to wash hands frequently.	Consistent hand hygiene is a proven method of removing pathogens from the skin that could otherwise cause infection and is especially important in patients whose immune systems are compromised. In the absence of hand washing opportunities, hand decontamination with an alcohol-based hand sanitizer provides adequate hand hygiene.
- Use of prophylactic antibiotics for any minor invasive procedures.	Prophylactic antibiotics reduce infection risk, which can occur in even minor procedures. Some health care providers encourage antibiotics for any minor invasive procedures, including dental cleaning.
- Avoiding working in soil for the first 6 months after transplantation.	This restriction minimizes the risk of acquiring *Aspergillus* infection.
- As indicated, quitting smoking; provide smoking cessation literature.	Smoking increases susceptibility to respiratory infection because it damages protective mechanisms such as cilia in the lungs. Smoking also causes detrimental changes to blood pressure (BP), HR, cholesterol levels, and clotting factors.

Nursing Diagnosis:

Deficient Knowledge

related to unfamiliarity with signs and symptoms of rejection, side effects of immunosuppressive agents, and transplantation complications.

Desired Outcome: Within the 24-hr period before hospital discharge, the patient verbalizes knowledge of signs and symptoms of rejection, side effects of immunosuppressive therapy, and complications of transplantation.

ASSESSMENT/INTERVENTIONS	RATIONALES
Assess the patient's health care literacy (language, reading, comprehension). Assess culture and culturally specific information needs.	This assessment helps ensure that information is selected and presented in a manner that is culturally and educationally appropriate.
Explain the importance of renal function monitoring: intake and output, daily weight, and BUN and serum creatinine values.	These tests evaluate kidney status and guide the therapeutic drug regimen and treatment plan: as renal function decreases, BUN and creatinine values will increase.
Teach signs and symptoms of rejection.	Signs and symptoms of rejection necessitate prompt intervention to save the kidney. These include oliguria, tenderness over the transplanted kidney (located in iliac fossa), sudden weight gain (2-3 lb), fever, malaise, hypertension, and increased BUN (greater than 20 mg/dL) and serum creatinine (greater than 1.5 mg/dL). In addition, the patient may have body aches, swelling in the legs or hands, and temperature greater than 100° F.
Instruct the patient to weigh self at the same time each day, using the same scale and wearing the same amount of clothing. Provide a notebook in which to record daily vital signs (VS) and weight measurements. Remind the patient to bring the notebook to all outpatient visits and to report abnormal values promptly should they occur.	These assessments monitor the trend of VS and weight measurements. Using the same standards daily ensures accuracy with weight measurements.
Teach the patient that if a rejection episode occurs, he or she will be removed from the antirejection medications and started on other agents until the creatinine level drops below 3 mg/dL.	Agents such as OKT3 and antithymocyte globulin are substitute antirejection medications that are less nephrotoxic. OKT3 requires a chest x-ray study to ensure no pulmonary edema occurs during administration, and patients will need VS monitored q4h to assess for temperature elevation after administration. Premedication is required to prevent dyspnea, chills, fever, and possible anaphylaxis.
Explain the importance of serial white blood cell (WBC) and platelet count monitoring.	Significant decreases in WBC and platelet counts can be a side effect of immunosuppressive agents, and therefore serial monitoring is essential.
Teach signs and symptoms of GI bleeding and the importance of reporting them promptly if they occur.	GI bleeding is a potential side effect of immunosuppressive agents and can be life threatening if it is excessive. Prompt reporting of the onset of these symptoms (e.g., tarry stools, "coffee-ground" emesis, orthostatic changes, dizziness, tachycardia, increasing fatigue and weakness) enables the health care provider to adjust medications or add medications such as antacids and H_2-receptor blockers to treat cause of the bleeding.
Teach the patient and/or significant others how to measure BP, and provide guidelines for values that would necessitate notification of the health care provider or staff member.	In a patient who has undergone renal transplantation, hypertension may develop for a variety of reasons, including cyclosporine or steroid use, rejection, or renal artery stenosis. In addition, the patient may have had hypertension before the transplant. A value that would necessitate notification of the health care provider is BP 20% above or below the patient's "normal" BP. This value and parameters for calling the health care provider are generally agreed on before the patient leaves the hospital.
Teach the importance of the medication regimen, including the appropriate timing of the medication and managing missed doses.	A large portion of rejection incidence can be attributed to missing drug doses due to non-adherence (approximately 20%), lack of knowledge, side effects, and/or improved health, during which patients no longer feel the need to take their medications. Missed doses need to be carefully evaluated. Patients need to take their medications as soon as they realize a dose has been missed, unless it is time for the next dose, at which time the missed dose can be omitted. Setting up a schedule is imperative to help avoid the number of missed doses.

ASSESSMENT/INTERVENTIONS	RATIONALES
Stress the need for continued medical evaluation of the transplant.	Continued evaluation will confirm that the kidney is working properly and the patient is not undergoing rejection.
Verify the patient's knowledge of immunosuppressive medication precautions and dosages.	A knowledgeable patient is likely to participate more effectively in the therapeutic regimen. *Antimetabolites (azathioprine and mycophenolate mofetil):* Dosage is adjusted or held based on the patient's WBC count. *Prednisone:* Some nondiabetic patients may develop glucose intolerance (new-onset diabetes mellitus) due to use. Patients with diabetes will find that their insulin requirements will need to be adjusted, typically needing more insulin as kidney function returns and appetite increases. *Calcineurin inhibitors (cyclosporine and tacrolimus):* These medications must not be mixed with grapefruit juice. Grapefruit juice has been known to potentiate medication, which could cause nephrotoxicity and/or loss of graft function. *"TOR" inhibitors (sirolimus and everolimus):* There is potential for nephrotoxicity; BUN and creatinine will require monitoring. The patient should be alert for decreased urine output and sudden weight gain (2-3 lb).

 PATIENT- FAMILY TEACHING AND DISCHARGE PLANNING

When providing patient-family teaching, focus on sensory information, avoid giving excessive information, and make appropriate referrals (e.g., visiting or home health nurse, community health resources) for follow-up teaching. Include verbal and written information about the following:

✓ Medications, including name; dosage; purpose; schedule; precautions; drug-drug, drug-herb, and food-drug interactions; and potential side effects. Provide guidelines for how to cope with medication side effects.

✓ The importance of never stopping medications, even if feeling better, because it is the medication that is keeping the kidneys functional and creating the feelings of wellness.

✓ Measures for preventing infection, including incision care. Stress to the patient that infections can be life threatening because of immunosuppression.

✓ Prescribed diet and activity level progression.

✓ Community resources for emotional and financial support.

✓ Importance of follow-up care to ensure long-term viability of the transplanted kidney.

✓ Telephone numbers to call in case problems or questions arise after discharge from care facility.

✓ Internet resources:
- United Network for Organ Sharing at *www.unos.org*
- National Kidney Disease Education Program at *www.nkdep.nih.gov*
- National Kidney Foundation at *www.kidney.org*
- The Kidney Foundation of Canada at *www.kidney.ca*
- Transplant Recipients International Organization (TRIO) at *www.trioweb.org*

Also see discussions in **Deficient Knowledge** related to signs and symptoms of rejection, side effects of immunosuppressive agents, and transplantation complications.

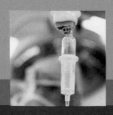

Ureteral Calculi 31

OVERVIEW/PATHOPHYSIOLOGY

Ureteral calculi (stones) constitute the third most common urologic condition after urinary tract infections (UTIs) and pathologic conditions of the prostate. Although the cause of stones is unknown in 50% of reported cases, it is believed that they originate in the kidney and are passed through the kidney to the ureter. About 90% of all stones pass from the ureter into the bladder and out of the urinary system spontaneously.

HEALTH CARE SETTING

Primary care; may require hospitalization for complications or surgery

ASSESSMENT

Signs and symptoms: Pain that is sharp, sudden, and intense or dull and aching; located in the flank area; and often radiating toward the groin. Pain may be intermittent (colic) as the stone moves along the ureter and may subside when it enters the bladder. Nausea, vomiting, diarrhea, abdominal pain, and paralytic ileus may occur. Patients may experience urgency and frequency, void in small amounts, and have hematuria. Fever may indicate an infected stone or secondary UTI.

Physical assessment: Pallor, diaphoresis, tachycardia, and tachypnea may be observed. Costovertebral angle (CVA) tenderness and guarding may be present. Bowel sounds may be absent secondary to ileus, and the abdomen may be distended and tympanic. The patient will be restless and unable to find a position of comfort.

History of: Sedentary lifestyle; residence in geographic area in which water supply is high in stone-forming minerals; vitamin A deficiency; vitamin D excess; hereditary cystinuria; inflammatory bowel disease; recurrent UTIs; prolonged periods of immobilization; gout or prophylactic therapy with allopurinol; use of indinavir sulfate, a protease inhibitor used in patients with human immunodeficiency virus (HIV) infection; decreased fluid intake; hyperparathyroidism; sarcoidosis;

and familial history of calculi or renal disease such as renal tubular acidosis.

DIAGNOSTIC TESTS

Serum tests: To assess calcium levels greater than 5.3 mEq/L, phosphorus levels greater than 2.6 mEq/L, and uric acid levels greater than 7.5 mg/dL, which have been implicated in stone formation.

Blood urea nitrogen (BUN) and creatinine tests: To evaluate renal-urinary function. Abnormalities are reflected by high BUN and serum creatinine and low urine creatinine levels.

> **Note:** *Be aware that BUN levels are affected by fluid volume excess and deficit. Volume excess will reduce BUN levels, whereas volume deficit will increase levels. For the older adult, serum creatinine level may not be a reliable measure of renal function because of reduced muscle mass and a decreased glomerular filtration rate (GFR). These tests must be evaluated based on an adjustment for the patient's age and hydration status and in comparison with other renal-urinary tests.*

Urinalysis: To provide baseline data on urinary system functioning, detect metabolic disease, and assess for the presence of UTI. A cloudy or hazy appearance; foul odor; pH greater than 7; and presence of red blood cells, leukocyte esterase, white blood cells (WBCs), and WBC casts signal UTI. A pH less than 5 is associated with uric acid calculi, whereas a pH of 7.5 or greater may signal presence of urea-splitting organisms (responsible for magnesium-ammonium-phosphate or struvite calculi).

Urine culture: To determine type of bacteria present in the genitourinary tract. To avoid contamination, a midstream specimen should be collected.

24-hr urine collection: To test for high levels of uric acid, cystine, calcium, magnesium, oxalate, calcium, phosphorus, or creatinine. A second 24-hr urine collection may be done after the patient has been on a diet restricted in sodium, oxalate, and calcium.

Note: *All urine samples should be sent to the laboratory immediately after they are obtained or refrigerated if this is not possible (specimens for culture are not refrigerated). Urine left at room temperature has greater potential for bacterial growth, turbidity, and alkaline pH, any of which can distort the reading.*

Kidney, ureter, and bladder (KUB) radiography: To monitor passage of a previously documented opaque stone.

Computed tomography (CT) scan with or without injection of contrast medium: To distinguish cysts, tumors, calculi, and other masses and determine presence of ureteral dilation and bladder distention.

Excretory urogram/intravenous pyelogram (IVP): Used to visualize kidneys, renal pelvis, ureters, and bladder. It can identify size of the stone and presence and severity of the obstruction. This test also outlines nonradiopaque stones within the ureters. Nonradiopaque stones (e.g., uric acid calculi) are seen as radiolucent defects in the contrast media.

Renal ultrasound: To identify ureteral dilation and presence of stones in the ureters.

Nursing Diagnosis

Acute Pain

related to the presence of a calculus or the surgical procedure to remove it

Desired Outcomes: The patient's subjective perception of pain decreases within 1 hr of intervention, as documented by a pain scale. Objective indicators, such as grimacing, are absent or diminished.

ASSESSMENT/INTERVENTIONS	RATIONALES
Assess and document the quality, location, intensity, and duration of pain. Devise a pain scale with the patient that ranges from 0 (no pain) to 10 (worst pain).	This assessment evaluates intensity and trend of pain and subsequent relief obtained.
Notify the health care provider of sudden and/or severe pain.	This is a sign that a stone is passing through the ureter.
Notify the health care provider of a sudden cessation of pain. Strain all urine for solid matter, and send to the laboratory for analysis.	This can signal passage of the stone.
Medicate the patient with prescribed analgesics, opioids, and antispasmodics; evaluate and document the response based on the pain scale.	Conservative therapy may consist of a trial of analgesia, dissolution agents, and normal fluid intake to 1500-2000 mL/day. Dissolution agents such as orange juice alkalinize urine and work to shrink stones so that they can pass through the ureter. **Note:** Morphine increases ureteral peristalsis, which aids in stone passage, but ureteral peristalsis can increase pain.
Encourage the patient to request medication before discomfort becomes severe.	Pain is easier to manage when it is treated before it gets too severe because prolonged stimulation of pain receptors increases sensitivity to painful stimuli and increases the amount of medication required to relieve pain.
Administer antiemetics (e.g., hydroxyzine, ondansetron, prochlorperazine, promethazine) as prescribed.	These agents promote comfort from nausea and vomiting.
Provide warm blankets or a heating pad to the affected area, or supply warm baths.	These measures increase regional circulation and relax tense muscles.
Provide back rubs.	Back rubs are especially helpful for postoperative patients who were in the lithotomy position during surgery.
See "Pain," p. 39, for other interventions.	

Nursing Diagnosis

Impaired Urinary Elimination

related to obstruction caused by the ureteral calculus

Desired Outcomes: The patient relates the return of a normal voiding pattern within 2 days. The patient demonstrates the ability to record intake and output (I&O) and strain urine for stones.

ASSESSMENT/INTERVENTIONS	RATIONALES
Assess and document the patient's normal voiding pattern.	This assessment establishes a baseline for subsequent assessment.
Assess quality and color of the urine.	Optimally, urine is straw colored and clear and has a characteristic odor. Dark urine is often indicative of dehydration, and blood-tinged urine can result from rupture of ureteral capillaries as the calculus passes through the ureter.
In patients for whom fluids are not restricted, encourage fluid intake of at least 2-3 L/day.	Increased hydration helps flush the calculus through the ureter into the bladder and out through the system.
Record accurate I&O; teach the patient how to record I&O.	Output that is less than input could signal an obstruction. Patients should participate in I&O documentation to ensure that all output and intake is being recorded.
Strain all urine for evidence of solid matter; teach the patient the procedure.	This intervention can detect passage of stones.
Send any solid matter to the laboratory for analysis.	The laboratory will test for high levels of uric acid, cystine, oxalate, calcium, or phosphorus, which would signal the presence and type of stones.

Nursing Diagnosis

Impaired Urinary Elimination

related to obstruction or postsurgical positional problems of the ureteral catheter

Desired Outcome: Following intervention, the patient has output from the ureteral catheter and is free of spasms or flank pain, which otherwise could signal obstruction or displacement.

ASSESSMENT/INTERVENTIONS	RATIONALES
If the patient has more than one catheter, label one *right* and the other *left;* keep all drainage records separate.	Occasionally, patients return from surgery with ureteral catheters. Ureteral catheters, also known as *stents,* are positioned postoperatively to enable healing and promote ureteral patency in the presence of edema. If the patient has two ureteral catheters, separate output records are used to identify how each ureter is functioning.
Monitor output from the ureteral catheter.	The amount will vary with each patient and will depend on catheter dimension.
If drainage is scanty or absent, milk the catheter and tubing gently. If this fails, notify the health care provider.	This action will help dislodge the obstruction.
Caution: Never irrigate a catheter without specific health care provider instructions to do so. If irrigation is prescribed, use gentle pressure and sterile technique. Always aspirate with a sterile syringe before instillation. Use another sterile syringe to insert instillation amounts of 3 mL or less.	There is potential for ureteral damage and infection during irrigation caused by overdistention and/or introduction of pathogens.

ASSESSMENT/INTERVENTIONS	RATIONALES
Explain to the patient that semi-Fowler's and side-lying positions are acceptable but that Fowler's position should be avoided.	Fowler's position should be avoided because sutures are seldom used and gravity can cause the catheter to move into the bladder. Typically, patients will require bedrest if the ureteral catheter is indwelling.
Carefully monitor the urethral catheter for movement, and ensure that it is securely attached to the patient.	Ureteral catheters are often attached to the urethral catheter after placement in the ureters. The urethral catheter should be monitored to detect movement and to ensure that it is securely attached to the patient.
Note: After ureteral catheters have been removed (usually simultaneously with the urethral catheter), monitor for flank pain, CVA tenderness, nausea, and vomiting.	These are indicators of ureteral obstruction, which necessitates prompt intervention.

Nursing Diagnosis

Risk for Impaired Skin Integrity

related to wound drainage after ureterolithotomy or procedures entering the ureter

Desired Outcome: The patient's skin surrounding the wound site remains nonerythremic and intact.

ASSESSMENT/INTERVENTIONS	RATIONALES
Assess incisional dressings frequently during the first 24 hr, and change or reinforce as needed. Note and document odor, consistency, and color of the drainage.	Immediately after surgery, drainage may be red. Flank approaches to the ureter require muscle-splitting incisions and result in significant postoperative oozing of blood. Because drainage will also include urine leaking from the entered ureter, excoriation can result from prolonged contact of urine with the skin.
Use Montgomery straps or net wraps (e.g., Surginet) rather than tape to secure the dressing.	This intervention facilitates frequent dressing changes without harming the skin with tape removal.
If drainage is copious after drain removal, apply a wound drainage or ostomy pouch with a skin barrier over the incision.	This measure prevents contact of wound drainage with the skin.
Use a pouch with an antireflux valve.	This valve prevents contamination from reflux.

Nursing Diagnosis

Deficient Knowledge

related to unfamiliarity with the dietary regimen and its relationship to calculus formation

Desired Outcome: Within the 24-hr period before hospital discharge, the patient verbalizes knowledge about foods and liquids to limit in order to prevent stone formation and demonstrates this knowledge by planning a 3-day menu that excludes or limits these foods.

ASSESSMENT/INTERVENTIONS	RATIONALES
Assess the patient's knowledge about diet and its relationship to stone formation.	This assessment will reveal the patient's baseline knowledge, which will enable formulation of an individualized teaching plan.
Advise nonrestricted patients to maintain a urine output of at least 2-3 L/day.	Increasing urine output reduces saturation of stone-forming solutes.

continued

ASSESSMENT/INTERVENTIONS	RATIONALES
Teach the patient to maintain adequate hydration of at least 2-3 L/day, especially after meals and exercise. **Caution:** Patients with cardiac, liver, or renal disease require special fluid intake instructions from their health care provider.	Good hydration after meals and exercise is important because a patient's solute load is highest at these times. These patients likely will need some degree of fluid restriction to prevent fluid overload.
Teach the technique for measuring urine specific gravity via a hydrometer.	In order to minimize stone formation, specific gravity should remain less than 1.010.
As appropriate, provide the following information.	
For uric acid stones:	
- Limit intake of foods such as lean meat, legumes, whole grains. Limit protein intake to 1 g/kg/day.	These foods are high in purines, which can lead to the formation of uric acid stones.
- Explain that allopurinol or sodium bicarbonate may be given.	These agents reduce uric acid production or alkalinize the urine, keeping pH at 6.5 or higher.
For calcium stones:	
- Limit intake of foods such as milk, cheese, green leafy vegetables, yogurt.	These foods are high in calcium content.
- Limit sodium intake.	A low-sodium diet helps reduce intestinal absorption of calcium.
- Limit intake of refined carbohydrates and animal proteins.	These foods can cause hypercalciuria.
- Encourage foods high in natural fiber content (e.g., bran, prunes, apples).	These foods provide phytic acid, which binds dietary calcium.
- Explain that sodium cellulose phosphate, 5 g, may be given three times a day before each meal.	Sodium cellulose phosphate, when used with calcium-restricted diet, reduces risk of stone formation by binding with intestinal calcium and thus increasing excretion of calcium. It should be used cautiously in postmenopausal women at risk for osteoporosis.
- Explain that orthophosphates (potassium acid phosphate and disodium and dipotassium phosphates) or thiazides also may be given for calcium stones.	These agents decrease urinary excretion of citrate and pyrophosphate and thus inhibit stone formation.
For oxalate stones:	
- Limit intake of foods such as chocolate, caffeine-containing drinks (including instant and decaffeinated coffees), beets, spinach, rhubarb, berries, draft beer, and nuts such as almonds, walnuts, pecans, and cashews.	These foods are high in oxalate content.
- Explain that large doses of pyridoxine may help with certain types of oxalate stones, and cholestyramine, 4 g four times daily, may be prescribed.	These agents bind with oxalate enterally.
- Explain that vitamin C supplements should be avoided.	As much as half of the vitamin C is converted to oxalic acid.
Ask the patient to plan a 3-day menu that includes or excludes appropriate foods.	This will demonstrate the patient's level of understanding of the prescribed diet and areas in which teaching should be reinforced. This effort by the patient also will reinforce learning.

ADDITIONAL NURSING DIAGNOSES/PROBLEMS:

"Perioperative Care"   p. 45

✓ **PATIENT-FAMILY TEACHING AND DISCHARGE PLANNING**

When providing patient-family teaching, focus on sensory information, avoid giving excessive information, and initiate a visiting nurse referral for necessary follow-up teaching. Include verbal and written information about the following:

✓ Medications, including drug name, purpose, dosage, schedule, precautions, and potential side effects. Also discuss drug-drug, herb-drug, and food-drug interactions.

✓ Indicators of UTI that necessitate medical attention: chills; fever; hematuria; flank, CVA, suprapubic, low back, buttock, scrotal, or labial pain; cloudy and foul-smelling urine; increased frequency, urgency; dysuria; and increasing or recurring incontinence.

✓ Care of incision, including cleansing and dressing. Teach signs and symptoms of local infection, including redness, swelling, local warmth, tenderness, and purulent drainage.

✓ Care of drains or catheters if the patient is discharged with them.

✓ Importance of daily fluid intake of at least 2-3 L/day in nonrestricted patients.

✓ Dietary changes as specified by the health care provider. Include fact sheets that list foods to restrict or add to the diet. Provide sample menus with examples of how dietary restrictions and requirements may be incorporated into daily meals.

✓ Activity restrictions as directed for the patient who has had surgery: avoid lifting heavy objects (more than 10 lb) for the first 6 wk, be alert to fatigue, get maximum rest, increase activities gradually to tolerance.

✓ Use of Nitrazine paper to assess pH of urine. Desired pH will be determined by the type of stone formation to which the patient is prone. Instructions for use are on the Nitrazine container.

✓ Importance of walking or other exercise to decrease risk of stone formation.

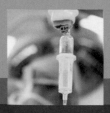

Urinary Diversions 32

OVERVIEW/PATHOPHYSIOLOGY

When the bladder must be bypassed or is removed, a urinary diversion is created. Urinary diversions most commonly are created for individuals with bladder cancer. However, malignancies of the prostate, urethra, vagina, uterus, or cervix may require creation of a urinary diversion if anterior, posterior, or total pelvic exenteration must be done. Individuals with severe, nonmalignant urinary problems, such as radiation or interstitial cystitis, or urinary incontinence that cannot be managed conservatively also are candidates for urinary diversion. Although most urinary diversions are permanent, some act as a temporary bypass of urine, and undiversion can be performed if the patient's condition changes.

The urinary stream may be diverted at multiple points: the renal pelvis (pyelostomy or nephrostomy), the ureter (ureterostomy), the bladder (vesicostomy), or via an intestinal "conduit." Vesicostomies are most commonly performed in children as a temporary diversion. While construction of a small bowel pouch (Kock procedure) or ileocolonic pouch (Indiana or Mainz procedure) is still the most common type of urinary diversion, the neobladder or orthotopic bladder is becoming the standard of definitive care. All these procedures reconstruct a new bladder from intestinal segments, resulting in a more normal urinary pattern. In addition, because males have an external urinary sphincter that can be left in place when the bladder is removed, men may undergo attachment of a reconstructed bladder to the urethra, which will enable urination without the use of catheterization. However, there is a 5%-10% risk of urethral reoccurrence of neoplasm with this procedure.

Continent urinary diversions: All continent urinary diversions are constructed with the following three components: a reservoir or reconstructed bladder, a continence mechanism, and an antireflux mechanism.

Orthotopic neobladder: This surgery involves use of the small intestine or small bowel–large bowel combination to create a low-pressure spherical reservoir that attaches to the patient's urinary sphincter. Additionally, a cystoprostatectomy is performed in men and a urethral-preserving anterior exenteration is performed in women. Similar to the Mainz and Kock techniques, the created "bladder" has the characteristics of low pressure, adequate volume, and control of urination without leakage or residual urine. The patient can sense a full bladder and urinate without catheterization. Normal continence is the goal for this procedure.

Indiana and Kock pouches: Both the Indiana and Kock pouches use the ileum to create a pouch and an antireflux valve. These types of continent urostomies require the patient to perform catheterizations to remove urine from the pouch.

Intestinal (ileal conduit): Any segment of bowel may be used to create a passageway for urine but the ileum conduit is most commonly used. A 15- to 20-cm section of ileum is resected from the intestine to form a passageway for the urine. The proximal end is closed, and the distal end is brought out through the abdomen, forming a stoma. The ureters are resected from the bladder and anastomosed to the ileal segment. The intestine is reanastomosed to the ileal segment, and therefore bowel function is unaffected. Occasionally, the jejunum is used for the conduit. However, jejunal-conduit syndrome (hyperkalemia, hyponatremia, hypochloremia) often occurs.

HEALTH CARE SETTING

Surgical unit; primary care

Nursing Diagnosis:

Anxiety

related to threat to self-concept, interaction patterns, or health status occurring with urinary diversion surgery

Desired Outcome: Before surgery, the patient communicates fears and concerns, relates attainment of increased psychologic and physical comfort, and exhibits a coping demeanor.

PART I: Medical-Surgical Nursing

ASSESSMENT/INTERVENTIONS	RATIONALES
Assess the patient's perception of his or her impending surgery and resulting body function changes. Listen actively.	This assessment provides an opportunity for the patient to express anxieties about the upcoming surgery and for the nurse to evaluate the response. For example, "You seem very concerned about next week's surgery." Anger, denial, withdrawal, and demanding behaviors may be coping responses.
Acknowledge the patient's concerns.	This will help focus attention on anxieties and concerns so that they can be dealt with.
Provide brief, basic information regarding physiology of the procedure and equipment that will be used after surgery, including tubes and drains.	Knowledge is one of the best means of decreasing anxiety.
Show the patient pouches that will be used after surgery. Assure the patient that the pouch usually cannot be seen through clothing and that it is odor resistant.	Patients may worry that others will be able to see and smell the pouch.
For the patient about to undergo a continent urostomy procedure of a Kock or Indiana pouch, explain that a pouching system may be needed for a short time after surgery. Reassure the patient that teaching about accessing the continent urostomy will be done in the surgeon's office or by the home care nurse.	This intervention likely will decrease anxiety by reassuring the patient that he or she will be taught necessary skills.
Discuss postsurgical activities of daily living (ADLs).	This information decreases anxiety that such ADLs as showers, baths, and swimming can continue and that diet is not affected after the early postoperative period.
As appropriate, ask the patient about the information that has been relayed by the surgeon about sexual implications of the surgery.	Patients may be very anxious about sexual implications of this surgery but afraid to ask. Asking this question will help establish an open relationship between the patient and nurse. For example, some men undergoing radical cystectomy with urinary diversion may become impotent, but recent surgical advances have enabled preservation of potency for others. The pelvic plexus, which innervates the corpora cavernosa (allowing penile erection), may be damaged permanently as a result of autonomic nerve damage. However, sensation and orgasm are mediated by the pudendal nerve (sensorimotor) and are not affected.
Arrange for a visit by the enterostomal therapy (ET) nurse during the preoperative period. Collaborate with the surgeon, ET nurse, and patient to identify and mark the most appropriate site for the stoma.	Showing patients the actual spot for placement may help alleviate anxiety by reinforcing that the impact on lifestyle and body image will be minimal.

Nursing Diagnosis:

Impaired Urinary Elimination

related to postoperative use of ureteral stents, catheters, or drains; and *related to* urinary diversion surgery

Desired Outcome: The patient's urinary output is 30 mL/hr or greater; urine is clear and straw-colored with normal, characteristic odor.

ASSESSMENT/INTERVENTIONS	RATIONALES
Assess intake and output, and record the total amount of urine output from the urinary diversion for the first 24 hr postoperatively. Differentiate and record separately amounts from all drains, stents, and catheters. Notify the health care provider of an output less than 60 mL during a 2-hr period.	This assessment checks for discrepancies between intake and output. In the presence of adequate intake a decreased output can signal a ureteral obstruction, a leak in one of the anastomotic sites, or impending renal failure. *Ureterostomy:* Urine is drained via the stoma and/or ureteral stents.

continued

ASSESSMENT/INTERVENTIONS	RATIONALES
	Intestinal conduit: Urine is drained via the stoma. Patients also may have ureteral stents and/or conduit catheter/stent in the early postoperative period to stabilize the ureterointestinal anastomoses and maintain drainage from the conduit during early postoperative edema.
	Continent urinary diversions or reservoirs: The Kock urostomy usually has a reservoir catheter and also may have ureteral stents. The Indiana (ileocecal) reservoir usually has ureteral stents exiting from the stoma, through which most of the urine drains and may have a reservoir catheter exiting from a stab wound, which serves as an overflow catheter. The neobladder has a urethral catheter in place that will drain urine, which initially will be light red to pink in color with mucus but should clear in 24-48 hr. This catheter generally remains in place for 21 days to ensure adequate healing of the anastomosis.
Also assess for flank pain, costovertebral angle (CVA) tenderness, nausea, vomiting, and anuria.	These are other indicators of ureteral obstruction.
Monitor functioning of the ureteral stents.	Ureteral stents, which exit from the stoma into the pouch, maintain ureteral patency and assist in healing of the anastomosis. Stents may become blocked with mucus, but as long as urine is draining adequately around the stent and the volume of output is adequate, this is not a problem. Right stents usually are cut at a 90-degree angle, and left stents are cut at a 45-degree angle. Each usually produces approximately the same amount of urine, although the amount produced by each is not important as long as each drains adequately and total drainage from all sources is 30 mL/hr or greater. Urine is usually red to pink for the first 24-48 hr and becomes straw-colored by the third postoperative day. Absent or lessening amounts of urine may indicate a blocked stent or problems with the ureter.
Monitor functioning of the stoma catheter.	Expect output from the stoma catheter to include pink or light red urine with mucus and small red clots for the first 24 hr. Urine should become amber colored with occasional clots within 3 postoperative days. Mucus production will continue but should decrease in volume.
	In continent urinary diversions, a catheter is placed in the reservoir to prevent distention and promote healing of suture lines. This new reservoir (i.e., resected intestine) exudes large amounts of mucus, necessitating catheter irrigation with 30-50 mL of normal saline, which is instilled gently and allowed to empty via gravity.
Monitor functioning of the drains.	Any urinary diversion may have Penrose drains or closed drainage systems in place to facilitate healing of the ureterointestinal anastomosis. Drainage from these systems may be light red to pink for the first 24 hr and then lighten to amber and decrease in amount. Excessive lymph fluid and urine can be removed via these drains to reduce pressure on anastomotic suture lines. In a continent urinary diversion, an increase in drainage after amounts have been low might signal an anastomotic leak, which necessitates notification of the health care provider.
Monitor drainage from the Foley (indwelling) catheter or urethral drain (if present). Note color, consistency, and volume of drainage, which may be red to pink with mucus.	Patients who have had a cystectomy may have a urethral drain, whereas those with a partial cystectomy will have an indwelling catheter in place.
⚠ Report a sudden increase or decrease in drainage to the health care provider.	A sudden increase would occur with hemorrhage; a sudden decrease can signal blockage that can lead to infection or, with partial cystectomy, hydronephrosis.
Encourage an intake of at least 2-3 L/day in the nonrestricted patient.	Increased hydration keeps the urinary tract well irrigated and helps prevent infection that could be caused by urinary stasis.

Nursing Diagnosis:

Risk for Infection

related to the invasive surgical procedure and potential for ascending bacteriuria with the urinary diversion

Desired Outcome: The patient is free of infection as evidenced by normothermia; white blood cell (WBC) count 11,000/mm^3 or less; and absence of purulent or excessive drainage, erythema, edema, warmth, and tenderness along the incision.

ASSESSMENT/INTERVENTIONS	RATIONALES
Assess the patient's temperature q4h during the first 24-48 hr after surgery. Notify the health care provider of fever (temperature greater than 101° F).	Elevated temperature is a sign that the body is mounting a defense against infection.
Inspect the dressing frequently after surgery. Change the dressing when it becomes wet, using sterile technique. Use extra care to prevent disruption of the drains.	Infection is most likely to become evident after the first 72 hr. The presence of purulent or excessive drainage on the dressing signals infection and the need to notify the health care provider promptly for timely intervention.
Assess the condition of the incision.	Erythema, tenderness, local warmth, edema, and purulent or excessive drainage are indicators of infection at the incision line.
Assess and record character of the urine at least q8h.	Urine should be yellow or pink tinged during the first 24-48 hr after surgery. Mucous particles are normal in urine of patients with ileal conduits and continent urinary diversions because of the nature of the bowel segment used. Cloudy urine, however, is abnormal and can signal infection.
Assess for flank or CVA pain, malodorous urine, chills, and fever.	These are indicators of urinary tract infection (UTI).
Note position of the stoma relative to the incision. If they are close together, apply the pouch first to avoid overlap of the pouch with the suture line.	Overlapping of the pouch with the suture line increases risk of infection.
If necessary, cut the pouch down on one side or place it at an angle.	This measure prevents contact of the pouch with drainage, which may loosen the adhesive.
Wash your hands thoroughly before and after caring for the patient.	Hand hygiene helps prevent contamination and cross-contamination.
Do not irrigate indwelling urethral catheters of patients with cystectomies.	Patients with cystectomies without anastomosis to the urethra may have an indwelling urethral catheter to drain serosanguineous fluid from the peritoneal cavity. Irrigation of this catheter can result in peritonitis.
Encourage fluid intake of at least 2-3 L/day.	Increased hydration helps flush urine through the urinary tract, removing mucous shreds, and preventing stasis that could result in infection.

Nursing Diagnosis:

Ineffective Protection

related to the potential for neurosensory, musculoskeletal, and cardiac changes occurring with hyperchloremic metabolic acidosis with hypokalemia

Desired Outcomes: The patient verbalizes orientation to person, place, and time (within the patient's normal range) and remains free of injury caused by neurosensory, musculoskeletal, and cardiac changes. Electrolytes remain within normal limits.

ASSESSMENT/INTERVENTIONS	RATIONALE
For patients with ileal conduits, assess for nausea and changes in level of consciousness (LOC) and muscle tone and irregular heart rate (HR).	Changes in neurosensory, musculoskeletal, and cardiac status are indicators of hypokalemia and metabolic acidosis that can occur secondary to the presence of Na^+ and Cl^- from the urine in the ileal segment, which results in compensatory loss of K^+ and HCO_3^-.
Monitor serum electrolyte studies.	K^+ less than 3.5 mEq/L signals hypokalemia, and HCO_3^- less than 7.40 signals metabolic acidosis.
If the patient displays confused behavior or exhibits signs of motor dysfunction, keep the bed in the lowest position and raise the side rails. If seizures appear imminent, pad the side rails. Notify the health care provider of significant findings.	These are standard safety precautions for patients who have confusion or motor dysfunction.
Encourage oral intake as directed, and assess fluid balance.	Maintaining fluid balance will help ameliorate acid-base and electrolyte imbalances.
If the patient is hypokalemic and allowed to eat, encourage foods high in potassium.	Foods high in potassium, such as potatoes, prune juice, pumpkin, spinach, sweet potatoes, Swiss chard, tomatoes, and watermelon will help reverse hypokalemia. The health care provider may prescribe intravenous (IV) fluids with potassium supplements to prevent or treat hypokalemia.
Encourage the patient to ambulate by the second day after surgery.	Mobility will help prevent urinary stasis, which would increase risk of electrolyte problems.

Nursing Diagnosis:

Risk for Impaired Skin Integrity

related to the presence of urine on the skin or sensitivity to appliance materials

Desired Outcome: The patient's peristomal skin remains nonerythematous and intact.

ASSESSMENT/INTERVENTIONS	RATIONALE
For patients with significant allergy history, patch-test the skin for a 24-hr period, at least 24 hr before surgery. If erythema, swelling, bleb formation, itching, weeping, or other indicators of tape allergy occur, document the type of tape that caused the reaction and note on the chart cover, "Allergic to _____ tape." Place an allergy armband on the patient.	This assessment evaluates for and documents allergies to different tapes that might be used on the postoperative appliance.
Assess integrity of the peristomal skin with each wafer change. Question the patient about itching or burning under the wafer. Change the wafer routinely (per agency or surgeon preference) or immediately if leakage is suspected.	Itching or burning can signal leakage of the pouch under the wafer. If the seal between the adhesive backing of the wafer and skin becomes compromised, leaking onto the peristomal skin can occur. **Note:** All pouches must be attached to a wafer and pouches are never placed directly over a stoma. The wafer covers the skin surrounding the stoma (peristomal skin). Pouches may come already attached to a wafer (one-piece system) or come separately (two-piece system).
Teach the patient how often to change the wafer and/or pouch if a **one-piece system** is used.	Routine wafer/pouch change is every 4-7 days. This schedule provides the consistency that usually avoids surprise leakage problems.
Teach the patient to monitor the skin for leakage and odor.	Leakage and odor indicate that the wafer and/or pouch must be changed.
Teach the patient to report signs of a rash to the health care provider.	A rash can occur with a yeast infection and will require a topical medication for treatment.
Assess the stoma, pouch, and skin for crystalline deposits.	These deposits are signals of alkaline urine, which can compromise skin integrity if exposure occurs.

ASSESSMENT/INTERVENTIONS	RATIONALE
In the presence of alkaline urine, teach the following: drink fluids that leave acid ash in the urine, such as cranberry juice, or take ascorbic acid in a dose consistent with the patient's size.	These actions help decrease urine pH, which will improve the peristomal skin condition.
When changing the wafer, measure the stoma with a measuring guide, and ensure that the skin barrier opening is cut to the exact size of the stoma.	
For a patient using a **two-piece system or pouch with a wafer:** Size the wafer to fit snugly around the stoma. For pouch placement, size the pouch to clear the stoma by at least $\frac{1}{8}$ inch.	These measures protect the peristomal area from maceration caused by pooling of urine on the skin.
For a patient using a **one-piece "adhesive only" pouch:**	
If the pouch has an antireflux valve, size the pouch to clear the stoma and any peristomal creases.	This helps ensure that the pouch adheres to a flat, dry surface. An antireflux valve prevents pooling of urine on skin.
If the pouch does not have an antireflux valve, size the pouch so that it clears the stoma by $\frac{1}{8}$ inch.	This will help prevent stomal trauma while minimizing the amount of exposed skin.
Use a copolymer film sealant wipe on the peristomal skin before applying the wafer or "adhesive-only" pouch and wafer system.	This will provide a moisture barrier and reduce epidermal trauma when the wafer is removed.
Wash the peristomal skin with water or a special cleansing solution marketed by ostomy supply companies. Dry the skin thoroughly before applying the skin barrier, wafer, and pouch.	Other products can dry out the skin, which would increase risk of irritation and infection.
When changing the pouch or wafer, instruct the patient to hold a gauze pad or clean small towel on (but not in) the stoma.	This will absorb urine and keep the skin dry.
After applying the pouch, connect it to a bedside drainage system if the patient is on bedrest. When the patient is no longer on bedrest, empty the pouch when it is one-third to one-half full, opening the spigot on the bottom of the pouch and draining urine into the patient's measuring container.	These interventions facilitate drainage of urine.
Do not allow the pouch to become too full. Instruct the patient accordingly.	An overly full pouch could break the seal of the wafer with the patient's skin.
Teach the patient to treat peristomal irritation as follows after hospital discharge:	
- Dry the skin with a hair dryer set on a cool setting.	This eliminates the necessity of wiping the skin, which would increase the irritation.
- Dust the peristomal skin with karaya powder or spread Stomahesive paste.	These agents absorb moisture.
- If desired, blot the skin with water or a sealant wipe or copolymer protectant that seals in the powder.	These agents provide a moisture barrier.
- Use a porous tape if tape is required.	Porous tape prevents trapping of moisture.
Notify the health care provider or wound, ostomy, and continence (WOC)/enterostomal therapy (ET) nurse of any severe or nonresponsive skin problems.	These problems call for skilled interventions.

Nursing Diagnosis:

Impaired Tissue Integrity: Stomal (or risk for same)

related to altered stomal circulation occurring with the urinary diversion procedure or improper appliance fit

Desired Outcomes: The patient's stoma is pink or bright red and shiny. The stoma of a cutaneous urostomy is raised, moist, and red.

ASSESSMENT/INTERVENTIONS	RATIONALES
Assess the stoma at least q8h and as indicated. Report significant findings promptly.	The stoma of an ileal conduit will be edematous and should be pink or red with a shiny appearance. The stoma formed by a cutaneous urostomy is usually raised during the first few weeks after surgery, red, and moist. A stoma that is dusky or cyanotic is indicative of insufficient blood supply and impending necrosis and must be reported to the health care provider for immediate intervention.
Also assess the degree of swelling. For patients with an ileal conduit, evaluate stomal height and plan accordingly (see **Risk for Impaired Skin Integrity**, p. 234).	The stoma should shrink considerably over the first 6-8 wk and less significantly over the next year. The stoma formed by a cutaneous ureterostomy is usually raised during the first few weeks after surgery, red in color, and moist.

Nursing Diagnosis:

Deficient Knowledge

related to unfamiliarity with self-care regarding the urinary diversion

Desired Outcome: The patient or significant other demonstrates proper care of the stoma and urinary diversion before hospital discharge.

ASSESSMENT/INTERVENTIONS	RATIONALES
Assess the patient's health care literacy (language, reading, comprehension). Assess culture and culturally specific information needs.	This assessment helps ensure that information is selected and presented in a manner that is culturally and educationally appropriate.
Also assess the patient's or significant other's readiness to participate in care.	A well-thought-out teaching plan is useless if individuals are unable or unwilling to understand/learn it.
Involve ET or WOC nurse in patient teaching if available.	An ET or WOC nurse is specially trained and skilled in teaching urinary diversion care.
Assist the patient with organizing the equipment and materials that are needed to accomplish home care.	Usually patients are discharged with disposable pouching systems. Most of these patients continue using disposable systems for the long term. Those who will use reusable systems usually are not fitted until 6-8 wk after surgery.
Teach how to remove and reapply the pouch; how to empty it; and how to use a gravity drainage system at night, including procedures for rinsing and cleansing the drainage system.	These are the basic skills the patient will need in order to accomplish self-care after hospital discharge.
Teach signs and symptoms of UTI, peristomal skin breakdown, and appropriate therapeutic responses, including maintenance of an acidic urine (if not contraindicated), importance of adequate fluid intake, and techniques for checking urine pH (which should be assessed weekly). Explain that urine pH should remain at 6.0 or less.	Persons with urinary diversion have a higher incidence of UTI than the general public, so it is important to keep their urinary pH acidic. If it is greater than 6.0, advise the patient to increase fluid intake and, with health care provider approval, to increase vitamin C intake to 500-1000 mg/day, which will increase urine acidity.
Teach patients with a continent urinary diversion the technique for reservoir catheter irrigation.	In continent urinary diversions, a catheter is placed in the reservoir to prevent distention and promote healing of suture lines. This new reservoir (i.e., resected intestine) exudes large amounts of mucus, necessitating catheter irrigation with 30-50 mL of normal saline, which is instilled gently and allowed to empty via gravity.
Teach patients with a continent urinary diversion with urethral anastomosis signals of the urge to void.	Feelings of vague abdominal discomfort and abdominal pressure or cramping are sensations of the need to void.
Instruct patients with a continent urinary diversion with urethral anastomosis about the procedure to void.	Relaxing the perineal muscles and employing Valsalva's maneuver help empty the diversion.

ASSESSMENT/INTERVENTIONS	RATIONALES
Emphasize the importance of follow-up visits, particularly for patients with a continent urinary diversion.	Follow-up visits, particularly for patients with continent urinary diversions who will be taught how to catheterize the reservoir and use a small dressing over the stoma rather than an appliance, help ensure that the patient can manipulate the pouch. Follow-up visits also facilitate answers to questions that ensue after hospital discharge.
Provide a list of ostomy support groups and ET nurses in the area.	Referrals such as this will assist the patient after hospital discharge.
Provide the patient with enough equipment and materials for the first week after hospital discharge.	The first postoperative visit is usually 1 wk after hospital discharge.
Remind the patient of the importance of proper cleansing of ostomy appliances.	This knowledge will help reduce the risk of bacterial growth and UTI after hospital discharge.

ADDITIONAL NURSING DIAGNOSES/PROBLEMS:

 PATIENT-FAMILY TEACHING AND DISCHARGE PLANNING

When providing patient-family teaching, focus on sensory information, avoid giving excessive information, and initiate a visiting nurse referral for necessary follow-up teaching. Include verbal and written information about the following:

✓ Medications, including drug name, dosage, schedule, precautions, and potential side effects. Also discuss drug-drug, herb-drug, and food-drug interactions.

✓ Indicators that necessitate medical intervention: fever or chills; nausea or vomiting; abdominal pain, cramping, or distention; cloudy or malodorous urine; incisional drainage, edema, local warmth, pain, or redness; peristomal skin irritation; or abnormal changes in stoma shape or color from the normal bright and shiny red.

✓ Maintenance of fluid intake of at least 2-3 L/day to maintain adequate kidney function.

✓ Importance of keeping urinary pH acidic. Individuals with urinary diversions have a higher incidence of UTI than the general public; therefore, it is important to keep their urinary pH acidic. Because many fruits and vegetables tend to make urine alkaline, the patient should drink cranberry juice rather than orange juice or other citrus juices or take vitamin C daily. (Check with the health care provider first.)

✓ Care of the stoma and application of urostomy appliances. Patients should be proficient in the application technique before hospital discharge.

✓ Care of urostomy appliances. Remind patients that proper cleansing will reduce the risk of bacterial growth, which would contaminate urine and increase risk of UTI.

✓ Importance of follow-up care with the health care provider and WOC/ET nurse. Confirm date and time of the next appointment.

✓ Telephone numbers to call in case questions or concerns arise about therapy after discharge. In addition, many cities have local support groups. Information for these patients can be obtained by contacting the following:

• United Ostomy Association at *www.uoa.org*
• United Ostomy Association of Canada at *www.ostomycanada.ca*
• American Cancer Society at *www.cancer.org*
• National Cancer Institute's Cancer Information Service (CIS) at *www.cis.nci.nih.gov*

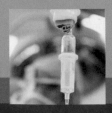

Urinary Tract Obstruction **33**

OVERVIEW/PATHOPHYSIOLOGY

Urinary tract obstruction usually is the result of blockage from pelvic tumors, calculi, and urethral strictures. Additional causes include neoplasms, benign prostatic hypertrophy, ureteral or urethral trauma, inflammation of the urinary tract, pregnancy, and pelvic or colonic surgery in which ureteral damage has occurred. Obstructions can occur suddenly or slowly, over weeks to months. They can occur anywhere along the urinary tract, but the most common sites are the ureteropelvic and ureterovesical junctions, bladder neck, and urethral meatus. The obstruction acts like a dam, blocking passage of urine. Muscles in the area contract to push urine around the obstruction, and structures behind the obstruction begin to dilate. The smaller the site of obstruction, the greater the damage. Obstructions in the lower urinary structures, such as the bladder neck or urethra, can lead to urinary retention and urinary tract infection (UTI). Obstructions in the upper urinary tract can lead to bilateral involvement of the ureters and kidneys, leading to hydronephrosis, renal insufficiency, and kidney destruction. Hydrostatic pressure increases, and filtration and concentration processes in the tubules and glomerulus are compromised.

HEALTH CARE SETTING

Primary care and acute care

ASSESSMENT

Signs and symptoms: Anuria, nausea, vomiting, local abdominal tenderness, hesitancy, straining to start a stream, dribbling, decreased caliber and force of urinary stream, hematuria, oliguria, and uremia. Pain may be sharp and intense or dull and aching; localized or referred (e.g., flank, low back, buttock, scrotal, labial pain).

Physical assessment: Bladder distention and "kettle drum" sound over the bladder with percussion (absent if obstruction is above the bladder) and mass in the flank area, abdomen, pelvis, or rectum.

History of: Recent fever (possibly caused by the obstruction), hypertensive episodes (caused by increased renin production from the body's attempt to increase renal blood flow).

DIAGNOSTIC TESTS

Serum K⁺ and Na⁺ levels: To determine renal function. Normal range for K^+ is 3.5-5.0 mEq/L; normal range for Na^+ is 137-147 mEq/L.

Blood urea nitrogen (BUN) and creatinine: To evaluate renal-urinary status. Normally, their values are elevated with decreased renal-urinary function. **Note:** These values must be considered based on the patient's age and hydration status. For the older adult, serum creatinine level may not be a reliable indicator because of decreased muscle mass and a decreased glomerular filtration rate. Hydration status can affect BUN: fluid volume excess can result in reduced values, whereas volume deficit can cause higher values.

Urinalysis: To provide baseline data on functioning of the urinary system, detect metabolic disease, and assess for the presence of UTI. A cloudy, hazy appearance; foul odor; pH greater than 8.0; and presence of red blood cells, leukocyte esterase, white blood cells (WBCs), and WBC casts are signals of UTI.

Urine culture: To determine the type of bacteria present in the genitourinary tract. To minimize contamination, a sample should be obtained from a midstream collection.

Hemoglobin (Hgb) and hematocrit (Hct): To assess for anemia, which may be related to decreased renal secretion of erythropoietin.

Kidneys, Ureters, and Bladder (KUB) radiography: To identify size, shape, and position of the KUB and abnormalities such as tumors, calculi, or malformations. This can be done in combination with ultrasonography.

Imaging studies: A variety of imaging studies may be used to identify the area and cause of obstructions:
- Ultrasonography: This is sensitive in revealing parenchymal masses, hydronephrosis, a distended bladder, and renal calculi.
- Computed tomography (CT) scans: To identify the degree and location of the obstruction, as well as cause in many situations.
- Excretory urography/intravenous pyelography: To evaluate the cause of urinary dysfunction by visualizing the kidneys, renal pelvis, ureters, and bladder.

- Antegrade urography: Involves placement of a percutaneous needle or nephrostomy tube through which radiopaque contrast is injected. Antegrade urography is indicated when the kidney does not concentrate or excrete intravenous (IV) dye.
- Retrograde urography: Radiopaque dye is injected through ureteral catheters placed during cystoscopy.
- Cystogram: Radiopaque dye is instilled via cystoscope or catheter. This enables visualization of the bladder and evaluation of the vesicoureteral reflex.

Bladder Scanner: Bladder scanners are designed to create a three dimensional image of the bladder and calculate the volume based on the image. The scan is frequently used to measure post-void residual (PVR) to evaluate the need for catheterization.

Maximal urinary flow rate: Less than 15 mL/sec indicates significant obstruction to flow.

Postvoid residual volume: Normal is less than 12 mL. Higher volume signals obstructive process.

Cystoscopy: To determine the degree of bladder outlet obstruction and facilitate visualization of any tumors or masses.

Nursing Diagnoses:

Risk for Deficient Fluid Volume
Risk for Shock
Risk for Electrolyte Imbalance

related to postobstructive diuresis

Desired Outcomes: The patient is normovolemic and free of signs of shock and electrolyte imbalance as evidenced by heart rate (HR) 100 bpm or less (or within the patient's normal range); blood pressure (BP) 90/60 mm Hg or greater (or within the patient's normal range); respiratory rate (RR) 20 breaths/min or less; no significant changes in mental status; and orientation to person, place, and time (within the patient's normal range). Within 2 days after bladder decompression, output approximates input, urinary output is normal for the patient (or 30-60 mL/hr or greater), and weight becomes stable.

ASSESSMENT/INTERVENTIONS	RATIONALES
Using sterile technique, insert a urinary catheter.	Catheterization will drain the bladder of the urine whose passage has been obstructed.
Assess the patient carefully during catheterization; clamp the catheter if the patient complains of abdominal pain or has a symptomatic drop in systolic blood pressure of 20 mm Hg or greater.	Although research has demonstrated that rapid bladder decompression of greater than 750-1000 mL does not result in shock syndrome as previously believed, this assessment/action could determine the presence of an electrolyte imbalance as a result of postobsructive diuresis.
Assess intake and output hourly for 4 hr and then q2h for 4 hr after bladder decompression.	This assessment monitors for postobstructive diuresis.
[!] Notify the health care provider if output exceeds 200 mL/hr or 2 L over an 8-hr period.	This can signal postobstructive diuresis, which can lead to major electrolyte imbalance. If this occurs, anticipate initiation of IV infusion.
[!] Assess vital signs for decreasing BP, changes in level of consciousness or mentation, tachycardia, tachypnea, and thready pulse.	These are signs of shock.
Anticipate need for urine specimens for analysis of electrolytes and osmolality and blood specimens for analysis of electrolytes.	Postobstructive diuresis can lead to major electrolyte imbalance.
Monitor for and report the following:	
- Abdominal cramps, lethargy, dysrhythmias.	These are signs of hypokalemia.
- Diarrhea, colic, irritability, nausea, muscle cramps, weakness, irregular apical or radial pulses.	These are signs of hyperkalemia.

continued

ASSESSMENT/INTERVENTIONS | RATIONALES

ASSESSMENT/INTERVENTIONS	RATIONALES
- Muscle weakness and cramps, complaints of tingling in fingers, positive Trousseau's and Chvostek's signs.	These are signs of hypocalcemia.
- Excessive itching.	This is a sign of hyperphosphatemia.
Monitor mentation, noting signs of disorientation.	Disorientation can occur with electrolyte disturbance.
Weigh the patient daily using the same scale and at the same time of day (e.g., before breakfast).	Weight fluctuations of 2-4 lb (0.9-1.8 kg) normally occur in a patient who is undergoing diuresis. Losses greater than this can result in dehydration and electrolyte imbalances. Weighing the patient in a consistent manner and under the same conditions helps ensure more precise measurements and comparisons.

Nursing Diagnosis:

Acute Pain

related to bladder spasms

Desired Outcomes: Within 1 hr of intervention, the patient's subjective perception of discomfort decreases, as documented by a pain scale. Objective indicators, such as grimacing, are absent or diminished.

ASSESSMENT/INTERVENTIONS	RATIONALES
Assess for and document complaints of pain in the suprapubic or urethral area. Devise a pain scale with the patient, rating pain from 0 (no pain) to 10 (worst pain).	This assessment establishes a baseline for subsequent assessment and evaluates degree of pain relief obtained. Spasms occur frequently with obstruction.
Medicate with antispasmodics or analgesics such as oxybutynin and flavoxate as prescribed. Document pain relief obtained, using the pain scale.	These medications relieve spasms and pain.
If the patient is losing urine around the catheter and has a distended bladder (with or without bladder spasms), check the catheter and drainage tubing for evidence of obstruction. Inspect for kinks and obstructions in the drainage tubing, compress and roll the catheter gently between your fingers to assess for gritty matter within the catheter, milk the drainage tubing to release obstructions, or instruct the patient to turn from side to side. Obtain a prescription for catheter irrigation if these measures fail to relieve the obstruction.	These assessments detect and manage obstructions in the catheter and tubing that may be contributing to spasms.
In nonrestricted patients, encourage intake of fluids to at least 2-3 L/day to help reduce frequency of spasms.	Increased hydration reduces the frequency of spasms. IV fluid therapy may be indicated for acutely ill, dehydrated patients, or to increase fluids in patients with calculi.
Teach nonpharmacologic methods of pain relief, such as guided imagery, relaxation techniques, and distraction.	These pain relief techniques augment pharmacologic interventions.

ADDITIONAL NURSING DIAGNOSES/PROBLEMS:

"Perioperative Care"   p. 45

"Ureteral Calculi" for **Risk for Impaired Skin Integrity**   p. 227
related to wound drainage

✓ PATIENT-FAMILY TEACHING AND DISCHARGE PLANNING

When providing patient-family teaching, focus on sensory information, avoid giving excessive information, and initiate a visiting nurse referral for necessary follow-up teaching. Include verbal and written information about the following:
✓ Medications, including drug name, dosage, purpose, schedule, precautions, and potential side effects. Also discuss drug-drug, herb-drug, and food-drug interactions.

✓ Indicators that signal recurrent obstruction and require prompt medical attention: pain, fever, decreased urinary output.

✓ Activity restrictions as directed for the patient who has had surgery: avoid lifting heavy objects (more than 10 lb) for first 6 wk, be alert to fatigue, get maximum rest, increase activities gradually to tolerance.

✓ Care of drains or catheters if the patient is discharged with them; care of the surgical incision if present.

✓ Indicators of wound infection: persistent redness, local warmth, tenderness, drainage, swelling, and fever.

✓ Indicators of UTI that necessitate medical attention: chills; fever; hematuria; flank, costovertebral angle, suprapubic, low back, buttock, scrotal, or labial pain; cloudy and foul-smelling urine; increased frequency, urgency; dysuria; and increasing or recurring incontinence. In older adults, confusion may be the first sign of a UTI.

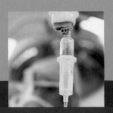

General Care of Patients with Neurologic Disorders 34

CARE OF PATIENTS WITH ACUTE NEUROLOGIC ISSUES

Nursing Diagnosis:

Decreased Intracranial Adaptive Capacity

related to increased intracranial pressure (IICP) and herniation occurring with positional factors or increased intrathoracic or intraabdominal pressure, fluid volume excess, hyperthermia, or discomfort occurring with brain injury

Desired Outcome: The patient becomes free of symptoms of IICP and herniation as evidenced by stable or improving Glasgow Coma Scale score; stable or improving sensorimotor functioning; blood pressure (BP) within the patient's normal range; heart rate (HR) 60-100 bpm; pulse pressure 30-40 mm Hg (difference between systolic blood pressure [SBP] and diastolic blood pressure [DBP]); orientation to person, place, and time; normal vision; bilaterally equal and normoreactive pupils; respiratory rate (RR) 12-20 breaths/min with normal depth and pattern (eupnea); normal gag, corneal, and swallowing reflexes; and absence of headache, nausea, nuchal rigidity, posturing, and seizure activity.

ASSESSMENT/INTERVENTIONS	RATIONALES
⚠ Assess for and report any of the following indicators of IICP or impending/occurring herniation:	Intracranial pressure (ICP) is the pressure exerted by brain tissue, cerebrospinal fluid (CSF), and cerebral blood volume within the rigid, unyielding skull. An increase in any one of these components without a corresponding decrease in another will increase ICP. Normal ICP is 0-10 mm Hg; IICP is greater than 15 mm Hg. Cerebral perfusion pressure (CPP) is the difference between mean arterial pressure and ICP. As ICP rises, CPP may decrease. Normal CPP is 70-100 mm Hg. If CPP falls below 40-60 mm Hg, ischemia occurs. When CPP falls to 0, cerebral blood flow ceases. Cerebral edema and IICP usually peak 2-3 days after injury and then decrease over 1-2 wk.
Early indicators of IICP: Declining Glasgow Coma Scale score; alterations in level of consciousness (LOC) ranging from irritability, restlessness, and confusion to lethargy; possible onset of or worsening of headache; beginning pupillary dysfunction, such as sluggishness; visual disturbances, such as diplopia or blurred vision; onset of or increase in sensorimotor changes or deficits, such as weakness; onset of or worsening of nausea.	The single most important assessment indicator of early IICP is a change in LOC.

ASSESSMENT/INTERVENTIONS	RATIONALES
Late indicators of IICP: Continuing decline in Glasgow Coma Scale score; continued deterioration in LOC leading to stupor and coma; projectile vomiting; hemiplegia; posturing; widening pulse pressure, decreased HR, and increased SBP; Cheyne-Stokes breathing or other respiratory irregularity; pupillary changes, such as oval-shaped, inequality, dilation, and nonreactivity to light; papilledema; and impaired brain stem reflexes (corneal, gag, swallowing).	Late assessment indicators of IICP signal impending or actual herniation and are generally related to brain stem compression and disruption of cranial nerves and vital centers.
Brain herniation: Deep coma, fixed and dilated pupils (first unilateral and then bilateral), posturing progressing to bilateral flaccidity, lost brain stem reflexes, and continuing deterioration in vital signs (VS) and respirations.	Brain herniation occurs when IICP causes displacement of brain tissue from one cranial compartment to another.
If changes occur, prepare for possible transfer of the patient to the intensive care unit (ICU).	Insertion of ICP sensors for continuous ICP monitoring, continuous bedside cerebral blood flow (CBF) monitoring (e.g., continuous transcranial Doppler), CSF ventricular drainage, vasopressor usage (e.g., dopamine), intubation, mechanical ventilation, propofol sedation, neuromuscular blocking, or barbiturate coma therapy may be necessary. Continuous cardiac monitoring for dysrhythmias also will be done. Intensive insulin therapy may be needed to maintain optimal serum glucose values. Testing (e.g., computed tomography [CT]) may be done, but lumbar puncture (LP) is contraindicated or used with caution in the presence of IICP.
⚠ Institute preventive measures for patients at risk for IICP. These include ensuring a patent airway, delivering O_2 as prescribed, and may include intubation and mechanical ventilation as necessary. Assess arterial blood gas (ABG) or pulse oximetry values.	Preventing hypoxia necessitates maintaining oxygen saturation at greater than 90% or PaO_2 at greater than 60 mm Hg. Therefore, it is important to preoxygenate before suctioning and limit suctioning to 10 sec. Prevention of CO_2 retention (and the resulting respiratory acidosis) is essential for preventing vasodilation of cerebral arteries, which can lead to cerebral edema.
Be aware that CBF measurements, continuous jugular venous oxygen saturation (SjO_2), and brain tissue oxygenation ($PbtO_2$) should be considered to assess for effectiveness (i.e., decreased IICP without decreased cerebral oxygen delivery) if hyperventilation is used as a treatment.	Mechanical hyperventilation, by lowering cerebral $PaCO_2$, results in an alkalosis, which causes cerebral vasoconstriction resulting in decreased CBF and ICP. The vasoconstriction also may cause decreased cerebral oxygen delivery, which could increase injury by increasing cerebral ischemia. Hyperventilation (e.g., with Ambu bag or if ventilated to keep $PaCO_2$ to 30-35 mm Hg) is now generally used only in cases of acute deterioration as a "quick fix" until other interventions can be instituted (e.g., mannitol) or in cases in which IICP is refractory and responds to nothing else.
⚠ Maintain head and neck alignment to avoid hyperextension, flexion, or rotation, ensuring that tracheostomy, endotracheal tube ties, or O_2 tubing does not compress the jugular vein, and avoiding Trendelenburg position for any reason.	These measures promote venous blood return to the heart to reduce cerebral congestion.
Ensure that pillows under the patient's head are flat.	This measure maintains head in a neutral rather than flexed position, thereby preventing backup of jugular venous outflow.
Keep head of bed (HOB) at whatever level optimizes CPP.	CPP needs to be at least 70 mm Hg or as prescribed to prevent ischemia. Without monitoring equipment, having the HOB at 30 degrees is considered safe and effective in promoting venous drainage and lowering ICP as long as patient is not hypovolemic, which could threaten CPP.
⚠ Take precautions against increased intraabdominal and intrathoracic pressures in the following ways:	Elevated intraabdominal and intrathoracic pressures interfere with cerebral venous drainage thus adding to IICP.
- Teach the patient to exhale when turning or during activity.	This action reduces intrathoracic pressure.
- Provide passive range-of-motion (ROM) exercises rather than allow active or assistive exercises.	This prevents increases in intraabdominal and intrathoracic pressures that could raise ICP.

continued

PART I: Medical-Surgical Nursing

ASSESSMENT/INTERVENTIONS	RATIONALES
- Administer prescribed stool softeners or laxatives; avoid enemas and suppositories.	These measures prevent straining at stool, which would increase intraabdominal and intracranial pressures.
- Instruct the patient not to move self in bed; to allow only passive turning; and use a pull sheet and avoid pushing against foot of bed or pulling against side rails. Avoid footboards; use high-top tennis shoes with toes removed to level of the metatarsal heads instead.	Movements involving pushing would increase intraabdominal and intrathoracic pressures.
- Assist the patient with sitting up and turning.	This action prevents increases in intraabdominal and intrathoracic pressures.
- Instruct the patient to avoid coughing and sneezing or, if unavoidable, to do so with an open mouth; provide antitussive for cough as prescribed and antiemetic for vomiting.	As above.
- Instruct the patient to avoid hip flexion. Do not place the patient in a prone position.	These positions increase intraabdominal pressure.
- Avoid using restraints.	Straining against restraints increases ICP.
- Rather than have the patient perform Valsalva's maneuver to prevent an air embolism during insertion of a central venous catheter, the health care provider should use a syringe to aspirate air from the catheter lumen.	Valsalva's maneuver increases intraabdominal and intrathoracic pressures.
Administer intravenous (IV) fluids with an infusion control device to prevent fluid overload. Keep accurate intake and output (I&O) records. (The patient usually has an indwelling urinary catheter.)	Isotonic or hypertonic IV fluids are given to maintain normovolemia and balanced electrolyte status. Fluid restrictions are avoided because resulting increased blood viscosity and decreased volume may lead to hypotension, thereby decreasing CPP.
When administering additional IV fluids (e.g., IV drugs) avoid using D_5W.	D_5W's hypotonicity can increase cerebral edema and hyperglycemia, which have been associated with inferior neurologic outcomes.
Help maintain the patient's body temperature within normal limits by giving prescribed antipyretics, regulating temperature of the environment, using a fan, limiting use of blankets, keeping the patient's trunk warm to prevent shivering, and administering tepid sponge baths or using a warming/cooling blanket or convection cooling units to reduce fever.	Hypothalamic dysfunction from swelling or injury may cause hyperthermia. In turn, fever increases the metabolic rate (5%-7% for each 1° C) and exacerbates IICP.
When using a hypothermia blanket, wrap the patient's extremities in blankets or towels, and if prescribed, administer chlorpromazine.	Both measures prevent shivering, which would increase ICP. Mild (e.g., 35° C) hypothermia treatment also may be attempted to minimize metabolic needs of the brain if ICP is increased.
Administer prescribed osmotic (e.g., mannitol) and loop diuretics (e.g., furosemide).	These agents reduce cerebral edema and blood volume, thereby lowering ICP.
Administer BP medications as prescribed.	These medications keep BP within prescribed limits that will promote optimal CBF without increasing cerebral edema. Hypotension is particularly detrimental inasmuch as it directly affects CBF. Hypertension may be allowed or treated first with drugs such as labetalol. Vasoactive drugs such as nitroprusside may worsen cerebral edema via vasodilation.
Administer prescribed analgesics promptly and as necessary.	Pain can increase ICP. Barbiturates and opioids usually are contraindicated because of the potential for masking the signs of IICP and causing respiratory depression. However, intubated, restless patients are usually sedated. A continuous propofol or midazolam drip has been demonstrated to decrease IICP. Lidocaine is sometimes used to block coughing before suctioning an endotracheal tube.
Administer antiepilepsy drugs (AEDs) as prescribed.	AEDs prevent or control seizures, which would increase cerebral metabolism, hypoxia, and CO_2 retention, which in turn would increase cerebral edema and ICP.
Monitor bladder drainage tubes for obstruction or kinks. Flush if an obstruction is suspected.	A distended bladder can increase ICP.

ASSESSMENT/INTERVENTIONS	RATIONALES
Provide a quiet and soothing environment. Control noise and other environmental stimuli. Use a gentle touch, and avoid jarring the bed. Try to limit painful procedures; avoid tension on tubes (e.g., urinary catheter); and consider limiting pain-stimulation testing. Avoid unnecessary touch (e.g., leave BP cuff in place for frequent VS; use automatic recycling BP monitoring devices); and talk softly, explaining procedures before touching to avoid startling the patient. Try to avoid situations in which the patient may become emotionally upset. Do not say anything in the presence of the patient that you would not say if he or she were awake. Limit visitors as necessary.	A quiet and soothing environment optimally will help keep BP and other pressures within therapeutic limits. Family discussions should take place outside the room.
Encourage significant others to speak quietly to the patient. If possible, arrange for the patient to listen to soft favorite music with earphones.	Hearing a familiar voice or listening to soft music may promote relaxation and decrease ICP.
Individualize care to ensure rest periods and optimal spacing of activities; avoid turning, suctioning, and taking VS all at one time. Plan activities and treatments accordingly so that the patient can sleep undisturbed as often as possible.	Multiple procedures and nursing care activities can increase ICP. For example, rousing patients from sleep has been shown to increase ICP.
Administer mild sedatives (e.g., diphenhydramine) or antianxiety agents (haloperidol, lorazepam, midazolam) as prescribed to a restless/agitated patient. Attempt to identify and relieve the cause (e.g., overstimulation, pain) before medicating.	These measures decrease restlessness or decrease/control agitation that may increase ICP.
Administer sedation and skeletal muscle relaxants (e.g., propofol, atracurium, pancuronium) as prescribed. (This therapy requires intubation and ventilation.)	These agents decrease the skeletal muscle tension that is seen with abnormal flexion and extension posturing, which can increase ICP. Bispectral index technology (BIS) may be used to guide administration of these drugs for sedation and neuromuscular blockade. BIS translates information from the electroencephalogram (EEG) into a single number that represents each patient's LOC. This number ranges from 100 (indicating an awake patient) to zero (indicating the absence of brain activity).

Nursing Diagnosis:

Risk for Aspiration

related to facial and throat muscle weakness, depressed gag or cough reflex, impaired swallowing, or decreased LOC

Desired Outcomes: The patient is free of the signs of aspiration as evidenced by RR 12-20 breaths/min with normal depth and pattern (eupnea), O_2 saturation greater than 92%, normal color, normal breath sounds, normothermia, and absence of adventitious breath sounds. Following instruction and on an ongoing basis, the patient or significant other relates measures that prevent aspiration.

ASSESSMENT/INTERVENTIONS	RATIONALES
For patients with new or increasing neurologic deficit, perform a dysphagia screening to assess for impaired swallowing. For more details, see the nursing diagnosis on p. 249.	Dysphagia screening will identify patients at risk for aspiration. These patients should be kept nothing by mouth (NPO) until a swallowing evaluation can be performed.
Assess lung sounds before and after the patient eats, effectiveness of the patient's cough, and quality, amount, and color of sputum.	New onset of crackles or wheezing can signal aspiration. Patients with a weak cough are at risk for aspiration. An increase in quantity or color change of sputum may indicate an infection from aspiration.

continued

ASSESSMENT/INTERVENTIONS	RATIONALES
Keep HOB elevated after meals or assist the patient into a right side-lying position.	This position facilitates flow of ingested food and fluids by gravity from the greater stomach curve to the pylorus, thereby minimizing the potential for regurgitation and aspiration.
If indicated, consult the health care provider about use of an upper gastrointestinal (GI) stimulant.	Stimulating upper GI tract motility and gastric emptying help to decrease the potential for regurgitation.
Provide oral hygiene after meals.	Oral hygiene removes food particles that could be aspirated.
Assess the mouth frequently, and suction prn.	These actions assess for particles or secretions that could be aspirated and removes them.
If the patient has nausea or vomiting or has secretions, turn on one side.	This position facilitates drainage and prevents their aspiration.
Anticipate need for an artificial airway if secretions cannot be cleared.	These measures help ensure a patent airway.
For general interventions, see this nursing diagnosis in "Older Adult Care," p. 93, and with **Impaired Swallowing**, later.	

Nursing Diagnosis (for patients who are ventilated):

Risk for Infection

related to inadequate primary defenses occurring with ventilator intubation in patients with neurologic disorders such as Guillain-Barré, bacterial meningitis, SCI, traumatic brain injury, and stroke

Desired Outcome: The patient exhibits reduced incidence/absence of ventilator-associated pneumonia as evidenced by normothermia, white blood cell count 11,000/mm^3 or less, sputum clear to whitish in color, lungs clear to auscultation, RR 14-20 breaths/min, and oxygen saturation greater than 92%.

ASSESSMENT/INTERVENTIONS	RATIONALES
Ensure the ventilator bundle discussed in the following interventions has been implemented on any patient who is mechanically ventilated.	This bundle is a series of interventions that, when implemented together (rather than individually), is associated with decreased incidence of ventilator-associated pneumonia (VAP). VAP is a leading cause of prolonged hospital stay and death.
Perform good hand hygiene before and after contact with the patient (even though gloves are worn).	Hand hygiene helps prevent spread of infection by removing pathogens from hands. Hand hygiene involves using alcohol-based waterless antiseptic agent (if hands are not visibly soiled) or soap and water.
Assess lung sounds, sputum characteristics, RR, HR, temperature, oximetry, ABG values, chest x-ray, and complete blood count (CBC). Report abnormal changes to the health care provider.	Assessing for and reporting early indicators of infection will enable prompt intervention and treatment.
Elevate HOB, preferably to 30 degrees if it is not contraindicated.	This elevated HOB position reduces risk of aspirating gastric contents by moving them away from the diaphragm, making ventilation easier. This position may be contraindicated in some patients.
Ensure frequent position changes.	Frequent turning facilitates drainage of secretions.
On a daily basis, attempt a spontaneous awakening trial ("sedation vacations") per facility protocol or as prescribed, and assess and document neurologic status and readiness to extubate. For example, "Patient awake, breathing at a sufficient rate and depth of breaths to maintain oxygenation, is able to cough and protect airway, and has adequate ABG values." Note prior documentation as a basis of comparison (e.g., improvement or deterioration) and notify the care provider as appropriate (e.g., if patient does not wake or respond despite sedation being turned off).	These measures promote early extubation and minimize sedation. A spontaneous awakening trial involves reducing sedation until the patient is awake and can follow simple commands or becomes agitated. During this "awake" time, a weaning trial may be done to test the patient's ability to breathe spontaneously. The patient's unsedated neurologic status also can be tested. If sedation is reinstated, it can be titrated to the minimal amount needed to achieve a calm, relaxed state. Decreasing sedation reduces the amount of time spent on mechanical ventilation and therefore the risk of VAP.

ASSESSMENT/INTERVENTIONS	RATIONALES
Ensure a closed endotracheal suction system, ideally one that allows for continuous subglottic secretion drainage.	A closed system reduces risk of contamination. A system that also allows for continuous subglottic secretion drainage will further reduce contamination of the lower airway by removing stagnant oropharyngeal secretions above the cuff that might otherwise be aspirated.
When possible, use oral tubes rather than nasal tubes.	Oral tubes reduce risk of sinusitis and aspiration of infected secretions.
Provide oral hygiene q2h or as recommended by facility protocol, possibly including use of a dental oral antibiotic rinse (e.g., chlorhexidine gluconate washes).	Oral hygiene reduces oral bacterial flora, which could be aspirated. Swabs and toothbrushes with built-in suction catheter capability may facilitate oral care.
As prescribed, implement other components that may be included in the bundle.	Many agencies also include peptic ulcer disease prophylaxis (to reduce mini-aspiration of acid secretions) and deep vein thrombosis prophylaxis.

Nursing Diagnosis:

Impaired Tissue Integrity: Corneal

related to irritation occurring with diminished blink reflex or inability to close the eyes

Desired Outcome: The patient's corneas become/remain clear and intact.

ASSESSMENT/INTERVENTIONS	RATIONALES
If the patient has a diminished blink reflex or is stuporous or comatose, assess eyes for irritation or presence of foreign objects.	Indicators of corneal irritation include red, itchy, scratchy, or painful eye; sensation of foreign object in eye; scleral edema; blurred vision; or mucous discharge.
Instill prescribed eye drops or ointment. Instruct coherent patients to make a conscious effort to blink eyes several times each minute. Apply eye patches or warm, sterile compresses over closed eyes.	These actions provide corneal lubrication and prevent corneal irritation. Normally, blinking occurs every 5-6 sec.
If the eyes cannot be completely closed, use caution in applying an eye shield or taping eyes shut. Consider use of moisture chambers (plastic eye bubbles), protective glasses, soft contacts, or humidifiers.	Semiconscious patients may open their eyes underneath the shield or tape and injure their corneas.
For chronic eye closure problems, consider use of special springs or weights on the upper lids. Surgical closure (tarsorrhaphy) also may be necessary.	These measures help ensure closure of the eyelid.
Teach the patient to avoid exposing eyes to talc or baby powder, wind, cold air, smoke, dust, sand, or bright sunlight. Instruct the patient not to rub the eyes. Advise wearing glasses to protect against wind and dust and to wear tight-fitting goggles when swimming.	These are irritants that could harm the corneas.

Nursing Diagnosis:

Risk for Deficient Fluid Volume

related to facial and throat muscle weakness, depressed gag or cough reflex, impaired swallowing, or decreased LOC affecting access to and intake of fluids

Desired Outcome: The patient is normovolemic as evidenced by balanced I&O, stable weight, good skin turgor, moist mucous membranes, BP within the patient's normal range, HR 100 bpm or less, normothermia, and urinary output at least 30 mL/hr with a specific gravity 1.030 or less.

ASSESSMENT/INTERVENTIONS	RATIONALES
Assess gag reflex, alertness, and ability to cough and swallow before offering fluids.	These assessments demonstrate if the patient has intact swallowing and gag reflexes, can cough, and is alert and therefore can safely ingest fluids.
Keep suction equipment at the bedside if indicated.	This enables immediate intervention in the event of aspiration.
Assess I&O. Involve the patient or significant others with keeping fluid intake records. Perform daily weight measurements if the patient is at risk for sudden fluid shifts or imbalances.	Patients with neurologic deficits may have difficulty attaining adequate fluid intake. Involving patients and significant others in record keeping optimally will keep them aware of the need for increased oral intake and influence their participation in fluid intake accordingly.
Alert the health care provider to a significant I&O imbalance.	This imbalance may signal the need for enteral or IV therapy to prevent dehydration.
Assess for and teach the patient and significant others such indicators as thirst, poor skin turgor, decreased BP, increased pulse rate, dry skin and mucous membranes, increased body temperature, concentrated urine (specific gravity more than 1.030), and decreased urinary output.	These are indicators of dehydration. Conditions such as fever and diarrhea increase fluid loss and risk of dehydration. A knowledgeable person is more likely to report these indicators promptly for timely intervention and will understand the need to increase fluid intake during conditions that promote dehydration.
Evaluate fluid preferences (type and temperature). Offer fluids q1-2h. Establish a fluid goal. For nonrestricted patients, encourage a fluid intake of at least 2-3 L/day.	Patients, especially if fatigued, will be more prone to consume preferred fluids in small volumes at frequent intervals. A fluid intake of 2-3 L/day will keep patients well hydrated. Renal and cardiac patients may have fluid restrictions.
Feed or assist very weak or paralyzed patients.	Such measures help ensure that fluid goals are met.
Instruct the patient to flex head slightly forward.	Flexing the head forward closes the airway and helps prevent aspiration.
Begin with small amounts of liquid. Instruct the patient to sip rather than gulp fluids. Do not hurry the patient.	Sipping small amounts tests and promotes a patient's ability to swallow the fluid without choking.
For patients at risk for aspiration, use thickened fluids. Maintain an appropriate upright position while the patient is eating/drinking and for at least 1½ hr after the meal.	Thickened liquids form a cohesive bolus that can be swallowed more readily. Gravity aids swallowing, and staying upright decreases risk of aspiration.
Provide periods of rest.	Rest prevents fatigue, which can contribute to decreased oral intake.
Provide oral care as needed.	Oral care promotes taste perception and prevents stomatitis, which otherwise may decrease oral intake.
If appropriate, provide assistive devices (e.g., plastic, unbreakable, special-handled, spill-proof cups or straws).	These devices promote independence, which is likely to increase fluid consumption. The individual who is paralyzed (e.g., with spinal cord injury [SCI]) may be able to drink independently via extra-long tubing or a straw connected to a water pitcher.
Teach patients with hemiparalysis or hemiparesis to tilt head toward the unaffected side.	Fluids will drain by gravity to the side of the face and throat over which the patient has control.
For patients with chewing or swallowing difficulties, see interventions under **Impaired Swallowing** p. 249, and **Risk for Aspiration**, p. 245.	

Nursing Diagnosis:

Risk for Imbalanced Body Temperature

related to illness or trauma affecting temperature regulation

Desired Outcome: Following intervention(s), the patient becomes/remains normothermic with core temperatures between 36.5° and 37.7°C (97.8° and 100°F).

ASSESSMENT/INTERVENTIONS	RATIONALES
Assess rectal, tympanic, or bladder core temperature q4h or, if the patient is in spinal shock, q2h.	Infection and hypothalamic dysfunction as a result of cerebral insult (trauma, edema) are two common causes of hyperthermia. Rapid development of spinal lesions (e.g., in SCI) breaks the connection between the hypothalamus and sympathetic nervous system (SNS), causing an inability to adapt to environmental temperature. In spinal cord shock, temperatures tend to lower toward the ambient temperature. Inability to vasoconstrict and shiver makes heat conservation difficult; inability to perspire prevents normal cooling. **Caution:** Steroids may mask fever or infection.
Assess for impaired ability to think, disorientation, confusion, drowsiness, apathy, and reduced HR and RR. Assess for complaints of being too cold, goose bumps (piloerection), and cool skin (in SCI patients, above the level of injury).	These are signs of hypothermia.
Assess for flushed face, malaise, rash, respiratory distress, tachycardia, weakness, headache, and irritability. Monitor for complaints of being too warm, sweating, or hot and dry skin (in SCI patients, above level of injury).	These are signs of hyperthermia.
Be alert to parched mouth, furrowed tongue, dry lips, poor skin turgor, decreased urine output, increased concentration of urine (specific gravity greater than 1.030), and weak, fast pulse.	These are signs of dehydration that can occur as a result of hyperthermia.
For hyperthermia: Maintain a cool room temperature (20° C [68° F]). Provide a fan or air conditioning. Remove excess bedding and cover the patient with a thin sheet. Give tepid sponge baths. Place cool, wet cloths at the patient's head, neck, axilla, and groin. Administer antipyretic agent as prescribed. Use a padded hypothermia blanket (wrap hands and feet in towels or blankets to prevent shivering) or convection cooling device if prescribed. Provide cool drinks. Evaluate for potential infectious cause.	These are measures that help prevent overheating.
For hypothermia: Increase environmental temperature. Protect the patient from drafts. Provide warm drinks. Provide extra blankets. Provide warming (hyperthermia) blanket or convection warming device.	These are measures that help increase body temperature.
Keep feverish patient dry. Change bed linens after diaphoresis. Provide careful skin care when the patient is on a hypothermia or hyperthermia blanket.	These actions prevent skin irritation and potential loss of skin integrity that could result from hyperthermia and diaphoresis.
Monitor I&O and maintain adequate hydration. Unless contraindicated, encourage increased fluid intake in febrile patients (e.g., more than 3000 mL/day).	Insensible water loss from fever should be a consideration when monitoring I&O because it may affect total hydration.
Increase caloric intake.	Patients with fever have increased metabolic needs.

CARE OF PATIENTS WITH SUB-ACUTE TO CHRONIC NEUROLOGIC ISSUES

Nursing Diagnosis:

Impaired Swallowing

related to decreased or absent gag reflex, decreased strength or excursion of muscles involved in mastication, perceptual impairment, or facial paralysis

Desired Outcome: Before oral foods and fluids are reintroduced, the patient exhibits ability to swallow safely without aspirating.

ASSESSMENT/INTERVENTIONS	RATIONALES
Assess for factors that affect the ability to swallow safely, including LOC, gag and cough reflexes, and strength and symmetry of tongue, lip, and facial muscles.	This assessment determines if swallowing deficits are present that necessitate aspiration precautions.
- Assess for coughing, regurgitation of food and fluid through the nares, drooling, food oozing from the lips, food trapped in buccal spaces, and development of a weak, "wet," or hoarse voice during or after eating.	These are signs of impaired swallowing.
- Check the swallow reflex by first asking the patient to swallow own saliva. Place a finger gently on top of the larynx. If the larynx elevates with the attempt, next ask the patient to swallow 3-5 mL of plain water. Document your findings.	Inability to swallow own saliva or a small amount of water and the presence of a stationary larynx during attempts to swallow signal the loss of the swallowing reflex.
Caution: The presence of the cough reflex is essential for the patient to relearn swallowing safely.	The cough reflex protects against aspiration and if delayed may signal silent aspiration.
Obtain a referral to a speech therapist for patients with a swallowing dysfunction.	The act of swallowing is complex, and interventions vary according to the phase of swallowing that is dysfunctional. Video fluoroscopy may be used to evaluate swallowing, and some patients with swallowing dysfunction are referred to speech therapists for evaluation and recommendations of appropriate interventions.
Encourage the patient to practice any prescribed exercises.	Exercises such as tongue and jaw ROM; sound phonation such as "gah-gah-gah" to promote elevation of the soft palate; puckering lips; and sticking the tongue out to touch the nose, chin, cheeks may be prescribed to facilitate swallowing ability.
Recognize that a nasogastric (NG) tube may hinder the patient's ability to relearn to swallow.	NG tubes may desensitize and impair reflexive response to food bolus stimulus.
Alert the health care provider to your findings.	Parenteral nutrition may be necessary for patients who cannot chew or swallow effectively or safely.
Keep suction equipment and a manual resuscitation bag with a face mask at the patient's bedside. Suction secretions in the patient's mouth as necessary.	This equipment enables immediate intervention in the event aspiration occurs.
Ensure that the patient is alert and responsive to verbal stimuli before attempting to swallow. Provide a rest period before meals or swallowing attempts.	Patients who are drowsy, inattentive, or fatigued have difficulty cooperating and are at risk of aspirating.
Initiate swallowing attempts with plain water (see earlier). Progressively add easy-to-swallow foods and liquids as the patient's ability to swallow improves. Determine and document which foods and liquids are easiest for the patient to swallow.	Generally, semisolid foods of medium consistency, such as puddings, hot cereals, and casseroles, tend to be easiest to swallow. Thicker liquids, such as nectars, tend to be better tolerated than thin liquids.
If indicated/prescribed, add commercially available powders (e.g., Thicket) to liquids.	Thickening foods increases their viscosity and makes them more easily swallowed. Gravy or sauce added to dry foods often facilitates swallowing as well.
Avoid giving peanut butter, chocolate, or milk.	Foods such as these may stick in the patient's throat or produce mucus.
Avoid nuts, hard candies, or popcorn.	These foods may be aspirated.
Reduce stimuli in the room (e.g., turn off television, lower radio volume, minimize conversation, and limit disruptions from phone calls). Caution the patient not to talk while eating.	These measures help patient focus on swallowing.
If the patient must remain in bed, use high Fowler's position if possible. Support the shoulders and neck with pillows.	Most patients swallow best when in an upright position. Sitting in a straight-back chair with feet on the floor is ideal.
Ensure that the patient's head is erect and flexed forward slightly, with the chin at midline and pointing toward the chest (i.e., the "chin tuck").	This head position minimizes the risk that food will go into the airway by forcing the trachea to close and the esophagus to open. In addition, stroking the anterior neck lightly may help some patients swallow.

ASSESSMENT/INTERVENTIONS	RATIONALES
Maintain the patient in an upright position for at least 30-60 min after eating.	This position helps prevent regurgitation and aspiration by facilitating flow of foods and fluids by gravity from the stomach to the pylorus.
Teach the patient to break down the act of chewing and swallowing into the following steps. - Take small bites or sips (approximately 5 mL each). - Place food on the tongue. - Use the tongue to transfer food so that it is directly under the teeth on the unaffected side of the mouth. - Chew food thoroughly. - Move food to the middle of tongue and hold it there. - Flex the neck and tuck the chin against the chest. - Hold the breath and think about swallowing. - Without breathing, raise the tongue to roof of mouth and swallow. - Swallow several times if necessary. - When the mouth is empty, raise the chin and clear the throat or cough purposefully once or twice.	Taking patients through these steps promotes concentration and focus, which will help ensure optimal swallowing.
Start with small amounts of food or liquid. Feed slowly.	For optimum safety, each bite should not exceed 5 mL (1 tsp).
Ensure that each previous bite has been swallowed. Check the mouth for pockets of food. After every few bites of solid food, provide a liquid to help clear the mouth.	Food may become pocketed in the affected side of the mouth, which could result in aspiration.
Avoid using a syringe.	The force of the fluid in the syringe, if sprayed, may cause aspiration.
Avoid use of drinking straws.	The act of sucking may add to the complexity of swallowing and allow too much liquid to enter the mouth, thereby increasing the risk of aspiration.
Tear a piece out of a Styrofoam cup to make a space for the nose so that the patient can drink with the neck flexed.	Having the neck in a flexed position minimizes the risk that food will go into the airway by forcing the trachea to close and the esophagus to open.
Teach the patient who has food that pockets in the buccal spaces to periodically sweep the mouth with the tongue or finger or to clean these areas with a napkin. Explain that applying external pressure to the cheek with a finger will help remove trapped food.	These actions help prevent aspiration of food particles, stomatitis, and tooth decay.
Teach the patient who has a weak or paralyzed side to place food on the side of the face that he or she can control.	Tilting the head toward the stronger side will allow gravity to help keep food or liquid on the side of the mouth patients can manipulate. However, some patients may find that rotating the head to the weak side will close the damaged side of the pharynx and facilitate more effective swallowing.
Serve only warm or cool foods to individuals with loss of oral sensation.	Patients with loss of oral sensation may be unable to identify foods or fluids of tepid temperature with the tongue or oral mucosa. Verbal cues and use of a mirror may help ensure that these patients keep their mouths clear after swallowing.
To facilitate movement of food in some patients, encourage repeated swallowing attempts. Evaluate swallowing ability at different times of the day. Reschedule mealtimes to times when the patient has improved swallowing, such as when well rested or in relationship to medications that may impact swallowing behavior (as seen in diseases such as Parkinson's disease [PD]).	Patients with a pathology that affects swallowing such as PD and stroke have difficulty getting the tongue to move a bolus of food into the pharynx for swallowing.
If decreased salivation is contributing to swallowing difficulties, perform one of the following before feeding: swab the patient's mouth with a lemon-glycerin sponge; have the patient suck on a tart-flavored hard candy, dill pickle, or lemon slice; teach the patient to move the tongue in a circular motion against the inside of the cheek; or use artificial saliva.	These actions stimulate salivation, which optimally will contribute to effective swallowing.

continued

ASSESSMENT/INTERVENTIONS	RATIONALES
Moisten food with melted butter, broth or other soup, or gravy. Dip dry foods such as toast into coffee or other liquid.	These actions moisten and soften food when salivation is decreased.
Rinse the patient's mouth as needed.	This intervention removes particles and lubricates the mouth.
Investigate medications the patient is taking for the potential side effect of decreased salivation.	Drugs such as anti-parkinsonian medications or those with extrapyramidal side effects may result in decreased salivation.
Consult with the health care provider regarding use of tablets, capsules, and liquids for patients with swallowing difficulties. Check with the pharmacist to confirm that crushing a tablet or opening a capsule does not adversely affect its absorption or duration (i.e., slow-release medications should not be crushed).	Tablets or capsules may be swallowed more easily when added to foods such as puddings or ice cream. Crushed tablets or opened capsules also mix easily into these types of foods. Liquid forms of medications also may be available through the pharmacy.
For patients taking anti-Parkinson's medications, assess the relationship of peak medication effect with swallowing.	Coordinating meals with peak medication effect may facilitate swallowing.
Teach significant others the Heimlich or abdominal thrust maneuver.	This information helps ensure intervention in the event of a patient's choking.

Nursing Diagnosis:

Risk for Falls

related to weakness, impaired balance, or unsteady gait occurring with sensorimotor deficit

Desired Outcomes: The patient is free of trauma caused by gait unsteadiness. Before hospital discharge, the patient demonstrates proficiency with assistive devices if appropriate.

ASSESSMENT/INTERVENTIONS	RATIONALES
Assess gait and monitor for weakness, difficulty with balance, tremors, spasticity, or paralysis.	These are indicators of motor deficits that could lead to falls.
Document baseline assessments.	Documentation helps ensure that changes in status can be detected and interventions made promptly to help prevent falls.
Incorporate a fall risk assessment tool into the patient's plan of care. Include appropriate interventions, specific-to-patient lifting/transferring/mobilization aids and techniques, and the appropriate amount of assistance. Update with changes in patient status.	Assessment and documentation of the patient's fall risk via an armband, identifying wall placard, and/or care plan provide added insurance in helping to prevent injury resulting from falls.
Assist the patient as needed when unsteady gait, weakness, or paralysis is noted. Instruct the patient to ask or call for assistance with ambulation. Frequently check on patients who may forget to call for assistance. Stand on the patient's weak side to assist with balance and support. Use a transfer belt for safety. Instruct the patient to use stronger side for gripping railing when stair climbing or using a cane.	These measures minimize risk of falls by providing assistance and surveillance.
Orient the patient to new surroundings. Keep necessary items (including water, snacks, phone, call light) within easy reach.	These measures minimize risk of falls as a result of strange environment, unfamiliarity with such items as call light, and the need to walk to get them.
Assess the patient's ability to use necessary items.	Patients who are very weak or partially paralyzed may require a tap bell or specially adapted call light.
Maintain an uncluttered environment with unobstructed walkways. Ensure adequate lighting at night (e.g., provide a night light) to help prevent falls in the dark. In addition, keep side rails up and bed in its lowest position with bed brakes on.	These measures promote safety by ensuring better sensory acuity.

ASSESSMENT/INTERVENTIONS	RATIONALES
Encourage the patient to use any needed hearing aids and corrective lenses when ambulating.	These measures minimize risk of tripping, falls in the dark, or injury from inability to see or hear.
For unsteady, weak, or partially paralyzed patients, encourage use of low-heel, nonskid, supportive shoes for walking. Teach use of a wide-based gait.	These measures minimize risk of falls in patients with special needs.
Instruct the patient to note foot placement when ambulating or transferring.	This action ensures that the foot is flat and in a position of support before the patient ambulates and transfers.
Teach, reinforce, and encourage use of an assistive device, such as a cane, walker, or crutches.	These devices provide added stability.
Teach exercises that strengthen arm and shoulder muscles for using walkers and crutches. Teach safe use of transfer or sliding boards. Teach patients in wheelchairs how and when to lock and unlock wheels.	These actions promote added stability and safety.
Demonstrate how to secure and support weak or paralyzed arms.	These actions help prevent subluxation and injury from falling into wheelchair spokes or wheels.
Suggest that patients with poor sitting balance may need a seat or chest belt, H-straps for leg positioning, and a wheelchair with an anti-tip device.	Such devices likely will prevent patients with poor sitting balance from falling or tipping the wheelchair.
Teach the patient to maintain sitting position before assuming standing position for ambulating.	Maintaining this position for a few minutes gives the patient time to get the feet flat and under self for balance and minimizes any dizziness that may occur because of rapid position changes.
Monitor spasticity, antispasmodic medications, and their effect on physical function.	Uncontrolled or severe spasms may cause falls, whereas mild to moderate spasms can be useful in activities of daily living (ADLs) and transfers if patients learn to control and trigger them.
Review with the patient and significant others potential safety needs at home.	Such measures include safety appliances (wall, bath, toilet grab rails; elevated toilet seat; nonslip surface in bathtub or shower). Loose rugs should be removed to prevent slipping and falling. Temperatures on hot water heaters should be turned down to prevent scalding in the event of a fall in the shower or tub. Furniture in the home may need to be moved to provide clear, safe pathways that avoid sharp corners on furniture, glass cabinets, or large windows the patient could fall against. Strategically placed additional lighting also may be needed. Edges of steps in the home may require taping with brightly colored strips to provide sufficient contrast so that edges can be recognized and more safely negotiated. Beds should be modified to prevent rolling. Activity should be balanced with rest periods because fatigue tends to increase unsteadiness and potential for falls. Ramps may need to be used instead of stairs.
Seek referral for a physical therapist (PT) as appropriate.	Patients may have special needs that cannot be met by the nursing staff.

Nursing Diagnosis:

Risk for Injury

related to impaired pain, touch, and temperature sensations occurring with sensory deficit or decreased LOC

Desired Outcomes: The patient is free of indicators of injury caused by impaired pain, touch, and temperature sensations. Before hospital discharge, the patient and significant other identify factors that increase the potential for injury.

ASSESSMENT/INTERVENTIONS	RATIONALES
Assess for decreased or absent vision and impaired temperature and pain sensation.	These sensory deficits could result in patient injury.
Document baseline neurologic and physical assessments.	These assessments enable rapid detection of deteriorating status so that changes can be detected and responded to promptly, thereby helping prevent injury.
Avoid use of heating pads. Encourage use of sunscreen when outside. Do not serve scalding hot foods and beverages.	These measures protect patients from exposure to hot items and sun that can burn the skin.
Always check temperature of heating devices and bath water before the patient is exposed to them. Teach the patient and significant other about these precautions.	Patients' tactile senses are altered and would not recognize if water or device is too hot.
Inspect skin twice daily for evidence of irritation. Teach coherent patients to perform self-inspection, and provide a mirror for inspecting posterior aspects of the body.	The patient is not able to feel skin irritation.
Use emollient lotions liberally on the patient's skin.	These lotions keep skin soft and pliable and less likely to break down.
Teach the patient to inspect placement of limbs with altered sensation.	This helps ensure that limbs are in a safe and supported position and avoids placing ankles directly on top of each other.
Pad wheelchair seat, preferably with a gel pad.	Padding evenly distributes weight and decreases pressure areas that could result in skin breakdown.
Teach the patient to change position q15-30min by lifting self and shifting position from side to side and forward to backward. Encourage frequent turning while in bed and, if tolerated and not contraindicated, periodic movement into prone position.	Changing positions and turning promote circulation and prevent pressure ulcers. Patients likely will not sense the need to do this and therefore should do it on a scheduled basis. Spending time in the prone position (if not contraindicated) with hips extended helps prevent hip flexion contractures.
Have the patient lift, not drag, self during transfers.	This action prevents shearing damage to skin.
Avoid injecting more than 1 mL into a flaccid muscle. If possible, give injections only in muscles with tone.	Injections into muscles with tone will enable better absorption with less risk of sterile abscess formation.

Nursing Diagnosis:

Imbalanced Nutrition: Less Than Body Requirements

related to chewing and swallowing deficits, fatigue, weakness, paresis, paralysis, visual neglect, or decreased LOC

Desired Outcome: The patient achieves adequate nutrition as evidenced by maintenance of or return to baseline body weight by hospital discharge.

ASSESSMENT/INTERVENTIONS	RATIONALES
Assess alertness, ability to cough and swallow, and gag reflexes before all meals. Keep suction equipment at the bedside if indicated.	Deficits found during this assessment signal that the patient is at risk for aspiration, which in turn could lead to imbalanced nutrition.
Assess for the type of diet that can be eaten safely. Request soft, semisolid, or chopped foods as indicated.	Although a pureed diet may be needed eventually, pureed food can be unappealing and may have a negative impact on self-concept as well as decrease the patient's intake.
Assess food preferences and offer small, frequent servings of nutritious food. Consider cultural or religious factors that may affect eating when evaluating food preferences. Encourage significant others to bring in the patient's favorite foods if not contraindicated. Plan meals for times when the patient is rested; use a warming tray or microwave oven to keep food warm and appetizing until the patient is able to eat. Serve cold foods while they are cold.	Optimally, these measures will promote eating.

ASSESSMENT/INTERVENTIONS	RATIONALES
Reduce stimuli in the room (e.g., turn off TV or radio). Minimize conversation and other disruptions such as phone calls. If the patient wears glasses, put them on the patient; ensure adequate lighting. As needed, redirect the patient's attention to eating.	These measures help the patient focus on eating.
Provide oral care before feeding. Clean and insert dentures before each meal, and ensure that they fit properly.	Oral care and good dentition promote comfort and the ability to taste and chew.
Encourage liquid nutritional supplements. Try different methods to make them more palatable (e.g., making a milkshake, serving over ice, or diluting with carbonated beverages).	Making supplements more appetizing may promote intake.
Cut up foods, unwrap silverware, and otherwise prepare the food tray.	This assistance helps ensure that patients with a weak or paralyzed arm can manage the tray one-handed.
For patients with visual neglect, place food within the unaffected visual field. Return during the meal to ensure the patient has eaten from both sides of the plate. Turn the plate around so that any remaining food is in the patient's visual field.	These actions help ensure that the patient eats all or most of the food on the plate.
Feed or assist very weak or paralyzed patients. If not contraindicated, position the patient in a chair or elevate HOB as high as possible. Ensure that the patient's head is flexed slightly forward. Begin with small amounts of food. Encourage chewing food on the unaffected side. Do not hurry the patient. Be sure that each bite is completely swallowed before giving another. Encourage patients with hemiplegia to consciously sweep the paralyzed side of the mouth with the tongue to clear it.	Raising HOB helps prevent aspiration by promoting drainage into the stomach and through the pylorus. Assisting the patient also helps conserve his or her energy and provides social interaction, which may promote eating. Flexing the head slightly forward closes the airway.
If appropriate, provide assistive devices such as built-up utensil handles, broad-handled spoons, spill-proof cups, rocker knife for cutting, wrist or hand splints with clamps to hold utensils, stabilized plates, and sectioned plates.	Assistive devices promote self-feeding and independence.
Provide materials for oral hygiene after meals. Give oral care to patients unable to do so for themselves.	Oral care minimizes risk of aspiration of food particles. Good oral hygiene will also help maintain integrity of mucous membranes to minimize risk of stomatitis, which otherwise may prevent adequate oral intake.
Document your assessment of the patient's appetite. Weigh the patient regularly (at least weekly) to assess for loss or gain. If indicated, notify the health care provider of the potential need for high-protein or high-calorie supplements.	The trend of the patient's weight is a good indicator of nutritional status. Calculation of weight enables determination of the percentage below ideal weight for height and frame.
Obtain dietitian consultation. For additional information, see "Providing Nutritional Support," p. 539.	The patient may need enteral or parenteral nutrition.
For weak, debilitated, or partially paralyzed patients, assess support systems, such as family or friends, who can assist the patient with meals. Consider referral to an organization that will deliver a daily meal to the patient's home.	These actions help ensure optimal nutritional status.
If appropriate for the patient's diagnosis (e.g., multiple sclerosis [MS]), consider referral to a speech pathologist.	This specialist will teach exercises that enhance the ability to swallow.
For patients with visual problems, assess their ability to see food. Identify utensils and foods, and describe their location. Arrange foods in an established pattern.	These measures promote independence with eating. Poor vision has been associated with lower caloric intake.
For patients with diplopia, consider patching one eye.	Patching one eye may enable better vision.
For patients with chewing or swallowing difficulties, see interventions in **Impaired Swallowing**, p. 249, and **Risk for Aspiration**, p. 245.	

Nursing Diagnosis:

Acute Pain

related to spasms, headache, or photophobia occurring with neurologic dysfunction

Desired Outcomes: Within 1 hr of intervention, the patient's subjective perception of discomfort decreases, as documented by a pain scale. Objective indicators, such as grimacing, are absent or diminished.

ASSESSMENT/INTERVENTIONS	RATIONALES
Assess characteristics (e.g., quality, severity, location, onset, duration, precipitating factors) of the patient's pain or spasms. Devise a pain scale with the patient, and document discomfort on a scale of 0 (no pain) to 10 (worst pain). Determine the patient's acceptable pain level and ways of coping with and relieving pain.	These assessments demonstrate the degree and type of discomfort, trend of the discomfort, and relief obtained after interventions. A graphic pain scale using facial expression may be used for patients who cannot use a numeric scale.
Respond immediately to the patient's complaints of pain. Administer analgesics and antispasmodics as prescribed. Consider scheduling doses of analgesia. Document effectiveness of the medication, using a pain scale, approximately 30 min after administration. Assess for untoward effects. Consult the health care provider if a dose or interval change seems necessary.	Prolonged stimulation of pain receptors results in increased sensitivity to painful stimuli and will increase the amount of medication required to relieve pain.
Teach the patient and significant others about the importance of timing the pain medication.	Providing this information helps ensure that analgesia is taken before pain becomes too severe and before major moves.
Teach about the relationship between anxiety and pain, as well as other factors that enhance pain and spasms (e.g., staying in one position for too long, fatigue, chilling).	This information gives patients control over some causes of pain.
Instruct the patient and significant others in use of nonpharmacologic pain management techniques.	Such techniques as repositioning; ROM; supporting painful extremity or part; back rubs, acupressure, massage, warm baths, and other tactile distraction; auditory distraction such as listening to soothing music; visual distraction such as television; heat applications such as warm blankets or moist compresses; cold applications such as ice massage; guided imagery; breathing exercises; relaxation tapes and techniques; biofeedback; and a transcutaneous electrical nerve stimulation (TENS) device may be effective when used to supplement pharmacologic treatment. These methods also promote a sense of focus and self-control.
Encourage rest periods. Try to provide uninterrupted sleep time at night.	Fatigue tends to exacerbate the pain experience. Pain may result in fatigue, which in turn may cause exaggerated pain and further exhaustion.
If patients have photophobia, provide a quiet and dark environment. Close the door and curtains, provide sunglasses, and avoid use of artificial lights whenever possible.	These actions eliminate painful light sources for patients with photophobia.
Recognize that pain in the spinal cord injury (SCI) patient often is poorly localized and may be referred.	In the SCI patient, intrascapular pain may be from the stomach, duodenum, or gallbladder. Umbilical pain may be from the appendix. Testicular or inner thigh pain may be from the kidneys (e.g., with pyelonephritis).
[!] If the patient's present complaint of pain varies significantly from previous pain or if interventions are ineffective, notify the health care provider.	These situations may signal a new or acute problem and should be reported promptly for timely intervention.
Evaluate patients with SCI for tachycardia, restlessness, urinary incontinence when it was previously controlled, and fever.	These are signs of infection or inflammatory processes that may or may not result in discomfort in the patient with SCI but should be reported promptly for timely intervention.

Also see "Pain," p. 39.

Nursing Diagnosis:

Impaired Verbal Communication

related to facial/throat muscle weakness, intubation, or tracheostomy

Desired Outcome: Following intervention and on an ongoing basis, the patient communicates effectively, either verbally or nonverbally, and relates decreasing frustration with communication.

ASSESSMENT/INTERVENTIONS	RATIONALES
Assess the patient's ability to speak, read, write, and comprehend.	This assessment helps determine the patient's communication abilities and interventions that would promote them.
If appropriate, obtain referral to a speech therapist or pathologist. Encourage the patient to perform exercises that increase the ability to control facial muscles and tongue.	These actions assist patients in strengthening muscles used in speech. Such exercises may include holding a sound for 5 sec; singing the scale; reading aloud; and extending the tongue and trying to touch the chin, nose, or cheek.
Provide a supportive and relaxed environment for the patient who is unable to form words or sentences or who is unable to speak clearly or appropriately. Provide enough time for the patient to articulate. Ask the patient to repeat unclear words. Observe for nonverbal cues; watch the patient's lips closely. Do not interrupt or finish sentences. Anticipate needs and phrase questions to allow simple answers, such as "yes" or "no."	Patients likely will be frustrated over inability to communicate. Maintaining a calm, positive, reassuring attitude and continuing to speak to patients using normal volume (unless hearing is impaired) will help ease frustrations.
Maintain eye contact.	This will help patients maintain focus.
If the patient is unable to speak, provide a language board, alphabet cards, picture or letter-number board, flash cards, pad and pencil. Other systems use eye blinks, tongue clicks, or hand squeezes; bell signal taps; or gestures such as hand signals, head nods, pantomime, or pointing. Use a communication board for urgent situations.	These are alternative methods of communication.
Document the method of communication used.	Documentation helps ensure that other health care team members use the same method(s).
If the patient's voice is weak and difficult to hear, reduce environmental noise.	This will enhance the listener's ability to hear and comprehend the patient's words.
Suggest that the patient take a deep breath before speaking; provide a voice amplifier if appropriate.	These measures project the patient's voice.
Encourage the patient to organize thoughts and plan what he or she will say before speaking. Encourage the patient to express ideas in short, simple phrases or sentences.	These measures help make efficient use of voice strength or breath the patient does have.
Remind the patient to speak slowly, exaggerate pronunciation, and use facial expressions.	Patients may have a flat affect in both pronunciation and facial expression. Exaggerating both may make the patient's conversation more engaging.
If the patient has swallowing difficulties that result in accumulation of saliva, suction the mouth.	Suctioning will promote clearer speech.
If indicated, massage facial and neck muscles before the patient attempts to communicate.	Massage promotes clearer speech in patients with muscle rigidity or spasms.
If the patient has a tracheostomy, ensure that a tap bell is within reach.	Tap bell sounds give patients the means to communicate and increase a sense of self-control and safety.
Teach patients with a temporary tracheostomy that ability to speak will return.	This provides reassurance about future ability to communicate.
For patients with a permanent tracheostomy, discuss learning alternate communication systems.	Alternate communication systems include sign language or esophageal speech, in which fenestrated tubes or covering the tracheostomy tube opening with a finger will enable speech.

continued

ASSESSMENT/INTERVENTIONS	RATIONALES
Establish a method of calling for assistance, and make sure the patient knows how to use it. Keep calling device where the patient can activate it (e.g., place call bell on nonparalyzed side). Depending on the deficit, use a tap bell for a weak patient, a pillow pad call light (triggered by arm or head movement), or a sip and puff device (triggered by the mouth).	These measures ensure that patients of varying abilities will be able to call for assistance.
Encourage patients with ability to write to keep a diary or write letters. If the patient has a weak writing arm, evaluate need for a splint or other device that will enable the patient to hold a pen or pencil.	These measures provide a means of ventilating feelings and expressing concerns. Felt-tip markers are useful because they require minimal pressure for writing. Large-barrel pens may be easier for grasping and writing. Patients also may be able to type. For patients able to speak, a computer voice recognition program may facilitate written and e-mail communication.

Nursing Diagnosis:

Constipation

related to inability to chew and swallow a high-roughage diet, side effects of medications, immobility, and neurologic (spinal cord) involvement

Desired Outcome: Within 2-3 days of intervention, the patient passes soft, formed stools and regains and maintains his or her normal bowel pattern.

ASSESSMENT/INTERVENTIONS	RATIONALES
Teach patients with chewing and swallowing difficulties that consuming 1 or 2 servings of applesauce with added bran, prune juice, or cooked bran cereal each day may be effective. Otherwise encourage use of natural fiber laxatives such as psyllium (e.g., Metamucil).	Although a high-roughage diet is ideal for patients who are immobilized or on prolonged bedrest, individuals with chewing and swallowing difficulties may be unable to consume such a diet.
As an alternative to psyllium, suggest polyethylene glycol (MiraLAX).	With MiraLAX, there is less risk of choking.
Encourage/promote a bowel elimination program. Keep a call bell within the patient's reach.	Elements that may be included in a successful bowel elimination program include the following: setting a regular time of day for attempting a bowel movement, preferably 30 min after eating a meal or drinking a hot beverage; using a commode instead of a bedpan for more natural positioning during elimination; using a medicated suppository 15-30 min before a scheduled attempt; bearing down by contracting abdominal muscles or applying manual pressure to the abdomen to help increase intraabdominal pressure; and drinking 4 oz of prune juice nightly.
As indicated, include abdominal and pelvic exercises in the patient's morning and evening routine.	These exercises will help promote bowel evacuation. For more detail, see **Risk for Activity Intolerance,** p. 61, in "Prolonged Bedrest."
Assess the patient's sitting balance and ability to assume a normal toileting position, and intervene accordingly.	This will help ensure the patient's safety while on the commode.
SCI patients with involvement at T8 and above should use extreme caution if using an enema or suppository. If either measure is unavoidable, use large amounts of anesthetic jelly in the rectum.	Either measure can precipitate life-threatening autonomic dysreflexia (AD). Using anesthetic jelly reduces that risk.
In addition, instruct patients at risk of IICP not to bear down with bowel movements.	This action can cause increased intraabdominal pressure, which in turn increases ICP. See **Decreased Intracranial Adaptive Capacity,** earlier.
Unless contraindicated, encourage fluid intake to at least 2500 mL/day or more, including liberal amounts of fresh fruit juices.	Adequate fluid intake helps prevent hard, dry stools that are difficult to evacuate.

ASSESSMENT/INTERVENTIONS	RATIONALES
If indicated by the patient's diagnosis (e.g., MS), provide instructions for anal digital stimulation.	This action promotes reflex bowel evacuation.
Avoid the above intervention for SCI patients with involvement at T8 or above.	At this level of involvement, anal digital stimulation can precipitate life-threatening AD.
For other interventions, see **Constipation**, p. 68, in "Prolonged Bedrest."	

Nursing Diagnosis:

Bathing, Dressing, Feeding, Toileting Self-Care Deficit

related to spasticity, tremors, weakness, paresis, paralysis, or decreasing LOC

Desired Outcome: At least 24 hr before hospital discharge, the patient performs care activities independently and demonstrates ability to use adaptive devices for successful completion of ADLs. (The totally dependent patient expresses satisfaction with activities that are completed for him or her.)

ASSESSMENT/INTERVENTIONS	RATIONALES
Assess the patient's ability to perform ADLs.	This assessment demonstrates performance barriers and degree to which patients need assistance with completing ADLs. These data will enable development of an individualized care plan.
As appropriate, demonstrate use of adaptive devices, such as long- or broad-handled combs; long-handled pickup sticks, brushes, and eating utensils; dressing sticks; stocking helpers; Velcro fasteners; elastic waistbands; nonspill cups; and stabilized plates. Also consider electric toothbrush and electric razor.	Adaptive devices may assist patients in maintaining independent care. For example, a flexor-hinge splint or universal cuff may aid in brushing teeth and combing hair.
Set short-range, realistic goals with the patient. Acknowledge progress. Encourage continued effort and involvement (e.g., in selection of meals, clothing).	These actions help decrease frustration and improve learning.
Provide care to totally dependent patients. Assist those who are not totally dependent according to the degree of disability. Encourage the patient to perform self-care to the maximum ability as defined by the patient. Encourage autonomy.	Promoting autonomy and positive self-image helps prevent learned helplessness.
Allow sufficient time for task performance; do not hurry the patient. Involve significant others with care activities if they comfortable doing so. Ask for the patient's input in planning schedules. Supervise activity until the patient can safely perform tasks without help.	Preserving energy by providing sufficient time for the task increases activity to tolerance.
Encourage use of electronically controlled wheelchair and other technical advances (e.g., environmental control system).	These devices help improve mobility and enable independent operation of electronic devices such as lights, radio, door openers, and window shade openers.
Provide privacy and a nondistracting environment. Place the patient's belongings within reach. Set out items needed to complete self-care tasks in the order they are to be used. Apply any needed adaptive devices such as hand splints.	These actions convey respect, simplify the task, and increase motivation.
Encourage the patient to wear any prescribed corrective eye lenses or hearing aids.	Enhanced vision and hearing may increase participation in self-care.
Provide prescribed analgesics to relieve pain.	Pain can hinder self-care.

continued

ASSESSMENT/INTERVENTIONS

RATIONALES

ASSESSMENT/INTERVENTIONS	RATIONALES
Provide a rest period before self-care activity, or plan activity for a time when the patient is rested.	Fatigue reduces self-care ability.
Encourage the patient or significant others to buy shoes without laces; long-handled shoe horns; front opening garments; wide-legged pants; and clothing that is loose-fitting with enlarged arm holes, front fasteners, zipper pulls, elastic waistbands, or Velcro closures. Avoid items with small buttons or tight buttonholes. Lay out clothing in the order it will be put on. Advise the patient to sit while dressing. Suggest that use of a dressing stick may help to pull up pants or retrieve clothing.	These products and devices facilitate dressing and undressing.
Place a stool in the shower.	A stool will help patients for whom sitting down will enhance self-care with bathing.
Explain that bathrooms should have nonslip mats and grab bars.	These mats and bars promote safety in self-care by preventing falls.
Suggest use of a handheld showerhead and a long-handled bath sponge or a washer mitt with a pocket that holds soap.	These devices and products facilitate autonomy in bathing.
Provide a commode chair, elevated toilet seat, or male or female urinal.	These chairs, seats, and urinals promote self-care with elimination.
Teach self-transfer techniques.	These techniques enable patients to get to the commode or toilet independently.
Keep call light within the patient's reach. Instruct the patient to call as early as possible.	Calling early provides time for the staff to respond and the patient will not have to rush because of urgency.
Offer toileting reminders q2h, after meals, and before bedtime.	Toileting schedules convey the message that continence is valued, optimally reducing episodes of incontinence.
Suggest use of a long-handled grasper that can hold tissues or washcloth for perineal care.	Some patients with limited hand or arm mobility may have difficulty with perineal care after elimination.
For patients with hemiparesis or hemiparalysis, teach use of the stronger or unaffected hand and arm for dressing, eating, bathing, and grooming. Instruct the patient to dress the weaker side first.	These measures simplify tasks and conserve energy.
For patients with visual field deficit, avoid placing items on their blind side. Encourage the patient to scan the environment for needed items by turning the head.	These measures enable visualization of the task at hand.
Suggest use of splints, weighted utensils, or wrist weights for patients with tremors.	Adaptive devices increase speed and safety of self-care and decrease exertion.
Teach the patient to rest the head against a high-backed chair.	Resting the head against a high-backed chair may reduce head tremors.
Obtain referral for an occupational therapist (OT) if indicated.	This referral will help determine the best method for performing activities.
Provide consistent caregiver and ADL routine for patients with cognitive deficits.	Individuals with cognitive defects need simple visual or verbal cues, increased gesture use, demonstration, reminders of next step, and gentle repetition.
If indicated teach the patient self-catheterization, or teach the technique to the caregiver.	At-home intermittent catheterization usually is done with clean (not sterile) technique and equipment. The catheter is washed after use in warm, soapy water; rinsed; and placed in a clean plastic sack. Catheter insertion guides are available commercially for females with limited upper arm mobility. Crusted catheters are soaked in a solution of half distilled vinegar and half water.
Teach the patient to assess for and notify the health professional of cloudy, foul-smelling, or bloody urine; urine with sediment; chills or fever; pain in lower back or abdomen; or a red or swollen urethral meatus.	These are indicators of urinary tract infection (UTI), which necessitates timely intervention.

ASSESSMENT/INTERVENTIONS | RATIONALES

ASSESSMENT/INTERVENTIONS	RATIONALES
Discuss, as appropriate, modifying the home environment.	Modifying the home environment (e.g., with extended sinks, grab bars, lower closet hooks, wheelchair-accessible shower, modified phones, lowered mirrors, and lever door handles that operate with reduced hand pressure) likely will promote independence and performance of ADLs at home.
Listen and provide opportunities for the patient to express self, and communicate that it is normal to have negative feelings about changes in autonomy. Discuss with the health care team ways to provide consistent and positive encouragement and strategies that increase independence progressively. Suggest a local support group.	Frustration can be decreased and coping skills increased when an individual expresses feelings in a supportive environment.

Nursing Diagnosis:

Impaired Oral Mucous Membrane
(or risk for same)

related to barriers to oral care (sensorimotor deficit or decreased LOC)

Desired Outcome: Before hospital discharge, the patient or significant others demonstrate ability to perform the patient's oral care.

ASSESSMENT/INTERVENTIONS | RATIONALES

ASSESSMENT/INTERVENTIONS	RATIONALES
Assess the patient's ability to perform mouth care.	This assessment enables identification of performance barriers (e.g., sensorimotor or cognitive deficits).
If the patient has decreased LOC or is at risk for aspiration, remove dentures and store them in a water-filled denture cup.	This action protects and prevents loss of dentures.
If the patient cannot perform mouth care, clean the teeth, tongue, and mouth at least twice daily with a soft-bristle toothbrush and nonabrasive toothpaste.	This intervention promotes oral hygiene and prevents accumulation of bacteria that can cause oral inflammation.
If the patient is unconscious or at risk for aspiration, turn to a side-lying position. Swab the mouth and teeth with sponge-tipped applicator (Toothette) moistened with diluted (half strength) mouthwash solution, and irrigate the mouth with a large syringe. If the patient cannot self-manage secretions, use only a small amount of liquid for irrigation each time, and, using a suction catheter or Yankauer tonsil suction tip, remove secretions.	These measures provide effective oral cleansing while preventing aspiration of oral solutions.
Perform this oral hygiene regimen at least q4h. As appropriate, teach the procedure to significant others.	Good oral hygiene helps prevent stomatitis and tooth decay and reduces risk of infections caused by an oral mucous membrane that is not intact.
Make toothbrush adaptations for patients with physical disabilities.	*For patients with limited hand mobility:* Enlarge the toothbrush handle by covering it with a sponge hair roller or aluminum foil (attaching with an elastic band) or by attaching a bicycle handle grip with plaster of Paris. *For patients with limited arm mobility:* Extend the toothbrush handle by overlapping another handle or rod over it and taping them together.

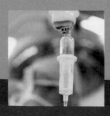

Bacterial Meningitis 35

OVERVIEW/PATHOPHYSIOLOGY

Bacterial meningitis is an infection that results in inflammation of the meningeal membranes covering the brain and spinal cord. Bacteria in the subarachnoid space multiply and cause an inflammatory reaction of the pia and arachnoid meninges. Purulent exudate is produced, and inflammation and infection spread quickly through the cerebrospinal fluid (CSF) that circulates around the brain and spinal cord. Bacteria and exudate can create vascular congestion, plugging the arachnoid villi. This obstruction of CSF flow and decreased reabsorption of CSF can lead to hydrocephalus, increased intracranial pressure (IICP), brain herniation, and death.

Meningitis generally is transmitted in one of four ways: (1) via airborne droplets or contact with oral secretions from infected individuals; (2) from direct contamination (e.g., from a penetrating skull wound; a skull fracture, often basilar, causing a tear in the dura; lumbar puncture (LP); ventricular shunt; or surgical procedure); (3) via the bloodstream (e.g., pneumonia, endocarditis); or (4) from direct contact with an infectious process that invades the meningeal membranes, as can occur with osteomyelitis, sinusitis, otitis media, mastoiditis, or brain abscess. Pneumonococcal meningitis, caused by *Streptococcus pneumoniae,* is the most common bacterial meningitis. Meningococcal meningitis, caused by *Neisseria meningitidis,* is the next leading cause. This organism can cause adrenal hemorrhage and insufficiency, leading to vascular collapse and death. Myocarditis also can occur. *Listeria monocytogenes* is less common and usually seen in such populations as newborns, those who are immune compromised, and in adults older than 50 yr. Outbreaks have been associated with consumption of contaminated dairy or undercooked fish, chicken, and meat. Any bacteria can cause meningitis, and some forms of meningitis, such as that caused by *Staphylococcus aureus,* can be difficult to treat because of their resistance to antibiotic therapy. Adhesions and fibrotic changes in the arachnoid layer and subspace may cause obstruction or reabsorption problems with CSF, resulting in hydrocephalus.

Risk factors: (1) age, (2) close community settings such as schools and college campuses, (3) medical conditions that either directly weaken the immune response or the treatment weakens the immune response, (4) work environments that may routinely expose one to causative pathogens, and (5) traveling to areas at higher risk for meningitis.

HEALTH CARE SETTING

Acute care

ASSESSMENT

Cardinal signs: Headache, fever, stiff neck, change in mental status, nausea, vomiting, and photophobia.

Infection: Fever, chills, malaise.

IICP and herniation: Decreased level of consciousness (LOC) (irritability, drowsiness, stupor, coma), nausea and vomiting, decreasing Glasgow Coma Scale score, vital sign (VS) changes (increased blood pressure [BP], decreased heart rate [HR], widening pulse pressure), changes in respiratory pattern, decreased pupillary reaction to light, pupillary dilation or inequality, severe headache.

Meningeal irritation: Back stiffness and pain, headache, nuchal rigidity.

Other: Generalized seizures and photophobia. In the presence of *Haemophilus influenzae,* deafness or joint pain may occur.

PHYSICAL ASSESSMENT

- Positive Brudzinski's sign may be elicited because of meningeal irritation: when the neck is passively flexed forward, both legs flex involuntarily at the hip and knee.
- Positive Kernig's sign also may be found: when the hip is flexed 90 degrees, the individual cannot extend the leg completely without pain.
- In the presence of meningococcal meningitis, a pink, macular rash; petechiae; ecchymoses; purpura; and increased deep tendon reflexes (DTRs) may occur. The rash signals septicemia and is associated with a 40% mortality rate, even with appropriate antibiotics. The rash can progress to gangrenous necrosis and may need débridement or even amputation.

DIAGNOSTIC TESTS

LP, CSF analysis, and Gram stain and culture: Gold star standard for diagnosing bacterial meningitis and identifying causative organism. Glucose is generally decreased, usually less than 40 mg/dL and protein is increased and can often be seen in the hundreds. Increased total lactate dehydrogenase (LDH) in CSF is a consistent finding. Presence or absence of C-reactive protein (CRP) in the CSF can differentiate

PART I: Medical-Surgical Nursing

between bacterial (positive for CRP) and nonbacterial (negative for CRP) meningitis. Typically, CSF will be cloudy or milky because of increased white blood cells (WBCs); CSF pressure will be increased because of the inflammation and exudate, causing an obstruction in outflow of CSF from the arachnoid villi. This test, in the presence of IICP, can cause brain herniation. If CSF pressure is elevated, check neurologic status and VS at frequent intervals for signs of brain herniation (decreased LOC; pupillary changes such as dilation, inequality, or decreased reaction; irregular respirations; hemiparesis). Neuroimaging should be done prior to LP to evaluate for evidence of IICP. If there is evidence of IICP, LP is contraindicated.

Xpert EV test: To distinguish between viral and bacterial meningitis rapidly (in less than 3 hr).

Culture and sensitivity testing of blood, sputum, urine, and other body secretions: To identify infective organism and/or its source and determine appropriate antibiotic.

Coagglutination tests: To detect microbial antigens in CSF and enable identification of the causative organism. Generally coagglutination tests have replaced counterimmunoelectrophoresis because results are obtainable much more rapidly.

Polymerase chain reaction: To analyze DNA in peripheral blood or CSF to identify causative infectious agents.

Radioimmunoassay, latex particle agglutination, or enzyme-linked immunosorbent assay: To detect microbial antigens in the CSF to identify causative organism.

Petechial skin scraping: For Gram stain analysis of bacteria.

Sinus, skull, and chest x-ray examinations: Taken after treatment is started to rule out sinusitis, pneumonia, and cranial osteomyelitis.

Computed tomography (CT) scan with contrast: To rule out hydrocephalus or mass lesions such as brain abscess and detect exudate in CSF spaces.

Magnetic resonance imaging (MRI): To rule out hydrocephalus or mass lesion and detect exudate in CSF spaces.

Nursing Diagnosis:
Deficient Knowledge

related to unfamiliarity with the rationale and procedure for Transmission-Based Precautions: Droplet

Desired Outcome: Before visitation, the patient and significant other verbalize knowledge about the rationale for Transmission-Based Precautions: Droplet and comply with prescribed restrictions and precautionary measures.

ASSESSMENT/INTERVENTIONS	RATIONALES
For patients with meningitis caused by *H. influenzae* or *N. meningitidis*, assess their knowledge base and explain, as indicated, the method of disease transmission via respiratory droplets generated by patients when coughing, sneezing, or talking or during performance of cough-inducing procedures (e.g., suctioning) and by contact with oral secretions; and the rationale for a private room and droplet precautions.	Patients with *N. meningitidis*, with *H. influenzae,* or in whom the causative organism is in doubt require observation with Transmission-Based Precautions: Droplet for 24 hr after initiation of appropriate antibiotic therapy. Patients should be placed in a private room if possible. If a private room is not available, an infected patient may be placed in a room with another patient who is at low risk for adverse outcome if transmission occurs, while ensuring that patients are physically separated (i.e., more than 3 ft) from each other.
Provide instructions for covering mouth before coughing or sneezing and properly disposing of tissue (Respiratory Hygiene/Cough Etiquette).	Infection may be spread by contact with respiratory droplets or oral secretions. Masks should be worn for close patient contact (e.g., within 3 ft), along with adherence to Standard Precautions (see p. 747).
Instruct patients with Transmission-Based Precautions: Droplet to stay in their room. If they must leave the room for a procedure or test, explain that a mask must be worn to protect others from contact with respiratory droplets.	As above.
For individuals in contact with the patient, explain importance of wearing a surgical mask and practicing good hand hygiene. Gloves should be worn when handling any body fluid, especially oral secretions. For more information, see Appendix A, "Infection Prevention and Control," p. 747.	As above.

continued

ASSESSMENT/INTERVENTIONS	RATIONALES
Reassure the patient that Transmission-Based Precautions: Droplet are temporary.	These precautions will be discontinued once patients have been taking the appropriate antibiotic for at least 24 hr.
Instruct individuals in contact with the patient that if symptoms of meningitis develop (e.g., headache, fever, neck stiffness, photophobia, change in mental status), they should report immediately to their health care provider.	This measure helps ensure prompt treatment. Mortality rate is high (70%-100%) in persons in whom meningitis is left untreated. However, in individuals in whom diagnosis and antibiotic treatment are established early, prognosis is good, and complete neurologic recovery is possible.

Nursing Diagnosis:

Acute Pain

related to headache, photophobia, and neck stiffness

Desired Outcomes: Within 1-2 hr of intervention, the patient's subjective perception of discomfort decreases, as documented by pain scale. Objective indicators, such as grimacing, are absent or diminished.

ASSESSMENT/INTERVENTIONS	RATIONALES
Assess the patient for pain and discomfort using an appropriate pain scale.	Using a pain scale provides a common language for assessing pain and relief obtained.
Provide a quiet environment, darkened room or sunglasses, and restrict visitors as necessary.	These measures reduce noise and help prevent photophobia.
Promote bedrest and assist with activities of daily living (ADLs) as needed.	These measures decrease movement that may cause pain.
Apply ice bag to head or cool cloth to eyes.	These actions help diminish headache.
Support the patient in a position of comfort. Keep the neck in alignment during position changes.	Many persons with meningitis are comforted in a position with the head in extension and the body slightly curled. Head of bed (HOB) elevated to 30 degrees also may help.
Provide gentle passive range of motion (ROM) and massage to neck and shoulder joints and muscles. If the patient is afebrile, apply moist heat to neck and back.	These measures help relieve stiffness, promote muscle relaxation, and decrease pain.
Keep communication simple and direct, using a soft, calm tone of voice. Avoid needless stimulation. Consolidate activities. Loosen constricting bed clothing. Avoid restraining the patient. Reduce stimulation to the minimal amount needed to accomplish required activity.	Patients tend to be hyperirritable with hyperalgesia. Sounds are loud, and even gentle touching may startle them.
Administer medications as prescribed.	Analgesics (e.g., acetaminophen, codeine) are given to relieve headache, myalgia, and other pain. Antipyretics (e.g., acetaminophen) are given for control of fever to reduce cerebral metabolism. Mild sedatives (e.g., diphenhydramine) are given to promote rest.
For other interventions see **Acute Pain** in "General Care of Patients with Neurologic Disorders," p. 256.	

Nursing Diagnosis:

Deficient Knowledge

related to unfamiliarity with the purpose, side effects, and precautions for the prescribed medications

Desired Outcome: Before beginning medication regimen, the patient and significant others verbalize knowledge about the purpose, potential side effects, and precautions for the prescribed medications.

ASSESSMENT/INTERVENTIONS	RATIONALES
Assess the patient's and significant others' health care literacy (language, reading, comprehension). Assess culture and culturally specific information needs.	This assessment helps ensure that information is selected and presented in a manner that is culturally and educationally appropriate.
Teach the patient and significant others about the prescribed antibiotic.	Because treatment cannot be delayed until culture results are known, high doses of parenteral antibiotics are started immediately, based on Gram stain results. The antibiotic must penetrate the blood-brain barrier into the CSF. Adjustments in therapy can be made after coagglutination test, counter immunoelectrophoresis (CIE), and culture and sensitivity test results are available. Antibiotics may include the following (usually in combination): penicillin G, ampicillin, cefotaxime, ceftriaxone, ceftazidime, chloramphenicol, gentamicin, and vancomycin.
As appropriate, teach the patient and significant others that sometimes intrathecal (i.e., in the subarachnoid space) antibiotics are used.	Intrathecal antibiotics may be used if it is believed that systemic antibiotics alone will not be curative in the presence of particular bacteria (e.g., *Pseudomonas, Enterobacter, Staphylococcus*).
As appropriate, teach the patient and significant others about the rationale for giving a glucocorticosteroid (e.g., dexamethasone) and its potential side effects.	Ideally it is given before or at same time as the first dose of antibiotics and then on an ongoing basis to reduce inflammation caused by toxic by-products released by bacterial cells as they are killed by antibiotics. In children, this therapy can reduce hearing loss caused by *H. influenzae*. **Caution:** Steroids can have side effects that can complicate the patient's clinical condition (e.g., increased glucose may make the patient more lethargic and may exaggerate emotional responses causing agitation and/or cause psychotic/hallucination type reactions).
For close contacts of the patient, explain the importance of taking the prophylactic antibiotic, including prescribed dose and schedule and symptoms to report.	Usually rifampin is administered. Other antibiotics, such as ciprofloxacin, ceftriaxone, chloramphenicol, sulfadiazine, or minocycline, may be used as well. It is important that all contacts be notified as soon as possible for treatment and know signs and symptoms of meningitis to report to the health care provider (e.g., headache, fever, stiff neck, change in mental state, nausea, vomiting, photophobia).
Explain that rifampin should be taken 1 hr before meals.	This ensures maximum absorption.
Teach the purpose of taking rifampin and its potential side effects.	Rifampin is taken as a preventive measure against meningitis. Potential side effects such as nausea, vomiting, diarrhea, orange urine, headache, and dizziness can occur.
Explain precautions when taking rifampin.	Persons taking this drug should avoid wearing contact lenses because the drug will permanently color them orange. In addition, rifampin reduces effectiveness of oral contraceptives and is contraindicated during pregnancy. Contacts who are taking rifampin also should report onset of jaundice (yellow skin or sclera), allergic reactions, and persistence of gastrointestinal side effects.

ADDITIONAL NURSING DIAGNOSES/PROBLEMS:

✓ PATIENT-FAMILY TEACHING AND DISCHARGE PLANNING

The extent of teaching and discharge planning will depend on whether the patient has any residual damage. When providing patient-family teaching, focus on sensory information, avoid giving excessive information, and initiate a visiting nurse referral for necessary follow-up teaching. Include verbal and written information about the following:

✓ Referrals to community resources, such as public health nurse, visiting nurses association, community support groups, social workers, psychologic therapy, vocational rehabilitation agency, home health agencies, and extended and skilled care facilities.

✓ Medications, including drug name, purpose, dosage, schedule, precautions, and potential side effects for patient's medications, as well as those for the prophylactic antibiotics taken by family and significant other. Also discuss drug-drug, herb-drug, and food-drug interactions. Close contacts taking prophylactic antibiotics should know signs and symptoms to report to the health care provider (e.g., headache, fever, neck stiffness).

✓ Vaccination: There are vaccines available against *S. pneumoniae*. *N. meningitidis* and *H. influenzae* Group B causing meningitis and other infections. *N. meningitidis* has several subgroup strains. For people at increased risk (e.g., travelers to countries with endemic infections), a meningococcal vaccine (group A, C, Y, W135) is available although it does not confer 100% protection. Centers for Disease Control and Prevention recommends this meningococcal vaccine for children 11-12 years of age, adolescents at high school entry, and college freshmen living in dormitories. In the United States the most common *N. meningitidis* is from Group B, and work is progressing on a Group B vaccine. *H. influenzae* Group B vaccine should be incorporated as part of all routine childhood inoculations.

✓ For patients with residual neurologic deficits, teach the following as appropriate: exercises that promote muscle strength and mobility; measures for preventing contractures and skin breakdown; transfer techniques and proper body mechanics; safety measures if patient has decreased pain and sensation or visual disturbances; use of assistive devices; indications of constipation, urinary retention, or urinary tract infection (UTI); bowel and bladder training programs; self-catheterization technique or care of indwelling catheters; and seizure precautions if indicated.

✓ Obtain additional information from the following: Meningitis Foundation of America, Inc., at *www.musa.org* and Centers for Disease Control and Prevention at *http://www.cdc.gov/meningitis/bacterial.html#prevention* and the Meningitis Research Foundation of Canada at *www.meningitis.ca*

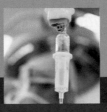

Guillain-Barré Syndrome 36

OVERVIEW/PATHOPHYSIOLOGY

Guillain-Barré syndrome (GBS) is a rapidly progressing polyneuritis of unknown cause. An inflammatory process enables lymphocytes to enter perivascular spaces and destroy the myelin sheath covering peripheral or cranial nerves. Posterior (sensory) and anterior (motor) nerve roots can be affected because of this segmental demyelination, and individuals may experience both sensory and motor losses. There is relative sparing of the axon. Respiratory insufficiency may occur in as many as half of affected individuals. Life-threatening respiratory muscle weakness can develop as rapidly as 24-72 hr after onset of initial symptoms. In about 25% of cases, motor weakness progresses to total paralysis.

Peak severity of symptoms usually occurs within 1-3 wk after onset of symptoms. A plateau stage follows that usually lasts 1-2 wk. The recovery stage starts with a return of function as remyelination occurs, but it may take months to years for a full recovery. Fifteen percent of patients have full neurologic recovery, and another 65% have mild deficits that do not interfere with activities of daily living (ADLs). Eighty percent to 90% of patients either recover completely or have only minor residual weakness or abnormal sensations, such as numbness or tingling. Of GBS patients, 5%-10% may have permanent severe disability. Deficits are the result of axonal nerve degeneration.

GBS is believed to be an autoimmune response triggered by a viral infection experienced by the patient 1-4 wk prior to its onset. Up to 75% of cases are proceeded by viral illnesses. Common viral illnesses include: (1) upper respiratory infection (URI), (2) gastroenteritis, (3) *Campylobacter jejuni*, (4) Cytomegalovirus, and (5) Epstein-Barr virus. Less commonly it may also be associated with vaccinations, HIV seroconversions, Hodgkin's lymphoma, SLE, sarcoidosis, thyroid disease, and lung cancer.

HEALTH CARE SETTING

The patient is likely to be in acute care (intensive care unit [ICU]) when the neurologic deficit is progressing and in an acute rehabilitation setting during the recovery phase.

ASSESSMENT

Progressive weakness and areflexia are the most common indicators. Typically, numbness and weakness begin bilaterally in the legs and ascend symmetrically upward, progressing to the arms and cranial nerves. Ascending GBS is most common. Variants of GBS include acute motor axonal neuropathy (primarily a motor component, with no sensory involvement), and descending GBS, in which cranial nerves are affected first and weakness progresses downward with rapid respiratory involvement. Other variants include Miller Fisher syndrome, which is characterized by a triad of abnormal muscle coordination (ataxia), paralysis of eye muscles (ophthalmoplegia), and absence of tendon reflexes (areflexia); and pharyngeal-cervical-brachial variant (rare) involving facial, oropharyngeal, cervical, and upper limbs with no lower limb involvement. Peak severity usually occurs within 10-14 days of onset. GBS does not affect level of consciousness (LOC), cognitive function, or pupillary function.

Anterior (motor) nerve root involvement: Weakness or flaccid paralysis that can progress to quadriplegia. Respiratory muscle involvement can be life threatening. There is loss of reflexes, muscle tension, and tone, but muscle atrophy usually does not occur.

Autonomic nervous system involvement: Sinus tachycardia, bradycardia, hypertension, hypotension, cardiac dysrhythmias, facial flushing, diaphoresis, inability to perspire, loss of sphincter control, urinary retention, adynamic ileus, syndrome of inappropriate antidiuretic hormone secretion, and increased pulmonary secretions may occur. Autonomic nervous system (ANS) involvement may occur unexpectedly and can be life threatening, but usually it does not persist for longer than 2 wk.

Cranial nerve involvement: Inability to chew, swallow, speak, or close the eyes.

Posterior (sensory) nerve root involvement: Presence of paresthesias, such as numbness and tingling, which usually are minor compared with the degree of motor loss. Ascending sensory loss often precedes motor loss. Muscle cramping, tenderness, or pain may occur.

Physical assessment: Symmetric motor weakness, impaired position and vibration sense, hypoactive or absent deep tendon reflexes, hypotonia in affected muscles, and decreased ventilatory capacity.

DIAGNOSTIC TESTS

Diagnostic tests are performed to rule out other diseases, such as acute poliomyelitis. Diagnosis of GBS is based on clinical presentation, history of recent viral illness, and cerebrospinal fluid (CSF) findings.

Lumbar puncture and CSF analysis: About 7 days after the initial symptoms, elevated protein (especially IgG) without an increase in white blood cell (WBC) count may be present. Although CSF pressure usually is normal, in severe disease it may be elevated.

Electromyography and nerve conduction studies: Reveal slowed nerve conduction velocities soon after paralysis appears because of demyelinization. Denervation potentials appear later.

Serum complete blood count (CBC): Will show presence of leukocytosis early in illness, possibly as a result of the inflammatory process associated with demyelinization.

Evoked potentials (auditory, visual, brain stem): May be used to distinguish GBS from other neuropathologic conditions.

Nursing Diagnosis:

Ineffective Breathing Pattern

related to neuromuscular weakness or paralysis of the facial, throat, and respiratory muscles (severity of symptoms peaks around wk 1-3)

Desired Outcome: Deterioration in the patient's breathing pattern (e.g., PaO_2 less than 80 mm Hg, vital capacity less than 800-1000 mL [or less than 10-12 mL/kg], tidal volume less than 75% of predicted value, or O_2 saturation 92% or less via oximetry) is detected and reported promptly, resulting in immediate and effective medical treatment.

ASSESSMENT/INTERVENTIONS	RATIONALES
As often as indicated, assess the patient's respiratory rate, rhythm, and depth. Auscultate for diminished breath sounds.	The frequency of assessment will depend on the patient's clinical condition. Accessory muscle use, nasal flaring, dyspnea, shallow respirations, diminished breath sounds, and apnea are signs of respiratory deterioration, which necessitates prompt notification of the health provider for rapid intervention.
On an ongoing basis, observe for changes in mental status, LOC, and orientation.	These changes may signal reduced oxygenation to the brain as a result of ineffective breathing pattern.
As indicated and at least once per shift during the acute phase, depending on the patient's clinical state, assess for ascending loss of sensation by touching the patient lightly with a pin or fingers at frequent intervals (hourly or more frequently initially). Assess from the level of the iliac crest upward toward the shoulders. Measure the highest level at which decreased sensation occurs.	Decreased sensation often precedes motor weakness; therefore, if it ascends to the level of the T8 dermatome, anticipate that intercostal muscles (used with respirations) soon will be impaired.
As indicated and at least once per shift during the acute phase, depending on the patient's clinical state, assess for the presence of arm drift and inability to shrug the shoulders. Alert the health care provider to significant findings.	Shoulder weakness is present if the patient cannot shrug the shoulders. Arm drift is present if one arm pronates or drifts down or out from its original position. Arm drift is detected in the following way: have the patient hold both arms out in front of the body, level with the shoulders and with palms up; instruct the patient to close the eyes while holding this position. If present, these findings need to be reported promptly because they are known to precede respiratory dysfunction.
Assess the patient's ability to take fluids orally. Assess q8h and before oral intake for cough reflexes, gag reflexes, and difficulty swallowing.	These assessments detect changes or difficulties that may indicate ascending paralysis.
As prescribed, keep patients with impaired reflexes and swallowing nothing by mouth (NPO).	Impaired swallowing and cough and gag reflexes likely will necessitate parenteral feedings to prevent aspiration until reflexes return to normal.
On an ongoing basis, assess the patient for breathlessness while speaking. To assess for breathlessness, ask the patient to take a deep breath and slowly count as high as possible on one breath. Alert the health care provider to significant findings.	A reduced ability to count to a higher number before breathlessness occurs may signal grossly reduced ventilatory function.

ASSESSMENT/INTERVENTIONS	RATIONALES
Monitor effectiveness of breathing by checking serial vital capacity and negative inspiratory force (NIF) results on pulmonary function tests.	If vital capacity is less than 1000 mL or is rapidly trending downward or if the patient exhibits signs of hypoxia such as tachycardia, increasing restlessness, mental dullness, cyanosis, decreased pulse oximetry readings, or difficulty handling secretions, these findings must be reported immediately to the health care provider to prevent further deterioration in status. If present, intubation is probable. Vital capacity initially is measured q2-4h and then more frequently if deterioration is present.
Assess arterial blood gas levels and pulse oximetry as per standard operational procedures or as prescribed.	These assessments detect hypoxia or hypercapnia ($Paco_2$ more than 45 mm Hg), a signal of hypoventilation. Pao_2 less than 80 mm Hg or O_2 saturation 92% or less usually signals need for supplemental oxygen.
Raise head of bed	This position promotes optimal chest excursion by taking pressure of abdominal organs off the lungs, which may increase oxygenation. This position also will reduce aspiration risk.
At least q4h and as indicated, encourage coughing and deep breathing to the best of the patient's ability.	These actions mobilize and enable expectoration of secretions to optimize breathing pattern.
Prepare the patient emotionally for life-saving procedures or for the eventual transfer to ICU or transition care unit for closer monitoring.	The patient may require tracheostomy, endotracheal intubation, or mechanical ventilation to support respiratory function.
For other interventions, see **Risk for Aspiration** in "Older Adult Care," p. 93.	

Nursing Diagnoses:

Risk for Ineffective Cerebral Tissue Perfusion
Risk for Decreased Cardiac Tissue Perfusion

related to blood pressure fluctuations occurring with autonomic dysfunction

Desired Outcomes: The patient has optimal cardiac and cerebral tissue perfusion as evidenced by systolic blood pressure (SBP) at least 90 mm Hg and less than 160 mm Hg; no significant mental status changes; and orientation to person, place, and time. Blood pressure (BP) fluctuations, if they occur, are detected and reported promptly.

ASSESSMENT/INTERVENTIONS	RATIONALES
As indicated, but no less frequently than q4h, assess LOC and BP, noting wide fluctuations. Report significant findings to the health care provider.	LOC will help determine the state of the patient's cerebral perfusion. Changes in BP that result in severe hypotension or hypertension may occur because of unopposed sympathetic outflow or loss of outflow to the peripheral nervous system, causing changes in vascular tone. The health care provider may prescribe a short-acting vasoactive agent for persistent hypotension or hypertension. Phenoxybenzamine may be used to treat paroxysmal hypertension, headache, sweating, anxiety, and fever.
On an ongoing basis, assess carefully for changes in heart rate (HR) and BP during activities such as coughing, suctioning, position changes, or straining at stool.	These are events that can trigger BP changes.
For patients with hypotension or postural hypotension, see these same nursing diagnoses, p. 318, in "Spinal Cord Injury."	

PART I: Medical-Surgical Nursing

Nursing Diagnoses:

Risk for Dysfunctional Gastrointestinal Motility

related to autonomic nervous system involvement

Imbalanced Nutrition: Less Than Body Requirements

related to NPO status occurring with adynamic ileus

Desired Outcome: The patient has adequate nutrition as evidenced by maintenance of base-line body weight.

ASSESSMENT/INTERVENTIONS	RATIONALES
Auscultate bowel sounds, noting presence, absence, or changes from baseline that may signal onset of ileus. Notify the health care provider of significant findings.	Bowel sounds are auscultated in all 4 quadrants for at least 2 min before determining that bowel sounds are not present. Abdominal distention or tenderness, nausea and vomiting, and absence of stool output are other signals of the onset of ileus. Also, GBS has been associated with *C. jejuni,* an infection that manifests as gastroenteritis. These findings should be reported promptly for timely intervention.
Initiate gastric, gastrostomy, or parenteral feedings as prescribed.	Patients with adynamic ileus generally require gastric decompression with a nasogastric tube. If the patient cannot chew or swallow effectively because of cranial nerve involvement, gastric, gastrostomy, or parenteral feedings may be initiated. The patient is advanced to a solid diet upon return of the gag reflex and swallowing ability. See "Providing Nutritional Support," p. 539.
Upon return of the gag reflex and swallowing ability, provide a high-fiber diet as prescribed.	Fiber provides bulk, which helps prevent constipation.
For general interventions, see **Imbalanced Nutrition**, p. 254, in "General Care of Patients with Neurologic Disorders."	

Nursing Diagnosis:

Anxiety

related to threat to biologic integrity and loss of control

Desired Outcome: Within 24 hr of this diagnosis, the patient expresses concerns regarding changes in life events, states anxiety is lessened or under control, and exhibits fewer symptoms of increased anxiety (e.g., less apprehension, decreased tension).

ASSESSMENT/INTERVENTIONS	RATIONALES
Assess need and arrange for transfer to a room close to the nurses' station for patients with progressing neurologic deficit.	This action will help alleviate the anxiety of being suddenly incapacitated and helpless.
Be sure the call light is within easy reach, and frequently assess the patient's ability to use it. Consider an easy-touch call bell to ensure the patient can call for help as needed.	These measures that promote patient's safety also will help allay anxiety.
Provide continuity of patient care through assignment of staff and use of care plan.	Familiarity may help reduce anxiety.
Perform assessments at frequent intervals, letting the patient know you are there. Provide care in a calm and reassuring manner.	Calm begets calm. Frequent assessments also reassure the patient that he or she is being watched out for.

ASSESSMENT/INTERVENTIONS

Allow time for the patient to vent concerns; provide realistic feedback regarding what the patient may experience. Determine past effective coping behaviors.

For other interventions, see **Anxiety**, p. 73, and **Fear**, p. 75, in "Psychosocial Support."

RATIONALES

Unexpressed concerns can contribute to frustration and stress. Information helps reduce anxiety caused by a lack of knowledge. Knowing past effective coping behaviors facilitates problem solving for ways in which these behaviors, or others, may prove useful in the current situation.

Nursing Diagnosis:

Deficient Knowledge

related to unfamiliarity with the therapeutic plasma exchange procedure

Desired Outcome: Before the scheduled date of the procedure, the patient verbalizes accurate information about the plasma exchange procedure.

ASSESSMENT/INTERVENTIONS

Assess the patient's health care literacy (language, reading, comprehension). Assess culture and culturally specific information needs.

Determine if the patient is taking angiotensin-converting enzyme (ACE) inhibitor medication and notify the health care provider accordingly.

Determine the patient's level of understanding of the health care provider's explanation of the plasma exchange procedure.

Explain in words the patient can understand the goal of plasma exchange.

Explain that if started within 1-2 wk of GBS symptoms, the exchange process seems to decrease disease duration and severity.

Assess the patient's experience with plasmapheresis, positive or negative effects, and nature of any fears or concerns. Document and communicate this information to other caregivers.

Answer any questions regarding potential complications.

RATIONALES

This assessment helps ensure that information is selected and presented in a manner that is culturally and educationally appropriate.

ACE inhibitor use is associated with flushing, hypotension, abdominal cramping, and other gastrointestinal symptoms while on plasmapheresis. These medications usually are held for 24 hr before the procedure to prevent these problems.

Before the plasma exchange procedure, the health care provider explains the reason for the procedure, its risks, and anticipated benefits or outcome and obtains a signed consent. The nurse's assessment of the patient's understanding provides an opportunity to clarify or reinforce information accordingly. Alternatives to plasma exchange include intravenous (IV) immunoglobulins, which may be given soon (1-5 days) after symptom onset to positively affect antibody response, or immunoadsorption therapy as an alternative to plasmapheresis for antibody removal. Informed consent is needed for invasive procedures.

The procedure is similar to hemodialysis. Blood is removed from the patient and separated into its components. The plasma is discarded; other blood components (e.g., red blood cells, WBCs, platelets) are saved and returned to the patient with donor plasma or replacement fluid. Multiple exchanges over a period of weeks can be expected.

Antibodies to the patient's peripheral and cranial nerve tissue are reduced by removal of the blood's plasma portion, which contains the circulating antibodies.

This will clarify the nurse's understanding of the patient's perspective, which in turn will enable further information gathering and clarification, optimally decreasing fears and concerns.

Although the following complications are rare, the patient is at risk during this procedure: deficient fluid volume, hypotension, fluid overload, hypokalemia (from dilution with albumin replacement), hypocalcemia (from free calcium binding to the citrate used during the procedure), cardiac dysrhythmias (from electrolyte shifts), clotting disorders (from decreased clotting factors with plasma removal), anemia, phlebitis, infection, hypothermia, and air embolism.

continued

ASSESSMENT/INTERVENTIONS	RATIONALES
Explain that the patient can expect the procedure to take 2-4 hr, although it may take considerably longer.	The length of time will depend on condition of the patient's veins, blood flow, and hematocrit level.
Explain that the patient can expect preprocedure and postprocedure blood work.	Blood will be assessed for clotting factors and electrolyte level, particularly of potassium and calcium, which can be reduced during this exchange procedure.
Explain that weight and vital signs (VS) will be taken before and after the procedure, with frequent VS checks during the procedure.	Hypotension and shift in fluid volume are possible.
Advise that calcium gluconate or potassium may be administered, based on laboratory values of calcium or potassium.	These agents will correct electrolyte imbalances.
Encourage the patient to report any unusual feelings or symptoms during plasma exchange.	Unusual feelings or symptoms may include chills, fever, hives, sweating, or lightheadedness, which may signal a reaction to donor plasma. Thirst, faintness, or dizziness can occur with hypotension or hypovolemia. Patients should take oral fluids during the procedure if possible. Numbness or tingling around lips or in the hands, arms, and legs; muscle twitching; cramping; or tetany can occur with hypocalcemia. Fatigue, nausea, weakness, or cramping may signal hypokalemia.
Inform the patient that medications (e.g., plasma-bound drugs) may be held until after the procedure.	Medications otherwise would be removed from the blood during the plasma exchange.
If the patient does not have a urinary catheter, remind him or her to void before and during the procedure, if necessary.	This measure prevents the mild hypotension caused by a full bladder.
Explain that intake and output will be monitored closely during the procedure.	Decreased urine output may signal hypovolemia.
Explain that the patient's temperature will be checked during the procedure and warm blankets will be provided.	These measures assess for and prevent hypothermia.
Explain that the patient probably will feel fatigued 1-2 days after the procedure. Encourage extra rest, a high-protein diet, and milk products during this time.	Fatigue could result from the decreased plasma protein level that occurs during the exchange.
Teach the patient to monitor the IV access site for warmth, redness, swelling, or drainage and to report significant findings.	These are signs of local infection.
Teach the patient to monitor for signs of bruising or bleeding. Caution the patient about avoiding cutting self or bumping into objects and to sustain pressure over cuts. Inform the patient that black, tarry stools usually signal the presence of blood and should be reported.	The anticoagulant citrate dextrose is used in the extracorporeal machine circuitry to prevent clotting. This may cause excessive bleeding at the access site. A pressure dressing may be kept in place over the access site for 2-4 hr after the procedure.

Nursing Diagnosis:

Acute Pain

related to muscle tenderness; hypersensitivity to touch; or discomfort in the shoulders, thighs, and back

Desired Outcomes: Within 1-2 hr of intervention, the patient's subjective perception of discomfort decreases, as documented by pain scale. Objective indicators, such as grimacing, are absent or diminished.

ASSESSMENT/INTERVENTIONS	RATIONALES
For patients with hypersensitivity, assess the amount of touch that can be tolerated, and incorporate this information into the plan of care.	This assessment facilitates development of an individualized plan of care and helps ensure that the patient is not touched more than necessary by all staff members.
For patients with muscle tenderness, consider use of massage, moist heat packs, cold application, or warm baths.	These measures may be very soothing for tender muscles.

ASSESSMENT/INTERVENTIONS

RATIONALES

ASSESSMENT/INTERVENTIONS	RATIONALES
Reposition the patient at frequent intervals.	Repositioning will help decrease muscle tension and fatigue. Some individuals find that a supine "frog-leg" position is particularly comfortable.
Provide passive range of motion and advise gentle stretching.	These measures reduce joint stiffness.
Administer pain medications as prescribed.	Opioids are often the most effective means of pain control, and a continuous morphine drip may be needed. Other medications that may be used to relieve uncomfortable paresthesias include anticonvulsants such as gabapentin and carbamazepine and tricyclics such as amitriptyline.

For other interventions, see **Acute Pain**, p. 256, in "General Care of Patients with Neurologic Disorders."

ADDITIONAL NURSING DIAGNOSES/PROBLEMS:

 PATIENT-FAMILY TEACHING AND DISCHARGE PLANNING

Most patients with GBS eventually recover fully or nearly so, but because the recovery period can be prolonged, the patient often goes home with some degree of neurologic deficit. Discharge planning and teaching will vary according to the degree of disability. When providing patient-family teaching, focus on sensory information, avoid giving excessive information, and initiate a visiting nurse referral for necessary follow-up teaching. Include verbal and written information about the following:

✓ Disease process, expected improvement, and importance of continuing in rehabilitation or physical therapy (PT) program to promote as full a recovery as possible.

✓ Safety measures relative to sensorimotor deficit.

✓ Exercises that promote muscle strength and mobility, measures for preventing contractures and skin breakdown, transfer techniques and proper body mechanics, and use of assistive devices.

✓ Indications of constipation, urinary retention, or urinary tract infection; implementation of bowel and bladder training programs; and, if appropriate, care of indwelling catheters or self-catheterization technique.

✓ Indications of URI; measures for preventing regurgitation, aspiration, and respiratory infection.

✓ Medications, including drug name, purpose, dosage, schedule, precautions, and potential side effects. Also discuss drug-drug, herb-drug, and food-drug interactions.

✓ Importance of follow-up care, including visits to the health care provider, PT, and occupational therapy.

✓ Referrals to community resources such as public health nurse, visiting nurse association, community support groups, social workers, psychologic therapy, home health agencies, and extended and skilled care facilities. Additional general information can be obtained by contacting the GBS/CIDP Foundation International at *www.gbs-cidp.org*.

Intervertebral Disk Disease 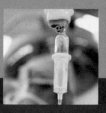 37

OVERVIEW/PATHOPHYSIOLOGY

The intervertebral disk is a semifluid-filled fibrous capsule that facilitates movement of the spine and acts as a shock absorber. The disk's ability to withstand stressors is not unlimited and diminishes with aging. Pressure on the disk eventually may force elastic material from the center of the disk, called the *nucleus pulposus*, to break (herniate) through the fibrous rim of the disk, called the *annulus*. Herniation usually occurs posteriorly because the posterior longitudinal ligament is inherently weaker than the anterior longitudinal ligament. The bulging or rupture (protrusion or extrusion) of an intervertebral disk causes its typical symptoms by pressing on and irritating the spinal nerve roots or spinal cord itself. Herniated nucleus pulposus usually is the result of injury or a series of insults to the vertebral column from lifting or twisting. When the disk ruptures without a known discrete injury, degenerative changes are the likely cause. Deterioration usually occurs suddenly with rupture, but it may happen gradually, with symptoms appearing months or years after the initial injury. Almost all herniated disks occur in the lumbar spine, with 90% of the problems occurring at L4-5 and L5-S1. Research is investigating the role of certain genes and environmental influences on lumbar disk disease. The spinal cord ends around L1, so lumbar herniated disks impinge on spinal nerves, which are more resilient than actual spinal cord tissue. The spinal nerves usually bounce back and function normally once the problem is relieved. Cervical disk problems most often occur at C5-6 and C6-7 and generally are caused by degenerative changes or trauma, such as whiplash or hyperextension. Cervical herniations may compress spinal nerves or impinge on the spinal cord itself. Thoracic disk problems are rare because of the rigid structure of the thoracic spine.

Herniated disks account for about 4% of back pain. Most back pain is related to muscle and ligament strain. Spondylolisthesis (slippage between two vertebrae) and degenerative changes such as stenosis; osteophyte (e.g., bone spur) formation, which can cause spinal nerve root compression; osteoporosis, which can lead to compression fractures; and osteoarthritis of the facet joints are other causes of non-disk back pain. Neoplasm and infection also can be sources of back pain.

HEALTH CARE SETTING

Primary care or acute care neurosurgery, neurology, or orthopedics; pain clinics

ASSESSMENT

General indicators: Onset can be sudden, with intense unilateral pain or with pain that is dull, diffuse, deep, and aching. Symptoms vary according to the level of injury and nerves involved. Usually, pain is increased with movement or activities that increase intraabdominal or intrathoracic pressure, such as sneezing, coughing, and straining. Often pain is improved by lying down. **Note:** Immediate medical attention is essential if there is any weakness or paralysis, extreme sensory loss, or altered bowel or bladder function, which indicate spinal cord compression in the lumbar back (e.g., cauda equina syndrome) and need for emergency decompression surgery. Indicators of cervical spinal cord compression (and need for early surgical treatment) include balance problems, unsteadiness when standing with eyes closed (Romberg's sign), hyperreflexes, and generalized numbness in the feet and legs.

Cervical disk disease: Pain or numbness in the upper extremities, shoulders, thorax, occipital area, or back of the head or neck. Pain can radiate down the forearms and into the hands and fingers. Interscapular aching or suboccipital headaches are commonly associated with cervical disk disease. Usually the neck has restricted mobility, and there can be cervical muscle spasm and loss of normal cervical lordosis. Patients may have upper extremity muscle weakness with abnormal biceps or triceps reflexes.

Lumbar disk disease: Pain in the lumbosacral area with possible radiculopathy (sciatica) to the buttock, down the posterior surface of the thigh and calf, and to the lateral border of the foot and toes. Sensory distribution for the L5 nerve root is the medial portion of the foot and the great toe, whereas sensory distribution for S1 is the lateral aspect of the foot, fifth toe, and sole of the foot. Often mobility is altered, as evidenced by decreased ability to stand upright, listing to one side, asymmetric gait, limited ability to flex forward, and restricted side movement caused by pain and muscle spasms. The individual walks cautiously, bearing little weight on the affected side, and often finds sitting or climbing stairs particularly painful. Reflex muscle spasms can cause bulging of the back with concomitant flattening of the lumbar curve and possible scoliosis at the level of the affected disk. Usually patellar and Achilles tendon reflexes are depressed due to nerve impingement. Sciatica usually is associated with intervertebral disk herniation.

Physical assessment: Possible findings include depressed reflexes, muscle atrophy, paresthesias (described as "pins and needles"), or anesthesia (numbness) in the dermatome of the involved nerves. The straight leg raise test and sciatic nerve test are two of several that are performed to confirm presence of lumbar disk disease.

Risk factors: Repetitive bending or lifting involving a twisting motion, continuous vibration, smoking, poor physical condition (especially weak abdominal muscles), poor posture, obesity, above-average height, osteoporosis, prolonged sitting, depression, severe scoliosis, spondylolisthesis, or genetic predisposition.

DIAGNOSTIC TESTS

In the absence of serious symptoms, diagnostic testing may not be done until 3 mo have passed and symptoms persist (90% of back pain resolves in less than 1 mo). Diagnostic testing should be done for pain that is constant, severe, unrelieved by rest or position, and is not calmed by antiinflammatory medication inasmuch as these symptoms may indicate presence of neoplasm or infection. Thoracic back pain also should be investigated because it may be caused by medical problems (e.g., aortic aneurysm).

Magnetic resonance imaging (MRI) scan: May reveal a disk impinging on the spinal cord or nerve root, or may show a related pathologic condition, such as a tumor or spondylosis.

A magnetic resonance (MR) neurogram helps image nerves after they leave the spinal column and can show compressions as they travel through the spinal foramina. MR myelogram helps view the cerebral spinal fluid sac without having to use a needle puncture. MRI has replaced computed tomography (CT) scan and myelogram as the test of choice in diagnosing herniated nucleus pulposus and is considered the "gold standard."

CT scan of the spine: May reveal disk protrusion/prolapse or a related pathologic condition, such as a bone spur, tumor, spondylosis, or spinal stenosis.

X-ray examination of the spine: May show narrowing of the vertebral interspaces in affected areas, loss of spine curvature, bone spur formation, and spondylosis.

Diskography: Identifies degenerated or extruded disks or annulus tear by means of contrast medium injected into the disk space using fluoroscopy. Often it is done in combination with CT and may differentiate between disk infection and rupture.

Myelogram: May show characteristic deformity and filling defect or a related pathologic condition; it is usually done in conjunction with a CT scan.

Electromyography: May show denervation patterns of specific nerve roots to indicate level and site of injury.

Evoked potential studies: For example, somatosensory studies may show slowed conduction due to nerve root compromise and can localize specific nerve root.

LABORATORY TESTS

Serum alkaline and acid phosphatase, glucose, calcium, erythrocyte sedimentation rate (ESR), and white blood cell count may rule out metabolic bone disease, metastatic tumors, diabetic mononeuritis, and disk space infection.

Nursing Diagnoses:

Deficient Knowledge
Acute Pain

related to unfamiliarity with pain control measures

Desired Outcome: Following instruction during outpatient treatment session or within the 24-hr period before hospital discharge, the patient verbalizes knowledge about pain control measures and demonstrates ability to initiate these measures when appropriate.

ASSESSMENT/INTERVENTIONS	RATIONALES
Teach methods of controlling pain and their individual applications.	Methods include distraction, use of counterirritants, massage, hydrotherapy, aquatherapy, acupressure, dorsal column stimulation, use of transcutaneous electrical nerve stimulation, behavior modification, relaxation techniques, hypnosis, music therapy, imagery, biofeedback, and diathermy. Whole body vibration exercise and spinal manipulation may be considered for uncomplicated back problems with no radiculopathy.

ASSESSMENT/INTERVENTIONS	RATIONALES
	In addition, applying intermittent heat may reduce muscle spasm, whereas icing may prevent further inflammatory swelling and provide some topical anesthesia. Icing should be done frequently, especially for the first 24-48 hr after surgery, and is often recommended after exercise. Continuous low-level heat wrap therapy reduces pain and improves function. Heat may be applied via warm/hot showers or heating pads. Cold can be achieved by freezing water in a paper cup, tearing off top of the cup to expose the ice, and massaging in a circular motion, using the remaining portion of the cup as a handle. A bag of frozen peas or corn may be used to apply continuous cold to the lower back. With any of these methods, a layer of cloth should be used so that ice does not touch the skin. A 20-min application of cold 4-6 times per day is recommended.
Suggest the patient use a stool to rest the affected leg when standing.	This measure will help relieve sciatica.
Advise the patient to sit in a straight-back chair that is high enough to get out of easily, including toilet seats that are raised.	Higher seats facilitate ease of movement in and out of chairs and provide comfort. Straddling a straight-back chair and resting arms on the chair back is comfortable for many individuals.
Encourage use of a moderately-firm to firm mattress and extra pillows as needed for positioning.	These measures support normal lumbar curvature. Some patients find the normal bed height too low and use blocks to raise it to a more comfortable height.
Instruct the patient on bedrest to roll rather than lift off the bedpan.	This action prevents straining of the back. The patient may find a fracture bedpan more comfortable than a regular bedpan.
Caution the patient to avoid sudden twisting or turning movements. Explain importance of logrolling when moving from side to side.	These measures prevent movements that could induce further back injury. Orthotics (e.g., splints, braces, girdles, cervical collars) also may be used to limit motion of the vertebral column. Temporary use of a back brace or corset may enable earlier return to activity with lumbar disk disease. Generally, long-term use of braces is discouraged because it prohibits development of necessary supporting musculature.
Advise the patient to avoid staying in one position too long, fatigue, chilling, and anxiety.	These factors can cause back spasms.
Suggest lying on the side with knees bent or lying supine with knees supported on pillows. Advise the patient that a small pillow supporting the nape of the neck may be helpful with cervical pain. Teach the patient to avoid prolonged periods of sitting, which stress the back.	These measures promote spinal comfort.
If appropriate, teach the patient to apply a heating pad to the back for 15-30 min before getting out of bed in the morning.	Heat will help allay stiffness and discomfort after a night in bed. Heating pads should be used only for short intervals and only if the patient's temperature sensations are intact.
Remind the patient to place a towel or cloth between the heating pad and skin.	This measure will help prevent burns.
Encourage the patient to rest when tired or stressed and not to exercise when in pain.	Tired muscles are more susceptible to injury. Usually patients resume normal activity as soon as possible, but pain is an indicator to limit the offending activity.
Instruct in use of cervical traction if prescribed.	Although infrequently prescribed, it may be used to help a cervical disk that has been bulging to slip back into place and unload the neck muscles and ligaments. Traditional method is a neck/head harness attached to a pulley and weight. A device for home use may include an inflatable collar that expands to push the head away from the shoulders.
Encourage a high-bulk diet, adequate or increased fluids, and stool softeners.	These measures prevent constipation, which would cause straining and pain.
Teach the purpose and potential side effects of the following medications for acute pain:	

continued

ASSESSMENT/INTERVENTIONS	RATIONALES
- Analgesics (e.g., acetaminophen and tramadol, and opioid combinations such as hydrocodone and acetaminophen or oxycodone and acetaminophen)	Sufficient medication is given to achieve pain relief or adequate pain reduction. Acetaminophen can cause serious skin reaction such as Steven-Johnson syndrome and can cause liver failure and death. Many opioids are combination medications with acetaminophen as well as OTCs (over 600 OTCs contain acetaminophen). Overdose of this medication is estimated at 55K-80K per year with at least 500 deaths. In addition, opioids are on the "high alert" medication list due to the possibility of serious consequences if accidentally given, and extra safeguards should be taken to reduce risk of error.
- Nonsteroidal antiinflammatory drugs (NSAIDs) and salicylates	These medications reduce inflammation and relieve pain. Dosing usually is scheduled initially to obtain a sustained antiinflammatory effect. Side effects include blood thinning and gastric irritation, and kidneys may be affected if these drugs are taken for a long time.
- Misoprostol or stomach protectants such as sucralfate or ranitidine	These agents may be considered to reduce gastric irritation caused by stress, medications, and steroids (if used).
- Muscle relaxants (e.g., cyclobenzaprine, carisoprodol, methocarbamol, diazepam)	These medications decrease muscle spasms, thereby reducing pain. Common side effects are drowsiness, fatigue, dizziness, dry mouth, and gastrointestinal (GI) upset.
- Corticosteroids (e.g., dexamethasone, prednisone, prednisolone)	Steroids may be given for a short period to reduce cord edema, if present, but use is controversial. These medications can have significant side effects such as increased blood sugar, agitation, and hallucinations. They need to be tapered while being discontinued.
Teach the patient about the following medications used for chronic pain:	
- Analgesics (e.g., NSAIDs, tramadol, gabapentin, amitriptyline)	Nonnarcotic analgesia such as NSAIDs is used for chronic pain. (See NSAID side effects, earlier.) Tramadol, a centrally acting analgesic, may be used long-term, especially for older adults. Tricyclic antidepressants (e.g., amitriptyline, desipramine, doxepin) also may help with chronic pain. Anticonvulsants such as gabapentin, carbamazepine, phenytoin, and levetracetam help with neuropathic pain caused by nerve injury.
- Local injection of anesthetic (lidocaine or bupivacaine) and/or cortisone into epidural spaces, facet joints, sacroiliac joint, or trigger points	These medications reduce pain and muscle spasms and increase function.
- Botulinum toxin injection into paravertebral regions	This injection relieves pain, probably through decreased muscle spasm, and improves function for 3-8 wk.
Teach the patient about the following techniques that may be effective in controlling chronic pain:	
- Souchard's global postural reeducation (GPR)	This French physical therapy (PT) technique has been effective in restoring function and relieving long-term chronic pain. It consists of a series of maneuvers in which patients are in supine, sitting, and standing positions and involves stretching the paraspinal muscles and those of the abdominal wall so that joints are relieved of the compression that is typically the source of pain.
- Percutaneous electrical nerve stimulation	This device uses acupuncture-like needle probes positioned in soft tissue and/or muscles to stimulate peripheral sensory nerves to relieve persistent back pain.
- Implantable epidural spinal cord stimulator	This stimulator may be used to aid in the control of chronic pain when all other measures (e.g., PT, medications, surgery) have failed.
Suggest alternative/complementary therapies such as chiropractic, acupuncture, and cranial-sacral massage.	Many people achieve pain relief from these therapies.

Nursing Diagnosis:

Deficient Knowledge

related to unfamiliarity with proper body mechanics and other measures that prevent back injury

Desired Outcome: Within the treatment session (outpatient) or within the 24-hr period before hospital discharge, the patient verbalizes knowledge of measures that prevent back injury and demonstrates proper body mechanics.

ASSESSMENT/INTERVENTIONS	RATIONALES
Teach the patient proper body mechanics: - Stand and sit straight with chin and head up and pelvis and back straight; avoid slouching. - Bend at knees and hips (squat) rather than at the waist, keeping back straight (not stooping forward). - When carrying objects, hold them close to the body, avoiding twisting when lifting or reaching. Spread feet for a wider base of support. Lift with legs, not the back. - Turn using the entire body instead of twisting. - Do not strain to reach things. If an object is overhead, raise oneself to its level, or move things out of the way if they are obstructing the object. - Avoid lifting anything heavier than 10-20 lb. - Encourage use of long-handled pickup sticks to pick up small objects. - Have the patient demonstrate proper body mechanics, if possible, before hospital discharge.	Using proper body mechanics avoids movements such as twisting, lifting with the back, and straining to reach that can cause back injury.
Teach about the following measures for keeping the body in alignment: - Sit close to the pedals when driving a car, and use a seat belt and firm back rest to support the back. - Support feet on a footstool when sitting so that knees are elevated to hip level or higher. - Obtain a firm mattress or bed board; use a flat pillow when sleeping to avoid strain on neck, arms, and shoulders; sleep in a side-lying position with knees bent or in a supine position with knees and legs supported on pillows; avoid sleeping in a prone position. - Avoid reaching or stretching to pick up objects. - Avoid sitting on furniture that does not support the back.	Keeping the body in proper alignment avoids strain on the back, thereby helping to prevent recurring back injury.
Encourage the patient to achieve and/or maintain proper weight for age, height, and gender; continue the exercise program prescribed by the health care provider; use thoracic and abdominal muscles when lifting; when standing for any length of time, stand with one foot on a step stool; sit in a firm chair for support.	Being overweight or obese can cause back strain and alteration in the center of balance, which can result in back pain and pressure. Exercise strengthens abdominal, thoracic, and back muscles. Using thoracic and abdominal muscles when lifting keeps a significant portion of weight off vertebral disks. Standing with one foot on a step stool helps relieve sciatica. Sitting in a firm chair provides support to the back.
Teach the rationale and procedure for Williams' back exercises:	
Pelvic tilt: Tighten stomach and buttock muscles, and tilt the pelvis while keeping the lower spine flat against the floor; that is, the hips and buttocks are kept on the floor.	*Pelvic tilt:* To strengthen abdominal muscles.
Knee-to-chest raise: Start with a pelvic tilt. Raise each knee individually to the chest and return to the starting position. Then raise each knee individually to the chest and hold them there (both knees on chest together).	*Knee-to-chest raise:* To help make a stiff back limber.
Nose-to-knee touch: Raise the knee to the chest, and then pull the knee to the chest with the hands. Raise the head, and try to touch nose to knee. Keep the lower back flat on floor.	*Nose-to-knee touch:* To stretch hip muscles and strengthen abdominal muscles.

continued

ASSESSMENT/INTERVENTIONS	RATIONALES
Half sit-ups: Slowly raise head and neck to top of the chest. Reach both hands forward to the knees, and hold for a count of 5. Repeat, keeping the lower back flat on the floor.	*Half sit-ups:* To strengthen abdomen and back.
Instruct the patient to wear supportive shoes with a low or moderate heel height for walking.	This measure helps maintain proper alignment of back and hips.
Encourage smoking cessation.	Smoking causes vasoconstriction thus reducing circulation to disks.
Teach the following technique for sitting up at the bedside from a supine position: Logroll to the side, then rise to sitting position by pushing against the mattress with the hands while swinging legs over side of the bed. Instruct the patient to maintain alignment of the back during the procedure.	This technique prevents strain on the back and promotes good body alignment.
Caution the patient that pain is the signal to stop or change an activity or position.	This precaution helps prevent additional back injury.
Encourage the patient to continue with a regular exercise and stretching program, including PT as indicated, walking, and exercising in water.	PT and a graded exercise program are initiated after acute symptoms subside and are the mainstay of therapy for low back pain. Exercise strengthens abdominal, thoracic, and back muscles to help prevent subsequent back injury. High-impact activities such as running may be limited until the injury is well healed.
Teach the patient that the following indicators necessitate medical attention: increased sensory loss, increased motor loss/weakness, and loss of bowel and bladder function.	These indicators signal disk herniation, which necessitates timely intervention to prevent further damage.

Nursing diagnosis for patients undergoing diskectomy with laminectomy or fusion procedure

Nursing Diagnosis:

Deficient Knowledge

related to unfamiliarity with diskectomy with laminectomy or fusion procedure

Desired Outcomes: Before surgery, the patient verbalizes knowledge about the surgical procedure, preoperative routine, and postoperative regimen. The patient demonstrates activities and exercises correctly.

ASSESSMENT/INTERVENTIONS	RATIONALES
For general interventions, see this nursing diagnosis in "Perioperative Care," p. 45.	Surgery is performed without delay if signs of spinal cord compression are present, such as significant motor or sensory loss or loss of sphincter control. Otherwise, surgery is considered only after symptoms fail to respond to conservative therapy.
Instruct the patient to expect the surgical team to confirm verbally and then mark the correct spinal level and correct side (e.g., anterior, posterior, right, left) of the surgical site.	These confirmations ensure that the appropriate surgery will be performed.
Reinforce the surgeon's explanation about the following:	
- Microdiskectomy	The herniated portion of the disk and small parts of the lamina are removed, using microsurgical techniques. Patients are usually out of bed the first day and may be released as outpatients or discharged the next day.

ASSESSMENT/INTERVENTIONS

RATIONALES

ASSESSMENT/INTERVENTIONS	RATIONALES
- Diskectomy with laminectomy	An incision is made, enabling removal of part of the vertebra (laminectomy) so that the disk's herniated portion can be removed (diskectomy). If multiple intervertebral disk spaces are explored, a wound drain may be present after surgery.
- Percutaneous lumbar disk removal	Ultrasonic nucleotome cannula or fiberoptic arthroscopic cannula can be inserted into the intervertebral space via fluoroscopy to enable fragmentation of the disk and its aspiration. A laser may be used to aid in disk excision. This is a relatively less-invasive method of relieving pain from herniated disk, is done under local anesthesia, and may be performed on an outpatient basis.
- Spinal fusion	Fusion may be indicated for patients with recurrent low back or neck pain, spondylolisthesis, subluxation of the vertebrae, or with multilevel disease. Bone chips are harvested from the iliac crest or tibia and placed between vertebrae in the prepared area of the unstable spine to fuse and stabilize the area. Internal fixation (e.g., rods, wiring, pedicle screws, lateral mass screws, fusion cages, interbody implants, bone rings, and plates) may be necessary to provide added stability until the fusion has healed fully. If the patient's own bone quality or quantity is inadequate, allograft (e.g., cadaver) bone or use of a recombinant human osteogenic protein preparation ("bone putty") as a bone graft substitute or supplement may be considered.
- Intradiskal electrothermal treatment (IDET)	IDET employs a probe that uses electricity to heat and shrink collagen tissue within the annulus wall to seal up painful tears. After healing, the disk toughens and desensitizes.
- Total intervertebral disk replacement with artificial disks such as the Charité	This procedure may help reduce need for spinal fusions and avoid premature degeneration at adjacent levels of the spine.
- Diskoplasty	This procedure reduces or reshapes a bulging disk via a small puncture, threading a probe into the center of the disc, and using a laser or radiofrequency to remove/evaporate the disk's center.
Teach the technique for deep breathing. Also teach use of incentive spirometry.	Deep breathing and incentive spirometry are performed immediately after surgery to help expand the alveoli and aid in mobilizing lung secretions. Coughing may be contraindicated in the immediate postoperative period to prevent disruption of the fusion or surgical repair.
Document baseline and serial neurovascular checks, including color, capillary refill, pulse, warmth, muscle strength, movement, and sensation.	Vital signs and neurologic status are assessed at frequent intervals after surgery and compared with baseline to monitor trend.
[!] Teach the following signs and symptoms and importance of reporting them promptly: paresthesias, weakness, paralysis, radiculopathy, and changes in bowel or bladder function.	These indicators of impairment necessitate immediate attention by the health care staff because they signal presence of autonomic stimulation—signs of cord compression caused by bleeding or hematoma formation.
[!] Teach the following signs and symptoms and importance of reporting them promptly: increased heart rate (HR), thirst, faintness, or dizziness.	These are signs, along with decreased blood pressure, of hypovolemia and may occur because of blood loss. Patients undergoing fusion lose more blood during surgery than do those undergoing laminectomy.
Explain that the surgical dressing will be inspected for excess drainage or oozing at frequent intervals and that a closed wound drainage device may be present for 1-3 days postoperatively with a fusion procedure.	Bleeding with a laminectomy usually is minimal. Patients with a fusion may have slight bloody oozing postoperatively. Serous drainage usually is checked with a glucose reagent strip. Presence of glucose is a signal of cerebrospinal fluid (CSF) leakage. Bulging in the area of the wound may also signal CSF leakage or hematoma formation and should be reported promptly.
Advise that dressings will be inspected for increased drainage after the patient has been up, and lumbar dressings will be checked after each bedpan use. Inform the patient undergoing fusions that he or she will have a second dressing at the donor site.	Wet or contaminated dressings require prompt changing to prevent infection.

continued

PART I: Medical-Surgical Nursing

ASSESSMENT/INTERVENTIONS	RATIONALES
Instruct the patient to report any nausea or vomiting.	This helps ensure that antiemetics are given promptly. Vomiting could cause increased intraspinal pressure, which would result in pain.
Explain that the patient will be assessed for bowel and bladder dysfunction after the procedure.	Nerve injury during surgery can contribute to paralytic ileus. The abdomen will be checked for bowel sounds and distention. Patients may be asked to void within 8 hr of the procedure to check for urinary retention.
Caution the patient to avoid straining at stool.	Straining could cause increased intraspinal pressure, which would result in pain. Stool softeners may be given for that purpose.
Explain that fever may occur during first few days postoperatively but that this does not necessarily signal an infection.	Early fever may be caused by drainage and contamination of CSF. Patients will be assessed for other indicators of infection, such as heat, redness, irritation, swelling, or drainage at wound site.
Instruct the patient to report headache, neck stiffness, or photophobia.	These are possible signs of meningeal irritation.
Inform the patient that pain may take days or weeks to resolve and does not indicate that surgery was unsuccessful.	Postoperative pain or tingling (paresthesia) often is caused by nerve root irritation and edema. Spasms are common on the third or fourth postoperative day and should not discourage the patient.
Teach the patient to request medication for pain as needed and not let pain get out of control. Instruct in use of 0-10 pain scale.	Pain is easier to manage before it becomes severe. Prolonged stimulation of pain receptors results in increased sensitivity to painful stimuli and will increase the amount of analgesic required to relieve pain. Patients who have had a fusion may expect significant pain from the bone graft donor site (commonly the iliac crest). The donor site may have extra padding. Muscle relaxants may be prescribed to supplement pain control. Patient-controlled analgesia (PCA) and NSAIDs also may be used for postoperative pain control. Use of the pain scale enables more accurate assessment of relief obtained.
Explain that in the immediate postoperative period the patient will follow the surgeon's activity restrictions and that new techniques and stabilization devices may enable earlier mobilization (some the same day) and fewer activity restrictions.	Patients may be required to lie supine for several hours to minimize the possibility of wound hematoma formation. After this period, the head of bead (HOB) of laminectomy patients usually can be raised to 20 degrees to facilitate eating and bedpan use. Patients undergoing spinal fusion may be kept flat and on bedrest longer than patients with laminectomies. Activity progression for spinal fusion patients is usually more cautious and slower than for laminectomy patients. Best practice regarding trapeze use is to restrict it during the initial 24-48 hr following lumbar and cervical procedures and avoid its use after thoracic procedures because of the torque and weight strain trapeze use can have on the spine.
Teach the following logroll technique for turning: position a pillow between legs, cross arms across chest while turning, and contract long back muscles to maintain shoulders and pelvis in straight alignment. Explain that, initially, the patient will be assisted in this procedure.	Only the logroll method is used for turning. This method stabilizes the spine and maintains alignment to enable healing and prevent dislodgement of the bone graft if a fusion is done. A turning sheet and sufficient help are used when logrolling patients.
Teach the following technique for getting out of bed: logroll to side, splint back, and rise to a sitting position by pushing against the mattress while swinging legs over side of bed.	This technique facilitates ease of getting out of bed and prevents disruption of the bone graft for fusion patients.
Explain that initially the patient will be helped to a sitting position and should not push against the mattress. Teach the patient with a cervical laminectomy not to pull self up with arms. When assisting patients with cervical laminectomy to a sitting position, caution them not to put their arms on the nurse's shoulders.	While in hospital with an electric bed, the HOB may be raised to facilitate a sitting position. These restrictions prevent neck flexion, extension, and hyperextension and strain on the operative site and incision. Pillows can be used to support arms for comfort.
Explain that antiembolism hose and possibly sequential compression devices (SCDs) will be applied after surgery.	These garments and devices promote venous return and prevent thrombus formation while patient is on bedrest. SCDs or hose should be worn until the amount of time out of bed ambulating is equal to the amount of time in bed.
Teach techniques for ankle circling and calf pumping.	These techniques promote leg circulation.

ASSESSMENT/INTERVENTIONS	RATIONALES
[!] Teach the patient to report calf pain, tenderness, or warmth.	These are signs of deep vein thrombosis.
Advise the patient that the health care provider will prescribe certain postoperative activity restrictions.	Sitting is commonly restricted or allowed for only limited, prescribed periods in a straight-back chair.
Teach the patient not to sit for long periods on edge of the mattress.	A mattress does not provide enough support to the spine.
Explain that weakness, dizziness, and lightheadedness may occur on a first walk.	These problems may occur secondary to orthostatic hypotension. For management, see discussion in **Risk for Ineffective Cerebral Tissue Perfusion**, p. 67, in "Prolonged Bedrest."
Explain that the patient will be encouraged to walk progressively longer distances.	This action will promote endurance.
[!] Instruct the patient to avoid stretching, twisting, flexing, or jarring the spine. Explain that the spine should be kept aligned and in a neutral position and that lifting and pulling/pushing objects are to be avoided.	These restrictions help prevent vertebral collapse, shifting of bone graft, or a bleeding episode.
If the patient is scheduled for a cervical laminectomy or fusion, caution not to pull with arms on objects such as side rails and avoid twisting, flexion, and extensions of the neck.	These restrictions prevent torque and strain on the spine that could cause misalignment.
Explain that a cervical collar may be worn postoperatively.	The collar aids in immobilizing the cervical spine.
Teach use of braces or corsets if prescribed.	Persons undergoing a fusion procedure often wear a supportive brace or corset for 3 mo or less to keep the operative site immobile so that the graft will heal and not dislodge. Braces should be applied while in bed.
Explain the importance of wearing cotton underwear under the brace, powdering the skin lightly with cornstarch, or providing additional padding under braces.	These measures help protect skin from irritation. Skin should be inspected daily for irritation or breakdown.
Explain that driving or riding in car (may be restricted for 6-8 wk up to several mo), sexual activity, lifting and carrying objects, tub bathing (generally, soaking the incision is avoided until about 1 wk after sutures are out), going up and down stairs, amount of time to spend in and out of bed, back exercises, and expected time away from work will be discussed by the health care provider before discharge.	These guidelines and activity restrictions promote patient safety and an uneventful recovery once he or she is at home.
[!] Explain that the patient should call the health care provider for symptoms such as increased weakness and numbness or change in bowel or bladder function.	These are indicators of spinal cord or nerve compression.
Teach the importance of reporting the following to the health care provider: swelling, discharge, drainage, persistent redness, local warmth, fever, and pain.	These signs and symptoms of postoperative wound infection require timely intervention.
Caution the patient to keep the incision dry and open to the air.	Moisture can promote infection. Wet dressings should be changed promptly. After 24-48 hr, the incision is usually undressed to promote "air" drying.

Nursing diagnosis for patients undergoing anterior cervical fusion

Nursing Diagnosis:

Impaired Swallowing (or Risk for Same)

related to postoperative edema or hematoma formation

Desired Outcome: The patient regains uncompromised swallowing ability (usually by the third postoperative day) as evidenced by normal breath sounds and absence of food in the oral cavity or choking/coughing.

PART I: Medical-Surgical Nursing

ASSESSMENT/INTERVENTIONS	RATIONALES
As part of preoperative teaching, instruct the patient in the potential for difficulty with swallowing or managing secretions after anterior cervical fusion and of the need to report these problems promptly.	Postoperative edema or bleeding causing difficulty with swallowing is related to retraction of the trachea and esophagus during surgery to gain access to the disk. An informed individual likely will report postoperative difficulties with swallowing promptly for timely intervention.
Explain that a soft diet and throat lozenges may be prescribed for 2-3 days postoperatively.	A sore throat can be expected after this surgery as a result of surgical manipulation and/or endotracheal tube.
After surgery, assess for edema of the face or neck or tracheal compression or deviation that could compromise respiratory function. Assess for complaints of excessive pressure in the neck or severe, uncontrolled incisional pain. Promptly report significant findings.	These indicators may be signs of hematoma or bleeding at the operative site that could cause airway compromise and therefore necessitate immediate intervention.
Listen for hoarseness. Encourage voice rest and facilitate alternative communication (e.g., provide storyboards, pen and pencil, flash cards).	Hoarseness can indicate laryngeal nerve irritation and signal ineffective cough or swallowing difficulty and necessitate choking and aspiration precautions. For most patients with hoarseness, the voice usually will return to normal as inflammation around the laryngeal nerve subsides.
Report immediately any respiratory distress, stridor, inability to speak, worsening hoarseness, or voice change.	These may be signs of aspiration, laryngeal nerve involvement/irritation, or increased edema or hematoma formation affecting the laryngeal nerve and vocal cords, any of which can be life threatening and necessitate immediate intervention.
Assess for and report diminished breath sounds compared with the patient's normal or preoperative status.	Diminished breath sounds could signal that aspiration has occurred and may result in pneumonia.
As indicated, assess oximetry as a quantitative measure of systemic oxygenation.	Values 92% or less may signal need for supplemental oxygen.
Monitor closed suction devices, and recharge suction device/chamber as indicated.	Recharging the closed suction device facilitates wound drainage.
Check for gag and swallowing reflexes before oral intake.	Absence of gag and swallowing reflexes indicates that patient cannot begin oral intake. A postoperative diet with clear fluids and progression to more solid foods may begin only after patient demonstrates ability to ingest fluids safely.
Position the patient in Fowler's position, or semi-Fowler's position at minimum, when initiating fluid intake.	These positions minimize risk of aspiration by promoting movement of fluids by gravity to the stomach and into the pylorus.
If not prohibited by surgery, encourage use of the chin tuck to lessen potential for aspiration.	A chin tuck forces the trachea to close and the esophagus to open, thereby decreasing risk of aspiration.
Also see **Risk for Aspiration**, p. 93, in "Older Adult Care."	

ADDITIONAL NURSING DIAGNOSES/PROBLEMS:

✓ PATIENT-FAMILY TEACHING AND DISCHARGE PLANNING

When providing patient-family teaching, focus on sensory information, avoid giving excessive information, and initiate a visiting nurse referral for necessary follow-up teaching. Include verbal and written information about the following:

✓ Prescribed exercise regimen, including rationale for each exercise, technique for performing the exercise, number of repetitions of each, and frequency of exercise periods. If possible, ensure that the patient demonstrates understanding of exercise regimen and proper body mechanics before hospital discharge.

✓ Wound incision care. Indicators of postoperative wound infection that necessitate medical attention include swelling, discharge, persistent redness, local warmth, fever, and pain.

✓ Review of use and application of cervical collar for patients who have had a cervical fusion and importance of wearing collar at all times.

✓ Use and care of a brace or immobilizer if appropriate.

✓ Medications, including drug name, rationale, dosage, schedule, precautions, and potential side effects. Also discuss drug-drug, herb-drug, and food-drug interactions.

✓ Anticonstipation routine, which should be initiated during hospitalization.

✓ Pain control measures.

✓ Telephone number of a resource person in case questions arise after hospital discharge.

✓ Postsurgical activity restrictions as directed by the health care provider. These may affect the following: driving and riding in a car, returning to work, sexual activity, lifting and carrying, tub bathing, going up and down steps, and amount of time spent in or out of bed.

✓ Signs and symptoms of worsening neurologic function and the importance of notifying health care provider immediately if they develop. These include numbness, weakness, paralysis, and bowel and bladder dysfunction.

✓ Additional general information, which can be obtained by contacting *www.spine-health.com* or the Canadian Spine Society *at www.spinecanada.ca*

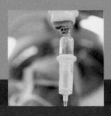

Multiple Sclerosis 38

OVERVIEW/PATHOPHYSIOLOGY

Multiple sclerosis (MS) has been classically thought of as an inflammatory disease characterized by remission and exacerbation. It is, however, an autoimmune/neurodegenerative disorder of the central nervous system (CNS) causing scattered and sporadic demyelination (plaques) and axonal damage (atrophy and black holes). In healthy individuals, myelin permits nerve impulses to travel quickly through the nerve pathways of the CNS. In response to the inflammation seen with MS, the myelin nerve sheaths scar, degenerate, or separate from the axon cylinders. This demyelination interrupts electrical nerve transmission and causes the wide variety of symptoms associated with MS. As less severe inflammation resolves, myelin function may regenerate, enabling electric nerve impulse transmission to be restored. If the inflammation is severe and/or repetitive, it causes irreversible destruction of myelin or axon degeneration. Involved areas are replaced by dense glial scar tissue that forms patchy areas of sclerotic plaque, which permanently damage conductive pathways of the CNS. Axon nerve fibers may degenerate. Axonal degeneration starts early in the disease process along with demyelination. Axonal damage is speculated to cause the permanent and progressive disability. Deficits presenting after 3 mo usually are permanent.

The course of MS is highly variable. Multifocal presentation and frequent attacks during the first year may imply a more aggressive course. Presently four forms of MS are considered. See Table 38-1.

Terms such as clinically isolated syndrome (CIS) and radiologic isolated syndrome (RIS) are now common in the literature. CIS refers to a single, acute neurologic event such as optic neuritis. RIS refers to MRI lesions consistent with MS but patients have not had a clinical event to date. It may be determined that these are actually the earliest forms of MS presentation. To date, patients are considered high risk for MS but do not carry that diagnosis.

Sometimes reference is made to " benign" MS (5%-10% of patients) in which full recovery occurs after a neurologic event.

Typically, an increasing number of symptoms occur with each exacerbation, with less complete clearing of symptoms and with deficits becoming cumulative. Over time, the relapsing-remitting form usually transitions to the secondary progressive form in which neurologic impairment progresses continuously with or without superimposed relapses. A small portion of patients (10%-20%) initially begin with the primary progressive form, characterized by gradual ongoing accumulation of symptoms and deficits, with absence of clear-cut exacerbations and remissions. The progressive relapsing form (5%) is characterized by a progressive disease course from onset, with clear acute exacerbations. Progression continues during the periods between disease exacerbations.

HEALTH CARE SETTING

Primary care, neurology clinic, physiatry/rehabilitation, psychiatry/mental health, pain clinic, or long-term care, with possible hospitalization resulting from complications

ASSESSMENT

Onset of MS can be extremely rapid, or it can be insidious, with exacerbations and remissions. Signs and symptoms vary widely, depending on site and extent of pathology and can change from day to day. Early symptoms can be vague, including fatigue, weakness, heaviness, clumsiness, numbness, and tingling. Optic neuritis is the most common presentation for MS diagnosis. Trigeminal neuralgia is also fairly common.

Damage to motor nerve tracts: Weakness, paralysis, and spasticity. Fatigue is common. Diplopia may occur secondary to ocular muscle involvement.

Damage to cerebellar or brain stem regions: Intention tremor, nystagmus, or other tremors; incoordination, ataxia; and weakness of facial and throat muscles resulting in difficulty chewing, dysphagia, dysarthria, dizziness, nausea, and vomiting.

Damage to sensory nerve tracts: Often, only sensory symptoms occur in the beginning and may include altered perception of pain, touch, and temperature; allodynia (pain caused by simple touch); paresthesias such as numbness and tingling ("pins and needles") or burning sensations; decrease or loss of proprioception; and decrease or loss of vibratory sense. Optic neuritis is a common early symptom, potentially causing partial or total loss of vision, visual clouding or shimmering, and pain with eye movement.

Damage to cerebral cortex (especially frontal lobes): Mood swings, inappropriate affect, euphoria, apathy, irritability,

Table 38-1   Forms of Multiple Sclerosis

Types of MS	Comments
Relapsing-remitting [RRMS]	Up to 85% of MS patients Marked by relapse/exacerbations followed by recovery and a period of stability.
Secondary-progressive [SPMS]	About 50% of RRMS patients will develop this over time Patients have gradual worsening over time; may have plateaus at times.
Progressive-relapsing [PRMS]	Acute relapses occur but disease progression continues between events.
Primary-progressive [PPMS]	Found in 10%-15% of patients; males outnumber females Gradual onset of symptoms that worsen with time. No definitive relapses/exacerbations.

depression, hyperexcitability, poor memory, judgment, foresight and planning, and abstract reasoning. There is often difficulty with word finding, concentration, attention, and processing or learning new information.

Damage to motor and sensory control centers: Urinary frequency, urgency, or retention; urinary and fecal incontinence; constipation.

Lower cord lesions (low thoracic and lumbar): Impotence; diminished sensations that result in inhibited sexual response.

Physical assessment: Motor or sensory impairment as discussed above. Lhermitte's sign may be present, in which an electrical sensation runs down the back and legs during neck flexion. Ophthalmoscopic inspection may reveal temporal pallor of optic disks. Reflex assessment may show increased deep tendon reflexes (DTRs) and diminished abdominal skin and cremasteric reflexes.

History/risk factors: Although the cause of MS is unknown, it is generally believed to result from a combination of environmental factors (e.g., geographic location of the individual pre-puberty; low vitamin D [sun] exposure), exposure to infectious agents (e.g., Epstein-Barr virus), and genetic predisposition. It is generally accepted that risk is 1 in 750 in the general population. If there is a family history, the risk is generally believed to be between 3% and 5%. MS is most common among people who have lived in cool, temperate climates before puberty. African Americans have half the incidence of white Americans. More females than males are affected (3:1). Onset ranges from pediatric ages to geriatric ages. It is most commonly diagnosed between 20 and 40 yr of age. Exacerbations may be fewer during pregnancy but increase postpartum up to 6 mo. Heat, fever, and infection tend to aggravate symptoms.

DIAGNOSTIC TESTS

Note: *MS is diagnosed by the classic "separation of time and space." This means there needs to be a distinction of two separate lesions at two distinct time intervals. MS is most commonly diagnosed using the McDonald criteria that rely heavily on MRI and to a lesser extent on paraclinical data to determine separation of time and space.*

MRI scan: Reveals presence of plaques and demyelination in the CNS. This is the test of choice when MS is suspected. Expanding MRI technology is becoming ever more sensitive and capable of identifying current sites of inflammation and demyelination and showing changes associated with disease progression. T1-weighted MRI may show hypointense lesions including black holes, which correlate with axonal loss and indicates old lesions. T2-weighted MRI can show old and new lesions and is most commonly used to follow response to treatment by many clinicians. Gadolinium enhancement shows areas of active demyelination. Fluid attenuated inversion recovery (FLAIR) is very helpful in detecting cerebral lesions specific to MS. All other forms of MRI are used strictly for research related to MS and can include MRI diffusion tensor imaging and magnetic resonance (MR) spectroscopy, which frequently reveal involvement of otherwise normal-appearing white matter. Magnetization transfer imaging may show indirect evidence of axonal loss. MR spectroscopy can measure decline in a brain chemical called N-acetylaspartate (NAA) as a marker of axonal damage and appears to predict disease severity. Functional MRI (fMRI) can show new lesions, and short tau inversion recovery (STIR) is useful in detecting demyelination.

EP studies: May be slow or absent because of interference of nerve transmission from demyelination or plaque formation. Visual EP (VEP) studies are most commonly used to evaluate optic nerve demyelination.

Lumbar puncture and cerebrospinal fluid (CSF) analysis: Evaluates CSF levels of oligoclonal bands and free kappa chains of immunoglobulin G (IgG), protein, gamma globulin, myelin basic protein, and lymphocytes, any of which may be elevated in the presence of MS. During acute MS attacks, destruction of the myelin sheath releases myelin basic protein into the CSF. Oligoclonal bands of IgG are seen in 85%-95% of patients with MS. This and the finding of free kappa chains in the CSF support a diagnosis of MS.

Computed tomography (CT) scan: Demonstrates presence of plaques and rules out mass lesions. This technique is less effective than MRI in detecting areas of plaque and demyelination and is no longer commonly used as part of the diagnostic workup if MRI is available.

Nursing Diagnosis:

Chronic Pain (and spasms)

related to motor and sensory nerve tract damage

Desired Outcomes: Within 1-2 hr of intervention, the patient's subjective evaluation of pain and spasms improves, as documented by pain scale. Objective indicators, such as grimacing, are absent or reduced.

ASSESSMENT/INTERVENTIONS	RATIONALES
Maintain a comfortable room temperature. Advise patients to keep the environment cool in warm weather and avoid hot baths or showers.	Heat tends to aggravate MS symptoms by increasing core body temperature.
Provide passive, assisted, or active range of motion q2h and periodic stretching exercises. Teach these exercises to the patient and significant others, and encourage their performance several times daily. Explain that sleeping in a prone position may help decrease flexor spasm of the hips and knees and that splints or cones for hands with elastic bands may help control hand spasms.	These interventions reduce muscle tightness and spasms, maintain joint function, and prevent contractures. Physical therapy (PT), occupational therapy (OT), and assistive devices or braces may be prescribed to maintain mobility and independence with activities of daily living (ADLs). Placing weights on the affected limbs may help with mild tremors.
Administer antispasmodics as prescribed.	These agents help decrease spasms, thus ultimately decreasing pain. In addition, there may be a secondary benefit with decrease in neuropathic pain. Classically used are baclofen and tizanidine. Dantrolene is an older medication that is still sometimes used, but it can cause sedation. Atypical medications are gabapentin and levetiracetam. They are usually well tolerated and cause little to no sedation. Severe spasticity may be treated with IM injections of botulinum toxin or intrathecal baclofen administered continually via a surgically implanted pump.
Administer tranquilizers (e.g., diazepam) as prescribed.	These medications may be given for both their anxiety-reducing and muscle relaxant effects, which may help spasms and tremors.
Administer analgesics (e.g., acetaminophen) and neuropathic pain medications as prescribed.	Neuropathic pain medications include anticonvulsants such as carbamazepine, gabapentin, topiramate, and lamotrigine (see "Seizures and Epilepsy," p. 309, for side effects/precautions), and tricyclic antidepressants (e.g., amitriptyline or imipramine). Uncontrolled pain may require nerve blocks or surgical intervention.
For other interventions, see "General Care of Patients with Neurologic Disorders," **Acute Pain,** p. 256.	

Nursing Diagnosis:

Deficient Knowledge

related to unfamiliarity with MS symptoms and factors that affect MS pathology.

Desired Outcome: By day 3 (or before hospital discharge), the patient and significant other verbalize factors that exacerbate, prevent, and ameliorate symptoms of MS.

ASSESSMENT/INTERVENTIONS	RATIONALES
Assess the patient's health care literacy (language, reading, comprehension). Assess culture and culturally specific information needs. Determine patient's knowledge base about MS.	This assessment helps ensure that materials are selected and presented in a manner that is culturally and educationally appropriate.
Teach the patient to avoid heat, both external (hot weather, bath) and internal (fever).	Heat tends to aggravate weakness, pain, and other symptoms of MS.

ASSESSMENT/INTERVENTIONS	RATIONALES
Teach preventive measures, such as avoiding hot baths or showers and using acetaminophen or aspirin to reduce fever, if present. Also suggest body cooling products such as vests, wrist wraps, or neck wraps or drinking ice cold water and using fan/air conditioning if available.	These measures aid in maintaining homeostasis of core body temperature.
Caution the patient to avoid exposure to persons known to have significant infections and take precautions against developing an infection.	Infection often precedes exacerbations. Some MS medications can make the patient more susceptible to infections. Patients should be given instructions in the proper technique for hand washing and hand antisepsis and the importance of avoiding vaccinations with live attenuated viruses, which could trigger an exacerbation.
Teach indicators of common infections and the importance of seeking prompt medical treatment in case they occur. Instruct the patient to check for typical signs/symptoms of UTI (increased frequency, urgency, or incontinence) and to check urine for changes in odor or presence of cloudiness or blood. Advise that an acute increase in spasticity can often signal an infection in MS. Also teach how to monitor for more serious infections such as pyelonephritis (e.g., fever, costovertebral angle tenderness, chills, flank pain).	A person with MS is especially susceptible to UTI because of bladder dysfunction. Because of the disease process, patients may not feel any pain with urination and therefore need to be alert to other signs of UTI. See "Care of the Renal Transplant Recipient," p. 220, for a discussion of common infections.
Teach the relationship between stress and fatigue to the exacerbations. Encourage the patient to reduce factors that cause stress. Encourage use of stress reduction techniques such as progressive relaxation, self-coaching, and guided imagery.	Avoiding stress and fatigue may prevent exacerbations.
Teach the patient and significant others the signs and symptoms of depression. If the patient is depressed, suggest that he or she discuss use of antidepressants (e.g., SSRIs, NSRIs) and counseling with a health care provider.	Depression rates in MS are significantly higher with a higher risk for suicide than the general population. It has an intrinsic cause from cerebral lesions resulting in a decrease in neurochemicals. It can also be caused by extrinsic factors such as loss of self-esteem and role within the family unit or career. Depression can compound fatigue, cognitive function, and sleep issues in MS.
Encourage the patient to get sufficient rest, stop activity short of fatigue, schedule activity and rest periods, and conserve energy in ADLs.	Patients can conserve energy during ADLs by sitting while getting dressed, rather than standing; sliding heavy objects along work surfaces, rather than lifting them; using a wheeled cart to transport items; having work surfaces at the proper height; and using assistive devices and delegating.
Suggest that the patient ask the health care provider about antifatigue medications and discuss possible contributing factors to fatigue such as depression, sleep difficulties, or metabolic issues.	Fatigue is the most common complaint in MS and does not correlate with the level of disability. Oftentimes co-morbidities (i.e., thyroid issues, low B12, anemia, sleep apnea, depression) can magnify the problem. Antifatigue drugs (e.g., amantadine, fluoxetine, modafinil) help relieve fatigue associated with MS. See "Parkinsonism," p. 299, for side effects and precautions when using amantadine.
Encourage the patient to plan each day, break projects into smaller tasks, distribute tasks throughout the day, rest before difficult tasks, take planned recovery time after tasks, identify priorities, and eliminate nonessential activities.	Conserving energy and decreasing fatigue are effective strategies for improving quality of life.
Discuss the need for family planning with both men and women. Provide information about birth control measures to female patients who desire counseling.	Patients are often on polypharmaceuticals. Drug-modifying therapies (DMTs) are contraindicated in pregnancy, and some of these medications can affect males as well as females. There may be a decreased relapse rate during pregnancy but increased exacerbations postpartum. Those planning a pregnancy should consult and work with their health care providers before pregnancy.
Encourage exercise, continued activity, and normal lifestyle even when limitations are necessary.	Deconditioning can contribute to a decreased functional level and quality of life. Exercise often decreases many MS symptoms, and a planned exercise program can be incorporated into a scheduled activity/rest plan.

Nursing Diagnosis:
Deficient Knowledge

related to unfamiliarity with MS exacerbations and medication management
of MS

Desired Outcome: By day 3 (or before hospital or clinic discharge), the patient verbalizes
accurate information about the prescribed medications.

ASSESSMENT/INTERVENTIONS	RATIONALES
Assess the patient's knowledge base about the prescribed medications. As indicated, provide verbal instructions and language-appropriate written handouts that describe name, purpose, dose, and schedule of the prescribed medications. Also discuss drug-drug, herb-drug, and food-drug interactions.	A well-informed patient is likely to follow the prescribed medication regimen, recognize side effects, and report those that necessitate prompt attention.
Educate the patient and significant others about DMTs: *glatiramer injections, interferon injections, infusion treatments, or oral therapies.*	DMTs are prescribed to help manage the disease process itself by reducing relapse rates, progression to disability, and MRI lesion accumulation. DMT treatment is long-term therapy and needs to be taken as prescribed on an ongoing basis.
❗ - Teach the side effect profile consistent with the patient's DMT.	DMTs have potentially very serious side effects. Patients and significant others need to know what and how to monitor for these and also when to notify their health care provider. Each DMT has specific resources available for this type of education. In addition there are many MS organizations that can help with this information.
- Notify the health care provider of any and all side effects.	Side effects need to be evaluated to determine the next course of action. Many side effects can be managed with minimal intervention. Some side effects warrant immediate discontinuation of the medication.
- Teach the specific issues related to the prescribed DMT.	Each DMT has very specific issues in maintaining efficacy, potency, and safety. For example, frequency, timing, and route of administration; screening/monitoring of blood work and other surveillance protocols; seriousness of non-adherence, which varies with DMTs and can be potentially fatal with certain DMTs.
Encourage the patient and significant others to become educated about MS, MS exacerbations, and MS symptoms. Encourage use of reputable web sites, MS organizations, and support groups; attending lectures from MS experts; and subscribing to MS publications (most are free).	MS is a complicated and dynamic disease process. Patients and significant others should understand the difference between MS symptoms and exacerbation, the importance of DMTs, the difference between DMTs vs. medication to manage symptoms and medications to treat exacerbations. Education helps maintain better adherence to treatments and interventions.
Teach about exacerbation treatment: use of high-dose steroids (i.e., prednisone, methylprednisolone, decadron) or similar products (e.g., ACTH).	The purpose of medications used to treat exacerbation is to reduce symptoms by decreasing inflammation and associated edema of the myelin, thereby hastening reduction of presenting symptoms.
- Educate the patient and significant others about the side effects of associated treatment.	Usually exacerbations are treated in the home environment. Therefore it is essential that side effects are understood and recognized so that they can be reported to the health care provider promptly.
❗ - Explain that tapering rather than abruptly stopping high-dose steroids when they are discontinued may be appropriate for some patients.	Tapering helps maintain the body's own cortisone sources. Abrupt discontinuation may result in adrenal crisis or psychosis.
- Teach symptoms of potassium deficiency, such as anorexia, nausea, and muscle weakness, and to eat foods high in potassium.	Hypokalemia is a common side effect of steroid use. Potassium supplements also may be prescribed.
- Teach the patient to eat a diet low in sodium and monitor for and report unusual weight gain or swelling of extremities.	A low-sodium diet minimizes the potential for fluid retention, which is a common occurrence with steroids. Diuretics may be prescribed to reduce fluid retention.

ASSESSMENT/INTERVENTIONS

ASSESSMENT/INTERVENTIONS	RATIONALES
- Teach the patient to measure blood pressure daily.	Hypertension is another side effect of steroid medications. Home blood pressure kits are available at most drug stores. Antihypertensives may be prescribed.
- Teach the patient to monitor blood glucose for hyperglycemia, report elevations, and as indicated, control glucose level with diet, oral agents, or insulin.	Hyperglycemia is a side effect of steroid use. In patients with known diabetes mellitus, a sliding scale insulin therapy is prescribed at the onset of treatment.
- Teach the patient to monitor for and report gastrointestinal (GI) symptoms, including tarry stools.	Tarry stools may signal occult blood, which can occur because of gastric ulcers, a common side effect of steroid use.
- Teach the patient to take the medication with food, milk, or buffering agents and to avoid aspirin, indomethacin, caffeine, or other GI irritants while taking this medication.	These measures help prevent stomach upset and gastric irritation. In addition to antacids, histamine H2-receptor blockers may be prescribed to prevent gastric ulcer.
- Teach the patient to monitor injuries and report wounds that are slow in healing.	Steroids can impair wound healing.
- Caution the patient to avoid contact with persons known to have infections and to monitor for and report fever, prolonged sore throat, and colds or other infections.	Steroids can mask infections, making them appear less severe; therefore, follow-up with the care provider is important.
- Advise the patient to be alert for and to report mood changes.	Antipsychotropic agents may be prescribed to help with mood changes associated with steroid use.

ADDITIONAL NURSING DIAGNOSES/PROBLEMS:

✓ PATIENT-FAMILY TEACHING AND DISCHARGE PLANNING

There are different forms of MS and the patient with MS may have a wide variety of symptoms. MS can cause disability ranging from mild to severe. When providing patient-family teaching, focus on treatment in terms of managing the disease itself via DMTs, treatment of exacerbation with steroids, and treatment of symptoms. Avoid giving excessive information, and initiate a visiting nurse referral for necessary follow-up

teaching. Include verbal and written information about the following:

✓ Exacerbation aspects of the disease process and progression. Explain effects of demyelination and neuronal injury on sensory and motor function and factors that aggravate symptoms. Explain that DMTs are proactive treatments that interfere with the natural history of the disease and have a positive impact on exacerbation rates, disability progression, and lesion activity. Additional treatment is symptomatic and supportive.

✓ Safety measures relative to decreased sensation, visual disturbances, and motor deficits.

✓ Medications, including drug name, purpose, dosage, frequency, precautions, and potential side effects. Also discuss drug-drug, herb-drug, and food-drug interactions.

✓ Exercises that promote muscle strength and mobility, measures for reducing spasticity and increasing strength, promote quality of life, and maintain safety. For more severe disabilities, preventing contractures and skin breakdown, transfer techniques and proper body mechanics, and use of assistive devices and other measures to maximize health and wellness are incorporated.

✓ Measures for relieving pain, muscle spasms, or other discomfort.

✓ Indications of constipation, urinary retention, or UTI; implementation of bowel and bladder training programs; and self-catheterization technique or care of indwelling urinary catheters.

✓ Indications of upper respiratory infection (URI); implementation of measures that help prevent regurgitation, aspiration, and respiratory infection.

✓ Measures for managing fatigue.

✓ Measures for fall prevention.

✓ Dietary adjustments that may be appropriate for neurologic deficit (e.g., soft, semisolid foods for patients with chewing difficulties or a high-fiber diet for patients experiencing constipation).

✓ Importance of follow-up care, including visits to the health care provider, PT, and OT, as well as speech, sexual, or psychologic counseling to help the patient and significant other cope and adapt to real or potential lifestyle changes functionally, emotionally, economically, and socially that are either a direct or an indirect result of the disease process.

✓ Referrals to community resources, such as local and national Multiple Sclerosis Society chapters, public health nurse, visiting nurse association, community support groups, social workers, psychologists, vocational rehabilitation agencies, home health agencies, extended and skilled care facilities, and financial counseling. Additional general information can be obtained by contacting the following:

• National Multiple Sclerosis Society at *www .nationalmssociety.org*

• Multiple Sclerosis Foundation at *www.msfacts.org*

• Multiple Sclerosis Association of America at *www .msaa.com*

• MS Views 7 News at *www.msviewsandnews.org*

• MS World at *www.msworld.org*

• Multiple Sclerosis International Federation at *www .msif.org*

• MS Perspectives at *www.MSperspectives.com*

• Multiple Sclerosis Society of Canada at *www .mssociety.ca*

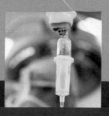

Parkinsonism 39

OVERVIEW/PATHOPHYSIOLOGY

Parkinson's disease (PD) is a slowly progressive degenerative disorder of the central nervous system (CNS) affecting the brain centers that regulate movement and balance. For unknown reasons, cell death occurs in the substantia nigra of the midbrain. When healthy, the substantia nigra projects dopaminergic neurons into the corpus striatum and releases the neurotransmitter dopamine in that area. Degeneration of these neurons leads to an abnormally low concentration of dopamine in the basal ganglia. The basal ganglia control muscle tone and voluntary motor movement via a balance between two main neurotransmitters, dopamine and acetylcholine. The deficit of dopamine, which has an inhibitory effect, allows the relative excess of acetylcholine. The excitatory effect of acetylcholine causes overactivity of the basal ganglia, which interferes with normal muscle tone and control of smooth, purposeful movement, causing the characteristic symptoms of PD: muscle rigidity, tremors, and slowness of movement. Nerve cell loss in the substantia nigra and accumulation of Lewy bodies in the brain stem and pigmented areas of the brain are the pathologic hallmarks of PD. Lewy bodies are tiny abnormal spherical alpha-synuclein protein deposits that accumulate inside the damaged nerve cells and disrupt the brain's normal functioning. Symptoms start when cell loss reaches about 80%.

Approximately 1% of all individuals older than 60 yr have this disease. PD is usually progressive, and death can result from aspiration pneumonia or choking. *Neuroleptic malignant syndrome,* a medical emergency, is usually precipitated by failure to take the prescribed medications. *Acute akinesia,* sometimes referred to as *parkinsonian crisis,* is another medical emergency and seems associated with infections or surgical procedures.

HEALTH CARE SETTING

Primary care, neurology clinic, rehabilitation facility, long-term care facility, and possible acute care hospitalization resulting from complications as the disease progresses

ASSESSMENT

Initially, symptoms are mild and include stiffness or slight hand tremors. They gradually increase and can become disabling. Cardinal features are tremors, rigidity, and akinesia/bradykinesia and postural disturbances/loss of reflexes. Presentation is ipsilateral and will become bilateral with progression. Clinical features most suggestive of idiopathic PD include unilateral onset, presence of resting tremor, and a clear-cut response to treatment with L-dopa. Assessment findings vary in degree and are highly individualized. PD is sometimes categorized as either tremor-dominant type or postural instability and gait disturbance (PIGD)-dominant type.

Tremors: Increase when the limb is at rest and completely supported against gravity, and stop with voluntary movement and during sleep (nonintentional "resting" tremor). "Pill-rolling" tremor of the hands and "to-and-fro" tremor of the head are typical.

Bradykinesia: Slowness of movement, stiffness of muscles, gait difficulty, and difficulty initiating movement. Patients may have a masklike, blank facial expression; "unblinking" stare; difficulty chewing and swallowing; drooling caused by decreased frequency of swallowing; and a high-pitched, monotone, weak voice. Speech may be slow and slurred. The patient also has loss of automatic associated movements, such as the normal arm-swing movement, difficulty getting out of a chair, and a small-step or shuffling gait when walking. Episodes of freezing are common and can be seen with gait initiation, in tight areas such as doorways, and in interrupted gait fluidity. Handwriting becomes progressively smaller, cramped, and tremulous (micrographia).

Increased muscle rigidity: Limb muscles become rigid on passive motion. Typically, this rigidity results in jerky ("cogwheel") motions or steady resistance to all movement ("lead-pipe" rigidity).

Loss of postural reflexes: Causes the typical stooped, forward-leaning, shuffling, propulsive gait with short, rapidly accelerating steps; stumbling; and difficulty maintaining or regaining balance, which makes the individual prone to stumbling and falling. Abnormal gait in which the body is bent backward (retropulsion) also may be present.

Autonomic: Excessive diaphoresis, seborrhea, postural hypotension, decreased libido, hypomotility of the gastrointestinal (GI) tract (causing constipation), and urinary hesitancy. Vision may blur as a result of lost accommodation.

Mental health/psychiatric: Dementia (e.g., forgetfulness, irritability, paranoia, hallucinations) is commonly associated with PD. However, not all patients develop impaired intellectual and mental functioning. Mental status testing may be complicated by the patient's movement disorder. Some patients may experience akathisia, a condition of motor restlessness, which can be as mild as a feeling of inner distress to a compelling need to walk about constantly. Depression is common. Psychosis is often drug-induced.

Neuroleptic malignant syndrome: The classic triad of symptoms includes fever (100%), rigidity (90%), and cognitive changes (e.g., drowsiness, confusion progressing to stupor and coma). Other symptoms include tremor, tachypnea, diaphoresis, and occasionally dystonia and chorea. Symptoms are associated with discontinuation or reduction in dopaminergic medications. This sudden and severe increase in muscle rigidity can cause inability to swallow or maintain a patent airway.

Acute akinesia: This sudden decrease in motor performance or inability to move ("frozen") lasts for more than 48 hr and is transiently unresponsive to dopaminergic rescue medication (e.g., apomorphine) or increases in dopaminergic medications. Triggering factors include infections, surgery, fractures, GI disease, and drug manipulations.

Oculogyric crisis: Fixation of eyes in one position, generally upward, sometimes for several hours. This is relatively rare.

Physical assessment: Usually a positive glabellar blink reflex (Myerson's sign) is elicited by tapping a finger between the patient's eyebrows. Normally individuals will blink several times before the reflex is extinguished. In PD the patient cannot extinguish the response and continues to blink until the stimulus (tapping) is removed. A positive palmomental (palm-chin) reflex can be elicited (ipsilateral muscles of the chin and corner of mouth contract when the patient's palm is stroked). Diminished postural reflexes are present on neurologic examination; however, there is risk of injury with this test because patients may quickly lose balance and fall.

History/risk factors: PD has many possible causes. Metabolic causes such as hypothyroidism need to be ruled out.

Long-term therapy with large doses of medications, such as haloperidol, phenothiazines, metoclopramide, methyldopa, reserpine, or chlorpromazine can produce extrapyramidal side effects known as pseudoparkinsonism. If caused by these medications, symptoms will disappear when the drug is discontinued, although it may take up to several months. The recreational drug "ecstasy" and an improperly synthesized heroin-like substance, 1-methyl-4-phenyl-1,2,3,6-tetrahydropyridine (MPTP), also have induced parkinsonism. Other causes include toxins (e.g., heavy metals, pesticides, lacquer thinner, and carbon monoxide), cerebrovascular disease, head injury (especially repeated injury), and viral encephalitis. Living in a rural area is associated with increased PD risk, while nicotine intake is associated with decreased PD risk. The vast majority of cases of PD occurs without an apparent or known cause, although genetic susceptibility is believed to play a role. Genetic factors appear to be more predominant when the disease begins before the age of 45-50, with the most common known forms of hereditary parkinsonism caused by mutations in the parkin gene (PARK2) and alpha-synuclein gene.

Unified PD rating scale: May be used as a standardized assessment tool and includes evaluation of self-reported disability (i.e., inability to perform activities of daily living) as well as clinical scoring by a health care provider.

Hoehn and Yahr stage scale: Simple and popular scale that establishes PD severity. The different stages of disease are classified from I (mild) to V (severe).

DIAGNOSTIC TESTS

Diagnosis usually is made on the basis of physical assessment of the characteristic symptoms, a ruling out of other causes of pathology, and a positive response to L-dopa therapy.

Nursing Diagnosis:

Risk for Falls

related to unsteady gait occurring with bradykinesia, tremors, rigidity, and postural instability

Desired Outcome: Following instruction, the patient demonstrates safe and effective ambulatory techniques and preventive measures against falls and remains free of trauma.

ASSESSMENT/INTERVENTIONS	RATIONALES
Assess ambulation and movement for deficit(s).	This assessment will help the nurse tailor interventions specific to the patient's deficit(s).
During ambulation, encourage the patient to deliberately swing the arms and raise the feet.	These actions assist gait, thereby helping to prevent falls.
Advise the patient to step over an imaginary object or line, practice taking long steps, and avoid shuffling.	This will help raise the feet higher and increase the stride, which will help prevent falls.

ASSESSMENT/INTERVENTIONS	RATIONALES
Have the patient practice movements that are especially difficult (e.g., turning). Teach the patient to walk in a wide arc ("U-turn") rather than pivot when turning.	These actions prevent crossing of one leg over the other and causing a fall.
Teach head and neck exercises.	These exercises promote good posture, which in turn helps the gait.
Remind the patient repeatedly to maintain an upright posture and look up, not down, especially when walking.	This is particularly important for patients with bifocal glasses inasmuch as a stooped posture promotes looking down through the reading portion of the bifocal lens where distant items are blurred.
Advise the patient to stop or consciously slow down periodically. Teach the patient to concentrate on listening to the feet as they touch the floor and to count cadence to prevent too fast a gait.	This will slow the walking speed, which is less likely to result in falls.
Encourage the patient to lift the toes and to walk with the heels touching the floor first.	This action keeps soles of the feet flat on the floor, which is less likely to cause tripping.
Remind the patient to maintain a wide-based gait.	This gait improves balance.
Provide a clear pathway while the patient is walking. Teach the patient to avoid crowds, scatter rugs, uneven surfaces, fast turns, narrow doorways, and obstructions.	These actions minimize the risk of tripping and falling.
Encourage range of motion and stretching exercises daily.	Exercising promotes flexibility, strength, gait, and balance, thereby decreasing the risk of falls. Routine exercises, along with the prescribed medications, may prevent or delay disability.
Advise the patient to wear leather-soled or smooth-soled shoes but to test shoes to ensure they are not too slippery.	Rubber-soled or crepe-soled shoes tend to catch on floors, especially carpeted floors, and may cause falls.
Encourage the patient not to hurry or rush.	Hurrying may precipitate falls.
Encourage males to keep a urinal at the bedside. A commode at the bedside may be helpful for females.	Slowness of gait and inability to get to the bathroom fast enough may cause incontinence or falls in an effort to get there.
Ask the physical therapy department to suggest exercises that improve balance.	Tai chi, for example, uses slow, graceful movements to relax and strengthen muscles and joints and may be encouraged as an option for some patients.
For other interventions, see **Risk for Falls,** p. 252, in "General Care of Patients with Neurologic Disorders."	

Nursing Diagnosis:

Impaired Physical Mobility

related to difficulty initiating movement

Desired Outcome: Following instruction, the patient demonstrates measures that enhance ability to initiate desired movement.

ASSESSMENT/INTERVENTIONS	RATIONALES
Assess mobility and movements.	This assessment will enable the nurse to tailor interventions to the patient's specific needs.
For patients having difficulty initiating movement, teach measures that may help.	Patients with PD often have difficulty initiating movement because their disease affects the brain centers that regulate movement and balance. Rocking from side to side may help initiate leg movement. Marching in place a few steps before resuming forward motion also may be helpful. Other measures include relaxing back on the heels and raising the toes; tapping the hip of the leg to be moved; bending at the knees and straightening up; raising the arms in a sudden, short motion; or humming a marching tune.
If the feet remain "glued" to the floor despite these measures, suggest that the patient think of something else for a few moments and then try again.	It might help also to try changing directions (e.g., move sideways if going forward is impossible).

continued

PART I: Medical-Surgical Nursing

ASSESSMENT/INTERVENTIONS	RATIONALES
Teach the patient to get out of a chair by getting to edge of seat, placing hands on arm supports, bending forward slightly, moving the feet back, and then rhythmically rocking in the chair a few times before trying to get up.	The deficit of dopamine, which has an inhibitory effect, allows the relative excess of acetylcholine. The excitatory effect of acetylcholine causes overactivity of the basal ganglia, which interferes with normal muscle tone and the control of smooth, purposeful movement, causing the characteristic symptoms of PD: muscle rigidity, tremors, and slowness of movement. These combined problems make it difficult to get out of a chair.
Advise the patient to sit in chairs with backs and arms and to purchase elevated toilet seats or sidebars in the bathroom.	These items will assist with rising from a sitting position and help prevent falls.
Teach measures that may help with getting out of bed: rocking to a sitting position, placing blocks under legs of the head of bed to elevate it, and tying a rope or sheet to the foot of bed to help the patient pull to a sitting position.	See discussion with getting out of a chair, above.
Teach the patient and significant others to recognize situations that can cause freezing episodes.	"Freezing" is variable and can fluctuate with stress or emotional state. For example, attempting two movements simultaneously, such as trying to change direction quickly while walking, can cause freezing. Distracting environmental, visual, or auditory stimuli also can precipitate a freezing episode. Doorways; narrow passages; or a change in floor color, texture, or slope can pose problems for many patients.
Provide a referral to an organization such as Canine Partners as indicated.	Specially trained dogs (e.g., Canine Partners) can help patients walk and get up after a fall and are trained to help break a "freeze" by tapping on the individual's foot.
Suggest that sexual relations be planned for when the prescribed drug is working to good effect and the person is rested. Being flexible about time; experimenting with positions; use of manual, oral, and vibrator stimulation; and use of sildenafil have proved beneficial.	PD makes it more difficult to move, which can affect intimacy.

Nursing Diagnosis:

Deficient Knowledge

related to unfamiliarity with side effects of and precautionary measures for taking anti-Parkinson medications

Desired Outcome: Following instruction and before hospital discharge, the patient and significant other verbalize knowledge about side effects of and necessary precautionary measures for taking anti-Parkinson medications.

> **Note:** *Teach the patient and significant other to report adverse side effects promptly because many side effects are dose related and can be controlled by a dosage adjustment.*

ASSESSMENT/INTERVENTIONS	RATIONALES
Issues Common to Most Anti-Parkinson Medications	
Assess the patient's understanding of the anti-Parkinson medications. As indicated, stress the importance of taking medication on schedule and not forgetting a dose. Advise the patient to carry extra dose(s) when leaving home.	Missing a dose may adversely affect mobility. The patient and health care provider can adjust the dose schedule so that the medication peaks at mealtime or at times when the patient needs mobility most.
Teach the patient or significant other how to premeasure doses in segmented or separate containers labeled with the date and time of dose.	This assists patients having difficulty with self-medication.

ASSESSMENT/INTERVENTIONS	RATIONALES
Teach the patient to take non–levodopa-containing medications with meals.	This will decrease the potential for nausea. If an antiemetic is needed for nausea, trimethobenzamide or domperidone may be prescribed. Promethazine, however, is avoided because it can worsen PD symptoms.
Encourage patients with anorexia to eat frequent small, nutritious snacks and meals.	Eating smaller meals rather than three larger meals is usually better tolerated in patients who are anorexic. Mirtazapine is sometimes used off label to act as an appetite stimulate. Megestrol is used and approved for anorexia/cachexia associated with cancer and HIV but can be used off label in PD.
Advise the patient to elevate head of bed and make position changes slowly and in stages. Teach the patient to dangle legs a few minutes before standing. Antiembolism hose may help as well. Advise avoiding dehydration especially in warm weather by increasing fluid intake to include 4-8 oz/day of a sport drink if not contraindicated by cardiac co-morbidity. Give tips for reducing morning orthostatic hypotension, including not limiting late evening fluid intake and keeping a glass of water at the bedside at night so it is available to drink in the morning before getting up. Encourage males to urinate from a sitting rather than standing position if possible. Provide a bedside commode for female patients. Suggest increasing dietary salt intake if not contraindicated by cardiac co-morbidity.	These measures counteract orthostatic hypotension, which is a potential side effect of these medications. (Orthostatic hypotension also may be a result of the autonomic neuropathy from the disease process itself.) Fludrocortisone or midodrine may be prescribed to prevent or reduce orthostatic hypotension.
Teach the patient to report dizziness to the health care provider.	This may be an indication of orthostatic hypotension. Medication adjustment may be needed.
Advise use of sugarless chewing gum or hard candy, frequent mouth rinses with water, or artificial saliva products.	These measures ease dry mouth, a common side effect of these medications, and help maintain integrity of oral mucous membrane. In the presence of drooling, however, an anticholinergic such as hyoscyamine or glycopyrrolate has a beneficial side effect of a reduction in secretions.
Advise the patient to report any urinary hesitancy or incontinence.	Either may signal urinary retention. Individuals taking anticholinergics may find that voiding before taking the medication eliminates this problem.
Teach the patient how to counteract constipation. For interventions, see **Constipation**, p. 68, in "Prolonged Bedrest."	Constipation is a common problem with these medications as well as the disease itself. Laxative and stool softeners as well as reduction in anticholinergic medications may help. If anorectal dysfunction is causing constipation, botulinum toxin injection into the puborectalis muscle may correct it.
Teach the patient to report mental status changes to the health care provider promptly.	Many of these drugs can cause or aggravate changes in mental status such as confusion; mental slowness or dullness; and even agitation, paranoia, and hallucinations. The health care provider may adjust the dose. Atypical antipsychotic agents such as quetiapine, olanzapine, and clozapine may be prescribed off label to decrease psychotic symptoms. Haloperidol may make PD symptoms worse and is therefore avoided.
Teach the patient to report feelings of depression to the health care provider promptly.	Depression can be a side effect of some drugs as well as a normal response to disability. It is also caused by the disease process itself due to alteration in neurochemical balance. Counseling or psychotherapy may help patients and significant others adapt to the disability and deal with emotions and feelings such as depression that are either a direct or an indirect result of the disease process or drug therapy. Antidepressants (e.g., fluoxetine, sertraline, paroxetine, venlafaxine) may be prescribed to treat depression as well as help some PD symptoms (may help to block reabsorption of dopamine and have some anticholinergic properties).

continued

ASSESSMENT/INTERVENTIONS	RATIONALES
Implement safety measures for patients with vision problems: orient to surroundings, identify self when entering room, keep walkways unobstructed, and encourage patients to ask for assistance when ambulating.	Blurred vision is a side effect of many anti-Parkinson medications.
Teach measures that promote sleep. See **Disturbed Sleep Pattern,** p. 73.	Insomnia is a side effect of many of these drugs. Reducing the evening dose may help promote sleep. Modafinil may be prescribed to reduce daytime sleepiness. Sleep disorder is also more common in PD then in the general population.
Side Effects Specific to Dopamine Replacement Therapy (Levodopa)	Levodopa, the metabolic precursor of dopamine, crosses the blood-brain barrier and restores dopamine levels in the extrapyramidal centers in the brain. Before levodopa crosses the blood-brain barrier, much of it is converted into dopamine by the peripheral metabolism (GI tract and liver), causing many of the drug's side effects. Dopamine is given in increasing amounts until symptoms are reduced or patient's tolerance to side effects is reached. It may be used as initial therapy or later when other medications can no longer control symptoms.
Teach patients with advanced PD that levodopa should be taken with a full glass of water on an empty stomach 30 min before meals or 2 hr after meals.	Levadopa is a protein-bound medication. Taking it with a high-protein meal will decrease absorption.
Instruct the patient to report muscle twitching, spasmodic winking, or other abnormal muscle movements.	These are signs of medication toxicity.
[!] Explain signs and symptoms of neuroleptic malignant syndrome and acute akinesia (see Assessment). Teach the patient that to avoid neuroleptic malignant syndrome, it is necessary to take levodopa as scheduled and not to stop this medication abruptly.	There is need for immediate medical intervention with these crises because respiratory and cardiac support may be necessary. In neuroleptic malignant syndrome, the dopaminergic drug needs to be restarted immediately and measures taken to treat fever and renal dysfunction. In acute akinesia, the triggering cause must be found and treated and the patient medically supported until this is resolved.
Explain signs of on-off response, wearing-off, other complications of therapy, interventions, and importance of working with the health care provider on fine-tuning the medication regimen.	Many of the problems with dopamine replacement therapy are related to fluctuating blood levels. Dose redistribution, use of adjunctive medications such as dopamine agonist [DA], catechol *O*-methyltransferase (COMT) inhibitor, and use of medication preparations in extended-release forms and transdermal forms should help downregulate these problems. Deep brain stimulation (DBS) should be considered as well as acute rescue injectable medication (apomorphine). *On-off response:* A rapid fluctuation or change in patient's condition. The individual is "on" one moment, in a state of relative mobility, and "off" the next, in a state of decreased mobility ranging from mild reduction in function to complete or nearly complete immobility. Although the cause is uncertain, it is believed that it is related to fluctuating dopamine blood levels in the brain. *"End-of-dose" wearing-off phenomenon:* Return of symptoms (bradykinesia, tremors, rigidity) before the next dose is given. *Other complications:* Choreiform or involuntary, spasmodic, jerking movements (e.g., facial grimacing, tongue protrusion, restlessness) and vivid dreaming. Medication adjustments usually help these side effects.
[!] Teach the patient and significant other to monitor for behavioral changes and report them to the health care provider promptly.	Severe depression with suicidal overtones can be caused by this drug and should be reported immediately. Patients can also develop severe obsessive behavior (e.g., gambling, impulsive buying, hypersexuality). The health care provider may prescribe a dose reduction.

ASSESSMENT/INTERVENTIONS	RATIONALES
Explain that the medication may cause changes in urine (dark or orange-colored).	Knowing what to expect may eliminate anxiety if these problems occur.
Caution the patient to avoid alcohol.	Alcohol impairs effectiveness of levodopa and worsens base symptoms related to gait and balance as well as worsens mental health and cognitive issues.
Side Effects Specific to Antiviral Agent (e.g., amantadine)	Although this drug is less effective than levodopa, it has fewer severe side effects. It may be used as initial therapy or as an adjunct. Effects diminish after a time; therefore, this drug may be used intermittently.
Teach the patient to take this medication early in the day.	This may prevent insomnia, which is one of its side effects.
❗ Teach the patient and significant other to monitor for and report any shortness of breath, peripheral edema, significant weight gain, or change in mental status.	These signs often signal heart failure, a possible side effect of this drug.
❗ Instruct the patient not to stop taking this medication abruptly.	Doing so may precipitate parkinsonian crisis (acute akinesia), a severe worsening of symptoms that can be life threatening.
Teach the patient to report a change in skin coloration if it occurs, but reassure that the condition is more cosmetic than serious.	A diffuse, rose-colored mottling of the skin, usually confined to the lower extremities, may develop. The condition may subside with continued therapy and will disappear in a few weeks to months after the drug is discontinued. Exposure to cold or standing may make the color more prominent.
Instruct the patient to monitor and promptly report to the health care provider a loss of seizure control.	Patients with history of seizures may have an increase in the number of seizures.
Caution the patient to avoid alcohol and CNS depressants.	These agents potentiate the effects of amantadine.
Explain that most side effects of amantadine are dose related.	Many side effects can be controlled by an adjustment in dosage.
Side Effects Specific to Dopamine Agonist (e.g., pramipexole, ropinirole, bromocriptine, pergolide, cabergoline, apomorphine)	These medications are administered with a concomitant reduction of dopamine replacement dosage or as initiation therapy independent of dopamine replacement. They may be used to reduce levodopa-induced dyskinesia (such as involuntary movements) and the frequency of "on-off" responses.
Caution the patient to avoid alcohol when taking this medication.	Alcohol tolerance will be lessened.
Teach the patient to avoid exposure to cold and to report onset of finger or toe pallor.	Bromocriptine can cause digital vasospasm.
❗ Teach patients taking bromocriptine, cabergoline, and pergolide to have regular follow-up evaluation of their lungs.	These medications have been associated with pulmonary fibrosis.
❗ Teach patients taking pergolide to have regular follow-up evaluations to monitor the heart.	Pergolide has the potential for promoting cardiac valve problems.
Teach the patient that changing the medication should help with acute obsessive behaviors such as gambling, impulsive buying, and hypersexuality.	Dopamine agonist (DA) therapy has been associated with potentially reversible pathologic gambling.
❗ Caution patients taking DAs against driving or using machinery until they know how they respond to the medications.	DAs are associated with abrupt onset of somnolence without warning.
❗ Teach the patient that despite its name, apomorphine does not contain morphine and is not addictive. Explain that an antiemetic (e.g., trimethobenzamide) needs to be taken before taking apomorphine, ideally on a prophylaxis basis 3 days before initiation of therapy. Teach the patient to implement safety precautions when taking apomorphine.	Apomorphine is a dopamine agonist given subcutaneously as a "rescue" drug for acute, intermittent treatment of hypomobility ("off" episodes). It needs to be initiated and titrated under monitored conditions. It frequently causes severe nausea and vomiting, although tolerance usually develops after about 8 wk. Dizziness or postural hypotension can occur.
Explain that the following can occur with apomorphine: injection site reactions including bruising, itching, and lumps that typically resolve on their own. Yawning, dyskinesia, somnolence, rhinorrhea, hallucination, and extremity edema also can occur.	These are common side effects.

continued

ASSESSMENT/INTERVENTIONS	RATIONALES
Explain that erections in men can occur spontaneously with apomorphine and should be reported to the health care provider if they last longer than 4 hr.	This side effect of apomorphine may be beneficial for selected patients. Presently it is only available in a subcutaneous formulation.
Side Effects Specific to Anticholinergic Medications (e.g., trihexyphenidyl, benztropine mesylate, ethopropazine, cycrimine, procyclidine, biperiden)	As a class, these medications are used less often due to side effects, mild to moderate efficacy, and availability of other medication choices. They are often used in conjunction with dopamine replacement therapy but may be used alone if the patient's symptoms are mild or if the patient cannot tolerate levodopa. They may improve tremors and rigidity but often do little for bradykinesia or balance problems.
Explain that the patient should avoid strenuous exercise and keep cool during summer to avoid heat stroke.	This medication may decrease perspiration.
Teach the patient not to stop taking this medication abruptly.	Doing so can result in parkinsonian crisis (acute akinesia), a severe worsening of symptoms that can be life-threatening.
Teach the patient to monitor for tachycardia or palpitation and to report either condition.	Many side effects such as these can be controlled by an adjustment in dosage.
Teach the patient and significant others to monitor for memory dysfunction and confusion and urinary hesitancy and retention (especially in older males) and to report symptoms to the health care provider.	As above.
Side Effects Specific to Monoamine Oxidase (MAO) Type B Inhibitor (e.g., selegiline, rasagiline)	This medication is used as an early intervention or as an adjunct with levodopa to inhibit the breakdown of levodopa, resulting in less fluctuation in blood levels.
Stress the importance of taking this medication only in prescribed dose and following dietary modifications to reduce intake of tyramine-containing foods.	These medications are MAO-B selective inhibitors, but they are in the MOA class. Therefore it is recommended to avoid foods containing tyramine at more than 150 mg.
Suggest avoidance of meperidine and other opioids.	At recommended doses, no drug interactions have been noted. However, fatal drug interactions have occurred with patients taking other nonselective MAO inhibitors and could conceivably occur if higher-than-recommended doses are taken.
Teach the patient to take the medication early in the day.	This may help prevent insomnia, a potential side effect.
Side Effects Specific to COMT Inhibitor (e.g., entacapone)	This medication reduces levodopa degradation in the GI tract, kidneys, and liver to minimize fluctuation in serum levels.
Teach the patient that this medication might cause urine discoloration (brownish orange), but it is not clinically important.	An informed patient is not likely to become anxious if urine discoloration occurs.
Explain that hallucinations, increased dyskinesia, persistent nausea, abdominal pain, and diarrhea should be reported promptly.	Many side effects are dose related and can be controlled by adjustment in dosage.

Nursing Diagnosis:

Deficient Knowledge

related to unfamiliarity with facial and tongue exercises that enhance verbal communication and help prevent choking

Desired Outcome: Following demonstration and within the 24-hr period before hospital discharge, the patient demonstrates facial and tongue exercises and states the rationale for their use.

ASSESSMENT/INTERVENTIONS

RATIONALES

ASSESSMENT/INTERVENTIONS	RATIONALES
Assess the patient's understanding of facial and tongue exercises. As indicated, explain that special exercises can help strengthen and control facial and tongue muscles, which in turn will improve verbal communication and help prevent choking. Refer the patient to a speech pathologist in order to design and individualize a speech program.	Routine exercises of facial and tongue muscles, along with prescribed medications, may prevent or delay disability.
Teach exercises that will improve verbal communication and help prevent choking. Have the patient return the demonstration.	Teaching, followed by return demonstration, is an effective way of helping patients understand and retain knowledge. Teaching patients how to hold a sound for 5 sec; sing the scale; recite the alphabet and days of the week; practice vowel breaths (ah, oh, oo) and nonsense syllables (ma, me, mi, pull, pill, pie), read aloud, and extend the tongue and try to touch the chin, nose, and cheek will help improve verbal communication skills and prevent choking.
Encourage the patient to practice increasing voice volume. Suggest that the patient read newspapers out loud and determine how many words can be said in one breath before volume decreases. Advise that the voice should vary from soft to loud.	This exercise will help combat monotone speech while promoting speech quality and understandability. This may be accomplished by having patients take a deep breath before speaking, open the mouth to let sound come out more, use shorter sentences, exaggerate the sound of every syllable, speak louder than others may think necessary, and use a tape recorder for feedback. Patients should practice reading or reciting out loud, focusing on breathing, and using a strong voice.
Teach the patient to raise the voice with a question and lower it with an answer.	These actions improve speech understandability.
Teach these tongue exercises: stick out the tongue as far as possible and hold; move the tongue slowly from corner to corner; stretch the tongue to the nose and then chin and then cheek; stick out the tongue and put it back in the mouth as quickly as possible; move the tongue in circles as quickly as possible.	These exercises will improve articulation.
Teach the patient to open and close the mouth slowly and then quickly; close the lips and press tightly; stretch the lips in a wide smile and hold; then pucker the lips and hold.	These are effective lip and jaw exercises for improving articulation.
Advise the patient to practice in front of a mirror.	This will enable patient to see and evaluate lip and tongue movement.
Provide a written handout that lists and describes the preceding exercises. Encourage the patient to perform them hourly while awake.	These measures reinforce the patient's knowledge.
Teach importance of stating feelings verbally. Encourage use of a mirror to practice expressing emotions such as happiness and displeasure.	Monotone speech and lack of facial expression impede nonverbal communication.
Advise patients to face the people to whom they are speaking and speak for themselves and not let others speak for them.	Individuals who have difficulty speaking often remain quiet and let others talk for them.

Nursing diagnosis for patients undergoing deep brain stimulation

Nursing Diagnosis:

Deficient Knowledge

related to unfamiliarity with deep brain stimulation

Desired Outcome: Following the explanation, the patient verbalizes accurate understanding of the deep brain stimulation (DBS) procedure and general follow-up care.

ASSESSMENT/INTERVENTIONS	RATIONALES
Assess the patient's understanding of DBS. As indicated, explain that the neurostimulator is an implantable pulse generator powered by a small battery that is implanted subcutaneously near the clavicle. The stimulation parameter is set to optimize symptom management with minimum adverse effects.	Deep brain electrostimulation is used preferentially over ablative procedures (e.g., stereotactic pallidotomy) because it has the same effect without actually destroying parts of the brain. Stimulation of the thalamus helps with tremors. Globus pallidus stimulation works better in controlling rigidity and balance and reduces medication side effects, leading to better tolerance, but it does not usually reduce the amount of medication given. Stimulation of the subthalamic nucleus (STN) helps with all parkinsonian symptoms and enables a reduction in medication. STN is the preferred target for deep brain stimulation. This does not replace oral medication management but sometimes the medications can be reduced, although medication reduction should not be an expectation. The patient can switch stimulation to on/off with a magnet.
Explain that health care provider follow-up is necessary.	Adverse effects may include paraesthesias, muscle contractions, double vision, and mood disturbances, all of which are usually transient. It is seldom possible to alleviate completely all PD symptoms with the stimulator alone. Therefore, medication may be needed and adjustments made for the first few months.
Advise that the sudden appearance of additional parkinsonian symptoms may be the only indicator of battery failure.	There are handheld devices that enable determination of the on/off status of the neurostimulator as well as battery charge status.
Advise that turning the neurostimulator off at night to conserve the battery is not recommended.	Some symptoms, such as rigidity, respond only to continuous stimulation.
Explain that ineffective stimulation may signal incorrect lead placement, poor anchoring, and drifting of leads.	This may necessitate removal for accurate repositioning of the electrodes.
Teach that adverse effects resulting from stimulation of nearby structures are corrected by adjusting the stimulation parameters.	Adverse effects include tingling of the head or hand, depression, slurred speech, loss of balance or muscle tone, and double vision. Patients should see health care providers for adjustments.
Explain that excessive STN stimulation may cause disabling dyskinesia.	This would be a valid reason for turning off the device until reprogramming can be performed.
Caution that some devices, such as theft detectors and screening devices found in airports, department stores, and public libraries can cause the neurostimulator to switch on or off. Ultrasonic dental equipment and electrocautery also may affect the device.	Usually, this only causes an uncomfortable sensation. However, symptoms could worsen suddenly. Patients always should carry the identification card given with the device and use it to request assistance to bypass those devices. Magnets and home programmers also should be carried in case the stimulator is accidentally switched off by such devices. The patient can then do a self assessment and turn it back on if needed. Computers and cellular phones do not interfere with the device.
Caution patients to avoid activities that may result in blunt trauma to the implanted device area.	This will help prevent loss of function of the implant generator or leads.
Caution patients they cannot undergo magnetic resonance imaging (MRI) scans because of possible movement of the leads or diathermy (shortwave or microwave).	MRI scans can heat up the wires and leads, resulting in serious injury or death.
Instruct in use of magnet to activate and deactivate the stimulator.	Magnets may damage televisions, credit cards, and computer disks and therefore should be kept at least 1 foot away from these items.

ADDITIONAL NURSING DIAGNOSES/PROBLEMS:

PATIENT-FAMILY TEACHING AND DISCHARGE PLANNING

When providing patient-family teaching, focus on sensory information, avoid giving excessive information, and initiate a visiting nurse referral for necessary follow-up teaching. Include verbal and written information about the following:

✓ Referrals to community resources, such as local and national Parkinson's Society chapters, public health nurse, visiting nurses association, community support groups, social workers, psychologic therapy, vocational rehabilitation agency, home health agencies, and extended and skilled care facilities. Additional general information can be obtained by contacting the following organizations:

- The American Parkinson Disease Association, Inc., at *www.apdaparkinson.com*
- Parkinson's Disease Foundation, Inc., at *www.pdf.org*
- National Parkinson Foundation, Inc., at *www.parkinson.org*
- Parkinson Society Canada at *www.parkinson.ca*

✓ Importance of avoiding certain medications that can worsen extrapyramidal symptoms. Examples include phenothiazines, prochlorperazine, metoclopramide, chlorpromazine, methyldopas, tetrabenazine, haloperidol, and reserpine. An exception is ethopropazine, which is a phenothiazine derivative that does not increase extrapyramidal effects and is used to treat PD symptoms.

✓ Speech therapy tips for communication related to dysarthria and for swallowing precautions.

✓ Related safety measures and fall prevention for patients with bradykinesia, muscle rigidity, and tremors.

✓ Emphasis that disability may be prevented or delayed through exercises and medications.

✓ Evaluation of home environment and tips for home accident prevention.

✓ Measures to prevent or lessen postural hypotension.

✓ Signs and symptoms of neuroleptic malignant and acute akinesia and the need for immediate medical attention.

✓ For other interventions, see "Patient-Family Teaching and Discharge Planning" (third through tenth entries only), in "Multiple Sclerosis," p. 292.

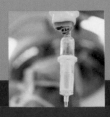

Seizures and Epilepsy 40

OVERVIEW/PATHOPHYSIOLOGY

Seizures result from an abnormal, uncontrolled electrical discharge from the neurons of the cerebral cortex in response to a stimulus. If the activity is localized in one portion of the brain, the individual will have a partial seizure, but when it is widespread and diffuse, a generalized seizure occurs. Symptoms vary widely, depending on the involved area of the cerebral cortex. Seizures are generally manifested as an alteration in sensation, behavior, movement, perception, or consciousness lasting from seconds to several minutes. A seizure can be an isolated incident that may not recur once the underlying cause is corrected (e.g., fever, alcohol withdrawal). *Epilepsy* or seizure disorder are the terms used for recurrent, unprovoked seizures.

Seizure threshold refers to the amount of stimulation needed to cause neural activity. Although anyone can have a seizure if the stimulus is sufficient, the seizure threshold is lowered in some individuals, and this may result in spontaneous seizures. Potential causes for lowered seizure threshold include congenital defects; craniocerebral trauma, particularly that from a penetrating wound; subarachnoid hemorrhage; stroke; intracranial tumors; infections, such as meningitis or encephalitis; exposure to toxins, such as lead; hypoxia; alcohol or other drug withdrawal; and metabolic and endocrine disorders, such as hypoglycemia, hypocalcemia, uremia, hypoparathyroidism, excessive hydration, and fever. Phenothiazine antidepressants and alcohol usage increase risk of seizure by lowering the seizure threshold. For susceptible individuals, triggers may include emotional tension or stress; physical stimulation, such as loud music, bright flashing lights, and some videos; lack of sleep or food; fatigue; menses or pregnancy; and excessive drug/alcohol use. If a trigger stimulus is identified, the individual has what is termed *reflex epilepsy*.

Although a seizure itself generally is not fatal, individuals can be injured by hitting their heads or breaking bones if they lose consciousness and fall to the ground. Seizure activity increases cerebral O_2 consumption by 60% and cerebral blood flow by 250%. Instances of prolonged and repeated generalized seizures, *status epilepticus (SE)*, can be life threatening because apnea, hypoxia, acidosis, cerebral edema, dysrhythmias, and cardiovascular collapse can occur.

HEALTH CARE SETTING

Primary care, neurology clinic, and possible acute care hospitalization for complications of therapy, continuous diagnostic video electroencephalogram (EEG) monitoring during pharmacologic or surgical interventions, or intensive care unit (ICU) for SE

ASSESSMENT

It is important to obtain an accurate description of seizure characteristics and duration, as well as any antecedent events, precipitating factors, and postictal phase. There are many clinical types of seizures, but the following are the most serious or common.

Generalized tonic-clonic (grand mal): Caused by bilateral electrical activity and can be symmetrical from onset, but in adults, it is usually preceded by an aura, indicating an initial focal onset followed by generalization. This is referred to as focal with secondary generalization. Generalized seizures always involve loss of consciousness. A possible prodromal phase of increased irritability, tension, mood changes, or headache may precede the seizure by hours or days. Patients may experience an aura (a sensory warning, such as a sound, odor, or flash of light) immediately preceding the seizure by seconds or minutes. The seizure activity, known as the ictal phase, usually does not last more than 2-5 min and includes the following:

- *Tonic (rigid/contracted muscles/extended limbs):* Often lasts only 15 sec, usually subsiding in less than 1 min. Symptoms include loss of consciousness, clenched jaws (potential for tongue to be bitten), apnea (may hear a cry as air is forced out of the lungs), and cyanosis. The patient may be incontinent, and pupils may dilate and become nonreactive to light.
- *Clonic (rhythmic contraction and relaxation of extremities and muscles):* May subside in 30 sec but can last 2-4 min. Eyes roll upward, and excessive salivation results in foaming at the mouth. During this phase, the potential is greatest for biting the tongue.
- *Postictal:* The first few minutes after the seizure, the individual may be limp and nonresponsive. Pupils begin to react to light and return to their normal size. After about

5 min, patients may be sleepy, semiconscious, confused, unable to speak clearly, and uncoordinated; have a headache; complain of muscle aches; and have no recollection of the seizure event. This phase usually lasts less than 15 min but can last for several hours. Temporary weakness, Todd's paralysis (post-ictal paralysis), dysphasia, or hemianopia lasting up to 48 hr after the seizure may be experienced.

Generalized absence (petit mal): Patients have momentary loss of awareness and consciousness with abrupt cessation of voluntary muscle activity. Patients may appear to be daydreaming with a vacant stare and may experience facial, eyelid, or hand twitching. Patients usually do not lose general body muscle tone and so do not fall. The individual resumes previous activity when the seizure ends. There is usually no memory of the seizure, and patients may have difficulty reorienting after the seizure event. This type of seizure can last 1-10 sec, may occur up to 100 times/day, and usually resolves by puberty.

Generalized myoclonic: Sudden, very brief contraction or jerking of muscles or muscle groups. Individuals may have a very brief, momentary loss of consciousness with some postictal confusion.

Partial simple motor (focal motor seizures): An irritative focus located in the motor cortex of the frontal lobe causes clonic movement in a particular part of the body, such as the hands or face. If the seizure activity spreads or marches in an orderly fashion to an adjacent area (e.g., hands to arms to shoulders), the seizure is termed a focal motor seizure with jacksonian march. The seizure usually lasts several seconds to minutes. There is no loss of consciousness. Other simple, partial seizures include those with somatosensory symptoms (e.g., smells, sounds), autonomic symptoms (e.g., tachycardia, tachypnea, diaphoresis, goose bumps (piloerection), pallor, flushing), or psychic symptoms (e.g., fear, déjà vu).

Partial complex seizure (psychomotor, "temporal lobe"): Generally lasts 1-4 min and involves impaired consciousness and a postictal state of confusion lasting several minutes. However, the individual does not fall to the ground, is able to interact with the environment, exhibits purposeful but inappropriate movements or behavior, and has no memory of the event. The individual will perform such automatisms as lip smacking, chewing, facial grimacing, picking, or swallowing movements. These patients may experience and remember various sensory or emotional hallucinations or sensations that occur immediately before the seizure, such as smells; ringing or hissing sounds; or feelings of déjà vu, fear, or pleasure.

Status epilepticus: State of continuous seizure activity lasting more than 5 min or two or more recurring seizures in which the individual does not completely recover baseline neurologic functioning between seizures. Individuals who suddenly stop taking their antiepilepsy medication are likely to develop this condition. Other common causes are drug withdrawal (e.g., alcohol, sedatives) and fever. This is a medical emergency, especially with tonic-clonic seizures, resulting in such potential complications as cerebral anoxia and edema, aspiration, rhabdomyolysis, hyperthermia, and exhaustion. Brain injury may occur in 20-30 min, and irreversible damage may occur in 60 min. Death may ensue. SE can occur in the absence of movement. The patient does not regain consciousness. This nonconvulsive SE may not be life threatening, but it can cause brain damage and will require continuous EEG monitoring. Expect patients in SE to be transferred to ICU.

Other classifications: Seizures also can be classified according to epileptic syndrome (e.g., generalized epilepsies, idiopathic with age-related onset). Establishing the correct diagnosis of seizure type and, when possible, epilepsy syndrome, will help tailor effective antiepilepsy drugs (AEDs) and treatment.

DIAGNOSTIC TESTS

Because a variety of problems can precipitate seizures, testing may be extensive. Common tests for initial workup include the following:

Laboratory tests: To rule out metabolic causes, such as hypoglycemia, hyponatremia, or hypocalcemia; kidney and liver problems; toxicology screens; and AED level.

EEG—both sleeping and awake: To reveal abnormal patterns of electrical activity, particularly with such stimuli as flashing lights or hyperventilation. Ambulatory EEGs may record brain activity for 48-72 hr, and 24-hr continuous EEG monitoring with video recording may show association of brain activity with the observed seizure. Generalized tonic-clonic seizures show up as high, fast-voltage spikes in all leads. A normal EEG does not rule out seizures.

Magnetic resonance imaging (MRI) scan: To show structural lesions causing seizures; also may reveal a space-occupying lesion such as a tumor or hematoma. Fast fluid attenuated inversion recovery (FLAIR) MRI may be particularly sensitive in finding tumors.

Positron emission tomography: To check for areas of cerebral glucose hypometabolism that correlate with the irritative seizure-causing focus. This test is useful in partial seizures but is available only in a few centers.

Computed tomography (CT) scan: To check for presence of a space-occupying lesion, such as a tumor or hematoma.

Skull x-ray examination: To reveal fractures, tumors, calcifications, or congenital anomalies (pineal shift, ventricular deformity).

Lumbar puncture and cerebrospinal fluid analysis: If infection such as meningitis is suspected. It also can rule out increased intracranial pressure and determine brain levels of gamma-aminobutyric acid (GABA).

Nursing Diagnosis:

Risk for Trauma

related to oral, musculoskeletal, and airway vulnerability occurring with seizure activity

Desired Outcomes: The patient exhibits no signs of oral or musculoskeletal tissue injury or airway compromise after the seizure. Before hospital discharge, the patient's significant others verbalize knowledge of actions necessary during seizure activity.

ASSESSMENT/INTERVENTIONS	RATIONALES
Seizure Precautions	
Assess the patient's environment. Pad side rails with blankets or pillows. Keep side rails up and bed in its lowest position when the patient is in bed. Keep bed, wheelchair, or stretcher brakes locked.	These actions promote safety and protect the patient from trauma in case a seizure occurs.
Keep suction and oxygen equipment readily available.	These measures enable a patent airway, prevent hypoxia, and protect patients from trauma in case a seizure occurs.
Consider a saline lock for intravenous (IV) access for high-risk patients.	Some AEDs must be administered IV, especially as a loading dose or in case of sustained seizure activity.
Use electronic tympanic thermometers for patients at high risk for seizure. If only breakable thermometers are available, take temperature via axillary or rectal route.	Glass or other breakable oral thermometers should be avoided when taking a patient's temperature because of the harm they could cause the patient if they break.
Caution patients to lie down and push the call button if they experience prodromal or aural warning. Keep the call light within reach.	Prodromal or aural warnings precede seizures in many patients.
Encourage the patient to empty the mouth of dentures or foreign objects.	This helps prevent choking in case a seizure occurs.
Do not allow unsupervised smoking.	This restriction prevents fire damage to the patient and surroundings if a seizure occurs.
Evaluate need for and provide protective headgear as indicated.	This protects the patient's head in case of a seizure.
During the Seizure	
Remain with the patient and stay calm. Assess for, record, and report type, duration, and characteristics of seizure activity and any postseizure response.	Seizure activity should be documented in detail to aid in management and differentiation of seizure type and identification of triggering factors. This should include, as appropriate, precipitating event, aura, initial location and progression, automatisms, type and duration of movement, changes in level of consciousness, eye movement (e.g., deviation, nystagmus), pupil size and reaction, bowel and bladder incontinence, head deviation, tongue deviation, or teeth clenching.
Prevent or break the fall and ease the patient to the floor if a seizure occurs while the patient is out of bed.	These actions promote the patient's physical safety.
Keep the patient in bed if a seizure occurs while there, and lower head of the bed to a flat position.	Flattening the patient's position reduces risk of falling out of bed during seizure activity.
NEVER insert anything into the patient's airway during a seizure.	Forcing objects into the patient's mouth can break teeth, lacerate the oral mucous membrane, or block the airway.
Never put your fingers in the patient's mouth.	The patient may bite your fingers.
Be sure the patient's head position does not occlude the airway. Turn the patient into a side-lying position or turn the head to the left. Remove from the environment objects (e.g., chairs) the the patient may strike. Pad floors to protect the patient's arms and legs. Remove the patient's glasses.	These measures protect the patient's airway from occlusion and the body from injury during the seizure. A towel folded flat or hands may be used to cushion the head from striking the ground.
Do not restrain the patient but rather guide the patient's movements gently.	This action helps prevent injury caused by flailing.

ASSESSMENT/INTERVENTIONS	RATIONALES
Roll the patient into a side-lying position. Use the head-tilt/chin-lift maneuver. Provide O₂ and suction as needed.	This promotes drainage of secretions, maintains a patent airway, and prevents hypoxia. During the tonic phase, respiratory muscles contract, and coordinated breathing does not occur.
Loosen tight clothing, collar, or belt.	This prevents trauma/hypoxia caused by constrictive clothing.
Maintain the patient's privacy. Clear nonessential people from the room.	Seizures likely are embarrassing for the patient.
Administer AEDs as prescribed.	IV administration of the prescribed AED can shorten the length and prevent reoccurrence of seizures.

⚠ After the Seizure

Determine if patient has had SE: that is, the seizure is continuous (longer than 5 min), longer than the patient's usual length of time by 1 or 2 min, or the patient has two or more seizures without recovering baseline neurologic functioning between seizures.	This condition is life threatening and can cause cerebral anoxia and edema, aspiration, hyperthermia, and exhaustion. Anticipate transfer to ICU but do not delay initial interventions, including administration of prescribed IV lorazepam or diazepam.
Reassure and gently reorient the patient. Check neurologic status and vital signs (VS).	During the postictal period that follows the seizure, the patient will need to be reoriented and reassured because some memory lapse will have occurred during the event.
Ask the patient if an aura preceded seizure activity. Record this information and postictal characteristics.	An aura is a sensory warning such as a sound, odor, or flash of light. It can be used in the future to warn the patient of an impending seizure.
Provide a quiet, calm environment. Keep talk simple and to a minimum. Speak slowly and with pauses between sentences.	Sounds and stimuli can be confusing to the awakening patient. Repetition may be necessary if the patient is confused.
Use room light that is behind, not above, the patient.	This prevents additional seizures triggered by the light and promotes comfort.
Do not offer food or drink until the patient is fully awake.	This prevents vomiting/aspiration.
Check the patient's tongue for lacerations and the body for injuries. Assess for weakness or paralysis, dysphasia, or visual disturbances.	These are potential occurrences during a seizure.
Assess urine for red or cola color.	Rhabdomyolysis or myoglobinuria may occur from muscle trauma.
If the patient has been incontinent, provide perineal care.	This will help prevent skin irritation.
If the patient vomited during the seizure, notify the health care provider.	This is a sign that aspiration can occur with subsequent seizures.
Check fingerstick blood glucose.	Hypoglycemia is a potential metabolic cause of the seizure.
Obtain serum laboratory tests as prescribed.	Electrolyte disorders such as hyponatremia and hypocalcemia can trigger a seizure.
Stay with patient for 15-20 min postseizure.	Sudden unexplained death in epileptic patients is not well understood, but it may be related to central respiratory apnea that can occur with a seizure.
Provide significant others with verbal and written information for the preceding interventions.	Significant others are likely to be in the patient's presence during subsequent seizures. If well informed, they will be able to protect the patient from trauma and life-threatening complications.

⚠ If SE Has Occurred:

Implement the ABCs: Assess airway, breathing, and circulation. Initiate O₂ therapy, oral airway suctioning, and intubation as needed.	These actions help maintain the airway and prevent hypoxia.
Place the patient in a side-lying position.	Positioning on the side reduces aspiration risk in case of vomiting.
Assess VS, pulse oximetry, heart rhythm, and arterial blood gas values.	This assessment enables early detection of hypoxia, dysrhythmias, and overall hemodynamics.
Obtain IV access.	IV access ensures administration of fluids and medications.
Ensure priority administration of IV lorazepam or diazepam within 3-10 min.	Initially the medication is given as a slow bolus. Sublingual lorazepam or rectal diazepam gel may be given if there is no IV access. If the seizure stops, this may be the extent of the interventions if the patient is already on AEDs.

continued

ASSESSMENT/INTERVENTIONS	RATIONALES
Assess blood glucose (fingerstick) and administer IV glucose (and thiamine) as appropriate.	This will reverse hypoglycemia, a potential cause of the seizure. If alcohol withdrawal is suspected or a possibility, thiamine should be given before dextrose to protect against an exacerbation of Wernicke's encephalopathy.
As indicated, draw blood for serum laboratory studies.	Hypoglycemia and electrolyte (e.g., hyponatremia, hypocalcemia, hypomagnesemia) or metabolic imbalances (kidney, liver) may be causing seizures. Serum drug screens are performed to assess serum AED level and determine presence of alcohol or other drugs that may be causing the seizures.
Ensure priority administration of IV fosphenytoin (loading dose).	This medication is given if the patient is not already on AEDs or if the seizure continues.
Administer loading dose of fosphenytoin no faster than 150 mg phenytoin equivalents/min.	This prevents hypotension caused by faster loading doses.
Administer IV phenobarbital if prescribed.	Phenobarbital is prescribed if diazepam and phenytoin are unsuccessful or if the patient is allergic to other medications.
Assess for signs of respiratory depression.	This is a possible side effect of phenobarbital.

Nursing Diagnosis:

Deficient Knowledge

related to unfamiliarity with life-threatening environmental factors and preventive measures for seizures

Desired Outcomes: Before hospital discharge, the patient verbalizes accurate information about measures that may prevent seizures and environmental factors that can be life threatening in the presence of seizures. The patient exhibits health care measures that reflect this knowledge.

ASSESSMENT/INTERVENTIONS	RATIONALES
Assess the patient's knowledge of measures that can prevent seizures and environmental hazards that can be life threatening in the presence of seizure activity. Provide or clarify information as indicated.	This assessment enables nurses to provide or clarify information as indicated and facilitates development of an individualized teaching plan.
Advise the patient to check into state regulations about automobile operation.	Most states require 3 months to 2 seizure-free years before an individual can obtain a driver's license.
Caution the patient to refrain from operating heavy or dangerous equipment, swimming, climbing excessive heights, and possibly even tub bathing until he or she is seizure free for an amount of time specified by the health care provider.	These restrictions prevent injury that can result while performing these activities in case a seizure occurs.
Advise the patient that some activities, such as climbing or bicycle riding, require careful risk/benefit evaluation.	The patient who decides to ride a bike should wear a helmet and avoid heavy traffic. Contact sports should be avoided.
Caution the patient never to swim alone regardless of amount of time he or she has been seizure free.	This makes rescue easier if a seizure occurs. Patients should swim only in shallow water and in the company of a strong swimmer.
Advise the patient to turn the temperature of hot water heaters down.	This prevents scalding if a seizure occurs in the shower.
Encourage stress management, progressive relaxation techniques, and diaphragmatic respiratory training.	These measures help control emotional stress and hyperventilation, which can trigger seizures.
Encourage vocational assessment and counseling.	The patient's epilepsy may place others at risk in some occupations, such as bus driver or airline pilot.
Advise female patients that seizure activity may change (increase or decrease) during menses or pregnancy (especially at 3-4 months' gestation).	Tonic-clonic seizures have caused fetal death. AEDs are associated with birth defects; however, 90% of women have normal pregnancies and healthy children.

ASSESSMENT/INTERVENTIONS | RATIONALES

ASSESSMENT/INTERVENTIONS	RATIONALES
Provide birth control information if requested.	Oral contraceptive effectiveness may be reduced by many AEDs. Intrauterine devices or other methods may be needed. When seizures in women worsen with hormonal changes, suppressing ovulation with medication may be recommended. Women wanting to get pregnant should consult with their health care provider. Monotherapy is preferred. They should be taking folic acid and receive vitamin K during the last 4 wk of pregnancy before delivery to avoid neonatal hemorrhage.
Teach that use of stimulants (e.g., caffeine) and depressants (e.g., alcohol) should be avoided.	Their use can change the seizure threshold, and withdrawal from stimulants and depressants can increase the likelihood of seizures.
Teach that getting adequate amounts of rest, avoiding physical and emotional stress, maintaining a nutritious and balanced diet and hydration status, and avoiding certain stimuli may help prevent seizure activity.	These are measures that may help prevent seizures. Meals should be spaced throughout the day to prevent hypoglycemia. Overhydration may precipitate seizure activity. Stimuli such as flashing lights, video or computer games, or loud music appear to trigger seizures, and patients should avoid environments that are likely to have these stimuli. Poorly adjusted TVs may trigger seizures and should be fixed. Patients should monitor for and treat fever early during an illness.
Encourage individuals who have seizures that occur without warning to avoid chewing gum or sucking on lozenges.	They may be aspirated during a seizure.
Encourage the patient to wear a medical alert bracelet or similar identification or to carry a medical information card.	They provide information to health care professionals if the patient is unable to.

Nursing Diagnosis:

Deficient Knowledge

related to unfamiliarity with purpose, precautions, and side effects of AEDs

Desired Outcome: Before hospital discharge, the patient verbalizes accurate knowledge about the prescribed AED.

ASSESSMENT/INTERVENTIONS	RATIONALES
Stress the importance of taking the prescribed AED regularly and on schedule, and not discontinuing medication without health care provider guidance.	Seizures will stop with drug treatment for 60% or more individuals with this disorder. Missing a scheduled dose can precipitate a seizure several days later. Abrupt withdrawal of any AED can precipitate seizures, and discontinuing these medications is the most common cause of SE.
Assist patients in finding methods that will help them remember to take their medication and monitor their drug supply to avoid running out.	AEDs may be necessary for the duration of the patient's life. Medications cannot be taken "as-needed," and absence of seizures does not mean the medication is unnecessary.
Explain the concept of drug half-life and steady blood levels.	It is important to maintain a therapeutic blood level of the AED to manage seizures.
Caution patients to consult the health care provider before changing from a trade name to a generic medication and to avoid abrupt withdrawal.	Medications differ in the amount of time they remain in the body and reach peak activity, and there may be differences in bioavailability. Medications are usually withdrawn slowly over 1-2 wk rather than abruptly stopped, which could result in seizures.
Stress importance of informing the health care provider about side effects and keeping appointments for periodic laboratory work.	Laboratory tests will reveal whether blood levels of AEDs are therapeutic. Many side effects are dose related, and medication can be adjusted based on AED blood levels and symptoms.

continued

ASSESSMENT/INTERVENTIONS	RATIONALES
Teach the patient to report immediately any bruising, bleeding, jaundice, or rash.	Many AEDs can cause blood dyscrasias or liver damage.
Advise the patient to supplement with vitamin K, vitamin D, and folic acid if prescribed.	Certain AEDs, such as phenytoin, decrease absorption of folic acid and metabolism of vitamins D and K, which can lead to deficiencies. For pregnant women, folic acid supplementation is critical to prevent birth defects. Vitamin K may be given to pregnant women 1 mo before and during delivery to prevent neonatal hemorrhage.
Teach the patient to avoid grapefruit juice.	It can inhibit hepatic metabolism of many AEDs and affect drug level.
Advise that calcium supplementation and antacids should not be taken within about 2 hr of AEDs.	AEDs taken at the same time as calcium supplements and antacids may decrease absorption and effects of both medicines. Vitamin D and calcium supplementation are used to prevent osteomalacia (soft bone) associated with some AEDs such as phenytoin, valproic acid, and carbamazepine. Periodic bone density monitoring is recommended.
Advise the patient to avoid activities that require alertness until the central nervous system (CNS) response to the medication has been determined.	AEDs may make people drowsy. Splitting the dose or giving the main dose at bedtime may help.
Teach the patient to take the AED with food or large amounts of liquid.	Nausea and vomiting are common side effects of most AEDs.
Advise patients taking valproic acid, topiramate, and zonisamide not to chew the medication.	These AEDs may irritate oral mucous membrane.
Advise patients taking valproic acid that this medication may produce a false-positive test for urine ketones.	It is important for patients, especially those with diabetes, to know this because ketone assessment is one aspect of managing their diabetes.
Advise the patient that any visual changes or pain should be reported immediately.	With valproic acid, a visual change may signal ocular toxicity. With topiramate, blurred vision or difficulty seeing may indicate glaucoma. Patients on vigabatrin must have periodic visual field testing because irreversible damage to the retina can occur. Prompt reporting and timely intervention may preserve vision.
Instruct the patient to notify the health care provider if a significant weight gain or weight loss occurs.	A change in dose or scheduling may be necessary.
Teach the patient to avoid alcoholic beverages and over-the-counter (OTC) medications containing alcohol.	Long-term alcohol use stimulates the body to metabolize phenytoin more quickly, thus lowering the seizure threshold because of decreased plasma phenytoin levels.
Caution patients taking phenobarbital or primidone to avoid alcohol.	Alcohol potentiates the CNS depressant effects of these medications.
Caution the patient to avoid OTC medications.	AEDs are potentiated or inhibited by many other drugs, including aspirin and antihistamines, and may affect potency of other medications as well.
Instruct the patient to report uncoordinated movement (ataxia), diplopia, nystagmus, and dizziness.	These are other side effects common to AEDs that may necessitate drug, dosage, or schedule change.
Teach patients who take carbamazepine, ethosuximide, or zonisamide to report immediately fever, mouth ulcers, sore throat, peripheral edema, dark urine, bruising, or bleeding.	These are possible side effects that may necessitate drug, dose, or schedule change.
Advise patients taking phenytoin to perform frequent oral hygiene with gum massage and gentle flossing and brush teeth 3-4 times/day with a soft-bristle toothbrush. Teach the patient to report immediately any measles-like rash.	Phenytoin can cause gingival hypertrophy and rash.
Caution patients taking phenytoin that there are two types of this drug and neither should be substituted for the other.	It is important not to confuse extended-release phenytoin (e.g., Dilantin Kapseal) with prompt-release phenytoin (e.g., Dilantin). Doing so may cause dangerous underdose or overdose.
Caution that generic phenytoin should not be substituted for Dilantin Kapseal.	Dilantin Kapseal is absorbed more slowly and is longer acting.
Monitor for increased body hair with phenytoin.	Hair removal creams can be used if increased hair is a problem.

ASSESSMENT/INTERVENTIONS	RATIONALES
Monitor for hyperglycemia with phenytoin.	Phenytoin blocks the release of insulin, which may cause increased blood sugar levels. Persons with diabetes in particular may need adjustments in their diabetic medications.
Encourage the patient to keep a drug and seizure chart diary.	This will help detect trend of the seizures, which will enable the health care provider to determine if current treatment is at a therapeutic level.
	Patients with intractable seizures that are not controlled by medication, excision, ablation of known epileptogenic areas (e.g., scar removal), or cortical resection (e.g., temporal lobectomy or corpus callosotomy) may undergo certain procedures in an attempt to obtain seizure control. One example is multiple subpial transections consisting of horizontal cuts to prevent spread of the seizure impulse. Implanted vagus nerve stimulation (VNS) may have an anticonvulsant effect on partial seizures. Surgical procedures require a craniotomy (see "Traumatic Brain Injury," p. 346).

Nursing Diagnosis:

Noncompliance: Therapy

related to denial of the illness, financial constraints, or perceived negative consequences of the treatment regimen

Desired Outcome: Before hospital discharge, the patient verbalizes knowledge about the disease process and treatment plan, acknowledges consequences of continued nonadhering behavior, explains the experience that caused altering of the prescribed behavior, describes appropriate treatment of side effects or appropriate alternatives, and exhibits health care measures that reflect this knowledge, following an agreed-on plan of care.

ASSESSMENT/INTERVENTIONS	RATIONALES
Assess the patient's understanding of the disease process, medical management, and treatment plan. Explain or clarify information as indicated.	This assessment enables nurses to explain or clarify information as indicated and facilitates development of an individualized care plan that promotes adherence.
Assess for causes of nonadherence, such as financial constraints, inconvenience, forgetfulness or memory problems, medication side effects, misunderstanding of instructions, or difficulty making significant lifestyle changes or following medication schedule.	Once causes are identified, the nurse can then focus the care plan accordingly.
Explain drug half-life and the concept of a steady blood level. Explain the importance of health care provider guidance if the medication is stopped for any reason. Instruct and provide written instructions for how to contact the health care provider and the importance of health care provider and laboratory follow-up. Explain what to do if a dose is missed and how to refill a prescription if the medication is lost or depleted.	Intermittent medication use may be informal experimentation or an effort to gain control. Explanation of consequences of nonadherence helps ensure awareness that stopping medications can be life threatening (e.g., cause SE).
Encourage the patient's expression of feelings (e.g., dependence, powerlessness, embarrassment, being different). In addition, evaluate the patient's perception of effectiveness or ineffectiveness of treatment.	This will help clarify the patient's perception of vulnerability to the disease process and signs of denial of the illness.
Confront myths and stigmas. Provide realistic assessment of risks, and counter misconceptions.	This will help determine if a value, cultural conflict, or spiritual conflict is causing nonadherence.
Discuss methods of dealing with common problems, such as obtaining insurance and job or workplace discrimination.	Helping to eliminate barriers and problems optimally will promote adherence.

continued

ASSESSMENT/INTERVENTIONS	RATIONALES
Assess the patient's support systems.	This will help determine if a family disruption pattern (whether or not it is caused by the patient's illness) is making adherence difficult and "not worth it."
After the reason for nonadherence is found, intervene accordingly. If it appears that changing the medical treatment plan (e.g., in scheduling medications) may promote adherence, discuss this possibility with the health care provider. Provide the patient with information about interventions that can minimize drug side effects (e.g., taking drug with food or large amounts of liquid to minimize gastric distress).	All may help facilitate adherence.
Encourage involvement with support systems such as the local epilepsy centers and national organizations.	Many people appreciate the support of others with the same condition. Feeling less alone and supported by others may promote adherence.
If indicated, suggest counseling or psychotherapy.	This may help patients with poor self-concept or coping difficulties related to the diagnosis that may be a cause of the nonadherence.

ADDITIONAL NURSING DIAGNOSES/PROBLEMS:

"Psychosocial Support" for **Ineffective Coping**   p. 75

Disturbed Body Image   p. 79

"Psychosocial Support for the Patient's Family and   p. 85
Significant Other" for **Interrupted Family Processes**

✓ PATIENT-FAMILY TEACHING AND DISCHARGE PLANNING

When providing patient-family teaching, focus on sensory information, avoid giving excessive information, and initiate a visiting nurse referral for necessary follow-up teaching. Include verbal and written information about the following:

✓ Reinforcement of knowledge of the disease process, pathophysiology, symptoms, and precipitating or aggravating factors.

✓ Medications, including drug name, purpose, dosage, schedule, precautions, and potential side effects. Also discuss drug-drug, herb-drug, and food-drug interactions and importance of adhering to medication routine. Some herbs (ginkgo, valerian root, evening primrose, ephedra) may be proconvulsant and should be avoided. Supplements such as taurine, selenium, and vitamin D and Asian herbs such as Saiko-keishi mixture are being investigated for possible benefit.

✓ Importance of follow-up care and keeping medical appointments. Stress that use of AEDs necessitates periodic monitoring of blood levels to ensure therapeutic medication levels and assessment for side effects. Instruct patient to keep emergency contact numbers for the health care provider.

✓ Seizure first aid. An uncomplicated convulsive seizure in an individual known to have epilepsy is not necessarily a medical emergency. On average, these people can continue about their business after a rest period. An ambulance should be called or medical attention sought if the seizure happens in water; if the individual is injured, pregnant, or diabetic; if the seizure lasts longer than 5 min; if a second seizure starts; if consciousness does not begin to return; or if there is any question the seizure may have been caused by something other than epilepsy.

✓ Environmental factors that can be life threatening in the presence of seizures, measures that may help prevent seizures, and safety interventions during seizures. Review state and local laws that apply to individuals with seizure disorders. Review home and personal safety tips.

✓ Employment or vocational counseling as needed. Discuss need to avoid overprotection and maintain, as possible, normal work and recreation. Review or provide information regarding the Americans with Disabilities Act.

✓ Risks of using AEDs during pregnancy. Provide birth control information or genetic counseling referral as requested.

✓ Benefits of joining local support groups. Provide the following addresses as appropriate:
- Epilepsy Foundation at *www.epilepsyfoundation.org*
- *www.epilepsy.com*
- Epilepsy Information Page: National Institute of Neurological Disorders and Stroke at *www.ninds .nih.gov/disorders/epilepsy/epilepsy.htm*
- Antiepileptic Drug Pregnancy Registry at *www .aedpregnancyregistry.org*
- American Epilepsy Society at *www.aesnet.org*
- Epilepsy Canada at *www.epilepsy.ca*

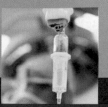

Spinal Cord Injury 41

OVERVIEW/PATHOPHYSIOLOGY

Spinal cord injuries (SCIs) are caused by vertebral fractures or dislocations that sever, lacerate, stretch, or compress the spinal cord and interrupt neuronal function and transmission of nerve impulses. Concussive trauma can cause damage from bruising, swelling, and inflammation. When blood supply to the spinal cord is interrupted, the spinal cord swells in response, and this, along with hemorrhage, can cause additional compression, ischemia, and compromised function. Neurologic deficits resulting from compression may be reversible if the resulting edema and ischemia do not lead to spinal cord degeneration and necrosis. Common causes of injury include motor vehicle accidents, diving or other sporting accidents, falls, and gunshot wounds. SCIs are classified in a number of different ways according to type (open, closed), cause (concussion, contusion, laceration, transection), site (level of spinal cord involved), mechanism of injury (compression, hyperflexion, hyperextension, rotational, penetrating), stability and degree of spinal cord function loss (complete, incomplete), or syndromes (central cord, Brown-Séquard [lateral], anterior cord, conus medullaris, cauda equina, and posterior cord). A *spinal cord concussion* involves a transient loss of cord function caused by a traumatic event, resulting in immediate flaccid paralysis that resolves completely in a matter of minutes or hours.

Prognosis: Any evidence of voluntary motor function, sensory function, or sacral sensation below the level of injury (lowest level in which motor function and sensation remain intact) indicates an incomplete SCI, with potential for partial or complete recovery. After an acute injury, the spinal cord usually goes into a condition called *spinal shock,* in which there can be total loss of spinal cord function below the level of injury. During spinal shock there is no reflex activity. Resolution of spinal shock with return of reflexes usually occurs within 1-2 wk, but may take 6 mo or more. If there is no evidence of returning motor function after local reflexes have returned, the spinal cord is considered irreversibly damaged. Generally, SCI does not cause immediate death unless it is at C1 through C3, which results in respiratory muscle paralysis. Individuals who survive these injuries require a ventilator for the rest of their lives. If the injury occurs at C4, respiratory difficulties may result in death, although some individuals who have survived the initial injury have been successfully weaned

from the ventilator. Injuries below C4 also can be life threatening because of ascending cord edema, which can cause respiratory muscle paralysis. Immediately after injury, common complications that require treatment include hypotension (systolic blood pressure [SBP] less than 80 mm Hg), bradycardia, paralytic ileus, urinary retention, pneumonia, and stress ulcers. Other long-term, life-threatening complications of SCI include autonomic dysreflexia (AD), pneumonia, decubitus ulcers, sepsis, urinary calculi, and urinary tract infection (UTI).

HEALTH CARE SETTING

Acute care, subacute care, rehabilitation center

ASSESSMENT

- There are a variety of neurologic assessment and functional outcome scales, including the American Spinal Injury Association (ASIA) Impairment scale, in which the impairment is described by whether it is complete, incomplete, or normal, with further differentiations for incomplete injuries.

  Acute indicators: Loss of sensation, weakness, or paralysis below level of injury, localized pain or tenderness over site of injury, headache, hypothermia or hyperthermia, and alterations in bowel and bladder function.

  Cervical injury: Possible alterations in level of consciousness (LOC); weakness or paralysis in all four extremities (tetraparesis or tetraplegia, previously termed *quadriparesis* or *quadriplegia*); and paralysis of respiratory muscles or signs of respiratory problems, such as flaring nostrils and use of accessory muscles for respirations. C4 and above injuries require ventilator support. Any cervical injury can result in low body temperature (to 96° F [35.5° C]), slowed pulse rate (less than 60 bpm) caused by vagal stimulation of the heart, hypotension (SBP less than 80 mm Hg) caused by vasodilation, and decreased peristalsis.

  Thoracic and lumbar injuries: Paraparesis/paraplegia or altered sensation in the legs; hand and arm involvement in upper thoracic injuries.

  Acute spinal shock: Can last from 2 days to 4-6 mo but usually resolves in 1-2 wk. Spinal shock results from loss of sympathetic nerve outflow and reflex function in all segments below level of injury. Indicators depend on injury severity and include total loss of spinal cord function, loss of skin sensation,

313

flaccid paralysis or absence of reflexes below level of injury, paralytic ileus and constipation secondary to atonic bowel, bladder distention secondary to atonic bladder, bradycardia, low/falling blood pressure (BP) secondary to loss of vasomotor tone and decreased venous return, and anhidrosis (absence of sweating and loss of temperature regulation) below level of injury. Autonomic instability is more dramatic in higher (e.g., cervical) lesions. Resolution of spinal shock is indicated by return of both the bulbocavernosus reflex (slight muscle contraction when glans penis is squeezed or urinary catheter is pulled, causing scrotal retraction) and the anal reflex (anal puckering on digital examination or gentle scratching around the anus). Remaining reflexes may take weeks to return.

Chronic indicators: As spinal shock resolves, muscle tone, reflexes, and some function may return, depending on severity and level of injury. Return of reflexes usually results in muscle spasticity. Chronic autonomic dysfunction may be manifested as fever; mild hypotension; anhidrosis; and alterations in bowel, bladder, and sexual function. Chronic neural pain may occur after SCI and tends to occur as either diffuse pain below level of injury or pain adjacent to level of injury. Injuries at or below L1 may result in permanent flaccid paralysis. Orthostatic hypotension is more typical of lesions above T7.

Upper motor neuron (UMN) involvement: UMNs are nerve cell bodies that originate in high levels of the central nervous system (CNS) and transmit impulses from the brain down the spinal cord. Injury interrupts this impulse transmission, causing muscle or organ dysfunction below level of injury. However, because the injury does not interrupt reflex arcs coming from those muscles or organs to the spinal cord, hypertonic reflexes, clonus paralysis, and spastic paralysis are seen. The patient will have a positive Babinski's reflex.

Lower motor neuron (LMN) involvement: LMNs are anterior horn cell bodies that originate in the spinal cord. LMNs transmit nerve impulses to muscles and organs and are involved in reflex arcs that control involuntary responses. Damage to LMNs will abolish voluntary and reflex responses of muscles and organs, resulting in flaccid paralysis, hypotonia, atrophy, and muscle fibrillations and fasciculations. The patient will have an absent Babinski's reflex. The spinal cord ends at the T12-L1 level. Below that level, a bundle of nerve roots from the spinal cord, called the *cauda equina*, fills the spinal canal. Injuries at or below L1 that damage nerve fiber after it leaves the spinal cord result in flaccid paralysis because of interrupted reflex arc activity.

Bowel and bladder dysfunction: Usually conscious sensation of the need to void or defecate is lost. UMN bowel and bladder involvement results in reflex incontinence. Flaccid LMN bladder involvement causes urinary retention with overflow incontinence. Flaccid LMN bowel involvement causes fecal retention/impaction.

Sexual dysfunction: Degree of dysfunction varies according to degree of completeness and whether injury is UMN or LMN. Males with complete UMN injuries have a loss of psychogenic erection but may have reflex erections. Ejaculation rates with complete UMN injuries are as low as 4%. Females have a loss of psychogenic lubrication but may have reflex lubrication. With complete LMN injuries, about 25% of males will have psychogenic erections but none will have reflex erections. About 50% of both sexes (by questionnaire) say they can experience orgasm regardless of injury level (possibly through other erogenous zones). Incomplete injuries will result in better sexual functioning that may include both erections and ejaculations.

Autonomic dysreflexia: Also known as *autonomic hyperreflexia*, AD is the exaggerated and unopposed sympathetic response to noxious stimuli below the SCI lesion and can be life threatening as reflex activity returns. AD is seen most commonly in patients with injuries at or above T6, but it has been reported with injuries as low as T8. Signs and symptoms include gross hypertension (BP more than 20 mm Hg above baseline, but BP can be as high as 240-300/150 mm Hg), pounding headache, blurred vision, bradycardia, nausea, and nasal congestion. Above level of injury, flushing and sweating may occur. Below level of injury, piloerection (goose bumps) and skin pallor, which signal vasoconstriction, may be present. Seizures, subarachnoid hemorrhage, stroke, or retinal hemorrhage also may occur.

PHYSICAL ASSESSMENT

Acute (spinal shock): Absence of deep tendon reflexes (DTRs) below level of injury, absence of cremasteric reflex (scratching or light stroking of inner thigh for male patients causes testicle on that side to elevate) for T12 and L1 injuries, absence of penile or anal sphincter reflex.

Chronic: Generally, increased DTRs occur when the spinal cord lesion is of the UMN type.

DIAGNOSTIC TESTS

Complete spine immobilization with a rigid cervical collar and backboard or other firm surface is essential until diagnostic tests rule out injury.

X-ray examination of spine: To delineate fracture, deformity, displacement of vertebrae, and soft tissue masses such as hematomas.

Magnetic resonance imaging (MRI) scan: To reveal changes in spinal cord and surrounding soft tissue. MRI scan evaluation is preferred and considered the "gold" standard for evaluation of degree of injury in patients who can tolerate it.

Computed tomography (CT) scan: To reveal changes in the spinal cord, vertebrae, and soft tissue surrounding the spine.

Arterial blood gas (ABG)/pulmonary function tests: To assess effectiveness of respirations and detect need for O_2 or mechanical ventilation.

Myelography: Used if other diagnostic examinations are inconclusive to show blockage or disruption of the spinal canal. Radiopaque dye is injected into the subarachnoid space of the spine, using a lumbar or cervical puncture.

Cystometry/urodynamic evaluation/external sphincter electromyogram: To assess bladder capacity and function after resolution of spinal shock for the best type of bladder training program.

Pulmonary fluoroscopy: To evaluate degree of diaphragm movement and effectiveness in individuals with high cervical injuries.

Evoked potential studies (e.g., somatosensory): To help locate level of spinal cord lesion by evaluating integrity of anatomic pathways and connections of the nervous system.

Stimulation of a peripheral nerve triggers a discrete electrical response along a neurologic pathway to the brain. Response or lack of response to stimulation is measured in this test.

Deep vein thrombosis (DVT) studies (e.g., venogram, duplex Doppler ultrasound, impedance plethysmography): To monitor for development of DVT.

Nursing Diagnosis:

Risk for Autonomic Dysreflexia

related to exaggerated unopposed autonomic response to noxious stimuli for individuals with SCI at or above T6

Desired Outcomes: On an ongoing basis, the patient is free of AD symptoms as evidenced by BP within the patient's baseline range, HR 60-100 bpm, and absence of headache and other clinical indicators of AD. Following instruction, the patient and significant others verbalize factors that cause AD, treatment and prevention, and when immediate emergency treatment is indicated.

ASSESSMENT/INTERVENTIONS	RATIONALES
Assess for indicators of AD, including hypertension (BP more than 20 mm Hg above baseline, but may go as high as 240-300/150 mm Hg), pounding headache, bradycardia, blurred vision, nausea, nasal congestion, flushing and sweating above the level of injury, and piloerection (goose bumps) or pallor below level of injury.	AD is a medical emergency that can occur after spinal shock resolution in patients with injuries at or above T6, but cases have been reported in patients with injuries as low as T8.
If AD is suspected, raise head of bed (HOB) immediately to 90 degrees or assist the patient into a sitting position.	These actions lower the patient's BP and decrease venous return. Seizures, subarachnoid hemorrhage, myocardial infarction (MI), stroke, or retinal hemorrhage can occur if severe hypertensive episode continues.
Call for someone to notify the health care provider; stay with the patient, and systematically search to identify and relieve the noxious stimulus. Speed is essential.	The noxious stimulus (e.g., distended bladder) must be found and alleviated as quickly as possible in order to remove the stimulus triggering AD.
Assess BP q3-5min during hypertensive episode.	This assesses trend of the BP.
Remain calm and supportive of the patient and significant other.	They will be very anxious.
Assess the following sites for causes, and implement measures for removing the noxious stimulus.	
Bladder: Distention, UTI, calculus and other obstructions, bladder spasms, catheterization, or bladder irrigations performed too quickly or with too cold a liquid.	Problems with the bladder are the most likely cause of AD.
Do not use Credé's method for a distended bladder.	The increased bladder pressure could further stimulate the reflex and worsen the condition.
Catheterize the patient (ideally using anesthetic jelly) if there is a possibility or question of bladder distention. Consult the health care provider *stat.*	Bladder distention is a potential cause of AD and requires immediate intervention. Anesthetic jelly prevents skin stimulation, which could trigger AD.
If a catheter is already in place, check tubing for kinks and lower drainage bag. For obstruction, such as sediment in tubing, slowly irrigate the catheter as indicated, using 30 mL or less of normal saline. If catheter patency is uncertain, recatheterize the patient using anesthetic jelly.	These interventions enable checking for catheter tube patency. Obstruction is a potential cause of AD.

continued

ASSESSMENT/INTERVENTIONS	RATIONALES
If the bladder is not distended, check for cloudy urine, hematuria, and positive laboratory or x-ray examination results.	These are signs of UTI and/or urinary calculi—two potential causes of AD.
Obtain a urine specimen.	Culture and sensitivity studies will show if UTI, a potential cause of AD, is present.
Instill tetracaine or lidocaine into the bladder if prescribed.	These agents will reduce bladder excitability.
Institute preventive measures as prescribed to prevent UTI and urinary calculi.	Future episodes may be caused by these factors.
Bowel: Constipation, impaction, insertion of suppository or enema, or rectal examination.	Problems with the bowel are the second most likely cause of AD. A good bowel regimen is a key factor in preventing the noxious stimuli that constipation may cause.
Do not attempt rectal examination without first anesthetizing the rectal sphincter and anal canal with anesthetic jelly.	Anesthetic jelly prevents skin stimulation, which could trigger AD.
Use large amounts of anesthetic jelly in the anus and rectum before disimpacting the bowel to remove potential stimulus.	Bowel impaction is a potential cause of AD.
Wait 5 minutes and check BP before disimpacting.	A lowered BP is a sign that anesthetic jelly has become effective.
Skin: Pressure, infection, injury, heat, pain, or cold.	These are possible causes of AD. A good skin integrity program is another key factor in preventing these noxious stimuli.
Loosen clothing and remove antiembolism hose, leg bandages, abdominal binder, or constrictive sheets as appropriate. For male patients, check for pressure source on penis, scrotum, or testicles and remove pressure if present.	Pressure on the skin is a potential cause of AD. Removal of hose, bandages, etc., also enables assessment of the skin for redness and other signs of pressure.
Check skin surfaces below the level of injury. Monitor for the presence of a pressure area or sore, infection, laceration, rash, sunburn, ingrown toenail, or infected area, or check skin for contact with a hard object. If indicated, apply a topical anesthetic.	Skin infection, pain, and injury are potential causes of AD.
Observe for and remove sources of heat or cold (e.g., ice pack, heating pad).	Topical heat or cold are two potential causes of AD.
Turn the patient on his or her side and ensure that bed linen is free of wrinkles. Consider adhering to a more frequent turning schedule.	These measures relieve other possible sources of pressure.
Additional causes: Surgical manipulation, incisional pain, sexual activity, menstrual cramps, labor, vaginal infection, or intraabdominal problems such as appendicitis.	
Administer antihypertensive agents such as nifedipine (oral, sublingual), nitroglycerin (sublingual, spray, or topical ointment), hydralazine, diazoxide, terazosin, or phenoxybenzamine as prescribed.	These medications lower BP.
Check for use of sildenafil, an erectile dysfunction medication, before giving nitroglycerin.	Sildenafil is contraindicated for people who are taking nitrates (e.g., nitroglycerin) because of the additive hypotensive effect.
Administer mecamylamine, prazosin, or clonidine if prescribed for recurrent AD.	These medications reduce severity of recurrent episodes.
On resolution of the crisis, answer the patient's and significant others' questions about AD. Discuss signs and symptoms, treatment, methods of prevention, and need for regular assessment of causative agents.	Prevention is the best way to deal with AD. A bowel regimen and skin integrity program are key factors in preventing the noxious stimuli that constipation and pressure areas may cause.
Encourage the patient to wear a medical alert bracelet or tag.	These items inform health care providers of the patient's condition in case the patient is unable to do so during AD.
Encourage keeping an AD kit on hand that includes a glove, lubricant jelly, straight catheter, electronic BP machine, and alert card.	This kit will help relieve and monitor this medical emergency when it occurs.

Nursing Diagnosis:

Ineffective Airway Clearance

related to neuromuscular paralysis/weakness; or related to restriction of chest expansion occurring with halo vest obstruction

Desired Outcome: Following intervention, the patient has a clear airway as evidenced by respiratory rate (RR) of 12-20 breaths/min with normal depth and pattern (eupnea) and absence of adventitious breath sounds.

ASSESSMENT/INTERVENTIONS	RATIONALES
Monitor ventilation capability by checking vital capacity, tidal volume, and pulmonary function tests. Monitor serial ABG values and/or pulse oximetry readings.	If vital capacity is less than 1 L or if the patient exhibits signs of hypoxia (Pao_2 less than 80 mm Hg, O_2 saturation 92% or less, tachycardia, increased restlessness, mental status changes or dullness, cyanosis), the health care provider should be notified immediately.
Provide oxygen as indicated.	Oxygen will help keep saturation greater than 92%.
Assess for increasing difficulty with secretions, coughing, respiratory difficulties, bradycardia, fluctuating BP, and increased motor and sensory losses at a higher level than baseline findings.	These signs may signal ascending cord edema secondary to the effects of contusion or bleeding. If present, the patient may require increased respiratory support.
Assess for loss of previous ability to bend arms at the elbows (C5-6) or shrug shoulders (C3-4). If these findings are noted, notify the health care provider immediately.	Changes from baseline or previous assessment may signal problems such as contusion, compression, bleeding, or damage to the blood supply, and they necessitate prompt intervention.
Keep the patient's head in neutral position, and suction as necessary. Be aware that suctioning may cause severe bradycardia in the patient with autonomic dysfunction. If indicated, prepare the patient for a tracheostomy, endotracheal intubation, and/or mechanical ventilation to support respiratory function. If appropriate, arrange for transfer to intensive care unit for continuous monitoring.	These actions maintain a patent airway and support respiratory function. Patients with injuries above C5 are intubated and put on a ventilator. Nasal intubation or tracheostomy may be used to prevent neck extension (and thus further damage) during intubation. An implanted phrenic nerve stimulator (e.g., diaphragm pacer) eventually may be inserted to enable selected patients on ventilators to be off the ventilator for short periods.
If the patient is wearing halo vest traction, assess respiratory status at least q4h or more frequently as indicated.	This action ascertains whether the vest is restricting chest expansion.
Assess ability to swallow for the patient in halo traction.	Inability to swallow may indicate improper position of the neck and chin or changes in cranial nerve function caused by cranial pin compression or irritation.
Teach use of incentive spirometry.	Spirometry promotes adequate ventilation and assesses quality of inspiratory abilities.
Assess for shortness of breath, hemoptysis, tachycardia, sudden shoulder pain, and diminished breath sounds.	These are indicators of venous thromboembolus (VTE)/pulmonary embolus (PE), which can occur because of impaired ventilation, altered vascular tone, and decreased mobility. Pain may or may not be present with VTE/PE, depending on the level of SCI. Sudden shoulder pain may be referred pain from VTE/PE.
Encourage coughing exercises. If the patient's cough is ineffective, implement the following technique, known as *assisted coughing:* place the heel of your hand under patient's diaphragm (below xiphoid process and above navel). Have the patient take several deep breaths, hold a deep breath, and then cough. As the patient exhales forcibly, quickly push up into the diaphragm to assist in producing a more forceful cough.	This technique enables production of a more forceful cough. An insufflation-exsufflation cough machine may be used to deliver breaths to patients in order to produce a more effective mechanically assisted cough. Caution: Assisted coughing may be contraindicated in patients with spinal instability.
Instruct the patient regarding intermittent positive pressure breathing, nebulizer treatments, and chest physiotherapy, if prescribed.	These therapies prevent and treat atelectasis. Respiratory therapy is ongoing past the acute stage. Noninvasive positive pressure ventilation may be used with some patients.

continued

ASSESSMENT/INTERVENTIONS	RATIONALES
Feed patients in Stryker frames, Foster beds, or similar mechanical beds in the prone position. Raise stable patients in halo traction to high Fowler's position if it is not contraindicated.	These actions minimize potential for aspiration.
For additional information, see **Risk for Aspiration,** p. 245.	

Nursing Diagnoses:

Risk for Ineffective Cerebral Tissue Perfusion
Risk for Decreased Cardiac Tissue Perfusion

related to relative hypovolemia occurring with decreased vasomotor tone

Desired Outcomes: By at least 24 hr before hospital discharge (or as soon as vasomotor tone improves), the patient has adequate cardiac and cerebral tissue perfusion as evidenced by SBP 90 mm Hg or higher and orientation to person, place, and time. For a minimum of 48 hr before hospital discharge, the patient is free of dysrhythmias.

ASSESSMENT/INTERVENTIONS	RATIONALES
Assess for hypotension (drop in SBP more than 20 mm Hg, SBP less than 90 mm Hg), lightheadedness, dizziness, fainting, and confusion.	Low/falling BP can occur secondary to loss of vasomotor tone and decreased venous return.
Assess oxygen saturation; administer oxygen as indicated.	Supplemental oxygen will help keep saturation at a level greater than 92%.
Assess heart rate (HR) and rhythm. Document dysrhythmias.	Sinus tachycardia/bradycardia may develop because of impaired sympathetic innervation or unopposed vagal stimulation. Atropine may be prescribed for symptomatic bradycardia.
Assess intake and output.	Adequate hydration and elimination are necessary to maintain stable hemodynamics.
Give prescribed intravenous (IV) fluids cautiously.	Impaired vascular tone can make the patient sensitive to small increases in circulating volume. Intravascular volume expanders or vasopressors (e.g., dopamine) may be required for hypotension.
Implement measures that prevent episodes of decreased cardiac output caused by postural hypotension.	Decreased cardiac output compromises cerebral and peripheral circulation. Postural hypotension is seen frequently in SCI, but it can be prevented and managed.
Change positions slowly.	This helps prevent postural hypotension.
Perform range-of-motion (ROM) exercises q2h. Prevent the patient's legs from crossing, especially when in a dependent position.	This prevents venous pooling and contractures.
If indicated, ensure that patients with SCI at higher levels, especially above T6, wear an abdominal binder in addition to antiembolic hose, leg wraps, and sequential compression devices or pneumatic foot pumps.	This helps prevent venous pooling. These individuals are prone to more severe hypotensive reactions, even with minor changes such as raising the HOB.
Work with the physical therapist to implement a gradual sitting program that will help the patient progress from a supine to an upright position.	The goal is to increase the patient's ability to sit upright while avoiding adverse effects, such as hypertension, dizziness, and fainting. This may include a bed that can rotate gradually from a horizontal position to a vertical position or a chair that has multiple positions progressing from flat to sitting.
Administer salt tablets and fludrocortisone as prescribed if nonmedication methods are ineffective.	These agents prevent orthostatic hypotension.
For additional information, see **Risk for Ineffective Cerebral Tissue Perfusion** in "Prolonged Bedrest," p. 67.	

Nursing Diagnoses:

Ineffective Peripheral Tissue Perfusion (or risk for same)
Risk for Decreased Cardiac Tissue Perfusion

related to venous stasis with corresponding risk of thrombophlebitis and VTE/PE occurring with immobility and decreased vasomotor tone

Desired Outcome: For at least 24 hr before hospital discharge and on an ongoing basis, the patient has adequate tissue perfusion as evidenced by absence of heat, erythema, and swelling in calves and thighs; HR 100 bpm or less; RR 20 breaths/min or less with normal depth and pattern (eupnea); and PaO_2 80 mm Hg or more or O_2 saturation greater than 92%.

ASSESSMENT/INTERVENTIONS	RATIONALES
⚠ Assess for erythema, warmth, decreased pulses, and swelling over area of inflammation and venous dilation, coolness, paleness, and edema distal to thrombus.	These are indicators of thrombophlebitis.
⚠ Measure calves and thighs daily while the patient is supine or before activity, and monitor for increased circumference.	An increase of 1.5 cm or more in 1 day is significant, as is calf diameter greater than 3 cm larger than the opposite calf.
Recognize that low-grade fever may be a more reliable signal of thrombophlebitis than pain. Notify the health care provider about significant findings.	The presence of pain or tenderness depends on the level of SCI.
⚠ Protect the patient's legs from injury during transfers and turning, and position them so they do not cross. Avoid intramuscular (IM) injections in the legs, and do not massage the legs.	SCI patients are prone to DVT, which can occur in the lower extremities because of immobility and changes in vascular tone.
Provide ROM to the legs qid; elevate legs 10-15 degrees.	These measures promote venous drainage.
⚠ Assess for tachycardia, shortness of breath, hemoptysis, decrease in PaO_2, O_2 saturation 92% or less, decreased or adventitious breath sounds, and chest or shoulder pain. Notify the health care provider about significant findings.	All are indicators of VTE/PE. Presence of pain depends on the level of injury. Sudden shoulder pain may represent referred pain from VTE/PE.
Consult the health care provider about use of antiembolism hose, sequential compression devices, pneumatic foot pumps, or prophylactic pharmacotherapy (e.g., acetylsalicylic acid [ASA], warfarin, low–molecular-weight or low-dose heparin).	These measures help prevent VTE/PE.
If indicated, explain use of a vena cava filter.	This filter helps prevent emboli from reaching the lungs in the presence of VTE/PE.
For other interventions, see **Ineffective Peripheral Tissue Perfusion** in "Prolonged Bedrest," p. 65.	

Nursing Diagnoses:

Urinary Retention or Reflex Urinary Incontinence

related to neurologic impairment (spasticity or flaccidity)

Desired Outcomes: The patient has urinary output without incontinence. The patient empties the bladder with residual volumes of less than 50 mL by the time of discharge. Following instruction, the patient demonstrates triggering mechanism and gains some control over voiding.

ASSESSMENT/INTERVENTIONS   RATIONALES

General Guidelines for Individuals with Bladder Dysfunction

Assess for evidence of bladder dysfunction or monitor cystometric test results.	Bladder dysfunction is complicated and should be assessed by cystometric testing to determine the best type of bladder program.
If intermittent catheterization is used and episodes of incontinence occur or more than 500 mL of urine is obtained, catheterize the patient more often.	Initially during acute spinal shock, patients will have an indwelling urinary catheter or scheduled intermittent catheterizations. As spinal reflexes return, intermittent catheterization or other bladder emptying technique is used. Indwelling catheters are avoided because of the potential for UTI.
Teach the patient and significant other the procedure for intermittent catheterization, care of indwelling catheters, and indicators of UTI (e.g., fever, chills, cloudy and/or foul-smelling urine, malaise, anorexia, restlessness, increased frequency or urgency, incontinence).	This teaching helps ensure readiness for self- or assisted care on discharge from the care facility.
Teach the patient and significant other that the habit/bladder scheduling program consists of gradually increasing the time between catheterizations or periodically clamping indwelling catheters.	The goal is a gradual increase in bladder tone. When the bladder can hold 300-400 mL of urine, measures to stimulate voiding are attempted. Bladder ultrasound may be used to determine fullness and aid in retraining.
Make sure the patient takes fluids at evenly spaced intervals throughout the day.	This promotes adequate hydration and increased bladder tone.
Restrict fluids before bedtime.	This helps prevent nighttime incontinence. Alcohol and caffeine-containing foods and beverages (e.g., cola, chocolate, coffee, tea) have a diuretic effect and may cause incontinence. In addition, caffeine-containing products may increase bladder spasms and reflex incontinence.
Instruct patients using bladder-emptying techniques to void at least q3h.	Maintaining a regular schedule prevents bladder distention. A wristwatch with timer alarm or an alarm clock can help patient maintain this schedule.
To obtain postvoid residual urine, catheterize the patient after an attempt to empty the bladder.	Residual amounts greater than 100 mL usually indicate need for a return to a scheduled intermittent catheterization program.
Assess response to measures that promote bladder training and continence, and obtain urinary specialist consult as appropriate.	A urinary diversion may be considered for patients whose bladders cannot be retrained. An artificial urinary sphincter or continent vesicotomy may be used to promote bladder continence. An external sphincterectomy may be done to reduce sphincter resistance, thereby producing continuous bladder emptying.

Guidelines for Patients with UMN-Involved Spastic Reflex Bladder

Explain to these patients that eventually they may be able to empty the bladder automatically and therefore may not require catheterization.	Lesions above conus medullaris (located at the lower two levels of the thoracic region, where the cord begins to taper) generally leave the S2, S3, and S4 spinal cord nerve segments intact. If this spinal reflex arc is intact, the patient will have UMN-involved bladder, resulting in a spastic bladder. This bladder has tone and occasional bladder contractions and periodically will empty on its own, resulting in reflex incontinence. The UMN-involved bladder is "trainable" with techniques that stimulate reflex voiding.
Teach tapping of the suprapubic area with the fingers, gently pulling pubic hair, digitally stretching the anal sphincter, stroking the glans penis, stroking the inner thigh, light pulsating pressure in the abdominal area just proximal to the inguinal ligaments, or using a hand-held vibration device against the lower abdomen. Advise the patient to perform the selected technique for 2-3 min or until a good urine stream has started. Explain that the patient should wait 1 min before trying another stimulation technique.	These techniques, which are described below, stimulate the voiding reflex and should be taught to patients accordingly. Stimulating reflex trigger zones accidentally may result in incontinence. Incontinence briefs will help control accidents.
	Bladder tapping: The patient positions self in a half-sitting position. Tapping is performed over the suprapubic area, and the patient may shift the site of stimulation within that area to find the most effective site. Tapping is performed rapidly (7-8 times/sec) with one hand for approximately 50 single taps. The patient continues tapping until a good stream starts. Explain that when the stream stops, the patient should wait about 1 min and repeat tapping until the bladder is empty. One or two tapping attempts without response indicate that no more urine will be expelled.

ASSESSMENT/INTERVENTIONS	RATIONALES
	Anal stretch technique (contraindicated in individuals with lesions at T8 or above because of the potential for AD): The patient positions self on a commode or toilet, leans forward on the thighs, and inserts 1 or 2 lubricated fingers into the anus to the anal sphincter. The patient then dilates the anal sphincter gently by spreading the fingers apart or pulling in a posterior direction. The patient maintains the stretching position, takes a deep breath, and holds the breath while bearing down to void. The patient relaxes and repeats until the bladder is empty.
Administer baclofen if it is prescribed.	Baclofen may be prescribed because it tends to promote more complete emptying of the bladder by reducing tone of the external urinary sphincter.

Guidelines for Patients with LMN-Involved Flaccid Bladders

Teach the patient that increasing intraabdominal pressure can overcome sphincter pressure, which may empty the bladder. Explain that this may be contraindicated, however, depending on the risk of ureteral reflux.	Lesions below the conus medullaris (T12) may injure S2, S3, and S4 nerve segments, which will disrupt the reflex arc, causing LMN-involved flaccid bladder. This bladder has no tone and will distend until it overflows, resulting in overflow incontinence.
	Bladder-emptying techniques (e.g., straining, Valsalva's maneuver) to increase intraabdominal pressure are controversial and generally not encouraged because of the potential for reflux past the vesicoureteral junction, thus increasing the potential for ascending UTIs.
Explain that the patient may be able to empty the bladder manually well enough to avoid catheterization.	Need for catheterization can be determined by checking residual urine volume.
If Credé's method is prescribed, teach the technique to the patient.	Credé's method is another technique for increasing intraabdominal pressure. It is performed as follows: The ulnar surface of the hand is placed horizontally along or just below the umbilicus; while the patient bears down with the abdominal muscles, the hand is pressed downward and toward the bladder in a kneading motion until urination is initiated. This is continued for 30 sec or until urination ceases. The patient then waits a few minutes and repeats the procedure to ensure complete emptying of the bladder.
Suggest alternative measures if the patient's bladder cannot be trained to empty completely.	Intermittent catheterization or external collection devices usually are indicated, and the patient may be a candidate for an artificial inflatable sphincter device or urinary diversion.

Nursing Diagnoses:

Dysfunctional Gastrointestinal Motility
Constipation

related to immobility, atonic bowel, and loss of sensation and voluntary sphincter control

Desired Outcome: The patient has bowel movements that are soft and formed every 1-3 days or within the patient's preinjury pattern.

ASSESSMENT/INTERVENTIONS	RATIONALES
Assess the patient's bowel function by auscultating for bowel sounds; inspecting for the presence of abdominal distention; and monitoring for nausea, vomiting, and fecal impaction. Notify the health care provider of significant findings.	During the acute phase of spinal shock, which usually resolves in 1-6 wk, constipation and paralytic ileus are common.
Manage a flaccid bowel with increased intraabdominal pressure technique (see below), manual disimpaction, and small-volume enemas.	Lesions below the conus medullaris (T12) may injure S3, S4, and S5 nerve segments, resulting in disruption of the reflex arc and causing LMN flaccid bowel and loss of anal tone.

continued

ASSESSMENT/INTERVENTIONS	RATIONALES
Administer small-volume enemas only.	The atonic intestine distends easily, and therefore only small volumes are recommended. In the presence of fecal impaction, gentle manual removal or a small cleansing enema may be prescribed.
Avoid long-term use of enemas.	Enemas may disrupt normal flora and affect peristalsis and sphincter tone.
For UMN reflex bowel, once bowel activity returns, teach the patient to attempt bowel movement 30 min after a meal or warm drink.	This regimen will enable the patient's gastrocolic and duodenocolic mass peristalsis reflexes to assist with evacuation. Lesions above the conus medullaris (located at the lower two levels of the thoracic region, where the cord begins to taper) generally leave S3, S4, and S5 spinal cord nerve segments intact. If this spinal reflex arc is intact, the patient will have UMN bowel and be capable of stimulating (training) reflex evacuation of the bowel.
In addition, teach the patient to sit, bear down, bend forward, or apply manual pressure to the abdomen. If allowed, provide a bedside commode. Check the patient's ability to maintain balance on a commode. If the patient is bedridden, turn the patient onto the side and use a pad rather than a bedpan to catch bowel movement.	These measures promote bowel movements by increasing intraabdominal pressure. An abdominal belt may be used if the patient is unable to strain at stool. Massaging the abdomen in a clockwise, circular motion also may help promote bowel evacuation. A prescribed, medicated suppository may be used if necessary.
For patients with injuries at T8 or above, promote adequate fluid intake (more than 2500 mL/day) and use of stool softeners and high-fiber diet.	These measures facilitate bowel evacuation by adding bulk and moisture to the stool.
⚠ Use suppositories and enemas only when essential and with extreme caution. Use anesthetic jelly liberally when performing a rectal examination or inserting a suppository or an enema.	Their use can precipitate AD. Anesthetic jelly prevents skin stimulation, which could otherwise trigger AD.
For patients with hand mobility (who are not at risk for AD), teach the technique for suppository insertion and digital stimulation of the anus.	These measures promote reflex bowel evacuation. Suppository inserters and rectal stimulation devices are available for patients with limited hand mobility.
For digital stimulation, teach the patient to insert a lubricated finger about 1½ inches into the rectum and gently rotate in a slow, circular motion, gently stretching the sphincter for about 30 sec (but no longer than 1 min at a time) until the internal sphincter relaxes. Restart the circular motion if the sphincter tightens, and remove the finger if the bowel movement begins. Stop if sphincter spasms are felt or if signs of AD occur. Repeat q5-10min several times until adequate evacuation occurs. If unsuccessful after 20-30 min of stimulation, insert a suppository.	Digital stimulation stretches and relaxes the internal sphincter to facilitate bowel movement.
Teach the patient to keep fingernails cut short.	This helps prevent injury to the rectal mucosa.
For other interventions, see **Constipation** in "Prolonged Bedrest," p. 68.	

Nursing Diagnosis:

Risk for Disuse Syndrome

related to paralysis, immobilization, or spasticity

Desired Outcomes: After stabilization of the injury, the patient exhibits complete ROM of all joints. By the time of discharge, the patient demonstrates measures that enhance mobility, reduce spasms, and prevent complications.

ASSESSMENT/INTERVENTIONS	RATIONALES
Once the injury is stabilized, assist the patient with position changes on a regular schedule.	This action alternates sites of pressure relief and decreases risk of contracture formation. For example, a prone position, if not contraindicated, helps prevent sacral decubiti and hip contractures.

ASSESSMENT/INTERVENTIONS	RATIONALES
For patients with spasticity, use hand splints or cones, keeping the fingers extended.	These devices assist with maintaining a functional grasp.
If the patient has spasticity, fit him or her with splints or high-top tennis shoes that are cut off at the toes so that each shoe ends just proximal to the metatarsal head.	This helps prevent foot contractures for patients with spasticity. These shoes help keep feet dorsiflexed but prevent contact of the balls of the feet with a hard surface, which can cause spasticity.
Avoid footboards for these patients.	Their hard surface may trigger spasticity and promote plantar flexion.
Teach the patient that some factors that trigger spasms are cold temperatures, anxiety, fatigue, emotional distress, infections (especially UTI), bowel or bladder distention, ulcers, pain, tight clothing, and lying too long in one position.	Controlling these factors may reduce the number of spasms experienced.
Teach patients with spasticity techniques such as proper positioning, ROM, and daily sustained stretching exercises.	Steady, continuous, directional stretching several times daily is especially important because it may decrease spasticity for several hours. Cooling and icing techniques, heat, light-pressure stroking massage, vibration therapy, and transcutaneous electrical nerve stimulation of spastic muscles also may be helpful.
When touch is necessary, do it in a firm, gentle, steady manner. Teach caregivers that touch may need to be limited.	Tactile stimulation may trigger spasms.
Administer prescribed muscle relaxants (e.g., diazepam) and antispasmodics (e.g., baclofen, tizanidine, or dantrolene).	These medications decrease spasms. Dantrolene causes muscle weakness, so it is generally reserved for patients on bedrest. More severe spasticity may be treated with IM injections of botulinum toxin or intrathecal baclofen pump. Intrathecal baclofen involves use of a programmable implanted pump to deliver a continuous dose of baclofen into the spinal canal sheath to control spasticity. Intrathecal baclofen must not be abruptly stopped because doing so may cause seizures and hallucinations.
Encourage participation in a physical therapy (PT) or occupational therapy program.	A therapy program is ongoing throughout the patient's rehabilitation. Passive ROM is started on all joints. After the injury is stabilized, an aggressive rehabilitation program is initiated, including muscle strengthening and conditioning exercises to develop alternative muscle groups needed for independence; a sitting program; massage; instruction in adaptive devices, equipment, and transfer techniques as appropriate; and instruction in orthotics and braces or splints to prevent contractures. Patients with sacral injuries have the potential to walk and should be instructed in the use of braces, crutches, or cane as appropriate. Functional electrical stimulation of paralyzed muscles assists some paraplegic patients with walking.
Assess the effectiveness of measures for spasticity.	Tenotomy, myotomy, peripheral neurectomy, and rhizotomy are some of the surgical approaches that may be used to treat spasticity that cannot be managed by medications or more conservative measures such as stretching or ROM.
Assess for pain, swelling, warmth, and decreased ROM function around joints, especially the hips.	These indicators may signal heterotopic ossification (HO), which is the abnormal formation of true bone within the extraskeletal soft tissues. Etidronate; nonsteroidal antiinflammatories, such as indomethacin; ROM exercises; and external beam radiation are prevention therapies. Once HO has formed, resection usually is necessary.
For additional interventions, see **Risk for Disuse Syndrome**, p. 63, in "Prolonged Bedrest."	

Nursing diagnoses for patients in halo vest traction

Nursing Diagnosis:

Risk for Trauma

related to incorrect neck position, irritation of cranial nerves, impaired lateral vision, and balancing difficulties

Desired Outcome: At the time of discharge (and ongoing during use of halo traction), the patient exhibits no adverse changes in motor, sensory, or cranial nerve function and is free of symptoms of injury caused by impaired vision or balancing difficulties.

ASSESSMENT/INTERVENTIONS	RATIONALES
Assess position of the patient's neck in relation to the body. Alert the health care provider to the presence of flexion or hyperextension. Caution the patient not to turn his or her head from side to side.	To ensure proper alignment and optimal healing, the patient's neck should be in a neutral position.
Assess any difficulty with swallowing.	Swallowing difficulty may signal improper position of neck and chin.
[!] Keep a torque screwdriver in a secure place.	This ensures that the health care provider can readily adjust tension on bars to return the patient's neck position to neutral.
Evaluate the degree of sensation and movement of the upper extremities, and assess cranial nerve function. Notify the health care provider of sudden changes in motor, sensory, or cranial nerve function (e.g., weakness, paresthesias, ptosis, difficulty chewing or swallowing).	Changes in cranial nerve function can occur if cranial pins compress or irritate a nerve. **Note:** Jaw pain may occur when chewing is attempted, and this needs to be differentiated from cranial nerve problems. A diet of soft foods, cut into small pieces, will help jaw pain.
Assess pins, bolts, and vest structure for looseness at least daily. Notify the health care provider if pins becomes loose or dislodged.	Clicking sounds may signal a loose pin, and if this occurs, it will be necessary to stabilize the patient's head to prevent misalignment.
[!] Never use the superstructure of halo traction in turning or moving the patient. Avoid putting pillows under support bars when the patient is lying down (e.g., to sleep).	This could result in misalignment of the patient's affected area.
Instruct the patient to avoid pulling clothes over top of the halo apparatus but rather to step into clothes and pull them up over feet and legs. Advise the patient to buy strapless bras, tube tops, or clothes that are several sizes too large, or to modify neck openings (e.g., with Velcro closures, ties).	These measures help prevent loosening of pins.
[!] Avoid loosening a buckle without the health care provider's directive.	The device must be worn correctly to maintain alignment, prevent skin breakdown, and prevent nerve injury. Buckle holes or straps should be marked so that they are always cinched correctly to the appropriate snugness.
If the patient is ambulatory, teach him or her to walk initially with assistance of two people and how to survey environment while walking, either by using a mirror, by turning eyes to their extreme lateral positions, or by turning the entire body.	The halo vest impairs lateral vision.
If indicated, suggest use of a cane.	A cane will help determine height of curbs and detect unseen objects or uneven walking surfaces.
Explain that trunk flexibility is limited and that achieving balance can be difficult. Teach the patient that bending over can be hazardous.	The vest's weight is top-heavy. Ambulating with a walker initially may help patients learn to adjust. Abdominal- and back-strengthening exercises may aid balance and walking.
Advise the patient to walk only in low-heeled shoes, use long-handled assistive devices to reach or pick up objects, and realize that extra space allowance may be needed when passing through doorways and to avoid bumping into objects.	These measures prevent falls and other injuries caused by wearing the vest.

ASSESSMENT/INTERVENTIONS	RATIONALES
Advise that a shower chair that rolls usually can fit over a toilet seat, providing an extra 3-6 inches in height.	This is the best method to promote safety and avoid straining to raise and lower the body onto a toilet seat.
To get out of bed, teach the patient to roll onto his or her side at the edge of the bed and then drop the legs over the side of the bed while pushing up the trunk sideways.	This technique promotes good alignment and body mechanics to prevent injury.
Recommend backing into car seat with the body bent forward when getting into a car.	This prevents hitting pins and device on car doorframe.
Caution the patient against driving.	Patients will have limited field of vision when wearing the vest.
Teach the patient to use high tables and swivel chairs at home.	A high table will help bring objects into view and a swivel chair will permit easier visualization of the environment.
Explain that the patient will need the assistance of another person to shampoo hair safely.	This promotes safety and helps prevent falling if water spills on the floor.
Advise that shampooing a short haircut is easiest, and hair should be blown dry.	Toweling hair may loosen the pins.
Teach caregivers and significant others how to release the vest in an emergency such as need for external cardiac compression.	Most vests have side straps that, when released, enable the vest to be opened to midline. If a wrench is required, it should be kept with the jacket (e.g., attached with Velcro).

Nursing Diagnoses:

Risk for Impaired Skin Integrity/Impaired Tissue Integrity

related to altered circulation and mechanical factors

Desired Outcome: At the time of discharge and on an ongoing basis, the patient's skin is nonerythremic and unbroken; and the tissue underlying and surrounding the halo vest blanches appropriately.

ASSESSMENT/INTERVENTIONS	RATIONALES
Assess the skin around vest edges for erythema and other signs of irritation. Keep the skin dry.	These are signs of impaired circulation caused by the vest. The skin is kept dry to prevent irritation.
Gently massage nonerythematous areas routinely.	Massage promotes circulation and helps prevent breakdown.
Teach skin inspection, which may require use of a mirror, flashlight, or another person.	For timely intervention, the patient should alert medical personnel if breakdown, sensitive spots, odor, dirty vest liner, or loose pins are present.
Investigate complaints of discomfort or uncomfortable fit. Pad the vest as needed until it can be properly adjusted or trimmed by the health care provider. Protect the vest from moisture and soiling.	A finger should be able to fit between the vest and the patient's skin. Weight loss or gain can affect fit.
Be alert to a foul odor from in or around the cast openings and to serosanguineous drainage on a pillowcase slipped through the vest from one side to another.	A foul odor can signal pressure necrosis beneath the vest, and serosanguineous drainage may indicate an area of skin breakdown.
Instruct/assist the patient with changing body position q2h. Support the vest while the patient is in bed, and use the logroll technique with sufficient help.	Changing positions promotes circulation and prevents skin and tissue breakdown by alternating sites of pressure relief.
Use soft padding. Use a small pillow under the patient's head at sleep time.	Padding helps prevent pressure on prominent body areas such as the forehead or shoulder and a small pillow promotes comfort and support for the neck.
Wash the skin under the vest with soap and warm water.	Usually, releasing one vest belt at a time as the patient is lying down is allowed for washing.

continued

ASSESSMENT/INTERVENTIONS	RATIONALES
Avoid use of lotion and powder under the vest.	These products can cake under the vest.
Replace soiled linens promptly. Dry perspiration with a hair dryer on a cool setting.	These actions prevent skin irritation and breakdown caused by moisture.
Inspect under both sides of the vest for redness, swelling, bruising, or chafing. Close the open side and repeat on the opposite side.	If a rash appears, the patient may be allergic to the vest's lining. A synthetic liner, knitted body stockinette, or T-shirt may correct this problem.
In the event of skin breakdown, keep the skin cleansed, dried, and covered with a transparent dressing. Notify the health care provider, wound, ostomy, continence/enterostomal therapy (WOC/ET) nurse, and orthotist accordingly.	At the first sign of skin breakdown, a WOC/ET nurse can implement a wound care regimen. An orthotist can make a brace adjustment to prevent further breakdown.
Place rubber corks over tips of the halo device.	This will diminish annoying sound vibrations if the apparatus is bumped and prevent lacerations from sharp edges.
Check tong placement (e.g., Crutchfield, Vinke, Gardner-Wells) at least daily.	If slippage has occurred, the patient's head should be immobilized with a sandbag and health care provider notified promptly to prevent misalignment of neck. Pain may signal erosion of bone and displacement into muscle.
Check drainage from tong sites for presence of cerebrospinal fluid (CSF) (see p. 344).	The presence of CSF indicates the tong has penetrated through the skull, and risk of meningitis and neurologic damage is possible.
Ensure that tong traction weights are hanging freely.	This helps ensure that traction is maintained as prescribed.
For a discussion of pin care, see "Fractures," p. 495, for **Deficient Knowledge** (function of external fixation, pin care, and signs and symptoms of pin site infection).	

Nursing Diagnosis:

Sexual Dysfunction

related to altered body function and deficient knowledge

Desired Outcome: Within the 24-hr period before hospital discharge, the patient discusses concerns about sexuality and verbalizes knowledge of alternative methods of sexual expression.

ASSESSMENT/INTERVENTIONS	RATIONALES
Evaluate your own feelings about sexuality. Refer the patient to someone (e.g., knowledgeable staff member, professional sexual therapy counselor) who can address the patient's sexual concerns if you are uncomfortable discussing these issues or unable to answer specific concerns and questions.	Nurses may not be able to answer all the patient's questions or may be uncomfortable discussing sexual issues. The nurse's discomfort would add to the patient's discomfort.
Provide a supportive, nonjudgmental environment that gives the patient permission to have and freely express sexual concerns. Elicit/assess the patient's knowledge, concerns, and questions.	Sexuality can be discussed as it relates to an erection that occurs during a bath or to objective findings noted during physical assessment.
Expect acting-out behavior related to the patient's sexuality.	This is a normal response to anxiety about the sexual response and prognosis. Such behaviors may include asking personal questions, sexual jokes or innuendoes, self-deprecating remarks, or flirting with the staff.

ASSESSMENT/INTERVENTIONS	RATIONALES
Provide information about the normal sexual response and changes caused by SCI.	Sexual functioning may be different but still possible with SCI. The general rule for men is the higher the lesion, the greater the chance of retaining the ability to have an erection (but with a lesser chance of ejaculation). Women may have problems with lubrication, and orgasm may be difficult to achieve because of decreased sensation. Women may also have a transient loss of ovulation; however, ovulation usually returns, and women can become pregnant and deliver vaginally.
	Sperm quality decreases in men after SCI, but they may still be capable of fathering a child naturally. Use of vibromassage or electroejaculation via electrical stimulation in the area of the prostate to obtain sperm, in utero insemination, in vitro fertilization, or intracytoplasmic sperm injection have improved fertility.
Provide information about birth control and oral contraception for women who desire it.	Uterine contractions of labor in women with SCI lesion at T8 or above may cause AD. Oral contraceptives may be contraindicated because of the risk of thrombophlebitis.
Provide specific suggestions that may provide gratification, including oral-genital sex, digital stimulation, vibrator stimulation, cuddling, mutual masturbation, anal eroticism, and massage. Provide specific suggestions for managing common problems, including decreasing fluid intake 2-3 hr before sexual encounter, emptying bladder and bowels (if necessary) before a sexual encounter, (for men) folding back indwelling catheter along the penis and holding it in place with a condom, (for women) taping catheter to the abdomen and leaving it in place, taking a warm bath before sexual activity to reduce spasticity, planning sexual activity for a time of day in which both partners are rested, experimenting with a variety of positions, and applying topical anesthetics to areas that are hypersensitive to touch.	Sexual activity may seem impossible to the SCI patient. These and the suggestions that follow may provide gratification and facilitate the act. Oral medications such as sildenafil generally have replaced other erectile dysfunction medications such as suppositories, penile injections, and topical applications. Patients with erections lasting longer than 4 hours should seek medical attention. Sublingual and nasally administered apomorphine (used in Europe and awaiting Food and Drug Administration approval in the United States) also may help obtain a long-lasting erection. Erection assistive techniques and devices (e.g., vacuum suction pump, penile prosthesis or implant) may help men with SCI attain erections.
Explain that water-soluble lubricants are useful, if needed, but that petroleum-based lubricants should be avoided.	Petroleum-based lubricants can cause UTI.
Explain that adductor spasms in women may pose a barrier but can be overcome if a rear entry is acceptable. Suggest that prolonged foreplay with stroking and light massage may also relax muscles. If AD occurs during sexual activity, suggest that the patient consult the health care provider about preventive measures (e.g., taking a ganglionic blocking agent before having sexual intercourse or applying a topical anesthetic).	These are guidelines for managing less common problems that can occur during a sexual encounter.
Suggest that the patient's partner be included in discussion about sexual concerns.	Explaining the physical condition caused by SCI and preparing the partner for scars, lack of muscle tone, atrophy, and the presence of a catheter will provide the partner with an opportunity to discuss sexual concerns.
For additional interventions, see **Ineffective Sexuality Pattern** in "Prolonged Bedrest," p. 71.	

ADDITIONAL NURSING DIAGNOSES/PROBLEMS:

✓ PATIENT-FAMILY TEACHING AND DISCHARGE PLANNING

When providing patient-family teaching, focus on sensory information, avoid giving excessive information, and initiate a visiting nurse referral for necessary follow-up teaching. Include verbal and written information about the following:

✓ Spinal cord functioning and the effects trauma has on how the body works.

✓ Referrals to community resources, such as public health nurse, visiting nurses association, community support groups, social workers, psychologic therapy, vocational rehabilitation agency, home health agencies, and extended and skilled care facilities. Additional general information can be obtained by contacting the following organizations:

- National Spinal Cord Injury Association at *www.spinalcord.org*
- Christopher and Dana Reeve Foundation at *www.christopherreeve.org*
- SCI Action Canada at *www.sciactioncanada.ca/*
- Spinal Cord Injury Ontario at http://www.sciontario.org/
- Paralyzed Veterans of American at *www.pva.org*
- Cure Paralysis Now at *www.cureparalysis.org*
- Rehabilitation Research Center at *www.tbi-sci.org*
- Paralinks at *www.paralinks.net*
- DisABILITY Information and Resources at *www.makoa.org*

✓ Safety measures relative to decreased sensation, motor deficits, orthostatic hypotension and symptoms, preventive measures, and interventions for AD.

✓ Use and care of a brace or immobilizer, medical equipment, and mobility aids as appropriate.

✓ What patient can expect if transferred to rehabilitation center.

✓ Techniques and devices for performing activities of daily living, including bathing, grooming, turning, feeding, and other self-care activities to patient's maximum potential. The patient may need a home accessibility evaluation and a driving evaluation and training.

✓ Indicators of ureteral calculi and dietary measures to prevent their formation (see p. 224).

✓ Indicators of VTE/DVT and measures to prevent it (see pp. 128, 186).

✓ Importance of participation in counseling and psychotherapy to help patient and significant other adjust to the disability. This should include addressing of sexual functioning and vocational rehabilitation.

✓ For additional information, see teaching and discharge planning interventions (the fourth through tenth entries only) as appropriate in "Multiple Sclerosis," p. 292.

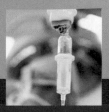

OVERVIEW/PATHOPHYSIOLOGY

A stroke, cerebrovascular accident (CVA), or brain attack is the sudden disruption of O_2 supply to the brain. This can be due to rupture in one or more of the blood vessels that supply the brain or loss of cerebral perfusion often resulting from hypoperfusion or reduction of O_2 supply. *Ischemic stroke* has three main mechanisms: thrombosis, embolism, and systemic hypoperfusion. Thrombosis or embolism results in a blockage of blood supply to the brain tissue. The resulting ischemia, if prolonged, causes brain tissue necrosis (infarction), cerebral edema, and increased intracranial pressure (IICP). Most thrombotic strokes are caused by blockage of large vessels as a result of atherosclerosis. Thrombi in small penetrating arteries result in "lacunar" strokes. Most embolic strokes are cardiogenic and the result of emboli produced from valve disease or during atrial fibrillation of the heart. Ischemic stroke caused by systemic hypoperfusion usually is the result of decreased cerebral blood flow owing to circulatory failure. Some causes of circulatory failure include hypovolemia, hypotension, and dysrhythmias. Hypoxia from any cause also can produce this syndrome.

A *transient ischemic attack (TIA)*, which is a temporary (less than 24 hr) neurologic deficit that resolves completely without permanent damage, occurs when the artery cannot deliver enough blood to meet the O_2 requirement of the brain. However, restoration of blood flow is timely enough to make the ischemia (and deficits) transient, thereby avoiding infarction and permanent damage. TIAs usually are associated with thrombosis but may be caused by any of the ischemic mechanisms just mentioned. TIAs may precede a permanent ischemic stroke by hours, days, months, or years. TIAs are a warning sign, and treatment may prevent a stroke. Most TIAs last an average of 5-10 min, although some can last longer than an hour. Many patients understand these as "mini strokes." A *reversible ischemic neurologic deficit (RIND)* lasts longer than 24 hr but otherwise is similar to a TIA.

Hemorrhagic stroke causes neural tissue destruction because of the infiltration and accumulation of blood. Ischemia and infarction may occur distal to the hemorrhage because of interrupted blood supply. Although a cerebral hemorrhage usually results from hypertension or an aneurysm, trauma also can cause hemorrhagic stroke. Bleeding may spread into the brain tissue itself, causing an intracerebral hemorrhage, or into the subarachnoid space. Usually there is a large rise in intracranial pressure (ICP) with a hemorrhagic stroke because of cerebral edema and the mass effect of blood.

A stroke may be classified as a *progressive stroke in evolution*, in which deficits continue to worsen over time, or as a *completed stroke*, in which maximum deficit has been acquired and has persisted for longer than 24 hr. Progressive strokes usually are the result of thrombus formation and often take 1-3 days to become "completed." Embolic strokes typically have sudden onset with maximal deficits. Presentation may be variable depending on scatter of the emboli. *Stroke syndromes* classically have been described according to distribution of the vessels (middle cerebral artery, anterior cerebral artery, posterior cerebral artery, vertebral, basilar) that supply particular regions of the brain and will have typical assessment findings. Stroke is the third most common cause of death and the most common cause of neurologic disability. Half the survivors are left permanently disabled or experience another stroke. Improvement may continue for 1-2 yr, but deficits at 6 mo usually are considered permanent.

A *brain attack*, also sometimes called a *code stroke* or *stroke alert*, is a sudden event and medical emergency with the same urgency as a heart attack. If the stroke is ischemic and the patient qualifies, "time-is-tissue," and the sooner the patient can be treated, the better the outcome. For appropriate patients, treatment with recombinant tissue plasminogen activator (rtPA), commonly referred to as TPA, needs to occur within 3 hr of symptom onset. To achieve this, all people should be educated to recognize warning signs of stroke and immediately call 911. Rapid transport to a hospital, preferably a stroke center, should occur, with the emergency medical technician starting the medical history, especially the time of symptom onset, and alerting the hospital before arrival so the stroke team (if available) can be assembled. Upon arrival at the hospital door, the time-to-treatment goal is 60 min and is further broken down into subgoals:

Time from arrival at hospital door to:
Evaluation by physician—10 min

Neurologic expert and "stroke team" (if available) contacted and patient assessed—15-25 min

Head computed tomography (CT) or magnetic resonance imaging (MRI) scan completed; other data (e.g., laboratory values) completed; decision to treat based upon data, contraindications—45 min

Start of treatment (e.g., rtPA) in appropriate patients —60 min

Intraarterial rtPA, collected—25 min

Available at some research centers, intraarterial rtPA may extend the window of opportunity to 6 hr. Thrombolytic therapy reverses symptoms of stroke by dissolving the clot(s) causing the ischemia before actual cell death. Use of a mechanical blood clot retrieval device (e.g., MERCI) may extend this time window further.

Stroke care can be differentiated into these basic types: thrombolytic ischemic stroke care, nonthrombolytic ischemic stroke care (including TIAs), and hemorrhagic stroke care. Care differences center mostly around BP management and use of anticoagulant and antiplatelet agents. Most hospitals, especially stroke centers, have protocols for stroke management.

HEALTH CARE SETTING

Critical care unit, step-down unit, acute rehabilitation unit, outpatient rehabilitation program

ASSESSMENT

Note: *Because of the narrow 3-hr window during which it may be possible to reverse permanent neurologic damage, it is critical to teach patients not to ignore symptoms and to call 911 without delay for the following:*

- Sudden numbness or weakness of the face, arm, or leg, especially on one side of the body
- Sudden confusion, trouble speaking or understanding
- Sudden trouble seeing in one or both eyes
- Sudden trouble walking, dizziness, loss of balance or coordination
- Sudden, severe headache with no known cause

A history to determine time of symptom onset is critical inasmuch as this may determine eligibility for treatment. Time of onset is when patient was last known to be "normal," so if the patient woke up after sleeping with symptoms, time of onset would be when the patient went to bed "normal" and not when he or she woke up symptomatic.

General findings: Classically, symptoms appear on the side of the body opposite the damaged site. For example, a stroke in the left hemisphere of the brain will produce symptoms in the right arm and leg. However, when the stroke affects the cranial nerves, symptoms of cranial nerve deficit will appear on the same side as the site of injury. Similarly, an obstruction of an anterior cerebral artery can produce bilateral symptoms,

as will severe bleeding or multiple emboli. Hemiplegia is fairly common. Initially, the patient usually has flaccid paralysis. As spinal cord depression resolves, more normal tone is seen and hyperactive reflexes occur.

Signs and symptoms: Vary with the size and site of injury and may improve in 2-3 days as the cerebral edema decreases. Changes in mentation, including apathy, irritability, disorientation, memory loss, withdrawal, drowsiness, stupor, or coma; bowel and bladder incontinence; numbness or loss of sensation; weakness or paralysis on part or one side of the body; aphasia; headache; neck stiffness and rigidity; vomiting; seizures; dizziness or syncope; ataxia; and fever may occur. A brain stem infarct leaving the patient completely paralyzed with intact cortical function is called *locked-in syndrome*. With *cranial nerve involvement*, visual disturbances include diplopia, blindness, and hemianopia. Inequality or fixation of the pupils, nystagmus, tinnitus, and difficulty chewing and swallowing also occur.

Physical assessment: Papilledema, arteriosclerotic retinal changes, or hemorrhagic retinal areas on ophthalmic examination. Hyperactive deep tendon reflexes (DTRs), decreased superficial reflexes, and positive Babinski's sign also may be present. To check for Babinski's response, stroke the lateral aspect of the sole of the foot (from the heel to the ball of the foot) with a hard object. Dorsiflexion of the great toe with fanning of the other toes is a positive sign. Positive Kernig's or Brudzinski's sign (see "Bacterial Meningitis," p. 262) indicates meningeal irritation.

TIA: Typical symptoms include temporary episodes of slurred speech, weakness, numbness or tingling, blindness in one eye, blurred or double vision, dizziness or ataxia, and confusion.

Risk factors: TIAs; hypertension; atherosclerosis; high serum cholesterol or triglycerides; high homocysteine levels; diabetes mellitus; gout; smoking; obesity; cardiac valve diseases, such as those that may result from rheumatic fever, valve prosthesis, and atrial fibrillation; cardiac surgery; blood dyscrasias; anticoagulant therapy; neck vessel trauma; oral contraceptive use; cocaine or methamphetamine use; family predisposition for arteriovenous malformation (AVM); aneurysm; advanced age; or previous stroke.

Assessment scales (e.g., GCS and NIHSS): The Glasgow Coma Scale (GCS) is helpful for quickly assessing level of consciousness (LOC). The National Institutes of Health Stroke Scale (NIHSS) not only assesses LOC but also assesses deficits and provides a standardized approach to neurologic examinations. An NIHSS total score of 0-1 is normal; 1-4 is a minor stroke; 5-15 is a moderate stroke; 15-20 is a moderately severe stroke; and more than 20 is a severe stroke. The NIHSS score also strongly predicts likelihood of recovery, with higher scores resulting in more disability and poorer outcomes. Use of thrombolytics (e.g., rtPA) is considered appropriate for ischemic stroke if the total score is more than 4-6 and there is sustained, nonimproving deficit. NIHSS is used for assessing effects of thrombolytic therapy and should, at minimum, be done initially as a baseline, 2 hr post treatment, 24 hr post onset of symptoms, and 7-10 days after symptom onset. The complete scale with instructions can be obtained from *www.strokecenter.org*.

DIAGNOSTIC TESTS

Selection, sequence, and urgency of the following tests will be determined by the patient's history and symptoms. For example, a patient whose symptoms have resolved from a TIA will have a different set or sequence of tests compared to the patient who is in coma. Because usage of rtPA is time limited, speed is essential in determining type of stroke (ischemic vs. hemorrhagic) and other contraindications to rtPA. Obtaining CT scan to determine type of stroke is a top priority along with laboratory tests to assess for contraindications.

CT scan: To reveal site of infarction, hematoma, and shift of brain structures. CT scan is of particular value in identifying blood released early during hemorrhagic strokes. CT scan is the test of choice for unstable patients. Generally, identifying ischemic areas is difficult until they start to necrose at around 48-72 hr. Xenon-enhanced CT may be done to study cerebral blood flow; CT angiography may be performed to evaluate blood vessels.

MRI scan: To reveal site of infarction, hematoma, shift of brain structure, and cerebral edema. MRI diffusion and perfusion-weighted studies are of particular value in identifying ischemic strokes early and in differentiating between acute and chronic lesions. Other magnetic resonance (MR) techniques include MR angiography to evaluate vessels and MR spectrography.

Laboratory tests: Certain tests (e.g., serum electrolytes, complete blood count including differential and platelet count, prothrombin time with international normalized ratio, and partial thromboplastin time) should be done immediately to assess for contraindications such as hypoglycemia or clotting abnormalities if the patient is a candidate for thrombolytic therapy. Other tests will be done depending on the patient (e.g., toxicology screen, pregnancy test, blood culture and erythrocyte sedimentation rate for endocarditis or vasculitis process, hemoglobin A_{IC} for diabetics). Lipid panel, C-reactive protein, and homocysteine levels also may be obtained.

Electrocardiogram: To evaluate for atrial fibrillation and myocardial ischemia.

Phonoangiography/Doppler ultrasonography: To identify presence of bruits if the carotid blood vessels are partially occluded. B-mode imaging and duplex scanning also may be done to evaluate the carotids to detect occlusive disease.

Dimensional ultrasound improves three-dimensional visualization and includes the potential for quantitative monitoring of plaque volume changes in all three directions —circumferential, length, and thickness.

Transcranial Doppler ultrasound: To provide information (noninvasively) about pressure and flow in the intracranial arteries.

Swallowing examination/videofluoroscopy: All patients should be screened for dysphagia. Videofluoroscopy identifies the problem or pathology, determines most appropriate treatment, and enables teaching of proper swallowing technique. This test is not performed for individuals known to aspirate saliva because it involves swallowing a barium-containing liquid, semisolid, and/or solid.

Positron emission tomography: To provide information on cerebral metabolism and blood flow characteristics. This test is useful in identifying ischemic stroke by showing areas of reduced glucose metabolism.

Single photon emission CT: To identify cerebral blood flow.

Electroencephalograph: To show abnormal nerve impulse transmission and indicate amount of brain wave activity present.

Lumbar puncture and cerebrospinal fluid (CSF) analysis: Not done routinely, especially in the presence of IICP, but may reveal increase in CSF pressure; clear to bloody CSF, depending on stroke type; and presence of infection or other nonvascular cause for bleeding. CSF glutamic oxaloacetic transaminase (GOT) will be increased for 10 days after injury. Blood in the CSF signals that a subarachnoid hemorrhage has occurred.

Cerebral and carotid angiography: If surgery is contemplated, this procedure is done to pinpoint site of rupture or occlusion and identify collateral blood circulation, aneurysms, or AVM.

Digital subtraction angiography: To visualize cerebral blood flow and detect vascular abnormalities, such as stenosis, aneurysm, and hematomas.

Echocardiography (e.g., transthoracic and transesophageal): To evaluate valvular heart structures for thrombus and myocardial walls for mural thrombi that may provide a source of emboli.

Evoked response test: Provides measurement of the brain's ability to process and react to different sensory stimuli. Responses from these sensory stimuli can indicate abnormal areas in the brain.

Electronystagmography: Evaluates patients who have dizziness, vertigo, or balance dysfunction and provides objective assessment of oculomotor and vestibular systems.

Nursing Diagnoses:

Impaired Physical Mobility
Risk for Disuse Syndrome

related to neuromuscular impairment with limited use of upper and/or lower limbs

Desired Outcomes: By at least 24 hr before hospital discharge, the patient and significant other demonstrate techniques that promote ambulating and transferring. The patient does not exhibit evidence of shoulder subluxation or shoulder-hand syndrome.

ASSESSMENT/INTERVENTIONS	RATIONALES
Assess for subluxation of the shoulder (e.g., shoulder pain and tenderness, swelling, decreased range of motion [ROM], altered appearance of bony prominences).	Shoulder subluxation occurs when weight of the affected arm is unable to be supported by the weakened shoulder muscles, causing separation of the shoulder joint.
Never pull on the affected arm. Guide the upper extremity movement from the scapula and not from the arm; use a lift sheet to reposition in bed. Ensure that the arm has a firm support surface when the patient is sitting.	These measures help prevent subluxation. When in bed the shoulder should be positioned slightly forward to counteract shoulder rotation. The affected arm should be placed in external rotation when the patient is supine or lying on affected side.
Teach methods for turning and moving, using the stronger extremity to move the weaker extremity.	For example, to move the affected leg in bed or when changing from a lying to a sitting position, slide the unaffected foot under the affected ankle to lift, support, and bring the affected leg along in the desired movement.
Encourage the patient to make a conscious attempt to look at extremities and check position before moving.	These are safety measures to prevent falling. For example, remind the patient to make a conscious effort to lift and then extend the foot when ambulating.
Instruct the patient with impaired sense of balance to compensate by leaning toward the stronger side as an attempt to ensure proper upright posture.	The tendency is to lean toward the weaker or paralyzed side. For example, the patient may need to be reminded to keep body weight forward over the feet when standing.
Recommend wearing well-fitting shoes.	Slippers, for example, tend to slide.
Prevent shoulder-hand syndrome with regular, gentle joint ROM exercises and proper arm positioning. Never place the arm under the body. When the patient is in bed, place the arm on the abdomen or pillow for support. Encourage repeated shoulder movement, elevation of the arm above cardiac level, and regular fist clenching and reclenching.	Shoulder-hand syndrome is a neurovascular condition characterized by pain, edema, and skin and muscle atrophy caused by impairment of the circulatory pumping action of the upper extremity.
Protect the impaired arm with a sling.	The sling will support the arm and shoulder when the patient is out of bed.
Position the patient in correct alignment, and provide a pillow or lapboard for support. Encourage active/passive ROM to improve muscle tone.	These measures will help maintain anatomic position.
Teach and implement the following: - Encourage weight bearing on the patient's stronger side. - Instruct the patient to pivot on the stronger side and use the stronger arm for support. - Teach the patient that transferring toward the unaffected side is generally easiest and safest. - Instruct the patient to place the unaffected side closest to bed or chair to which he or she wishes to transfer. - Explain that when transferring, the affected leg should be under the patient with the foot flat on the ground. - Position a braced chair or locked wheelchair close to the patient's stronger side.	These are general principles to follow when transferring patients with impaired physical mobility. These transfer principles emphasize using the stronger or unaffected side to help support patients for safe transfers to reduce the risk of falling.
If the patient requires assistance from a staff member, teach the patient not to support self by pulling on or placing hands around the assistant's neck.	Staff members should use their own knees and feet to brace the feet and knees of patients who are very weak.

ASSESSMENT/INTERVENTIONS	RATIONALES
Obtain physical therapy (PT) and occupational therapy (OT) referrals as appropriate. Reinforce special mobilization techniques (e.g., Bobath, constraint-induced [CI] movement therapy, proprioceptive neuromuscular facilitation [PNF]) per the patient's individualized rehabilitation program.	These techniques may vary from the general principles mentioned. For example, Bobath focuses on use of the affected side in mobility training so that patients try to bear weight on their affected side and move toward their affected side to relearn normal movement patterns and position. CI movement therapy involves restraining the functioning arm to induce "rewiring of the brain," thereby improving amount and quality of functional movement.

Nursing Diagnosis:

Impaired Verbal Communication

related to aphasia occurring with cerebrovascular insult

Desired Outcome: At least 24 hr before hospital discharge, the patient demonstrates improved self-expression and relates decreased frustration with communication.

ASSESSMENT/INTERVENTIONS	RATIONALES
Assess nature and severity of the patient's aphasia. When doing so, avoid giving nonverbal cues. Assess the patient's ability to speak clearly without slurring words, use words appropriately, point or look toward a specific object, follow simple directions, understand yes/no questions, understand complex questions, repeat both simple and complex words, repeat sentences, name objects that are shown, demonstrate or relate purpose or action of objects, fulfill written requests, write requests, and read. When evaluating for aphasia, be aware that the patient may be responding to nonverbal cues and may understand less than you think. Document this assessment with simple descriptions and specific examples of aphasia symptoms. Use it as the basis for a communication plan.	Aphasia is the partial or complete inability to use or comprehend language and symbols and may occur with dominant (left) hemisphere damage. It is not the result of impaired hearing or intelligence. There are many different types of aphasias. Generally, patients have a combination of types that vary in severity. Fluent aphasia (e.g., Wernicke's, sensory, or receptive aphasia) is characterized by inability to recognize or comprehend spoken words. It is as if a foreign language were being spoken or the patient has word deafness. The patient often is good at responding to nonverbal cues. In nonfluent aphasia (e.g., Broca's, motor, or expressive aphasia) the ability to understand and comprehend language is retained but the patient has difficulty expressing words or naming objects. Gestures, groans, swearing, or nonsense words may be used.
Ask the patient to repeat unclear words by speaking slowly in short phrases. If this is unsuccessful, ask the patient to use another word or give a nonverbal clue.	Do not pretend you understand if you do not. Say so. Nonverbal cues, pointing, flash cards of basic needs, pantomime, paper/pen, spelling, or picture board may help communication.
Obtain referral to a speech therapist or pathologist as needed. Provide the therapist with a list of words that would enhance the patient's independence and/or care. In addition, ask for tips that will help improve communication with the patient.	Patients may need the expertise of a specialist to facilitate ability to communicate.
When communicating with the patient, try to reduce distractions in the environment, such as television or others' conversations.	This focuses the patient's attention on communication.
Ensure that the patient is well rested.	Fatigue affects the ability to communicate.
Communicate with the patient as much as possible. Use gestures, facial expressions, and pantomime to supplement and reinforce your message. Give short, simple directions, and repeat as needed to ensure understanding. Use concrete terms (e.g., "water" instead of "fluid" or "leg" instead of "limb"). If the patient does not understand after repetition, try different words.	These are general principles for patients who may not recognize or comprehend the spoken word. Other suggestions include the following: face the patient and establish eye contact, speak slowly and clearly, give the patient time to process your communication and answer, keep messages short and simple, stay with one clearly defined subject, avoid questions with multiple choices but rather phrase questions so that they can be answered "yes" or "no," and use the same words each time you repeat a statement or question (e.g., "pill" vs. "medication" and "bathroom" vs. "toilet").
When helping the patient regain use of symbolic language, start with nouns first and progress to more complex statements as indicated, using verbs, pronouns, and adjectives.	Progression from simple to complex helps facilitate comprehension. For continuity, it is a good plan to keep at the bedside a record of words to be used (e.g., "pill" rather than "medication").

continued

Neurologic Care Plans

ASSESSMENT/INTERVENTIONS	RATIONALES
Treat the patient as an adult. Be respectful.	It is not necessary to raise the volume of your voice unless the patient is hard of hearing.
When the patient has difficulty expressing words or naming objects, encourage the patient to repeat words after you. Begin with simple words such as "yes" or "no," and progress to others, such as "cup." Progress to more complex statements as indicated.	These measures enable practice in verbal expression.
Listen and respond to the patient's communication efforts. If the patient makes an error, do not criticize the patient's effort but rather compliment it by saying, "That was a good try." Praise accomplishments.	Otherwise the patient may give up.
Be prepared for labile emotions. Do not react negatively to emotional displays. Address and acknowledge the patient's frustration over the inability to communicate. Maintain a calm and positive attitude.	These patients become frustrated and emotional when faced with their impaired speech.
When improvement is noted, let the patient complete your sentence (e.g., "This is a _____"). Keep a list of words the patient can say, and add to the list as appropriate. Avoid finishing the patient's sentences.	This list then can be used when formulating questions the patient is known to be able to answer.
Avoid labeling the patient as "belligerent" or "confused" when the problem is aphasia and frustration. Listen for errors in conversation, and provide feedback.	Patients who have lost the ability to monitor their verbal output may not produce sensible language but may think they are making sense and not understand why others do not comprehend or respond appropriately to them.
Avoid instructing the patient to "wait 5 min" because this may not be meaningful.	Patients who have lost the ability to recognize number symbols or relationships will have difficulty understanding time concepts or telling time.
Point to an object and clearly state its name. Watch signals the patient gives you.	This facilitates practice in receiving word images.
Bring patients with nondominant (right) hemisphere damage back to the subject by saying, "Let's go back to what we were talking about."	Patients with nondominant (right) hemisphere damage often have no difficulty speaking; however, they may use excessive detail, give irrelevant information, and get off on a tangent. These patients tend to respond better to verbal, rather than nonverbal, encouragement.
Observe for nonverbal cues, and anticipate the patient's needs. Allow time to listen if the patient speaks slowly.	This validates the patient's message without rushing him or her, which would cause frustration.
Ensure that the call light is available and the patient knows how to use it.	The call light is the first step in communicating a need for assistance.
For additional interventions for patients with dysarthria, see **Impaired Verbal Communication** in "General Care of Patients with Neurologic Disorders," p. 257.	Dysarthria can complicate aphasia.

Nursing Diagnosis:

Unilateral Neglect

related to brain injury affecting the right hemisphere

Desired Outcome: Following intervention and on an ongoing basis, the patient scans the environment and responds to stimuli on the affected side.

ASSESSMENT/INTERVENTIONS	RATIONALES
Assess the patient's ability to recognize objects to the right or left of his or her visual midline; perceive body parts as his or her own; perceive pain, touch, and temperature sensations; judge distances; orient self to changes in the environment; differentiate left from right; maintain posture sense; and identify objects by sight, hearing, or touch. Document specific deficits.	This assessment enables the nurse to develop a plan of care individualized for the patient. Neglect of and inattention to stimuli on the affected side occur more often with right hemisphere injury. Neglect cannot be totally explained on the basis of loss of physical senses (e.g., both ears are used in hearing, but with auditory neglect, patients may ignore conversations or noises that occur on the affected side).
Arrange the environment by keeping necessary objects, such as call light, on the patient's unaffected side.	This will facilitate performance of activities of daily living (ADLs).
Perform activities on the unaffected side unless you are specifically attempting to stimulate the patient's neglected side.	Communicating and performing activities on the patient's unaffected side will engage and be less confusing to the patient.
If you must approach the affected side, announce yourself first.	This announcement avoids startling the patient.
Inform significant others about the patient's deficit and compensatory interventions.	This enables significant others to be informed participants in the patient's care plan.
Visual Neglect:	Patients do not turn their head to see all parts of an object. For example, patients may read only half of a page or eat from only one side of the plate.
Continuously cue the patient to the environment. Initially place the patient's unaffected side toward the most active part of room, but as compensation occurs, reverse this. As the patient begins to compensate, place additional items out of his or her visual field, thereby gradually increasing stimuli on the affected side. Place the patient's food on the neglected side, encouraging the patient to look to the neglected side and name the food before eating.	While communicating with the patient, physically moving across the patient's visual boundary and standing on that side will shift the patient's attention to the neglected side. Encouraging patients to turn their head past the midline and scan the entire environment, especially while ambulating, will help to prevent injury from falls or bumping into things.
Self-Neglect:	The patient does not perceive the affected arm or leg as being a part of the body. For example, when combing or brushing hair, the patient attends to only one (unaffected) side of the head. Inadequate self-care and injury may occur.
Periodically refer to the patient's body parts on the neglected side. Encourage the patient to touch or massage and look at the affected side and make a conscious effort to care for neglected body parts first when performing ADLs.	This promotes the patient's self-recognition. For example, have the patient use the unaffected arm to perform ROM on the affected side and provide a mirror so the patient can watch self while shaving and brushing teeth and hair.
Encourage consciously monitoring the affected side for position and checking for exposure to sharp objects, irritants, and hot or cold items.	This helps prevent contractures and skin breakdown or injury. For example, position the affected arm on the bedside table or wheelchair lapboard with the hand or arm past the midline, where the patient can see it.
Provide structured tactile stimulation on the affected side.	Stimulate with a warm washcloth, cold ice chip, rough or soft-surfaced cloth, or similar item.
When the patient is in bed or sitting up in a chair, provide side rails and restraints.	These are necessary safety measures because the patient is unaware of the affected side and may attempt to get up.
Auditory Neglect:	The patient ignores individuals who approach and speak from the affected side but communicates with those who approach or speak from the unaffected side.
Move across the auditory boundary while speaking, and continue speaking from the patient's neglected side to bring the patient's attention to that area.	This stimulates the patient's attention to the affected side.

Nursing Diagnosis:

Risk for Injury

related to altered sensory reception, transmission, and/or integration

Desired Outcome: Following intervention and on an ongoing basis, the patient interacts appropriately with his or her environment and does not exhibit evidence of injury caused by sensory/perceptual deficit.

ASSESSMENT/INTERVENTIONS	RATIONALES
Assess type and degree of hemisphere injury the patient exhibits.	See details, below, which describe right and left hemisphere injuries.
Remind patients who have a dominant (left) hemisphere injury to scan their environment.	These patients may lack or have decreased pain sensation and position sense and have visual field deficit on the right side of the body. They may need reminders to scan their environment but usually do not exhibit unilateral neglect.
Give short, simple messages or questions and step-by-step directions. Keep conversation on a concrete level (e.g., say "water," not "fluid"; "leg," not "limb").	These individuals may have poor abstract thinking skills. They tend to be slow, cautious, and disorganized when approaching an unfamiliar problem and benefit from frequent, accurate, and immediate feedback on performance. They may respond well to nonverbal encouragement, such as a pat on the back.
Encourage patients with nondominant (right) hemisphere injury to slow down and check each step or task as it is completed.	Patients with nondominant (right) hemisphere injury also may have decreased pain sensation and pain sense and visual field deficit but typically are unconcerned or unaware of or deny deficits or lost abilities. They tend to be impulsive and too quick with movements. Typically, they have impaired judgment about what they can and cannot do and often overestimate their abilities. These individuals are at risk for burns, bruises, cuts, and falls and may need to be restrained from attempting unsafe activities. They also are more likely to have unilateral neglect than individuals with dominant (left) hemisphere injury (see **Unilateral Neglect**, earlier).
Have patients with apraxia return your demonstration of the task or see if they are able to be talked through a task or may be able to talk themselves through a task step-by-step.	Patients with apraxia have an inability to carry out previously learned motor tasks, although they may be able to describe them in detail.
Encourage making a conscious effort to scan the rest of the environment by turning head from side to side.	Patients may have visual field deficits in which they can physically see only a portion (usually left or right side) of the normal visual field (homonymous hemianopsia).
Intervene as follows for patients with nondominant (right) hemisphere injury:	Patients may have the following sensory perceptual alterations:
- Direct the patient's attention to a particular sound (e.g., if a cat meows on the television, state that it is the sound a cat makes and point to the cat on the screen).	*Impaired ability to recognize, associate, or interpret sounds* (e.g., voice quality, animal noises, musical pieces, types of instruments).
- Provide a structured, consistent environment. Mark outer aspects of the patient's shoes or tag inside sleeve of a sweater or pair of pants with "L" and "R."	*Visual-spatial misconception:* The patient may have trouble judging distance, size, position, rate of movement, form, and how parts relate to the whole. For example, the patient may underestimate distances and bump into doors or confuse inside and outside of an object, such as an article of clothing. These patients may lose their place when reading or adding up numbers and therefore never complete the task.
- Assist these individuals with eating. Monitor the environment for safety hazards, and remove unsafe objects such as scissors from the bedside.	*Difficulty recognizing and associating familiar objects:* Patients may not know the purpose of silverware. These patients may not recognize dangerous or hazardous objects because they do not know the purpose of the object or may not recognize subtle distinctions between objects (e.g., the difference between a fork and spoon may become too subtle to detect).
- Provide these patients with a restraint or wheelchair belt for support.	*Inability to orient self in space:* They may not know if they are standing, sitting, or leaning.
- Teach the patient to concentrate on body parts (e.g., by watching feet carefully while walking). Provide a mirror to help them adjust.	*Misconception of own body and body parts:* These patients may not perceive their foot or arm as being a part of their body.
- Keep the patient's environment simple to reduce sensory overload and enable concentration on visual cues. Remove distracting stimuli.	*Impaired ability to recognize objects by means of senses of hearing, vibration, or touch:* These patients rely more on visual cues.

Nursing diagnosis for patients having carotid procedures

Nursing Diagnosis:

Deficient Knowledge

related to unfamiliarity with carotid endarterectomy or carotid angioplasty/ stent procedure

Desired Outcome: Before surgery, the patient verbalizes understanding of the carotid endarterectomy procedure, including the purpose, risks, expected benefits or outcome, and postsurgical care.

ASSESSMENT/INTERVENTIONS	RATIONALES
After the health care provider has explained the procedure to the patient, assess the patient's level of understanding and facility with language; employ an interpreter or language-appropriate written materials; and reinforce or clarify information as needed.	This enables development of an individualized teaching plan in the preoperative stage that the patient understands.
Obtain baseline neurologic and cranial nerve function test results.	These assessments will be the basis of comparison postoperatively.
For Patients Undergoing Carotid Endarterectomy As indicated, explain the procedure.	Carotid endarterectomy is removal of plaque in the obstructed artery to increase blood supply to the brain.
Describe the following postsurgical assessments:	
- There will be assessment of vital signs (VS) and neurologic status at least hourly.	Pupils will be checked with a light and hands and legs will be tested for weakness and equality.
- The patient may be asked to swallow, move the tongue, smile, speak, and shrug shoulders to determine facial drooping, tongue weakness, hoarseness, speech difficulty, dysphagia, shoulder weakness, or loss of facial sensation.	Deficits in these abilities are signs of cranial nerve impairment. Stretching of the cranial nerves during surgery can occur, causing edema, and may leave a temporary deficit.
- The patient will be asked to report any numbness, tingling, or weakness.	These signs may indicate carotid occlusion.
- Superficial temporal and facial pulses will be palpated for strength, quality, and symmetry.	This will evaluate patency of the external carotid artery.
- There will be periodic assessments of the neck for edema, hematoma, bleeding, or tracheal deviation from midline. The patient should report immediately any respiratory distress, difficulty managing secretions, or sensation of neck tightness.	Any bleeding or excess edema at the surgical site can cause neck edema, which can deviate the trachea and compromise the airway. This can result in an emergent situation that necessitates airway management and surgical evacuation of the hematoma.
- Pulse oximetry may be continuously monitored and O_2 will most likely be supplied, even without respiratory distress or airway compromise.	Manipulation of the carotid sinus may cause temporary loss of normal physiologic response to hypoxia.
- Frequent BP checks may be performed and the patient may need vasoactive medications. The patient will be monitored for orthostatic hypotension when first getting up.	Temporary carotid sinus dysfunction may cause BP problems (usually hypertension). Vasoactive drugs may be given to keep systolic blood pressure (SBP) within a specified range (usually 100-150 mm Hg) to maintain cerebral perfusion while preventing disruption of graft or sutures as well as hyperperfusion syndrome.
Keep head of bed (HOB) in the prescribed position (flat or elevated) and the patient positioned off the operative side.	HOB may be elevated to promote wound drainage, particularly if a closed suction drain is left in place. (A closed drainage system with suction may be left in the neck for a day.) Positioning also enables visibility of the wound site and promotes comfort.
If prescribed, keep ice packs on the incision.	Ice will reduce edema and pain.
Administer anticoagulant/antiplatelet therapy as prescribed.	Anticoagulant/antiplatelet therapy (e.g., aspirin, warfarin) may be instituted for 3-6 mo after the procedure and may continue longer, depending on patient's needs.

continued

ASSESSMENT/INTERVENTIONS	RATIONALES
Include home instructions for the following: incision care (wash gently with soap and water), signs of infection (incision red, swollen, and painful; drainage, fever greater than 100.5° F); activity restrictions (no heavy lifting, no driving while neck turning is uncomfortable), and changes in neurologic status (alterations in speech, swallowing, vision, and numbness or weakness in arm or leg, especially on opposite side).	Following these instructions will decrease risk of infection and promote the patient's physiologic safety.

For Patients Undergoing Carotid Angioplasty and Stenting

ASSESSMENT/INTERVENTIONS	RATIONALES
Teach the patient about angioplasty and stenting.	Angioplasty is the opening of a stenosed artery via a slender catheter that is passed through the narrow spot with balloon inflation to open up the obstruction. A stent, which will physically hold the newly unblocked vessel open, also may be placed.
Explain that frequent VS and neurology checks (as described previously) will be performed.	Cranial nerve problems are less frequent with this procedure because nerves have not been stretched, but they still will be included in the neurologic examination.
BP medications may be given to keep BP within specified parameters.	Temporary carotid sinus dysfunction may cause BP problems (usually hypertension), but this is less common than with endarterectomy. Maintaining systolic BP at less than 150 mm Hg may prevent hyperperfusion syndrome.
Advise the patient that groin and distal pulses will be assessed for bleeding and patency.	The femoral artery is the usual vessel accessed.
Explain that the HOB is usually elevated after a predetermined period of time immediately postprocedure and that this requires the patient to lie flat.	This position may help prevent headache.
Advise that patients are usually discharged the next day and go home on anticoagulants such as aspirin or ticlopidine.	Anticoagulants will help prevent clots forming in the stent and angioplasty area.

ADDITIONAL NURSING DIAGNOSES/PROBLEMS:

✓ PATIENT-FAMILY TEACHING AND DISCHARGE PLANNING

When providing patient-family teaching, focus on sensory information, avoid giving excessive information, and initiate a visiting nurse referral for necessary follow-up teaching. Include verbal and written information about the following:

- ✓ Symptoms that necessitate prompt attention: sudden weakness, numbness (especially on one side of the body), vision loss or dimming, trouble talking or understanding speech, unexplained dizziness, unsteadiness, or severe headache. To help families remember, teach the "FAST" acronym whereby "F" = face (have patient smile, look for weakness/numbness), "A" = arms (check for arm drift/strength/numbness), "S" = speech (have the patient say a simple sentence and watch for slurred or difficulty speaking/understanding), and "T" = Time (call 911 if any of these is present because "time is tissue"). **Note:** *http://www.stroke.org/site/PageServer?pagename=symp.* This site lists more information in relation to FAST and is intended to be a layperson's assessment.
- ✓ Interventions for safe swallowing and aspiration prevention.
- ✓ Importance of minimizing or treating the following risk factors: diabetes mellitus, hypertension, high cholesterol, high sodium intake, obesity, inactivity, smoking, prolonged bedrest, and stressful lifestyle.
- ✓ Interventions that increase effective communication in the presence of aphasia or dysarthria. Additional patient information can be obtained by contacting the National Aphasia Association at *www.aphasia.org.*
- ✓ Referrals to the following as appropriate: public health nurse, visiting nurses association, psychologic therapy, vocational rehabilitation agency, home health agencies, and extended and skilled care facilities.
- ✓ For patient information pamphlets, contact the National Institute of Neurological Disorders and Stroke (NINDS) at *www.ninds.nih.gov.*
- ✓ Additional general information can be obtained by contacting the following organizations:
  - American Stroke Association at *www.strokeassociation.org*
  - Stroke Center at *www.strokecenter.org*
  - National Stroke Association at *www.stroke.org*
  - Heart and Stroke Foundation of Canada at *www.heartandstroke.com* 🍁

See Also: Teaching and discharge planning (third through tenth entries only) under "Multiple Sclerosis," p. 292.

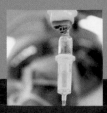

Traumatic Brain Injury 43

OVERVIEW/PATHOPHYSIOLOGY

Traumatic brain injury (TBI) can cause varying degrees of damage to the skull and brain tissue. Primary injuries occur at the time of impact and include skull fracture, concussion, contusion, scalp laceration, brain tissue laceration, and tear or rupture of cerebral vessels. Secondary problems that arise soon after and are the result of the primary injury include hemorrhage and hematoma formation from tear or rupture of vessels, ischemia from interrupted blood flow, cerebral swelling and edema, infection (e.g., meningitis or abscess), and increased intracranial pressure (IICP) or herniation, any of which can interrupt neuronal function. These secondary injuries or events increase the extent of initial injury and result in poorer recovery and higher risk of death. Cervical neck injuries are commonly associated with TBIs. Because of the potential for spinal cord injury, all TBI patients should be assumed to have cervical neck injury until it is conclusively ruled out by cervical spine x-ray examination.

Most TBIs result from direct impact to the head. Depending on force and angle of impact, the brain may suffer injury directly under the point of impact (coup) or in the region opposite the point of impact (contrecoup) because of brain rebound action within the skull, or tissue tearing or shearing may occur elsewhere because of the rotational action of the brain within the cranial vault. TBI may be classified by location, severity, extent, or mechanism (contact, acceleration, deceleration, rotational). Common causes include motor vehicle accidents; falls; and sports-related injuries, such as those occurring in football or boxing. Acts of violence, such as gunshot or stab wounds, often result in missile or impalement TBIs. This is especially true related to military TBI. This population represents a special subset of TBI patients because recovery also includes managing comorbid states such as posttraumatic stress syndrome (PTSD). These patients are often managed by the VA, but due to changes in the health care arena, this population is sometimes being managed outside the VA.

HEALTH CARE SETTING

Mobile ICU, flight units, acute care (trauma center, intensive care, neurology floors, medical-surgical floors), rehabilitation unit

ASSESSMENT

The Glasgow Coma Scale (GCS) standardizes observations for objective assessment of a patient's level of consciousness (LOC). GCS 13-15 is mild, 9-12 is moderate, and 3-8 is severe. This or some other objective scale should be used to prevent confusion with terminology and to quickly detect changes or trends in the patient's LOC. LOC is the most sensitive indicator of overall brain function.

Concussion: Mild diffuse TBI in which there is temporary, reversible neurologic impairment may involve loss of consciousness and possible amnesia of the event. No damage to brain structure is visible on computed tomography (CT) scan or magnetic resonance imaging (MRI) examination. Pathology is believed to occur at the axonal levels.

TBI concussions have been given the following grades:
- Grade I: No loss of consciousness
  - Transient confusion
  - Symptoms resolve in less than 15 min
- Grade II: No loss of consciousness
  - Transient confusion
  - Symptoms last more than 15 min
  - If symptoms last more than 1 wk, imaging may be needed
- Grade III: Any loss of consciousness

After concussion, patients may have headache, dizziness, nausea, lethargy, difficulty focusing, and irritability, especially to bright lights or loud noises. Although full recovery usually occurs in a few days, a postconcussion syndrome with headache; dizziness; irritability; emotional lability; lethargy; sleep disturbance; and decreased attention, judgment, concentration, and memory abilities may continue for several weeks or months.

Diffuse axonal injury: Diffuse brain injury caused by stretching and tearing of the neuronal projections because of a rotational, shearing type of injury. Diffuse microscopic damage occurs. No distinct focal lesion, such as infarction, ischemia, contusion, or intracerebral bleeding, is noted, but patients have an immediate and prolonged unconsciousness of at least 6-hr duration. CT scan may show small hemorrhagic areas in the corpus callosum, cerebral edema, and small midline ventricles. Brain stem injury may be associated with diffuse axonal injury (DAI), resulting in autonomic dysfunction. *Mild DAI* is coma lasting 6-24 hr with the patient beginning to follow commands by 24 hr. Full recovery is expected. *Moderate DAI* is coma lasting longer than 24 hr but without prominent brain stem signs. *Severe DAI* is prolonged coma with prominent brain stem signs, such as decortication or decerebration, and usually predicts severe disability, possible vegetative state, or death.

Contusion: Bruising of brain tissue, which produces a longer-lasting neurologic deficit than concussion. Size and severity of bruising vary widely, and the bruise or a small, diffuse venous hemorrhage usually is visible on CT scan. Traumatic amnesia often occurs, causing loss of memory not only of the trauma, but also of events occurring before the incident. Loss of consciousness is common, and it is generally more prolonged than that with concussion. Changes in behavior, such as agitation or confusion, can last for several hours to days. Headache, nausea, lethargy, motor paralysis, paresis, and possibly seizures can occur as well. Depending on extent of damage, there is potential for either full recovery or permanent neurologic deficit, such as seizures, paralysis, paresis, or even coma and death.

Brain laceration: Actual tearing of the brain's cortical surface, resulting in direct mechanical disruption of neural function and causing focal deficits. Blood vessel tearing causes hemorrhage, resulting in contusion, edema, or hematoma formation. Seizures often occur as well. Brain lacerations usually result from depressed skull fractures, penetrating injuries, missile or impalement injuries, or rotational shearing injury within the skull. Shock waves from a bullet's high energy produce additional damage. A knife or other impalement object should be supported and left in the wound to control bleeding until it can be removed during surgery. Contusions and lacerations often are found together. The consequences of a laceration usually are more serious than those with a contusion because of the increased severity of trauma.

Skull fracture: Can be *closed* (simple, with skin intact) or *open* (compound), depending on whether the scalp is torn, thereby exposing the skull to the outside environment. Skull fractures are further classified as *linear* (hairline), *comminuted* (fragmented, splintered), or *depressed* (pushed inward toward the brain tissue). A blow forceful enough to break the skull is capable of causing significant brain tissue damage, and therefore close observation is essential. With a penetrating wound or basilar fracture (see below), there is potential for cerebrospinal fluid (CSF) leakage, meningitis, encephalitis, brain abscess, cellulitis, or osteomyelitis.

- *Basilar fractures:* Fractures of the base of the skull do not show up easily on skull/cervical x-ray examination. Indicators include blood from the nose, throat, ears; serous or serosanguineous drainage from the nose (rhinorrhea), throat, ears (otorrhea), eyes; Battle's sign (bruising noted behind the ear); "raccoon's eyes" (bruising around eyes in the absence of eye injury); and bleeding behind the tympanum (eardrum) noted on otoscopic examination. Glucose in serous drainage signals the presence of CSF. CSF leakage indicates a tear in the dura, making the patient particularly

susceptible to meningitis. Basilar fractures may damage the internal carotid artery and cranial nerves. Hearing loss also may occur.
- *Temporal fractures:* May result in deafness or facial paralysis.
- *Occipital fractures:* May cause visual field and gait disturbances.
- *Sphenoidal fractures:* May disrupt the optic nerve, possibly causing blindness.

Rupture of cerebral blood vessels

- *Epidural (extradural) hematoma or hemorrhage:* Usually, bleeding between the dura mater (outer meninges) and skull causes hematoma formation. This creates pressure on the underlying brain and produces a local mass effect, causing IICP and shifting of tissue, which leads to brain stem compression and herniation. Indicators are primarily those of IICP: altered LOC, headache, vomiting, unilateral pupil dilation (on same side as the lesion), and possibly hemiparesis. Although some individuals never regain consciousness, most patients lose consciousness for a short period immediately after injury, regain consciousness, and have a lucid period lasting a few hours or 1-2 days. However, because arterial bleeding causes a rapid rise in intracranial pressure (ICP), a rapid decrease in LOC often ensues. The bleeding site often is the middle meningeal artery or vein because of temporal bone fracture. These patients are at risk for brain stem herniation. A unilateral dilated fixed pupil is a sign of impending herniation and is a neurosurgical emergency. Patients should not be left alone because respiratory arrest may occur at any time.
- *Subdural hematoma or hemorrhage:* Accumulation of venous blood between the dura mater (outer meninges) and arachnoid membrane (middle meninges) that is not reabsorbed. Hematoma formation creates pressure on the underlying brain and produces a local mass effect, causing IICP and shifting of tissue, leading to brain stem compression and herniation. This type of hematoma is classified as acute, subacute, or chronic depending on how quickly indicators arise. In acute subdural hematomas, indicators appear within 24-48 hr, resulting from focal neurologic deficit (hemiparesis, pupillary dilation) and IICP (decreased LOC, falling GCS score, nausea, vomiting, headache). When indicators occur 2-14 days later, the hematoma is considered subacute. When indicators occur more than 2 wk later, it is considered chronic. Early indicators can include headache, progressive personality changes, decreased intellectual functioning, slowness, confusion, and drowsiness. Later indicators may include unilateral weakness or paralysis, loss of consciousness, and occasionally seizures. Patients with cerebral atrophy (e.g., older persons, long-term alcohol users) are more prone to subdural hematoma formation.
- *Intracerebral hemorrhage:* Arterial or venous bleeding into the brain's white matter. Signs of IICP may develop early if the bleeding causes a rapidly expanding space-occupying lesion. If the bleeding is slower, signs of IICP can take 36-72 hr to develop. Indicators depend on hematoma

location and size and can include altered LOC, headache, aphasia, hemiparesis, hemiplegia, hemisensory deficits, pupillary changes, and loss of consciousness.

- *Subarachnoid hemorrhage:* Bleeding into the subarachnoid space below the arachnoid membrane (middle meninges) and above the pia mater (inner meninges next to brain). The patient often has a severe headache. Other general indicators include vomiting, restlessness, seizures, and loss of consciousness. Signs of meningeal irritation include nuchal rigidity and positive Kernig's and Brudzinski's signs (see p. 262). This patient may be a candidate for a shunt because of hemorrhagic interference with CSF circulation and reabsorption and is at particular risk of cerebral vasospasm.

Indicators of IICP

- *Early indicators:* Alteration in LOC ranging from irritability, restlessness, and confusion to lethargy (LOC is the most sensitive, reliable indicator of neurologic dysfunction); possible onset or worsening of headache; beginning pupillary dysfunction, such as sluggishness; visual disturbances, such as diplopia or blurred vision; onset of or increase in sensorimotor changes or deficits, such as weakness; onset or worsening of nausea.
- *Late indicators:* Continued deterioration of LOC leading to stupor and coma; projectile vomiting; hemiplegia; posturing; alterations in vital signs (VS) (typically increased systolic blood pressure [SBP], widening pulse pressure, decreased pulse rate); respiratory irregularities, such as Cheyne-Stokes breathing; pupillary changes, such as inequality, dilation, and nonreactivity to light; papilledema; and impaired brain stem reflexes (corneal, gag, swallowing).

Note: *The single most important early indicator of IICP is a change in LOC. Late indicators of IICP usually signal impending or occurring brain stem herniation. Signs generally are related to brain stem compression and disruption of cranial nerves and vital centers. Hypotension and tachycardia in the absence of explainable causes, such as hypovolemia, usually are seen as a terminal event in TBI. IICP usually peaks around 72 hr after initial insult and then gradually subsides over 2-3 wk.*

Brain herniation: Brain herniation occurs when IICP causes displacement of brain tissue from one intracranial compartment to another, resulting in compression, destruction, and laceration of brain tissue. See late indicators of IICP for signs of impending or initial herniation. In the presence of actual brain herniation, the patient is in a deep coma, pupils become fixed and dilated bilaterally, posturing may progress to bilateral flaccidity, brain stem reflexes generally are lost, and respirations and VS deteriorate and may cease.

Brain death: Criteria for determining brain death are not universally agreed upon. Check state and institutional guidelines. General criteria include absent brain stem reflexes (e.g., apnea, pupils nonreactive to light, no corneal reflex, no oculovestibular reflex to ice-water calorics), absent cortical activity (e.g., several flat electroencephalogram [EEG] tracings spaced over time), and coma irreversibility continued over a specific timeframe (e.g., 24 hr). Brain stem auditory-evoked responses and cerebral blood flow studies (e.g., transcranial Doppler, angiography, brain scan with a cerebral perfusion agent) also may be used to help confirm brain death.

DIAGNOSTIC TESTS

Cervical spine and skull x-ray examinations: To locate neck and skull fractures. Because of the close association between TBIs and spinal or vertebral injuries, cervical immobilization is essential until cervical x-ray examination rules out fracture and potential SCI.

CT scan: Used with acute injury to identify type, location, and extent of injury, such as accumulation of blood or a shift of midline structure caused by IICP.

MRI scan: To identify type, location, and extent of injury. Although not usually performed in acute, unstable patients, this test is the study of choice for subacute or chronic TBI. It is superior to CT scan for detecting isodense chronic subdural hematomas or evaluating contusions and shearing injuries, especially in the brain stem area. MRI techniques such as fluid attenuated inversion recovery (FLAIR) are particularly sensitive to detecting DAI and small hemorrhages.

Cerebral blood flow studies (transcranial Doppler, xenon inhalation enhanced CT): To determine focal areas of low blood flow or spasm, possibly indicating ischemic areas, by noninvasively measuring cerebral blood flow velocities.

EEG: To reveal abnormal electrical activity indicating neuronal damage caused by ischemia or hemorrhage. EEG may be used to establish brain death in conjunction with other tests and may be done serially to assess development of pathologic waves.

Evoked potentials: To evaluate integrity of the anatomic pathways and connections of the brain. Stimulation of a sense organ, such as an ear, triggers a discrete electrical response (i.e., evoked potential) along a neurologic pathway to the brain. Measurement of the brain's response to auditory, visual, and/or somatosensory stimulation also aids in predicting neurologic outcome.

Positron emission tomography: To evaluate tissue metabolism of glucose and oxygen.

Single photon emission CT: To determine low cerebral blood flow and areas at risk for ischemic tissue perfusion.

Infrared spectroscopy: To continuously and noninvasively assess cerebral O_2 saturation.

Cerebral angiography: To reveal presence of a hematoma and status of blood vessels secondary to rupture or compression. Angiography usually is performed only if CT scan or MRI scan is unavailable or to evaluate possible carotid or vertebral artery dissection.

Cisternogram: To identify dural tear site with basilar skull fracture.

CSF analysis: To evaluate for infection, if indicators are present.

Nursing diagnosis (for patients going home with a concussion):

Deficient Knowledge

related to unfamiliarity with caretaker's responsibilities for observing a patient who is sent home with a concussion

Desired Outcome: Following instruction, the caretaker verbalizes understanding about the observation regimen and of patient presentations that necessitate return to the hospital for evaluation.

ASSESSMENT/INTERVENTIONS	RATIONALES
Assess the caretaker's health care literacy (language, reading, comprehension). Assess culture and culturally specific information needs.	This assessment helps ensure that materials are selected and presented in a manner that is culturally and educationally appropriate.
⚠ Give the following instructions:	
- Manage headache pain by stratified protocol: give the mildest analgesic prescribed to manage the level of pain. Do not exceed maximum dose or strength.	A possible exception is codeine for pain control. Otherwise, opioids and other medications that alter mentation are avoided because they can mask neurologic indicators of IICP and cause respiratory depression. Aspirin is usually contraindicated because it can prolong bleeding if it occurs.
- Assess the patient at least q1-2h for the first 24 hr or as prescribed, and as follows: awaken the patient; ask the patient's name, location, and the caretaker's name; monitor for twitching or seizure activity.	This information gives the caretaker the necessary information for returning the patient to the hospital. The caretaker should return the patient to the hospital immediately if the patient becomes increasingly difficult to awaken; cannot answer questions appropriately; cannot answer at all; becomes confused, restless, or agitated; develops slurred speech; develops twitching or seizures; develops or reports worsening headache or nausea/vomiting; has visual disturbances (e.g., blurred or double vision); develops weakness, numbness, or clumsiness or has difficulty walking; has clear or bloody drainage from nose or ear; or develops a stiff neck.
- Ensure that the patient rests and eats lightly for the first day or so after concussion or until he or she feels well.	Nausea and vomiting occur with IICP.
- Over the next several days, caution the patient to avoid activities that are physically taxing or take a high degree of concentration. Avoid alcohol and taking medication for headache or nausea without calling the health care provider. Examples of activities to avoid: driving, contact sports, swimming, using power tools.	These restrictions help ensure the patient's safety. There is potential for neurologic deterioration at this time. For this reason, the patient should return to a full schedule slowly.
⚠ Inform the patient and significant other that some individuals may have postconcussion syndrome. Explain the importance of reporting these problems to the health care provider, especially if they worsen.	Some individuals may continue to have headaches, dizziness, or lethargy for several weeks or months after a concussion. Patients also may experience sleep disturbance, difficulty concentrating, poor memory, irritability, emotional lability, difficulty with judgment or abstract thinking, and may be very distractible with hypersensitivity to noise and light. These problems should be reported promptly for timely evaluation and intervention. Additional testing may be done to ensure other processes (e.g., chronic subdural hematoma) are not occurring, and medications may be prescribed to help with some symptoms (e.g., pain, sleep problems).

PART I: Medical-Surgical Nursing

Nursing diagnoses for patients who are hospitalized

Nursing Diagnosis:

Risk for Infection

related to inadequate primary defenses occurring with basilar skull fractures, penetrating or open TBIs, or surgical wounds

Desired Outcomes: The patient is free of symptoms of infection as evidenced by normothermia; stable or improving LOC; and absence of headache, photophobia, or neck stiffness. The patient verbalizes knowledge about signs and symptoms of infection and the importance of reporting them promptly.

ASSESSMENT/INTERVENTIONS	RATIONALES
Assess the injury site or surgical wounds for indicators of infection. Notify the health care provider of significant findings.	Persistent erythema, local warmth, pain, hardness, and purulent drainage are indicators of localized infection that can occur as a result of loss of skin integrity.
Assess for indicators of meningitis or encephalitis.	Meningitis or encephalitis (fever, chills, malaise, back stiffness and pain, nuchal rigidity, photophobia, seizures, ataxia, sensorimotor deficits) can occur after a penetrating, open TBI, or cerebral surgical wound. For more detail, see "Bacterial Meningitis," p. 262.
When examining scalp lacerations and assessing for foreign bodies or palpable fractures, wear sterile gloves and follow sterile technique. Cleanse the area gently, and cover scalp wounds with sterile dressings.	These measures reduce the possibility of infection, which can be serious if the TBI has created a breach directly into the nervous system.
Document drainage and its amount, color, and odor.	If the patient has clear or bloody drainage from the nose, throat, or ears, it should be assumed the patient has a dural tear with CSF leakage until proven otherwise and the health care provider should be notified accordingly. Complaints of a salty taste or frequent swallowing may signal CSF dripping down the back of the throat. Bending forward may produce nasal drainage that can be tested for CSF.
Inspect the dressing and pillowcases for a halo ring (blood encircled by a yellowish stain).	A halo ring may indicate CSF drainage.
Test clear drainage with a glucose reagent strip. Drainage may be sent to the laboratory to test for Cl^-.	The presence of glucose and Cl^- (CSF Cl^- is greater than serum Cl^-) in nonsanguineous drainage indicates that the drainage is CSF rather than mucus or saliva.
If CSF leakage occurs, do not clean the ears or nose unless prescribed by the health care provider. Position the patient so that fluids can drain. Place a sterile pad over the affected ear or under the nose to catch drainage, but do not pack them. Change dressings when they become damp, using sterile technique.	These measures prevent introducing bacteria into the nervous system from the breach created by the TBI.
If not contraindicated, place the patient in semi-Fowler's position.	This position helps reduce cerebral congestion and edema and promotes venous drainage.
With CSF leakage or possible basilar fracture, avoid nasal suction.	Nasal suction could introduce bacteria into the nervous system.
Instruct the patient to avoid Valsalva's maneuver, straining with bowel movement, and vigorous coughing. Caution the patient not to blow nose, sneeze, or sniff in nasal drainage.	These actions could tear the dura and increase CSF flow.
Be aware that if the gastric tube is to be placed nasally, the health care provider usually performs the intubation.	Nasogastric (NG) tubes have been known to enter the fracture site and curl up into the cranial vault during insertion attempts. **Note:** The tube for gastric decompression may be placed through the mouth for patients with basilar skull fractures to avoid passing the tube via the nose through the fracture area and into the brain.

ASSESSMENT/INTERVENTIONS

RATIONALES

ASSESSMENT/INTERVENTIONS	RATIONALES
[!] Check tube placement via x-ray before applying suction. Visually check the back of the patient's throat for the NG tube to help confirm placement.	These measures help confirm the tube's proper placement and avoid causing harm to the patient.
As prescribed, keep individuals with basilar skull fractures flat in bed and on complete bedrest.	This position helps decrease pressure and amount of CSF draining from a dural tear.
Administer antibiotics as prescribed.	Patients are given antibiotics to prevent infection and observed for healing and sealing of the dural tear within 7-10 days.
Teach the patient that a CSF leak will be a source of infection until healed or repaired and that most CSF leaks from dural tears heal themselves in 5-10 days.	If a CSF leak does not heal, serial lumbar punctures or a lumbar subarachnoid drain may be needed to drain CSF, reduce CSF pressure, and promote healing. Acetazolamide or dexamethasone may be given to decrease CSF production. Radionuclide-labeled materials may be injected into the subarachnoid space and pledgets placed in the nose and ears to find the site of the CSF leak. A blood patch may be used. Surgical repair (e.g., duraplasty) may be required if other methods prove ineffective. Basilar fractures are a common site of CSF leaks and make surgical repair difficult because of location inaccessibility.
[!] For patients with a lumbar drain, explain that they will be on bedrest with the head of bed (HOB) elevated up to 15-20 degrees. Teach the patient to call for assistance and not to cough, sneeze, or strain. Explain that VS and neurologic checks will be monitored for any deterioration and the patient should call for problems such as new-onset weakness, numbness, difficult swallowing, and headache.	Deterioration of neurologic signs may indicate possible meningitis (see p. 262) or a pneumocranium resulting from too-rapid drainage of CSF, which causes air to siphon in through the dural tear, creating an intracranial mass effect. If neurologic signs deteriorate, the care provider should be called promptly. Clamping the lumbar drain tubing and placing the patient in a flat or in a slight Trendelenburg position with supplemental O_2 will promote absorption of intracranial air.
Explain that glucose may be closely monitored and kept under strict control.	Hyperglycemia is associated with poorer outcomes, including higher infection rates. Intensive insulin therapy may be used during the acute phase when patients are in intensive care unit (ICU), with insulin drips and frequent monitoring to keep glucose at less than 120 mg/dL. After stabilization, sliding scale or rainbow coverage to keep glucose at less than 150 mg/dL is usually instituted.

Nursing Diagnoses:

Excess Fluid Volume
Risk for Electrolyte Imbalance

related to compromised regulatory mechanisms with increased antidiuretic hormone (ADH); and increased renal resorption occurring with syndrome of inappropriate ADH secretion (SIADH)

Desired Outcome: By hospital discharge (or within 3 days of injury), the patient is normovolemic as evidenced by stable weight; balanced intake and output (I&O); urinary output 30 mL/hr or more; urine specific gravity 1.010-1.030; BP within the patient's baseline limits; absence of fingerprint edema over the sternum; and orientation to person, place, and time.

ASSESSMENT/INTERVENTIONS   RATIONALES

ASSESSMENT/INTERVENTIONS	RATIONALES
Differentiate between SIADH and cerebral salt wasting (CSW) syndrome, whose treatments are different.	While both syndromes involve hyponatremia (Na^+ less than 137 mEq/L), SIADH results in hypervolemia and CSW results in hypovolemia. In CSW syndrome, the kidneys are unable to conserve Na^+, and a true serum hyponatremia occurs with decreased plasma volume, weight loss, high blood urea nitrogen level, decreased serum osmolality, and hypernatruria. CSW is treated with fluid replacement (intravenous [IV] normal saline), volume expanders, salt tablets, and occasionally fludrocortisone to inhibit Na^+ excretion and induce Na^+ retention. If serum Na^+ is very low, a hypertonic saline may be used. Usually both syndromes resolve in a week or two.

continued

ASSESSMENT/INTERVENTIONS	RATIONALES
Monitor serum Na⁺, I&O, and weight and notify the health care provider of significant findings.	In the presence of SIADH, a potential complication of TBI, the patient will have inappropriate urinary concentration causing excessive water retention and a dilutional hyponatremia. Expect seizure activity when the serum Na⁺ level drops below 118 mEq/L. Serum Na⁺ level less than 115 mEq/L may result in loss of reflexes, coma, and death. Seizure activity would increase the metabolic rate in the central nervous system (CNS) and further compromise the patient's neurologic status.
Assess for fingerprint edema over the sternum.	This reflects cellular edema. Because fluid is not retained in the interstitium with SIADH, peripheral edema will not necessarily occur.
Be aware that depending on the serum Na⁺ value, fluids may be restricted to an amount as low as 500-1000 mL/24 hr. Intervene accordingly and as prescribed.	Fluid restriction helps achieve homeostasis by increasing osmolarity, thereby decreasing risk of hyponatremia.
If indicated and prescribed, enable free use of salt or salty foods in the patient's diet.	This measure helps normalize the Na⁺ level.
For other interventions, see these nursing diagnoses in "Syndrome of Inappropriate Antidiuretic Hormone," p. 393.	

Nursing Diagnosis:

Acute Pain

related to headaches occurring with TBI

Desired Outcome: Within 1 hr of intervention, the patient's subjective perception of pain decreases, as documented by a pain scale.

ASSESSMENT/INTERVENTIONS	RATIONALES
Assess and document duration and character of the patient's pain, rating it on a scale of 0 (no pain) to 10 (worst pain). Assess for nonverbal indicators of pain such as facial grimacing, muscle tension, guarding, restlessness, increased or decreased motor activity, irritability, anxiety, or sleep disturbance.	This assessment provides a baseline for subsequent comparison and quantifies the degree of pain and pain relief obtained.
Administer analgesics as prescribed.	Patients with TBI generally do not have much pain, and it is usually relieved by analgesics, such as acetaminophen. Sometimes codeine is prescribed, but as a rule, other opioids are contraindicated because they can mask neurologic indicators of IICP and cause respiratory depression.
Assess for pain, swelling, warmth, and decreased range of motion (ROM) around joints, especially the hips.	These signs may indicate heterotopic ossification (HO), which is abnormal formation of true bone within the extraskeletal soft tissues and can occur after a fracture. Etidronate, nonsteroidal antiinflammatory drugs (such as indomethacin), ROM exercises, and external beam radiation are prevention therapies. Once HO has formed, resection usually is necessary.
For additional interventions, see **Acute Pain,** p. 256, in "General Care of Patients with Neurologic Disorders."	

Nursing diagnosis (for patients undergoing craniotomy):

Deficient Knowledge

related to unfamiliarity with the craniotomy procedure

Desired Outcome: Following the explanation, the patient verbalizes accurate understanding of the craniotomy procedure, including presurgical and postsurgical care, risks, and expected outcomes.

ASSESSMENT/INTERVENTIONS	RATIONALES
After the health care provider's explanation of the procedure, assess the patient's level of understanding of the purpose, risks, and anticipated benefits or outcome. Reinforce the health care provider's explanation as appropriate. Provide and review language-appropriate printed material if available.	This assessment enables development of an effective teaching plan. A craniotomy is a surgical opening into the skull to remove a hematoma or tumor, repair a ruptured aneurysm, apply arterial clips or wrap the involved vessel to prevent future rupture, control hemorrhage, remove bone fragment or foreign objects, debride necrotic tissue, elevate depressed fractures, or decompress the brain. Trephination ("burr" holes) may be used to evacuate hematomas or insert intracranial monitoring devices. Cranioplasty is done to repair traumatic or surgical defects in the skull.
Obtain informed consent. Encourage questions and discuss fears and anxiety as it relates to risks of the procedure discussed in the informed consent.	There is the possibility of cognitive and behavioral changes related to the site of surgery, which frequently diminish or disappear in 6 wk to 6 mo.
As appropriate, explain that the bone flap may be left open postoperatively.	This enables accommodation of cerebral edema and prevents compression. When the bone is removed, the procedure is called a *craniectomy*.
Explain that before surgery, antiseptic shampoos may be given and the patient may be started on corticosteroids, such as dexamethasone, and antiepilepsy drugs.	Hair can be a major source of microorganisms. Dexamethasone may be given for cerebral edema; antiepilepsy drugs may be given prophylactically.
Explain that a baseline neurologic assessment will be performed.	This provides a basis for comparison with postoperative neurologic checks.
During the immediate postoperative period, the patient is in ICU. Explain the following considerations and interventions that are likely to occur:	
- VS and neurologic status will be assessed at least hourly. Emphasize the importance of performing these tasks to the best of the patient's ability.	Patients will be asked to perform a variety of assessment measures, including squeezing the tester's hand, moving the extremities, extending the tongue, and answering questions.
- Changes in body image can occur because of loss of hair, presence of a head dressing, and potential for and expected duration of facial edema.	Patients may consider use of headpiece, scarf, or wig for concerns regarding changes in body image.
- Presence of sequential compression devices on the legs and possibly an arterial line for continuous BP monitoring as well as other devices such as ICP monitoring equipment and external ventriculostomy.	This equipment will be used to prevent thrombophlebitis and pulmonary emboli, for continuous BP monitoring, and to detect changes in ICP. Typically patients are on a cardiac monitor for 24-48 hr because dysrhythmias are not unusual after posterior fossa surgery or when blood is in CSF.
- Possible need for respiratory and airway support, including O_2, intubation, or ventilation.	Respirations will be monitored for irregularity (a sign of bleeding and brain stem compression).
Presence of a large head dressing and drains. Stress the importance of not pulling or tugging on the dressing or drains. Advise that the patient should report a sweet or salty taste in mouth because this may indicate a CSF leak.	Dressing and incisions will be inspected periodically for bleeding or CSF leakage, which will be reported to the health care provider for prompt intervention.
- The patient will be given nothing by mouth (NPO) for the first 24-48 hr.	There is risk of vomiting and choking. Patients may experience a dry throat at this time and will be assessed for swallowing difficulties, which may signal cranial nerve compression from IICP.
- Possible presence of periorbital swelling and interventions if it is present.	This usually occurs within 24-48 hr of supratentorial surgery. Relief is obtained with applications of cold or warm compresses around the eyes. Having HOB raised with patient lying on the nonoperative side also may help reduce edema.
- Insertion of an indwelling urinary catheter.	This enables accurate measurement of I&O and monitors for potential problems such as diabetes insipidus (DI).
- Measurement of core temperature (e.g., rectal, tympanic, bladder) at frequent intervals.	A rectal probe or bladder catheter temperature probe may be used for continuous monitoring so that fever can be evaluated and treated promptly. Oral temperatures are avoided during the period in which cognitive function is decreased.

continued

ASSESSMENT/INTERVENTIONS	RATIONALES
Teach the patient that postsurgical positioning is a key factor during recovery, as discussed in the following procedures:	Patients usually are maintained with the HOB elevated to 30 degrees (or as prescribed). Patients are assisted with turning and usually will be kept off the operative site, especially if the lesion was large. The head and neck are kept in good alignment.
- *Supratentorial craniotomy*	HOB is kept flat or as prescribed. Sitting may increase risk of venous air embolus with posterior fossa surgery. Pressure usually is kept off the operative site, especially with a craniectomy; therefore, these patients are kept off their backs for 48 hr. In posterior fossa surgery, the supporting neck muscles are altered. Patients are logrolled to alternate sides, keeping the head in good alignment. A soft cervical collar may be used to prevent anterior or lateral angulation of the neck. A small pillow may be used for comfort.
- *Infratentorial craniotomy (for cerebellar or brain stem surgery)*	Patients are not positioned onto the operative side immediately after surgery because this could cause shifting inside the space.
- *For areas of evacuation causing large intracranial space*	Turning onto the side from which bone was removed is avoided. Staff will label on the chart and bed the location of the missing bone.
- *After craniectomy*	This may involve a gradual elevation of HOB to prevent cerebral hemorrhage. For example, HOB may be flat for 24 hr, 15 degrees for the next 24 hr, 30 degrees for the next 24 hr, 45 degrees for the next 24 hr, and then 90 degrees.
- *Ventricular shunts and chronic subdural hematomas*	HOB may be flat while the drain is in place and for 24 hr after removal to prevent air from being pulled into the subdural space.
If a subdural drain is placed:	
Explain that bedrest is usually maintained for the first 24 hr.	Bedrest enables the effects of anesthesia to wear off fully, reduces activity that may increase ICP, and helps ensure stability of VS.
Explain that patients having supratentorial surgery near the area of the pituitary gland or hypothalamus may develop transient DI.	Supratentorial surgery may cause localized edema around the pituitary stalk, which could cause DI. See "Diabetes Insipidus," p. 353, for details.
Teach patients undergoing infratentorial surgery that they are likely to experience the following:	
- A longer period of bedrest.	These patients are likely to experience an extended period of dizziness and hypotension.
- Nausea, which should be reported as soon as it is noted.	This ensures that antiemetics (e.g., metoclopramide, trimethobenzamide) are given promptly.
- Swallowing difficulties, extraocular movements, or nystagmus, any of which should be reported promptly.	These problems are the result of cranial nerve edema.
Teach the patient the following precautions that are taken to prevent increased intraabdominal and intrathoracic pressure: exhaling when being turned; not straining at stool; not moving self in bed, but rather letting staff members do all moving; importance of deep breathing and avoiding coughing and sneezing (if coughing and sneezing are unavoidable, they must be done with an open mouth to minimize pressure buildup); and avoiding hip flexion and lying prone.	Increased intraabdominal and intrathoracic pressures can cause IICP, which could result in brain edema and ischemia, neurologic changes, and brain herniation. For additional precautions against IICP, see **Decreased Intracranial Adaptive Capacity,** p. 242.
Explain that precautions are taken for seizures.	See **Risk for Trauma** related to oral, musculoskeletal, and airway vulnerability secondary to seizure activity, p. 306.
Teach wound care and indicators of infection: fever; redness; drainage from surgical site, nose, or ears; and increased headache.	Generally, a surgical cap is worn after removal of the head dressing. Patients must avoid scratching the wound, staples, or sutures and must keep the incision dry. When sutures or staples are removed, hair can be shampooed, being careful not to scrub around the incision line. Hair dryers are avoided until hair is regrown to prevent tissue damage caused by heat. For more information, see **Risk for Infection**, p. 344.

PART I: Medical-Surgical Nursing

ASSESSMENT/INTERVENTIONS	RATIONALES
Explain that patients undergoing acoustic neuroma excision may have nausea; hearing loss; facial weakness or paralysis; diminished or absent blinking; eye dryness; tinnitus; vertigo; headache; and occasionally swallowing, throat, taste, or voice problems.	Acoustic neuromas can wrap around cranial nerve VII, and surgery may damage this cranial nerve and cause localized edema. Other cranial nerves whose nuclei are in the brain stem also may be affected.
	Nausea and dizziness may be profound problems after surgery. Prescribed antiemetics will be given, and patients should be turned and moved slowly. Patients should be spoken to on the unaffected side for best hearing, and the phone and call light should be placed on that side of the bed. Contralateral routing of signal hearing aids may improve hearing by directing sound from the deaf ear to the hearing ear via a tiny microphone and transmitter. Background music or other white noise may mask tinnitus. Awareness of tinnitus eventually should lessen. Balance exercises and walking with assistance will start the compensation process by the functioning vestibular system.
	Watching television or reading may be difficult because of vertigo; listening to books on tape or the radio are good alternatives. Eye dryness, from impaired eyelid function, may require use of eye drops or ointment.
For additional interventions, see **Deficient Knowledge** (surgical procedure), p. 45, in "Perioperative Care."	

Nursing diagnosis (for patients undergoing ventricular shunt procedure):

Deficient Knowledge

related to unfamiliarity with the ventricular shunt procedure

Desired Outcome: Following explanation, the patient verbalizes accurate information about the ventricular shunt procedure, including presurgical and postsurgical care.

ASSESSMENT/INTERVENTIONS	RATIONALES
Assess the patient's understanding of the procedure after the health care provider's explanation, including purpose, risks, and anticipated benefits or outcome. Intervene accordingly. Also assess the patient's facility with language; provide an interpreter or language-appropriate written materials as indicated.	This assessment enables development of an effective teaching plan. A ventricular puncture, or ventriculostomy, is a temporary procedure used to remove excess CSF.
As indicated, reinforce the purpose of the procedure.	A ventricular shunt procedure is performed to enable permanent drainage of CSF when flow is obstructed (e.g., because of presence of a tumor or blood) through a one-way pressure gradient valve.
Explain that the patient may have a cranial dressing, as well as a dressing on the neck, chest, or abdomen.	Shunt types vary but can extend from the lateral ventricle of the brain to one of the following: subarachnoid space of the spinal canal, right atrium of the heart, a large vein, or the peritoneal cavity.
Explain that it is important to avoid lying on the insertion site after the procedure.	This restriction prevents pressure on the shunt mechanism, which could decrease CSF drainage.
Advise that the head and neck are kept in alignment.	This prevents kinking and compression of the shunt catheter.
Explain that there is a shunt valve for controlling CSF drainage or reflux.	Most shunts have a valve that is preset to open at a particular pressure to permit CSF flow and does not require "pumping." There also are valves that have adjustable programmable opening pressures that are adjusted externally by using a magnet or programming device. Pumping is usually contraindicated for these new shunts, depending on manufacturer recommendations.

continued

ASSESSMENT/INTERVENTIONS	RATIONALES
Explain that the valve, which is usually located behind or above the ear and is the approximate diameter of a pencil, can be felt to empty and then refill.	Malfunction may be noted by either deterioration in neurologic status or failure of the reservoir to refill when pumped.
Reassure the patient and significant other that before hospital discharge, specific instructions will be given about shunt care, recognition of shunt site infection and malfunction, and steps to take should they occur. Teach signs and symptoms of IICP (i.e., headache; change in LOC such as drowsiness, lethargy, irritability, nausea, personality changes) that should be reported to the health care provider and may indicate shunt malfunction.	Kinked tubing, obstructed tubing or valve, and movement of the cannula can result in inadequate drainage of the ventricles. Cannula movement also can result in abdominal viscus perforation or subdural hematoma formation. For ventriculoatrial shunts, emboli or endocarditis may occur. For ventriculoperitoneal shunts, ascites may occur.
If the patient is to have an endoscopic third ventriculostomy, explain the procedure and its purpose.	This procedure may be tried as an alternative to a standard shunt in order to provide drainage of CSF in cases of obstructive hydrocephalus. A small hole or holes are made in the third ventricle to enable CSF to flow into the basal cistern for absorption.
For additional interventions, see **Risk for Infection,** p. 344, and **Deficient Knowledge** (Surgical Procedure), p. 45, in "Perioperative Care."	

ADDITIONAL NURSING DIAGNOSES/PROBLEMS:

✓ PATIENT-FAMILY TEACHING AND DISCHARGE PLANNING

The patient with TBI can have varying degrees of neurologic deficit, ranging from mild to severe. When providing patient-family teaching, focus on sensory information, avoid giving excessive information, and initiate a visiting nurse referral for necessary follow-up teaching. Include verbal and written information about the following:

✓ Referrals to community resources, such as cognitive retraining specialist, head injury rehabilitation centers, visiting nurses association, community support groups, social workers, psychologic therapy, vocational rehabilitation agency, home health agencies, and extended and skilled care facilities. Additional general information can be obtained by contacting the following organizations:

- Brain Injury Association, Inc., at *www.biausa.org*
- Brain Trauma Foundation at *www.braintrauma.org*
- Brain Injury Association of Canada at *biac-aclc.ca*
- The Rehabilitation and Research Center at *www.tbi-sci.org*

✓ Safety measures related to decreased sensation, visual disturbances, motor deficits, and seizure activity.

✓ Measures that promote communication in the presence of aphasia.

✓ Wound care and indicators of infection. Instruct patient to avoid scratching sutures and shampoo only after sutures are out.

✓ Indicators of ICP, which include change in LOC, lethargy, headache, nausea, and vomiting and should be reported to health care provider promptly.

✓ Measures that deal with cognitive or behavioral problems. As appropriate, include home evaluation for safety. Caution significant other that personality can change drastically after TBI. Patient may demonstrate inappropriate social behavior, inappropriate affect, hallucination, delusion, and altered sleep pattern.

✓ Cognitive rehabilitation goals (e.g., Rancho Los Amigos Hospital) for appropriate patients to promote highest level of cognitive functioning. Family can be instructed in and participate in coma stimulation techniques (usually for short periods 2-4 times/day). Most cognitive recovery occurs in the first 6 mo.

✓ If the patient had a concussion, a description of problems that may occur at home and necessitate prompt medical attention (see **Deficient Knowledge,** p. 343).

✓ For other information, see teaching and discharge planning interventions (fourth through tenth entries only) in "Multiple Sclerosis," p. 292, as appropriate.

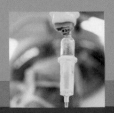

Diabetes Insipidus 44

OVERVIEW/PATHOPHYSIOLOGY

Diabetes insipidus (DI) is a condition that can result from one of several problems. *Central (neurogenic) DI* is caused by a defect in the synthesis of antidiuretic hormone (ADH) by the hypothalamus or release from the posterior pituitary. *Nephrogenic DI* results from a defect in the renal tubular response to ADH, causing impaired renal conservation of water. The primary problem is excessive output of dilute urine. Neurogenic DI may be the result of primary DI (i.e., a hypothalamic or pituitary lesion or dominant familial trait), secondary DI (following injury to the hypothalamus or pituitary stalk), or vasopressinase-induced DI, which is seen in the last trimester of pregnancy (caused by a circulating enzyme that destroys vasopressin). Nephrogenic DI either occurs as a familial X-linked trait or is associated with pyelonephritis, renal amyloidosis, Sjögren's syndrome, sickle cell anemia, myeloma, potassium depletion, effects of certain drugs such as lithium or demeclocycline, or chronic hypercalcemia. A rare form of DI, termed *psychogenic diabetes insipidus,* is associated with compulsive water drinking. Another form of water consumption related to DI is *dipsogenic diabetes insipidus,* caused by an abnormality in hypothalamic control of the thirst mechanism. This condition is most often idiopathic but has been associated with chronic meningitis, granulomatous diseases, multiple sclerosis, and other widely diffuse brain diseases. Patients with this disorder have severe polydipsia and polyuria. *Gestagenic diabetes insipidus* is caused by an enzyme secreted by the placenta that destroys vasopressin. The condition may be treated with desmopressin (a synthetic form of ADH) if severe, but generally resolves 6-8 wk following delivery.

Except for when it follows infection or trauma, DI onset is usually insidious, with progressively increasing polydipsia and polyuria. DI following trauma or infection has three phases. In the first phase, polydipsia and polyuria immediately follow the injury and last 4-5 days. In the second phase, which lasts about 6 days, the symptoms disappear. In the third phase, the patient experiences continued polydipsia and polyuria. Depending on the degree of injury, the condition can be either temporary or permanent.

DI must be differentiated from other syndromes resulting in polyuria. History, physical examination, and simple laboratory procedures assist in diagnosis. Other causes of polyuria include recent lithium or mannitol administration; renal transplantation; renal disease; hyperglycemia; hyperosmolality (early); hypercalcemia; and potassium depletion, including primary aldosteronism.

HEALTH CARE SETTING

Acute care (either medical-surgical or intensive care unit) or outpatient care depending on seriousness of the condition.

ASSESSMENT

Signs and symptoms: Polydipsia, polyuria (2-20 L/day) with dilute urine (specific gravity less than 1.007).

Physical assessment: Usually within normal limits, but the patient may show signs of dehydration if fluid intake is inadequate. Individuals with cranial injury, disease, or trauma may exhibit impairment of neurologic status, including altered level of consciousness (LOC) and sensory or motor deficits.

History of: Cranial injury, especially basilar skull fracture; meningitis; primary or metastatic brain tumor; surgery in the pituitary area; cerebral hemorrhage; encephalitis; syphilis; or tuberculosis (TB). Familial incidence rarely is a factor.

DIAGNOSTIC TESTS

Urine osmolality: Decreased (less than 200 mOsm/kg) in the presence of disease.

Specific gravity: Decreased (less than 1.007) in the presence of disease.

Serum osmolality: Increased (300 mOsm/kg or greater) in the presence of disease.

Vasopressin (DDAVP) challenge test: After administration of vasopressin subcutaneously or desmopressin by nasal spray, urine is collected q15-30 min for 2 hr. Quantity and specific gravity are then measured. Normally, individuals will show a concentration of urine but not as pronounced as that of persons with DI; a person with kidney disease will have a lesser response to vasopressin. **Note:** One serious side effect of this test is precipitation of heart failure in susceptible individuals.

Hypertonic saline infusions: NaCl 3% solution is infused intravenously (IV) to assess for subsequent water conservation. Although this test seldom is necessary for diagnosis of DI, it does help document changes in the osmotic threshold for ADH release.

Water deprivation (dehydration) test: Although less commonly used today, some health care providers do use it as a marker. Baseline measurements of body weight, serum and urine osmolalities, and urine specific gravity are obtained. Fluids are not permitted, and measurements are repeated hourly. Test is terminated when urine osmolality exceeds 300 mOsm/kg (normal responses) or plasma osmolality or sodium concentration increases to above normal. If sodium or plasma osmolality increases before urine osmolality exceeds 300 mOsm/kg, the diagnoses of primary polydipsia, partial neurogenic DI, and partial nephrogenic DI are excluded, and a vasopressin challenge test should be done to determine whether the patient has severe neurogenic or severe nephrogenic DI. Because the most serious side effect of this test is severe dehydration, the test should be performed early in the day so that patients can be more closely monitored. Before a firm diagnosis of DI can be made from an abnormal water deprivation test, it is also necessary to demonstrate that the kidneys can respond to vasopressin.

Magnetic resonance imaging (MRI) scan of the brain: MRI scan is used to identify pituitary lesions that may have caused the DI. If the patient has the "bright spot" or hyperintense emission from the posterior pituitary gland, the patient likely has primary polydipsia. If the "bright spot" is small or absent, the patient likely has nephrogenic or neurogenic DI.

Nursing Diagnoses:

Deficient Fluid Volume
Risk for Shock

related to active loss occurring with polyuria

Desired Outcome: The patient becomes normovolemic within 7 days of onset of symptoms as evidenced by stable weight, balanced intake and output (I&O), good skin turgor, moist tongue and oral mucous membrane, blood pressure (BP) 90-120/60-80 mm Hg (or within the patient's normal range), heart rate (HR) 60-100 bpm, urine specific gravity greater than 1.010, and central venous pressure (CVP) 8-12 mm Hg.

ASSESSMENT/INTERVENTIONS	RATIONALES
Assess for hypovolemia by monitoring I&O, specific gravity, and vital signs (VS) hourly. Check weight daily.	Signs of hypovolemia include weight loss, inadequate fluid intake to balance output, thirst, poor skin turgor, decreased specific gravity, furrowed tongue, hypotension, and tachycardia.
If available, monitor CVP.	CVP may decrease to less than 2 mm Hg in the presence of profound hypovolemia.
Immediately report the following to the health care provider: (1) urinary output more than 200 mL in each of 2 consecutive hr, (2) urinary output more than 500 mL in any 2-hr period, or (3) urine specific gravity less than 1.002.	These are signs of extreme diuresis. Diuresis may result in hypotension, hypokalemia, and dehydration leading to highly viscous blood. The patient is at increased risk of hypovolemic shock, stroke, dysrhythmias, and heart attack.
Provide unrestricted fluids: keep the water pitcher full and within easy reach of the patient. Explain importance of consuming as much water as can be tolerated.	The chief danger to patients with DI is dehydration from the inability to take in adequate fluids to balance the excessive output of urine. Water is the best replacement, and patients should avoid excessive ingestion of salt, sugar, and artificial sweeteners.
Administer vasopressin and antidiuretic agents (or thiazide diuretic for patients with nephrogenic DI) as prescribed.	These measures are instituted to prevent extreme diuresis. Several vasopressin preparations are available, and it is important to read package inserts carefully to ensure proper administration. Potential side effects of exogenous vasopressin include hypertension secondary to vasoconstriction, myocardial infarction secondary to constriction of coronary vessels, uterine cramps, and increased peristalsis of the gastrointestinal (GI) tract. A mild antidiuretic effect may be achieved with thiazide diuretics (e.g., hydrochlorothiazide), nonsteroidal antiinflammatory drugs (NSAIDs), and other medications that increase the action (desired effect for nephrogenic DI) or release of ADH (desirable for central DI). **Note:** Although it may seem antithetical to treat diuresis with a diuretic, one of the side effects of the thiazide diuretics and NSAIDs in patients with DI is reducing the excretion of free water.

continued

ASSESSMENT/INTERVENTIONS	RATIONALES
For unconscious patients, administer IV fluids as prescribed. Unless otherwise directed, for every mL of urine output, deliver 1 mL of IV fluid.	To promote rehydration, lost water is replaced with IV hypotonic (e.g., 0.45% NaCl) solution. Initial replacement is rapid, necessitating close monitoring of BP, HR, and urine output to prevent overhydration. IV normal saline may be used following initial fluid resuscitation.

Nursing Diagnoses:

Ineffective Protection
Risk for Electrolyte Imbalance

related to potential for side effects of vasopressin

Desired Outcomes: Optimally, the patient demonstrates normal mental acuity; verbalizes orientation to person, place, and time; and is free of signs of injury caused by side effects of vasopressin. As appropriate, the patient or significant other demonstrates administration of coronary artery vasodilators by the time of hospital discharge.

ASSESSMENT/INTERVENTIONS	RATIONALES
Assess VS and report significant changes.	Significant changes such as systolic blood pressure (SBP) elevated more than 20 mm Hg over baseline SBP or HR increased more than 20 bpm over baseline HR are signs of vasoconstriction, which is an undesirable effect when vasopressin is used solely as an ADH.
Assess for changes in mental status or LOC, confusion, weight gain, headache, convulsions, and coma.	These are signs of water intoxication caused by fluid retention.
[!] If these signs develop, stop the vasopressin, restrict fluids, and notify the health care provider. Institute safety measures accordingly, and reorient the patient as needed.	Water intoxication causes significant dilution of circulating electrolytes, resulting in effects seen with such electrolyte disorders as hyponatremia, hypokalemia, and hypochloremia.
[!] For older adults or persons with vascular disease, keep prescribed coronary artery vasodilators (i.e., nitroglycerin) at the bedside for use if angina occurs. Teach patients and significant others how to administer these medications.	Angina may result from coronary vasoconstriction induced by vasopressin. Vasopressin dose should be reduced if angina occurs.

✓ **PATIENT-FAMILY TEACHING AND DISCHARGE PLANNING**

When providing patient-family teaching, speak slowly and simply, avoid giving excessive information, and initiate a visiting nurse referral for necessary follow-up teaching. Include verbal and written information about the following:

  ✓ Importance of medical follow-up; confirm date and time of next visit to the health care provider.
  ✓ Medications, including drug name, purpose, dosage, schedule, precautions, and potential side effects. Also discuss drug-drug, food-drug, and herb-drug interactions.
  ✓ Importance of seeking immediate medical attention if signs of dehydration or water intoxication occur. See *Ineffective Protection/Risk for Electrolyte Imbalance*, earlier.
  ✓ Recommendations for fluid replacement: guidelines on type and amount of replacement fluids prescribed for the patient.
  ✓ Additional information available from
    • Diabetes Insipidus Foundation, Inc., at *www .diabetesinsipidus.org*
    • The Canadian Diabetes Association at *www .diabetes.ca*

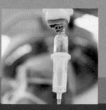

Diabetes Mellitus 45

OVERVIEW/PATHOPHYSIOLOGY

Diabetes mellitus (DM) is a worldwide epidemic of chronic hyperglycemia affecting more than 7.8% (24 million) of the total U.S. population. There are 1.6 million new cases of DM diagnosed in the United States each year. While 18 million cases are diagnosed, more than 6 million remain undiagnosed. An additional 57 million Americans are at risk of DM.

Hispanic, Native American, and African American populations have a higher incidence than Caucasians and other groups and are the most likely to be undiagnosed. Prevalence has increased in a direct relationship with increasing incidence of obesity.

Metabolic, vascular, and neurologic disorders ensue from dysfunctional glucose transport into body cells. Insulin facilitates glucose transport into cells for oxidation and energy production. Food intake, glycogen breakdown, and gluconeogenesis increase the serum glucose level, which stimulates the beta islet cells of the pancreas to release needed insulin for transport of glucose from the bloodstream into the cells. At the cellular level, insulin receptors control the rate of transport of glucose into the cells. As glucose leaves the blood, serum levels return to normal (70-100 mg/dL).

Individuals with DM have impaired glucose transport because of decreased or absent insulin secretion and/or ineffective insulin receptors. Carbohydrate, fat, and protein metabolism are abnormal, and patients are unable to store glucose in the liver and muscle as glycogen, store fatty acids and triglycerides in adipose tissue, or transport amino acids into cells normally. DM is classified into the following four clinical classes including prediabetes.

Type 1 (5%-10%): Complete lack of effective endogenous insulin, causing hyperglycemia and ketosis resulting from beta islet cell destruction. This type is precipitated by altered immune responses, genetic factors, and environmental stressors. Certain human leukocyte antigens have been strongly associated with type 1 DM. These individuals depend on insulin for survival and prevention of life-threatening diabetic ketoacidosis (DKA).

Type 2 (90%-95%): Metabolic disorder that may range from insulin resistance with moderate insulin deficiency to a severe defect in insulin secretion with insulin resistance that results in severe hyperglycemia without ketosis. Untreated hyperglycemia can result in hyperglycemic hyperosmolar syndrome (HHS). Most individuals with type 2 DM are obese.

Other types: Formerly termed *secondary diabetes*, these include the following:

- *Diseases of the exocrine pancreas:* Pancreatitis, cystic fibrosis, hemochromatosis, trauma, infection, pancreatic cancer, and pancreatectomy may result in destruction of beta islet cells. All diseases except cancer generally involve extensive pancreatic destruction.
- *Drug-induced by insulin antagonists:* Many drugs impair insulin secretion, including phenytoin, steroids (hydrocortisone, dexamethasone), hormones (estrogen), intravenous (IV) pentamidine, nicotinic acid, thyroid hormone, thiazides, alpha-interferon, and rat poison.
- *Endocrine dysfunction/hormonal diseases:* Growth hormone, epinephrine, cortisol, and glucagons antagonize insulin and may be increased when diseases such as acromegaly, Cushing's syndrome, pheochromocytoma, or glucagonoma are present. Presence of excess antagonistic hormones results in reduced insulin action, and with somatostatinoma and aldosteronoma, insulin secretion may be reduced.
- *Genetic defects of the beta cell:* An autosomal dominant pattern results in severely impaired insulin secretion, most often characterized by hyperglycemia beginning before 25 years of age; it is also termed *maturity onset diabetes of the young.*
- *Genetic defects in insulin action:* A genetic defect manifested as abnormal insulin action is reflected by hyperinsulinemia with mild to severe hyperglycemia. Persons with acanthosis nigricans and women with polycystic ovaries may have this type of insulin resistance. Leprechaunism and Rabson-Mendenhall syndrome are two pediatric syndromes in this category.
- *Infections:* Presence of several different viruses, including rubella, coxsackievirus B, cytomegalovirus (CMV), adenovirus, and mumps has resulted in beta cell destruction.
- *Uncommon immune-mediated diabetes:* Antiinsulin receptor antibodies bind to insulin receptors and can either block or increase binding of insulin, resulting in either hyperglycemia or hypoglycemia. Systemic lupus erythematosus and "stiff-man" syndrome are examples of implicated disorders.
- *Other genetic syndromes*: Hyperglycemia has been linked to patients with Down's syndrome, Klinefelter's syndrome, Turner's syndrome, and Wolfram's syndrome.

Many of these "secondary" causes have recently become subclassified under type 1 and type 2 DM as possible primary causes of these diseases.

Gestational diabetes mellitus (GDM): Glucose intolerance with hyperglycemia that develops during pregnancy in approximately 4% of pregnant women, resulting in increased perinatal risk to the child and increased risk (25%) of the mother developing chronic DM during the next 10-15 yr. This type does not include *previously* diabetic pregnant women. Deterioration of glucose tolerance is considered "normal" during the third trimester of pregnancy.

Prediabetes with impaired glucose tolerance and impaired fasting glucose: Certain individuals may manifest chronic hyperglycemia without meeting other criteria for DM and are classified as having impaired glucose tolerance (IGT) or impaired fasting glucose (IFG), with fasting blood glucose levels 100 mg/dL or more but less than 126 mg/dL or 2-hr oral glucose tolerance test (OGTT) of 140 mg/dL or more but less than 200 mg/dL. These persons are at risk for developing DM and cardiovascular disease. IGT was formerly termed *borderline, chemical, latent, subclinical,* or *asymptomatic* DM. At least 20.1 million people in the United States, ages 40 to 74, have prediabetes. Some long-term damage to the body, especially the heart and circulatory system, already may be occurring during prediabetes. If blood glucose is controlled when prediabetes is identified, development of type 2 DM can be prevented.

HEALTH CARE SETTING

Primary care, with possible hospitalization to treat complications

ASSESSMENT

Metabolic signs of chronic hyperglycemia: Fatigue, weakness, weight loss, paresthesias, mild dehydration, and symptoms of hyperglycemia (polyuria, polydipsia, polyphagia). These indicators are seen in the early stages of illness.

Impending type 1 crisis—DKA: Profound dehydration and hyperglycemia, electrolyte imbalance, metabolic acidosis caused by ketosis, altered mental status, Kussmaul's respirations (paroxysmal dyspnea), acetone breath, possible hypovolemic shock (hypotension, weak and rapid pulse), abdominal pain, and possible strokelike symptoms.

Impending type 2 crisis—HHS: Severe dehydration, hypovolemic shock (hypotension, weak and rapid pulse), severe hyperglycemia, shallow respirations, altered mental status, slight lactic acidosis or normal pH, possible strokelike symptoms.

COMPLICATIONS

Potential for acute crisis: *For type 1,* include DKA and hypoglycemia; *for Type 2,* include HHS and hypoglycemia. All individuals with DM are at higher risk for developing cardiovascular disease. These complications should be preventable and are discussed as follows.

Long-term complications: The most important factor in delaying progression to long-term complications is stabilization of blood glucose levels to normal range.

Macroangiopathy: Patients are at higher risk for heart attack and stroke caused by vascular disease affecting the coronary arteries and larger vessels of the brain and lower extremities (peripheral vascular disease [PVD]). Risk factors are hyperglycemia, hypertension, hypercholesterolemia, smoking, aging, and extended duration of DM.

Microangiopathy: Patients are at higher risk for blindness and renal failure caused by thickening of capillary basement membranes resulting in retinopathy and nephropathy. Early symptoms include increased leakage of retinal vessels and microalbuminuria.

Neuropathy: Patients are at higher risk for gastroparesis (impaired gastric emptying), lack of sensation (especially in the feet), and neurogenic bladder caused by deterioration of peripheral and autonomic nervous systems, resulting in impaired or slowed nerve transmission.

Morning hyperglycemia: Blood glucose elevation found on awakening. Causes include each of the following or a combination of the effects of their interactions.

Insufficient insulin: The most common cause of hyperglycemia before breakfast is probably inadequate levels of circulating insulin. The patient may need a higher dosage, a mixture of insulins, or longer-acting insulin.

Dawn phenomenon: Glucose remains normal until approximately 3 AM, when the effect of nocturnal growth hormone may elevate glucose in type 1 DM. It may be corrected by changing time of the evening dose of intermediate-acting insulin injection to bedtime instead of dinnertime.

Somogyi phenomenon: The patient becomes hypoglycemic during the night. Compensatory mechanisms to raise glucose levels are activated and result in overcompensation. It may be corrected by decreasing evening dose of intermediate-acting insulin and/or eating a more substantial bedtime snack.

Problems with insulin

Insulin resistance: A problem experienced by most individuals with DM and other diseases at some point in the illness, when the daily insulin requirement to control hyperglycemia and prevent ketosis exceeds 200 Units. It is characterized as one of the following anomalies:

- *Prereceptor:* Insulin abnormal or insulin antibodies present.
- *Receptor:* Number of insulin receptors decreased or insulin binding to the receptors diminished.
- *Postreceptor:* Receptors not appropriately activated by insulin.

Local allergic reactions: Soreness, erythema, or induration at the insulin injection site within 2 hr after injection. Reactions are decreasing in frequency with the evolution of more purified insulins. Beef and beef/pork insulins are no longer commercially available in the United States. Pork insulin is used in less than 10% of patients. Use of human insulin has decreased the number of reactions significantly.

Systemic allergic reactions: With the advent of primarily human insulin and insulin analogues, systemic allergic reactions are extremely rare. The episode begins with a localized skin reaction, which evolves into generalized urticaria or anaphylaxis. Patients must be desensitized to insulin by progression from minuscule to more normal doses over the course of 1 day, using a series of subcutaneous injections.

Lipodystrophy: Local disturbance in fat metabolism resulting in loss of fat (lipoatrophy) or development of abnormal fatty masses at the injection sites (lipohypertrophy). Lipoatrophy rarely has been seen since the development of 100 U and human source insulins. Rotation of injection sites helps prevent lipohypertrophy. Individuals experiencing lipohypertrophy should use alternate injection sites until the condition resolves.

DIAGNOSTIC TESTS

Testing for DM should be considered for persons of any age who are overweight or obese and have at least one other risk factor for DM (hypertension [blood pressure (BP) greater than 130/80 mm Hg], high-density lipoprotein [HDL] cholesterol of less than 35 mg/dL or triglycerides more than 250 mg/dL, history of vascular disease or other diseases associated with hyperglycemia, history of IFG/IGT, or polycystic ovarian syndrome), and persons older than 45 yr who are overweight or obese (body mass index greater than 25 kg/m^2). If results are normal, testing should be repeated at least every 3 yr. For those who are overweight or obese with risk factors, the American Diabetes Association (ADA) recommends all patients be counseled about considering weight loss and increasing exercise. For those overweight who are younger than age 60, lifestyle counseling is suggested, along with metformin being recommended for blood glucose control. Those who exhibit any signs of prediabetes should be rescreened annually. The ADA also recommends screening women for type 2 DM who developed gestational diabetes. Screening is done between 6-12 wk postpartum and at least every 3 yr thereafter. Clinical guidelines vary among the ADA, American Academy of Family Practitioners (AAFP), and United States Preventive Service Task Force (USPSTF), largely due to levels of evidence required to place a recommendation in a guideline coupled with the population served by more specialized physicians versus the general population.

The World Health Organization (WHO) and ADA define the following diagnostic criteria for DM in nonpregnant adults.

Fasting plasma glucose/blood sugar: The preferred diagnostic test, a value greater than 126 mg/dL is indicative of DM. Fasting is defined as no calories consumed or infused for 8 hr before testing.

Oral glucose tolerance test: The 2-hr sample during the test is 200 mg/dL or more. The test is poorly reproducible and not performed often in practice. The patient is given a high glucose solution and undergoes multiple blood sample testings over the following 2 hr.

Casual/random plasma glucose: Measurement is 180 mg/dL or more on at least two occasions. The blood is drawn regardless of food/beverage consumption at any time during the day.

Hemoglobin A$_{1c}$/glycosylated hemoglobin (glycohemoglobin): Normal range is 4%-6%. Individuals with DM will have values greater than 6%. A target of 4%-6% is appropriate unless patients have frequent hypoglycemia when trying to adhere to the guideline. Less stringent guidelines may be acceptable for more complex patients, such as those with comorbid conditions who have long-standing diabetes with minimal or stable microvascular complications, those with limited life expectancy, children, and those who have manifested severe hypoglycemia. This value is measured to assess control of blood glucose over a preceding 2- to 3-mo period. The larger the percentage of glycosylated Hgb, the poorer the blood glucose control. Reducing glycohemoglobin levels to less than 6% may further reduce complications in less complex patients. Kits are now available to monitor this value in the home.

Once the diagnosis of diabetes mellitus is made

Fasting lipid profile: If total and low-density lipoprotein (LDL) cholesterol values are elevated, triglyceride value is elevated, or HDL cholesterol level is decreased, the patient is at high risk for developing cardiovascular disease.

Urinalysis for presence of microalbuminuria, ketones, protein, and sediment: If present, may indicate early renal disease caused by hyperglycemia. This test should be performed with routine checkups every 3 mo.

Serum creatinine: If elevated, may indicate renal disease.

12-lead electrocardiogram (ECG): If the patient has symptoms of cardiovascular disease, an ECG can identify areas of myocardial ischemia, infarction, and active injury.

Nursing Diagnosis:

Risk for Unstable Blood Glucose Level

related to inadequate blood glucose monitoring, dietary intake, and/or medication management

Desired Outcomes: Optimally, the patient has a blood glucose reading of less than 180 mg/dL at all times; fasting blood glucose readings less than 140 mg/dL when hospitalized; hemoglobin A$_{1C}$ level of less than 7; adequate tissue perfusion as evidenced by warmth, sensation, brisk capillary refill time (less than 2 sec), and peripheral pulses greater than 2+ on a 0-4+ scale in the extremities; BP within his or her optimal range; urinary output 30 mL/hr or more; baseline vision; good appetite; and absence of nausea and vomiting. The patient demonstrates adherence to the therapeutic regimen (essential for promoting optimal tissue perfusion).

ASSESSMENT/INTERVENTIONS	RATIONALES
Assess blood glucose before meals and at bedtime.	This monitors effectiveness of blood glucose control at times when the patient's glucose is not increased by food being digested. The American Diabetes Association and American Association of Clinical Endocrinologists (2013) have determined that both morbidity and mortality could be reduced for thousands of patients if hyperglycemia is diagnosed at admission and treated throughout hospitalization. Guidelines state that in critically ill patients, blood sugar level should be maintained at 140-180 mg/dL. Non–intensive care patients should be maintained at a premeal level of no more than 140 mg/dL and a maximum level of 180 mg/dL. Previously accepted tight glycemic control guidelines were changed following the NICE Sugar Trial, published in 2009. The trial revealed that benefits of tight control did not outweigh any potential negative outcomes of low blood sugar.
! Assess for changes in mentation, apprehension, erratic behavior, trembling, slurred speech, staggering gait, and seizure activity. Treat hypoglycemia as prescribed.	These are signs of hypoglycemia. Patients with hypoglycemia may experience vasodilation and diminished myocardial contractility, which decrease cerebral circulation and impair cognition.
In addition to sensation, assess capillary refill, temperature, peripheral pulses, and color.	This assessment monitors the patient's peripheral perfusion to detect macroangiopathy or PVD.
Administer basal, prandial, and correction doses of insulin as prescribed.	Adherence to the therapeutic regimen is essential for promoting optimal tissue perfusion. Progression of vascular disease and neuropathy, including blindness, kidney failure, gastroparesis, heart attack, and stroke, is the root cause of all complications of DM. By keeping serum glucose in a more normal range, the vascular endothelium receives better nourishment within the cells and will be less likely to deteriorate.
Encourage and teach the patient how to perform regular home blood glucose monitoring.	Blood glucose is generally monitored before meals, at bedtime, and possibly during the night (3:00 AM) in order to assess whether a correction dose of short-acting insulin is needed. Self-monitoring by patients is extremely useful in reducing complications.
Check BP every 4 hr. Alert the health care provider to values outside the patient's normal range. Administer antihypertensive agents as prescribed and document response.	Hypertension is commonly associated with diabetes. Careful control of BP is critical in preventing or limiting development of heart disease, stroke, retinopathy, and nephropathy.
! Monitor for orthostatic hypotension after administering blood pressure medications. For more information, see discussion later in this nursing diagnosis.	Orthostatic hypotension is a potential side effect of antihypertensive agents and of autonomic neuropathy in which the patient's compensatory mechanisms may be impaired.
Protect patients with impaired peripheral perfusion from injury caused by sharp objects or heat (e.g., avoid use of heating pads; always wear shoes outdoors and slippers at home).	Patients may experience decreased sensation in the extremities because of peripheral neuropathy.
Teach the patient to avoid pressure at the back of the knees by not crossing legs or "gatching" bed under the knees. Caution the patient to avoid garments that constrict circulation to the extremities and lower body. For additional information, see **Risk for Impaired Skin Integrity, p. 360.**	These actions could cause venous stasis and reduction in arterial perfusion in patients with macroangiopathy or impending PVD.
As indicated, orient the patient to locations of such items as water, tissues, glasses, and call light.	This orientation provides necessary information and a safe environment for patients with diminished eyesight caused by diabetic retinopathy.

ASSESSMENT/INTERVENTIONS	RATIONALES
Monitor laboratory values for changes in renal function.	Laboratory values that would signal changes in renal function include increases in blood urea nitrogen (more than 20 mg/dL) and creatinine (more than 1.5 mg/dL). Approximately half of all persons with type 1 DM develop chronic kidney disease (CKD) and end-stage renal disease. Protelnuria (protein more than 8 mg/dL in a random sample of urine) or microalbuminuria are early indicators of developing CKD. (See "Chronic Kidney Disease," p. 205, for more information.)
Also monitor urine output, especially after exposure to contrast medium. Observe these patients for indicators of acute renal failure (ARF). (See "Acute Renal Failure," p. 190, for more information.)	Individuals with DM and with reduced renal function are at significant risk for dehydration and development of ARF after exposure to contrast medium. Patients who will receive contrast medium should be well hydrated and possibly receive several doses of oral acetylcysteine or an IV bicarbonate infusion to protect the kidneys from contrast-related deterioration.
In Addition Assess for the Following:	
	Individuals with DM may experience multiple problems resulting from autonomic neuropathy.
Orthostatic hypotension: - Check BP while the patient is lying down, sitting, and then standing. Alert the health care provider to significant findings.	BP decreased from the patient's normal, along with lightheadedness, dizziness, diaphoresis, pallor, tachycardia, and syncope, are signals of orthostatic hypotension. A drop in systolic blood pressure (SBP) 20 mm Hg or more signals the need to return the patient to a supine position.
- Assist patients when getting up suddenly or after prolonged recumbency.	This action helps prevent falls caused by orthostatic hypotension.
Gastroparesis/impaired gastric emptying with nausea and vomiting:	Progressive autonomic neuropathy may cause a delay in gastric emptying, resulting in nausea and vomiting.
Administer metoclopramide before meals if prescribed.	Metoclopramide is an antiemetic that also promotes gastric emptying.
- Assess for a change in level of consciousness.	Usage has become infrequent due to its prompting of new-onset confusion and disorientation.
- Keep a record of all stools.	Diarrhea is a potential problem in patients with DM who have autonomic neuropathy and are taking metoclopramide to increase gastrointestinal motility.
Neurogenic bladder:	Neurogenic bladder is caused by deterioration of peripheral and autonomic nervous systems, resulting in impaired or slowed nerve transmission.
- Encourage the patient to void every 3-4 hr during the day.	Intermittent catheterization may be necessary in severe cases of neurogenic bladder secondary to autonomic neuropathy.
- Avoid use of indwelling urinary catheters.	Infection risk is increased with use of indwelling catheters.

Nursing Diagnosis:

Risk for Infection

related to chronic disease process (e.g., hyperglycemia, neurogenic bladder, poor circulation)

Desired Outcome: The patient is asymptomatic for infection as evidenced by normothermia, negative cultures, and white blood cell count 11,000/mm^3 or less.

ASSESSMENT/INTERVENTIONS	RATIONALES
Assess temperature every 4 hr. Alert the health care provider to elevations.	Infection is the most common cause of DKA. Fever can signal presence of an infection.
Maintain meticulous sterile technique when changing dressings, performing invasive procedures, or manipulating indwelling catheters.	Nonintact skin and invasive procedures and catheters place patients at risk for ingress of bacteria.

continued

ASSESSMENT/INTERVENTIONS — RATIONALES

ASSESSMENT/INTERVENTIONS	RATIONALES
Monitor for indicators of infection, including the following:	
- Fever, chills, cough productive of sputum, crackles, rhonchi, dyspnea, inflamed pharynx, and sore throat.	These are indicators of upper respiratory infection.
- Burning or pain with urination, cloudy or malodorous urine, tachycardia, diaphoresis, nausea, vomiting, and abdominal pain.	These are indicators of urinary tract infection (UTI). Patients with DM often have a neurogenic bladder, which increases the chance of UTI caused by urinary retention.
- Hypothermia, flushed skin, and hypotension.	These are indicators of systemic sepsis.
- Erythema, swelling, purulent drainage, and warmth at IV sites.	These are indicators of localized infection.
Consult the health care provider about obtaining culture specimens for blood, sputum, and urine during temperature spikes or for wounds that produce purulent drainage.	Infection can be present in blood (sepsis), urine, sputum (lungs/respiratory tract), or wounds. Occult infection also can be present outside these sources.

Nursing Diagnosis:

Risk for Impaired Skin Integrity

related to altered circulation and sensation occurring with peripheral neuropathy and vascular pathology

Desired Outcomes: The patient's lower extremity skin remains intact. Within the 24-hr period before hospital discharge, the patient verbalizes and demonstrates knowledge of proper foot care.

ASSESSMENT/INTERVENTIONS	RATIONALES
Assess integrity of the skin and evaluate reflexes of the lower extremities by checking knee and ankle deep tendon reflexes, proprioceptive sensations, two-point discrimination, and vibration sensation (using a tuning fork on the medial malleolus).	These assessments monitor presence/degree of neuropathy and vascular pathology. In addition to higher-risk areas on the extremities and pressure points, skin on the legs is at highest risk and typically is the first to exhibit problems. If sensations are impaired, the patient likely will be unable to respond appropriately to stimuli.
Monitor peripheral pulses, comparing quality bilaterally.	Peripheral pulses 2+ or less on a 0-4+ scale signal poor circulation that could compromise skin integrity.
Use a foot cradle on the bed, space boots for ulcerated heels, elbow protectors, and pressure-relief mattress.	These measures prevent pressure points and promote patient comfort.
Minimize patient activities and incorporate progressive passive and active exercises into the daily routine. Discourage extended rest periods in the same position.	These measures alleviate acute discomfort while preventing hemostasis.
Teach the patient the following steps for foot care:	
- Wash feet daily with mild soap and warm water; check water temperature with water thermometer or elbow.	Patients with decreased sensation are at risk for burns if they are unaware that water temperature is too hot. Hot water and strong soaps also can promote dry skin, which can become irritated and break down.
- Inspect feet daily for the presence of erythema, discoloration, or trauma, using mirrors as necessary for adequate visualization.	These are signs the skin needs vigilant assessment and preventive care. When the skin is no longer intact, the patient is at risk for infection that eventually can lead to amputation.
- Alternate between at least two pairs of properly fitted shoes.	This measure eliminates the potential for pressure points that can occur by wearing one pair only.
- Change socks or stockings daily and wear white cotton or wool blends.	These measures prevent infection from moisture or dirt in contact with nonintact skin. The white fabric enables patients more readily to see any blood or exudates from nonintact skin.

ASSESSMENT/INTERVENTIONS	RATIONALES
- Use gentle, unscented moisturizers.	These products soften and lubricate dry skin. Moisturizers with scent contain alcohol, which may increase skin dryness.
- Avoid putting moisturizer between the toes.	Moisturizer between the toes may macerate the skin, causing skin breakdown.
- Cut toenails straight across after softening them during a bath. File nails with an emery board.	These actions help prevent ingrown toenails, which could lead to infection.
- Do not self-treat corns or calluses; visit a podiatrist regularly. Do not go barefoot indoors or outdoors.	These measures minimize risk for trauma, which could lead to infection and ultimately to amputation.
- Attend to any foot injury immediately, and seek medical attention.	Diabetes can cause slow wound healing. Prompt care can prevent a small injury from becoming worse.

Nursing Diagnosis:

Deficient Knowledge

related to unfamiliarity with proper insulin administration, dietary precautions, and exercise for promoting normoglycemia

Desired Outcome: Within the 24-hr period before hospital discharge, the patient verbalizes and demonstrates knowledge of proper insulin administration, symptoms and treatment of hypoglycemia, the prescribed dietary regimen, and the role of exercise in promoting normoglycemia.

ASSESSMENT/INTERVENTIONS	RATIONALES
Assess the patient's health care literacy (language, reading, comprehension). Assess culture and culturally specific information needs.	This assessment helps ensure that information is selected and presented in a manner that is culturally and educationally appropriate.
Teach the patient to check expiration date on the insulin vial and to avoid using it if outdated.	Insulin may lose potency if the bottle has been open for more than 30 days.
Also teach proper storage of insulin and the importance of avoiding temperature extremes.	Extreme temperatures destroy insulin.
Teach the patient to use U-100 insulin with U-100 syringes as needed. Insulin pens are preferred to use of insulin syringes.	The patient must be aware there are differences in strengths of insulin suspensions, and each strength must be given using the appropriate syringe.
Suggest that the patient ask his or her health care provider if the prescribed insulin is available in an insulin pen.	An insulin pen eliminates the chance for errors since the pen is a self-enclosed dosing system, wherein the patient applies a new needle and sets the dose using a dial on the pen.
Explain that some intermediate- and long-acting insulins require mixing. Demonstrate rolling the insulin vial between your palms to mix contents.	Insulin separates when the bottle sits, and the molecules must be remixed to ensure appropriate concentration throughout the vial.
Explain that long-acting analogue insulins (glargine/Lantus and detemir/Levemir) work differently from older long-acting insulins and may need to be administered only once or twice daily, depending on the dose.	Long-acting insulin analogues do not have a profound peak action. Once glargine is injected and absorbed, the action is consistent over 24 hr, while the duration of action of detemir is approximately 20 hr.
Caution the patient to avoid shaking the vial of insulin.	Shaking produces air bubbles that can interfere with accurate dose measurement.
Explain that regular prandial insulin (e.g., NovoLin or HumuLin) should be injected 30 min before eating a meal; newer insulin analogues (NovoLog, HumaLog, Apidra) may be injected immediately before or directly after eating.	Time of onset/peak of older, regular insulins is slightly delayed compared with that of the newer insulins. If patients are unable to finish at least half of a meal, they may be advised to hold their prandial insulin if receiving an analogue (e.g., NovoLog, HumaLog, Apidra). Because analogues can be given after a meal, dosage is more flexible than with regular human insulins, which should be injected well before eating a meal.

· continued

ASSESSMENT/INTERVENTIONS	RATIONALES
Explain that either making a change in insulin type or withholding a dose of insulin may be required under various circumstances.	These instances include the following: when fasting for studies or surgery, when not eating because of nausea/vomiting, or when hypoglycemic. Stress from illness or infection can increase insulin requirements (or necessitate insulin therapy for one whose condition is normally controlled with oral hypoglycemics), and increased exercise will necessitate additional food intake to prevent hypoglycemia when no change is made in insulin dose. Adjustments are always individually based and require clarification with the patient's health care provider.
Provide a chart that depicts injection site rotations. Explain that injection sites should be at least 1 inch apart.	Injections in or near the same site each time may result in development of hard lumps or extra fatty deposits. Both of these problems are unsightly and make the insulin action less reliable.
Explain the importance of inserting the needle perpendicular to the skin rather than at an angle.	This ensures deep subcutaneous administration of insulin. Very thin persons may need to use a 45-degree angle.
Ensure the patient understands and demonstrates the technique and timing for home monitoring of blood glucose using a commercial kit.	A commercial kit provides ongoing data reflecting degree of control and may identify necessary changes in diet and medication before severe metabolic changes occur. Self-monitoring by patients is extremely useful in reducing complications, especially in type 1 DM patients who require more stringent control of serum glucose levels. Self-monitoring also enables the patient's self-control and psychologic security.
Teach the patient the importance of following a diet that is controlled in simple carbohydrates, consistent in complex carbohydrates, low in fat, and high in fiber.	Adequate nutrition, along with controlled carbohydrates and calories, is essential to maintaining normoglycemia in these individuals. A diet low in fat and high in fiber is an effective means of controlling blood fats, especially cholesterol and triglycerides. Complex carbohydrates are metabolized more slowly than simple carbohydrates. Consistent consumption of complex carbohydrates prevents "spikes" in blood glucose following consumption. Diet is the sole method of control for many individuals with type 2 DM. Typically, three daily meals and an evening snack are prescribed. Some fat and protein should be present in all meals and snacks to slow down the elevation of postprandial blood glucose. Adding 10-15 g of fiber will slow the digestion of monosaccharides and disaccharides. For all types of diabetes, refined and simple sugars and carbohydrates (white bread, any crackers made with processed flour) should be reduced and complex carbohydrates (whole grain products including breads, cereals, pasta, legumes, beans, and lentils) encouraged. Carbohydrate counting is preferred to the use of exchange lists.
Teach the patient how to count carbohydrates.	The "magic number" used for counting carbohydrates generally is 15, because 15 g of carbohydrates = one serving of carbohydrates. Many carbohydrate-controlled diets allow four servings of carbohydrates per meal. Complex carbohydrates are preferred to simple because they have a lower glycemic index; thus, complex carbohydrates raise blood glucose more gradually than do simple carbohydrates.
For patients who experience low blood glucose at night, discuss commercially available long-acting carbohydrate sources.	Long-acting carbohydrate sources may decrease risk of nighttime low blood glucose levels.
Teach the patient to be alert to changes in mentation, apprehension, erratic behavior, trembling, slurred speech, staggering gait, and seizure activity.	These are indicators of hypoglycemia.
Explain that oral hypoglycemics should be omitted several days before planned surgery. Teach the patient to treat hypoglycemia as prescribed.	Hypoglycemia involving oral hypoglycemics can be severe and persistent. Monitoring must be diligent. Any condition, situation, or medication that enhances the hypoglycemic effects of these drugs requires close monitoring of blood glucose when symptoms of hypoglycemia arise. Common factors in the development of hypoglycemia are fasting for diagnostic purposes, skipping meals, unplanned increase in activity, malnourishment related to illness or nausea and vomiting, and other medication therapy (any of which adds to the hypoglycemic action of the oral hypoglycemics). Use of oral hypoglycemic agents in hospitalized patients is discouraged because the potential for unstable blood glucose is great. Inpatient hyperglycemia may be best managed with insulin until the patient stabilizes.

ASSESSMENT/INTERVENTIONS	RATIONALES
Teach signs, symptoms, and reasons for hyperglycemia.	Hyperglycemia can occur with increased food intake, too little insulin, decreased exercise, infection or illness, and emotional stress. Signs and symptoms of hyperglycemia (polydipsia, polyuria, polyphagia, fatigue, fruity smelling breath) can appear within hours or even several days. Hyperglycemia will be detected during routine self-testing of blood glucose.
Teach that the following herbal remedies may cause changes in blood glucose levels if used along with prescribed medications: aloe vera, banaba, bitter melon, chia, cinnamon longa, fenugreek, ginseng, *Gymnema,* sylvestre, milk thistle, nopal, salacia oblonga, stevia.	All herbal remedies listed promote lowering of the blood glucose level, except for stevia, which is used as a sugar substitute. Stevia is not a sugar and cannot be used when patients experience hypoglycemia.
Explain the role that exercise has in patients with DM.	Exercise is as important as diet and insulin in treating DM. It lowers blood glucose levels, helps maintain normal cholesterol levels, and decreases insulin resistance at the sites of muscle receptors. These effects increase the body's ability to metabolize glucose and help reduce the therapeutic dose of insulin for most patients. The exercise program must be consistent and individualized (especially for individuals with type 1 DM). Patients should be given a complete physical examination and encouraged to incorporate acceptable activities as part of their daily routine. **Note:** If blood glucose level is greater than 250 mg/dL, exercise may act as a stressor in patients who are not used to exercise, causing blood glucose to increase rather than decrease. Patients should monitor blood glucose levels with a monitoring device before beginning an exercise program.

ADDITIONAL NURSING DIAGNOSES/PROBLEMS:

✓ PATIENT-FAMILY TEACHING AND DISCHARGE PLANNING

The American Association of Diabetes Educators (AADE) recommends that all patients with diabetes have access to self management information, focusing on the AADE 7™ Self-Care Behaviors: (1) healthy eating, (2) being active, (3) monitoring, (4) taking medication, (5) problem solving, (6) healthy coping, and (7) reducing risks. For additional information regarding the recommended content of the teaching, see Guidelines for the Practice of Diabetes Education at *http://www.diabeteseducator.org/export/sites/aade/_resources/pdf/PracticeGuidelines2009.pdf.* Focus on sensory information, avoid giving excessive information, and initiate a visiting nurse referral for necessary follow-up teaching. Ask about existing knowledge of the disease, ability for self-management, and acceptance of the disease during initial assessment. Include verbal and written information about the following:

✓ Importance of carrying a diabetic identification card, wearing a medical alert bracelet or necklace, and having identification card outline diagnosis and emergency treatment. For information contact MedicAlert Foundation at *www.medicalert.org.*

✓ Recognizing warning signs of both hyperglycemia and hypoglycemia, treatment, and factors that contribute to both conditions. Emphasize the importance of disclosing all alternative and complementary health practices being used because some may affect blood glucose or possibly lead to adverse drug reactions. Remind the patient that stress from illness or infection can increase insulin requirements (or necessitate insulin therapy for one who is normally controlled with oral hypoglycemics) and that increased exercise will necessitate additional food intake to prevent hypoglycemia when no change is made in insulin dosage under normoglycemic conditions. Blood glucose at a level greater than 250 mg/dL at the beginning of exercise may make the exercise a stressor that elevates rather than decreases the glucose level.

✓ Drugs that cause hyperglycemia: estrogens, corticosteroids, thyroid preparations, beta-adrenergic agonists (many respiratory aerosols or inhalers), diuretics, phenytoin, glucagon, drugs containing sugar (e.g., cough syrup), and certain antibiotics. Drugs that cause hypoglycemia: salicylates, sulfonamides, tetracyclines, methyldopa, anabolic steroids, acetaminophen, monoamine oxidase (MAO) inhibitors, ethanol, haloperidol, and marijuana. Propranolol and other beta-adrenergic blocking agents may mask the signs of and inhibit recovery from hypoglycemia. For a list of herbal remedies that affect blood glucose, see **Deficient Knowledge**, p. 361.

✓ Home monitoring of blood glucose using commercial kits, which provide ongoing data reflecting degree of control and may identify necessary changes in diet and medication before severe metabolic changes occur. These tests also provide a means for the patient's self-control and psychologic security. In addition, kits for monitoring glycohemoglobin (Hemoglobin A_{1C}) are available for home use and may assist patients in determining overall effectiveness of their diabetes management regimen. New, smaller lancets allow more frequent blood glucose testing by decreasing pain from fingersticks. Stress need for careful control of blood glucose as a means of decreasing risk of or minimizing long-term complications of DM. Encourage the patient to rotate sites as much as possible to avoid possibility of injuring any one site.

✓ Importance of daily exercise, maintenance of normal body weight, and yearly medical evaluation. Explain that exercise is as important as diet in treating DM. Exercise lowers blood glucose, helps maintain normal cholesterol levels, and increases circulation. These effects increase the body's ability to metabolize glucose and help reduce the therapeutic dose of insulin for most patients. Stress that each exercise program must be individualized (especially for persons with type 1 DM) and implemented consistently. The patient should have a complete physical examination and then be encouraged to incorporate acceptable exercise activities into his or her daily routine.

✓ Review of diet that is consistent in carbohydrates, low in fat, and high in fiber as an effective means of controlling blood fats, especially cholesterol and triglycerides. Stress that diet is the sole method of control for many individuals with type 2 DM. Adequate nutrition with controlled carbohydrates and calories is essential to maintaining normoglycemia in these individuals. Patients who gained weight before developing type 2 DM are sometimes able to normalize their blood glucose by losing weight and maintaining ideal body weight.

✓ Mixing insulins properly by drawing up the regular first, followed by the intermediate- or long-acting insulin. Insulin analogues (HumaLog, NovoLog, Apidra, glargine [Lantus], and detemir [Levemir]) should not be mixed with other insulin preparations.

✓ Use of syringe magnifiers that can be used by patients with poor visual acuity. Other products that permit safe and accurate filling of syringes are also available.

✓ Rotating injection sites and injecting insulin at room temperature. Provide a chart showing possible injection sites, and describe the system for site rotation. Complications related to insulin injections, including lipodystrophy, insulin resistance, and allergic reactions, should be discussed thoroughly.

✓ Importance of daily meticulous skin, wound, and foot care.

✓ Necessity of annual eye examination for early detection and treatment of retinopathy.

✓ Scheduling dental checkups at least every 6 mo to help prevent periodontal disease, a major problem for individuals with DM. The mouth often is the primary site of origination for low-grade infections.

✓ Inserting the needle perpendicular to the skin rather than at an angle to ensure deep subcutaneous administration of insulin. Individuals who are very thin may need to use a 45-degree angle.

✓ Medications, including purpose, dosage, schedule, precautions, interactions, and potential side effects for all medications used. Also discuss drug-drug, food-drug, and herb-drug interactions.

✓ Identifying available resources for ongoing assistance and information, including nurses, dietitian, the patient's health care provider, and other individuals with DM in patient care unit. Other resources include the local chapter of ADA, the local chapter of the American Association of Diabetes Educators (AADE), and local library for free access to current materials on diabetes. The following is a list of resources available to patients:
- American Diabetes Association at *www.diabetes.org*
- American Association of Diabetes Educators at *www.diabeteseducator.org*
- Canadian Diabetes Association at *www.diabetes.ca*
- Juvenile Diabetes Research Foundation International at *www.jdrf.org*
- Joslin Diabetes Center at *www.joslin.org*
- National Diabetes Information Clearinghouse at *www.niddk.nih.gov/health/diabetes/ndic.htm*
- American Heart Association, National Center, at *www.americanheart.org*
- Can-Am-Care (Diabetes care store brand availability guide) at *www.canamcare.com*

The following is a list of journals available for patients:
- Diabetes Forecast at *http://forecast.diabetes.org/*
- Diabetes Health Magazine at *www.diabeteshealth.com*
- Diabetes Self-Management at *www.diabetesselfmanagement.com*

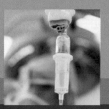

Diabetic Ketoacidosis 46

OVERVIEW/PATHOPHYSIOLOGY

Diabetic ketoacidosis (DKA) is a life-threatening condition caused by severe lack of effective insulin, resulting in major hyperglycemia and metabolic, anion-gap acidosis from abnormal carbohydrate, fat, and protein metabolism resulting in production of ketones. The intracellular environment is unable to receive necessary glucose for oxidation and energy production without insulin to facilitate transport of glucose from the bloodstream across the cell membrane. Impairment of glucose uptake results in hyperglycemia, while the intracellular environment continues to lack necessary nutrients. Glucagon secretion increases, causing available body stores of food substances to be broken down in an attempt to provide cell nourishment. Impaired amino acid transport, protein synthesis, and protein degradation facilitate protein catabolism with a resultant increase in serum amino acids, while fat breakdown results in elevated free fatty acids (FFAs) and glycerol. The liver converts the newly available amino acids, fatty acids, and glycerol into glucose (gluconeogenesis) in an attempt to provide nourishment for the cells, but instead the hyperglycemia worsens because of the lack of insulin to transport glucose into the cells. The liver also produces ketone bodies from available FFAs, causing mild to severe acidosis. As ketone bodies increase in the extracellular fluid, the hydrogen ions within the ketones are exchanged with K ions from within the cells. Thus, intracellular K^+ is released into the extracellular fluid and therefore to circulating fluid, where it is excreted by the kidneys into the urine. Hyperglycemia acts as an osmotic diuretic, causing severe fluid and electrolyte losses, leading to hypovolemic shock if untreated. Individuals with severe DKA may lose nearly 500 mEq of Na^+, Cl^-, and K^+, along with approximately 7 L of water in 24 hr.

HEALTH CARE SETTING

Acute care (intensive care unit)

ASSESSMENT/DIAGNOSTIC TESTS

Clinical Findings: Comparison of Diabetic Ketoacidosis (DKA), Hyperglycemic Hyperosmolar Syndrome (HHS), and Hypoglycemia

	DKA	HHS	Hypoglycemia
Type of diabetes	Usually type 1	Usually type 2	
Signs, symptoms/physical assessment	Symptoms are a result mainly of hyperglycemia, intracellular hypoglycemia, hypotension or impending hypovolemic shock, and fluid-electrolyte imbalance with possible acid-base imbalance	Same as DKA	Symptoms result from intracellular hypoglycemia and hypotension/impending "insulin" shock (vasogenic)
Neurologic	Altered LOC (confusion, lethargy, irritability, coma), strokelike symptoms (unilateral/bilateral weakness, paralysis, numbness, paresthesia), fatigue	Same as DKA; also possible seizures and tremors	Tremors, trembling, shaking, confusion, apprehension, erratic behavior; may be same as DKA
Respiratory	Deep, rapid Kussmaul's respirations	Shallow, rapid (tachypneic) breathing	Usually rapid (tachypneic) breathing
Cardiovascular	Tachycardia, hypotension, ECG changes	Same as DKA	Same as DKA, possibly with diaphoresis

continued

Clinical Findings: Comparison of Diabetic Ketoacidosis (DKA), Hyperglycemic Hyperosmolar Syndrome (HHS), and Hypoglycemia—*cont'd*

	DKA	HHS	Hypoglycemia
Metabolic/GI/endocrine	Polyuria, polyphagia, polydipsia, fruity "acetone" breath, abdominal pain, weight loss, fatigue, generalized weakness, nausea, vomiting	Polyuria, polyphagia, polydipsia, fatigue, generalized weakness, nausea, vomiting	Hunger, nausea, eructation (belching)
Integumentary	Dry, flushed skin; poor turgor; dry mucous membranes	Same as DKA	Cool, clammy, pale skin
VS monitoring	BP low (more than 20% below normal), HR more than 100 bpm, CVP less than 2 mm Hg (less than 5 cm H_2O), temperature normal	BP low (more than 20% below normal), HR more than 100 bpm, CVP less than 2 mm Hg (less than 5 cm H_2O), temperature possibly elevated	BP normal to low, HR more than 100 bpm, CVP usually unchanged
Diagnostic tests/laboratory values	Values reflect dehydration/metabolic acidosis (ketosis) secondary to hyperglycemia, abnormal lipolysis, and osmotic diuresis; fluid loss 6.5 L or more. Anion gap: more than 10	Values reflect dehydration secondary to hyperglycemia, osmotic diuresis, and possible lactic acidosis from hypoperfusion; fluid loss 9 L or more. Anion gap: normal	Values reflect hypoglycemia, possibly with vasodilation owing to insulin shock
Hgb/Hct	Elevated	Same as DKA	Unchanged to slightly decreased
Serum BUN/creatinine	Elevated	Same as DKA	Normal
Serum electrolytes	Initially elevated, then decreased	Same as DKA	Usually unchanged
Serum glucose	250-800 mg/dL (+ ketones)	400-1800 mg/dL (− ketones)	15-50 mg/dL
Serum ketones	Elevated	Normal; rarely slightly elevated	Normal
ABGs	pH 6.8-7.3, HCO_3^- 12-20 mEq/L, CO_2 15-25 mEq/L	pH 7.3-7.5, HCO_3^- 20-26 mEq/L, CO_2 30-40 mEq/L	pH 7.3-7.5, HCO_3^- 20-26 mEq/L, CO_2 30-40 mEq/L
Serum osmolality	300-350 mOsm/L	More than 350 mOsm/L	Less than 280 mOsm/L
Urine glucose/acetone	Positive/positive	Positive/negative	Negative/negative
Onset	Hours to days	More than 1 day	Minutes to hours
History/risk factors for development of crisis	Undiagnosed DM, infections, acute pancreatitis, uremia, insulin resistance *Medications:* digitalis intoxication; omission/reduction of insulin dosage; failure to increase insulin to compensate for stress of infections; injury, emotional problems, or surgery	Undiagnosed DM; infections, especially gram-negative; acromegaly; Cushing's syndrome; thyrotoxicosis; acute pancreatitis; hyperalimentation; pancreatic carcinoma; cranial trauma/subdural hematoma; uremia, hemodialysis, peritoneal dialysis; burns, heat stroke; pneumonia; MI; stroke *Medications:* loop and thiazide diuretics (i.e., hydrochlorothiazide, chlorthalidone, furosemide), diazoxide; glucocorticoids (i.e., hydrocortisone, dexamethasone), propranolol (Inderal); phenytoin (Dilantin), sodium bicarbonate	Excessive dose of insulin, excessive dose of sulfonylureas/oral hypoglycemic agents, skipping meals, too much exercise with controlled blood glucose without extra food intake *Medications:* insulin, sulfonylureas and all medications used to reduce blood glucose in patients with diabetes, especially when food intake is reduced or changed
Mortality	10% or less	10%-25%	Less than 0.1%

ABGs, arterial blood gases; *BP,* blood pressure; *BUN,* blood urea nitrogen; *CVP,* central venous pressure; *DM,* diabetes mellitus; *ECG,* electrocardiogram; *GI,* gastrointestinal; *Hct,* hematocrit; *Hgb,* hemoglobin; *HR,* heart rate; *LOC,* level of consciousness; *MI,* myocardial infarction; *VS,* vital signs.

Nursing Diagnoses:

Deficient Fluid Volume
Risk for Electrolyte Imbalance
Risk for Shock

related to failure of regulatory mechanisms or decreased circulating volume occurring with hyperglycemia

Desired Outcomes: The patient becomes normovolemic within 10 hr of treatment, as evidenced by BP 90/60 mm Hg or more (or within the patient's normal range), HR 60-100 bpm, CVP 6-8 mm Hg, good skin turgor, moist and pink mucous membranes, specific gravity less than 1.020, balanced intake and output (I&O), and urinary output at least 30 mL/hr or 0.5 mL/kg/hr. Electrolyte levels are within normal limits.

ASSESSMENT/INTERVENTIONS	RATIONALES
Assess for signs and symptoms of hypovolemic shock, including changes in VS, q15min until the patient remains stable for 1 hr. Notify the health care provider promptly of significant findings.	Hyperglycemia acts as an osmotic diuretic, causing severe fluid and electrolyte losses that can lead to hypovolemic shock if untreated. HR greater than 120 bpm, BP less than 90/60 mm Hg or decreased 20 mm Hg or more from baseline, and CVP less than 2 mm Hg are signs of hypovolemia and will need prompt intervention.
Assess for poor skin turgor, dry mucous membranes, sunken and soft eyeballs, tachycardia, and orthostatic hypotension.	These are physical indicators of hypovolemia and will need prompt intervention.
Measure I&O accurately and weigh the patient daily. Monitor urinary specific gravity and report findings of more than 1.020 in the presence of other indicators of dehydration. Report to the health care provider if urine output is less than 30 mL/hr or less than 0.5mL/kg/hr for 2 consecutive hr.	Decreasing urinary output may signal diminishing intravascular fluid volume or impending renal failure. Loss of weight and output that exceeds intake may signal dehydration. However, loss of weight is unlikely in the setting of aggressive rehydration. To ensure accuracy, weight should be measured on the same scale if possible.
Administer intravenous (IV) fluids as prescribed.	This ensures adequate rehydration. Usually, normal saline or 0.45% saline is administered until plasma glucose falls to 200-300 mg/dL. After that, dextrose-containing solutions usually are given to prevent rebound hypoglycemia. Initially, IV fluids are administered rapidly (i.e., up to 2000 mL infused during the first 2 hr of treatment and 150-250 mL/hr thereafter until BP stabilizes).
Be alert to indicators of fluid overload, particularly in elders or in patients with a history of heart failure or renal failure.	Indicators of fluid overload (jugular vein distention, dyspnea, crackles, CVP more than 12 mm Hg) can occur with rapid infusion of fluids.
Administer insulin as prescribed.	Insulin usually is given by continuous IV infusion for rapid action and because poor tissue perfusion caused by dehydration sometimes makes the subcutaneous route less effective. Numerous protocols for IV insulin infusion are available and vary widely in the dosing regimen. Infusion protocols usually require a dosage increase when the blood glucose fails to decrease. Safer, more effective protocols should take into consideration the patient's level of insulin sensitivity and/or insulin resistance. The continuous infusion is administered through a separate IV tubing and controlled with an infusion control device. Computerized insulin dosing systems, dosing tables, and dosing algorithms are available. Dosage is adjusted based on serial glucose levels and resolution of ketosis. When formulas are used, the insulin sensitivity number is reflected as a variable multiplier that increases with higher levels of insulin resistance. Insulin analogues (i.e., NovoLog, HumaLog, Apidra) may be used in place of regular insulin to lower blood glucose levels.
Before initiating treatment, flush the tubing with at least 30 mL of the insulin-containing IV solution.	Insulin, when added to IV solutions, may be absorbed by the container and plastic tubing. Flushing the tubing ensures that maximum adsorption of the insulin by the container and tubing has occurred before it is delivered to the patient.

continued

ASSESSMENT/INTERVENTIONS	RATIONALES
If connecting the insulin infusion into another IV line, use the port closest to the patient to avoid unnecessary insulin dosage increases.	Using the port closest to the patient ensures the insulin is entering the bloodstream, rather than making the journey down lengthy tubing when "point of care" blood glucose readings are done.
Monitor laboratory results for abnormalities. Promptly report to the health care provider serum K⁺ levels less than 3.5 mEq/L. Observe for clinical manifestations of the electrolyte, glucose, and acid-base imbalances associated with DKA as follows: - *Hypokalemia:* Muscle weakness, hypotension, anorexia, drowsiness, hypoactive bowel sounds. - *Hyponatremia:* Headache, malaise, muscle weakness, abdominal cramps, nausea, seizures, coma. - *Hypophosphatemia:* Muscle weakness, progressive encephalopathy possibly leading to coma. - *Hypomagnesemia:* Anorexia, nausea, vomiting, lethargy, weakness, personality changes, tetany, tremor or muscle fasciculations, seizures, confusion progressing to coma. - *Hypochloremia:* Hypertonicity of muscles, tetany, depressed respirations. - *Hypoglycemia:* Headache, impaired mentation, agitation, dizziness, nausea, pallor, tremors, tachycardia, diaphoresis. - *Metabolic acidosis:* Lassitude, nausea, vomiting, Kussmaul's respirations, lethargy progressing to coma.	Before treatment there is risk of hyperkalemia from excess transport of intracellular K⁺ to extracellular spaces as a result of the acidosis. Na⁺ and Cl⁻ are replaced with IV normal saline. K⁺ must be monitored and corrected carefully. After initiation of treatment, K⁺ returns to the intracellular compartment through accelerated transport into cells via insulin and following correction of acidosis, and therefore the patient is at risk for becoming hypokalemic. Use of phosphorus replacement is controversial, but if phosphorus levels remain low, potassium phosphate solutions can be used to assist with K⁺ and phosphate replacement. Proper rehydration and insulin dosing should correct ketoacidosis, and lactic acidosis resulting from hypoperfusion due to hypovolemia and/or hypovolemic shock.

Nursing Diagnosis:

Risk for Infection

related to inadequate secondary defenses (suppressed inflammatory response) occurring with protein depletion

Desired Outcome: The patient is free of infection as evidenced by normothermia, HR 100 bpm or less, BP within the patient's normal range, white blood cell (WBC) count 11,000/mm³ or less, and negative culture results.

ASSESSMENT/INTERVENTIONS	RATIONALES
Assess for evidence of infection. Monitor laboratory results for increased WBC count; culture purulent drainage as prescribed.	Infection is the most common cause of DKA in adults, whereas nonadherence to treatment regimen is more likely responsible for DKA in children and teenagers. Indicators of infection include fever, chills, pain with urination, vomiting, erythema and swelling around IV sites, and increased WBC count.
Use meticulous hand hygiene when caring for the patient.	Patients are at increased risk for bacterial infection because of suppressed inflammatory response.
Manage invasive lines carefully. Schedule dressing changes according to agency policy.	Peripheral IV sites should be rotated at least q96h and dressings changed, depending on agency policy. Central lines should be discontinued as soon as feasible and when in place should be handled carefully.
Inspect insertion sites for erythema, swelling, or purulent drainage. Document the presence of any of these indicators, and notify the health care provider.	These are signs of local infection that should be reported promptly for timely intervention.
Provide good skin care.	Intact skin is a first line of defense against infection.
Provide a pressure-relief mattress or pressure redistribution surface on the patient's bed.	These surfaces help prevent skin breakdown, which could lead to infection.

ASSESSMENT/INTERVENTIONS	RATIONALES
Use meticulous sterile technique when caring for or inserting indwelling urinary catheters.	This minimizes the risk of bacterial entry into the body.
Note: Limit use of indwelling urethral catheters to patients who are unable to void in a bedpan or when continuous assessment of urine output is essential.	There is increased risk of infection with indwelling catheters. Nationally recognized nurse-sensitive indicators recommend that, if an indwelling catheter is inserted, every effort be made to remove it within 48 hr.
Encourage hourly use of incentive spirometry while the patient is awake, along with deep-breathing and coughing exercises. When the patient stabilizes, enable the patient to get out of bed, which also helps mobilize secretions and reduces the potential for deep vein thrombosis (DVT) or venous thromboembolus (VTE).	Deep inhalations with incentive spirometry along with deep breathing exercises expand alveoli and help mobilize secretions to the airways. Coughing further mobilizes and clears the secretions. These exercises help prevent pulmonary infection.

Nursing Diagnoses:

Acute Confusion
Risk for Injury

related to altered cerebral function occurring with dehydration or cerebral edema associated with DKA

Desired Outcomes: The patient verbalizes orientation to person, place, and time and does not demonstrate significant change in mental status; and normal breath sounds are auscultated over the patient's airway. In the event of a seizure, the patient's oral cavity and musculoskeletal system remain intact.

ASSESSMENT/INTERVENTIONS	RATIONALES
[!] Assess the patient's mental status; orientation; LOC; and respiratory status, especially airway patency, at frequent intervals.	With DKA, cerebral function may be altered because of dehydration or cerebral edema.
[!] Keep an appropriate-size oral airway, manual resuscitator and mask, and supplemental oxygen at the bedside.	In older patients, the increased work of breathing may exceed their ability to compensate, and this can result in respiratory arrest. In very rare instances, increased intracranial pressure caused by cerebral edema may impinge upon the brain stem, prompting respiratory arrest.
[!] Maintain bed in the lowest position, monitor the patient closely, and keep side rails up at all times.	These measures reduce the likelihood of injury from falls resulting from the patient's altered cerebral function.
As prescribed, insert a gastric tube in comatose patients. Attach the gastric tube to low, intermittent suction; assess patency q4hr.	These actions decrease the likelihood of aspiration. All tubes are a portal for entry of bacteria and thus a potential source of infection.
Ensure that the tube is removed as soon as the patient's LOC improves.	Timely removal reduces the chance of infection and skin breakdown related to securing the tube or movement of the tube at the insertion site.
Elevate head of the bed to 45 degrees.	This elevation minimizes risk of aspiration.
[!] Initiate seizure precautions. For details, see "Seizures and Epilepsy," p. 304.	

PART I: Medical-Surgical Nursing

Nursing Diagnosis:

Ineffective Peripheral Tissue Perfusion (or risk for same)

related to interrupted venous or arterial flow occurring with increased blood viscosity, increased platelet aggregation/adhesiveness, and patient immobility

Desired Outcomes: Optimally, the patient has adequate peripheral perfusion as evidenced by peripheral pulses greater than 2+ on a 0-4+ scale; warm skin; brisk capillary refill (less than 2 sec); and absence of swelling, bluish discoloration, erythema, and discomfort in the calves and thighs. Alternatively, if signs of altered peripheral tissue perfusion occur, they are detected and reported promptly.

ASSESSMENT/INTERVENTIONS	RATIONALES
Assess for hemoconcentration by monitoring hematocrit results.	Hemoconcentration is reflective of dehydration. Normal values are 40%-54% (male) or 37%-47% (female). With proper fluid replacement, results should return to normal within 24 hr.
Assess for increasing urine output and a reduction in BUN and creatinine values.	Normal BUN value is 6-20 mg/dL. Normal creatinine is 0.6-1.1 mg/dL. An increasing or normalizing urine output coupled with decreasing BUN and creatinine values is an indicator of improved renal perfusion.
Assess peripheral pulses q2-4h and report significant findings.	Significant decreases in amplitude or absence of pulse(s) should be reported to the health care provider promptly as it may signal DVT/VTE or other cause of perfusion deficit (e.g., hypovolemia).
[!] Be alert to erythema, pain, tenderness, warmth, and swelling over area of thrombus and bluish discoloration, paleness, coolness, and dilation of superficial veins in distal extremities, especially lower extremities.	These are indicators of DVT/VTE. For more information, see "Venous Thrombosis/Thrombophlebitis," p. 186.
[!] Also be alert to pain, paresthesias (especially loss of sensation of light touch and two-point discrimination), cyanosis with delayed capillary refill, mottling, and coolness of the extremity.	These are indicators of arterial thrombosis, which can lead to profound limb ischemia and tissue hypoxia and eventually to tissue anoxia and death.
Report significant findings to the health care provider immediately.	When untreated, limb ischemia may result in loss of limb and/or digits.
Encourage the patient to exercise extremities q2h.	Exercise increases blood flow to the tissues. Calf pumping and ankle circles should be encouraged at least q2h in patients susceptible to DVT/VTE.
Unless contraindicated, encourage fluid intake to more than 1000 mL/day.	Increased hydration decreases the potential for hemoconcentration, which could lead to DVT/VTE.
Apply pneumatic alternating pressure stockings or pneumatic foot pumps as prescribed.	These garments and devices promote venous return and aid in prevention of thrombosis.

Nursing Diagnosis:

Deficient Knowledge

related to unfamiliarity with the cause, prevention, and treatment of DKA

Desired Outcome: Within the 24-hr period before hospital discharge, the patient verbalizes understanding of the cause, prevention, and treatment of DKA.

ASSESSMENT/INTERVENTIONS	RATIONALES
Assess the patient's health care literacy (language, reading, comprehension). Assess culture and culturally specific information needs.	This assessment helps ensure that information is selected and presented in a manner that is culturally and educationally appropriate.

ASSESSMENT/INTERVENTIONS

RATIONALES

ASSESSMENT/INTERVENTIONS	RATIONALES
Determine the patient's knowledge about DKA and its treatment.	This will enable, as needed, further explanation of the disease process of DM and DKA and common early symptoms of worsening hyperglycemia, including polyuria, polydipsia, polyphagia, dry and flushed skin, and increased irritability.
Assess the patient's ability to engage in self-management of blood glucose monitoring and control. Explore whether the patient psychologically accepts the disease as a significant health challenge.	This information will enable individualized teaching that will facilitate adherence to the prescribed management regimen designed to maintain normoglycemia.
Stress the importance of maintaining a consistent controlled carbohydrate diet, exercise, and insulin regimen.	This regimen helps ensure optimal control of serum glucose levels and prevention of adverse physical effects of DM, such as peripheral neuropathies and increased atherosclerosis.
Explain the importance of blood glucose monitoring during episodes of stress, injury, and illness. Caution that DKA necessitates professional medical management and cannot be self-treated.	Increased stress impacts metabolism of carbohydrates, fats, and proteins, causing increased blood glucose.
Discuss "sick day management," which includes continuing the same insulin regimen: *not* stopping insulin or skipping doses, testing urine ketones if ill or vomiting, and increasing the frequency of blood glucose testing to monitor more closely for hyperglycemia.	Testing urine ketones may be advised. Blood glucose greater than 250 mg/dL and the appearance of large amounts of urine ketones should be reported to the health care provider so that insulin dose can be increased.
Remind the patient of the importance of maintaining adequate oral fluid intake during illness despite anorexia or nausea.	Anorexia or nausea may limit food intake, but patients should make every effort to continue fluid intake to avoid dehydration, hypovolemia, and possible hypotension.
Review testing and insulin administration procedure as indicated.	Insulin or insulin analog must be taken 1-4 times/day as prescribed, and lifetime insulin therapy is necessary to achieve control of blood glucose.
! Teach the importance of receiving prompt treatment if such indicators as dizziness, impaired mentation, irritability, pallor, and tremors occur.	These are signs of insulin or insulin analogue excess (hypoglycemia).
! Caution the patient to get prompt treatment if the following indicators occur: polyuria, polydipsia, polyphagia, or increasingly dry and flushed skin.	These are signs of insulin deficiency (hyperglycemia).
Explain the consequences of not receiving prompt treatment.	If untreated, these conditions could lead to coma and death.
Explain the importance of dietary changes as prescribed by the health care provider.	Typically patients are put on a consistent carbohydrate diet composed of 60% carbohydrates, 20%-30% fats, and 12%-20% proteins. Counting carbohydrates and prescribing insulin dosage according to the amount of carbohydrates consumed is a newer strategy of blood glucose management.
Advise that fats should be polyunsaturated and proteins chosen from low-fat sources.	Reducing saturated fat intake reduces risk of developing coronary artery and peripheral vascular disease.
Teach the importance of eating three meals per day at regularly scheduled times and a bedtime snack.	Such a diet affords the best opportunity for maintaining a physiologically normal blood glucose level rather than "roller coaster" values of alternating hyperglycemia and hypoglycemia. Meals and insulin administration must be linked together, especially when insulin analogues such as HumaLog, NovoLog, or Apidra are given before meals and in conjunction with snacks. Analogues are quicker acting than regular insulins.
Explain causes for adjustments in insulin dose. Instruct the patient to monitor blood glucose and urine ketone levels closely during periods of increased emotional stress and periods of increased or decreased exercise and to adjust insulin dose accordingly.	Adjustments in insulin dose include increased or decreased food or carbohydrate intake and any physical (e.g., exercise) or emotional stress. Exercise and emotional stress may increase release of glucose from the liver or increase insulin resistance.
Remind the patient that alternative and complementary health strategies may alter blood glucose levels and prompt a need for adjustment of medications.	For example, certain herbal preparations can alter metabolism and may increase or decrease blood glucose. All methods used should be reported to the health care provider. For a list of herbal remedies that alter blood glucose, see **Deficient Knowledge** in "Diabetes Mellitus," p. 361.

continued

PART I: Medical-Surgical Nursing

ASSESSMENT/INTERVENTIONS	RATIONALES
Explain that good hygiene and meticulous daily foot care are necessary to prevent infection. Stress the importance of avoiding exposure to communicable diseases, and explain that the following indicators of infection necessitate prompt medical treatment: fever, chills, increased HR, diaphoresis, nausea, and vomiting. In addition, teach the patient and significant other to be alert to wounds or cuts that do not heal, burning or pain with urination, and a productive cough.	Persons with diabetes are susceptible to infection because of decreased immune response.
Instruct the patient to implement the following therapy when ill for any reason:	
- Do not alter insulin (NovoLin, HumuLin), insulin analogue (HumaLog, NovoLog, Apidra), or oral diabetes or hyperglycemia medication dosage unless the health care provider has prescribed a supplemental regimen.	Altering the insulin regimen increases risk for hypoglycemia if medication dosage is increased.
- Perform blood glucose monitoring and urine ketone checks at least q4h, and promptly report glucose greater than 250 mg/dL and positive ketones to the health care provider.	If the insulin dose is decreased for persistent incidences of hypoglycemia, the blood glucose should increase to the normal range with proper dosage. The stress associated with illness alters metabolism and glucose uptake. Hyperglycemia can ensue quickly when patients become ill.
- Eat small, frequent meals of soft, easily digestible, nourishing foods if regular meals are not tolerated.	If carbohydrate intake falls significantly, insulin dosage may need to be reduced to prevent hypoglycemia. Smaller, more frequent meals may help maintain more normal intake.
- Maintain adequate hydration, particularly if diarrhea, vomiting, or fever is persistent.	Dehydration can lead to hypovolemia, which in turn can lead to shock if left untreated.
- Use a balance of sugar-containing beverages and water to ensure adequate calories yet prevent hyperosmolality caused by sugars in the beverages.	Intake of carbohydrates must be maintained unless insulin dose is altered to avoid hypoglycemia. Water must be consumed to maintain intravascular volume. There are too many carbohydrates in juice or soda to use either as a primary source of volume. If carbohydrate intake is not appropriately balanced with water intake, glucose may increase, prompting polyuria, which increases the risk for hypovolemia or, if severe, hypovolemic shock.
Provide the following address of the American Diabetes Association (ADA): *www.diabetes.org* or the Canadian Diabetes Association at *www.diabetes.ca*. See "Diabetes Mellitus," p. 364, for a complete listing of organizations that can supply information regarding DM.	The ADA website is the original source of information for pamphlets and magazines related to the disease, its complications, and appropriate treatment. Other sources of information are now available.

ADDITIONAL NURSING DIAGNOSES/PROBLEMS:

"Psychosocial Support"   p. 72

PATIENT-FAMILY TEACHING AND DISCHARGE PLANNING

See **Deficient Knowledge** related to unfamiliarity with cause, prevention, and treatment of DKA, p. 370.

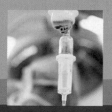

Hyperglycemic Hyperosmolar Syndrome 47

OVERVIEW/PATHOPHYSIOLOGY

Hyperglycemic hyperosmolar syndrome (HHS), also known as *hyperosmolar hyperglycemic nonketotic syndrome* (HHNK), *hyperosmolar coma, nonketotic hyperosmolar coma, hyperosmolar nonketotic syndrome, hyperosmolar hyperglycemic nonketotic coma,* and *nonketotic hyperglycemic hyperosmolar coma,* is a life-threatening emergency resulting from a lack of effective insulin, or severe insulin resistance, causing extreme hyperglycemia. Often HHS is precipitated by a stressor such as trauma, injury, or infection that increases insulin demand. It is believed there is enough insulin to prevent acidosis and formation of ketone bodies at the cellular level, but there is not enough insulin to facilitate transportation of all the glucose into the cells. Thus glucose molecules accumulate in the bloodstream, causing serum hyperosmolality with resultant osmotic diuresis and simultaneous loss of electrolytes, most notably potassium, sodium, and phosphate.

Caution: Patients may lose up to 25% of their total body water. Fluids are pulled from individual body cells by increasing serum hyperosmolality and extracellular fluid loss, causing intracellular dehydration and body cell shrinkage. Neurologic deficits (e.g., slowed mentation, confusion, seizures, stroke-like symptoms, coma) can occur as a result. Loss of extracellular fluid stimulates aldosterone release, which facilitates sodium retention and prevents further loss of potassium. However, aldosterone cannot halt severe dehydration. As extracellular volume decreases, blood viscosity increases, causing slowing of blood flow. Thromboemboli are common because of increased blood viscosity, enhanced platelet aggregation and adhesiveness, and possibly patient's immobility. Cardiac workload is increased and may lead to myocardial infarction. Renal blood flow is decreased, potentially resulting in renal impairment or failure. Stroke may result from thromboemboli or decreased cerebral perfusion. Mortality rate of HHS ranges from 10%-50%, which is higher than that of diabetic ketoacidosis (DKA) (1.2%-9%). Mortality data are difficult to interpret because of the high incidence of coexisting diseases or comorbidities.

Historically, HHS and DKA were described as distinct syndromes; but one third of patients exhibit findings of both conditions. HHS and DKA may be at opposite ends of a range of decompensated diabetes, differing in time of onset, degree of dehydration, and severity of ketosis. HHS occurs most commonly in older people with type 2 diabetes mellitus (DM), but with the recent obesity epidemic, occasionally obese children and teenagers with both diagnosed and undiagnosed type 2 DM manifest HHS. The cascade of events in HHS begins with osmotic diuresis. Glycosuria impairs the ability of the kidney to concentrate urine, which exacerbates the water loss. Normally, the kidneys eliminate glucose above a certain threshold and prevent a subsequent rise in blood glucose level. In HHS, the decreased intravascular volume or possible underlying renal disease decreases the glomerular filtration rate (GFR), causing the glucose level to increase. More water is lost than sodium, resulting in hyperosmolarity. Insulin is present, but not in adequate amounts to decrease blood glucose levels, and with type 2 DM, significant insulin resistance is present.

Unlike DKA, in which ketoacidosis produces severe symptoms requiring fairly prompt hospitalization, symptoms of HHS develop more slowly and often are nonspecific. The anion gap is normal, versus widened with DKA due to ketone production. The cardinal symptoms of polyuria and polydipsia are noted first but may be ignored by older persons or their families. Neurologic deficits may be mistaken for senility. The similarity of these symptoms to those of other disease processes common to this age group may delay differential diagnosis and treatment, allowing progression of pathophysiologic processes with resultant hypovolemic shock and multiple organ failure. As shock progresses, lactic acidosis may ensue due to poor perfusion.

HEALTH CARE SETTING

Acute care (usually intensive care) unless the condition is not severe

ASSESSMENT

See Table in "Diabetic Ketoacidosis," p. 365.

Note: *Patients with HHS may be older than 50 yr and have preexisting cardiac or pulmonary disorders. The incidence of type 2 DM is increasing in children, teenagers, and young adults, so younger people are now presenting with HHS. Assessment results often cannot be evaluated based on accepted normal values. Evaluate results based on what is normal or optimal for the individual patient. Central venous pressure (CVP), heart rate (HR), and blood pressure (BP) should be evaluated in terms of deviations from the patient's baseline and concurrent clinical status.*

DIAGNOSTIC TESTS

Serum glucose: From 400 to 1800 mg/dL is diagnostic of HHS.

Serum chemistry: Serum values change as osmotic diuresis progresses. At late stages, the patient may reflect the following electrolyte values/losses:

- Na^+: 125-160 mEq/L. Although the patient has lost large quantities of Na^+, osmotic diuresis causes abnormally high blood concentration. The Na^+ value may appear high despite probable Na^+ deficits.
- K^+: less than 3.5 mEq/L.
- Cl^-: less than 95 mEq/L.
- *Phosphorus:* less than 1.7 mEq/L.
- *Magnesium:* less than 1.5 mEq/L.

Serum osmolality: Will be greater than 350 mOsm/L. A quick bedside calculation of serum osmolality can be obtained by using the following formula:

$$2(Na^+ + K^+) + BUN\,(mg/dL)/2.8 + Glucose\,(mg/dL)/18 = mOsm/L$$

For example: $Na^+ = 140$; $K^+ = 4.5$; $BUN = 20$; $Glucose = 120$

$$2(140 + 4.5) + 20/2.8 + 120/18 = 2(144.5) + 7 + 6.7$$

$$289 + 7 + 6.7 = 302.7\,mOsm/L$$

Anion gap: normal

COMPLICATIONS

Complications of HHS include arterial thrombosis, stroke, renal failure, heart failure, multiple organ failure, cerebral edema, malignant dysrhythmias (due to fluid volume deficiency, which prompts poor end-organ perfusion), and gram-negative sepsis (from infection that may have caused the problem to ensue).

Nursing Diagnosis:

Deficient Knowledge

related to unfamiliarity with causes, prevention, and treatment of HHS

Desired Outcome: Within the 24-hr period before hospital discharge, the patient and significant other verbalize understanding of causes, prevention, and treatment of HHS.

ASSESSMENT/INTERVENTIONS	RATIONALES
Assess the patient's health care literacy (language, reading, comprehension). Assess culture and culturally specific information needs.	This assessment helps ensure that information is selected and presented in a manner that is culturally and educationally appropriate.
Determine the patient's understanding of HHS and its treatment. Enable verbalization of fears and feelings about the diagnosis; correct any misconceptions.	This enables the nurse to reinforce, as needed, information about the disease process of DM and HHS and common early symptoms of worsening DM, including polyuria, polydipsia, polyphagia, dry and flushed skin, and increased irritability.
⚠ Caution the patient that fluid resuscitation may be a critical component in his or her recovery from HHS.	Patients may lose up to 25% of their total body water. Fluids are pulled from individual body cells by increasing serum hyperosmolality and extracellular fluid loss, causing intracellular dehydration and body cell shrinkage. For details, see "Diabetic Ketoacidosis" for **Deficient Fluid Volume/Risk for Electrolyte Imbalance/Risk for Shock,** p. 367.
Teach the importance of testing blood glucose levels as prescribed before meals and at bedtime. As indicated, review testing procedure with the patient.	Blood glucose monitoring is essential for calculating appropriate basal, mealtime, and supplemental insulin dosages.

ASSESSMENT/INTERVENTIONS	RATIONALES
Explain that fasting morning blood glucose greater than 140 mg/dL should be reported to the health care provider.	Reporting this value enables prompt adjustment in insulin dose based on blood glucose levels.
Stress the importance of dietary changes as prescribed by the health care provider. Provide a referral to a dietitian as needed.	Typically, the person with type 2 DM is obese and will be on a reduced-calorie diet with fixed amounts of carbohydrate, fat, and protein. Fats should be polyunsaturated and proteins chosen from low-fat sources.
Teach the importance of eating three meals per day at regularly scheduled times and a bedtime snack and information related to type(s) of insulin being administered.	Mealtime insulin should be administered within the 30 min before a meal (regular insulin) or 15 min before or after a meal (analogue short-acting insulins such as Humalog, Novolog, or Apidra). If meals are not spaced appropriately, patients may experience hyperglycemia or hypoglycemia between meals. Analogue insulin is more commonly administered at mealtime. Mixed insulin such as 70/30 is used in lieu of requiring another injection of mealtime insulin. Patients not receiving analogue insulin should be considered candidates if glucose is fluctuant.
Explain that increased or decreased food intake will necessitate adjustment in insulin dosage.	Mealtime insulin dose is calculated based on the average amount of carbohydrates in the patient's diet. If meal consumption changes, the insulin dose must change accordingly to ensure adequate control of blood glucose.
Caution about the importance of taking oral hypoglycemic agents as prescribed.	Oral hypoglycemic agents must be taken as prescribed or the patient may become hypoglycemic or hyperglycemic.
In addition, explain that exogenous insulin or insulin analogues may be required during periods of physical and emotional stress and that blood glucose levels should be monitored closely during these times.	Increased stress creates insulin resistance, which may prompt hyperglycemia even though the patient's food intake remains constant.
For patients with type 2 DM, explain benefits of regular exercise for maintaining blood glucose levels.	Exercise increases insulin effectiveness and reduces serum triglyceride and cholesterol levels, thus also decreasing risk of atherosclerosis. Aerobic exercises, such as walking or swimming, are most effective in lowering blood glucose levels.
Caution the patient to always monitor blood glucose levels before exercise.	A level greater than 250 mg/dL is indicative of inadequate blood glucose management. In this case, exercise could be a stressor in patients not used to exercise, resulting in further elevation of blood glucose.
Explain need for measures to prevent infection, such as good hygiene and meticulous daily foot care. Stress the importance of avoiding exposure to communicable diseases. Explain that the following indicators of infection necessitate prompt medical treatment: fever, chills, tachycardia, diaphoresis, and nausea and vomiting. In addition, teach the patient and significant other to be alert to wounds or cuts that do not heal, burning or pain with urination, and cough that is productive of sputum.	Immune system dysfunction results from the lack of energy production at the cellular level of all components of the immune system. Hyperglycemia indicates glucose has not been transported from the bloodstream into the cells. Without normal levels of intracellular glucose, cellular energy production is impaired. All body system functions, including the immune system, are dysfunctional because cells involved with cellular and humoral immunity are unable to do 100% of the work required. The inability of glucose to "power" the cells suppresses the immune system, thereby increasing the risk of infection.
Provide the following address of the American Diabetes Association (ADA): www.diabetes.org or the Canadian Diabetes Association: www.diabetes.ca. See "Diabetes Mellitus," p. 364, for a complete listing of information sources.	Patients may acquire pamphlets and magazines related to diabetes, its complications, and treatment.

ADDITIONAL NURSING DIAGNOSES/PROBLEMS:

✓ PATIENT-FAMILY TEACHING AND DISCHARGE PLANNING

See **Deficient Knowledge** related to unfamiliarity with causes, prevention, and treatment of HHS, p. 374.

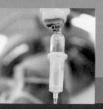

Hyperthyroidism 48

OVERVIEW/PATHOPHYSIOLOGY

Hyperthyroidism is a clinical syndrome caused by excessive circulating thyroid hormone. Because thyroid activity affects all body systems, excessive thyroid hormone exaggerates normal body functions and produces a hypermetabolic state. *Lymphocytic* ("painless") and *postpartum thyroiditis* are autoimmune disorders that result in thyroid inflammation with release of stored thyroid hormone into systemic circulation. Postpartum thyroiditis may ensue several months after delivery and remain active for several months, sometimes followed by hypothyroidism lasting several months. *Subacute (granulomatous) thyroiditis* is considered a viral syndrome, and it results in a painful, enlarged thyroid with overactive thyroid until the virus is controlled, which may in turn prompt transient hypothyroidism. Hyperthyroid symptoms also result from ingestion of too much thyroid replacement medication.

Graves' disease (diffuse toxic goiter) accounts for approximately 85% of reported cases of hyperthyroidism. It is characterized by spontaneous exacerbations and remissions that appear to be unaffected by therapy. The cause of Graves' disease is unknown, but recent advances in diagnostic techniques have isolated an immunoglobulin known as *long-acting thyroid stimulator* in a majority of patients with this disorder, suggesting that Graves' disease is an autoimmune response.

The most severe form of hyperthyroidism is *thyrotoxic crisis,* or *thyroid storm,* which results from a sudden surge of large amounts of thyroid hormones into the bloodstream, causing an even greater increase in body metabolism. This is a *medical emergency.* Precipitating factors include infection, trauma, and emotional stress, all of which increase demands on body metabolism. Thyrotoxic crisis also can occur following thyroidectomy because of manipulation of the gland during surgery.

HEALTH CARE SETTING

Primary care with possible hospitalization resulting from complications

ASSESSMENT

Signs and symptoms: Nervousness, irritability, alteration in appetite, weight loss or gain, rapid pulse (usually noted by the patient), irregular heartbeats, menstrual irregularities, fatigue, heat intolerance, increased perspiration, frequent defecation or diarrhea, anxiety, restlessness, tremor, and insomnia. Patients bordering on thyroid storm may be confused and possibly psychotic.

Physical assessment: Tachycardia, palpitations, widened pulse pressure, exophthalmos, diplopia, hyperpyrexia, enlargement of the thyroid gland, dependent lower extremity edema, muscle weakness, hyperreflexia, fine tremor, fine hair, thin skin, hypercholesterolemia, impaired glucose tolerance, and stare and/or lid lag. Occasionally males may present with gynecomastia.

Thyrotoxic crisis (thyroid storm): Acute exacerbation of some or all the above signs, marked tachycardia, hyperpyrexia, central nervous system (CNS) irritability, and sometimes coma or heart failure. Cardiovascular collapse and shock are occasionally how patients present. Various clinical syndromes also produce hyperthyroidism, but thyroid storm is most often associated with Graves' disease.

History/risk factors: Family history of hyperthyroidism is a significant factor for development of this disorder. Another important factor is presence of thyroid nodules or nodular toxic goiters in which one or more thyroid adenomas hyperfunction autonomously. Amiodarone use has caused thyroid dysfunction in 14%-18% of individuals taking this commonly used antidysrhythmic drug. Patients should have thyroid studies done before the drug is initiated and be monitored serially afterward. For thyrotoxic crisis, patients with hyperthyroidism resulting from Graves' disease, thyroid nodules, or toxic goiter may have undergone a recent stressful experience, including severe infection, trauma, major surgery, thromboembolism, diabetic ketoacidosis, preeclampsia, pregnancy, labor, and/or delivery.

DIAGNOSTIC TESTS

Serum thyroid-stimulating hormone (thyrotropin): Most commonly used test to detect thyroid dysfunction. It is decreased in the presence of disease.

Serum T_4 (thyroxine) or free T_4: Elevated in the presence of disease. It may be more accurate than thyroid-stimulating hormone (TSH) if patients have been recently treated for hyperthyroidism or if receiving high doses of thyroid replacement therapy. Thyroxine should be monitored along with TSH for the first year of therapy, especially in older adults.

Serum T_3 (thyroxine triiodothyronine) radioimmunoassay or free T_3: Elevated in the presence of disease.

Serum thyroid autoantibodies: Can detect TSH receptor antibodies and thyroid-stimulating immunoglobulins, which may be present if autoimmune disease is present.

Thyroid binding globulin: Measures the level of the protein that binds with circulating thyroid hormones. Abnormal T_4 or T_3 measurements are often caused by binding protein abnormalities rather than abnormal thyroid function.

Thyroid scan ^{123}I (preferably) or ^{99m}Tc pertechnetate: Helps determine the cause of the hyperthyroidism. The scan also may be useful in assessing functional status of any palpable thyroid irregularities or nodules associated with a toxic goiter.

Doppler ultrasonography: To diagnose size of the gland and abnormal densities, which can indicate presence of nodules.

Radioiodine (^{131}I) uptake and thyroid scan: Clarifies gland size and detects presence of hot or cold nodules.

^{123}I scintiscan/thyroid scintigraphy: Defines functional characteristics of the gland to help determine cause of hyperthyroidism.

Nursing Diagnosis:

Ineffective Protection

related to potential for thyrotoxic crisis (thyroid storm) occurring with emotional stress, trauma, infection, or surgical manipulation of the gland

Desired Outcomes: The patient is free of symptoms of thyroid storm as evidenced by normothermia; blood pressure (BP) 90/60 mm Hg or more (or within the patient's baseline range); heart rate (HR) 100 bpm or less; and orientation to person, place, and time. If thyroid storm occurs, it is detected promptly and reported immediately.

ASSESSMENT/INTERVENTIONS	RATIONALES
⚠ Assess for hyperthermia and report rectal or core temperature greater than 38.3° C (101° F).	An increased temperature often is the first sign of impending thyroid storm.
⚠ Assess for signs of heart failure. Immediately report significant findings to the health care provider, and prepare to transfer the patient to the intensive care unit if they are noted.	Signs of heart failure (jugular vein distention, crackles, decreased amplitude of peripheral pulses, peripheral edema, and hypotension) can occur as an effect of thyroid storm. If not aggressively monitored and managed, thyroid storm can lead to lethal cardiac and hemodynamic compromise.
Assess vital signs hourly in patients in whom thyroid storm is suspected.	These assessments may reveal evidence of hypotension and increasing tachycardia and fever, which may reflect increasing severity of heart failure associated with thyroid storm.
Provide a cool, calm, protected environment. Reassure the patient and explain all procedures before performing them. Limit the number of visitors.	These measures minimize emotional and physical stress, which can precipitate thyroid storm.
Ensure good hand hygiene and meticulous aseptic technique for dressing changes and invasive procedures. Advise visitors who have contracted or been exposed to a communicable disease either not to enter the patient's room or to wear a surgical mask, if appropriate.	These measures reduce risk of infection, which is a precipitating factor in the development of thyroid storm.
In the Presence of Thyroid Storm	
Assess for hyperthermia and administer acetaminophen as prescribed.	Acetaminophen will decrease temperature secondary to the fever associated with thyroid storm.
⚠ Avoid giving aspirin.	Aspirin is contraindicated because it releases thyroxine from protein-binding sites and increases free thyroxine levels, which would exacerbate symptoms of thyroid storm.
Provide cool sponge baths, or apply ice packs to the patient's axilla and groin area. If high temperature continues, obtain prescription for a hypothermia blanket.	These actions will decrease the fever caused by thyroid storm.
Administer thioamides such as propylthiouracil (PTU) and methimazole as prescribed.	Thioamides will prevent further synthesis and release of thyroid hormones.

ASSESSMENT/INTERVENTIONS	RATIONALES
! Monitor complete blood count values, particularly the WBC counts.	The most severe side effect of thioamides is leukopenia, which increases the possibility that patients may acquire an infection. Patients should discontinue thioamides at the first sign of infection and obtain a complete blood count. If the blood count is normal, medication is promptly resumed. Rash, another side effect, can be treated easily with antihistamines. Methimazole may have a lower rate of these effects. PTU is more effective than methimazole in thyroid storm.
Administer propranolol as prescribed.	Propranolol will block sympathetic nervous system (SNS) effects. It reduces HR and BP, which are elevated as a result of hyperthyroidism.
Administer intravenous (IV) fluids as prescribed.	Fluid volume deficit may occur because of increased fluid excretion by the kidneys or excessive diaphoresis. IV fluids will provide adequate hydration and prevent vascular collapse.
Carefully monitor intake and output (I&O) hourly.	Hourly assessment of I&O will reveal fluid overload or inadequate fluid replacement, either of which necessitates prompt intervention. Decreasing output with normal specific gravity may indicate decreased cardiac output, whereas decreasing output with increased specific gravity can signal dehydration.
! If sodium iodide is prescribed, wait 1 hr after administering PTU before giving the sodium iodide.	Iodine is necessary for subsequent production of thyroid hormones following resolution of the crisis. However, if given before PTU, sodium iodide can exacerbate symptoms in susceptible persons.
Administer small doses of insulin as prescribed.	This will help control hyperglycemia. Hyperglycemia can occur as an effect of thyroid storm because of the release of stress hormones as part of the body's response to the hypermetabolic state. Stress hormones create insulin resistance.
Administer prescribed supplemental O_2 as necessary.	O_2 demands are increased as metabolism increases.

Nursing Diagnosis:

Imbalanced Nutrition: Less Than Body Requirements

related to the hypermetabolic state and/or inadequate nutrient absorption

Desired Outcomes: By a minimum of 24 hr before hospital discharge, the patient has adequate nutrition as evidenced by stable weight and a positive nitrogen balance. Within 24 hr of the instruction, the patient lists types of foods that are necessary to restore a normal nutritional state.

ASSESSMENT/INTERVENTIONS	RATIONALES
Assess for weight loss by weighing the patient daily, and report significant losses to the health care provider. Assess daily nutritional intake.	Daily weight assessment is a useful indicator of nutritional status. Weight loss may indicate the patient is not receiving appropriate nutritional support for the accelerated metabolic rate. The patient's needs (e.g., as indicated by continued weight loss) will help determine the amount and type of nutritional intake.
Assess for and manage diarrhea with prescribed antidiarrheal medications.	These medications increase absorption of nutrients from the gastrointestinal tract.
Provide foods high in calories, protein, carbohydrates, and vitamins. Teach about foods that will provide optimal nutrients.	This will help restore a normal nutritional state for patients with hyperthyroidism.
Provide between-meal snacks.	Snacks will help maximize the patient's consumption and provide needed calories.
Administer vitamin supplements as prescribed, and explain their importance to the patient.	Vitamins provide essential nutrients to facilitate appropriate digestion/absorption of foods that contribute to energy production.

Nursing Diagnosis:

Disturbed Sleep Pattern

related to accelerated metabolism

Desired Outcome: Within 48 hr of hospital admission, the patient relates the attainment of sufficient rest and sleep.

ASSESSMENT/INTERVENTIONS	RATIONALES
Assess the patient's sleep pattern and adjust care activities to the patient's tolerance.	It may be necessary to alter the care regimen to comply with the patient's rest/sleep disturbance.
Assess activity tolerance and provide frequent rest periods of at least 90-min duration. If possible, arrange for the patient to have bedrest in a quiet, temperature-controlled room with nonexertional activities such as reading, watching television, working crossword puzzles, or listening to soothing music.	Patients will have difficulty relaxing. Therefore, all efforts must be made to provide a calm, quiet environment to promote rest/sleep. Setting the temperature of the room to the patient's comfort level will assist with relaxation.
Assist with walking up stairs or other exertional activities if needed.	If the patient is tired, more assistance is needed until rest/sleep pattern normalizes.
Administer short-acting sedatives (e.g., lorazepam) as prescribed. After administering these agents, raise the side rails if the patient is hospitalized.	These medications promote rest. This will help protect the patient, who will be drowsy after taking these sedatives.

Nursing Diagnosis:

Anxiety

related to SNS stimulation

Desired Outcomes: Within 24 hr of hospital admission, the patient is free of harmful anxiety as evidenced by an HR of 100 bpm or less, respiratory rate (RR) 12-20 breaths/min with normal depth and pattern (eupnea), and absence of or decrease in irritability and restlessness. The patient and significant others verbalize knowledge about the causes of the patient's behavior.

ASSESSMENT/INTERVENTIONS	RATIONALES
Assess for signs of anxiety; administer short-acting sedatives as prescribed. Assess the effectiveness of sedatives in controlling the anxiety.	Short-acting sedatives (e.g., alprazolam or lorazepam) reduce anxiety.
Administer propranolol as prescribed.	Propranolol reduces symptoms of anxiety, tachycardia, and heat intolerance.
Provide a quiet environment away from loud noises or excessive activity.	This will help reduce stress and anxiety.
Limit the number of visitors and the amount of time they spend with the patient. Advise significant others to avoid discussing stressful topics and refrain from arguing with the patient.	These measures will help reduce stress and anxiety.
Inform significant others that the patient's behavior is physiologic and should not be taken personally.	Reassuring family members helps them regain emotional control/reduce their stress regarding the patient's unusual behaviors.
Reassure the patient that anxiety symptoms are related to the disease process and that treatment decreases their severity.	Reassurance helps patients regain emotional control/reduce emotional stress through better understanding of the cause and treatment.

Nursing Diagnosis:

Impaired Tissue Integrity: Corneal

related to dryness that can occur with exophthalmos in persons with Graves' disease

Desired Outcome: Within 24 hr of admission, the patient's corneas are moist and intact.

ASSESSMENT/INTERVENTIONS	RATIONALES
Assess for dry eyes and administer lubricating eye drops as prescribed.	Eye drops will supplement lubrication and decrease SNS stimulation, which can cause lid retraction.
Teach the patient to wear dark glasses.	This will help protect the corneas. Dark glasses also protect those individuals who are photosensitive.
If appropriate, apply eye shields or tape the eyes shut at bedtime.	Hyperthyroidism can result in severe exophthalmos that prevents eyelids from closing fully, making the corneas vulnerable to injury.
Administer thioamides as prescribed.	Thioamides maintain a normal metabolic state and halt progression of exophthalmos.

Nursing Diagnosis:

Disturbed Body Image

related to exophthalmos or surgical scar on the neck

Desired Outcome: Within the 24-hr period before hospital discharge, the patient verbalizes measures for disguising exophthalmos or the surgical scar and exhibits self-acceptance.

ASSESSMENT/INTERVENTIONS	RATIONALES
Assess for indicators of body image disturbance.	Patients may exhibit nonverbal indicators (avoiding looking at self in the mirror, keeping eyes fully or partially closed when speaking, bowing head when speaking to minimize exposure of the throat) or verbal indicators (expressing negative feelings about facial appearance or surgical scar on throat/neck.)
Encourage the patient to communicate feelings of frustration.	Such communication may help patients relieve stress that would otherwise further stimulate the hypophyseal/thyroid/adrenal axis.
Advise the patient to wear dark glasses.	Dark glasses will disguise exophthalmos while also protecting the corneas from photosensitivity.
Suggest measures that can disguise the scar.	Customized jewelry, high-necked clothing such as turtlenecks, and loose-fitting scarves are examples of measures that will help disguise the scar.
Suggest that after the incision has healed, the patient can use makeup colored in his or her skin tone.	This will decrease visibility of the scar.
Caution the patient that creams are contraindicated until the incision has healed completely, and even then may not minimize scarring.	This is standard postoperative teaching for most surgical procedures. Patients are advised by some health care providers to increase vitamin C intake up to 1 g/day to promote healing. Some surgeons also advise against direct sunlight to the operative site for 6-12 mo to avoid hyperpigmentation of the incision. Instruct the patient accordingly.
For additional information, see this nursing diagnosis in "Psychosocial Support," p. 79.	

Nursing Diagnosis:

Deficient Knowledge

related to unfamiliarity with the potential for side effects from iodides and thioamides or stopping thioamides abruptly

Desired Outcome: Within the 24-hr period before hospital discharge, the patient verbalizes knowledge about the potential side effects of the prescribed medications, signs and symptoms of hypothyroidism and hyperthyroidism, and the importance of following the prescribed medical regimen.

ASSESSMENT/INTERVENTIONS	RATIONALES
Assess the patient's health care literacy (language, reading, comprehension). Assess culture and culturally specific information needs.	This assessment helps ensure that materials are selected and presented in a manner that is culturally and educationally appropriate.
Explain the importance of taking antithyroid medications daily, in divided doses, and at regular intervals as prescribed.	A knowledgeable patient is more likely to adhere to the treatment regimen.
Teach indicators of hypothyroidism and the signs and symptoms that necessitate medical attention.	Indicators of hypothyroidism (e.g., early fatigue, weight gain, anorexia, constipation, menstrual irregularities, muscle cramps, lethargy, inability to concentrate, hair loss, cold intolerance, and hoarseness) may occur from excessive medication. Signs and symptoms that necessitate medical attention because the medications that cause them may require dose adjustment include cold intolerance, fatigue, lethargy, and peripheral or periorbital edema.
⚠ Teach the side effects of thioamides and symptoms that necessitate medical attention.	Appearance of a rash, fever, or pharyngitis can occur in the presence of agranulocytosis, a recognized side effect of thioamides. This necessitates medical attention to adjust the dose or change the medication.
⚠ Alert patients taking iodides to signs of worsening hyperthyroidism and the need to report them promptly.	Signs of worsening hyperthyroidism (high body temperature, palpitations, rapid HR, irritability, anxiety, and feelings of restlessness or panic) may signal need for medication dosage adjustment to manage the problem and should be reported promptly for timely intervention.

Nursing diagnoses for the patient who has undergone subtotal thyroidectomy

Nursing Diagnosis:

Acute Pain

related to subtotal thyroidectomy surgical procedure

Desired Outcomes: Within 2 hr of surgery, the patient's subjective perception of pain decreases, as documented by a pain scale. Objective indicators, such as hesitation before turning or moving the head, are absent or diminished.

ASSESSMENT/INTERVENTIONS	RATIONALES
Assess and document the degree and character of the patient's pain, including precipitating events. Devise a pain scale with the patient, rating pain on a scale of 0 (no pain) to 10 (worst pain).	This assessment will enable the nurse to determine trend of the pain and degree of pain relief obtained.
Advise the patient to clasp hands behind the neck when moving.	This measure will minimize stress on the incision.

ASSESSMENT/INTERVENTIONS	RATIONALES
After the health care provider has removed surgical clips and drain, teach the patient to perform gentle range-of-motion (ROM) exercises for the neck.	While the surgical clips and drain are in place, mobility of the neck is limited, leading to tight neck muscles. Following removal of these devices, gentle ROM is done to help relax the neck muscles and decrease pain.
For other interventions, see "Pain," p. 39.	

Nursing Diagnosis:

Impaired Swallowing (or risk for same)

related to edema or laryngeal nerve damage resulting from the surgical procedure

Desired Outcomes: The patient reports swallowing with minimal difficulty, has minimal or absent hoarseness, and is free of symptoms of respiratory dysfunction as evidenced by RR 12-20 breaths/min with normal depth and pattern (eupnea) and absence of inspiratory stridor. Laryngeal nerve damage, if it occurs, is detected promptly and reported immediately.

ASSESSMENT/INTERVENTIONS	RATIONALES
Assess for dysphagia by monitoring for inability to swallow, choking, and coughing while drinking or eating and respiratory status for dyspnea and inspiratory stridor.	These are signs of postsurgical edema. Edema in the neck may impinge on the pharynx or esophagus, making swallowing more difficult.
[!] Assess the patient's voice. Promptly report persisting hoarseness.	Although slight hoarseness is normal after surgery, hoarseness that persists is indicative of laryngeal nerve damage and should be reported to the health care provider promptly. If bilateral nerve damage is present, upper airway obstruction and dysphagia can occur.
Elevate head of bed (HOB) 30-45 degrees.	Elevating HOB enables gravity to facilitate swallowing and promotes edema reduction.
Support the patient's head with flat or cervical pillows so that it is in a neutral position with the neck (does not flex or hyperextend).	This position minimizes incisional stress and reduces the chance of choking and dysphagia.
[!] Keep a tracheostomy set and O₂ equipment at the bedside at all times.	This equipment will be used for emergency treatment in the event upper airway obstruction occurs.
Gently suction the upper airway as needed.	Patients can aspirate retained secretions if edema and/or laryngeal nerve problems are present. Using gentle, rather than aggressive, suctioning avoids stimulating laryngospasm.
Administer analgesics promptly and as prescribed.	This will minimize pain and anxiety and enhance the patient's ability to swallow.

ADDITIONAL NURSING DIAGNOSES/PROBLEMS:

"Perioperative Care"   p. 45

✓ **PATIENT-FAMILY TEACHING AND DISCHARGE PLANNING**

When providing patient-family teaching, focus on sensory information, avoid giving excessive information, and initiate a visiting nurse referral for necessary follow-up teaching. Part of the initial assessment should include asking about existing knowledge of the disease, ability for self-management, and psychologic acceptance. Include verbal and written information about the following:

✓ Diet high in calories, protein, carbohydrates, and vitamins. Inform the patient that as a normal metabolic state is attained, the diet may change.

✓ Medications, including drug name, purpose, dosage, schedule, precautions, and potential side effects. Also discuss drug-drug, food-drug, and herb-drug interactions. Herbal interactions that may change the effectiveness of prescribed medications are more common with the following agents: eleuthero, echinacea, bugleweed, bladderwrack, ashwagandha, adrenal complex, and Rehmannia complex.

✓ Changes that can occur as a result of therapy, including weight gain, normalized bowel function, increased strength of skeletal muscles, and a return to normal activity levels.

✓ Importance of continued and frequent medical follow-up; confirm date and time of next appointment.

✓ Indicators that necessitate medical attention, including fever, rash, or sore throat (side effects of thioamides), and symptoms of hypothyroidism (see p. 385) or worsening hyperthyroidism.

✓ For patients receiving radioactive iodine, importance of not holding children to the chest for 72 hr following therapy because children are more susceptible to the effects of radiation. Explain that there is negligible risk for adults.

✓ Importance of avoiding physical and emotional stress early in the recuperative stage and maximizing coping mechanisms for dealing with stress.

✓ Additional information and educational information may be found at. The American Thyroid Association at *www.thyroid.org*

• Thyroid Foundation of America at *www.tsh.org*
• The Hormone Foundation at *www.hormone.org*
• Thyroid Association of Canada at *www.thyroid.ca*

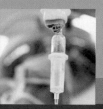

OVERVIEW/PATHOPHYSIOLOGY

Hypothyroidism is a condition in which there is an inadequate amount of circulating thyroid hormone, causing a decrease in metabolic rate that affects all body systems.

Primary hypothyroidism accounts for 90% of cases of hypothyroidism and is caused by pathologic changes in the thyroid itself. The most common cause of the disease in the United States is chronic autoimmune thyroiditis (Hashimoto's disease). Postpartum thyroiditis and granulomatous thyroiditis related to inflammatory conditions or viral syndromes also occur.

Secondary hypothyroidism is caused by dysfunction of the anterior pituitary gland, which results in decreased release of thyroid-stimulating hormone (TSH). *Tertiary hypothyroidism* is caused by a hypothalamic deficiency in the release of thyrotropin-releasing hormone (TRH).

When hypothyroidism is untreated, or when a stressor such as infection affects an individual with hypothyroidism, a life-threatening condition known as *myxedema coma* can occur. Hypothyroidism is eight times more likely to occur in women than men, and it frequently presents in the later years; older women are the most likely candidates to present with myxedema. The clinical picture of myxedema coma is that of exaggerated hypothyroidism, with dangerous hypoventilation, hypothermia, hypotension, and shock. Coma and seizures can occur as well. Myxedema coma usually develops slowly, has a greater than 50% mortality rate, and requires prompt and aggressive treatment.

HEALTH CARE SETTING

Primary care with possible hospitalization resulting from complications

ASSESSMENT

Signs and symptoms can progress from mild early in onset to life threatening.

Signs and symptoms: Early fatigue, weight gain from fluid retention, anorexia, lethargy, cold intolerance, hoarseness, ataxia, memory and mental impairment, decreased concentration, menstrual irregularities or heavy menses, infertility, constipation, depression, and muscle cramps. Signs and symptoms may be life threatening in a patient with history of hypothyroidism who has experienced a recent stressful event.

Physical assessment: Possible presence of goiter, bradycardia, hypothermia, deepened voice, hyperlipidemia, and obesity. Skin may appear yellow and dry, cool, and coarse, and hair may be thin, coarse, and brittle. The tongue may be enlarged (macroglossia), and reflexes may be slowed.

Myxedema coma: Hypoventilation, hypoglycemia, hypothermia, hypotension, hyponatremia, bradycardia, and shock.

History/risk factors: *Primary hypothyroidism:* Dietary iodine deficiency, thyroid gland radioablation for hyperthyroidism management, thyroid atrophy or fibrosis of unknown cause, radiation therapy to the neck, surgical removal of all or part of the gland, drugs that suppress thyroid activity including propylthiouracil and iodides, invasion of the thyroid gland by tumor (e.g., lymphoma), drugs including lithium and interferon, or a genetic dysfunction resulting in inability to produce and secrete thyroid hormone.

Secondary hypothyroidism: Pituitary tumors, postpartum necrosis of the pituitary gland, hypophysectomy.

DIAGNOSTIC TESTS

TSH: Most commonly used test to detect thyroid dysfunction. It will be elevated unless the disease is long-standing or severe.

Free thyroxine index and T_4 (thyroxine) levels: Decreased with hypothyroidism.

^{131}I scan and uptake: Will be less than 10% in a 24-hr period. In secondary hypothyroidism, uptake increases with administration of exogenous TSH.

Doppler ultrasonography: To diagnose gland size and abnormal densities, which may be present if nodules are present.

Thyroid autoantibodies: Presence of thyroperoxidase autoantibodies or antithyroglobulin autoantibodies signals chronic autoimmune thyroiditis.

Thyroid binding globulin: Measures the level of the protein that binds with circulating thyroid hormones. Abnormal T_4 or T_3 measurements often occur because of binding protein abnormalities rather than abnormal thyroid function.

Thyroid scan ^{131}I and radioactive iodine uptake: Identifies thyroid nodules. In primary hypothyroidism, uptake will be less than 10% in a 24-hr period. In secondary hypothyroidism, uptake increases with administration of exogenous TSH.

Nursing Diagnosis:

Ineffective Breathing Pattern (or risk for same)

related to upper airway obstruction occurring with enlarged thyroid gland and/ or decreased ventilatory drive caused by greatly decreased metabolism

Desired Outcomes: The patient has an effective breathing pattern as evidenced by respiratory rate (RR) 12-20 breaths/min with normal depth and pattern (eupnea), normal skin color, O_2 saturation 95% or more, and absence of adventitious breath sounds. Alternatively, if an ineffective breathing pattern occurs, it is detected, reported, and treated promptly.

ASSESSMENT/INTERVENTIONS	RATIONALES
Assess rate, depth, and quality of breath sounds, and be alert to the presence of adventitious sounds or decreasing or crowing sounds.	This enables the nurse to be alert to the presence of adventitious sounds (e.g., from developing pleural effusion) or decreasing or crowing sounds (e.g., from swollen tongue or glottis).
Assess for signs of inadequate ventilation. Immediately report significant findings to the health care provider.	Decreased respiratory rate, shallow breathing, and circumoral or peripheral cyanosis are signs of inadequate ventilation. Ventilatory insufficiency in a patient with hypothyroid condition can indicate onset of heart failure secondary to impending myxedema coma or hypothyroid crisis.
Assess for hypoxemia by measuring O_2 saturation intermittently or continuously in patients with increased work of breathing or decreased respiratory rate or depth. Administer oxygen as prescribed.	Decreasing O_2 saturation (92% or less) may signal need for oxygen supplementation in symptomatic patients.
Teach the patient coughing, deep breathing, and use of incentive spirometer. Suction upper airway prn.	These measures help clear secretions that may increase with hypoventilation.
For the patient experiencing respiratory distress, be prepared to assist the health care provider with intubation or tracheostomy and maintenance of mechanical ventilatory assistance or transfer to the intensive care unit (ICU).	The patient likely will need emergency treatment and intensive care.

Nursing Diagnosis:

Excess Fluid Volume

related to compromised regulatory mechanisms occurring with adrenal insufficiency

Desired Outcome: By a minimum of 24 hr before hospital discharge, the patient is normovolemic as evidenced by urinary output 30 mL/hr or more, stable weight, nondistended jugular veins, presence of eupnea, and peripheral pulse amplitude 2+ or more on a 0-4+ scale.

ASSESSMENT/INTERVENTIONS	RATIONALES
Assess intake and output hourly for evidence of decreasing output.	Decreasing output signals fluid retention leading to hypervolemia.
Assess for weight gain by weighing the patient at the same time every day, with the same clothing, and using the same scale. Report increasing weight to the health care provider.	Increasing weight signals fluid retention, which can lead to hypervolemia/volume overload. Weighing the patient at the same time and under the same conditions avoids discrepancies that could reflect inaccurate losses or gains.
Assess for indicators of heart failure. Report significant findings to the health care provider.	Indicators of heart failure include jugular vein distention, crackles, shortness of breath, dependent edema of extremities, and decreased amplitude of peripheral pulses. Lack of thyroid hormones can decrease the heart rate and force of contractions, leading to heart failure. Associated fluid retention worsens the problem.
Restrict fluid and sodium intake as prescribed.	This helps prevent fluid retention that could lead to volume overload.
Use a rate control device to administer intravenous (IV) fluids.	This will prevent accidental fluid overload.

Nursing Diagnosis:

Activity Intolerance

related to weakness and fatigue occurring with slowed metabolism and decreased cardiac output caused by pericardial effusions, atherosclerosis, and decreased adrenergic stimulation

Desired Outcome: During activity the patient rates perceived exertion at 3 or less on a 0-10 scale and exhibits cardiac tolerance to activity as evidenced by heart rate (HR) 20 bpm or less over resting HR; systolic blood pressure (SBP) 20 mm Hg or less over or under resting SBP; warm and dry skin; and absence of crackles (rales), murmurs, chest pain, and new dysrhythmias.

ASSESSMENT/INTERVENTIONS	RATIONALES
Assess for complications of a decreased metabolic rate by taking vital signs and apical pulse at frequent intervals.	This enables the nurse to be alert to hypotension, slow pulse, dysrhythmias, decreasing urine output, and changes in mentation, which along with complaints of chest pain or discomfort may signal heart failure/impending pulmonary edema.
Assess activity tolerance by asking the patient to rate perceived exertion (RPE). See **Risk for Activity Intolerance** in "Prolonged Bedrest," p. 62, for details.	An RPE more than 3 on a 0-10 scale is a signal of cardiac intolerance during exertion and also a sign that the patient should stop or modify the activity causing the exertion.
Promptly report significant changes to the health care provider.	This will help prevent progression of heart failure to cardiac arrest.
As prescribed, administer IV isotonic solutions such as normal saline.	Isotonic solutions help prevent or ameliorate hypotension. Hypotension ensues as a result of reduced sympathetic nervous system stimulation, which causes decreased cardiac output and hypotension.
Balance activity with adequate rest.	Rest decreases workload of the heart.
Assist the patient with range of motion and other in-bed exercises and consult with the health care provider about implementation of exercises that require greater cardiac tolerance. For details, see **Risk for Activity Intolerance,** p. 61, and **Risk for Disuse Syndrome,** p. 63.	Exercise prevents problems caused by immobility.

Nursing Diagnosis:

Risk for Infection

related to compromised immunologic status occurring with alterations in adrenal function

Desired Outcome: The patient is free of infection as evidenced by normothermia, absence of adventitious breath sounds, normal urinary pattern and characteristics, and well-healing wounds.

ASSESSMENT/INTERVENTIONS	RATIONALES
Assess for early indicators of infection. Notify the health care provider of significant findings.	Fever; erythema, swelling, or discharge from wounds or IV sites; urinary frequency, urgency, or dysuria; cloudy or malodorous urine; presence of adventitious sounds on auscultation of lung fields; and changes in color, consistency, and amount of sputum are early indicators of infection. Prompt assessment and treatment can halt their progression to prevent complications such as myxedema coma, a life-threatening condition.

continued

ASSESSMENT/INTERVENTIONS	RATIONALES
Provide meticulous care of indwelling urinary catheters.	This minimizes risk of urinary tract infection. Guidelines recommend indwelling urinary catheters be removed within 48 hr of insertion.
Use sterile technique when performing dressing changes and invasive procedures.	Nonintact skin and invasive procedures can lead to bacterial ingress.
Provide good skin care.	Open sores are sites of ingress for bacteria.
Advise visitors who have contracted or been exposed to a communicable disease not to enter the patient's room or to wear a surgical mask, if appropriate.	This will minimize risk of systemic infection in patients who are immunocompromised.

Nursing Diagnosis:

Risk for Imbalanced Nutrition: More Than Body Requirements

related to slowed metabolism

Desired Outcomes: The patient does not experience weight gain. Within the 24-hr period before hospital discharge, the patient verbalizes understanding of the rationale and measures for the dietary regimen.

ASSESSMENT/INTERVENTIONS	RATIONALES
Assess for weight gain by weighing the patient at the same time every day, with the same clothing, and using the same scale. Report increasing weight to the health care provider.	Increasing weight may signal fluid retention or excessive calorie intake for activity level and decreased metabolic rate. Weighing patients at the same time and under the same conditions avoids discrepancies that could reflect inaccurate losses or gains.
Provide a diet that is high in protein and low in calories.	This diet will promote weight loss.
As prescribed, restrict or limit sodium intake and foods high in sodium content.	This measure decreases edema caused by fluid retention.
Teach the patient about foods to augment and foods to limit or avoid.	Foods high in protein and low in calories and sodium will help with weight control while the patient is in a hypometabolic/fluid-retaining state.
Provide small, frequent meals of appropriate foods the patient particularly enjoys.	This promotes weight control and decreases the chance of patients overeating if allowed to get too hungry.
Encourage foods that are high in fiber content (e.g., fruits with skins, vegetables, whole grain breads and cereals, nuts).	Adding bulk to the diet improves gastric motility, which will help elimination that may be decreased as a result of slowed metabolism.
Administer vitamin supplements as prescribed.	Vitamins will help patients who are unable to consume appropriate recommended daily allowance minimum requirements on their restricted diets.

Nursing Diagnoses:

Constipation
Dysfunctional Gastrointestinal Motility

related to inadequate dietary intake of roughage and fluids, prolonged bedrest, and/or decreased peristalsis occurring with slowed metabolism

Desired Outcome: Prior to discharge, the patient has a bowel movement at least every third day with no evidence of abdominal distention.

ASSESSMENT/INTERVENTIONS	RATIONALES
Assess for decreasing bowel sounds and the presence of distention and increases in abdominal girth.	These indicators can occur with ileus or fecal impaction and lead to an obstructive process, which is fairly common in hypothyroidism, especially in older adults.
Encourage the patient to maintain a diet with adequate roughage and fluids. Ensure that fluid intake in persons without underlying cardiac or renal disease is at least 2-3 L/day.	Such foods as fruits with skins, fruit juices, cooked fruits, vegetables, whole grain breads and cereals, and nuts provide bulk, which will promote bowel elimination by increasing peristalsis and, coupled with increased fluid intake, add moisture to keep stool moving through the intestines/colon.
Administer stool softeners and laxatives as prescribed.	These agents minimize constipation by moistening stool and increasing peristalsis. **Caution:** Suppositories are contraindicated because of risk of stimulating the vagus nerve, which would further decrease HR and blood pressure (BP).
Advise the patient to increase amount of exercise.	Exercise promotes regularity by increasing peristalsis. Exercise also tones gastrointestinal muscles to hold intestines/colon in place, which seems to facilitate bowel elimination.

Nursing Diagnosis:

Acute Confusion

related to altered sensory reception, transmission, or integration occurring with cerebral retention of water

Desired Outcomes: The patient verbalizes orientation to person, place, and time. Alternately, if signs of myxedema coma appear, they are detected, reported, and treated promptly.

ASSESSMENT/INTERVENTIONS	RATIONALES
[!] Assess the patient's mental status at frequent intervals by assessing orientation to person, place, and time.	Increasing lethargy or confusion can signal onset of myxedema coma, which necessitates immediate medical attention.
Reorient the patient frequently. Have a clock and calendar visible, and use radio or television for orientation.	This ensures that the patient has information necessary to answer neurologic assessment questions appropriately.
Clearly explain all procedures to the patient before performing them. Provide adequate time for the patient to ask questions.	This promotes better understanding of procedures for a patient who may have memory impairment.
If necessary, remind the patient to complete activities of daily living such as bathing and brushing hair.	As above.
Encourage visitors to discuss topics of special interest to the patient.	This will enhance the patient's alertness.
Administer thyroid replacement hormones as prescribed.	Thyroid replacement increases metabolic rate, which in turn promotes cerebral blood flow. Patients are started on low doses that are increased gradually, based on serial laboratory tests (TSH and T_4), and adjusted until the TSH is in a normal range. Dose titration prevents hyperthyroidism caused by too much exogenous hormone. Therapy is continued for the patient's lifetime.
[!] For patients with secondary hypothyroidism, avoid administering thyroid supplements.	Thyroid supplements can promote acute symptoms in patients with secondary hypothyroidism and therefore are contraindicated.

PART I: Medical-Surgical Nursing

Nursing Diagnosis:

Ineffective Protection

related to potential for myxedema coma occurring with inadequate response to treatment of hypothyroidism or stressors such as infection

Desired Outcomes: The patient is free of symptoms of myxedema coma as evidenced by HR 60 bpm or greater; BP 90/60 mm Hg or greater (or within the patient's normal range); RR 12 breaths/min or more with normal depth and pattern; and orientation to person, place, and time. Alternatively, if myxedema coma occurs, it is detected, reported, and treated promptly.

ASSESSMENT/INTERVENTIONS	RATIONALES
Assess the patient for hypoxia. Immediately report significant findings to health care providers.	Circumoral or peripheral cyanosis and decrease in level of consciousness (LOC) are signs of hypoxia, which may signal that the patient is about to experience cardiac arrest.
Check medication doses carefully before administration, especially barbiturates and sedatives.	Because of decreased metabolism, drug action times are prolonged. Patients with hypothyroidism do not tolerate barbiturates and sedatives, and therefore central nervous system depressants are contraindicated unless absolutely necessary to manage the patient during a crisis.
Monitor for signs of toxicity if sedatives or barbiturates are administered.	Signs of toxicity include decreased LOC and decreases in BP or ventilatory effort.
Monitor laboratory work, including complete metabolic panel, complete blood count, lipids, and glucose.	If in a coma, the patient should be evaluated for the following abnormalities, which are associated with myxedema coma: anemia, elevated CPK, elevated creatinine, elevated transaminases, hypercapnia, hyperlipidemia, hypoglycemia, hyponatremia, hypoxia, leukopenia, respiratory acidosis
In the presence of myxedema coma, implement the following:	
Restrict fluids or administer hypertonic saline as prescribed.	This will correct hyponatremia. A too-rapid correction could cause central pontine myelinolysis, which is brain cell dysfunction caused by destruction of the myelin sheath covering nerve cells in the brainstem (pons). The rate of correction should not exceed 0.5-1 mEq/L/hour, with a total increase not to exceed 12 mEq/L/day. It is necessary to correct the hyponatremia to a safe range (usually to no greater than 120 mEq/L) rather than to a normal value.
Use an infusion control device.	This device maintains accurate infusion rate of IV fluids.
As prescribed, administer and carefully monitor IV thyroid replacement hormones with IV hydrocortisone and IV glucose.	In the treatment of hypoglycemia, rapid IV administration of thyroid hormone can precipitate hyperadrenalism. This can be avoided by concomitant administration of IV hydrocortisone. Although concomitant administration of IV hydrocortisone helps prevent adrenal problems, it may cause hypoadrenalism if not carefully monitored.

ASSESSMENT/INTERVENTIONS	RATIONALES
Monitor for signs of heart failure. Notify the health care provider of any significant findings.	Jugular vein distention, crackles (rales), shortness of breath, peripheral edema, weakening peripheral pulses, and hypotension are signs of heart failure, which can occur secondary to hypothyroidism and lead to myxedema coma. Hypotension is treated with administration of IV isotonic fluids, such as normal saline and lactated Ringer's solution. Hypotonic solutions, such as 5% dextrose in water, are contraindicated because they can decrease serum Na^+ levels further. Because of altered metabolism, these patients respond poorly to vasopressors.
Prepare to transfer the patient to ICU. Keep oral airway and manual resuscitator at the bedside in the event of seizure, coma, or the need for ventilatory assistance	This enables emergency treatment for a decreased ventilatory drive.

✓ PATIENT-FAMILY TEACHING AND DISCHARGE PLANNING

When providing patient-family teaching, focus on sensory information, avoid giving excessive information, and initiate a visiting nurse referral for necessary follow-up teaching. Part of the initial assessment should include asking about existing knowledge of the disease, ability for self-management, and psychologic acceptance. Include verbal and written information about the following:

✓ Medications, including drug name, purpose, dosage, schedule, precautions, and potential side effects. Also discuss drug-drug, food-drug, and herb-drug interactions. Herbal interactions change the effectiveness of thyroid medications and are more common with the following remedies: eleuthero, echinacea, bugleweed, bladderwrack, ashwagandha, adrenal complex, and Rehmannia complex.

✓ Reminder that thioamides, iodides, and lithium are contraindicated because they decrease thyroid activity. Be sure the patient is aware that thyroid replacement medications are to be taken for life.

✓ Dietary requirements and restrictions, which may change as hormone replacement therapy takes effect.

✓ Expected changes that can occur with hormone replacement therapy: increased energy level, weight loss, and decreased peripheral edema. Neuromuscular problems should improve as well.

✓ Importance of continued, frequent medical follow-up; confirm date and time of next medical appointment.

✓ Importance of avoiding physical and emotional stress, and ways for the patient to maximize coping mechanisms for dealing with stress.

✓ Signs and symptoms that necessitate medical attention, including fever or other symptoms of upper respiratory, urinary, or oral infections and signs and symptoms of hyperthyroidism, which may result from excessive hormone replacement.

✓ Available resources:
  • The American Thyroid Association at *www.thyroid.org*
  • Thyroid Foundation of America at *www.tsh.org*
  • The Hormone Foundation at *www.hormone.org*
  • Thyroid Association of Canada at *www.thyroid.ca*

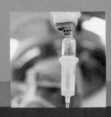

Syndrome of Inappropriate Antidiuretic Hormone 50

OVERVIEW/PATHOPHYSIOLOGY

Syndrome of inappropriate antidiuretic hormone (SIADH) or syndrome of inappropriate antidiuresis (SIAD) is a condition of abnormal release of antidiuretic hormone (ADH, vasopressin [VP]) in response to changes in plasma osmolality that result in hyponatremia. Hyponatremia is defined as an excess of water in relation to the amount of sodium in the extracellular fluid. SIADH is the most frequent cause of hyponatremia, which is the most common electrolyte imbalance in hospitalized patients. Mild hyponatremia (serum sodium less than 135 mEq/L) occurs in 15%-22% of hospitalized patients and 7% of ambulatory patients, while moderate hyponatremia (serum sodium less than 130 mEq/L) occurs in 1%-7% of hospitalized patients. Hyponatremia is often caused by extracellular fluid volume depletion associated with many diuretics that cause a significant loss of sodium along with water. Hyponatremia is important to manage because of its potential morbidity and should be recognized as an indicator of underlying disease.

ADH (VP) is produced in the hypothalamus, stored in the posterior pituitary, and regulates free water volume in the kidney. Hyponatremia resulting from chronic SIADH is not always caused by reduced water excretion or volume overload. Plasma ADH level may not be high and measurement is often not helpful in establishing the diagnosis. Findings may reflect dilute (hypoosmolar) plasma and hyponatremia with a normal circulating blood volume. Morbidity and mortality of hyponatremia associated with SIADH stem from cerebral edema and abnormal nerve function. Values of serum sodium less than 100 mEq/L are life threatening.

ADH is a key component in the regulation of fluid and electrolyte balance through direct effects on renal water regulation. Water is reabsorbed in the distal nephron, where the kidney both concentrates and dilutes urine in response to the ADH level. VP stimulates the nephron to produce aquaporin (AQP), a specific water channel protein, on the surface of the interstitial cells lining the collecting duct. The presence of AQP in the wall of the distal nephron allows resorption of water from the duct lumen according to the osmotic gradient and excretion of concentrated urine.

HEALTH CARE SETTING

Acute care

ASSESSMENT

Signs and symptoms: Decreased urine output with concentrated urine. Signs of water intoxication may appear, including altered level of consciousness (LOC), fatigue, headache, diarrhea, anorexia, nausea, vomiting, and seizures. **Note:** Because of loss of Na+, edema will not accompany the fluid volume excess.

Physical assessment: Weight gain without edema, elevated blood pressure (BP), altered mental status. Laboratory values must be correlated with physical findings. The goal of assessment is to differentiate between SIADH and a compensatory response of ADH release in patients with chronic, mild volume depletion/dehydration.

History of: Cancers of the lung, pancreas, duodenum, and prostate, which can secrete a biologically active form of ADH. Other common causes include pulmonary disease (e.g., tuberculosis, pneumonia, chronic obstructive pulmonary disease, empyema), acquired immunodeficiency syndrome, head trauma, brain tumor, intracerebral hemorrhage, meningitis, and encephalitis. Positive-pressure ventilation, physiologic stress, chronic metabolic illness, and a wide variety of medications (chlorpropamide, acetaminophen, oxytocin, narcotics, general anesthetic, carbamazepine, thiazide diuretics, tricyclic antidepressants, neuroleptics, angiotensin-converting enzyme inhibitors, cancer chemotherapy agents) all have been linked to SIADH.

DIAGNOSTIC TESTS

Serum Na+ level: Decreased to less than 130 mEq/L.
Serum osmolality: Decreased to less than 275 mOsm/kg.
Urine osmolality: Elevated disproportionately relative to plasma osmolality.
Urine Na+ level: Increased to more than 20 mEq/L. Increases to more than 60 mEq/L are common. Urine Na+ level (e.g., increased) is best evaluated in comparison with serum Na+ level (e.g., decreased).
Urine specific gravity: More than 1.030.

Serum arginine vasopressin (ADH) level: May be normal to elevated, depending on the type of SIADH present.

Water load test: Excretion of water or urine output may be reduced to 30%-40% of the ingested load in the presence of VP production. Normal urine output is 78%-82% of the ingested water load during the 4-hr test. In SIADH, low plasma osmolality is present with highly concentrated urine, with decreased plasma sodium indicating abnormal secretion of ADH/VP.

Urinary aquaporin-2 (AQP-2): May be useful in the differentiation of SIADH from other causes of hyponatremia.

Nursing Diagnoses:

Excess Fluid Volume
Risk for Electrolyte Imbalance

related to hyponatremia or its management

Desired Outcomes: Within 72 hr of initiating treatment, the patient verbalizes orientation to time, place, and person; has stable weight; BP is 90-140/60-85 mm Hg or within the patient's normal range; and heart rate (HR) is 60-100 bpm. Na+ levels are within normal limits.

ASSESSMENT/INTERVENTIONS	RATIONALES
! Assess for clinical signs of hyponatremia and possible hypervolemia. Promptly report significant findings or changes to the health care provider.	Hyponatremia causes changes in neurologic/neuromuscular symptoms including lethargy, coma, seizures, headache, confusion, and weakness. Sodium levels of less than 120 mEq/L can cause life-threatening symptoms. Decreasing LOC, elevated BP and central venous pressure (CVP), urine output less than 30 mL/hr, and weight gain are signs of excess fluid volume that may occur with SIADH.
Monitor laboratory results for hyponatremia and indicators of water intoxication. Report significant findings to the health care provider.	Normal values are as follows: urine specific gravity, 1.010-1.020; serum Na+, 137-147 mEq/L; urine osmolality, 300-1090 mOsm/kg; serum osmolality, 280-300 mOsm/kg. Decreased serum Na+ and plasma osmolality, urine osmolality elevated disproportionately in relation to plasma osmolality, and increased urine Na+ are values that may be seen with SIADH. Water retention may occur secondary to increased ADH secretion that dilutes the blood and results in reduced amounts of more concentrated urine.
Initiate fluid restriction, if needed and prescribed, to prevent hypervolemia. Explain necessity of this treatment to the patient and significant other. Do not keep water or ice chips at the bedside. Ensure precise delivery of fluid administered intravenous (IV) by using a monitoring device.	Restricting fluids to the amount manageable by the kidneys will allow restoration of normal serum Na+ levels and osmolality without complications from pharmacotherapy.
Elevate head of bed (HOB) 10-20 degrees, especially if hypervolemia is present.	A slightly elevated HOB promotes venous return and thus reduces ADH release. Excess fluid volume can sometimes result in cerebral edema, which may add to problems with neural regulation of ADH secretion.
Administer demeclocycline, conivaptan, tolvaptan, and furosemide as prescribed; carefully observe and document the patient's response.	These medications promote normalization of hyponatremia.
! Administer hypertonic (3%) saline as prescribed.	This may be given if the patient has severe hyponatremia. Rate of administration is usually based on serial serum Na+ levels. To minimize the risk of too rapid correction of hyponatremia, ensure that laboratory specimens are drawn on time. *Serum Na+ should not be allowed to increase more than 10 mEq/L in 24 hr* because of the risk of neurologic damage (osmotic demyelination), particularly if the hyponatremia is chronic rather than acute.
Make sure that specimens for laboratory tests are drawn on time and results are reported to the health care provider promptly.	Serum blood levels of Na+ are assessed to determine if the patient has hypernatremia as a result of aggressive treatment.
! Institute seizure precautions as indicated and per agency policy. For more information, see "Seizures and Epilepsy," p. 304.	Seizures can occur in the presence of hyponatremia associated with SIADH.

Nursing Diagnosis (for patients undergoing intracranial surgery):

Ineffective Protection

related to the potential for increased intracranial pressure (IICP), hemorrhage, and infection (if SIADH occurs after intracranial surgery)

Desired Outcomes: Optimally, the patient demonstrates normal level of mental acuity; verbalizes orientation to person, place, and time; and is free of indicators of injury caused by complications of intracranial surgery. Immediately after instruction, the patient and significant other verbalize understanding of the importance of avoiding Valsalva-type maneuvers and describe signs and symptoms of IICP and infection.

ASSESSMENT/INTERVENTIONS	RATIONALES
⚠ Assess for changes in mental status or LOC, sluggish or unequal pupils, and changes in respiratory rate or pattern.	These are indicators of IICP. Neurologic deterioration may necessitate computed tomography (CT) scan.
Monitor for decreased vision, eye muscle weakness, abnormal extraocular eye movements, double vision, and airway obstruction. Report significant findings to the health care provider.	The surgery may interfere with cranial nerves governing eye movements and visual acuity—II, III, IV, and VI.
⚠ Measure intake and output hourly for 24 hr, and monitor urine specific gravity q1-2h. Monitor weight daily for evidence of weight gain or loss.	Intracranial surgical procedures may prompt either SIADH or diabetes insipidus caused by swelling or tissue integrity disturbances in the area of the pituitary gland or hypothalamus.
⚠ In the presence of suspected cerebrospinal fluid (CSF), elevate HOB and immediately report any suspicious drainage.	Raising the HOB decreases the potential for bacteria entering the brain. The presence of CSF represents a serious breach in cranial integrity.
Elevate the HOB 30 degrees.	This elevation will help decrease intracranial pressure (ICP) and swelling. Dexamethasone may be prescribed to reduce cerebral swelling.
⚠ Explain that coughing, sneezing, and other Valsalva-type maneuvers must be avoided.	These actions can stress the operative site and increase ICP.
As indicated, obtain prescription for a mild cathartic or stool softener.	This will help prevent straining with bowel movements.
Be alert to and teach the following signs and symptoms of infection, which necessitate medical attention: fever, nuchal rigidity, moderate to severe headache, and photophobia.	These signs of infection also may signal impending meningitis. However, periorbital edema, mild headache, and tenderness over the sinuses for 2-3 days are common and can be relieved by cold compresses.

ADDITIONAL NURSING DIAGNOSES/PROBLEMS:

"Diabetic Ketoacidosis" for **Risk for Injury** related to   p. 369
altered cerebral function

✓ PATIENT-FAMILY TEACHING AND DISCHARGE PLANNING

When providing patient-family teaching, speak slowly and simply, avoid giving excessive information, and initiate a visiting nurse referral for necessary follow-up teaching. Include verbal and written information about the following:

✓ Importance of fluid restriction for the prescribed period if the patient was hypervolemic. Assist the patient with planning permitted fluid intake (e.g., by saving liquids for social and recreational situations as indicated).

✓ How to safely enrich diet with Na^+ and K^+ salts, particularly if ongoing diuretic use is prescribed.

✓ How to use daily weight measurements to assess hydration status.

✓ Signs of hyponatremia and hypervolemia: altered LOC, fatigue, headache, nausea, vomiting, and anorexia, any of which should be reported promptly to the health care provider.

✓ Medications, including drug name, dosage, route, purpose, precautions, and potential side effects. Also discuss drug-drug, food-drug, and herb-drug interactions. Encourage the patient to report to the health care provider all alternative and complementary health strategies being used.

✓ Importance of continued medical follow-up; confirm date and time of next medical appointment.

✓ How to obtain a medical alert bracelet and identification card outlining diagnosis and emergency treatment by contacting MedicAlert Foundation at *www.medicalert.org* or the Medic Alert Foundation (Canada) at *www.medicalert.ca*

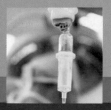

Abdominal Trauma 51

OVERVIEW/PATHOPHYSIOLOGY

Abdominal trauma accounts for nearly 7 million emergency department visits in the United States annually and often causes serious injury to major organs and blood vessels. It is essential to understand the mechanism of the injury (blunt, penetrating, or combination) and the abdominal organs and blood vessels affected to avoid complications in the recovery period. Astute serial assessments in the posttraumatic period may prevent serious consequences and avoid life-threatening situations. Abdominal injuries often are associated with multisystem trauma. See also discussions in "Pneumothorax/Hemothorax," p. 122; "Spinal Cord Injury," p. 313; and "Traumatic Brain Injury," p. 340.

Knowledge of the injury mechanism and location assists the nurse in anticipating specific injuries to abdominal organs and vessels. Abdominal trauma, along with thoracic and musculoskeletal trauma, especially below the fourth rib, is an indicator that specific abdominal organs are at risk of injury. Solid organs (liver, kidneys, and spleen) tend to fracture and bleed with trauma; hollow organs (stomach and intestines) may collapse or rupture, releasing caustic substances into the peritoneum. Injury also may result from movement of organs within the body, particularly at the transition between rigidly fixed and mobile organs. Injury to the urinary bladder is not common but may be associated with pelvic fractures. Rectal and vaginal examinations are necessary to assess for injury and bleeding.

Blunt trauma may be caused by falls, assaults, motor vehicle collisions, or sports injuries and involve direct transmission of energy to solid or hollow organs, most commonly affecting the spleen and liver. Splenic injury should be suspected in the presence of left lower rib fractures. Rupture may not be immediately obvious, reinforcing the need for ongoing assessments. Pain radiating to the left shoulder (Kehr's sign) may indicate blood beneath the diaphragm from splenic bleeding. Pain radiating to the right shoulder may indicate injury to the liver. Other organs that may be affected by blunt trauma include the kidneys and, occasionally, the pancreas and small and large intestines. Bleeding is the most common complication, resulting in increased morbidity and mortality. Abdominal vessels are sometimes injured when blunt abdominal trauma occurs, and this may lead to shock and death if not recognized early. Signs of blood loss may not be evident initially; therefore, continual assessment is essential.

Gunshot, stabbing, or impalement may cause penetrating trauma, and the external appearance of the wound often does not accurately represent internal damage. If the lower esophagus, stomach, or intestines are injured by penetration, complications from release of irritating gastric and intestinal fluids into the peritoneum and free air below the diaphragm may occur. Penetrating injuries to the solid organs may cause fatal damage if not identified early.

HEALTH CARE SETTING

Emergency care, trauma center, acute care surgical unit, rehabilitation center

ASSESSMENT

As with all trauma patients, immediate life-threatening problems must be identified and treatment initiated before the more detailed secondary assessments are completed.

Caution: Recently injured patients should be evaluated for peritoneal signs (generalized abdominal pain or tenderness, guarding of abdomen, abdominal wall rigidity, rebound tenderness, abdominal pain with movement or coughing, abdominal distention, and decreased or absent bowel sounds) frequently. These signs are evidence of bleeding, and the health care provider must be notified immediately of these signs as well as evidence of shock, gastric or rectal bleeding, or gross hematuria.

Vital signs (VS) and hemodynamic measurements: VS should be assessed continually to detect changes early. Gradual or sudden changes may signal hemorrhage following trauma, with tachycardia, impaired capillary refill, and hypotension key indicators of bleeding or shock. Respiratory assessment is also essential because ventilatory excursion may be diminished due to pain, thoracic injury, or limited diaphragmatic movement caused by abdominal distention, which may impede oxygenation.

Pain: Mild tenderness to severe abdominal pain may be present, with pain either localized to the site of injury or diffuse. Blood or fluid collection within the peritoneum causes irritation and may cause guarding, distention, rigidity, and rebound tenderness.

Gastrointestinal symptoms: Nausea and vomiting may be present following blunt or penetrating trauma secondary to bleeding or obstruction.

> **Note:** *Absence of signs and symptoms, especially in patients who have sustained head or spinal cord injury, does not exclude presence of major abdominal injury.*

Inspection: Abrasions and ecchymoses are suggestive of underlying injury. For example, ecchymosis over the left upper quadrant (LUQ) suggests possible splenic injury. Ecchymotic areas around the umbilicus or flanks are suggestive of retroperitoneal bleeding. Erythema and ecchymosis across the lower abdomen suggest intestinal or bladder injury caused by lap belts. Ecchymoses may take hours to days to develop, depending on rate of blood loss. Abdominal distention may signal bleeding, free air, or inflammation.

Auscultation: Bowel sounds should be auscultated frequently, especially in the first 24-48 hr after injury. Auscultate before percussion and palpation to avoid stimulating the bowel and confounding assessment findings. Bowel sounds may be decreased or absent with abdominal organ injury and intraperitoneal bleeding. However, the presence of bowel sounds does not exclude significant abdominal injury. Bowel sounds in the chest could indicate a ruptured diaphragm with small bowel herniation into the thorax. Absence of bowel sounds is suggestive of ileus or other complications, such as bleeding, peritonitis, or bowel infarction. Presence of an abdominal bruit (turbulent blood flow through vessels) could indicate arterial injury.

> **Note:** *Percuss and palpate painful areas last. If the patient's pain is severe, do not percuss or palpate because more advanced studies are indicated for evaluation.*

Percussion: Tympany suggests the presence of gas. Percussion may reveal unusually large areas of dullness over ruptured blood-filled organs (e.g., a fixed area of dullness in the LUQ suggests a ruptured spleen).

Palpation: Tenderness or pain to palpation suggests abdominal injury. Blood or fluid in the abdomen can result in signs and symptoms of peritoneal irritation.

DIAGNOSTIC TESTS

White blood cell (WBC) count: Leukocytosis is expected immediately after injury. Splenic injuries in particular result in rapid development of a moderate to high WBC count. A later increase in WBCs or a shift to the left reflects an increase in the number of neutrophils, which signals inflammatory response and possible intraabdominal infection.

Platelet count: Mild thrombocytosis is seen immediately after traumatic injury. Thrombocytopenia may be present following massive hemorrhage.

Glucose: Glucose is initially elevated because of catecholamine release and insulin resistance associated with major trauma. Glucose metabolism is abnormal after major hepatic resection, and patients should be monitored to prevent hypoglycemic episodes.

Amylase: Elevations reflect pancreatic or upper small bowel injury.

Liver function tests: Elevations reflect hepatic injury.

Arterial blood gases: Essential in respiratory distress to determine presence of hypoxemia, hypercapnia, and respiratory or metabolic acidosis or alkalosis.

Type and cross match: If blood replacement is anticipated.

X-ray examination: Initially, flat and upright chest x-ray examinations exclude chest injuries (commonly associated with abdominal trauma) and establish a baseline. Subsequent chest x-ray examinations aid in detecting complications, such as atelectasis and pneumonia. In addition, chest and pelvic x-ray examinations may reveal fractures, missiles, foreign bodies, free intraperitoneal air, hematoma, or hemorrhage. Plain abdominal films are not useful in blunt trauma because they cannot define blood in the peritoneum.

Ultrasound: A rapid, noninvasive assessment tool for detecting intraabdominal hemorrhage. The Focused Assessment Sonogram for Trauma (FAST) is a rapid bedside examination that has a sensitivity, specificity, and accuracy rate of more than 90% in detecting 100 mL or more of intraabdominal blood or fluid. Four areas are evaluated: the perihepatic and hepatorenal space, the perisplenic area, the pelvis, and the pericardium. A single negative FAST cannot absolutely exclude intraabdominal bleeding. FAST is used in conjunction with the full trauma evaluation.

Computed tomography (CT) scan: Reveals organ-specific blunt abdominal injury and quantifies the amount of blood and source of hemorrhage in the abdomen. CT images the ureters and can detect extravasation of urine. Disadvantages are the expense and time required to perform the examination. Patients with positive CT scan require diagnostic laparotomy. **Caution:** A patient in unstable condition always must be accompanied by a nurse during the CT scan.

Diagnostic peritoneal lavage: Involves insertion of a peritoneal dialysis catheter into the peritoneum to check for intraabdominal bleeding. This procedure is much less common since FAST and CT scan have become available. It may be indicated for confirmed or suspected blunt abdominal trauma for any patient with signs and symptoms of abdominal injury obscured by intoxication, head or spinal cord trauma, opioids, or unconsciousness. Diagnostic peritoneal lavage is unnecessary for patients who have obvious intraabdominal bleeding or other indications for immediate laparotomy.

Laparotomy: The "gold standard" for intraabdominal injuries, this procedure enables complete evaluation of the abdomen and retroperitoneum. It is recommended in all patients with severe hypotension, penetration of the abdominal wall, peritonitis, air in the abdomen, and in most cases of organ-specific injury noted on CT scan.

Occult blood: Gastric contents, urine, and stool must be tested for occult blood because bleeding can occur as a result of direct injury, causing significant complications.

Angiography: Performed to evaluate injury to spleen, liver, pancreas, duodenum, and retroperitoneal vessels. **Caution:** Ensure adequate hydration and monitor urine output closely for 24-48 hr following angiography because the large amount of contrast used may cause renal failure, especially in older adults or in patients with preexisting cardiovascular or renal disease. Decreased urinary output and increased blood urea nitrogen (BUN) and creatinine may indicate contrast-associated acute tubular necrosis.

Nursing Diagnosis:

Ineffective Breathing Pattern

related to pain from injury or surgical incision, chemical irritation of blood or bile on pleural tissue, and diaphragmatic elevation caused by abdominal distention

Desired Outcome: Within 24 hr of admission or surgery, the patient is eupneic with respiratory rate (RR) 12-20 breaths/min and clear breath sounds.

ASSESSMENT/INTERVENTIONS	RATIONALES
Assess quality of breath sounds, RR, presence/absence of cough, and sputum characteristics.	Individuals sustaining abdominal trauma are likely to be tachypneic, with poor ventilatory effort.
Report significant findings to the health care provider.	If not reversed, this breathing pattern could result in atelectasis and pneumonia.
Monitor oximetry readings q2-4h.	O₂ saturation 92% or less usually signals need for supplemental oxygen.
Report significant findings.	Oxygen is essential to recovery.
Administer supplemental oxygen as prescribed. Monitor and document effectiveness.	Supplemental O₂ is delivered until the patient's arterial blood gas or oximetry values while breathing room air are acceptable.
Encourage and assist the patient with coughing, deep breathing, incentive spirometry, and turning q2-4h.	These measures help prevent pneumonia and atelectasis.
Administer analgesics at dose and frequency that relieves pain and associated impaired chest excursion.	Reducing pain will enable full chest excursion for better oxygenation.
Instruct the patient in methods to splint the abdomen.	This information will help the patient reduce pain on movement, coughing, and deep breathing, which in turn will aid the respiratory effort.
For additional interventions, see "Perioperative Care" in **Ineffective Breathing Pattern,** p. 50.	

Nursing Diagnoses:

Risk for Bleeding
Risk for Shock

related to potential (or actual) decrease in blood volume occurring with trauma

Desired Outcome: Within 4 hr of admission or on definitive repair (e.g., surgery), the patient is normovolemic as evidenced by systolic blood pressure (SBP) 90 mm Hg or higher (or within the patient's baseline range), heart rate (HR) 60-100 bpm, urinary output at least 30 mL/hr, warm extremities, brisk capillary refill (2 sec or less), distal pulses at least 2+ on a 0-4+ scale, and absence of orthostasis.

ASSESSMENT/INTERVENTIONS	RATIONALES
In *recently injured* patients, assess BP continually in the presence of obvious bleeding or unstable VS.	Even a small but sudden decrease in SBP signals need to notify the health care provider, especially with a trauma patient in whom extent of injury is unknown. Most trauma patients are young, and excellent neurovascular compensation results in a near normal blood pressure (BP) until there is large intravascular volume depletion.
Be alert to and report increasing diastolic blood pressure (DBP) and decreasing SBP. In *stable postoperative* patients, perform routine VS assessment.	Increasing diastolic pressure with decreasing systolic pressure is a sign of hypovolemic shock. The difference between the systolic blood pressure and the diastolic blood pressure is termed *pulse pressure*. When the pulse pressure is narrowed (less than 25% of SBP), this signals decreasing cardiac output and increasing peripheral vascular resistance in the presence of hypovolemic shock.
Assess extremities for temperature, color, capillary refill, and strength of distal pulses. Report significant findings.	Pallor, coolness, delayed capillary refill (2 sec or more), and decreased or absent peripheral pulses are physical indicators of bleeding/hemorrhage/shock.
Assess HR and RR and for anxiety (early) and confusion, lethargy, and coma (later). Immediately report significant findings.	Tachycardia (HR more than 100 bpm) and tachypnea (RR more than 20 breaths/min) are clinical indicators of bleeding/hemorrhage/ shock as are anxiety, confusion, lethargy, and coma. Early detection and treatment of shock are essential to prevent irreversible cardiovascular collapse and death.
Monitor HR and cardiovascular status continually until the patient's condition is stable. Report dramatic changes to the health care provider.	Tachycardia and hypotension occur with bleeding. VS should be assessed continually to detect changes early for prompt intervention.
Administer prescribed fluids rapidly through large-caliber (18-gauge or larger) intravenous (IV) catheters in patients with evidence of active blood loss.	Massive blood loss is frequently associated with abdominal injuries. Restoration and maintenance of adequate intravascular volume are essential. Ringer's lactate or an isotonic solution is administered. Packed red blood cells are administered to replace blood loss, especially with hemoglobin less than 8.0 g/dL. Patients with abdominal trauma must have two large-bore IV lines inserted peripherally or centrally for rapid replacement of volume.
Evaluate IV flow rate frequently during rapid volume resuscitation, and monitor the patient closely.	These assessments will help prevent fluid volume overload and complications such as heart failure.
Titrate IV fluid therapy to maintain SBP greater than 90 mm Hg.	Maintaining SBP greater than 90 mm Hg is essential for adequate peripheral perfusion.
Ensure that large volumes of fluid are warmed before they are infused.	Warming is necessary to prevent hypothermia.
Be alert to decreasing urinary output and to infrequent voiding. Report significant findings.	Deficient fluid volume is an indicator that renal perfusion may be severely compromised.
Measure urinary output hourly if a catheter is in place or when the patient voids.	Low urine output reflects inadequate intravascular volume and decreased renal perfusion.
Note and report significant increases in the amount of drainage, especially if it is sanguineous.	An increase in sanguineous drainage signifies bleeding, and immediate intervention may be required to maintain hemodynamic stability.
Measure all output from drainage tubes and catheters, noting color, consistency, and odor (e.g., "coffee grounds," burgundy, bright red). Monitor and measure quantity of bloody stools.	These measurements provide an estimate of ongoing blood loss.
Note frequency/number of dressings used in performing dressing changes due to saturation with blood.	This assessment estimates the amount of blood lost via the wound site.

Nursing Diagnosis:

Acute Pain

related to irritation caused by intraperitoneal blood or secretions, trauma or surgical incision, or manipulation of organs during surgery

Desired Outcomes: Within 4 hr of admission, the patient's subjective perception of pain decreases, as documented by pain scale. Nonverbal indicators, such as grimacing, are absent or diminished. The patient's pain is controlled without sedation.

ASSESSMENT/INTERVENTIONS	RATIONALES
Assess for the presence and location of traumatic, preoperative, and postoperative pain. Use a pain scale, rating discomfort from 0 (no pain) to 10 (worst pain).	Pain related to trauma is an indicator of the extent of injury. Preoperative pain is anticipated and is a vital diagnostic aid. Location and character of postoperative pain also can be important. For example, incisional and some visceral pain can be anticipated, but intense or prolonged pain, especially when accompanied by other peritoneal signs, can signal bleeding, bowel infarction, infection, or other complications. Autonomic nervous system response to pain can complicate assessment of abdominal injury and hypovolemia. A pain scale helps quantify pain and determine subsequent relief obtained.
Administer analgesics as prescribed and indicated.	An alert patient should not suffer severe pain while awaiting surgical evaluation. Postoperatively prescribed analgesics should be administered on a continual or regular schedule promptly with additional analgesia as needed, or provide patient-controlled analgesia (PCA). Analgesics are helpful in relieving pain and in aiding the recovery process by promoting greater ventilatory excursion. As the severity of pain lessens, alternative analgesics such as nonsteroidal antiinflammatory drugs (NSAIDs) (e.g., ketorolac, ibuprofen) may be prescribed if not contraindicated by patient history of gastric bleeding.
Encourage the patient to request analgesic before the pain becomes severe.	Prolonged stimulation of pain receptors results in increased sensitivity to painful stimuli and will increase the amount of drug required to relieve pain.
Try to obtain an accurate drug and alcohol use history.	Intoxication often is involved in traumatic events. Patients may be drug or alcohol users, with a higher-than-average tolerance for opioids, requiring adjusted dosage for adequate pain relief. (Opioids can decrease gastrointestinal [GI] motility and may delay return to normal bowel function.) These individuals may suffer symptoms of alcohol withdrawal (tremors, weakness, tachycardia, elevated BP, delusions, agitation, hallucinations) or narcotic withdrawal (lacrimation, rhinorrhea, anxiety, tremors, muscle twitching, mydriasis, nausea, abdominal cramps, vomiting), and this will necessitate prompt recognition and treatment.
Use withdrawal scales if needed.	Withdrawal scales enable standardized assessment and treatment.
Monitor PCA, if prescribed, and document effectiveness, using pain scale.	For this and other interventions/rationales, see discussions in "Pain," p. 39.
Incorporate nonmedication pain relief measures such as positioning, massage, music, and distraction to aid in pain reduction. Provide these instructions to the patient and family members.	Nonpharmacologic maneuvers support analgesia therapy in reducing pain.

Nursing Diagnosis:

Risk for Infection

related to inadequate primary defenses occurring with disruption of the GI tract (particularly of the terminal ileum and colon) and traumatically inflicted open wound, multiple indwelling catheters and drainage tubes, and compromised immune state caused by blood loss and metabolic response to trauma

Desired Outcome: The patient is free of infection as evidenced by temperature less than 37.7°C (100°F); HR 100 bpm or less; no significant changes in mental status; orientation to person, place, and time; and absence of unusual erythema, edema, tenderness, warmth, or drainage at surgical incisions or wound sites.

ASSESSMENT/INTERVENTIONS	RATIONALES
Wash your hands before and after all patient encounters.	Handwashing is the number one defense against infection.
Assess VS for temperature increases and associated increases in heart and respiratory rates. Notify the health care provider of sudden temperature elevations.	These signs are indicators of infection.
Assess mental status, orientation, and level of consciousness (LOC) as frequently as needed.	Mental status changes, confusion, or deterioration from baseline LOC can signal infection.
Evaluate incisions and wound sites for unusual erythema, warmth, tenderness, edema, delayed healing, and purulent or unusual drainage.	These signs are evidence of localized infection.
Assess the amount, color, character, and odor of all drainage, and report significant findings.	Foul-smelling or abnormal drainage can occur with infection and should be reported for prompt intervention.
Ensure patency of all surgically placed tubes or drains. Irrigate or attach to low-pressure suction as prescribed. Maintain continuity of closed drainage systems; use sterile technique when emptying drainage and recharging suction containers. Promptly report loss of tube patency.	Blocked drainage systems may promote infection and abscess formation. Maintaining a closed drainage system and using sterile technique decrease risk of infection.
Administer antibiotics on time. Reschedule parenteral antibiotics if a dose is delayed more than 1 hr. Check blood levels as indicated (e.g., with vancomycin and gentamicin).	Failure to administer antibiotics on schedule may result in inadequate blood levels and treatment failure.
Administer pneumococcal vaccine to patients with total splenectomy, as prescribed.	This measure minimizes risk of postsplenectomy sepsis.
Administer tetanus immune globulin and tetanus toxoid as prescribed.	Risk for tetanus following trauma increases if the patient has not been immunized within the past 10 years.
Change dressings as prescribed, using sterile technique; change one dressing at a time.	These interventions prevent infection and cross-contamination from various wounds.
Use drains, closed drainage systems, or drainage bags to remove and collect GI secretions.	These measures prevent contamination of the surgical incision site.
If the patient has or develops an evisceration, do not reinsert tissue or organs. Place sterile, saline-soaked gauze over the evisceration, and cover with a sterile towel until the surgeon can evaluate the evisceration.	Evisceration is an emergent, life-threatening situation. Preventing infection and maintaining homeostasis is essential until a surgical intervention can be made.
Keep the patient on bedrest in semi-Fowler's position with knees bent.	This position reduces strain on eviscerated organs. Bedrest minimizes disruption to the abdominal organs, preventing further tissue damage and risk of infection.
Maintain nothing by mouth (NPO) status for the patient.	The patient may need emergency surgery.

Nursing Diagnosis:

Risk for Ineffective Gastrointestinal Perfusion

related to interrupted blood flow to the abdominal viscera occurring with vascular disruption or occlusion, or *related to* moderate to severe hypovolemia caused by hemorrhage

Desired Outcomes: The patient has adequate GI tissue perfusion as evidenced by normoactive bowel sounds; soft, nondistended abdomen; and return of bowel elimination. Gastric secretions, drainage, and excretions are negative for occult blood.

ASSESSMENT/INTERVENTIONS	RATIONALES
[!] Auscultate for bowel sounds hourly in recently injured patients and at least q8h during the recovery phase. Report significant findings.	Absent or diminished bowel sounds may be anticipated for up to 72 hr after trauma or surgery. Prolonged or sudden absence of bowel sounds may signal bowel ischemia or infarction and must be reported promptly for intervention.
[!] Assess the patient for peritoneal signs and report significant findings.	Signs of peritoneal irritation (generalized abdominal pain or tenderness, guarding, abdominal wall rigidity, rebound tenderness, abdominal pain with movement or coughing, abdominal distention, and decreased or absent bowel sounds) may occur acutely secondary to injury or may not develop until days or weeks later if complications caused by slow bleeding or other mechanisms occur.
Evaluate laboratory data for evidence of bleeding (e.g., serial hematocrit [Hct]) and Hgb; elevated liver or pancreatic enzymes) and report significant findings.	Decreases in Hgb and Hct signify bleeding. Increases in liver or pancreatic enzymes indicate hepatic or pancreatic inflammation or injury.
[!] Document the amount and character of GI secretions, drainage, and excretions and report significant findings.	Changes suggestive of bleeding (presence of frank or occult blood), infection (e.g., increased or purulent drainage), or obstruction (e.g., failure to eliminate flatus or stool within 72 hr after surgery) may signal the presence of a complication that necessitates timely intervention.
Ensure adequate intravascular volume (see discussion in **Risk for Bleeding/Risk for Shock,** earlier).	Adequate intravascular volume optimizes organ perfusion.

Nursing Diagnoses:

Risk for Impaired Skin Integrity

related to potential for exposure to irritating GI drainage

Impaired Tissue Integrity

related to direct trauma and surgery, catabolic posttraumatic state, and altered circulation

Desired Outcome: The patient exhibits wound healing, and the skin remains nonerythremic and intact.

ASSESSMENT/INTERVENTIONS	RATIONALES
Assess wounds, fistulas, and drain sites at routine intervals and report significant findings.	These measures identify signs of irritation, infection, and ischemia (i.e., erythema, edema, purulent drainage) for prompt intervention.
Identify infected and devitalized tissue. Aid in their removal by irrigation, wound packing, or preparing the patient for surgical debridement.	Removal of devitalized tissue is essential for wound healing to progress.

continued

ASSESSMENT/INTERVENTIONS	RATIONALES
Promptly change all dressings that become soiled with drainage or blood. Protect skin surrounding tubes, drains, or fistulas, keeping the areas clean and free from drainage.	Gastric and intestinal secretions and drainage are irritating and can lead to skin excoriation.
If necessary, apply ointments, skin barriers, or drainage bags. Apply reusable dressing supports such as Montgomery straps or tubular mesh gauze.	These measures prevent excessive injury to surrounding skin.
Consult a wound, ostomy, continence (WOC)/enterostomal therapy (ET) nurse for complex or involved cases, and follow evidence-based recommendations.	Consulting with experts and following evidence-based recommendations can substantially aid in preventing skin damage.
Consult the dietitian to ensure adequate protein and calorie intake (see **Imbalanced Nutrition,** following).	Adequate nutrition is necessary for tissue healing to occur.
For more information, see "Managing Wound Care," p. 533.	

Nursing Diagnosis:

Imbalanced Nutrition: Less Than Body Requirements

related to decreased intake occurring with disruption of GI tract integrity (traumatic or surgical) and increased need due to hypermetabolic posttrauma state

Desired Outcome: By at least 24 hr before hospital discharge, the patient has adequate nutrition as evidenced by maintenance of baseline body weight and positive or balanced nitrogen (N) state.

ASSESSMENT/INTERVENTIONS	RATIONALES
Collaborate with the health care provider, dietitian, and pharmacist to assess the patient's metabolic needs based on type of injury, activity level, and nutritional status before injury.	Patients with abdominal trauma have complex nutritional needs because of the hypermetabolic state associated with major trauma and traumatic or surgical disruption of normal GI function. Often, infection and sepsis contribute to a negative nitrogen (N) state and increased metabolic needs. Prompt initiation of enteric feedings and administration of supplemental calories, proteins, vitamins, and minerals are essential for healing. Parenteral feedings are given if enteral feedings cannot be used. If patients are tube-fed enterally, the feeding tube must be placed distal to the injury.
Monitor laboratory values, including prealbumin, albumin, total protein, and blood glucose.	Prealbumin, albumin, and total protein are indicators of nutritional stores and guide nutritional replacement. Patients with hepatic or pancreatic injury may be unable to regulate blood sugar levels.
Assess patency of gastric or intestinal tubes.	Gastric decompression requires a patent gastric/intestinal tube in order to prevent accumulation of gas or fluid in the stomach and reduce the chance of aspiration while promoting healing and return of bowel function. The tube usually remains in place until bowel function returns, as detected by positive bowel sounds, passage of flatus, and decreased gastric output via the tube.
Confirm placement of the feeding tube before each tube feeding. After initial insertion, check x-ray film for position of the tube. Mark to determine tube migration, secure the tubing in place, and reassess q4h and before each feeding.	Determining correct placement of the feeding tube before instilling medications or feedings is essential to prevent aspiration or instillation of liquids or medications into the lungs. Insufflation with air and aspiration of stomach contents do not always confirm placement of small-bore feeding tubes.
Use caution and consult the surgeon before irrigating nasogastric (NG) or other tubes that have been placed in or near recently sutured organs.	Some NG tubes are sutured in place; irrigation or movement of the tube could disrupt sutures and cause bleeding.

ASSESSMENT/INTERVENTIONS

Assess pH of gastric aspirate.

Avoid opioid analgesics if possible; administer prescribed nonnarcotic analgesics (e.g., ketorolac).

For more information, see "Providing Nutritional Support," p. 539.

RATIONALES

A pH less than 5 usually signals gastric placement. However, acid blockade medications may alter pH.

Opioid analgesics decrease GI motility and may contribute to nausea, vomiting, abdominal distention, and ileus.

Nursing Diagnosis:

Posttrauma Syndrome

related to life-threatening accident or event resulting in trauma

Desired Outcomes: By at least 24 hr before hospital discharge, the patient verbalizes aspects of the psychosocial impact of the event and does not exhibit signs of severe stress reaction, such as display of inconsistent affect, suicidal or homicidal behavior, or extreme agitation or depression. The patient cooperates with the treatment plan.

ASSESSMENT/INTERVENTIONS

Assess the patient's mental status at regular intervals. Be alert to indicators of severe stress reaction, such as display of affect inconsistent with statements or behavior, suicidal or homicidal statements or actions, extreme agitation or depression, and failure to cooperate with instructions related to care.

Assess for organic causes that may contribute to the posttraumatic response.

Consult specialists such as a psychiatrist, psychologist, psychiatric nurse practitioner, or pastoral counselor if the patient displays signs of severe stress reaction described previously.

For other interventions, see "Psychosocial Support," p. 72, and "Substance-Related and Addictive Disorders," p. 739.

RATIONALES

Many victims of major abdominal trauma sustain life-threatening injury. The patient is often aware of the situation and fears death. Even after the physical condition stabilizes, the patient may have a prolonged or severe reaction triggered by recollection of the trauma.

Severe pain, alcohol intoxication or withdrawal, electrolyte imbalance, metabolic encephalopathy, and impaired cerebral perfusion are potential contributors to the posttraumatic response and should be treated accordingly.

Specialized intervention supports the patient and may prevent long-term suffering or suicide.

ADDITIONAL NURSING DIAGNOSES/PROBLEMS:

✓ PATIENT-FAMILY TEACHING AND DISCHARGE PLANNING

Anticipate extended physical and emotional rehabilitation for the patient and significant other. When providing patient-family teaching, focus on sensory information, avoid giving excessive information, and initiate a visiting nurse referral for necessary follow-up teaching. Include verbal and written information about the following:

✓ Self-management: Assessment of the patient's ability to manage own care should be completed before hospital discharge. Identification of support persons to assist with care should be initiated early.

✓ Probable need for emotional care, even for patients who have not required extensive physical rehabilitation. Provide referrals to support groups for trauma patients and family members.

✓ Availability of rehabilitation programs, extended care facilities, and home health agencies for patients unable to accomplish self-care on hospital discharge.

✓ Availability of rehabilitation programs for substance abuse, as indicated. Immediately after the traumatic event, patient and family members are very impressionable, making this period an ideal time for patients with substance abuse issues to begin to resolve the problem.

✓ Medications, including drug name, purpose, dosage, schedule, precautions, and potential side effects. Also discuss drug-drug, herb-drug, and food-drug interactions. Encourage patients taking antibiotics to take medications for prescribed length of time, even though they may be asymptomatic. If the patient received a tetanus immunization, ensure that he or she receives documentation of the immunization.

✓ Wound and catheter care and dressing changes. Have the patient or caregiver describe and demonstrate proper technique before hospital discharge. Reinforce the importance of handwashing before and after all care activities to prevent infection.

✓ Activity: Restrictions and recommendations should be reviewed thoroughly with the patient and caregivers. An at-home assessment may be necessary if activity is severely limited or adaptations are necessary. Consider

referral to an occupational therapist (OT) or physical therapist (PT).

✓ Diet/nutrition: Review diet recommendations with the patient/family. If enteral or parenteral feeding is necessary, have the patient or caregiver describe and demonstrate correct technique before hospital discharge. Home health care services may be warranted for support and evaluation.

✓ Importance of seeking medical attention if indicators of infection or bowel obstruction occur (e.g., fever, severe or unusual abdominal pain, nausea and vomiting, unusual drainage from wounds or incisions, a change in bowel habits).

✓ Injury prevention: Following traumatic injury, the patient and family members are especially likely to respond to injury prevention education. Provide instructions on proper seatbelt applications (across pelvic girdle rather than across soft tissue of lower abdomen), safety for infants and children, and other factors suitable for individuals involved.

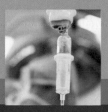

Appendicitis 52

OVERVIEW/PATHOPHYSIOLOGY

Appendicitis is the most commonly occurring inflammatory lesion of the bowel and one of the most common reasons for abdominal surgery. Appendicitis occurs most often in adolescents and young adults, and is more common in males than females. The appendix is a blind, narrow tube that extends from the inferior portion of the cecum and does not serve any known useful function. Appendicitis can be caused by obstruction of the appendiceal lumen by a fecalith (hardened bit of fecal material), inflammation, a foreign body, or a neoplasm. Obstruction prevents drainage of secretions that are produced by epithelial cells in the lumen, thereby increasing intraluminal pressure and compressing mucosal blood vessels. This tension eventually impairs local blood flow, which can lead to necrosis and perforation. Inflammation and infection result from normal bacteria invading the devitalized wall. Mild cases of appendicitis can heal spontaneously, but severe inflammation can lead to a ruptured appendix, which can cause local or generalized peritonitis.

HEALTH CARE SETTING

Acute care surgical unit. Inpatient status for ruptured appendix with peritonitis; 1-day length of stay for suspected acute appendicitis without complications

ASSESSMENT

Signs and symptoms vary because of differences in anatomy, size, and age. The sequence of symptoms can be significant in the differential diagnosis. Abdominal discomfort, indigestion, and bowel irregularity occur first.

Early stage: Pain usually occurs in either the epigastric or umbilical area and may be vague and diffuse or associated with mild cramping. Nausea and vomiting are not always present, but if they occur, they follow the onset of pain. Fever and leukocytosis occur later.

Intermediate (acute) stage: Over a period of a few hours, pain shifts from the midabdomen or epigastrium to the right lower quadrant (RLQ) at McBurney's point (approximately 2 inches from the anterior superior iliac spine on a line drawn from the umbilicus) and is aggravated by walking, coughing, and movement. Pain may be accompanied by a sensation of constipation (gas-stoppage sensation). Anorexia, malaise, occasionally diarrhea, and diminished peristalsis also can occur.

On physical assessment, the patient may experience pain in the RLQ elicited by light palpation of the abdomen; presence of rebound tenderness; RLQ guarding, rigidity, and muscle spasms; tachycardia; low-grade fever; and pain elicited with rectal examination. A palpable, tender mass may be felt in the peritoneal pouch if the appendix lies within the pelvis.

> **Note:** Physical assessment is performed in four steps—inspection, auscultation, percussion, and palpation—in that order, to avoid stimulating the abdomen by palpation and percussion, which can affect bowel sounds.

Acute appendicitis with perforation: Increasing, generalized pain; recurrence of vomiting. On physical assessment, the patient usually exhibits temperature increases to more than 38.5°C (101.4°F) and generalized abdominal rigidity. Typically, the patient remains rigid with flexed knees. Presence of abscess can result in a tender, palpable mass. The abdomen may be distended.

DIAGNOSTIC TESTS

Abdominal computed tomography (CT) scan: Has accuracy rate of 95% overall and should be performed before a laparotomy.

White blood cell count with differential: Reveals presence of leukocytosis and an increase in neutrophils. A shift to the left with more than 75% neutrophils is a consistent finding in later stages of appendicitis.

Abdominal ultrasound: May be done to rule out appendicitis or conditions that mimic it, such as Crohn's disease, diverticulitis, or gastroenteritis. Higher success rate for diagnosis is found in children.

Abdominal x-ray examination: May reveal presence of a fecalith. About half of these patients may have x-ray findings of localized air-fluid levels, increased soft tissue density in the RLQ, and indications of localized ileus. If perforation has occurred, the presence of free air is noted.

Urinalysis: To rule out genitourinary conditions mimicking appendicitis; may reveal microscopic hematuria and pyuria. This test result usually is normal.

Intravenous (IV) pyelogram: May be performed to rule out ureteral stone or pyelitis.

Nursing Diagnosis:

Risk for Infection

related to inadequate primary defenses (danger of rupture, peritonitis, abscess formation) occurring with inflammatory process

Desired Outcomes: The patient is free of infection as evidenced by normothermia, heart rate (HR) 100 bpm or less, blood pressure (BP) at least 90/60 mm Hg, respiratory rate (RR) 12-20 breaths/min with normal depth and pattern (eupnea), absence of chills, soft and nondistended abdomen, and bowel sounds 5-34/min in each abdominal quadrant. Following instruction, the patient verbalizes rationale for not administering enemas or laxatives preoperatively and enemas postoperatively and demonstrates compliance with the therapeutic regimen.

ASSESSMENT/INTERVENTIONS	RATIONALES
Assess and document quality, location, and duration of the pain; presence of nausea; and the patient's positioning.	Signs of worsening appendicitis that can lead to rupture include pain that becomes accentuated; recurrent vomiting; and the patient assuming a side-lying or supine position with flexed knees. Pain that worsens and then disappears is a signal that rupture may have occurred.
Monitor vital signs for elevated temperature, increased pulse rate, hypotension, and shallow/rapid respirations; assess the abdomen for presence of rigidity, distention, and decreased or absent bowel sounds. Report significant findings to the health care provider.	Any of these indicators can occur with rupture.
Monitor for ambulation with a limp or pain with hip extension.	Retrocecal abscess may irritate the psoas muscle as it traverses the area of posterior RLQ of the abdomen and results in pain with hip extension.
Caution the patient about the danger of preoperative self-treatment with enemas and laxatives.	Enemas and laxatives increase peristalsis, which increases risk of perforation and hence peritonitis and sepsis. Enemas should be avoided until approved by the health care provider (usually several weeks after surgery). If constipation occurs postoperatively, the health care provider may prescribe laxatives/stool softeners at bedtime after the third day.
Teach postoperative incisional care, as well as care of drains if the patient is to be discharged with them.	Maintaining a clean incision and avoiding contamination of drains help prevent infection in areas in which the skin is no longer intact. An incisional drain may be inserted in the presence of abscess, rupture, or peritonitis to facilitate drainage of exudate and peritoneal fluid and avoid complications of infection.
Provide instructions for prescribed antibiotics if the patient is to be discharged with them.	Antibiotics prevent or treat systemic infection from a ruptured appendix. See "Peritonitis," p. 454, for more information.

Nursing Diagnoses:

Acute Pain
Nausea

related to the inflammatory process

Desired Outcomes: Within 1-2 hr of pain-relieving interventions, the patient's subjective perception of pain and nausea decreases, as documented by pain scale. Objective indicators, such as grimacing, are absent or diminished.

ASSESSMENT/INTERVENTIONS	RATIONALES
Assess and document quality, location, and duration of the pain. Devise a pain scale with the patient, rating discomfort from 0 (no pain) to 10 (worst pain). Assess and document nausea in the same way.	These characteristics of discomfort may be seen during the following stages of appendicitis: *Early stage:* Abdominal pain (either epigastric or umbilical) that may be vague and diffuse, nausea and vomiting, fever, and sensitivity over appendix area. *Intermediate (acute) stage:* Pain that shifts from the epigastrium to the RLQ at McBurney's point (approximately 2 inches from the anterior superior iliac spine on a line drawn from the umbilicus) and is aggravated by walking or coughing. The pain may be accompanied by a sensation of constipation (gas-stoppage sensation). Anorexia, malaise, occasional diarrhea, and diminished peristalsis also can occur. *Acute appendicitis with perforation:* Increasing, generalized pain; recurrence of vomiting; increasing abdominal rigidity.
Medicate with antiemetics, sedatives, and analgesics as prescribed; evaluate and document the patient's response, using the pain scale.	These agents reduce nausea and pain. Opioids are avoided until diagnosis is certain because they mask clinical signs and symptoms.
Encourage the patient to request medication *before* symptoms become severe.	Prolonged stimulation of pain receptors results in increased sensitivity to painful stimuli and will increase the amount of drug required to relieve the discomfort.
Keep the patient nothing by mouth (NPO) before surgery.	Being NPO helps prevent aspiration during anesthesia when the gag reflex is compromised. After surgery, nausea and vomiting usually disappear.
If prescribed, insert a gastric tube.	A gastric tube enables decompression in preoperative patients with severe nausea and vomiting.
Teach the technique for slow, diaphragmatic breathing.	This technique reduces stress and helps promote comfort by relaxing tense muscles.
Help position the patient for optimal comfort.	Many patients find comfort from a side-lying position with knees bent, whereas others find relief when supine with pillows under the knees (avoiding pressure on popliteal area). These positions help to reduce pain by decreasing traction on the abdomen.

Nursing Diagnosis:

Risk for Adverse Reaction to Iodinated Contrast Media

related to administration during CT scan procedures

Desired Outcome: Following completion of the CT scan procedure, the patient has no significant changes in vital signs, no adverse reactions, and is able to tolerate increased fluid intake and void at least 30 mL/hr to excrete contrast dye.

ASSESSMENT/INTERVENTIONS

RATIONALES

ASSESSMENT/INTERVENTIONS	RATIONALES
Before the procedure, assess the patient for allergies to iodine, shellfish, and previous allergic reaction to iodinated or other contrast media. If these allergies exist, notify the health care provider.	An iodine-based contrast medium may cause an anaphylactic response in patients allergic to these substances.
Obtain prescribed laboratory tests, such as blood urea nitrogen (BUN) and creatinine levels.	If levels are elevated, notify the health care provider, because the patient is at increased risk for renal failure secondary to the contrast media.
Administer preprocedure medication as prescribed	Premedication with prednisone and diphenhydramine may be prescribed to decrease or prevent contrast media reaction. A nonionic, hypoallergenic contrast dye may be used instead.
Instruct the patient to increase fluids and report any decrease in urinary output from his or her normal range.	Increased fluid intake promotes contrast dye excretion and prevents dye-induced renal failure.
Instruct the patient to contact the health care provider immediately if rash, hives, tachycardia, or dyspnea occurs.	Reactions to contrast media can occur starting from 2-6 hr postprocedure and to within 7 days after contrast dye injection.

ADDITIONAL NURSING DIAGNOSES/PROBLEMS:

"Perioperative Care"   p. 45

✓ PATIENT-FAMILY TEACHING AND DISCHARGE PLANNING

When providing patient-family teaching, focus on sensory information, and avoid giving excessive information. Include verbal and written information about the following:

✓ Medications, including drug name, dosage, purpose, schedule, precautions, and potential side effects. Also discuss drug-drug, food-drug, and herb-drug interactions.

✓ Care of incision, including dressing changes and bathing restrictions if appropriate.

✓ Indicators of infection: fever, chills, incisional pain, redness, swelling, and purulent drainage.

✓ Postsurgical activity precautions: avoid lifting heavy objects (more than 10 lb) for the first 6 wk or as directed, be alert to and rest after symptoms of fatigue, get maximum rest, gradually increase activities to tolerance.

✓ Importance of avoiding enemas for the first few postoperative weeks. Caution the patient about need to check with the health care provider before having an enema.

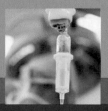

Cholelithiasis, Cholecystitis, and Cholangitis 53

OVERVIEW/PATHOPHYSIOLOGY

Gallstones may be found anywhere in the biliary system. They may cause pain and other symptoms or remain asymptomatic for years. Of the people who have gallstones, 70% or more have no symptoms; however, these individuals have a 1%-4% chance of developing symptoms or complications at some point in time. *Cholelithiasis* is characterized by the presence of stones in the gallbladder. *Choledocholithiasis* is the term used to describe gallstones that have migrated to the common bile duct. Gallstones are classified as cholesterol or pigment stones. Cholesterol stones are more common in the United States and represent approximately 80% of cases. These stones originate in the gallbladder. Black-pigment stones also originate in the gallbladder and result from an increase of calcium and unconjugated bilirubin and are associated with cirrhosis and chronic hemolysis. Brown-pigment stones are the predominant type found in native Asians and may be associated with bacterial infection of the bile. These stones originate in the bile duct. Precipitating factors for stone formation include disturbances in metabolism, biliary stasis, obstruction, hypertriglyceridemia, and infection. Gallstones are especially prevalent in women who are multiparous, are taking estrogen therapy, or use oral contraceptives. Other risk factors include obesity, dietary intake of fats, sedentary lifestyle, and familial tendencies. The incidence increases with age, and it is estimated that one of every three persons who reach 75 yr of age has gallstones. Cholelithiasis is commonly seen in disease states such as diabetes mellitus, regional enteritis, and certain blood dyscrasias. Usually cholelithiasis is asymptomatic until a stone becomes lodged in the cystic tract. If the obstruction is unrelieved, biliary colic causes acute, sharp pain when the gallbladder contracts while a stone is lodged in the cystic duct. Biliary colic eventually leads to acute cholecystitis.

Acute cholecystitis is most commonly associated with cystic duct obstructions caused by impacted gallstones; however, it may also result from stasis, bacterial infection, or ischemia of the gallbladder. When the cystic tract becomes obstructed, the gallbladder becomes distended. Structural changes such as swelling and thickening of the gallbladder walls can occur. Additionally, serosal edema, mucosal sloughing, and congestion within the venous and lymphatic systems occur. Ultimately, ischemia can occur, resulting in gangrene or perforation.

With chronic cholecystitis, stones almost always are present and the gallbladder walls are thickened and fibrosed.

Ascending cholangitis or acute cholangitis is the most serious complication of gallstones and is more difficult to diagnose than either cholelithiasis or cholecystitis. It is caused by an impacted stone in the common bile duct, resulting in bile stasis, bacteremia, and septicemia if left untreated. Cholangitis is most likely to occur when an already infected bile duct becomes obstructed. Bacteria enter the duct easily due to the adjacent duodenum. It is believed that chronic bacteremia within the bile duct can eventually cause *primary sclerosing cholangitis* with the hallmarks, including biliary duct fibrosis (intra- and extrahepatic) and inflammatory changes of the portal and periportal liver. Mortality rate is high if not recognized and treated early.

HEALTH CARE SETTING

Primary care; acute care

ASSESSMENT

Cholelithiasis: History of occasional discomfort after eating. As the stone moves through the duct or becomes lodged, a sudden onset of mild, aching pain occurs in the midepigastrium after eating (especially after a high-fat meal) and increases in intensity during a colic attack, potentially radiating to the right upper quadrant (RUQ), right subscapular region, or right shoulder. Nausea, vomiting, tachycardia, mild fever, and diaphoresis also can occur. Many individuals with gallstones are entirely asymptomatic. The patients who develop gallstone pancreatitis may be completely asymptomatic of their gallstones until they develop the symptoms of pancreatitis.

Acute cholecystitis: Marked by right upper quadrant pain, fever, and leukocytosis. There may be a history of discomfort after eating, including regurgitation, flatulence, belching, epigastric heaviness, indigestion, heartburn, chronic upper abdominal pain, and nausea. Amber-colored urine, clay-colored stools, pruritus, jaundice, steatorrhea, fever, and bleeding tendencies can be present if there is biliary obstruction. Symptoms may be vague. An acute attack may last 7-10 days, but it usually resolves in several hours.

Cholangitis: Fever is present in nearly all the patients with bacterial cholangitis. Jaundice, chills, mild and transient

RUQ pain, mental confusion, and lethargy are part of the presenting symptoms. Leukocytosis and elevated bilirubin are present in 80% of cases.

PHYSICAL ASSESSMENT

Cholelithiasis: Palpation of the RUQ reveals a tender abdomen during episodes of biliary colic. Otherwise, between episodes of pain, the examination is usually normal.

Acute cholecystitis: Palpation elicits tenderness localized behind the inferior margin of the liver. With progressive symptoms, a tender, globular mass may be palpated behind the lower border of the liver. Rebound tenderness and guarding also may be present. With the patient taking a deep breath, palpation over the RUQ elicits Murphy's sign (pain and inability to inspire when the examiner's hand comes in contact with the gallbladder).

Cholangitis: RUQ tenderness is present in 90% of cases. Peritoneal signs (abdominal pain, tenderness, guarding, decreased or absent bowel sounds, nausea) are not common and only occur in 15% of patients. Hypotension and mental confusion are present in severe cases.

> **Note:** *Cholangitis is a surgical emergency requiring prompt decompression of the biliary tract.*

DIAGNOSTIC TESTS

Ultrasonography: With its 95% sensitivity and specificity, ultrasonography is the preferred test for confirming the presence of gallstones, as well as their number, size, and location. Ultrasound can also identify gallbladder wall changes such as thickening and edema, as well as the presence of sludge and fluid collection Ultrasonography is readily available, does not expose the patient to radiation, and is inexpensive.

Hydroxyliminodiacetic acid (HIDA) scan or cholescintigraphy: Obtained if the diagnosis of acute cholecystitis remains uncertain following ultrasonography. HIDA is injected intravenously, absorbed in the liver, and then excreted in the biliary system. If an obstructing stone is present in the cystic duct, HIDA is prevented from filling the gallbladder. HIDA scan is not the preferred test for diagnosing gallstones and should be reserved for situations such as uncertain diagnosis or in ruling out cholecystitis. False-positive HIDA scans can occur.

Endoscopic retrograde cholangiopancreatography (ERCP): Visualization and evaluation of the biliary tree or pancreatic duct. ERCP is useful to both diagnose and treat common bile duct stones and can also help with evaluation of anatomic structures. ERCP does have its risks, because complications such as ERCP-induced pancreatitis, hemorrhage, perforation, and cholangitis are possible.

Magnetic resonance imaging (MRI) and magnetic resonance cholangiopancreatography (MRCP): MRI and MRCP also can be used to diagnose common bile duct stones; however, unlike ERCP, common bile duct stones cannot be removed with MRCP. MRCP is a more costly test, so its use is likely limited, although it can be a helpful study to assess RUQ pain in pregnancy.

Computed tomography (CT) scan: Although ultrasonography is preferred over CT scanning for suspected gallbladder disease, CT scanning of the abdomen is used in cases of uncertain diagnosis or suspicion of additional pathologies.

Complete blood count with differential: To assess for presence of infection or blood loss. Infection and inflammation cause leukocytosis. WBC counts greater than 20,000 suggest possible gangrene or gallbladder perforation.

Bilirubin tests (serum and urine) and urobilinogen tests (urine and fecal): May be performed to differentiate among hemolytic disorders, hepatocellular disease, and obstructive disease. Usually there is an increase of bilirubin in the plasma and urine with biliary disease.

Serum liver enzyme test: Usually normal in cholecystitis but often becomes abnormal in the presence of prolonged cholecystitis or common duct stones. If elevated in cholecystitis, it is usually associated with worse outcomes.

Prothrombin time: To assess for prolonged clotting time secondary to faulty vitamin K absorption.

Electrocardiogram: To rule out cardiac disease.

Nursing Diagnoses:

Acute Pain
Nausea

related to obstructive or inflammatory process

Desired Outcomes: The patient's subjective perception of discomfort decreases within 1 hr of intervention, as documented by a pain scale. Nonverbal indicators, such as grimacing, are absent or diminished.

ASSESSMENT/INTERVENTIONS

RATIONALES

ASSESSMENT/INTERVENTIONS	RATIONALES
Monitor the patient for pain or other discomfort. Devise a pain scale with the patient, rating discomfort on a scale of 0 (no pain) to 10 (worst pain).	Using a pain scale enables a more objective measurement of discomfort and subsequent relief obtained.
Explain that a low Fowler's position will minimize discomfort.	This position decreases tension on abdominal contents to promote comfort.
Teach about the prescribed diet.	The prescribed diet will prevent nausea and spasms and varies according to the patient's condition. During an acute attack, nothing by mouth (NPO) status with intravenous (IV) fluids may be instituted in preparation for possible surgery. With severe nausea and vomiting, a gastric tube is inserted and attached to low, intermittent suction. The diet advances to the patient's tolerance, and small, frequent feedings of a low-fat diet are recommended for both the acute and chronic conditions. This diet minimizes the secretion of bile salts and subsequent gallbladder spasms. After cholecystectomy, a low-fat diet is used initially, and fatty foods may be introduced gradually to the patient's level of tolerance.
Administer a bile salt–binding agent (e.g., cholestyramine) as prescribed.	Cholestyramine and colestipol bind with bile salts in the intestine to facilitate their excretion and may also provide relief from pruritus caused by prolonged obstructive jaundice.
Provide cool Alpha Keri baths and cold water or ice for topical application; use soft linens on the bed.	These measures help control itching. Using Alpha Keri as a bath oil and avoiding soap help minimize the potential for dryness and itching.
Administer analgesics as prescribed and report significant side effects.	Nonsteroidal antiinflammatory drugs or opioid analgesics may be indicated, depending on pain severity. For postoperative patients, epidural, continuous IV, and patient-controlled infusions of opioid analgesics are used with increasing frequency and superior efficacy (see "Pain," p. 39, for more information). IV ketorolac q6h for 4-8 doses has shown benefit in controlling postoperative pain with these patients, reducing need for opioid analgesics. It should not be used for more than 5 days because of its toxic effects. Although meperidine has long been used as the opioid of choice to prevent sphincter of Oddi spasms, there is risk of severe respiratory depression associated with its cumulative effects. Meperidine can be used alone or in conjunction with nonopioid medications.
Administer acid suppression therapy if prescribed.	This therapy neutralizes gastric hyperacidity and reduces associated pain. H₂ blockers (e.g., famotidine, cimetidine) and antacids should be used as first line therapy. Ginger is an alternative remedy for digestive upset and nausea.
Administer antiemetics as prescribed.	Antiemetics (e.g., hydroxyzine, ondansetron, prochlorperazine, promethazine) are given to control nausea and vomiting. Ginger is an alternative remedy for digestive upset and nausea.

Nursing Diagnosis:

Risk for Injury

related to potential for postsurgical perforation or recurrence of biliary obstruction

Desired Outcomes: The patient is free of symptoms of postsurgical perforation as evidenced by diminishing dark brown drainage of less than 1000 mL/day and the presence of a soft and nondistended abdomen. The patient is free of symptoms of recurring biliary obstruction as evidenced by normal skin color, brown-colored stools, and straw-colored urine.

ASSESSMENT/INTERVENTIONS | RATIONALES

ASSESSMENT/INTERVENTIONS	RATIONALES
Monitor color of the skin, sclera, urine, and stool.	If obstruction recurs and bile is forced back into the bloodstream, the skin becomes jaundiced (yellow), urine is amber colored, and stools are clay colored (clay color is normal if bile is drained via a T-tube). Brown color should return to the stools once the bile begins to drain normally into the duodenum.
If a T-tube is present, note and record color, amount, odor, and consistency of drainage from T-tube or wound drain q2h on day of surgery and at least every shift thereafter.	Initially drainage will be dark brown with small amounts of blood and can amount to 500-1000 mL/day. Greater amounts of blood or drainage should be reported to the health care provider. The amount should subside gradually as swelling diminishes in the common duct and drainage into the duodenum normalizes. **Note:** Laparoscopic surgery for common bile duct exploration often does not necessitate insertion of a T-tube. Disadvantages of T-tube insertion include a 2-wk period of insertion; the fact that the patient may not be as inclined to move and ambulate postoperatively due to its presence and fear of dislodgement or obstructing drainage; and infection, obstruction, and risk of prolonged recovery and increased mortality.
Ensure that drainage collection devices are positioned lower than the level of the common bile duct.	This will prevent reflux of drainage when the patient is ambulating.
Be alert to abdominal distention, rigidity, and complaints of diaphragmatic irritation (caused by inflammation or bleeding and in this case is pain referred to the right shoulder) along with cessation or significant decrease in the amount of drainage. If these signs occur, notify the health care provider immediately and anticipate tube replacement with a 14-French catheter.	These are indicators of a dislodged or clogged drainage tube causing bile leakage into the abdomen or backup of bile, necessitating timely intervention.

ADDITIONAL NURSING DIAGNOSES/PROBLEMS:

"Perioperative Care"	p. 45
"Hepatitis" for **Risk for Impaired Skin Integrity** related to pruritus	p. 439

✓ PATIENT-FAMILY TEACHING AND DISCHARGE PLANNING

When providing patient-family teaching, focus on sensory information, avoid giving excessive information, and initiate a visiting nurse referral for necessary follow-up monitoring of postoperative patients. Include verbal and written information about the following:

✓ Notifying health care provider if the following indicators of recurrent biliary obstruction occur: dark urine, pruritus, jaundice, clay-colored stools. Inform the patient that loose stools may occur for several months as the body adjusts to the continuous flow of bile.

✓ Medications, including drug name, dosage, schedule, purpose, precautions, and potential side effects. Also discuss drug-drug, food-drug, and herb-drug interactions.

✓ Care of dressings and tubes if applicable at hospital discharge, and monitoring of incision and drain sites for signs of infection (e.g., fever, persistent redness, pain, purulent discharge, swelling, increased local warmth). The patient should not submerge the abdomen in the bathtub with incisions and drain sites present.

✓ Importance of maintaining a diet low in fat and eating frequent, small meals for medically managed patients.

✓ Importance of follow-up appointments with the health care provider; reconfirm time and date of next appointment.

✓ Avoiding alcoholic beverages during first 2 postoperative months to minimize risk of pancreatic involvement.

✓ Necessity of postsurgical activity precautions: avoid lifting heavy objects (more than 10 lb) for first 4-6 wk or as directed, rest after periods of fatigue, get maximum amounts of rest, and gradually increase activities to tolerance. Postsurgical patients may experience fatty food intolerance (e.g., flatulence, cramps, diarrhea) for several months postoperatively until the body acclimates to loss of the gallbladder.

✓ For more information contact the following organizations:
- National Institute of Diabetes & Digestive & Kidney Diseases at *www.niddk.nih.gov*
- American Gastroenterological Association at *www.gastro.org*
- Canadian Association of Gastroenterology at *www.cag-acg.org*
- Canadian Liver Foundation at *www.liver.ca*

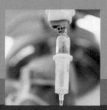

Cirrhosis 54

OVERVIEW/PATHOPHYSIOLOGY

Cirrhosis is a chronic, serious disease in which normal configuration of the liver is changed, resulting in cell death. As cells die, they are replaced with nonfunctioning fibrous tissue. Hepatomegaly, or liver enlargement, results from fibrous tissue, nodules, and fat build-up. Hepatomegaly leads to abdominal distention and shortness of breath due to pressure on the diaphragm. Eventually blood flow to the liver is impaired as the portal vein becomes obstructed. As a result of impaired blood flow, essential functions of the liver become disrupted, including digestion, metabolism, glycogen storage, protein synthesis, blood coagulation, hormone metabolism, fluid and electrolyte balances, and detoxification of chemicals. The liver holds approximately 13% of the body's total blood supply, and as the portal vein becomes obstructed, blood flow backs up into the spleen and GI tract. Patients with cirrhosis are at high risk for serious bleeding.

Alcoholic (Laënnec's) cirrhosis: Alcohol is a major cause of liver disease. Oftentimes other liver insults, such as chronic viral hepatitis or nonalcoholic fatty liver disease, increase the risk factors for liver disease in alcohol users. The spectrum of the disease starts with fatty liver and progresses to alcoholic hepatitis, and ultimately to chronic hepatitis with fibrosis or cirrhosis. In most cases, simple, uncomplicated fatty liver can be reversed by abstaining from alcohol for 4 to 6 wk; however, in 5%-15% of individuals who abstain, the fatty liver can progress to irreversible fibrosis or cirrhosis.

Cirrhosis also can be caused by any chronic liver disease: chronic hepatitis B, chronic hepatitis C, hereditary hemochromatosis, nonalcoholic fatty liver disease (NAFLD), autoimmune hepatitis, Wilson's disease, or alpha-1-antitrypsin deficiency.

The presence of cirrhosis places the patient at risk for the development of hepatocellular carcinoma (primary liver cancer) as well as decompensated liver disease (liver failure).

Biliary cirrhosis: Associated with chronic retention of bile and inflammation of the bile ducts and accounts for 15% of all cirrhosis cases. It may be further classified as follows.

Primary biliary cirrhosis (PBC): An inflammatory disease of intrahepatic bile ducts. This chronic, slowly progressive disease is believed to be autoimmune in origin. Small and medium bile ducts are destroyed by activated CD4 and CD8 lymphocytes. Eventually, end-stage liver disease occurs.

Patients may first note fatigue, as well as pruritus and right upper quadrant (RUQ) pain.

Secondary biliary cirrhosis: Results from chronic obstruction to bile flow, usually from an obstruction outside the liver, such as bile duct strictures after gallbladder surgery, chronic pancreatitis, pericholangitis, idiopathic sclerosing cholangitis, cystic fibrosis, calculi, neoplasms, or biliary atresia. Bile builds up in the liver as a result of damage to the bile ducts and eventually, the liver will fail.

HEALTH CARE SETTING

Primary care, acute care

ASSESSMENT

Signs and symptoms: Many patients with cirrhosis have no symptoms. Others exhibit symptoms in varying degrees, depending on the degree of impaired hepatocellular function. Symptoms may include weakness, fatigability, weight loss, pruritus, fever, anorexia, nausea, occasional vomiting, abdominal pain, diarrhea, menstrual abnormalities, sterility, impotence, loss of libido, and hematemesis. Urine may be dark (brownish) because of the presence of urobilinogen, and stools may be pale and clay colored because of the absence of bilirubin.

Physical assessment: Jaundice, hepatomegaly, ascites, peripheral edema, pleural effusion, and fetor hepaticus (a musty, sweetish odor on the breath). There may be slight changes in personality and behavior, which can progress to coma (a result of hepatic encephalopathy); spider angiomas, testicular atrophy, gynecomastia, pectoral and axillary alopecia (a result of hormonal changes); splenomegaly; hemorrhoids (a result of portal hypertension complications); spider nevi; purpuric lesions; and palmar erythema. Asterixis (i.e., jerking movements of the hands and wrists when the wrists are dorsiflexed with the fingers extended) may be present in advanced cirrhosis.

History of: Excessive alcohol ingestion, chronic hepatitis B or C infection, exposure to hepatotoxic drugs or chemicals, biliary or metabolic disease.

DIAGNOSTIC TESTS

Hematologic: Red blood cells may be decreased in hypersplenism and decreased with hemorrhage. White blood cells and platelet counts may be decreased with hypersplenism and increased with infection.

Serum biochemical tests

Bilirubin levels: Elevated because of failure in hepatocyte metabolism and obstruction in some instances. Very high or persistently elevated levels are considered a poor prognostic sign, reflective of the poor excretory function of the liver.

Alkaline phosphatase levels: Normal to mildly elevated in most cases. In PBC it is elevated 2-3 times normal, reflective of biliary tract dysfunction.

Aspartate aminotransferase (AST) and alanine aminotransferase (ALT) levels: Usually elevated to more than 300 U with acute liver failure and normal or mildly elevated with chronic liver failure. ALT is more specific than AST for hepatocellular damage.

Albumin levels: Reduced, especially with ascites. Persistently low levels suggest a poor prognosis. This test is not a perfect indicator of liver function because it is affected by poor nutrition and fluid status.

Gamma glutamyl transpeptidase (GGT): Levels likely will be elevated, especially in patients who use alcohol or other substances toxic to the liver.

Globulins: Important in forming antibodies, proteins, and clotting factors. There are three types of globulins: alpha, beta, and gamma. Elevated gamma globulin levels occur in advanced cirrhosis.

Na^+ levels: Normal to low. Na^+ is retained but is associated with water retention, which results in normal serum Na^+ levels or even a dilutional hyponatremia. Often severe hyponatremia is present in the terminal stage and is associated with tense ascites and hepatorenal syndrome.

K^+ levels: Slightly reduced unless the patient has renal insufficiency, which would result in hyperkalemia. Chronic hypokalemic acidosis is common in patients with chronic alcoholic liver disease.

Glucose levels: Hypoglycemia possible because of impaired gluconeogenesis and glycogen depletion in patients with severe or terminal liver disease.

Blood urea nitrogen levels: May be slightly decreased because of failure of Krebs cycle enzymes in the liver or elevated because of bleeding or renal insufficiency.

Ammonia levels: May be elevated because of inability of the failing liver to convert ammonia to urea and shunting of intestinal blood via collateral vessels. Gastrointestinal (GI) hemorrhage, infection, or an increase in intestinal protein from dietary intake increases ammonia levels.

Note: *Serum ammonia sample must be transported to the lab immediately for processing.*

Coagulation: Prothrombin time (PT)/international normalized ratio (INR) is elevated and, in severe liver disease, unresponsive to vitamin K therapy. The failing liver is unable to synthesize clotting factors. Coagulation abnormalities usually include factor V but also factors II, VII, IX, and X. These tests are more sensitive in reflecting synthesis function of the liver.

Urine tests: Urine bilirubin is increased; urobilinogen is normal or increased; and proteinuria may be present.

Liver biopsy: Performed for three reasons: to establish a diagnosis, assess disease prognosis, and as a tool to assist in disease management. There are four methods of obtaining a liver biopsy: percutaneous, including the techniques of palpation/percussion guided, image guided, and real-time image guided; transvenous (transjugular or transfemoral); surgical/laparoscopic; and plugged biopsy. Plugged biopsy is a modification of the percutaneous method; the biopsy area is plugged with collagen or thrombin as the needle is removed, but the sheath remains in place. This technique may be safer for those cirrhosis patients with coagulopathy or thrombocytopenia. Preparation for liver biopsy includes patient teaching and education related to the disease and procedure; placement of an intravenous catheter; preparation for oral anxiolysis or conscious sedation; and type and crossmatching in the event of hemorrhage. Liver biopsy produces a tissue specimen for histological analysis. It is considered the definitive test for determining the extent of disease in cirrhosis.

Radiologic studies: Ultrasound may be used to assess size of the liver and spleen, screen for liver tumors (particularly hepatocellular carcinoma), and assess for signs of biliary obstruction. A Doppler study can also be performed to assess blood flow through the portal vessels. Computed tomography (CT) scan of the abdomen and magnetic resonance imaging (MRI) can show great detail related to assessment of hepatic vasculature and any masses. With MRI, a cholangiogram can be performed, eliminating the need for endoscopic retrograde cholangiopancreatography (ERCP).

Angiographic studies: Establish portal vein patency and visualize portosystemic collateral vessels to determine cause of and effective treatment for variceal bleeding. Portal venous anatomy must be established before such operations as portal systemic shunt or hepatic transplantation. In patients with previously constructed surgical shunts, loss of patency may be confirmed as a factor leading to the present bleeding episode. The most common procedure is portal venography by indirect angiography. The femoral artery is catheterized, and contrast material is injected into the splenic artery. Contrast material flows through the spleen into the splenic and portal veins.

- Hepatic vein wedge pressure is measured by introducing a balloon catheter into the femoral vein and threading it into a hepatic vein until it becomes wedged in a venule by a balloon. This pressure reading represents the hepatic sinusoidal pressure.

Esophagogastroduodenoscopy (EGD or upper endoscopy): Visualizes the esophagus and stomach directly via a fiberoptic endoscope. Varices in the esophagus and upper portion of the stomach are identified, and attempts are made to identify the exact source of bleeding. Variceal bleeding may be treated by band ligation, sclerotherapy, electrocautery, laser, vasoconstrictive agents, or other methods during the endoscopic procedure.

Critical flicker frequency: In the past, psychometric testing has been used to detect minimal hepatic encephalopathy (MHE). MHE can affect the patient's quality of life and ability to safely carry out activities of daily living. Psychometric testing is affected by variables such as age, educational level, and learning. Critical flicker frequency (CFF) testing can be used in place of psychometric testing because it is not affected by the variables that affect psychometric testing. CFF is a neurophysiologic test to assess the ability of the central nervous system to detect flickering light. In addition to assessing presence of MHE, the tool can also assess the level of recovery from MHE after treatment has been initiated.

Nursing Diagnosis:

Impaired Gas Exchange

related to alveolar hypoventilation due to shallow breathing occurring with ascites or hepatic hydrothorax; altered oxygen-carrying capacity of the blood occurring with anemia; and possible ventilation/perfusion mismatching

Desired Outcome: Within 24 hr of admission, the patient has adequate gas exchange as evidenced by $PaCO_2$ 45 mm Hg or less, PaO_2 80 mm Hg or more, O_2 saturation greater than 92%, and respiratory rate (RR) 12-20 breaths/min with normal depth and pattern (eupnea).

ASSESSMENT/INTERVENTIONS	RATIONALES
Monitor arterial blood gas (ABG) values and pulse oximetry; notify the health care provider of PaO_2 less than 80 mm Hg or O_2 saturation 92% or less. Administer oxygen as prescribed.	These lower than normal values usually signal the need for supplemental oxygen.
Obtain baseline abdominal girth measurement, and measure girth either daily or every shift. Measure around the same circumferential area each time, marking the site with indelible ink. Report significant findings to the health care provider.	An increase in abdominal girth indicates increased ascitic fluid accumulation, which can cause pressure on the diaphragm with subsequent dyspnea.
During complaints of dyspnea or orthopnea, assist the patient into semi-Fowler's or high Fowler's position.	These positions promote gas exchange, which is likely to be altered by pressure of ascitic fluid on the diaphragm.
Encourage position changes and deep breathing at frequent intervals. Teach use of incentive spirometry.	Deep breathing expands the alveoli and aids in mobilizing secretions to the airway.
Include ambulation and movement from bed to chair as a part of position changes and deep breathing exercises.	Getting the patient out of bed will prevent deconditioning of the muscles and enable the patient to better perform incentive spirometry.
If secretions are present, ensure that the patient coughs frequently.	Coughing further promotes mobilization and clearing of secretions.
! Notify the health care provider if the patient has fever, chills, diaphoresis, and adventitious breath sounds.	These are indicators of respiratory infection, which can lead to complications such as pneumonia and respiratory distress. Patients with severe cirrhosis are weak and, with poor maintenance of secretions, are more susceptible to infections.
! Position the patient in a side-lying position during episodes of vomiting.	This position decreases risk of aspiration, which could result in respiratory complications such as pneumonia.

Nursing Diagnosis:

Risk for Bleeding

related to portal hypertension and altered clotting factors

Desired Outcomes: The patient is free of bleeding/hemorrhage as evidenced by blood pressure (BP) at least 90/60 mm Hg; heart rate (HR) 100 bpm or less; warm extremities; distal pulses greater than 2 on a 0-4 scale; brisk capillary refill (less than 2 sec); and orientation to person, place, and time. Bruising, melena, and hematemesis are absent.

ASSESSMENT/INTERVENTIONS	RATIONALES
Assess vital signs (VS) q4h (or more frequently if VS are outside of the patient's baseline values).	Upper GI hemorrhage is common in patients with chronic liver disease and can result from esophageal varices, portal hypertensive gastropathy, duodenal or gastric ulcers, or Mallory-Weiss tear (mucosal laceration at the juncture of the distal esophagus and proximal stomach). Early diagnosis is essential to enable appropriate intervention. Hypotension and increased HR, as well as cool extremities, delayed capillary refill, decreased amplitude of distal pulses, mental status changes, and decreasing level of consciousness (LOC), are indicators of hypovolemia and hemorrhage.
Assess for signs of bleeding and notify the health care provider of significant findings.	Bruising, melena, and hematemesis are signs of bleeding. Altered VS, irritability, air hunger, pallor, and weakness are signs of significant bleeding and necessitate prompt intervention.
Inspect stools for the presence of blood; perform stool occult blood test as indicated.	This is an assessment for bleeding within the GI tract.
Monitor PT and INR for abnormality.	INR: Normal range is less than 2.0 sec for patients not receiving anticoagulant therapy. PT: Normal range is 10.5-13.5 sec. A PT that is prolonged signals the patient is at risk for bleeding.
Teach the patient to avoid swallowing foods that are chemically or mechanically irritating.	Rough or spicy foods, hot foods, hot liquids, and alcohol may be injurious to the esophagus and result in bleeding.
Teach the importance of avoiding actions such as sneezing, lifting, or vomiting.	These actions increase intraabdominothoracic pressure, which can result in bleeding.
Administer stool softeners as prescribed.	Stool softeners help prevent straining with defecation, which puts patients at risk for bleeding.
As appropriate, encourage intake of foods rich in vitamin K (e.g., spinach, cabbage, cauliflower, liver).	These foods may help decrease PT.
As often as possible, avoid invasive procedures such as giving injections and taking rectal temperatures.	If clotting is altered, invasive procedures could result in prolonged bleeding.
Monitor the patient undergoing band ligation or injection sclerotherapy of varices for increased HR, decreased BP, pallor, weakness, and air hunger.	These are signs of esophageal perforation caused by the treatment of varices, whether by injection, cautery, or the scope itself.
If signs of perforation occur, notify the health care provider immediately, keep the patient nothing by mouth (NPO), and prepare for gastric suction. Administer antibiotics as prescribed to prevent infection.	NPO status and gastric suction prevent leakage of fluid, secretions, or food through the perforation into the mediastinum. This emergency situation necessities immediate intervention.

Nursing Diagnoses:

Excess Fluid Volume
Risk for Electrolyte Imbalance

related to compromised regulatory mechanism with sequestration of fluids occurring with portal hypertension and hepatocellular failure

Desired Outcome: By at least 24 hr before hospital discharge, the patient is normovolemic as evidenced by stable or decreasing abdominal girth, RR 12-20 breaths/min with normal depth and pattern (eupnea), HR 100 bpm or less, edema 1 or less on a 0-4 scale, and absence of crackles (rales).

ASSESSMENT/INTERVENTIONS	RATIONALES
Obtain baseline abdominal girth measurement.	A baseline assessment enables comparison for subsequent assessments. Girth measurements indicate amount of ascitic fluid in the abdomen and provide information regarding effectiveness of medical treatment.
Place the patient in a supine position and mark the abdomen with indelible ink. Measure girth daily or every shift as appropriate.	These measures ensure accurate serial measurements from the same circumferential site.
⚠ Monitor and record weight and I&O.	Output should be equal to or exceed intake. Weight loss should not exceed 0.5 kg/day (1.1 lb/day) except in the presence of massive edema or ascites, which would permit a greater loss. Rapid diuresis from diuretics can lead to loss or shifts in electrolytes, particularly sodium, leading to encephalopathy and elevated creatinine.
⚠ Assess the degree of edema from 1 (barely detectable) to 4 (deep, persistent pitting), and document accordingly.	The presence of edema signals excess sodium intake or low serum albumin. Low albumin levels are associated with ascites; persistently low levels suggest a poor prognosis.
⚠ Monitor serum Na$^+$ and K$^+$ values and report abnormalities to the health care provider.	Optimal values are serum Na$^+$ 137-147 mEq/L and serum K$^+$ 3.5-5 mEq/L. Na$^+$ is retained but is associated with water retention, which results in normal serum Na$^+$ levels or even a dilutional hyponatremia. Severe hyponatremia is present in the terminal stage and is associated with tense ascites and hepatorenal syndrome. K$^+$ may be slightly reduced unless the patient has renal insufficiency, which would result in hyperkalemia. Chronic hypokalemic acidosis is common in patients with chronic alcoholic liver disease.
⚠ Be alert to dyspnea, basilar crackles that do not clear with coughing, orthopnea, and tachypnea. Report significant findings to the health care provider.	These are clinical indicators of pulmonary edema, which occurs from excess fluid volume in the circulatory system. Symptoms also may be present with pleural effusion caused by a small defect in the right hemidiaphragm, which develops with acute, rapid shortness of breath as the abdomen decompresses.
Give frequent mouth care, and provide ice chips to help minimize thirst.	These measures help minimize thirst while not compounding problems with fluid volume excess.
As indicated, remind the patient to avoid food and nonfood items that contain sodium, such as antacids, baking soda, and some mouthwashes.	Sodium may be restricted because of retention by the kidneys.
Elevate the lower extremities.	This will decrease peripheral edema.
Apply antiembolism hose or support stockings, sequential compression devices, or pneumatic foot compression devices as prescribed.	These garments/devices decrease peripheral edema by external compression of the extremities.
⚠ Monitor for signs of variceal hemorrhage (see **Risk for Bleeding,** earlier).	Rapid increases in intravascular volume can precipitate variceal hemorrhage in susceptible individuals.

Nursing Diagnosis:

Imbalanced Nutrition: Less Than Body Requirements

related to anorexia, nausea, or malabsorption

Desired Outcome: By at least 24 hr before hospital discharge, the patient demonstrates progress toward adequate nutritional status as evidenced by stable weight, balanced intake and output, stable blood glucose levels, and normal electrolyte values.

ASSESSMENT/INTERVENTIONS	RATIONALES
Assess and record intake and output (I&O); weigh the patient daily.	These measures help assess adequacy of diet/nutritional intake and measure effectiveness of diuretic therapy for ascites.
Explain dietary restrictions. Encourage the patient to eat foods that are permitted within dietary restrictions.	With fluid retention and ascites, sodium and fluids are restricted. Sodium intake should be less than 2000 mg daily in the presence of ascites/edema. Fluid restriction of 1.5 L/day may be required in the presence of ascites/edema. 25%-30% of calories should be from fat. Malnourished patients may need 30-40 kcal/kg/day of protein.
Monitor glucose levels.	Patients with cirrhosis may have glucose intolerance or diabetes. No more than 5-6 g/kg/day of glucose should be given.
Encourage small, frequent meals, including a bedtime snack or late evening meal, and caution the patient to avoid missing meals.	This helps ensure adequate nutrition without causing bloating from large meals.
Or administer parenteral or enteral nutrition if prescribed (see "Providing Nutritional Support," p. 539).	Parenteral nutrition is administered only if nutritional needs cannot be met via oral or enteral routes. Enteral nutrition may be used in patients with a functional gut who cannot meet their protein energy needs via the oral route.
Encourage significant others to bring desirable foods as permitted.	Patients are more likely to consume foods they like.
Administer vitamin and mineral supplements as prescribed.	For example, folic acid may be given for macrocytic anemia and vitamin K for a prolonged PT.
Teach the patient about the potential use of milk thistle.	Milk thistle *(Silybum marianum)* has been found to diminish complications associated with cirrhosis.
Administer the following prescribed medications: acid suppression agents, antiemetics, and cathartics.	These agents decrease gastric distress, which may facilitate intake.
Manage prescribed therapies such as diuresis, colloid replacement, and paracentesis.	These therapies relieve/mobilize ascites and decrease pressure on intraabdominal structures, which may decrease a sense of early satiety caused by severe ascites.
Encourage abstinence of alcohol in patients with alcoholic cirrhosis.	This remains the primary intervention in patients with alcohol-induced cirrhosis. Abstinence can result in healing of reversible factors of alcoholic liver disease over a period of months. Continued use of alcohol will further damage the liver to the point of irreversibility.

Nursing Diagnosis:

Acute Confusion (or risk for same)

related to neurosensory changes occurring with cerebral accumulation of ammonia or GI bleeding

Desired Outcome: The patient verbalizes orientation to person, place, and time; exhibits intact signature; and is free of symptoms of injury caused by neurosensory changes.

ASSESSMENT/INTERVENTIONS	RATIONALES
Perform a baseline assessment of the patient's personality characteristics, LOC, and orientation. Enlist aid of the patient's significant others to help determine slight changes in personality or behavior.	Having a baseline assessment will help determine subsequent changes in personality or behavior, which could progress to hepatic coma if left unchecked.
Have the patient demonstrate signature daily.	If writing deteriorates, hepatic encephalopathy may be worsening.
Be alert to generalized muscle twitching and asterixis (flapping tremor induced by dorsiflexion of wrist and extension of fingers). Report significant findings to the health care provider.	Asterixis may be present in advanced cirrhosis.

ASSESSMENT/INTERVENTIONS

RATIONALES

ASSESSMENT/INTERVENTIONS	RATIONALES
⚠ Monitor for indicators of GI bleeding, including melena or hematemesis. Report bleeding promptly to the health care provider.	GI bleeding can precipitate hepatic encephalopathy.
⚠ Keep side rails up and the bed in its lowest position, and assist with ambulation when need is determined.	These measures protect the patient from injury that could be precipitated by a confused state. Because of the patient's encephalopathy and resulting neurosensory changes, reminders and reorientation are necessary to help ensure the patient's safety. Additionally, the patient may be experiencing alcohol withdrawal (in cases of alcohol cirrhosis), which would place the patient at risk for seizures.
⚠ Avoid opioid analgesics and phenothiazines. Use caution when administering sedatives, antihistamines, and other agents affecting the central nervous system.	Opioids and sedatives are metabolized by the liver and therefore are contraindicated. Small doses of benzodiazepines with a short half-life may be administered if absolutely necessary.

ADDITIONAL NURSING DIAGNOSES/PROBLEMS:

"Hepatitis" for **Deficient Knowledge** (causes of hepatitis and modes of transmission)   p. 438

✓ PATIENT-FAMILY TEACHING AND DISCHARGE PLANNING

When providing patient-family teaching, focus on sensory information, avoid giving excessive information, and initiate a visiting nurse referral for necessary follow-up teaching of any skilled care needed after discharge. Include verbal and written information about the following:

- ✓ Medications, including drug name, purpose, dosage, schedule, precautions, and potential side effects. Also discuss drug-drug, food-drug, and herb-drug interactions.
- ✓ Dietary restrictions, in particular those of sodium, protein, and ammonia.
- ✓ Potential need for lifestyle changes, including avoiding alcoholic beverages. Stress that alcohol cessation is a major factor in survival of this disease. Include

appropriate referrals (e.g., to Alcoholics Anonymous, Al-Anon, and Alateen). As appropriate, provide referrals to community nursing support agencies.
- ✓ Awareness of hepatotoxic agents, especially over-the-counter drugs, including acetaminophen, aspirin, and many popular complementary and alternative use medications, such as herbals, dietary supplements, and vitamins.
- ✓ Importance of deep breathing exercises when ascites is present.
- ✓ Indicators of variceal bleeding/hemorrhage (i.e., vomiting blood, change in LOC) and need to inform the health care provider if they occur.
- ✓ Telephone numbers to call in case questions or concerns arise about therapy or disease after discharge. Additional general information can be obtained by contacting National Institute of Diabetes & Digestive & Kidney Diseases at *www.niddk.nih.gov*
- ✓ For patients awaiting transplantation, provide the following information: United Network for Organ Sharing at *www.unos.org*
- ✓ As an additional information source, refer patients to American Liver Foundation at *www.liverfoundation.org* or Canadian Liver Foundation at *www.liver.ca*

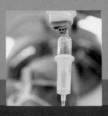

Crohn's Disease 55

OVERVIEW/PATHOPHYSIOLOGY

Crohn's disease (CD), also known as *regional enteritis, granulomatous colitis,* or *transmural colitis,* is a chronic inflammatory disease that can involve any part of the gastrointestinal (GI) tract from the mouth to the anus. Usually the disease occurs segmentally, demonstrating discontinuous areas of disease with segments of healthy bowel in between. In 45%-50% of cases, the end of the ileum and cecum/ascending colon are involved (ileocolitis); in 35% of cases, the terminal ileum is affected (ileitis); and in 20% of cases, the colon alone is affected (Crohn's colitis). A small number of patients have involvement of the jejunum, duodenum, stomach, esophagus, and mouth; in these cases, the ileum, colon, or both are also involved. Approximately 30%-35% of patients have perianal fistulas, fissures, or abscesses. The disease affects all layers of the bowel: the mucosa, submucosa, circular and longitudinal muscles, and serosa, predisposing to intestinal strictures and fistulas. A family history of this disease or ulcerative colitis occurs in 15%-20% of affected patients.

The cause of CD is unknown, but theories include infection, immunologic factors, environmental factors, and genetic predisposition. In a genetically susceptible subject, an outside agent or substance, such as a bacterium, virus, or other antigen, interacts with the body's immune system to trigger the disease or may cause damage to the intestinal wall, initiating or accelerating the disease process. The resulting inflammatory response continues unregulated by the immune system. As a result, inflammation continues to damage the intestinal wall, causing the symptoms of CD. It is a chronic disease that has no cure. However, there are effective treatments to aid in controlling the disease. Initial treatment is nonoperative, individualized, and based on symptomatic relief. Surgery is reserved for complications rather than used as a primary form of therapy.

Since the end of World War II, the incidence of CD has increased steadily, whereas that of ulcerative colitis (UC) has stabilized. This rise may reflect increased diagnostic awareness rather than increased incidence of CD. There is a 20-fold increase in risk of inflammatory bowel disease (IBD) in first-degree relatives of individuals with CD. CD is generally diagnosed between the ages of 15 and 35, but it also can occur in young children and in people 70 years of age or older.

Prevalence is essentially equal in women and in men. CD, like UC, is seen more frequently in the Caucasian population and in Ashkenazi Jews than in nonwhite populations and in people of non-Jewish descent. It is more prevalent in urban, developed countries with temperate climates than in rural, more southern countries. However, increasing incidence is being observed in African American populations and in Japan and South America. Cigarette smoking has been shown to increase the risk of developing CD and is associated with resistance to medical therapy and recurrence of disease after surgery.

HEALTH CARE SETTING

Primary care, with possible hospitalization resulting from complications

ASSESSMENT

Signs and symptoms: Clinical presentation varies as a direct reflection of the location of the inflammatory process and its extent, severity, and relationship to contiguous structures. Sometimes onset is abrupt, and the patient can appear to have appendicitis, UC, intestinal obstruction, or a fever of obscure origin. Acute symptoms include right lower quadrant (RLQ) pain, tenderness, spasm, flatulence, nausea, fever, and diarrhea. A more typical picture is insidious onset with more persistent but less severe symptoms, such as vague abdominal pain, unexplained anemia, and fever. Diarrhea—liquid, soft, or mushy stools—is the most common symptom. The presence of gross blood is rare. Abdominal pain is a common symptom, and it may be colicky or crampy, initiated by meals, centered in the lower abdomen, and relieved by defecation because of chronic partial obstruction of the small intestine, colon, or both. As the disease progresses, anorexia, malnutrition, weight loss, anemia, lassitude, malaise, and fever can occur in addition to fluid, electrolyte, and metabolic disturbances.

Physical assessment: In early stages, examination is often normal but may demonstrate mild tenderness in the abdomen over the affected bowel. In more advanced disease, a palpable mass may be present, especially in the RLQ with terminal ileum involvement. Persistent rectal fissure, large ulcers, perirectal abscess, or rectal fistula is the first indication of disease in 15%-25% of patients with small bowel involvement and in 50%-75% of patients with colonic involvement.

Rectovaginal, abdominal, and enterovesical fistulas also can occur. Extraintestinal manifestations characteristic of UC do occur, but less commonly (10%-20%).

DIAGNOSTIC TESTS

Stool examination: Usually reveals occult blood; frank blood may be noted in stools of patients with colonic involvement or with ulcerations and fistulas of the rectum. A few patients have a presenting symptom of bloody diarrhea. Stool cultures and smears rule out bacterial and parasitic disorders. Specimens are also examined for fecal fat. Stool also is examined for the presence of white blood cells and certain proteins, the presence of which suggests inflammation.

Sigmoidoscopy: Evaluates possible colonic involvement and obtains rectal biopsy. The finding of granulomas on mucosal biopsy argues strongly for the diagnosis of CD. However, because granulomas are more numerous in the submucosa, suction biopsy of the rectum provides deeper, larger, and less traumatized specimens for a better diagnostic yield than mucosal biopsy obtained through an endoscope.

Colonoscopy: May help differentiate CD from UC. Characteristic patchy inflammation (skip lesions) rules out UC. However, colonoscopy usually does not add useful diagnostic information in the presence of positive findings from sigmoidoscopy or radiologic examination. When diagnosis is unclear and there is a question of malignancy, colonoscopy provides the means of directly visualizing mucosal changes and obtaining biopsies, brushings, and washings for cytologic examination. Colonoscopy also may assist in planning for surgery by documenting the extent of colonic disease. The evolving techniques of high-resolution and high-magnification endoscopy have the potential for detecting subtle mucosal changes.

Note: *Because of risk of perforation, this procedure may be contraindicated in patients with acute phases of Crohn's colitis or when deep ulcerations or fistulas are known to be present.*

Endoscopic ultrasonography: Aids in diagnosis of perirectal fistula and abscesses and in detecting transmural depth of inflammation in the bowel or esophagus, using an endoscopically placed ultrasound probe.

Small bowel enteroscopy: Permits visualization of the upper GI tract to identify areas of inflammation and bleeding to the level of the midjejunum.

Wireless capsule: Permits visualization of the small intestine to identify abnormalities. The patient swallows a large capsule that contains a small disposable camera; images are transmitted to a receiver on the patient's waist. New capsules that contain light filters to enhance mucosal abnormalities are under development and study.

Note: *Use is contraindicated if strictures exist, because strictures can prevent the capsule from progressing through the intestine; surgical removal of the capsule may be required.*

Barium enema and upper GI series with small bowel follow-through: Contribute to diagnosis of CD. Involvement of only the terminal ileum or segmental involvement of the colon or small intestine almost always indicates CD. Thickened bowel wall with stricture (string sign) separated by segments of normal bowel, cobblestone appearance, and presence of fistulas and skip lesions are common findings. A double-contrast barium enema technique may increase sensitivity in detecting early or subtle changes.

Note: *Barium enema may be contraindicated in patients with acute phases of Crohn's colitis because of risk of perforation. Upper GI barium series is contraindicated in patients in whom intestinal obstruction is suspected.*

Computed tomography (CT) scan: Complements information gathered via endoscopy and conventional radiography. In advanced disease, CT scanning clearly delineates extraluminal complications (e.g., abscess, phlegmon, bowel wall thickening, mesenteric inflammation). CT scan has been used also to percutaneously drain fistulas (colovesicular, enterovesicular, colovaginal, enterocolonic) and to evaluate perirectal disease, enterocutaneous fistula, and sinus tracts.

CT enterography (CTE): An emerging modality for specialized visualization of the small intestine and lumen and for depicting inflammatory changes.

Magnetic resonance imaging (MRI) and MR enterography (MRE): Imaging techniques used to evaluate extraluminal complications (e.g., perirectal fistula, sinus tracts, and abscesses) and the small intestine. Because they use a magnetic field and radio waves, their advantage is not exposing predominantly young patients to x-ray radiation as would occur with CT and CTE.

Serum antibody testing: In difficult to diagnose cases, may be helpful in differentiating CD from UC.

Radionuclide imaging: Intravenous (IV) indium-111– or technetium-99–labeled leukocytes migrate to areas of active inflammation and are then identified by scans performed after 4 and 24 hr. This procedure aids in differentiating CD from UC and evaluating abscess and fistula formation.

Blood tests: Are nonspecific for diagnosis of CD but help determine whether the inflammatory process is active and evaluate the patient's overall condition. Anemia may be present and may be microcytic because of iron deficiency from chronic blood loss and bone marrow depression secondary to chronic inflammatory process or megaloblastic because of folic acid or vitamin B_{12} deficiency (usually seen only in patients with extensive ileitis causing malabsorption). Increased white blood cell (WBC) count, sedimentation rate, and C-reactive protein reflect disease activity and inflammation. Hypoalbuminemia corresponds with disease activity and results from decreased protein intake, extensive malabsorption, and significant enteric loss of protein. Hypokalemia is seen in patients with chronic diarrhea; hypophosphatemia and hypocalcemia are seen in patients with significant malabsorption. Liver function studies may be abnormal secondary to pericholangitis.

Urinalysis and urine culture: May reveal urinary tract infection secondary to enterovesicular fistula.

Tests for malabsorption: Because patients with active, extensive disease (especially when it involves the small intestine) may develop malabsorption and malnutrition, the following tests are clinically significant: D-xylose tolerance test (for upper jejunal involvement); Schilling test (for ileal involvement); serum albumin, carotene, calcium, and phosphorus levels; and fecal fat (steatorrhea).

Nursing Diagnoses:

Deficient Fluid Volume
Risk for Electrolyte Imbalance

related to active loss occurring with diarrhea or presence of GI fistula

Desired Outcomes: The patient is normovolemic within 24 hr of admission as evidenced by balanced intake and output (I&O), urinary output 30 mL/hr or more, specific gravity 1.010-1.030, blood pressure (BP) 90/60 mm Hg or higher (or within the patient's normal range), respiratory rate (RR) 12-20 breaths/min, stable weight, good skin turgor, and moist mucous membranes. The patient reports that diarrhea is controlled. Serum electrolytes potassium, sodium, and chloride are all within optimal values as outlined in the first Rationales section, below.

ASSESSMENT/INTERVENTIONS	RATIONALES
Assess I&O and urinary specific gravity, weigh the patient daily, and monitor laboratory values to evaluate fluid and electrolyte status.	These assessments monitor for fluid loss and electrolyte imbalance. GI fluid losses (nasogastric [NG] suction, vomiting, diarrhea, fistula) can lead to hyponatremia, hypokalemia, and hypochloremia. Optimal values are serum K^+ 3.5-5.0 mEq/L, serum Na^+ 137-147 mEq/L, and serum Cl^- 95-108 mEq/L. Critical values: K^+ less than 2.5 or more than 6.5 mEq/L, Na^+ less than 120 or more than 160 mEq/L, Cl^- less than 80 or more than 115 mEq/L.
Assess frequency and consistency of stools. Keep a stool count, and measure the volume of liquid stools.	These assessments monitor for the presence and amount of blood, mucus, fat, and undigested food, which occur secondary to the underlying inflammatory process.
Assess for the presence of thirst, poor skin turgor, dryness of mucous membranes, fever, and concentrated (specific gravity greater than 1.030) and decreased urinary output.	These are indicators of dehydration.
Maintain the patient on parenteral replacement of fluids, electrolytes, and vitamins as prescribed.	Patients with involvement of the small intestine often require supplementation of vitamins and minerals, especially calcium, iron, folate, and magnesium secondary to malabsorption or to compensate for foods excluded from the diet. Patients with extensive ileal disease or resection often require vitamin B_{12} replacement, and if bile salt deficiency exists, cholestyramine and medium-chain triglycerides may be needed to control diarrhea and reduce fat malabsorption and steatorrhea. Vitamin D deficiency is common in these patients and may require replacement with cholecalciferol.
When the patient is taking food orally, provide the prescribed diet. Assess tolerance to the diet by determining incidence of cramping, diarrhea, and flatulence. Modify the diet plan accordingly.	Bland diets low in residue, roughage, and fat but high in protein, calories, carbohydrates, and vitamins provide good nutrition and reduce excessive stimulation of the bowel. A diet free of milk, milk products, gas-forming foods, alcohol, and iced beverages reduces cramping and diarrhea. Elemental diets (e.g., Vivonex, Ensure) that are free of bulk and residue, low in fat, and digested in the upper jejunum provide good nutrition with low fecal volume to enable bowel rest in selected patients. Use of elemental diets is being investigated for effectiveness as a primary therapy as an alternative to steroids and bowel rest in treating patients with acute CD.

Nursing Diagnoses:

Risk for Injury
Risk for Infection

related to potential complications caused by the intestinal inflammatory disorder

Desired Outcome: The patient is free from indicators of infection and intraabdominal injury/dysfunction as evidenced by normothermia; heart rate (HR) 60-100 bpm; RR 12-20 breaths/min; normal bowel sounds; absence of abdominal distention, rigidity, or localized pain and tenderness; absence of nausea and vomiting; negative culture results; no significant change in mental status; and orientation to person, place, and time.

ASSESSMENT/INTERVENTIONS	RATIONALES
Assess for abdominal distention, abdominal rigidity, and increased episodes of nausea and vomiting.	These are indicators of intestinal obstruction. Contributing factors to the development of intestinal obstruction include use of opioids and prolonged use of antidiarrheal medication.
Assess for fever, increased RR and HR, chills, diaphoresis, and increased abdominal discomfort.	These indicators can occur with intestinal perforation, abscess or fistula formation, or generalized fecal peritonitis and septicemia. **Note:** Systemic therapy with corticosteroids and antibiotics can mask development of these complications.
Evaluate mental status, orientation, and level of consciousness q2-4h.	Mental cloudiness, lethargy, and increased restlessness can occur with peritonitis and septicemia.
Obtain cultures of blood, urine, fistulas, or other possible sources of infection, as prescribed, if the patient has a sudden temperature elevation. Monitor culture reports, and notify the health care provider promptly of any positive results.	Abscesses or fistulas to the abdominal wall, bladder, or vagina are common in CD and are potential sources of infection, as are abscesses or fistulas to other loops of the small bowel and colon.
If draining fistulas or abscesses are present, change dressings and pouching system or irrigate tubes or drains as prescribed. Note color, character, and odor of all drainage. Refer to wound, ostomy, continence (WOC)/enterostomal therapy (ET) nurse for fistula management as needed.	Foul-smelling or abnormal drainage, which can signal infection, or loss of tube/drain patency should be reported to the health care provider promptly for intervention.
Administer antibiotics as prescribed and on the prescribed schedule.	Maintaining the therapeutic serum level of antibiotics will help control suppurative complications (e.g., bacterial overgrowth) and perianal fistulas in patients with mild to moderate colonic or ileocolonic CD. In patients who are allergic, intolerant, or unresponsive to sulfasalazine, metronidazole appears to be effective in colonic disease and in promoting healing of perianal disease. Long-term use of metronidazole is limited because of the potential for peripheral neuropathy and other side effects. Patients with bacterial overgrowth in the small intestine may be treated with broad-spectrum antibiotics. Ciprofloxacin may be useful in treating patients who are intolerant or unresponsive to metronidazole therapy.
Administer immunomodulators and biologic agents as prescribed.	These agents aid in healing, especially with refractory disease or active disease unresponsive to conventional therapy; reduce drainage of perianal and cutaneous fistulas; reduce steroid dosage; and maintain remission.
Use good hand hygiene before and after caring for the patient, and dispose of dressings and drainage using proper infection control techniques (see Appendix A, p. 747).	These measures prevent transmission of potentially infectious organisms. Since immunomodulators, steroids, and biologic agents can reduce the response of the immune system, the patient can be at increased risk for infection, and therefore should be monitored closely.

Nursing Diagnoses:

Acute Pain
Nausea

related to the intestinal inflammatory process

Desired Outcomes: The patient's subjective perception of discomfort decreases within 1 hr of intervention, as documented by a pain scale. Objective indicators, such as grimacing, are absent or diminished.

ASSESSMENT/INTERVENTIONS	RATIONALES
Assess and document the characteristics of discomfort, and assess whether it is associated with ingestion of certain foods or with emotional stress. Devise a pain scale with the patient, rating discomfort from 0 (no pain) to 10 (worst pain). Eliminate foods that cause cramping and discomfort.	The discomfort of pain, nausea, and abdominal cramping may be associated with certain foods or emotional stress. A pain scale will help determine the degree of relief obtained after interventions have been implemented.
As prescribed, keep the patient nothing by mouth (NPO) and provide parenteral nutrition.	These measures allow bowel rest, which will help alleviate discomfort.
Administer antidiarrheal medications and analgesics as prescribed.	These medications are given to reduce abdominal discomfort, often with a concomitant decrease in abdominal cramping.
Assess the patient's response to these medications. Report significant findings to the health care provider.	If the patient does not respond appropriately to standard antidiarrheal medications and mild sedation, the presence of obstruction, bowel perforation, or abscess formation is suspected.
Assess the patient's level of discomfort at frequent intervals, using the pain scale as above. Also, instruct the patient to request analgesia before pain becomes severe.	Prolonged stimulation of pain receptors results in increased sensitivity to painful stimuli and increases the amount of medication required to relieve discomfort.
Provide nasal and oral care at frequent intervals.	These measures lessen discomfort from NPO status and presence of an NG tube.
Administer antiemetic medications before meals.	These agents enhance appetite when nausea is a problem.
For additional information, see "Pain," p. 39.	

Nursing Diagnoses:

Diarrhea
Dysfunctional Gastrointestinal Motility

related to the intestinal inflammatory process

Desired Outcome: The patient reports a reduction in frequency of stools and a return to more normal stool consistency within 3 days of hospital admission.

ASSESSMENT/INTERVENTIONS	RATIONALES
Assess the patient's bowel pattern. If the patient is experiencing frequent and urgent passage of loose stools, provide a covered bedpan or commode or be sure the bathroom is easily accessible and ready to use at all times.	Providing easy access to a bedpan, commode, or bathroom promotes patient safety, reduces stress, and enables patients to cope with diarrhea more effectively.
Empty the bedpan or commode promptly.	This intervention will control odor and decrease the patient's anxiety and self-consciousness.
Administer antidiarrheal medications as prescribed.	These agents decrease fluidity and the number of stools, inhibit gastrointestinal peristaltic activity, and increase transit time and stool consistency.

ASSESSMENT/INTERVENTIONS	RATIONALES
Administer cholestyramine as prescribed.	This agent controls diarrhea if bile salt deficiency (because of ileal disease or resection) is contributing to this problem.
Eliminate or decrease fat content in the diet.	Fat can increase diarrhea in individuals with malabsorption syndromes.
Restrict raw vegetables and fruits; whole-grain cereals; condiments; gas-forming foods; alcohol; iced and carbonated beverages; and, in lactose-intolerant patients, milk and milk products.	These foods and beverages also can precipitate diarrhea and cramping. When remission occurs, a less restricted diet can be tailored to the individual patient, excluding foods known to precipitate symptoms.

Nursing Diagnosis:

Activity Intolerance

related to generalized weakness occurring with the intestinal inflammatory process

Desired Outcome: The patient adheres to the prescribed rest regimen and sets appropriate goals for self-care as the condition improves (optimally within 3-7 days of admission).

ASSESSMENT/INTERVENTIONS	RATIONALES
Keep the patient's environment quiet.	This will facilitate needed rest.
Assist with activities of daily living (ADLs), and plan nursing care to provide maximum rest periods.	Adequate rest is necessary to sustain remission.
Facilitate coordination of health care providers. Provide 90 min for undisturbed rest.	This enables rest periods between care activities.
As prescribed, administer sedatives and tranquilizers.	These agents promote rest and reduce anxiety.
As the patient's physical condition improves, encourage self-care to the greatest extent possible and assist the patient with setting realistic, attainable goals.	These measures enable the patient to increase endurance incrementally to his or her tolerance and prevent problems associated with prolonged bedrest.
For additional information, see **Risk for Activity Intolerance**, p. 61, in "Prolonged Bedrest."	

Nursing Diagnoses:

Deficient Knowledge

related to unfamiliarity with medications used for the treatment of CD

Risk for Allergy Response

related to immunomodulator and biologic/anti-TNF medications

Desired Outcome: Immediately following teaching, the patient verbalizes accurate information about the medications used during exacerbations of CD.

ASSESSMENT/INTERVENTIONS	RATIONALES
Teach the patient about the following, referring to the therapeutic agent or combination of agents prescribed:	Treatment is customized based upon type and severity of symptoms.
Aminosalicylates: Sulfasalazine and 5-Aminosalicytic Acid (5-ASA) Preparations	
	These medications work on the intestinal lining to decrease inflammation.

continued

ASSESSMENT/INTERVENTIONS | RATIONALES

Sulfasalazine

	This medication is given to treat acute exacerbations of colonic and ileocolonic disease. Although sulfasalazine does not prevent recurrence of CD, patients who respond tend to benefit from long-term therapy and relapse when the agent is discontinued. It appears to be more effective in patients with mild to moderate disease limited to the colon than in those with disease limited to the small bowel.
- Folic acid supplements are necessary during treatment.	Sulfasalazine impairs folate absorption.
- Have blood count done within the first 4 mo of treatment.	WBCs may be lowered with this medication, and anemia can occur (uncommon).
- Have liver enzymes checked within the first year of treatment.	Hepatitis, though uncommon, has occurred.
- Notify the health care provider immediately if discoloration of the skin or urine occurs.	Sulfasalazine may produce orange-yellow discoloration of the skin and urine and could cause contact lenses to turn yellow.
- Men may want to check for infertility by sperm analysis.	Infertility has occurred in some men, though it reverses when patients stop taking the medication.
- Be alert to the following side effects: fever, skin rash, joint pain, nausea, headache, or fatigue when the dose exceeds 4 tablets/day.	Most side effects are sulfa related and caused by the sulfa component of the drug.

5-Aminosalicylic Acid (5-ASA) Preparations

	5-ASA is used in patients unable to tolerate sulfasalazine. Extended-release mesalamine (Pentasa®) and delayed-released mesalamine (Asacol®) are used for mildly to moderately active ileocolonic and ileal disease and for maintenance therapy in selected patients. They may delay or prevent postoperative recurrence when initiated soon after ileal and colonic resection.
- Patients on prolonged treatment must have an annual kidney profile and urine examination, including blood urea nitrogen (BUN) and creatinine.	There is risk of kidney damage with high doses (above 4000 mg/day).

Corticosteroids

	These agents reduce the active inflammatory response by depressing the immune system, decreasing edema in moderate to severe forms, and controlling exacerbations in chronic disease. The oral route is most effective for disease limited to the small intestine.
- Check BP during each clinic/office visit.	Secondary hypertension is a potential side effect.
- Test blood glucose after 1 mo of therapy, then q3mo.	Increased blood glucose level can occur.
- Schedule an eye examination annually. However, notify the health care provider immediately if experiencing eye pain or vision changes because some complications may result in permanent vision loss.	There is potential for cataract formation, glaucoma, and temporary vision changes during treatment with steroids. Also, extraintestinal manifestations of CD can involve the eye.
- Schedule bone mineral density scanning if on more than 3 consecutive mo of corticosteroid treatment or if on recurrent courses of corticosteroids.	Bone loss can occur with prolonged use of steroids, as well as occur as a result of chronic inflammation.
- Be alert to rounding of face (moon face), acne, increased appetite and weight gain, red marks/blotches on skin, facial hair, severe mood swings, weakness, and leg cramps.	These are typical side effects with steroids.
- As active disease subsides, prednisone is tapered.	The goal is eventual elimination of the medication in order to prevent complications from long-term usage.
- In some cases of chronic disease, continuous corticosteroid therapy may be necessary.	Many patients with CD become steroid dependent, meaning they are symptomatic with low-dose therapy (5-15 mg/day) or with total discontinuation of the drug.

ASSESSMENT/INTERVENTIONS	RATIONALES
- A nonsystemic steroidal agent, budesonide, is approved for treatment of mild to moderate disease involving the ileum and cecum or ascending colon.	It provides benefits of traditional therapy with reduced side effects, since it is nonsystemic and therefore primarily released in the GI tract. It is used for flare-ups but not commonly for maintenance therapy.
- Avoid grapefruit and grapefruit juice when taking budesonide.	They may increase drug effects.
- Topical therapy is an effective route.	Topical therapy with hydrocortisone has controlled inflammation via retention enemas for patients with proctosigmoiditis (involvement to 40 cm); suppositories have been used for patients with Crohn's proctitis.

Immunomodulators
Azathioprine
6-mercaptopurine (6-MP)
Methotrexate

	These agents modify or "quiet down" the immune system in order to decrease inflammation. They may take several months to be effective. Once they do take effect, they allow dosage reduction or withdrawal of corticosteroids in steroid-dependent patients, are used for maintenance therapy with a lower relapse rate, and aid in healing and reducing drainage of perianal fistulas.
- If taking azathioprine or 6-MP check blood cell counts every other week until dose has been stable for 6 mo. Then monitor every month for 3 mo, then once every 3 mo.	Lowered WBC count, anemia, low platelet levels, low hemoglobin levels, and abnormal liver enzyme levels can occur.
- Be alert to and report the following when taking azathioprine or 6-MP: allergic reaction (fever, skin rash, joint aches), pancreatitis (severe abdominal pain typically radiating through the back), and infection.	These are possible side effects/allergic reactions.
- Methotrexate is used with extreme caution in people with preexisting liver disease or who consume significant quantities of alcohol. Blood cell counts and liver enzymes are checked monthly for first 3 mo, then at 3-mo intervals.	This drug can affect liver function.
- Methotrexate is contraindicated during pregnancy. In women anticipating pregnancy, methotrexate should be discontinued for at least 3 mo prior to planned conception.	It may cause fetal death and congenital abnormalities and can be transferred via breast milk.
- There is risk of malignancy with immunomodulators.	Lymphoma has occurred, but risk is considered to be low.

Biologic/Anti-TNF Agents
Adalimumab
Certolizumab pegol
Infliximab
Natalizumab

	These genetically engineered agents are designed to block inflammation or to stimulate antiinflammatory processes in the body. They are used intravenously (infliximab and natalizumab) or subcutaneously (adalimumab and certolizumab pegol) to treat and maintain remission of moderate to severe active disease unresponsive to conventional therapy. Infliximab also is used to treat and maintain remission in fistulizing disease.
- The patient should be alert to and report sore throat, upper respiratory infection, abscesses, sinusitis, and bronchitis.	There is risk of altered immune response with these medications; therefore, risk for infection is increased.
- There is risk of malignancy.	Lymphoma has occurred in some patients.
- Infusion- and injection site–related reactions that occur during or shortly after administration include fever, chills, headache, low BP, rash, muscle and joint pain, chest pain, itching, and shortness of breath. Teach the patient to watch for reactions during and up to 2 hours after infusion.	These reactions usually are of short duration and almost always respond to treatment with acetaminophen, antihistamines, corticosteroids, or epinephrine as prescribed.
- A tuberculosis skin test should be performed before therapy is initiated.	Treatment of latent tuberculosis infection is needed before starting infliximab therapy.
- The patient needs to inform the health care providers of use of biologic/anti-TNF agents, and also use of immunomodulatory agents and corticosteroids, before receiving vaccines.	Live-virus vaccines should not be administered until therapy stops because these agents may affect normal immune response. However, immune status of the individual should be assessed on a case-by-case basis to determine risks versus benefits.

continued

Gastrointestinal Care Plans

ASSESSMENT/INTERVENTIONS	RATIONALES
Combination Therapy	
- Immunomodulators and biologic/anti-TNF agents	Both may be more effective in combination to maintain remission.
- Ensure that the patient verbalizes accurate knowledge about the purpose, precautions, and potential side effects of any prescribed medication he or she will be taking. Refer to the sections above that describe the potential side effects/allergic reactions that can occur with both types of medications.	A knowledgeable individual is more likely to adhere to the therapeutic regimen and promptly report untoward side effects to the health care provider.

ADDITIONAL NURSING DIAGNOSES/PROBLEMS:

✓ PATIENT-FAMILY TEACHING AND DISCHARGE PLANNING

When providing patient-family teaching, focus on sensory information, avoid giving excessive information, and initiate a visiting nurse referral for necessary follow-up teaching. Include verbal and written information about the following:

- ✓ Medications, including drug name, rationale, dosage, schedule, route of administration, precautions, and potential side effects. Also discuss drug-drug and food-drug interactions.
- ✓ Discuss herbal/alternative therapies, such as vitamins, herbs, dietary supplements, minerals, homeopathy, and probiotics, in order to minimize interactions with prescribed medications and adverse effects.
- ✓ Importance of taking medications as prescribed in order to maintain remission and prevent flares.
- ✓ Importance of tobacco cessation, since smoking is associated with resistance to medical therapy, recurrence of disease after surgery, and shortened duration of remission.
- ✓ Signs and symptoms that necessitate medical attention, including fever, nausea and vomiting, abdominal discomfort, any significant change in appearance and frequency of stools, or passage of stool through the vagina or stool mixed with urine, any of which can signal recurrence or complications of CD.

- ✓ Importance of dietary management to promote nutritional and fluid maintenance and prevent abdominal cramping, discomfort, and diarrhea.
- ✓ Importance of perineal/perianal skin care after bowel movements.
- ✓ Importance of balancing activities with rest periods, even during remission, because adequate rest is necessary to sustain remission.
- ✓ Referral to community resources, including the following organization: Crohn's & Colitis Foundation of America, Inc., at www.ccfa.org; Crohn's and Colitis Foundation of Canada at www.ccfc.ca; the website: UC and Crohn's Teen Site at www.ucandcrohns.org; and the following social media: Online Community at www.ccfacommunity.org, Facebook at https://www.facebook.com/ccfafb, and Twitter at http://twitter.com/ccfa
- ✓ Importance of follow-up medical care, including supportive psychotherapy, because of the chronic and progressive nature of CD.

In addition, if the patient has a fecal diversion (colostomy or ileostomy):

- ✓ Care of the incision, dressing changes, and bathing.
- ✓ Care of the stoma and peristomal skin, use of ostomy equipment, and method for obtaining supplies.
- ✓ Gradual resumption of ADLs, excluding heavy lifting (more than 10 lb), pushing, or pulling for 6-8 wk to prevent incisional herniation.
- ✓ Referral to community resources, including home health care agency, WOC/ET nurse, local ostomy association, the United Ostomy Association of America at uoaa.org, and the Young Ostomate and Diversion Alliance of America (for young adults ages 18 to 35 years) found under Affiliate Support Groups at uoaa.org
- ✓ Importance of reporting signs and symptoms that require medical attention, such as change in stoma color from the normal bright and shiny red; lesions of stomal mucosa that may indicate recurrence of disease; peristomal skin irritation; diarrhea or constipation, fever, chills, abdominal pain, distention, nausea, and vomiting; and incisional pain, local increased temperature, drainage, swelling, or redness.

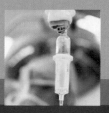

Fecal Diversions: Colostomy, Ileostomy, and Ileal Pouch Anal Anastomoses

56

OVERVIEW/PATHOPHYSIOLOGY

For a discussion of ulcerative colitis (UC), see p. 459; for a discussion of Crohn's disease (CD), see p. 420.

HEALTH CARE SETTING

Acute care on surgical unit, primary care, home care after hospital discharge

SURGICAL INTERVENTIONS

It is sometimes necessary to interrupt continuity of the bowel because of intestinal disease or its complications. A fecal diversion may be necessary to divert stool around a diseased portion of the bowel or, more commonly, out of the body. A fecal diversion can be located anywhere along the bowel, depending on location of the diseased or injured portion, and it can be permanent or temporary. The most common sites for fecal diversion are the colon and ileum.

Colostomy: Created when the surgeon brings a portion of the colon to the surface of the abdomen. An opening in the exteriorized colon permits elimination of flatus and stool through the stoma. Any part of the colon may be diverted into a colostomy.

Transverse colostomy: Most commonly created stoma to divert feces on a temporary basis. Surgical indications include relief of bowel obstruction before definitive surgery for tumors, inflammation, or diverticulitis and colon perforation secondary to trauma. Stool can be liquid to pastelike or soft and unformed, and bowel elimination is unpredictable. A temporary colostomy may be double barreled, with a proximal stoma through which stool is eliminated, and a distal stoma, called a *mucus fistula*, adjacent to the proximal stoma. More commonly, a loop colostomy is created with a supporting rod placed beneath it until the exteriorized loop of colon heals to the skin.

Descending or sigmoid colostomy: Usually a permanent fecal diversion. Rectal cancer is the most common cause for surgical intervention. Stool is usually formed, and some individuals may have stool elimination at predictable times. In a permanent colostomy, the surgeon brings the severed end of the colon to the abdominal skin surface. The diseased or injured portion of the colon and/or rectum is resected and

removed. To create the stoma, the colon above the skin surface is rolled back on itself to expose the mucosal surface of the intestine. The end of the cuff is sutured to the subcutaneous tissues with absorbable sutures to hold it in place as it heals.

Temporary colostomy: Typically created when there is significant inflammation in the diseased portion of the bowel (e.g., perforated diverticulum or ulcerative colitis) or when rectum-sparing surgery is performed for colorectal cancer. When a temporary colostomy is created, the severed end of the colon is brought through the abdominal wall as for a permanent colostomy. The diseased or injured portion of colon is resected and removed. The remaining rectum or rectosigmoid is oversewn and left in the peritoneal cavity; it is referred to as *Hartmann's pouch*. After the inflammatory process has resolved (e.g., 3-6 mo), the colostomy is taken down and reattached to the bowel of Hartmann's pouch, thus reconstructing continuity of the bowel and normal bowel elimination.

Cecostomy or ascending colostomy: Not a common procedure. A temporary diverting colostomy is used to bypass an unresectable tumor. The stool from an ascending colostomy is soft, unformed, pastelike, semiliquid, or liquid, and bowel elimination is unpredictable. Surgical procedure is similar to that with transverse colostomies.

Ileostomy:

Conventional (Brooke) ileostomy: Created by bringing a distal portion of the resected ileum through the abdominal wall. A permanent ileostomy is created by the same procedure discussed with a permanent colostomy. Surgical indications include ulcerative colitis (UC), Crohn's disease (CD), and familial adenomatous polyposis (FAP) requiring excision of the entire colon and rectum. For any ileostomy, the output is usually liquid (or, more rarely, pastelike) and is eliminated continually. The more proximal the ileostomy, the more active are digestive enzymes within the effluent (stool) and the greater their potential for irritation to exposed skin around the stoma. A collection pouch is worn over the stoma on the abdomen to collect gas and fecal discharge.

Temporary ileostomy: Usually a loop stoma with or without a supporting rod in place beneath the loop of the ileum until the exteriorized loop of ileum heals to the skin.

The purpose is to divert the fecal stream away from a more distal anastomotic site or fistula repair until healing has occurred.

Continent (Kock pouch) ileostomy: An intraabdominal pouch constructed from approximately 30 cm of distal ileum. Intussusception of a 10-cm portion of ileum is performed to form an outlet nipple valve from the pouch to the skin of the abdomen, where a stoma is constructed flush with the skin. The intraabdominal pouch is continent for gas and fecal discharge and is emptied approximately four times daily by inserting a catheter through the stoma. No external pouch is needed, and a Band-Aid or small dressing is worn over the stoma to collect mucus. Surgical indications include UC and FAP requiring removal of the colon and rectum. CD is generally a contraindication for this procedure because the disease can recur in the pouch, necessitating its removal. A long-term complication of Kock pouch is pouchitis. See under ileal pouch anal anastomosis (IPAA) next, with the exception that tenesmus is not a symptom for a patient with a Kock pouch.

Ileal pouch anal anastomosis (IPAA) or restorative procto-colectomy: A two-stage surgical procedure developed to preserve fecal continence and prevent the need for a permanent ileostomy. During the first stage after total colectomy and removal of the rectal mucosa, an ileal reservoir or pouch is constructed and lowered into position in the pelvis just above the rectal cuff. Then the ileal outlet from the pouch is brought down through the cuff of the rectal muscle and anastomosed to the anal canal. The anal sphincter is preserved, and the resulting ileal pouch provides a storage place for feces. A temporary diverting ileostomy is required for 2-3 mo to allow healing of the anastomosis. The second stage occurs when the diverting ileostomy is taken down and fecal continuity is restored. Initially, the patient experiences fecal incontinence and 10 or more bowel movements per day. After 3-6 mo, the patient experiences decreased urgency and frequency with 4-8 bowel movements per day. This procedure is an option for patients requiring colectomy for UC or FAP. Its use is controversial in patients with CD. It is contraindicated with incontinence problems. Pouchitis is a long-term complication of IPAA. Its cause is unknown but may be due to stasis of bacteria in the ileal pouch. Symptoms include increased stool frequency, cramping, tenesmus, and bleeding. Pouchitis is effectively treated with metronidazole or ciprofloxacin. Probiotics also may be effective in preventing and maintaining remission in patients with recurrent pouchitis.

Note: *Consult a wound, ostomy, continence (WOC)/enterostomal therapy (ET) nurse, if available, since he or she has expertise in all aspects of fecal diversion management and the related patient care.*

Nursing Diagnoses:

Risk for Impaired Skin Integrity: Peristomal

related to exposure to stool/small bowel effluent, soaps, solvents, or appliance material (irritant contact dermatitis)

Risk for Allergy Response: Peristomal

related to hypersensitivity to chemical elements contacting the peristomal skin (allergic contact dermatitis [occurs rarely])

Impaired Tissue Integrity: Stomal (or risk for same)

related to improperly fitted appliance resulting in damage to stomal tissue and/or impaired circulation

Desired Outcomes: The patient's peristomal skin remains nonerythremic and intact. The patient's stoma remains red, moist, viable, and intact.

ASSESSMENT/INTERVENTIONS	RATIONALES
After Colostomy or Conventional Ileostomy (Permanent or Temporary)	
Assess the stoma for viability q8h.	The stoma should be red, moist, and shiny with mucus. A stoma that is pale, dark purple to black, or dull in appearance may indicate circulatory impairment and should be documented and reported to the health care provider immediately.

ASSESSMENT/INTERVENTIONS	RATIONALES
Apply a pectin, gelatin, methylcellulose-based, or synthetic solid-form skin barrier around the stoma.	This barrier will protect peristomal skin from irritation caused by contact with stool or small bowel effluent.
Cut an opening in the skin barrier the exact circumference of the stoma or as recommended by the manufacturer. Remove the release paper and apply the sticky surface directly to the peristomal skin.	For some pouching systems, the skin barrier may be a separate barrier to be used with an adhesive-backed pouch, part of a two-piece system, or an integral part of a one-piece pouch system. Pectin-based paste also may be used to "caulk" around the barrier and compensate for irregular surfaces on the peristomal skin. A pectin-based paste may prevent undermining of the barrier with effluent and protect the skin immediately adjacent to the stoma.
Remove the skin barrier and inspect the skin q3-4d. Monitor peristomal skin for erythema, erosion, serous drainage, bleeding, and induration. Carefully document abnormal findings, and report them to the health care provider.	These indicators may signal infection, irritation, or sensitivity to the materials placed on the skin. With irritant dermatitis, erythema, erosion, and skin damage are confined to areas of stool or irritant contact. In allergic dermatitis, margins of contact are more blurred, may extend beyond the area of contact, and are pruritic.
Discontinue use of irritating materials, and substitute other materials.	This will help heal and protect irritated and/or denuded skin.
Patch-test the patient's abdominal skin.	This will determine sensitivity to suspected materials. A dermatology consult may be required.
Recalibrate the skin barrier opening to the size of the stoma with each change.	Stomas become less edematous over a period of 6-8 wk after surgery, necessitating changes in the size of the skin barrier opening. The skin barrier opening should be the exact circumference of the stoma, or as recommended by the manufacturer, to prevent contact of stool with the skin and to prevent constriction of the stoma, which can result in increased edema of and decreased blood flow to the stoma. Commercial templates are available to aid in estimating size of the opening needed for the skin barrier.
Teach the patient to report immediately any burning or itching under the skin barrier or any fecal odor.	Burning, itching, and odor are signs that stool or effluent may have contacted the skin. In order to prevent skin irritation or breakdown, the skin barrier should be changed immediately.
Empty the pouch when it is one-third to one-half full of stool and/or gas.	This helps ensure maintenance of a secure pouch seal. A pouch with a larger amount of stool and/or gas could break the seal.

After Continent Ileostomy (Kock Pouch)

Assess the site for erythema, induration, drainage, or erosion around the stoma. Report significant findings to the health care provider.	These are signs of infection, irritation, or sensitivity to materials placed on the skin.
Assess catheter q2h for patency, and irrigate with sterile saline (30 mL). Notify the health care provider if solution cannot be instilled, if there are no returns from the catheter, or if leakage of irrigating solution or pouch contents appears around the catheter.	These measures check for and help prevent catheter obstruction. Instilling 30 mL of saline will clear the catheter and liquefy the secretions/effluent without adding unnecessary pressure on the pouch walls and areas of anastomosis.
Avoid stress on the ileostomy catheter and its securing suture.	This will prevent tissue destruction and catheter dislodgement.
As prescribed, maintain the catheter on low, continuous suction or gravity drainage.	The catheter was inserted through the stoma into the continent ileostomy pouch during surgery to prevent stress on the nipple valve and maintain pouch decompression so that suture lines are allowed to heal without stress or tension.
Change the 4 × 4 dressing around the stoma q2h or as often as it becomes wet.	This will help prevent peristomal skin irritation.
Report frank bleeding to the health care provider.	Normally, drainage will be serosanguineous at first and mixed with mucus.
Assess the stoma for viability with each dressing change.	The stoma should be red and moist and shiny with mucus. A stoma that is pale, dark purple to black, or dull in appearance may indicate circulatory impairment and should be documented and reported to the health care provider immediately.

continued

ASSESSMENT/INTERVENTIONS	RATIONALES
After Ileal Pouch Anal Anastomosis (IPAA)	
After the first stage of the operation, perform routine care for the temporary diverting ileostomy.	See earlier discussion for "After colostomy or conventional ileostomy (permanent or temporary)."
Maintain perineal/perianal skin integrity by gently cleansing the area with water and cotton balls or soft tissues.	After the first stage of the operation, the patient may have incontinence of mucus.
Avoid soap.	Soap can cause itching and irritation.
Use an absorbent pad at night.	This will absorb oozing mucus from the anus.
After the second stage of the operation (when the temporary diverting ileostomy is taken down), assess the patient's defecation pattern.	The patient likely will experience frequency and urgency of defecation.
Assess perineal/perianal skin for erythema and denuded areas.	Proteolytic enzymes present in effluent can cause skin breakdown.
Wash perineal/perianal area with warm water or commercial perineal/perianal cleansing solution, using a squeeze bottle, cotton balls, or soft tissues.	This will promote comfort and cleanse the perineal/perianal area to ensure skin integrity.
Do not use toilet paper. If desired, dry the area with hair dryer on a cool setting.	Toilet paper can cause skin irritation. A hair dryer on a cool setting will prevent skin irritation potentially caused by other materials.
Provide sitz baths.	These will promote comfort and help clean the perineal/perianal area.
Apply protective skin sealants or ointments.	This will help maintain skin integrity. **Note:** Skin sealants containing alcohol should not be used on irritated or denuded skin because the high alcohol content would cause a painful burning sensation; apply only to intact skin.

Nursing Diagnosis:

Bowel Incontinence

related to disruption of normal function with a fecal diversion

Desired Outcomes: Within 2-4 days after surgery, the patient has bowel sounds and eliminates gas and stool via the fecal diversion. Within 3 days after teaching has been initiated, the patient verbalizes understanding of measures that will maintain a normal elimination pattern and demonstrates care techniques specific to the fecal diversion.

ASSESSMENT/INTERVENTIONS	RATIONALES
After Colostomy and Conventional Ileostomy (Permanent and Temporary)	
Assess intake and output (I&O). Empty stool from the bottom opening of the pouch, and assess quality and quantity of stool. Record the volume of liquid stool and its color and consistency.	This assessment documents return of normal bowel function and its quality and quantity. Expect serosanguineous to serous liquid drainage and flatus initially. Colostomy output of clear brown, liquid stool usually begins within 3-4 days. Ileostomy output of liquid, bilious effluent usually begins within 24-48 hours. Output consistency thickens as solid food is ingested and varies with the type of ostomy.
If the colostomy is not eliminating stool after 3-4 days and bowel sounds have returned, gently insert a gloved, lubricated finger into the stoma.	This may reveal the presence of a stricture at skin or fascial levels and the presence of any stool within reach of the examining finger. To stimulate elimination of gas and stool, the health care provider may prescribe colostomy irrigation. (For the procedure, see **Deficient Knowledge** [colostomy irrigation procedure], p. 434.)

ASSESSMENT/INTERVENTIONS | RATIONALES

After Continent Ileostomy (Kock Pouch)

ASSESSMENT/INTERVENTIONS	RATIONALES
Assess I&O, and record amount, color, and consistency of output.	The patient likely will have bright red blood or serosanguineous liquid drainage from the Kock pouch during the early postoperative period.
As gastrointestinal (GI) function returns after 3-4 days, assess and document the color and character of output.	Usually, drainage changes from blood-tinged to greenish brown liquid. When ileal output appears, suction (if used) is discontinued and the pouch catheter is connected to or maintained on gravity drainage.
Check and irrigate the catheter q2h and as needed.	This will maintain catheter patency. As the patient's diet progresses from clear liquids to solid food, ileal output thickens. If the patient reports abdominal fullness in the area of the pouch along with decreased fecal output, catheter placement and patency should be assessed.
When the patient is alert and taking food by mouth, teach the catheter irrigation procedure, which should be performed q2h; demonstrate how to empty pouch contents through the catheter into the toilet.	Irrigation liquefies effluent for easier flow through the catheter. Frequent irrigations prevent overdistention of the pouch.
Before hospital discharge, teach the patient how to remove and reinsert the catheter.	Teaching, followed by a return demonstration, helps ensure that learning has occurred and facilitates retention of that information.

After Ileal Pouch Anal Anastomosis (IPAA)

ASSESSMENT/INTERVENTIONS	RATIONALES
Assess the patient for temperature elevation accompanied by perianal pain and discharge of purulent, bloody mucus from drains and anal orifice. Report significant findings to the health care provider.	These are signs of infection or anastomotic leak, which should be reported for prompt intervention.
If drains are present, irrigate them as prescribed.	Irrigation helps maintain patency, decrease stress on suture lines, and decrease incidence of infection.
Assess output from IPAA.	This assessment monitors quantity, quality, and consistency of output. Also see earlier discussion, "After colostomy or conventional ileostomy (permanent or temporary)," for the monitoring of output from a temporary diverting ileostomy.
After the first stage of the operation, advise the patient to wear a small pad in the perianal area to absorb mucus drainage.	This will prevent soiling of outer garments. After the first stage of the operation, the patient may experience oozing of mucus from the anus.
After the second stage of the operation (when the temporary diverting ileostomy is taken down), assess the patient's output.	The patient likely will have incontinence and 15-20 bowel movements per day with urgency when on a clear-liquid diet. The number of bowel movements decreases to 6-12/day and the consistency thickens when the patient is eating solid foods.
Assist with perianal care, and apply protective skin care products.	This helps maintain perineal/perianal skin integrity. If nocturnal incontinence is especially troublesome, the catheter can be placed in the reservoir and connected to a gravity drainage bag overnight.
Administer hydrophilic colloids and antidiarrheal medications as prescribed.	These agents decrease frequency and fluidity of stools.
Provide a diet consultation.	The patient can learn about foods that cause liquid stools (spinach, raw fruits, highly seasoned foods, green beans, broccoli, prune and grape juices, alcohol) and increase intake of foods that cause thick stools (cheese, ripe bananas, applesauce, creamy peanut butter, gelatin, pasta).
Reassure the patient that frequency and urgency are temporary and that as the reservoir expands and absorbs fluid, bowel movements should become thicker and less frequent.	This reassurance may decrease anxiety about the disruption of the patient's usual bowel pattern.

Nursing Diagnosis:

Disturbed Body Image

related to the presence of a fecal diversion

Desired Outcome: Within 5-7 days after surgery, the patient demonstrates actions that reflect beginning acceptance of the fecal diversion and incorporates changes into his or her self-concept as evidenced by acknowledging body changes, viewing the stoma, and participating in care of the fecal diversion.

ASSESSMENT/INTERVENTIONS	RATIONALES
Assess the patient for expressed fears about the fecal diversion.	Many fears may be expressed by patients experiencing a fecal diversion. Some patients view incontinence as a return to infancy. The following fears may be expected: physical, social, and work activities will be curtailed significantly; rejection, isolation, and feelings of uncleanliness will occur; everyone will know about the altered pattern of fecal elimination; and loss of voluntary control may occur.
Assess carefully for and listen closely to expressed or nonverbalized needs.	Each patient will react differently to the surgical procedure.
Encourage the patient to discuss feelings and fears; clarify any misconceptions. Involve family members in discussions because they too may have anxieties and misconceptions.	Fears and anxieties about body image may be reduced by talking about them. Such discussions also enable clarification about misconceptions.
Provide a calm and quiet environment for the patient and significant other to discuss the surgery. Initiate an open, honest discussion.	An open discussion enables understanding of the patient's perspective of the impact the diversion will have and assists in development of an individualized plan of care that will help the patient.
Encourage the patient to participate in care.	Optimally, this will promote acceptance of the fecal diversion and enhance a sense of control.
Assure the patient that physical, social, and work activities will not be affected by the presence of a fecal diversion.	Resuming the previous lifestyle with minimal disruption is an essential component of the rehabilitation. It helps rebuild a sense of independence and self-esteem.
Expect the patient to have fears about sexual acceptance. If you are uncomfortable talking about sexuality with patients, be aware of these potential concerns and arrange for a consultation with someone who can speak openly and honestly about these problems.	Although these fears usually are not expressed overtly, concerns center on change in body image; fears about odor and the ostomy appliance interfering with intercourse; conception, pregnancy, and discomfort from the perianal wound and scar in women; and impotence and failure to ejaculate in men, especially after more radical dissection of the pelvis in patients with cancer.
Consult the patient's health care provider about a visit by another person with an ostomy.	Patients gain reassurance and build positive attitudes and body image by seeing a healthy, active person who has undergone the same type of surgery, and it expands their support systems as well.

Nursing Diagnosis:

Deficient Knowledge

related to unfamiliarity with the colostomy irrigation procedure

Desired Outcome: Within 3 days after initiation of teaching, the patient demonstrates proficiency with the procedure for colostomy irrigation.

> **Note:** *Teach the patient to irrigate the colostomy per facility policy and procedures. If this protocol is not available, teach the patient how to perform the irrigation procedure as outlined below.*

ASSESSMENT/INTERVENTIONS	RATIONALES
Teach the following steps and have the patient return the demonstration:	The prescribed colostomy irrigation is taught to patients with permanent descending or sigmoid colostomy. Colostomy irrigation is performed daily or every other day so that wearing a pouch becomes unnecessary. An appropriate candidate is a patient who has one or two formed stools each day at predictable times (same as normal stool elimination pattern before illness). In addition, the patient must be able to manipulate the equipment, remember the technique, and be willing to spend approximately 1 hr/day performing the procedure. It may take 4-6 wk for the patient to have stool elimination regulated with irrigation. A return demonstration with explanation for each step will enable the nurse to determine the patient's knowledge level and facilitate learning retention for the patient.
Position the irrigating sleeve over the colostomy, centering the stoma in the opening. Secure the sleeve in place with an adhesive disk on the sleeve or with a sleeve belt.	The irrigation sleeve provides controlled diversion of stool and irrigation solution into the toilet.
Fill the enema/irrigation container with 500-1000 mL (1-2 pints) warm water. With the patient in a sitting position on the toilet or on a chair facing the toilet, position the sleeve so that it empties into the toilet. Hang the enema/irrigation container so that the bottom surface is at the patient's shoulder level.	The volume of water must be titrated for each patient to effect colon distention without causing cramping or excessive stretching of the colon wall.
Open the slide or roller clamp and flush the tubing; reclamp the tubing.	This removes air from the tubing.
Gently dilate the stoma with a gloved finger lubricated with water-soluble lubricant.	This enables the patient to identify the direction of the intestinal lumen and presence or absence of obstructing stool or stomal stenosis.
Lubricate the cone, with or without the attached catheter, and slowly insert into the stoma.	This prevents bowel perforation. If the cone has an attached catheter, the catheter should be inserted no more than 3 in.
Hold the cone gently, but firmly, in place against the stoma.	This prevents backflow of irrigant.
Let water slowly enter the stoma from the container through the tubing; allow 15 min for fluid to enter the colon.	This prevents cramping caused by too rapid an infusion.
Note: If cramping occurs while water is flowing, stop the flow and leave the cone in place until the cramping passes. Then the flow of water may be resumed.	This likely will stop the cramping. If cramping does not resolve, the colon is probably ready to evacuate and should be allowed to do so.
After water has entered the colon, advise the patient to hold the cone in place for a few seconds and then gently remove it.	This ensures complete infusion of the water.
Leave the sleeve in place for 30-40 min.	This enables water and stool to be eliminated.
When elimination is complete, remove the irrigation sleeve and cleanse and dry the peristomal area.	Cleaning and drying the skin help prevent skin irritation.
Apply a small dressing or security pouch over the colostomy between irrigations.	This collects mucus drainage from the stoma. **Note:** During initial adaptation period, a drainable pouch is worn between irrigations to collect the expected spillage of stool.

ADDITIONAL NURSING DIAGNOSES/PROBLEMS:

"Perioperative Care" p. 45

"Psychosocial Support" p. 72

 PATIENT-FAMILY TEACHING AND DISCHARGE PLANNING

When providing patient-family teaching, focus on sensory information, avoid giving excessive information, and initiate a visiting nurse referral for necessary follow-up teaching. Include verbal and written information about the following:

✓ Medications, including drug name, rationale, dosage, schedule, route of administration, precautions, and potential side effects. Also discuss drug-drug, herb-drug, and food-drug interactions.

✓ Importance of dietary management to promote nutritional and fluid maintenance.

✓ Care of incision, dressing changes, and permission to take baths or showers once sutures and drains are removed.

✓ Care of stoma, care of peristomal and perianal skin, use of ostomy equipment, and method for obtaining supplies.

✓ Gradual resumption of activities of daily living, excluding heavy lifting (more than 10 lb), pushing, or pulling for 6-8 wk to prevent development of incisional herniation.

✓ Referral to community resources including home health care agency, WOC/ET nurse, local ostomy association, and the United Ostomy Association of America at *www.uoaa.org* and the Young Ostomate and Diversion Alliance of America (for young adults ages 18 to 35 yr) found under Affiliate Support Groups at *uoaa.org*; or the United Ostomy Association of Canada at *www.ostomycanada.ca*.

✓ Importance of follow-up care with the health care provider and WOC/ET nurse; confirm date and time of next appointment.

✓ Importance of reporting signs and symptoms that necessitate medical attention, such as change in stoma color from normal bright and shiny red; peristomal or perianal skin irritation; any significant changes in appearance, frequency, and consistency of stools; fever, chills, abdominal pain, or distention; and incisional pain, increased local warmth, drainage, swelling, or redness; and signs and symptoms of pouchitis, including diarrhea, cramping, tenesmus, and bleeding.

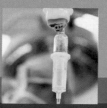
OVERVIEW/PATHOPHYSIOLOGY

Viral hepatitis may be caused by one of five viruses that are capable of infecting the liver: hepatitis A (HAV), B (HBV), C (HCV), D or delta (HDV), or E (HEV). HDV is not a stand-alone hepatitis. HDV does not exist outside the presence of HBV. A sixth virus, hepatitis G (HGV), has been isolated in a few cases of hepatitis caused by other viruses of the five common strains. It is not known what the role of HGV is in liver disease, nor are clinical manifestations, natural history, or pathogenesis known. Although symptomatology is similar among all the hepatitis viruses, immunologic and epidemiologic characteristics are different. When hepatocytes are damaged, necrosis and autolysis can occur, which in turn lead to abnormal liver functioning. Generally these changes are completely reversible after the acute phase. In some cases, however, massive necrosis can lead to acute liver failure and death.

Chronic hepatitis is inflammation of the liver for more than 6 months. Forms of chronic hepatitis are associated with infection from HBV, HCV, and HDV; viral infections such as cytomegalovirus (CMV); excessive alcohol consumption; inflammatory bowel disease; and autoimmunity (chronic active lupoid hepatitis).

Alcoholic hepatitis occurs as a result of tissue necrosis caused by alcohol abuse; it is nonviral and noninfectious. Generally it is a precursor to cirrhosis (see p. 413), but it may occur simultaneous with cirrhosis.

Jaundice is discoloration of body tissues from increased serum levels of bilirubin (total serum bilirubin more than 2.5 mg/dL) and can occur with any hepatitis. Jaundice may be seen in any patient with impaired hepatic function and occurs as bilirubin begins to be excreted through the skin. There is also an increased excretion of urobilinogen and bilirubin by the kidneys, resulting in darker, almost brownish, urine. Jaundice is classified as follows.

Prehepatic (hemolytic): Caused by increased production of bilirubin following erythrocyte destruction. Prehepatic jaundice is implicated when the indirect (unconjugated) serum bilirubin is more than 0.8 mg/dL.

Hepatic (hepatocellular): Caused by dysfunction of the liver cells (hepatocytes), which reduces their ability to remove bilirubin from the blood and form it into bile. Hepatic jaundice is also implicated with indirect serum bilirubin and is associated with acute hepatitis.

Posthepatic (obstructive): Caused by obstruction of the flow of bile out of the liver and resulting in backed-up bile through the hepatocytes to the blood. Posthepatic jaundice is implicated when direct serum bilirubin is more than 0.3 mg/dL.

HEALTH CARE SETTING

Primary care, with possible brief hospitalization resulting from complications

ASSESSMENT

Signs and symptoms: Nausea, vomiting, malaise, anorexia, epigastric discomfort, aversion to smoking, muscle or joint aches, fatigue, irritability, pruritus, slight to moderate temperature increases, dark urine, clay-colored stools, and jaundice.

Acute hepatic failure: Nausea, vomiting, and abdominal pain tend to be more severe. Jaundice is likely to appear earlier and deepen more rapidly. Mental status changes (possibly progressing to encephalopathy), coma, seizures, ascites, sharp rise in temperature, significant leukocytosis, coffee-ground emesis, gastrointestinal (GI) hemorrhage, purpura, shock, oliguria, and azotemia all may be present.

Physical assessment: Presence of jaundice; palpation of lymph nodes and abdomen may reveal lymphadenopathy, hepatomegaly, and splenomegaly. Liver size usually is small with acute hepatic failure.

History of/risk factors: Clotting disorders, multiple blood transfusions, excessive alcohol ingestion, parenteral drug use, exposure to hepatotoxic chemicals or medications (including over-the-counter medications or herbal supplements), travel to developing countries, men who have sex with men, prostitutes/heterosexuals with multiple sexual partners, injection drug users.

DIAGNOSTIC TESTS

Immunoglobulins: Chronic infection markers are present for HBV, HCV, and HDV. They are HBsAg, anti-HBc IgG for hepatitis B; anti-HCV (enzyme-linked immunosorbent assay) and HCV RNA quantitation for hepatitis C; and anti-HDV IgG for hepatitis D.

Serum enzymes: Aspartate aminotransferase (AST) and alanine aminotransferase (ALT) are initially elevated and then drop. Gamma-glutamyl transpeptidase (GGT) is elevated early in liver disease and persists as long as cellular damage continues.

Other hematologic tests: Total bilirubin may be elevated, and prothrombin time (PT) may be prolonged. Differential white blood cell (WBC) count reveals leukocytosis, monocytosis, and atypical lymphocytes.

Urine tests: Reveal elevation of urobilinogen, mild proteinuria, and mild bilirubinuria.

Liver biopsy: Although this procedure is performed to obtain a definitive diagnosis of hepatitis, clinically it is not always advisable because of the high risk of bleeding. When performed, a biopsy is obtained percutaneously or via laparoscopy to collect a specimen for histologic examination to confirm differential diagnosis.

Nursing Diagnosis:

Fatigue

related to decreased metabolic energy production occurring with faulty absorption, metabolism, and storage of nutrients

Desired Outcome: By at least 24 hr before hospital discharge, the patient relates decreasing fatigue and increasing energy.

ASSESSMENT/INTERVENTIONS	RATIONALES
Take a diet history to determine food preferences. Consult the dietitian regarding increased intake of carbohydrates or other high-energy food sources within prescribed dietary limitations. Encourage significant others to bring in desirable foods if permitted. Monitor and record intake.	In general, dietary management consists of giving palatable meals as tolerated without overfeeding. If oral intake is substantially decreased, parenteral or enteral nutrition may be initiated. Sodium restrictions may be indicated in the presence of fluid retention. Protein is moderately restricted, or eliminated, depending on the degree of mental status changes (i.e., encephalopathy). If no mental status changes are noted, normal amounts of high biologic value protein are indicated to facilitate tissue healing, promote energy, and decrease fatigue. All alcoholic beverages are strictly forbidden. When appetite and food selection are poor, vitamins may be given to supplement dietary intake.
Encourage small, frequent feedings, and provide emotional support during meals.	Smaller and more frequent meals are usually better tolerated in patients who are fatigued, nauseated, and anorexic.
Provide rest periods of at least 90 min before and after activities and treatments.	Rest facilitates recovery after the body has experienced stress and may be indicated when symptoms are severe, with a gradual return to normal activity as symptoms subside.
Advise the patient to avoid exercise immediately after meals.	Exercise after meals increases the potential for nausea and vomiting, which could cause loss of nutrients and exacerbate fatigue.
Keep frequently used objects within easy reach.	This will help conserve the patient's energy.
Decrease environmental stimuli; provide back massage and relaxation tapes; and speak with the patient in short, simple terms.	These measures promote rest and sleep and decrease sensory overload.
Administer acid suppression therapy, antiemetics, antidiarrheal medications, and cathartics as prescribed.	These agents minimize gastric distress and promote absorption of nutrients, which will help provide energy and reverse feelings of fatigue.

Nursing Diagnosis:

Deficient Knowledge

related to unfamiliarity with causes of hepatitis and modes of transmission

Desired Outcome: Within the 24-hr period before hospital discharge, the patient verbalizes knowledge about the causes of hepatitis and measures that help prevent transmission.

ASSESSMENT/INTERVENTIONS	RATIONALES
Assess the patient's health care literacy (language, reading, comprehension). Assess culture and culturally specific information needs.	This assessment helps ensure that information is selected and presented in a manner that is culturally and educationally appropriate.
Assess the patient's knowledge about the disease process, and educate as necessary.	Determining a patient's level of knowledge will facilitate development of an individualized teaching plan.
Make sure the patient knows you are not making moral judgments about alcohol/drug use or sexual behavior.	This will promote the patient's confidence in you.
Teach the patient and significant others the importance of wearing gloves and using good hand hygiene if contact with body fluids such as urine, blood, wound exudate, or feces is possible.	These measures help prevent spread of infection.
If appropriate, advise patients with HAV that crowded living conditions with poor sanitation should be avoided.	This information may prevent recurrence.
☒ Remind patients with HBV and HCV that they should modify sexual behavior as directed by the health care provider. Explain that blood donation is no longer possible.	For patients with HBV and HCV, contact with blood is a likely mode of transmission, and blood contact can occur with some types of sexual activities. For patients with HBV, sexual contact is a likely mode.
☒ Advise patients with HBV that their sexual partners should receive HBV vaccine.	For patients with HBV, sexual contact is a likely mode of transmission.
Refer the patient to drug treatment programs as necessary.	Drug use is not only a causative factor but can also further damage the liver.

Nursing Diagnosis:

Risk for Impaired Skin Integrity

related to pruritus occurring with hepatic dysfunction

Desired Outcome: The patient's skin remains intact.

ASSESSMENT/INTERVENTIONS	RATIONALES
Keep the patient's skin moist by using tepid water or emollient baths, avoiding alkaline soap (which is a stronger soap; use transparent soaps such as a glycerin soap), and applying emollient lotions at frequent intervals.	Hot water and alkaline soaps can dry the skin and may cause irritation in patients with sensitive skin. Emollients and lipid creams (i.e., Eucerin) are used to keep skin moist and supple.
Encourage the patient not to scratch skin and to keep nails short and smooth.	These measures help prevent skin breakdown and infection.
Suggest use of knuckles if the patient must scratch. Wrap or place gloves on the patient's hands (especially comatose patients).	Knuckles and gloved hands are less traumatic to the skin and tissue than fingernails.
Treat any skin lesion promptly.	This will help prevent infection. Pathogens can enter the body through nonintact skin.
Administer antihistamines as prescribed; observe closely for excessive sedation.	Antihistamines may be used for symptomatic relief of pruritus. However, if used, they are administered with caution and in low doses because they are metabolized by the liver.
Encourage the patient to wear loose, soft clothing; provide soft linens (cotton is best).	These measures help prevent abrasions caused by tight clothing or rough material on skin that is already compromised.
Keep the environment cool.	Cool temperatures help prevent further skin irritation caused by perspiration.
Change soiled linen as soon as possible.	This measure helps prevent further irritation caused by waste products or fluids having constant skin contact.

Nursing Diagnosis:

Risk for Bleeding

related to decreased vitamin K absorption, thrombocytopenia

Desired Outcome: The patient is free of bleeding as evidenced by negative tests for occult blood in the feces and urine and absence of ecchymotic areas and bleeding at the gums and injection sites.

ASSESSMENT/INTERVENTIONS	RATIONALES
Monitor PT levels daily.	These assessments detect prolonged PT. Optimal range for PT is 10.5-13.5 sec. In hepatitis, PT is prolonged because of inability of the liver to produce coagulation factors.
Monitor platelet count daily.	These assessments detect thrombocytopenia. Optimal range is 150,000-400,000/mm^3. In hepatitis, platelet count is decreased because of the decrease in production of thrombopoietin or platelet pooling caused by splenomegaly and portal hypertension.
Monitor hematocrit (Hct) and hemoglobin (Hgb) daily.	These assessments detect decreases that may indicate occult bleeding. Optimal ranges are Hct 40%-54% (male) and 37%-47% (female) and Hgb 14-18 g/dL (male) and 12-16 g/dL (female).
Handle the patient gently (e.g., when turning or transferring).	This measure helps minimize risk of bleeding within the tissues.
Minimize intramuscular (IM) injections. Rotate sites, and use small-gauge needles. Administer medications orally or intravenously when possible.	Bleeding may result from use of large-bore needles. Rotating sites helps prevent tissue damage caused by frequent injections in same tissue.
Apply moderate pressure after an injection, but do not massage the site.	These measures minimize bleeding at the injection site while preventing excessive pressure on the tissue.
Observe for ecchymotic areas. Inspect gums, and test urine and feces for bleeding. Report significant findings to the health care provider.	These assessments detect early signs of bleeding potential and abnormal bleeding sources.
Teach the patient to use an electric razor and soft-bristle toothbrush.	These measures minimize risk of bleeding from cuts or abrasions caused by a razor or hard bristles.
Administer vitamin K as prescribed.	For patients with prolonged PT, vitamin K is a cofactor that modifies clotting factors to provide a site for calcium binding—an essential part of the clotting function. Patients with severe hepatic failure may not respond to vitamin K and may require transfusions of fresh frozen plasma before invasive procedures.

ADDITIONAL NURSING DIAGNOSES/PROBLEMS:

"Cirrhosis" **for Risk for Bleeding**, if the patient develops encephalopathy   p. 415

☑ **PATIENT-FAMILY TEACHING AND DISCHARGE PLANNING**

When providing patient-family teaching, focus on sensory information, avoid giving excessive information, and initiate a visiting nurse referral for necessary follow-up teaching. Include verbal and written information about the following:

✓ Importance of rest and getting adequate nutrition. When appropriate, provide a list of high–biologic value protein food sources or protein foods to avoid and sample menus to demonstrate how these foods may be incorporated into or excluded from the diet. Instruct the patient to eat frequent, small meals; to eat slowly; and to chew all food thoroughly. Teach the patient to rest for 30-60 min after meals. Initiate dietitian consult as needed for diet instruction.

✓ Importance of avoiding hepatotoxic agents, including over-the-counter (OTC) drugs and herbal supplements. Examples of OTC drugs include aspirin and other salicylates, nonsteroidal antiinflammatory drugs (NSAIDs), acetaminophen, alcohol, and vitamin A.

✓ Prescribed medications (e.g., multivitamins), including drug name, purpose, dosage, schedule, potential side effects, and precautions. Also discuss drug-drug, food-drug, and herb-drug interactions.

✓ Importance of informing health care providers, dentists, and other health care workers of the hepatitis diagnosis.

✓ Potential complications, including delayed healing, skin injury, and bleeding tendencies.

✓ Importance of avoiding alcohol during recovery.

✓ Referral to alcohol/drug treatment programs as appropriate.

✓ Provide information about organizations available for education:

- American Liver Foundation at *www.liverfoundation.org*
- Canadian Liver Foundation at *www.liver.ca*
- Hepatitis Foundation International at *www.hepfi.org*
- Centers for Disease Control and Prevention at *www.cdc.gov/ncidod/diseases/hepatitis/index.htm*
- National Digestive Diseases Information Clearinghouse (NDDIC) at *http://digestive.niddk.nih.gov/resources/patient.htm*

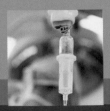

Pancreatitis 58

OVERVIEW/PATHOPHYSIOLOGY

The pancreas serves both endocrine (hormonal) and exocrine (nonhormonal) functions. (Pancreatic endocrine function is discussed in "Diabetes Mellitus," p. 355.) The exocrine portion comprises 98% of its tissue mass. Exocrine secretions, which are produced by the acini cells, empty through a series of lobular ducts into the main pancreatic duct, where they are released into the duodenum. Exocrine function is the secretion of potent enzymes, proteases, lipases, and amylases that act to reduce proteins, fats, and carbohydrates, respectively, into simpler chemical substances. Pancreatic proteases (trypsin, chymotrypsin, carboxypeptidases A and B, elastase, and phospholipase A) aid in protein digestion. Pancreatic lipase acts on fats to produce glycerides, fatty acids, and glycerol; pancreatic amylase acts on starch to produce disaccharides. The pancreas also secretes sodium bicarbonate to neutralize the strongly acidic gastric content as it enters the duodenum. The resultant mixture of acids and bases provides an optimal pH of 8.3 for activation of pancreatic enzymes.

Pancreatitis, which can be acute or chronic, is an inflammation of the pancreas with varying degrees of edema, hemorrhage, and necrosis. The damage can lead to fibrosis, stricture, and calcifications. Acute pancreatitis occurs when pancreatic ductal flow becomes obstructed and digestive enzymes escape from the pancreatic duct into surrounding tissue. Self-destruction of the pancreas produces edema, hemorrhage, and necrosis of pancreatic and surrounding tissue. Biochemical abnormalities and disruption of cardiopulmonary, renal, metabolic, and gastrointestinal (GI) function are likely. Pancreatitis has been associated with gallstones, alcoholism, surgical manipulation, abdominal trauma, abdominal vascular disease, heavy metal poisoning, infectious agents (viral, bacterial, mycoplasmal, parasitic), medications, and some allergic reactions. Pancreatitis also is associated with familial hyperlipidemia and can be induced by endoscopic retrograde cholangiopancreatography (ERCP). The majority of acute pancreatitis cases are mild, require a short hospitalization, and leave no long-term adverse effects. Severe acute pancreatitis involving multiple organ failure occurs in approximately 25% of cases but accounts for 98% of deaths associated with acute pancreatitis. Complications of acute pancreatitis include pancreatic abscess, hemorrhage, pancreatic pseudocyst, fistula formation, and transient hypoglycemia. Acute, life-threatening complications include renal failure, hemorrhagic pancreatitis, septicemia, adult respiratory distress syndrome (ARDS), shock, and disseminated intravascular coagulation (DIC).

Chronic pancreatitis is characterized by varying degrees of pancreatic insufficiency, which results in decreased production of enzymes and bicarbonate and malabsorption of fats and proteins. The digestion of fat is affected most severely. As a result, a high-fat content in the bowel stimulates water and electrolyte secretion, which produces diarrhea. The action of bacteria on fecal fat produces flatus, fatty stools (steatorrhea), and abdominal cramps. Often diabetes mellitus (DM) occurs as a result of chronic pancreatitis because of damage to the insulin-producing beta cells and resultant deficient insulin production. Chronic pancreatitis is also associated with complications of DM, chronic pain, maldigestion, pseudocysts, and bleeding.

HEALTH CARE SETTING

Primary care with hospitalization for acute pancreatitis and complications of chronic pancreatitis

ASSESSMENT

Acute pancreatitis: Symptoms vary according to severity of the attack. Sudden onset of constant, severe epigastric pain often occurs after a large meal or alcohol intake. Pain frequently radiates to the back or left shoulder and is somewhat relieved by a sitting position with the spine flexed. It is caused by biliary tree obstruction, enzymes irritating pancreatic and surrounding tissue, and the resulting edema. Nausea and vomiting, sometimes with persistent retching, usually occur and are caused by bowel hypermotility or ileus. Pain may be increased after vomiting because of increased pressure on the ducts, leading to further obstruction of secretions and tissue damage. Fever is usually present as well as hypotension and tachycardia. Jaundice suggests biliary tree obstruction. Extreme malaise, restlessness, respiratory distress, and diminished urinary output may be present. Hypovolemic shock may be present with hemorrhagic events, or distributive shock may occur secondary to systemic inflammatory response syndrome.

Physical assessment: Diminished or absent bowel sounds, suggesting presence of ileus; mild to moderate ascites; generalized abdominal tenderness; tachypnea, crackles (rales) at lung bases related to atelectasis, and interstitial fluid accumulation;

diminished ventilatory excursion related to splinting and guarding with pain; low-grade fever (37.7°-38.8°C [100°-102°F]) or pronounced fever with abscess or sepsis; and agitation, confusion, and altered mental status may occur because of electrolyte/metabolic abnormalities or acute alcohol withdrawal. Gray-blue discoloration of the flank (Grey Turner's sign) or blue-red discoloration around the umbilicus (Cullen's sign) sometimes is present with pancreatic hemorrhage.

Chronic pancreatitis: Constant, dull epigastric pain; steatorrhea resulting from malabsorption of fats and protein; weight loss; and onset of symptoms of DM (polydipsia, polyuria, polyphagia).

History of: Biliary tract disease; chronic excessive alcohol consumption; physical trauma to the abdomen (especially in young people); peptic ulcer disease; viral infection; ERCP; cystic fibrosis; neoplasms; shock; and use of certain medications, such as estrogen-containing oral contraceptives, glucocorticoids, sulfonamides, chlorothiazides, and azathioprine.

DIAGNOSTIC TESTS

Serum amylase: When significantly elevated (more than 500 units/dL), rules out acute abdomen conditions, such as cholecystitis, appendicitis, bowel infarction/obstruction, and perforated peptic ulcer and confirms presence of pancreatitis. These levels return to normal 48-72 hr after onset of acute symptoms, even though clinical indicators may continue. Sensitivity is limited in patients with alcoholic pancreatitis and hypertriglyceridemia.

Serum lipase: Has higher specificity and sensitivity than serum amylase. It rises more slowly than serum amylase and persists longer. Both lipase and amylase levels reflect the degree of necrotic pancreatic tissue.

Blood glucose: Hyperglycemia occurs because of interference with beta cell function. It is transient with acute pancreatitis but common with chronic pancreatitis, during which DM is likely to develop.

Ultrasound, magnetic resonance imaging (MRI), computed tomography (CT) scan: May reveal an enlarged and edematous pancreatic head or abscess, pseudocyst, or calcification.

MR cholangiopancreatography (MRCP): Used to visualize pancreatic and common bile ducts and may be used if an ERCP is not feasible.

ERCP: A combined endoscopic-radiographic tool that is used to study the degree of pancreatic disease via assessment of biliary-pancreatic ductal systems. It allows direct visualization of the ampulla of Vater, diagnoses biliary stones and duct stenosis, and distinguishes cancer of the pancreas from pancreatic calculi. ERCP is not performed until the acute episode has subsided.

Potassium: Hyperkalemia will occur in the presence of tissue damage, metabolic acidosis, and renal failure in severe cases.

Serum calcium and magnesium: May be lower than normal. On electrocardiogram, hypocalcemia is evidenced by prolonged QT segment with a normal T wave.

Complete blood count: Elevated white blood cell (WBC) count caused by inflammatory process. Polymorphonuclear bodies may increase if bacterial peritonitis is present secondary to duodenal rupture. Hematocrit (Hct) may be elevated or decreased.

Blood urea nitrogen (BUN) and serum creatinine: To evaluate renal function.

Urinalysis: May show presence of glycosuria, which can signal the onset of DM. Elevated urine amylase levels are useful diagnostically when serum levels have dropped off. An elevated specific gravity reflects the presence of dehydration.

Abdominal x-ray examination: May show dilation of the small or large bowel and presence of pancreatic calcification in chronic pancreatitis.

Nursing Diagnosis:

Acute Pain

related to inflammatory process of the pancreas

Desired Outcomes: Within 6 hr of intervention, the patient's subjective perception of discomfort decreases, and it is controlled within 24 hr, as documented by pain scale. Nonverbal indicators, such as grimacing and splinting of abdominal muscles, are absent or diminished.

ASSESSMENT/INTERVENTIONS	RATIONALES
Assess for and document the degree and character of the patient's discomfort. Devise a pain scale with the patient, rating discomfort on a scale of 0 (no pain) to 10 (worst pain).	Pain characteristics may signal varying problems (see Assessment section). Baseline and subsequent use of a pain scale helps determine effectiveness of pain relief.
Assess the patient's previous responses to pain and previously effective pain relief measures.	The patient's previous history of pain and how well it was managed influence perceptions and trust in present pain relief measures.
Consider possible cultural and spiritual influences that may affect the patient's beliefs regarding pain.	Some cultures allow less outward show of pain, whereas others do not prohibit expressions of pain.

continued

PART I: Medical-Surgical Nursing

ASSESSMENT/INTERVENTIONS	RATIONALES
Ensure that the patient maintains limited activity or bedrest.	Rest helps minimize pancreatic secretions and pain.
Maintain nothing by mouth (NPO) status, and monitor nasogastric (NG) tube function if it is used.	NPO status is initiated early in the course of illness to decrease the stimulus for pancreatic secretions and reduce stress in the GI tract. NG suction is generally used only in more severely ill patients who have unrelieved vomiting. After acute pain and ileus have resolved, the patient is given clear liquids and the diet is advanced as tolerated.
Administer analgesics, steroids, histamine H₂-receptor blockers, antiemetics, and other medications as prescribed. Be alert to the patient's response to medications, using the pain scale.	Analgesics reduce discomfort associated with pancreatitis. Steroids may be given to reduce inflammation in certain types of pancreatitis when infection is not a problem. Histamine H₂-receptor blockers are given to reduce gastric acid secretion, which stimulates pancreatic enzymes. Antiemetics (e.g., hydroxyzine, ondansetron, prochlorperazine, promethazine) are given for nausea and vomiting. Antacids are given to neutralize gastric acid and reduce associated pain.
⚠ Avoid use of meperidine (Demerol) and its metabolites as well as pentazocine (Talwin).	**Note:** Although morphine has been believed to cause spasm to the sphincter of Oddi, it is now considered an acceptable alternative due to the potential side effects of meperidine. The metabolite of meperidine, normeperidine, can cause CNS side effects such as seizures. Pentazocine, once used as an alternative analgesic, is 25% as potent as morphine and can cause psychotomimetic effects and cardiovascular side effects.
Instruct the patient to request an analgesic before pain becomes severe.	Pain is more easily managed when it is treated before it becomes severe. If the analgesic is ineffective, the health care provider should be notified because the patient may require another intervention. Optimally, analgesics are administered via patient-controlled pumps.
⚠ Avoid intramuscular (IM) injections in individuals with clotting or bleeding complications.	Transdermal analgesics or small, frequent doses of intravenous (IV) opioids usually are more effective than IM injections, which also increase the risk of bleeding in individuals with bleeding/clotting complications.
Assist the patient in attaining a position of comfort.	A sitting or supine position with the knees flexed often helps relax abdominal muscles.
Emphasize nonpharmacologic pain interventions (e.g., relaxation techniques, distraction, guided imagery, massage).	These interventions are especially important for patients in whom chronic pancreatitis develops and who are prone to chemical dependence.
Prepare significant others for personality changes and behavioral alterations associated with extreme pain and opioid analgesic. Reassure them that these are normal responses.	Pancreatitis can be very painful. Family members sometimes misinterpret the patient's lethargic or unpleasant disposition and may even blame themselves.
Monitor the patient's respiratory pattern and level of consciousness (LOC) closely.	Both may be depressed by the large amount of opioids usually required to control pain. **Note:** Opioid analgesics also decrease intestinal motility and delay return to normal bowel function.
Report O₂ saturation of 92% or less.	Continuous pulse oximetry identifies decreasing oxygen saturation associated with hypoventilation. Values of 92% or less often signal need for supplemental oxygen.
Consider referral to a pain management team.	A pain management team can help with conventional pain control measures during acute pain situations in patients with chronic or frequent bouts of pancreatitis or with low pain tolerance. Less conventional measures, such as nerve blocks that interfere with transmission of pain sensations along visceral nerve fibers, are effective in the relief of pancreatic pain. Bilateral splanchnic nerve or left celiac ganglion blocks may be performed as well.

For additional pain interventions, see "Pain," p. 39.

Nursing Diagnosis:

Risk for Infection

related to the potential for tissue destruction with resulting necrosis occurring with release of pancreatic enzymes

Desired Outcome: The patient remains free of infection as evidenced by body temperature less than 37.7°C (less than 100°F); negative culture results; heart rate (HR) 60-100 bpm; respiratory rate (RR) 12-20 breaths/min; blood pressure (BP) within the patient's normal range; and orientation to person, place, and time.

ASSESSMENT/INTERVENTIONS	RATIONALES
Assess the patient's temperature q4h.	An increase may signal infection. **Note:** Hypothermia may precede hyperthermia in some individuals, particularly older adults.
If there is a sudden elevation in temperature, obtain specimens for culture of blood, sputum, urine, wound, drains, and other sites as indicated. Monitor culture reports, and report findings promptly to the health care provider.	Cultures enable detection of a developing necrotic pancreas or presence of an abscess. The body may be developing systemic inflammatory response syndrome (SIRS), which is a precursor to sepsis. SIRS is manifested by two or more of the following: body temperature higher than 38°C (100.4°F) or lower than 36°C (98.6°F), RR more than 20 breaths/min or CO_2 less than 32 mm Hg, HR greater than 90 bpm, WBC count greater than 12,000 mm^3 or less than 4000 mm^3, or presence of more than 10% immature neutrophils ("bands").
Assess BP, HR, and RR q4h.	Increases in HR (up to 100-140 bpm) and RR are associated with infection of the necrotic pancreatic tissue and SIRS. BP may be either transiently high or low with significant orthostatic hypotension.
Monitor all secretions and drainage for changes in appearance or odor that may signal infection.	Sputum, for example, can become more copious and change in color from clear to white to yellow to green in the presence of infection.
Assess mental status, orientation, and LOC q4-8h. Document and report significant deviations from baseline.	Impairments may occur with alcohol withdrawal, hypotension, electrolyte imbalance, hypoxia, and from the sepsis associated with the necrotic, infected pancreas.
Administer parenteral antibiotics in a timely fashion.	These measures help maintain bacteriocidal serum levels.
Reschedule antibiotics if a dose is delayed for more than 1 hr.	Failure to administer antibiotics on schedule can result in inadequate blood levels and treatment failure.
Use good hand hygiene before and after caring for the patient, and dispose of dressings and drainage carefully.	These measures help prevent transmission of potentially infectious agents.

Nursing Diagnoses:

Risk for Imbalanced Fluid Volume
Risk for Electrolyte Imbalance

related to active loss occurring with NG suctioning, vomiting, diaphoresis, or pooling of fluids in the abdomen and retroperitoneum; or related to fluid gain occurring with aggressive fluid replacement

Desired Outcomes: The patient is normovolemic within 8 hr of hospital admission as evidenced by HR 60-100 bpm, central venous pressure (CVP) 2-6 mm Hg (5-12 cm H_2O), brisk capillary refill (less than 2 sec), peripheral pulse amplitude greater than 2+ on a 0-4+ scale, urinary output at least 30 mL/hr, and stable weight and abdominal girth measurements. Electrolytes K$^+$ and Ca^{2+} are within normal limits.

ASSESSMENT/INTERVENTIONS	RATIONALES
Assess vital signs (VS) q2-4h.	This assessment enables detection of a falling BP and increasing HR (100-140 bpm), which can occur with moderate to severe fluid loss.
Assess intake and output (I&O) and monitor CVP, if available, q2-4h. Weigh the patient daily, and note trends.	CVP less than 2 mm Hg can occur with volume-related hypotension, and output greater than intake signals fluid loss. Weight decreases when fluid is lost or intake is insufficient.
Correlate weight measurements with I&O ratios.	Fluid loss requires immediate replacement to prevent shock and acute renal failure. Approximately 1 kg weight = 1 L fluid.
Measure orthostatic VS initially and q8h.	This enables detection of decreasing BP and increasing HR on standing, which suggests need for crystalloid and/or colloid volume expansion.
Administer parenteral solutions (lactated Ringer solution is preferred) and plasma volume expanders as prescribed.	These measures help maintain adequate circulating blood volume. Fluid resuscitation reduces morbidity among patients with acute pancreatitis. Examples of blood volume expanders include albumin and plasma protein fraction.
Monitor closely for adventitious breath sounds, increased weight, and drop in Hct without concomitant blood loss.	These are signs of fluid overload and potentially of pulmonary edema as a result of overly aggressive fluid resuscitation. In cases of severe, acute pancreatitis, patients develop a profound loss of circulating blood volume and need adequate fluid resuscitation quickly, sometimes as much as 5-6 L/day. This increases risk for fluid overload, especially if the patient has been hypotensive and the kidneys are not functioning well enough to handle the large amounts of fluid. The fluid overload can lead to pulmonary edema and respiratory failure. In fact, respiratory dysfunction is the most frequent complication of severe, acute pancreatitis and one of the main causes of early death.
Monitor values of the following for irregularities: Hct, hemoglobin (Hgb), WBC count, Ca^{2+}, glucose, BUN, creatinine, and K^+.	Irregularities can occur in patients with infection, inflammatory response, and bleeding caused by necrotic pancreas and would be outside the following normal values: Hct 40%-54% (male) and 37%-47% (female), Hgb 14-18 g/dL (male) and 12-16 g/dL (female), Ca^{2+} 8.5-10.5 mg/dL (4.3-5.3 mEq/L), glucose 145 mg/dL (2-hr postprandial) and 65-110 mg/dL (fasting), BUN 6-20 mg/dL, K^+ 3.5-5 mEq/L, and WBC count 4500-11,000 mm^3.
Be alert to positive Chvostek's sign (facial muscle spasm) and Trousseau's sign (carpopedal spasm), muscle twitching, tetany, or irritability.	These signs are indicators of hypocalcemia, which can occur with electrolyte loss.
Administer electrolytes (K^+, Ca^{2+}) as prescribed.	Replacement of these electrolytes helps prevent cardiac dysrhythmias, tetany, and other problems caused by their specific decreases.

Nursing Diagnosis:

Impaired Gas Exchange

related to ventilation-perfusion mismatching occurring with atelectasis or accumulating pulmonary fluid

Desired Outcome: Following interventions, the patient has adequate gas exchange as evidenced by RR 12-20 breaths/min with normal depth and pattern (eupnea); oxygen saturation greater than 92%; no significant changes in mental status; orientation to person, place, and time; and breath sounds that are clear and audible throughout the lung fields.

ASSESSMENT/INTERVENTIONS	RATIONALES
Assess and document RR q2-4h as indicated by the patient's condition. Note pattern, degree of excursion, and whether the patient uses accessory muscles of respiration. Report significant deviations from baseline to the health care provider.	Irregular pattern, decreased chest excursion, and use of accessory muscles of respiration occur with impending respiratory compromise (can occur with ARDS and respiratory failure) and may be a sign of inadequate pain control or worsening pancreatitis.

ASSESSMENT/INTERVENTIONS	RATIONALES
Auscultate both lung fields q4-8h.	Presence of abnormal (crackles, rhonchi, wheezes) or diminished breath sounds can occur with fluid overload (see discussion in **Risk for Imbalanced Fluid Volume,** earlier) or atelectasis.
Assess sputum production, and promptly report to the health care provider an increase or color change (from clear to white to yellow to green) in respiratory secretions.	Copious secretions that change color can indicate respiratory tract infection; copious secretions without color changes can occur with pulmonary edema.
Assess for changes in mental status, restlessness, agitation, and alterations in mentation.	These are early signs of hypoxia.
Monitor pulse oximetry q8h or as indicated (report oxygen saturation 92% or less). Monitor arterial blood gas results as available (report Pao$_2$ less than 80 mm Hg).	These decreased values usually signal need for supplementary oxygen.
Administer oxygen as prescribed. Monitor oxygen delivery system at regular intervals.	Hypoxia is an early sign of impending respiratory failure and necessitates oxygen delivery.
Elevate head of bed 30 degrees or higher, depending on the patient's comfort level.	This position optimizes ventilation and oxygenation.
If pleural effusion or other defect is present on one side, position the patient with the unaffected lung dependent.	This position maximizes ventilation-perfusion relationship, which optimizes oxygenation.
Avoid overaggressive fluid resuscitation.	This could lead to hypoxia, heart failure, pleural effusions, and respiratory failure. See discussion in **Risk for Imbalanced Fluid Volume,** earlier.
Explain to the patient and significant others that the patient is at risk for hypostatic pneumonia.	Pancreatitis results in decreased production of surfactant, and pain limits adequate respiratory excursion, increasing the potential for hypostatic pneumonia.
Teach use of a hyperinflation device (e.g., incentive spirometer) followed by coughing exercises. Explain that emphasis of this therapy is on inhalation to expand the lungs maximally. Ensure that the patient inhales slowly and deeply 2 times normal tidal volume and holds the breath at least 5 sec at the end of inspiration. Monitor the patient's progress and document in nurses' notes.	Deep breathing expands alveoli and helps mobilize secretions to the airways, while coughing further mobilizes and clears secretions. Ten breaths/hr is recommended to maintain adequate alveolar inflation.
When appropriate, teach methods of splinting wounds or upper abdomen.	Splinting helps reduce pain and enable effective cough.
Teach the cascade cough (i.e., a succession of more short and forceful exhalations) to patients who cannot cough effectively.	A cascade cough helps keep lungs expanded when abdominal pain would not otherwise enable deep cough.
Encourage activity as prescribed.	Activity helps mobilize secretions and promote effective airway clearance.

Nursing Diagnosis:

Dysfunctional Gastrointestinal Motility

related to bowel dysfunction occurring with electrolyte disturbance

Desired Outcome: Following interventions, GI motility normalizes as evidenced by the presence of bowel sounds and flatus and absence of nausea, vomiting, and abdominal distention.

ASSESSMENT/INTERVENTIONS	RATIONALES
Assess for the absence of flatus/bowel sounds or change in bowel sounds and the presence of abdominal cramping or pain.	These findings may be present with bowel dysfunction, which can occur with an electrolyte imbalance (particularly hypokalemia) resulting directly from severe pancreatitis. Although serious, it is not a major complication.

continued

ASSESSMENT/INTERVENTIONS	RATIONALES
Assess for bowel sounds in all four abdominal quadrants.	Bowel dysfunction may occur at any point along the GI tract. Diminished or absent bowel sounds suggest the presence of ileus and therefore must be auscultated in all four quadrants before NPO can be rescinded. Hypoactive sounds (3-5/min) indicate decreased motility; hyperactive sounds (more than 34/min) can be caused by anxiety, infectious diarrhea, irritation of intestinal mucosa from blood, or gastroenteritis. High-pitched tinkling sounds (hyperperistalsis) occur during intestinal obstruction, usually accompanied by cramping pain.
In the absence of bowel sounds, keep the patient NPO.	Fluids and food are not tolerated until the bowel returns to normal function, as evidenced by bowel sounds.
Following recommencement of fluids and food, monitor for bowel movements and emesis.	Absence of emesis and the presence of bowel movements indicate return of normal GI function.

Nursing Diagnosis:

Imbalanced Nutrition: Less Than Body Requirements

related to anorexia, dietary restrictions, and digestive dysfunction

Desired Outcome: The patient attains baseline body weight and exhibits a positive or balanced nitrogen (N) state on N studies by the 24-hr period before hospital discharge.

ASSESSMENT/INTERVENTIONS	RATIONALES
Assess for dysphagia, polydipsia, and polyuria.	These indicators of a hyperglycemic state reflect the need for health care provider evaluation and intervention to ensure proper metabolism of carbohydrates if endocrine function is impaired. Hyperglycemia occurs because of interference with beta cell function. It is transient with acute pancreatitis but common with chronic pancreatitis, during which DM is likely to develop.
Monitor capillary blood sugar levels for the presence of hyperglycemia. Adjust insulin amounts according to capillary blood glucose levels, as prescribed.	Laboratory values of fasting blood sugar and bedside monitoring of blood glucose may reveal abnormalities in blood glucose levels and direct the appropriate insulin therapy (see "Diabetes Mellitus," p. 355, for more information).
Note the amount and degree of steatorrhea (foamy, foul-smelling stools high in fat content).	This is an indicator of fat malabsorption, which is common with chronic pancreatitis. Steatorrhea can indicate recurrence of the disease process or ineffectiveness of drug therapy and should be reported to the health care provider.
Weigh the patient daily to assess gain or loss.	Progressive weight loss may signal the need to change the diet or provide enzyme replacement therapy.
Deliver enteral or parenteral nutrition as prescribed.	Enteral feedings are being used with increasing frequency but should be infused past the ligament of Treitz to avoid pancreatic stimulation. Parenteral nutrition likely is instituted if distal enteral feedings are unobtainable or unsuccessful within 5-7 days.
Monitor blood glucose level q4h if administering parenteral nutrition.	Blood glucose needs to be monitored with parenteral nutrition due to the high glucose level in the fluids.
Provide oral hygiene at frequent intervals.	This measure enhances appetite and minimizes nausea.
When the gastric tube is removed, provide the diet as prescribed.	Small, high-carbohydrate, low-fat meals at frequent intervals (six per day) with protein added according to tolerance is the usual diet for patients with pancreatitis.
Instruct the patient to avoid coffee, tea, alcohol, and nicotine or other gastric irritants.	These are stimulants that increase pancreatic enzyme secretion.

ASSESSMENT/INTERVENTIONS

RATIONALES

ASSESSMENT/INTERVENTIONS	RATIONALES
As prescribed, administer pancreatic enzyme supplements.	Pancreatic enzyme supplements are given before introducing fat into the diet to enable its digestion.
If prescribed, administer other dietary supplements that support nutrition and caloric intake.	These supplements, which may include products that consist of medium-chain triglycerides (MCTs) such as MCT oil, do not require pancreatic enzymes for absorption.
Avoid administering pancreatin with hot foods or drinks.	Heat deactivates its enzyme activity.
Provide meals in small feedings throughout the day.	Smaller, more frequent meals may help alleviate bloating, nausea, and cramps experienced by some patients.

ADDITIONAL NURSING DIAGNOSES/PROBLEMS:

✓ PATIENT-FAMILY TEACHING AND DISCHARGE PLANNING

When providing patient-family teaching, focus on sensory information, avoid giving excessive information, and initiate a visiting nurse referral for necessary follow-up teaching. Include verbal and written information about the following:

- ✓ Cause for current episode of pancreatitis, if known, so that recurrence may be avoided.
- ✓ Alcohol consumption, which can cause or exacerbate acute or chronic pancreatitis.
- ✓ Diet: frequent, small meals that are high in carbohydrates and protein. Food should be bland until gradual return to normal diet is prescribed. Remind the patient to avoid enzyme stimulants, such as coffee, tea, nicotine, and alcohol.
- ✓ Medications, including drug name, purpose, dosage, schedule, precautions, and potential side effects.

Also discuss drug-drug, food-drug, and herb-drug interactions.

- ✓ Signs and symptoms of DM, including fatigue, weight loss, polydipsia, polyuria, and polyphagia.
- ✓ Necessity of medical follow-up; confirm time and date of next medical appointment.
- ✓ Potential for recurrence of steatorrhea as evidenced by foamy, foul-smelling stools that are high in fat content.
- ✓ Weighing daily at home; importance of reporting weight loss to the health care provider.
- ✓ If surgery was performed, instruct the patient on how to prevent infection and on the indicators of wound infection: redness, swelling, discharge, fever, pain, or increased local warmth.
- ✓ Availability of chemical dependency programs to prevent/treat drug dependence, which is a common occurrence with chronic pancreatitis; or to treat alcoholism. Discuss availability of community support groups, such as the following:
  - Alcoholics Anonymous at *www.alcoholics-anonymous .org*
  - Alcoholics Anonymous Canada at *aacanada.com*
  - Narcotics Anonymous at *www.na.org*
- ✓ For more information, contact the National Institute of Diabetes & Digestive & Kidney Diseases at *www .niddk.nih.gov*

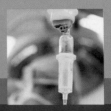

Peptic Ulcer Disease 59

OVERVIEW/PATHOPHYSIOLOGY

Peptic ulcers are erosions of the upper gastrointestinal (GI) tract mucosa, potentially extending through the muscularis mucosa and into the muscularis propria. They may occur anywhere the mucosa is exposed to the erosive action of gastric acid and pepsin. Commonly, ulcers are gastric or duodenal, but the esophagus, surgically created stomas, and other areas of the upper GI tract may be affected. Autodigestion of mucosal tissue and ulceration are associated with increased acidity of the stomach juices or increased sensitivity of the mucosal surfaces to erosion. Erosions can penetrate deeply into the mucosal layers and become a chronic problem, or they can be more superficial and manifest as an acute problem resulting from severe physiologic or psychologic trauma, infection, or shock (stress ulceration of the stomach or duodenum). The most common causes of peptic ulcer disease are use of nonsteroidal antiinflammatory drugs (NSAIDs) and infection with *Helicobacter pylori* (*H. pylori*). Duodenal and gastric ulcers also can occur in association with high-stress lifestyle, smoking, use of irritating drugs, as well as secondary to other diseases. Ulceration may occur as a part of Zollinger-Ellison syndrome, in which gastrinomas (gastrin-secreting tumors) of the pancreas or other organs develop. Gastric acid hypersecretion and ulceration subsequently occur.

H. pylori, a gram-negative, spiral-shaped bacterium with four to six flagella on one pole, was first isolated from gastric biopsies in 1983. *H. pylori* can reside below the mucosa of the stomach because it produces the enzyme *urease*, which hydrolyzes urea to ammonia and carbon dioxide, providing a buffering alkaline halo. Infection can go undetected for years because there may be no symptoms until gastric or duodenal ulceration or gastritis occurs. Transmission of *H. pylori* has been determined to be by fecal-oral and oral-oral routes. A high duodenal acid load is one of the characteristics of duodenal ulcer disease inasmuch as it reduces concentration of bile acids that normally inhibit growth of *H. pylori*. Gastric ulcers tend to occur on the lesser curvature of the stomach. Ulcers in both locations are characterized by slow healing leading to metaplasia. In turn, a greater colonization with *H. pylori* causes slow healing and results in a vicious cycle.

Serious and disabling complications, such as hemorrhage, GI obstruction, perforation, peritonitis, or intractable ulcer pain, are common. With treatment, ulcer healing usually occurs within 4-6 wk (gastric ulcers can take as long as 12-16 wk to heal), but there is potential for recurrence in the same or another site.

HEALTH CARE SETTING

Primary care; acute care for complications

ASSESSMENT

Signs and symptoms: Burning, gnawing, dull pain typically 1-3 hr after eating. Discomfort occurs more often between meals and at night. With duodenal ulcer, eating usually alleviates discomfort; with gastric ulcer, pain often worsens after meals. Older adults have less sensory perception in the stomach and may not experience pain as a symptom. In addition, 40% of patients with active ulcers deny abdominal pain. However, on evaluation there may be findings of ulcers, gastritis, and other conditions. Even so, pain symptoms warrant further investigation.

Hematemesis, melena, dizziness, and syncope are associated with an actively bleeding ulcer. Sudden, severe epigastric pain, often radiating to the right shoulder, suggests perforation of an ulcer. Pain described as piercing through to the back suggests penetration of the ulcer into adjacent posterior structures in the abdomen.

Physical assessment: Tenderness over the involved area of the abdomen. With perforation, there is severe pain (see "Peritonitis" for more information) and rebound tenderness. With penetration, the pain is usually altered by changes in back position (extension or flexion).

History and risk factors: NSAID use; smoking; use of irritating agents such as caffeine, alcohol, corticosteroids, salicylates, reserpine, indomethacin, or phenylbutazone; disorders of the endocrine glands, pancreas, or liver; and hypersecretory conditions, such as Zollinger-Ellison syndrome.

DIAGNOSTIC TESTS

Endoscopy: Allows visualization of the stomach (gastroscopy), duodenum (duodenoscopy), both stomach and duodenum (gastroduodenoscopy), or the esophagus, stomach, and duodenum (esophagogastroduodenoscopy) via passage of a lighted, fiberoptic, flexible endoscope. Patients are given nothing by mouth (NPO) for 8-12 hr before the procedure, and written consent is required. Before the test, a sedative is administered to relax the patient, and an opioid analgesic may be given to prevent pain. Local anesthetic may be sprayed into the posterior pharynx to ease passage of the tube. A biopsy may be performed as part of the endoscopy procedure. Biopsied tissue may be sent for histologic examination and for culture and sensitivity to identify *H. pylori* infection. Postprocedure care involves maintaining NPO status for ½-1 hr; ensuring return of the gag reflex before allowing the patient to eat (if local anesthetic was used); administering throat lozenges or analgesics as prescribed; and monitoring for complications, such as bleeding or perforation (e.g., hematemesis, pain, dyspnea, tachycardia, hypotension).

H. pylori *testing*: Serum antigen testing identifies exposure to *H. pylori* bacteria; this is the least expensive means of identifying *H. pylori* infection. However, antibody tests remain positive many months after successful therapy and are not reliable for assessing therapy effectiveness. A breath test is available to identify *H. pylori* infection by detecting carbon dioxide and ammonia as by-products of the action of the bacterium's urease in the patient's expired air. Histologic identification of the microorganism and culture are other direct tests for *H. pylori*. Direct tests and stool antigen testing require discontinuation of all drugs that suppress *H. pylori* for 2 wk before testing.

Barium swallow: Uses contrast agent (e.g., barium) to detect abnormalities. The patient should maintain NPO status and not smoke for at least 8 hr before the test. Postprocedure care involves administration of prescribed laxatives and enemas to facilitate passage of the barium and prevent constipation and fecal impaction.

Complete blood count (CBC): Reveals a decrease in hemoglobin (Hgb), hematocrit (Hct), and red blood cells when acute or chronic blood loss accompanies ulceration.

Stool for occult blood: Positive if bleeding is present.

Nursing Diagnoses:

Ineffective Protection
Risk for Bleeding

related to the potential for obstruction and perforation occurring with the ulcerative process

Desired Outcome: The patient is free of signs and symptoms of bleeding, obstruction, perforation, and peritonitis as evidenced by negative results for occult blood testing, passage of stool and flatus, soft and nondistended abdomen, good appetite, and normothermia.

ASSESSMENT/INTERVENTIONS	RATIONALES
⚠ Assess for hematemesis and melena. Check all NG aspirate, emesis, and stools for occult blood. Report positive findings.	Bleeding can occur with an ulcerative process.
Monitor results of CBC and coagulation studies.	Hct less than 40% (male) or less than 37% (female) and Hgb less than 14 g/dL (male) or less than 12 g/dL (female) are indicators of bleeding and should be reported promptly. The incidence of peptic ulcers is increased in cirrhosis patients, in whom clotting factors are altered. Partial thromboplastin time (PTT) greater than 70 sec or prothrombin time (PT) greater than 12.5 sec are longer than normal clotting times.
If indicated, insert a gastric tube.	A gastric tube will enable evacuation of blood from the stomach, monitoring of bleeding, and gastric lavage as prescribed.
⚠ Do not use gastric tubes in patients who have or are suspected of having esophageal varices.	Trauma from tube insertion could result in hemorrhage.
Monitor O₂ saturation via oximetry and report O₂ saturation 92% or less.	Usually patients with O₂ saturation 92% or less require oxygen supplementation.
If the patient is actively bleeding or if Hct is low, administer prescribed O₂.	A low Hct or Hgb indicates an anemic state, which means there is less available Hgb for oxygen transport.
⚠ Assess for and note abdominal pain, abnormal (increased peristalsis, "rushes," or "tinkles") or absent bowel sounds, distention, anorexia, nausea, vomiting, and inability to pass stool or flatus.	These are indicators of obstruction, a serious complication of peptic ulcers, which necessitates prompt notification of the health care provider for rapid intervention.

continued

ASSESSMENT/INTERVENTIONS	RATIONALES
Be alert to sudden or severe abdominal pain, distention, and rigidity; fever; nausea; and vomiting. Notify the health care provider immediately of significant findings.	These are indicators of perforation and peritonitis, serious complications of peptic ulcers that necessitate prompt notification of health care provider for rapid intervention. See "Peritonitis," p. 454, for more information.
Teach signs and symptoms of GI complications and the importance of reporting them promptly to the staff or the health care provider if they occur.	A knowledgeable patient likely will report these signs promptly, which will enable rapid treatment.

Nursing Diagnosis:

Impaired Tissue Integrity

related to GI exposure to chemical irritants (gastric acid, pepsin)

Desired Outcomes: The patient verbalizes knowledge of necessary lifestyle alterations within the 24-hr period before hospital discharge and demonstrates compliance with medical recommendations for peptic ulcer throughout the hospital stay. Gastric and duodenal mucosal tissues heal and remain intact as evidenced by reduced or absent pain and absence of bleeding.

ASSESSMENT/INTERVENTIONS	RATIONALES
Encourage the patient to avoid foods that seem to cause pain or increase acid secretion.	Although this response is highly individualized, foods that cause pain or increase acid secretion worsen mucosal erosion.
Advise the patient to avoid NSAIDs, aspirin, coffee, caffeine, and alcohol.	These foods and drugs are associated with increased acidity and GI erosions.
If applicable, recommend strategies for smoking cessation.	Smoking impairs ulcer healing and has been associated with a higher incidence of complications and the need for surgical repair of the ulcer.
Administer *H. pylori* eradication therapy for *H. pylori*–associated ulceration.	Highest eradication rates are obtained with a triple-drug regimen of proton pump inhibitor (PPI), clarithromycin, and amoxicillin. Metronidazole is substituted for amoxicillin in those patients who are allergic to penicillin. Treatment is given for 7 to 14 days. Some patients may receive a four-drug regimen, with the addition of bismuth.
Administer acid suppression therapy as prescribed.	This therapy is given for acute episodes of ulceration.
- PPIs (e.g., omeprazole, esomeprazole, lansoprazole, pantoprazole, rabeprazole, dexlansoprazole)	PPIs deactivate the enzyme system that pumps hydrogen ions (H^+) from the parietal cells, thus inhibiting gastric acid secretion. They are used for short-term treatment of active duodenal and gastric ulcers and for long-term treatment of gastroesophageal reflux disease and hypersecretory conditions. Omeprazole and lansoprazole are now available over the counter (OTC).
- Histamine H2-receptor blockers (e.g., cimetidine, ranitidine, nizatidine, famotidine)	These agents are administered by mouth (PO) or intravenous (IV) to suppress secretion of gastric acid and facilitate ulcer healing. They also can be used prophylactically for limited periods of time, especially in patients susceptible to stress ulceration. They are administered with meals at least 1 hr apart from antacids because antacids can reduce their absorption. They are available both through prescription and OTC, and although time to relief obtained is longer than with antacids, their effects last longer.
- Sucralfate	This is an antiulcer agent that coats the ulcer with a protective barrier so that healing can occur. It must be taken before meals and at bedtime. It should not be taken within 30 min of antacids because acid facilitates adherence of sucralfate to the ulcer.

ASSESSMENT/INTERVENTIONS

RATIONALES

ASSESSMENT/INTERVENTIONS	RATIONALES
- Antacids	Antacids are administered orally or through an NG tube to provide quick, symptomatic relief, facilitate ulcer healing, and prevent further ulceration. They can be administered prophylactically in patients who are especially susceptible to ulceration. Antacids are administered after meals and at bedtime or given periodically via NG tube for patients who are intubated.
Avoid or use misoprostol cautiously in women of childbearing age.	Because it can cause abortion this medication is used with caution in women of childbearing years who could be pregnant.
- Misoprostol	This is a synthetic prostaglandin E_1 analogue that enhances the body's normal mucosal protective mechanisms and decreases acid secretion. The drug may be used in the healing and prevention of NSAID-induced ulcers for people requiring high doses of NSAIDs for treatment of arthritis and other chronic pain conditions.
Stress the importance of taking medications at prescribed intervals, not just for symptomatic relief of pain.	Initial pain relief does not mean the ulcer is completely healed.
Refer the patient to community resources and support groups for assistance in smoking cessation or abstinence from drinking.	Smoking increases acid secretions and decreases mucosal blood flow, thereby inhibiting ulcer healing. Alcohol also slows the healing process.

ADDITIONAL NURSING DIAGNOSES/PROBLEMS:

"Perioperative Care"	p. 45
"Crohn's Disease" for **Acute Pain**, **Nausea**	p. 424

PATIENT-FAMILY TEACHING AND DISCHARGE PLANNING

When providing patient-family teaching, focus on sensory information, avoid giving excessive information, and initiate a visiting nurse referral for necessary follow-up teaching of skilled needs. Include verbal and written information about the following:

✓ Importance of following prescribed diet to facilitate ulcer healing, prevent exacerbation or recurrence, or control postsurgical dumping syndrome. If appropriate, arrange consultation with dietitian.

✓ Medications, including drug name, rationale, dosage, schedule, precautions, and potential side effects. Also discuss drug-drug, food-drug, and herb-drug interactions.

✓ Signs and symptoms of exacerbation and recurrence, as well as potential complications.

✓ Care of incision line and dressing change technique, as necessary.

✓ Signs of wound infection, including persistent redness, swelling, purulent drainage, local warmth, fever, and foul odor.

✓ Role of lifestyle alterations in preventing exacerbation or recurrence of ulcer, including smoking cessation, stress reduction, decreasing or eliminating consumption of alcohol, and avoidance of irritating foods and drugs. Note that histamine H2-receptor blockers are more effective in individuals who are nonsmokers.

✓ Referral to a health care specialist for assistance with stress reduction as necessary.

✓ Referrals to community support groups, such as Alcoholics Anonymous at *www.alcoholics-anonymous.org*

✓ Referrals to other reliable websites:
- National Digestive Diseases Information Clearinghouse at *www.digestive.niddk.nih.gov*
- American Gastroenterologic Association at *www.gastro.org* (use Patient Center link)
- Canadian Association of Gastroenterology at *www.cag-acg.org*

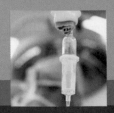

Peritonitis 60

OVERVIEW/PATHOPHYSIOLOGY

Peritonitis is the inflammatory response of the peritoneum to offending chemical and bacterial agents invading the peritoneal cavity. The inflammatory process can be local or generalized and may be classified as primary, secondary, or tertiary, depending on pathogenesis of the inflammation. Primary peritonitis, such as spontaneous bacterial peritonitis, occurs without a recognizable cause. Secondary peritonitis is caused by abdominal injury or rupture of abdominal organs. Common events include abdominal trauma, postoperative leakage of gastrointestinal (GI) content or blood into the peritoneal cavity, intestinal ischemia, ruptured or inflamed abdominal organs, poor sterile techniques (e.g., with peritoneal dialysis), and direct contamination of the bloodstream. Tertiary peritonitis is a persistent abdominal sepsis without a focus of infection, and it may follow treatment of a previous episode of peritonitis. The peritoneum responds to invasive agents by attempting to localize the infection with a shift of the omentum (the "guardian of the abdominal cavity") to wall off the inflamed area. Inflammation of the peritoneum results in tissue edema, development of fibrinous exudate, and hypermotility of the intestinal tract. As the disease progresses, paralytic ileus occurs, and intestinal fluid, which then cannot be reabsorbed, leaks into the peritoneal cavity. As a result of the fluid shift, cardiac output and tissue perfusion are reduced, leading to impaired cardiac and renal function. If infection or inflammation continues, respiratory failure and shock can ensue. Peritonitis often is progressive and can be fatal. It is the most common cause of death following abdominal surgery, and mortality is dictated by the patient's overall health, including nutritional and immune status and organ function.

HEALTH CARE SETTING

Acute care surgical unit, critical care unit

ASSESSMENT

Signs and symptoms

Early findings: Acute abdominal pain with movement, anorexia, nausea, vomiting, chills, fever, rigor, malaise, weakness, hiccoughs, diaphoresis, absence of bowel sounds, and abdominal distention and rigidity (often described as boardlike).

Later findings: Dehydration (e.g., thirst, dry mucous membranes, oliguria, concentrated urine, poor skin turgor).

Physical assessment: Presence of tachycardia, hypotension, and shallow and rapid respirations caused by abdominal distention and discomfort. Often the patient assumes a supine position with knees flexed or side-lying with knees drawn up toward the chest. Palpation usually reveals peritoneal irritation as shown by distention, abdominal rigidity with general or localized tenderness, guarding, and rebound or cough tenderness. However, as many as one fourth of these patients will have minimal or no indications of peritoneal irritation. Auscultation findings include hyperactive bowel sounds during the gradual development of peritonitis and absence of bowel sounds or infrequent high-pitched sounds ("tinkling" or "squeaky") during later stages if paralytic ileus occurs. Ascites may be present as demonstrated by shifting areas of dullness on percussion.

History of: Abdominal surgery, cirrhosis, peptic ulcer disease, cholecystitis, acute necrotizing pancreatitis, other GI disorders, acute salpingitis, ruptured appendix or diverticulum, trauma, peritoneal dialysis.

DIAGNOSTIC TESTS

Serum tests: May reveal presence of leukocytosis, usually with a shift to the left (may be the only sign of tertiary peritonitis); hemoconcentration; elevated blood urea nitrogen (BUN); and electrolyte imbalance, particularly hypokalemia. Hypoalbuminemia and prolonged prothrombin time (PT), in combination with leukocytosis, are especially characteristic.

Arterial blood gas (ABG) values: May reveal hypoxemia (PaO$_2$ less than 80 mm Hg) or acidosis (pH less than 7.40).

Urinalysis: Often performed to rule out genitourinary involvement (e.g., pyelonephritis).

Paracentesis for peritoneal aspiration with culture and sensitivity and cell count: May be performed to determine presence of blood, bacteria, bile, pus, and amylase content and identify causative organism. Gram stain of ascitic fluid is positive in only about 25% of these patients. Diagnosis of bacterial peritonitis is confirmed by positive culture of ascitic fluid and cell count and differential of the ascitic fluid notable for elevated polymorphonuclear (PMN) count of 250 cells/mm^3 or greater. Ascitic fluid also may be tested for total protein, glucose concentration, and lactate dehydrogenase to differentiate spontaneous bacterial peritonitis from secondary bacterial peritonitis.

Abdominal x-ray examination: To determine presence of distended loops of bowel and abnormal levels of fluid and gas, which usually collect in the large and small bowel in the presence of a perforation or obstruction. "Free air" under the diaphragm also may be visualized, which indicates a perforated viscus.

Computed tomography (CT) scan, ultrasound, and magnetic resonance imaging (MRI): May be used to evaluate abdominal pain and more clearly delineate nondistinct areas found by plain abdominal x-ray examination.

Chest x-ray examination: Abdominal distention may elevate the diaphragm. Pain from peritonitis may limit respiratory excursion and lead to associated infiltrates in the lower lobes. In later stages, changes in serum osmolality allow for pleural effusions to occur.

Contrast x-ray examination: May be used to identify specific intestinal pathologic conditions. Water-soluble contrast (e.g., meglumine diatrizoate) may be used to evaluate suspected upper GI perforation.

Radionuclide scans: Gallium, hepatoiminodiacetic acid (HIDA) (lidofenin), and liver-spleen scans may be used to identify intraabdominal abscess.

Nursing Diagnoses:

Risk for Infection
Risk for Shock

related to the potential for worsening/recurring peritonitis or development of an inflammatory process

Desired Outcome: The patient is free of symptoms of worsening/recurring peritonitis or septic shock as evidenced by normothermia, blood pressure (BP) at least 90/60 mm Hg (or within the patient's normal range), heart rate (HR) 100 bpm or less, absence of chills, presence of eupnea, urinary output at least 30 mL/hr, central venous pressure (CVP) 2-6 mm Hg (5-12 cm H_2O), decreasing abdominal girth measurements, and minimal tenderness to palpation.

ASSESSMENT/INTERVENTIONS	RATIONALES
[!] Assess the abdomen q1-2h during the acute phase and q4h once the patient is stabilized.	Bowel sounds initially may be frequent but later are absent as peritonitis advances. The patient may have decreased/absent bowel sounds with an ileus; intermittent loud, rushing bowel sounds with an obstruction; abdominal rigidity, distention, rebound tenderness; hyperresonance/tympany with an ileus or free air in the abdomen; and loss of dullness over the liver (free air in the abdomen).
[!] *Lightly* palpate the abdomen for evidence of increasing rigidity or tenderness.	This would signal disease progression. If the patient experiences increased pain on removal of your hand, rebound tenderness is present.
[!] Measure abdominal girth. Notify the health care provider of significant findings.	Girth measurements monitor for increasing distention, which would signal development of ascites.
Use a permanent marker to identify placement of tape measure.	This ensures consistent site of measurement by caregivers.
[!] Assess vital signs (VS) and skin at least q2h and more frequently if the patient's condition is unstable. Be alert to signs of septic shock: increased temperature, hypotension, tachycardia, shallow and rapid respirations, urine output less than 30 mL/hr, and CVP less than 2 mm Hg (less than 5 cm H_2O).	In the early stage of shock (preshock or warm shock), skin usually is warm, pink, and dry secondary to peripheral venous pooling, and BP and CVP begin to drop. In the late stage of shock, extremities become pale and cool because of decreasing tissue perfusion.
If prescribed, insert a gastric tube and connect it to suction.	Suction prevents or decreases distention.
Administer antibiotics as prescribed; ensure close adherence to schedules for maintenance of bacteriocidal serum levels.	Combination broad-spectrum antibiotic therapy is rapidly begun to ensure treatment of gram-negative bacilli and anaerobic bacteria. Common agents include cephalosporins (cefotaxime, cefepime), aminoglycosides (gentamicin), ampicillin, floxacin (Floxin), and metronidazole. Antibiotics are commonly administered intravenously and may also be directly instilled into the peritoneal cavity via surgically placed catheters.

continued

ASSESSMENT/INTERVENTIONS	RATIONALES
Collect peak and trough antibiotic determinations as prescribed.	Peak and trough levels are drawn at specific times around the antibiotic dose. Peak levels indicate if there is enough medication in the bloodstream and the dose is high enough. The trough level indicates if the kidneys/liver are clearing the medication adequately.
Monitor CBCs for the presence of leukocytosis, which signals infection, and hemoconcentration (increased hematocrit [Hct] and hemoglobin [Hgb]), which occurs with decreased plasma volume. Notify the health care provider of significant findings.	Normal values are as follows: white blood cell (WBC) count 4500-11,000/mm³; Hgb 14-18 g/dL (male) or 12-16 g/dL (female); Hct 40%-54% (male) or 37%-47% (female). With peritonitis, WBC count usually is greater than 20,000/mm³.
Maintain sterile technique with dressing changes and all invasive procedures.	This prevents/reduces spread of infection.
Teach signs and symptoms of recurring peritonitis and the importance of reporting them promptly if they occur: fever, chills, abdominal pain, vomiting, and abdominal distention.	An informed individual likely will report these signs promptly for rapid treatment.

Nursing Diagnoses:

Acute Pain
Nausea

related to the inflammatory process, fever, and tissue damage

Desired Outcomes: The patient's subjective perception of pain decreases within 1 hr of intervention, as documented by a pain scale. Nonverbal indicators, such as grimacing and abdominal guarding, are absent or diminished.

ASSESSMENT/INTERVENTIONS	RATIONALES
Assess and document the character and severity of discomfort q1-2h. Devise a pain scale with the patient, rating discomfort on a scale of 0 (no pain) to 10 (worst pain).	This assessment will not only define the type of pain but it will monitor relief of discomfort obtained to determine effectiveness of the treatment.
After diagnosis has been made, administer opioids, other analgesics, and sedatives as prescribed.	These medications relieve severe pain and discomfort once the diagnosis has been confirmed. Because potent analgesics can mask diagnostic symptoms, opioids should not be administered until surgical evaluation has been completed.
Encourage the patient to request analgesic *before* pain becomes severe. Document relief obtained, using the pain scale.	Pain management is more effective when analgesia is given before pain becomes too severe. Prolonged stimulation of pain receptors results in increased sensitivity to painful stimuli and will increase the amount of analgesia required to relieve pain.
Keep the patient on bedrest. Provide a restful and quiet environment.	Rest minimizes pain, which can be aggravated by activity and stress.
Instruct the patient in methods to splint the abdomen.	Splinting reduces pain on movement, coughing, and deep breathing.
Keep the patient in a position of comfort, usually semi-Fowler's position with the knees bent.	This position promotes fluid shift to the lower abdomen, which will reduce pressure on the diaphragm and enable deeper and easier respirations. Raising the knees will decrease stress on the abdominal wall.
Describe and explain the illness, all procedures, and the treatment plan to the patient.	Information helps minimize anxiety, which can exacerbate discomfort.
Offer mouth care and lip moisturizers at frequent intervals.	Oral care helps relieve discomfort from continuous or intermittent suction, dehydration, and nothing by mouth (NPO) status.
Administer antiemetics (e.g., hydroxyzine, ondansetron, prochlorperazine, promethazine) as prescribed; instruct the patient to request medication *before* nausea becomes severe.	These medications, when given early, combat nausea and vomiting before they become more difficult to control.
See "Pain," p. 39, for other pain interventions.	

Nursing Diagnoses:

Impaired Gas Exchange

related to alveolar hypoventilation

Ineffective Breathing Pattern

related to decreased depth of respirations occurring with guarding

Desired Outcomes: The patient has an effective breathing pattern and optimal gas exchange as evidenced by PaO_2 at least 80 mm Hg; oxygen saturation greater than 92%; BP at least 90/60 mm Hg (or within the patient's baseline range); HR 100 bpm or less; and orientation to person, place, and time. Eupnea occurs within 1 hr after pain-relieving intervention(s).

ASSESSMENT/INTERVENTIONS	RATIONALES
Monitor VS, ABG, and oximetry results for evidence of hypoxemia.	The following are indicators of hypoxemia and usually signal the need for supplemental oxygen: PaO_2 less than 80 mm Hg, low oxygen saturation (92% or less), and the following clinical signs: hypotension, tachycardia, tachypnea, restlessness, confusion or altered mental status, central nervous system depression, and possibly cyanosis.
Auscultate the lung fields. Note and document the presence of adventitious breath sounds.	This assessment monitors ventilation and detects pulmonary complications, such as pleural effusion. Pleural effusion, an accumulation of fluid in the pleural space, can develop in later stages of peritonitis because of changes in serum osmolality. Decreased breath sounds and pleural friction rub are diagnostic of pleural effusion.
Keep the patient in semi-Fowler's or high Fowler's position; encourage deep breathing and coughing. Assist with and monitor the effects of incentive spirometry.	These positions and exercises aid respiratory effort and promote deep breathing to enhance oxygenation and coughing to clear pulmonary secretions.
Instruct the patient in splinting the abdomen.	Splinting enables better chest excursion to facilitate respiratory hygiene.
Administer oxygen as prescribed.	Oxygen supports increased metabolic needs and treats hypoxia.

Nursing Diagnosis:

Imbalanced Nutrition: Less Than Body Requirements

related to vomiting and intestinal suctioning

Desired Outcome: By at least 24 hr before hospital discharge, the patient demonstrates optimal progress toward adequate nutritional status as evidenced by stable weight and balanced or positive nitrogen (N) state.

ASSESSMENT/INTERVENTIONS	RATIONALES
Keep the patient NPO as prescribed during the acute phase.	Oral fluids are not resumed until the patient has passed flatus and the gastric/intestinal tube has been removed. If the patient has an ileus, a nasogastric tube will be inserted to decompress the abdomen.
Reintroduce oral fluids gradually once motility has returned, as evidenced by bowel sounds, decreased distention, and passage of flatus.	This ensures the patient will tolerate fluids through the intestines, which may have become irritated from the inflammatory process.
Support the patient with peripheral parenteral nutrition or total parenteral nutrition (TPN), as prescribed, depending on duration of the acute phase (usually by day 5).	If the GI tract is nonfunctioning, TPN usually is initiated in the early stages to promote nutrition and protein replacement.

continued

ASSESSMENT/INTERVENTIONS	RATIONALES
Administer replacement fluids, electrolytes, and vitamins as prescribed.	This maintains hydration and restores electrolytes and nutrients lost in gastric/intestinal tube output and fluid shifts. Daily measurements of serum electrolytes and calculations of fluid volume are performed to determine necessary types of fluid and electrolyte replacement. Crystalloids, colloids (albumin, Plasmanate), blood, and blood products may be administered to correct hypovolemia, hypoproteinemia, and anemia.
Teach the patient the rationale for tube placement and NPO status; underlying pathologic condition (as appropriate); need for close monitoring of fluid intake and output; and, eventually, diet advancement.	A knowledgeable patient likely will adhere to the treatment regimen and report symptoms that would necessitate timely intervention.

ADDITIONAL NURSING DIAGNOSES/PROBLEMS:

 PATIENT-FAMILY TEACHING AND DISCHARGE PLANNING

When providing patient-family teaching, focus on sensory information, avoid giving excessive information, and initiate a visiting nurse referral for necessary monitoring of wound care and follow-up teaching. Include verbal and written information about the following:

✓ Medications, including drug name, dosage, schedule, purpose, precautions, and potential side effects. Also discuss drug-drug, food-drug, and herb-drug interactions.

✓ Activity alterations as prescribed by the health care provider, such as avoiding heavy lifting (more than 10 lb), resting after periods of fatigue, getting maximum amounts of rest, and gradually increasing activities to tolerance.

✓ Notifying the health care provider of the following indicators of recurrence: fever, chills, abdominal pain, vomiting, abdominal distention.

✓ If the patient has undergone surgery, indicators of wound infection: fever, pain, chills, incisional swelling, persistent erythema, purulent drainage.

✓ Importance of follow-up medical care; confirm date and time of next medical appointment.

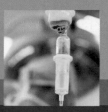

Ulcerative Colitis 61

OVERVIEW/PATHOPHYSIOLOGY

Ulcerative colitis (UC) is a nonspecific, chronic inflammatory disease of the mucosa and submucosa of the colon. Generally the disease begins in the rectum and sigmoid colon, but it can extend proximally and uninterrupted as far as the cecum. In 30%-50% of cases, the rectum (proctitis) or rectosigmoid (proctosigmoiditis) is affected; in 30%-40% of cases, the disease extends to the splenic flexure (left-sided or distal colitis); and in 20%-30% of cases, the disease extends proximally to involve the entire colon (pancolitis). In some instances, a few centimeters of distal ileum are affected. This is sometimes referred to as *backwash ileitis*, and it occurs in only about 10% of patients with UC involving the entire colon. In the majority of patients, extent of colonic involvement is maintained from onset through the disease course, with the patient experiencing flare-ups and remissions. UC initially affects the mucosal layer. Eventually small mucosal layer abscesses form that ultimately penetrate the submucosa, spread horizontally, and allow sloughing of the mucosa, creating ulcerative lesions. The muscular layer (muscularis) generally is not affected, but the serosal layer may have congested and dilated blood vessels.

The cause of UC is unknown, but theories posit an interaction of external agents, host responses, and genetic immunologic factors creating the pathogenic responses. In a genetically susceptible subject, an outside agent or substance, such as a bacterium, virus, or other antigen, interacts with the body's immune system to trigger the disease or may cause damage to the intestinal wall, initiating or accelerating the disease process. The resulting inflammatory response continues unregulated by the immune system. As a result, inflammation continues damaging the intestinal wall, causing symptoms of UC. Medical therapy is based on symptomatic relief. The goals are to terminate the acute attack, induce and maintain remission, maintain quality of life, and prevent complications, both disease related and therapy related. Surgical intervention is indicated only when the disease is intractable to medical management or when the patient develops a disabling complication. Total proctocolectomy cures UC and results in construction of a permanent fecal diversion.

The most firmly established risk factor for developing inflammatory bowel disease (IBD) is a positive family history. There is a 10-fold increase in risk of IBD in first-degree relatives of patients with UC. Individuals with UC develop colonic adenocarcinomas at 10 times the rate of the general population. UC can occur at any age but is generally diagnosed in the third decade of life with a second peak in the fifth and sixth decades. There is no difference in gender distribution; however, men are more likely than women to be diagnosed in the fifth and sixth decades of life. Incidence is higher in the Caucasian population and in Ashkenazi Jews than in nonwhite populations and in people of non-Jewish descent. UC is more prevalent in urban, developed countries with temperate climates than in rural, more southern countries. It is more common in nonsmokers and former smokers, suggesting that smoking has a protective effect and may decrease severity of symptoms. Appendectomy before age 20 may reduce risk.

HEALTH CARE SETTING

Primary care; acute care for complications

ASSESSMENT

Signs and symptoms:

Bloody diarrhea (the cardinal symptom): The clinical picture can vary from acute episodes with frequent discharge of watery stools mixed with blood, pus, and mucus, accompanied by fever, abdominal pain, rectal urgency, and tenesmus, to loose or frequent stools, to formed stools coated with a little blood. However, nearly two thirds of patients have crampy abdominal pain and varying degrees of fever, vomiting, anorexia, weight loss, and dehydration. Remissions and exacerbations are common. Extracolonic manifestations also can occur, including polyarthritis, skin lesions (erythema nodosum, pyoderma gangrenosum), liver impairment, and ophthalmic complications (iritis, uveitis). Extracolonic manifestations may precede overt bowel disease, and their clinical activity may be related or unrelated to the clinical activity of the bowel disease.

Physical assessment: With mild disease, there is no significant abdominal tenderness; left lower quadrant (LLQ) cramps are commonly relieved by defecation. With moderate disease, abdominal pain and tenderness may be present; mild fever (temperature 99°-100° F), anemia (hematocrit [Hct] 30%-40%), and hypoalbuminemia (3.0-3.5 g/dL) may be present. With severe disease, abdominal pain and tenderness are present, especially in the LLQ; distention and a tender, spastic anus also may be present; fever (temperature greater than 100° F), severe anemia (Hct less than 30%), and impaired nutrition with hypoalbuminemia (less than 3.0 g/dL) and weight loss are present. With rectal examination, the mucosa may feel gritty and the examining gloved finger may be covered with blood, mucus, or pus.

Risk factors: Duration of active disease more than 10 yr, pancolitis, and family history of colonic cancer.

DIAGNOSTIC TESTS

Stool examination: Reveals presence of frank or occult blood. Stool cultures and smears rule out bacterial and parasitic disorders. Stool is examined also for white blood cells (WBCs) and certain proteins, the presence of which suggests inflammation.

> **Note:** *Collect specimens before barium enema is performed.*

Sigmoidoscopy: Reveals red, granular, hyperemic, and extremely friable mucosa; strips of inflamed mucosa undermined by surrounding ulcerations, which form pseudopolyps; and thick exudate composed of blood, pus, and mucus.

> **Note:** *Enemas should not be given before the examination because they can produce hyperemia and edema and may cause exacerbation of the disease. A limited prep may be given to facilitate visualization during examination.*

Colonoscopy: Will help determine extent of the disease and differentiate UC from Crohn's disease (CD) through both endoscopic appearance and histologic examination of biopsy tissues. Serial colonoscopy is also performed to monitor patients with chronic UC at risk for colon carcinoma. The evolving techniques of high-resolution and high-magnification endoscopy have the potential for detecting subtle mucosal changes. *Chromoendoscopy* is a staining technique used during surveillance colonoscopy in which a blue dye is used to improve detection of flat neoplastic lesions or polyps.

> **Note:** *Colonoscopy may be contraindicated in patients with acute disease because of risk of perforation or hemorrhage.*

Rectal biopsy: Helps differentiate UC from carcinoma and other inflammatory processes.

Barium enema: Reveals mucosal irregularity from fine serrations to ragged ulcerations, narrowing and shortening of the colon, presence of pseudopolyps, loss of haustral markings, and presence of spasms and irritability. Double-contrast technique may facilitate detection of superficial mucosal lesions. With a double-contrast technique, barium is instilled into the colon as with a conventional barium enema, but most of the barium is then withdrawn and the colon is inflated with air, which causes a thin coating of barium to line the intestinal wall. The double-contrast technique has become the "gold standard" for evaluating patients for colitis.

> **Note:** *Because they produce hyperemia and edema and may cause exacerbation of the disease, irritant cathartics and enemas should not be given before the examination.*

Abdominal plain films (flat plate): An important tool for screening severely ill patients when colonoscopy and barium enema are contraindicated. An abdominal flat plate may reveal fecal residue, appearance of mucosal margins, widening or thickening of visible haustra, and colonic wall diameter. In patients with suspected ileus, obstruction, or perforation, the flat plate film reveals abnormal gas and fluid levels or presence of free air in the peritoneal cavity.

Computed tomography (CT) scan: Used to identify suspected complications of UC (e.g., toxic megacolon, pneumatosis coli).

Serum antibody testing: Several serum antibodies are being evaluated for aiding in the development of noninvasive diagnostic techniques for UC. Some of these tests have been found to be useful in differentiating UC from CD.

Radionuclide imaging: To identify extent of disease activity, especially when colonoscopy and barium enema are contraindicated. Injections of indium-111–labeled autologous leukocytes are used to identify areas of active inflammation.

Blood tests: Anemia, with hypochromic microcytic red blood indices in severe disease, usually is present because of blood loss, iron deficiency, and bone marrow depression. WBC count may be normal to markedly elevated in severe disease. Sedimentation rate usually is increased according to illness severity. C-reactive protein elevation reflects degree of inflammation. Hypoalbuminemia and negative nitrogen (N) state occur in moderately severe to severe disease and result from decreased protein intake, decreased albumin synthesis in the debilitated condition, and increased metabolic needs. Electrolyte imbalance is common; hypokalemia is often present because of colonic losses (diarrhea) and renal losses in patients taking high doses of corticosteroids. Bicarbonate may be decreased because of colonic losses and may signal metabolic acidosis.

Nursing Diagnoses:

Deficient Fluid Volume
Risk for Bleeding
Risk for Electrolyte Imbalance

related to active loss occurring with diarrhea and gastrointestinal (GI) disorder/surgery

Desired Outcomes: The patient is normovolemic within 24 hr of admission as evidenced by balanced intake and turgor, moist mucous membranes, stable weight, blood pressure (BP) 90/60 mm Hg or more (or within the patient's normal range), and respiratory rate (RR) 12-20 breaths/min. Serum electrolytes, Hct, hemoglobin (Hgb), and red blood cells (RBCs) are all within optimal values as outlined in the third rationale, below.

ASSESSMENT/INTERVENTIONS	RATIONALES
Assess for hypotension, increased heart rate (HR) and RR, pallor, diaphoresis, and restlessness. Assess stool for quality (e.g., is it grossly bloody and liquid?) and quantity (e.g., is it mostly blood or mostly stool?). Report significant findings to the health care provider.	These are signs of hemorrhage.
Assess for thirst, poor skin turgor (may not be a reliable indicator of hydration in the older adult), dryness of mucous membranes, fever, and concentrated (specific gravity greater than 1.030) and decreased urinary output.	These are indicators of dehydration.
Assess I&O and urine specific gravity; weigh the patient daily; and assess laboratory values to evaluate fluid, electrolyte, and hematologic status.	These assessments evaluate fluid, electrolyte, and hematologic status. Optimal values are serum K^+ 3.5-5.0 mEqL, Hct 40%-54% (male) and 37%-47% (female), Hgb 14-18 g/dL (male) and 12-16 g/dL (female), and RBCs 4.5-6.0 million/mm^3 (male) and 4.0-5.5 million/mm^3 (female). Critical values: K^+ less than 2.5 or greater than 6.5 mEq/L, Hct less than 15% or greater than 60%, Hgb less than 5.0 g/dL or greater than 20 g/dL. Hypokalemia is common because of the prolonged diarrhea. Prolonged anemia may result in decreased Hct, Hgb, and RBCs.
Assess frequency and consistency of stool. For frequent bowel movements, keep a stool count; measure liquid stools. Assess and record presence of blood, mucus, fat, and undigested food.	Although bloody diarrhea is most commonly seen, the patient may experience acute episodes with frequent discharge of watery stools mixed with blood, pus, and mucus, accompanied by fever, abdominal pain, rectal urgency, and tenesmus; loose or frequent stools; or formed stools coated with a little blood.
Provide parenteral replacement of fluids, electrolytes, and vitamins as prescribed.	These measures maintain the acutely ill patient and are guided by laboratory test results.
Administer blood products and iron as prescribed.	This will help correct existing anemia and losses caused by hemorrhage.
Double-check blood product and type with a colleague.	These precautions help ensure that the patient receives the correct blood product and type, which otherwise could result in transfusion reaction.
Monitor for and report chills, back pain, dyspnea, hives, and wheezing.	These are signs of a transfusion reaction.
Provide a bland, high-protein, high-calorie, low-residue diet as prescribed, when the patient is taking food by mouth (PO).	Nutritional management varies with the patient's condition. In severely ill patients, total parenteral nutrition (TPN) along with nothing by mouth (NPO) status are prescribed to replace nutritional deficits while allowing complete bowel rest and improving nutritional status before surgery. For less severely ill patients, a low-residue elemental diet provides good nutrition with low fecal volume to allow bowel rest. A bland, high-protein, high-calorie, low-residue diet with vitamin and mineral supplements and excluding raw fruits and vegetables provides good nutrition and decreases diarrhea. Milk and wheat products are restricted to reduce cramping and diarrhea in patients with lactose and gluten intolerance.
Assess tolerance to the diet.	Cramping, diarrhea, and flatulence are signs the patient is not tolerating the diet.

Nursing Diagnoses:

Risk for Injury
Risk for Infection

related to potential for perforation occurring with deeply inflamed colonic mucosa

Desired Outcome: The patient is free of signs of perforation as evidenced by normothermia; HR 60-100 bpm; RR 12-20 breaths/min with normal depth and pattern (eupnea); normal bowel sounds; absence of abdominal distention, tympany, or rebound tenderness; negative culture results; no mental status changes; and orientation to person, place, and time.

ASSESSMENT/INTERVENTIONS	RATIONALES
Assess for fever, chills, increased respiratory and heart rates, diaphoresis, and increased abdominal discomfort.	These indicators can occur with perforation of the colon and potentially result in localized abscess or generalized fecal peritonitis and septicemia. **Note:** Systemic therapy with corticosteroids and antibiotics can mask the development of this complication.
Report any evidence of sudden abdominal distention associated with the preceding symptoms.	Together these indicators can signal toxic megacolon. Factors contributing to development of this complication include hypokalemia, barium enema examinations, and use of opioids and anticholinergics. Surgery to prevent perforation is indicated in patients with fulminant disease or toxic megacolon whose condition worsens or does not improve in 48-72 hr.
Assess mental status, orientation, and level of consciousness q2-4h.	Mental cloudiness, lethargy, and increased restlessness can signal impending or actual septic shock.
If the patient has a sudden temperature elevation, culture blood and other sites as prescribed. Assess culture reports, notifying the health care provider promptly of any positive cultures.	A temperature spike can signal septicemia; a culture will identify causative organism if present.
Assess WBC counts.	Patients with severe UC can have markedly elevated WBC counts—greater than 20,000/mm^3 and occasionally as high as 50,000/mm^3. Critical values are less than 2500/mm^3 and greater than 30,000/mm^3.
Administer antibiotics as prescribed and in a timely fashion.	This measure ensures optimal blood levels of the effective therapeutic dose in order to kill the bacteria and control infection in the patient with acute pancolitis or toxic megacolon because secondary bacterial infection of deeply inflamed mucosa is likely. Antibiotics are not indicated in the management of mild to moderate disease because infectious agents are not believed to be responsible for UC.

Nursing Diagnoses:

Acute Pain
Nausea

related to the intestinal inflammatory process

Desired Outcomes: Within 1 hr of intervention, the patient's subjective perception of discomfort decreases as documented by pain scale. Objective indicators, such as grimacing, are absent or diminished.

ASSESSMENT/INTERVENTIONS	RATIONALES
Assess and document characteristics of the discomfort, and assess whether it is associated with ingestion of certain foods or medications or with emotional stress. Devise a pain scale with the patient, rating discomfort from 0 (no pain) to 10 (worst pain). Eliminate foods that cause cramping and discomfort.	These assessments help determine the discomfort trigger and degree to which discomfort is alleviated following intervention.
[!] Assess for intensification of symptoms. Notify the health care provider of significant findings.	This can indicate the presence of complications, which should be treated promptly.
As prescribed, maintain the patient NPO or on TPN to provide bowel rest.	These measures provide bowel rest, which should help alleviate symptoms.
Provide nasal and oral care at frequent intervals.	These measures lessen discomfort from NPO status, nausea, or presence of a nasogastric (NG) tube.
Keep the patient's environment quiet. Facilitate coordination of health care providers to provide rest periods between care activities. Allow 90 min for undisturbed rest.	Rest promotes healing.
Administer sedatives and tranquilizers as prescribed.	These agents promote rest and reduce anxiety, which optimally will lessen symptoms.
[!] Administer hydrophilic colloids, anticholinergics, and antidiarrheal medications as prescribed.	These agents relieve cramping and diarrhea. **Caution:** Opioids and anticholinergics should be administered with extreme caution because they contribute to the development of toxic megacolon.
Instruct the patient to request medication before discomfort becomes severe.	Cramping and diarrhea are more easily controlled if they are treated before they become severe.

Nursing Diagnoses:

Diarrhea
Dysfunctional Gastrointestinal Motility
Risk for Electrolyte Imbalance

related to the inflammatory process of the intestines

Desired Outcome: The patient's stools become normal in consistency, and frequency is lessened within 3 days of admission.

ASSESSMENT/INTERVENTIONS	RATIONALES
Assess and record the amount, frequency, and character of stools. When possible, measure liquid stools.	Although bloody diarrhea is the cardinal symptom, the clinical picture can vary from acute episodes with frequent discharge of watery stools mixed with blood, pus, and mucus, accompanied by fever, abdominal pain, rectal urgency, and tenesmus, to loose or frequent stools, to formed stools coated with a little blood.
Assess serum electrolytes, particularly K^+, for abnormalities. Alert the health care provider to K^+ less than 3.5 mEq/L. (Critical value: K^+ less than 2.5 mEq/L.)	Hypokalemia is often present because of colonic losses (diarrhea) and renal losses in patients taking high doses of corticosteroids.
Provide a covered bedpan, commode, or bathroom that is easily accessible and ready to use at all times.	This will control odor and decrease the patient's anxiety and self-consciousness. Easy access promotes patient safety and enables the patient to cope with diarrhea more effectively.
Empty the bedpan and commode promptly.	This will remove the source of odor and decrease the patient's anxiety about incontinence.

continued

ASSESSMENT/INTERVENTIONS	RATIONALES
Administer hydrophilic colloids, anticholinergics, and antidiarrheal medications as prescribed.	These agents decrease fluidity and number of stools as well as inhibit GI peristaltic activity. **Caution:** Opioids and anticholinergics should be administered with extreme caution because they contribute to the development of toxic megacolon.
Administer topical corticosteroid or aminosalicylate preparations and antibiotics via retention enema, as prescribed.	These agents reduce mucosal inflammation in patients with mild disease limited to the rectum and sigmoid colon. In patients with acute moderate to severe disease and with more extensive (pancolonic) disease, oral or intravenous (IV) corticosteroid therapy is initiated. In patients not responding to steroids or aminosalicylates, immunosuppressive immunomodulatory therapy may be initiated to reduce inflammation.
If the patient has difficulty retaining the enema for the prescribed amount of time, consult the health care provider about use of corticosteroid foam.	Corticosteroid foam is easier to retain and administer.
Administer probiotics or fish oil, as prescribed.	Probiotics are beneficial bacteria that restore balance to the intestinal environment, with resulting reduction in inflammation. Omega-3 fatty acids found in fish oil appear to benefit patients with active UC by decreasing inflammation; they must be taken in large quantity.

Nursing Diagnosis:

Risk for Impaired Skin Integrity: Perineal/Perianal

related to persistent diarrhea

Desired Outcome: The patient's perineal/perianal skin remains intact with no erythema.

ASSESSMENT/INTERVENTIONS	RATIONALES
Provide materials or assist the patient with cleansing and drying the perineal area after each bowel movement. Use a nonirritating cleansing agent.	These measures help keep skin clean and intact.
Apply protective skin care products (skin preparations, gels, or barrier films).	These products prevent irritation caused by frequent liquid stools and maintain perianal skin integrity. Skin care products containing alcohol should not be used on broken or denuded skin because the alcohol content causes a painful burning sensation.
Administer hydrophilic colloids, anticholinergics, and antidiarrheal medications as prescribed.	These agents decrease fluidity and number of stools and inhibit GI peristaltic activity. **Caution:** Opioids and anticholinergics should be administered with extreme caution because they contribute to the development of toxic megacolon.

Nursing Diagnosis:

Deficient Knowledge

related to unfamiliarity with the purpose and precautions for medications used with UC

Desired Outcome: Immediately following teaching (if the patient is not hospitalized) or within the 24-hr period before hospital discharge, the patient verbalizes accurate information about medications used with UC, including their purpose and necessary precautions.

ASSESSMENT/INTERVENTIONS	RATIONALES

Note: Treatment is customized based upon the type and severity of symptoms. Teach patients the following:

⚠ Corticosteroids

	Corticosteroids reduce mucosal inflammation by depressing the immune system.
Dosage and routes of administration vary with the severity and extent of the disease.	In patients with mild disease limited to the rectum and sigmoid colon, rectal instillation of steroids via enema (topically treats inflammation in the sigmoid colon as well as rectum) and via foam or suppository (topically treats inflammation in the rectum) may induce or maintain remission. In patients with more extensive (pancolonic) and acute active disease, oral corticosteroid therapy with prednisone or prednisolone usually is initiated. In severely ill patients with fulminant disease, IV corticosteroids are given.
Once clinical remission is achieved, IV and oral corticosteroids are tapered until discontinuation.	These medications have not been shown to prolong remission or prevent future exacerbations.
For additional information on side effects and precautions, see "Crohn's Disease," **Deficient Knowledge** (Corticosteroids).	

Aminosalicylates: Sulfasalazine and 5-Aminosalicytic Acid (5-ASA) Preparations

	These medications work at the intestinal lining to decrease inflammation. They do not suppress the immune system.

Sulfasalazine (Azulfidine)

This oral agent helps maintain remissions and is effective in the treatment of mild to moderate attacks of UC and appears to decrease frequency of subsequent relapse.	Sulfasalazine is considered inferior to corticosteroids in the treatment of severe attacks of disease; once remission has been attained by use of corticosteroid therapy, sulfasalazine appears to be superior to systemic corticosteroids in the maintenance of remission.

5-Aminosalicytic Acid (5-ASA) Preparations

These preparations are effective in treating mild to moderately active UC and for maintenance therapy.	They are used if patients are unable to tolerate sulfasalazine. These medications have a variety of delivery mechanisms that allow release of the active therapeutic agent directly into the colon or ileum.
	For oral use, mesalamine is available in delayed-release tablets (Asacol® and Lialda®) and extended-release capsule (Pentasa®) so that any part of the colon can be treated; also see topical therapy below.
	For oral use, olsalazine (Dipentum®) capsule allows 5-ASA to be absorbed slowly, resulting in high local concentration in the colon.
	For oral use, balsalazide (Colazal®) remains intact until reaching the colon.
Topical therapy with mesalamine is an effective route for proctitis or proctosigmoiditis.	Mesalamine suppository (Canasa®) is used for proctitis because this form topically treats inflammation located in the rectum; mesalamine retention enema (Rowasa®) is used for proctosigmoiditis because the enema form can treat inflammation located in the sigmoid colon as well as the rectum.
Combination therapy of mesalamine enema and oral mesalamine may be used.	Combination therapy may be more effective than using oral form alone.
For additional information on side effects and precautions, see "Crohn's Disease," **Deficient Knowledge** (Aminosalicylates).	

⚠ Immunomodulators

These agents modify or "quiet down" the immune system in order to decrease inflammation.	This therapy reduces inflammation in patients not responding to steroids and sulfasalazine; in patients unwilling or unable to undergo colectomy; or as an alternative to steroid dependency. Azathioprine and 6-mercaptopurine have been used alone and in combination with steroids. Cyclosporine has been used cautiously in severe UC because it is toxic and associated with many side effects. Its use has been diminished with the advent of the biologic agent infliximab.

continued

ASSESSMENT/INTERVENTIONS	RATIONALES
Immunomodulatory therapy has been used to maintain remission in patients with frequent relapses.	These agents may have steroid-sparing and steroid-enhancing effects and are used with the goal of gradually withdrawing, or substantially reducing, the dosage of corticosteroids.
Advise the patient of the need to be closely monitored.	Therapy may be necessary for 3-6 mo to achieve therapeutic response, and this amount of time can result in hematologic toxicity.
For additional information on side effects and precautions, see "Crohn's Disease," **Deficient Knowledge** (Immunomodulators) and **Risk for Allergy Response** *related to* immunomodulator and biologic/anti-TNF drugs.	
Biologic/Anti-TNF agent Infliximab (Remicade®)	This genetically engineered agent blocks inflammation. It is used intravenously to treat and maintain remission and to achieve mucosal healing in patients with moderately to severely active disease unresponsive to conventional therapy.
For additional information on side effects and precautions, see "Crohn's Disease," **Deficient Knowledge** (Biologic/Anti-TNF Agents), and **Risk for Allergy Response** *related to* immunomodulator and biologic/anti-TNF drugs.	

ADDITIONAL NURSING DIAGNOSES/PROBLEMS:

✓ PATIENT-FAMILY TEACHING AND DISCHARGE PLANNING

When providing patient-family teaching, focus on sensory information, avoid giving excessive information, and initiate a visiting nurse referral for necessary follow-up teaching. Include verbal and written information about the following:

✓ Medications, including drug name, rationale, dosage, schedule, route of administration, precautions, and potential side effects. Also discuss drug-drug and food-drug interactions. **Note:** Caution patients receiving high-dose steroid therapy to avoid abrupt discontinua-tion of steroids to prevent precipitation of adrenal crisis. Withdrawal symptoms include weakness, lethargy, restlessness, anorexia, nausea, and muscle tenderness. Instruct the patient to notify the health care provider if these symptoms occur.

✓ Herbal/alternative therapies, such as vitamins, herbs, dietary supplements, minerals, and homeopathy in order to minimize interactions with prescribed medications and adverse effects. Discuss with the patient that even though a probiotic (VSL#3) is indicated for dietary management of UC, it should be used under supervision of the prescribing health care provider.

✓ Importance of taking medications as prescribed in order to maintain remission and prevent flares.

✓ Signs and symptoms that necessitate medical attention, including fever, nausea and vomiting, diarrhea or constipation, and any significant change in appearance and frequency of stools, any of which can signal exacerbation of the disease.

✓ Dietary management to promote nutritional and fluid maintenance and prevent abdominal cramping, discomfort, and diarrhea.

✓ Importance of perineal care after bowel movements.

✓ Enteral or parenteral feeding instructions if the patient is to supplement diet or is NPO.

✓ Referral to community resources, including the Crohn's & Colitis Foundation of America, Inc., at *www.ccfa.org*; the Website: UC and Crohn's Teen Site at *www.ucandcrohns.org* ; the Crohn's and Colitis Foundation of Canada at *www.ccfc.ca*; and the following social media: Online Community at *www.ccfacommunity.org*, Facebook at *https://www.facebook.com/ccfafb*, and Twitter at *http://twitter.com/ccfa*

✓ Importance of follow-up medical care, particularly for patients with long-standing disease because so many of them develop colonic adenocarcinoma.

✓ Referral to a mental health specialist if recommended by the health care provider.

In addition, if the patient has a fecal diversion (colostomy, ileostomy, or ileal pouch anal anastomosis):

✓ Care of incision, dressing changes, and permission to take baths or showers once sutures and drains are removed.

✓ Care of stoma, peristomal/perianal skin, or perineal wound; use of ostomy equipment; and method for obtaining supplies. Sitz baths may be indicated for perineal wound.

✓ Medications that are contraindicated (e.g., laxatives) or that may not be well tolerated or absorbed (e.g., antibiotics, enteric-coated tablets, long-acting tablets).

✓ Gradual resumption of activities of daily living, excluding heavy lifting (more than 10 lb), pushing, or pulling for 6-8 wk to prevent incisional herniation.

✓ Referral to community resources, including home health care agency, wound, ostomy, continence (WOC)/enterostomal therapy (ET) nurse, the local ostomy association, and the United Ostomy Association of America at *www.uoaa.org*, and the Young Ostomate and Diversion Alliance of America (for young adults ages 18 to 35 years) found under Affiliate Support Groups at *uoaa.org*.

✓ Importance of reporting signs and symptoms that require medical attention, such as change in stoma color from the normal bright and shiny red; peristomal or perianal skin irritation; diarrhea; incisional pain, local increased temperature, drainage, swelling, or redness; signs and symptoms of fluid and electrolyte imbalance; and signs and symptoms of mechanical or functional obstruction.

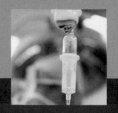
Anemias of Chronic Disease 62

OVERVIEW/PATHOPHYSIOLOGY

Erythropoietin (EPO) is a naturally occurring protein hormone produced and released by the kidneys (90%) and liver (10%). The kidneys are stimulated to release EPO in response to low blood oxygenation. EPO then stimulates stem cells in the bone marrow to develop and produce red blood cells (RBCs). Individuals with decreased renal function (e.g., chronic kidney disease [CKD]) often become anemic because their kidneys cannot produce EPO. In other chronic conditions (cancer, congestive heart failure, human immunodeficiency virus [HIV], rheumatologic disorders), elevated cytokines (such as interleukin 6) may reduce bone marrow erythrocyte production, reduce erythropoietic response in the bone marrow, restrict iron recycling from the liver, reduce iron absorption from the gut, and shorten erythrocyte survival. Recombinant human erythropoietin (epoetin alpha) has provided some benefits for patients with CKD, some patients receiving chemotherapy for cancer, and patients undergoing treatment for infection with HIV, but it may pose risks of life-threatening cardiovascular events. Because anemia may be caused by other conditions, including blood loss, hemolysis, and inadequate dietary intake of iron, vitamin B_{12} (cobalamine), or folate, these conditions must be ruled out before the ultimate cause of anemia can be identified.

HEALTH CARE SETTING

Primary care; acute care for blood transfusion or treatment for sequelae of chronic diseases

ASSESSMENT

Chronic indicators: The patient may be asymptomatic or have brittle hair and nails and pallor. In the presence of severe and chronic disease, shortness of breath, dizziness, and fatigue may be present even at rest. The patient may have a history of CKD, dialysis therapy, cancer within the bone marrow (e.g., leukemia), cancer chemotherapy, or other chronic conditions (e.g., HIV, congestive heart failure, diabetes).

Acute indicators: Fatigue, decreased ability to concentrate, cold sensitivity, menstrual irregularities, and loss of libido.

Physical assessment: Tachycardia, palpitations, tachypnea, exertional dyspnea, pale mucous membranes, pale nail beds, and vertigo.

DIAGNOSTIC TESTS

Blood count: Usually RBCs and hemoglobin (Hgb) are decreased, and hematocrit (Hct) is low because the percentage of RBCs in the total blood volume is decreased. The mean corpuscular volume (MCV) may be normal or slightly decreased. In iron-deficiency anemia, the MCV will be decreased; in cobalamine and folic acid deficiencies, the MCV will be increased.

Ferritin: Normal or increased. However, if it is less than 30 mcg/L, there is a coexisting iron deficiency.

Peripheral blood smear to examine RBC indices: Morphology reveals normocytic and normochromic erythrocytes (normal or slightly low mean corpuscular volume [MCV]).

Total iron-binding capacity: Decreased.

Reticulocyte count: Normal to slightly decreased.

Bilirubin: Normal.

Serum iron levels: Normal to decreased.

Transferrin: Normal to decreased.

Cobalamine, folate: Normal.

Nursing Diagnosis:

Activity Intolerance

related to anemia and decreased oxygen-carrying capacity of the blood occurring with decreased RBCs

Desired Outcome: After treatment, Hgb and Hct levels are within medical goals, and the patient perceives exertion at 3 or less on a 0-10 scale and tolerates activity as evidenced by respiratory rate (RR) 12-20 breaths/min, presence of eupnea, heart rate (HR) 100 bpm or less, and absence of dizziness and headaches.

ASSESSMENT/INTERVENTIONS	RATIONALES
Assess for signs of activity intolerance. Ask the patient to rate perceived exertion on a 0-10 scale (see "Prolonged Bedrest" for **Risk for Activity Intolerance,** p. 62).	Dyspnea on exertion, dizziness, palpitations, headaches, and verbalization of increased exertion level (rated perceived exertion [RPE] more than 3) are signs of activity intolerance and decreased tissue oxygenation, and the patient should stop or modify the activity until signs of increased exertion are no longer present with the activity.
[!] Assess risk of falling and implement appropriate strategies.	Because of the potentially slow, progressive nature of this anemia, patients may not be aware of weaknesses and limitations leading to reductions in strength and balance. Patient falls can result in severe injury, prolonged hospitalization, and even death.
Monitor oximetry; report O_2 saturation 92% or less.	O_2 saturation 92% or less may signal need for supplementary oxygen.
Administer oxygen as prescribed; encourage deep breathing.	Both measures augment oxygen delivery to the tissues.
Facilitate coordination of care providers, allowing time for at least 90 min of undisturbed rest.	Fewer interruptions in rest enable patients to benefit from the undisturbed rest/sleep they need until the anemia is resolved.
Encourage gradually increasing activities to tolerance as the patient's condition improves.	This promotes endurance while preventing problems caused by prolonged bedrest. An effective measure is setting mutually agreed on goals with the patient (e.g., "Let's plan this morning's activity goals. Do you think you could walk up and down the hall once, or twice?" or appropriate amount, depending on the patient's tolerance).
Administer blood components (usually packed RBCs) through an intravenous catheter as prescribed.	This will increase the number of circulating RBCs, which in turn will increase the blood's oxygen-carrying capacity.
[!] Double-check type and crossmatching and the patient identifiers with a colleague, and monitor for and report signs of transfusion reaction.	These measures reduce the risk of delivering the wrong type of blood to the patient and enable rapid treatment if transfusion reaction occurs.
Reassure the patient that symptoms usually are relieved and tolerance for activity increased with the treatment plan.	Treatment may include packed red blood cells or erythropoietin replacement (recombinant EPO [epoetin-α]), 150 units/kg IV 3 times each week, or 600 units/kg subcutaneously once each week, or darbepoietin alfa 200 mcg every 2 weeks. Red cell production is improved through additional EPO (red cells are not responsive to normal EPO levels in chronic conditions). Iron and other supplements (cobalamine, folate) may be given to replenish Hgb and depleted iron and other deficiencies if needed. People with chronic disease, especially older individuals, may not have normal dietary intake of these substances. Supplements will maximize normal erythropoiesis. Improvements in dietary intake and strength also may help reduce symptoms.

ADDITIONAL NURSING DIAGNOSES/PROBLEMS:

See "Cancer Care" for **Risk for Infection** related to   p. 16
myelosuppression

✓ **PATIENT-FAMILY TEACHING AND DISCHARGE PLANNING**

When providing patient-family teaching, focus on sensory information, avoid giving excessive information, and initiate a visiting nurse referral for necessary follow-up teaching. Include verbal and written information about the following:

✓ Importance of a well-balanced diet, especially iron intake, if appropriate, which is found in foods such as red meat, dark green vegetables, legumes, and certain fruits (apricots, figs, raisins). Refer to clinical dietitian as prescribed.

✓ Importance of safety during mobility when experiencing weakness and fatigue. Instruct the patient and family/caregivers on safety strategies; recommend referral to physical therapy as appropriate.

✓ Special instructions for taking iron (and its concomitant risk of constipation), if appropriate, depending on the type prescribed. Therapy may need to be continued for 4-6 mo to replace iron stores adequately.

✓ Necessity and consent for EPO replacement therapy to be continued for duration of the underlying condition.

✓ When self-administering EPO, importance of *not* shaking medication vial before taking it. Shaking the vial may denature glycoprotein in the solution and render it biologically inactive. Any discolored solution or solution with particulate matter should not be used.

✓ Other medications, including drug name, dosage, purpose, schedule, precautions, and potential side effects. Also discuss drug-drug, herb-drug, and food-drug interactions.

✓ Risks and benefits for RBC transfusion (as explained by the health care provider) and necessity for signed consent to the transfusion.

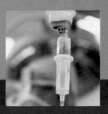

Disseminated Intravascular Coagulation 63

OVERVIEW/PATHOPHYSIOLOGY

Disseminated intravascular coagulation (DIC) is an acute coagulation disorder characterized by paradoxical clotting and hemorrhage. The sequence usually progresses from massive clot formation, depletion of clotting factors, and activation of diffuse fibrinolysis to hemorrhage. DIC occurs secondary to widespread coagulation factors in the bloodstream caused by extensive surgery, burns, shock, sepsis, neoplastic diseases, or abruptio placentae; extensive destruction of blood vessel walls caused by eclampsia, anoxia, or heat stroke; or damage to blood cells caused by hemolysis, sickle cell disease, or transfusion reactions. Although clotting and bleeding occur simultaneously, organ failure related to thromboses of vital organs (e.g., kidneys, lungs, central nervous system, liver) is usually the primary life-threatening concern. Prompt assessment of the disorder can result in a good prognosis. Usually, affected patients are transferred to the intensive care unit (ICU) for careful monitoring and aggressive therapy. DIC may be classified as low-grade (compensated or chronic) or fulminant (acute).

HEALTH CARE SETTING

Acute care/critical care unit

ASSESSMENT

Clinical indicators: Bleeding of abrupt onset; oozing from venipuncture sites or mucosal surfaces; bleeding from surgical sites; and presence of hematuria, blood in stool (melena or hematochezia), hemoptysis, spontaneous ecchymosis (bruising), petechiae, purpura fulminans (extensive skin hemorrhagic necrosis), pallor, or mottled skin. The patient also may bleed from the vagina (menometrorrhagia), nose (epistaxis), and oral mucous membranes. Joint pain and swelling may signal bleeding into joints. Complaint of headache or mental status changes may indicate intracranial hemorrhage and/or stroke. Symptoms of hypoperfusion can occur, including decreased urine output and abnormal behavior.

Physical assessment: Abdominal assessment may reveal signs of gastrointestinal (GI) bleeding, such as guarding;

distention (increasing abdominal girth measurements); hyperactive, hypoactive, or absent bowel sounds; and a rigid, boardlike abdomen. With significant hemorrhage, patients may exhibit the following: systolic blood pressure (SBP) less than 90 mm Hg and diastolic blood pressure (DBP) less than 60 mm Hg; heart rate (HR) greater than 100 bpm; peripheral pulse amplitude 2+ or less on a 0-4+ scale; respiratory rate (RR) greater than 22 breaths/min; shortness of breath; urinary output less than 30 mL/hr; secretions and excretions positive for blood; cool, pale, clammy skin; lack of orientation to person, place, and time; or changes in mental status.

Risk factors: Infection, burns, trauma, hepatic disease, hypovolemic shock, severe hemolytic reaction, malignancy, obstetric complications, and hypoxia.

DIAGNOSTIC TESTS

Oxygen saturation (Spo₂): Low (less than 92%) indicating a tissue perfusion problem.

Serum fibrinogen: Low because of abnormal consumption of clotting factors in the formation of fibrin clots.

Platelet count: Less than 100,000/mm^3 indicating increased utilization by bleeding and/or sequestration in large clots

Fibrin split products: Increased, indicating widespread dissolution of clots. Fibrinolysis produces fibrin split products (FSPs), also known as *fibrin degradation products (FDPs)*, as an end product.

D-dimers: The byproducts of fibrinolysis, D-dimers are increased in DIC and, along with increased FDPs, are considered diagnostic of DIC.

Prothrombin time: Normal, low, or possibly increased because of depletion of clotting factors.

Partial thromboplastin time: Normal, low, or possibly high because of depletion of clotting factors.

Protein C: Low because normal anticoagulation is impaired. Protein C is a coagulation inhibitor.

Peripheral blood smear: Shows fragmented red blood cells (RBCs; schistocytes).

Nursing Diagnoses:

Ineffective Peripheral Tissue Perfusion (or risk for same)
Risk for Ineffective Cerebral Tissue Perfusion
Risk for Ineffective Renal Tissue Perfusion
Risk for Decreased Cardiac Tissue Perfusion

related to coagulation/fibrinolysis processes

Desired Outcome: Following treatment, the patient has adequate tissue perfusion as evidenced by blood pressure (BP) 90/60 mm Hg or greater and HR 100 bpm or less (or within the patient's baseline range); SpO₂ greater than 92%; peripheral pulse amplitude 2+ or greater on a 0-4+ scale; urinary output 30 mL/hr or more; equal and normoreactive pupils; normal/baseline motor function; orientation to person, place, and time; and no mental status changes.

Note: *Risk for Bleeding,* *which follows, discusses the hemorrhagic component in greater depth.*

ASSESSMENT/INTERVENTIONS	RATIONALES
⚠ Assess for coagulation and bleeding as follows:	DIC is an acute coagulation disorder characterized by paradoxical clotting and hemorrhage.
- Monitor vital signs (VS), particularly BP, HR, and peripheral pulses.	Decreased BP, increased HR, and decreased amplitude of peripheral pulses may signal that coagulation and thrombus formation are occurring. This in turn can lead to digital ischemia and gangrene.
- Perform neurologic checks, including orientation, mental status assessments, pupillary reaction to light, level of consciousness (LOC), and motor response.	Deficits may signal that cerebral perfusion is ineffective and should be reported promptly. Signs may be general, such as increased confusion, agitation, or seizures, and become more focal, such as a unilateral widened pupil. If signs of impaired cerebral perfusion occur, it is important to protect the patient from injury caused by cerebral impairment by implementing fall precautions as appropriate.
- Monitor intake and output (I&O); report significant findings.	Urine output less than 30 mL/hr in the presence of adequate intake may indicate renal vessel thrombosis.
- Monitor for hemorrhage from intravenous catheters, surgical wounds, GI and genitourinary (GU) tracts, and mucous membranes.	Hemorrhage is a potential risk after fibrinolysis. See **Risk for Bleeding,** which follows.
- Monitor oxygen saturation via pulse oximetry q4h or as indicated; report oxygen saturation 92% or less.	Oxygen perfusion may be compromised by pulmonary emboli and/or pulmonary hemorrhage. Oxygen saturation 92% or less often signals need for supplement oxygen.
Monitor laboratory work for values suggestive of DIC.	Increased D-dimer values, low serum fibrinogen (less than 200 mg/dL), low platelet count (less than 100,000/mm³), increased FSPs (9 mcg/mL or greater), possible increased prothrombin time (PT) (greater than 11-15 sec), and possible increased partial thromboplastin time (PTT) (greater than 40-100 sec) are common with DIC.
⚠ Report significant findings to the patient's health care provider; prepare for emergent blood product transfusion, medical support, and transfer to ICU if the condition worsens.	The patient may require careful monitoring and aggressive therapy.
Administer anticoagulant agents as prescribed.	Heparin may be of value in some cases to prevent clotting-related ischemia; recombinant protein C and antithrombin may be used for their anticoagulant and antiinflammatory effects. Close monitoring and frequent blood draws may be needed so that excessive bleeding does not occur.

ASSESSMENT/INTERVENTIONS	RATIONALES
Administer blood products as prescribed.	Packed red blood cells replace blood volume; platelets may be needed to restore hemostasis for severe bleeding; fresh frozen plasma and/or cryoprecipitate also may be used for severe bleeding and low fibrinogen levels.
Double-check blood product and type with a colleague, and monitor for and report signs of transfusion reaction, including chills, back pain, dyspnea, hives, and wheezing.	These precautions help ensure the patient receives the correct blood product and type, which otherwise could result in transfusion reaction.
Make sure the patient has been informed of risks and benefits of all blood product transfusions by the health care provider and that the patient signs consent to the transfusion.	Although risk of life-threatening reactions and infections is low, patients must be informed as to the risks and benefits by the health care provider according to the Paul Gann Act.

Nursing Diagnosis:

Risk for Bleeding

related to hemorrhagic component of DIC

Desired Outcome: The patient is free of signs of bleeding as evidenced by SBP 90 mm Hg or greater; HR 100 bpm or less (or within the patient's normal range); RR 12-20 breaths/min with normal depth and pattern (eupnea); urinary output 30 mL/hr or more; secretions and excretions negative for blood; stable abdominal girth measurements; orientation to person, place, and time; and no changes in mental status.

ASSESSMENT/INTERVENTIONS	RATIONALES
Assess LOC and monitor VS at frequent intervals; report significant changes.	Hypotension, tachycardia, dyspnea, disorientation, and changes in mental status can signal hemorrhage.
Be careful of pressure used with BP cuffs. Inflate cuff only as high as needed to obtain reading. Alternate arms with each BP check.	Frequent BP readings may cause bleeding under the cuff. Alternating arms reduces repeated tissue trauma.
Assess for abdominal pain, abdominal distention, changes in bowel sounds, and a boardlike abdomen.	These are signs of GI bleeding.
Check stool, urine, emesis, and nasogastric drainage for blood using point of care testing or send to the laboratory STAT.	A positive test signals presence of blood in the GI/GU tracts and should be reported to the health care provider promptly for rapid intervention.
Assess puncture sites regularly.	This assessment will detect external bleeding or oozing.
When possible, treat bleeding sites with ice, pressure, rest, and elevation.	In addition, some health care providers promote use of thrombin-soaked gauze, such as Gelfoam, or topical thrombin powder.
Be alert to visual changes, headache, and joint pain.	Visual changes may signal retinal hemorrhage. Joint pain and headache are other signs that bleeding may be occurring and could be life threatening.
Monitor coagulation and other hematologic laboratory values.	Increased PT (more than 11-15 sec) is a sign that clotting factors are depleted and the patient is at risk for hemorrhage.
Prevent or promptly control retching, vomiting, coughing, and straining with bowel movements. Avoid giving intramuscular (IM) injections, and minimize venipunctures as appropriate.	These measures minimize the potential for bleeding.
Post "Bleeding Precautions" signs.	This will notify all health care providers that venipuncture sites may require additional manual pressure to stop bleeding.
Administer blood products (packed RBCs, platelets, fresh frozen plasma [FFP]), and intravenous (IV) fluids as prescribed. See precautions listed with the previous nursing diagnosis.	These products help counteract deficiencies causing the bleeding and support blood volume. Cryoprecipitate or FFP may be used if fibrinogen is low; platelets may be given if they are less than 10,000/mm³ or if there is bleeding.

continued

ASSESSMENT/INTERVENTIONS	RATIONALES
Teach patients to use electric shaver and soft-bristle toothbrush and avoid forceful nose blowing (dab instead), bending down (head lower than the heart), and potentially traumatic procedures (e.g., enemas, rectal temperatures).	These precautions reduce the risk of bleeding. Razors, hard bristles, rectal thermometers, and enema nozzles, for example, could break the skin and mucous membranes, causing bleeding.
Report significant findings to the patient's health care provider. Prepare for emergent blood product transfusion, medical support, and transfer to ICU if the condition worsens.	The patient may require aggressive therapy and careful monitoring.

Nursing Diagnoses:

Risk for Impaired Skin Integrity
Impaired Tissue Integrity

related to altered circulation occurring with hemorrhage and thrombosis

Desired Outcome: The patient's skin and tissue remain nonerythremic and intact.

ASSESSMENT/INTERVENTIONS	RATIONALES
Assess the patient's skin, noting changes in color, temperature, and sensation.	Erythema that does not clear after removal of pressure or changes in color, sensation, and temperature may signal decreased perfusion that can lead to tissue damage.
Ensure that the patient turns q2h, and consider use of protective measures on elbows and heels and enhanced pressure-distribution mattress padding. Do not pull on extremities when turning the patient.	These measures eliminate or minimize pressure points that could damage the skin/tissue.
As prescribed, encourage active range of motion (ROM) of all extremities q2h.	ROM exercise reduces tissue pressure and promotes circulation.
Keep the patient's extremities warm.	Warmth helps prevent tissue hypoxia, which would increase risk of tissue damage/necrosis.
Use alternatives to tape to hold dressings in place, such as gauze wraps or net gauze if tape causes injury.	Tape removal could damage fragile skin and tissue.
If the patient has areas of breakdown, see "Managing Wound Care," p. 533	

ADDITIONAL NURSING DIAGNOSES/PROBLEMS:

"Pulmonary Embolus" for **Risk for Bleeding**   p. 130
   related to anticoagulation therapy

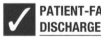 **PATIENT-FAMILY TEACHING AND DISCHARGE PLANNING**

See the patient's primary diagnosis.

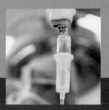

OVERVIEW/PATHOPHYSIOLOGY

Polycythemia is a chronic disorder characterized by excessive production of red blood cells (RBCs), platelets, and myelocytes. As these increase, blood volume, blood viscosity, and hemoglobin (Hgb) concentration increase, causing excessive workload for the heart and congestion of organs (e.g., liver, kidney), hemorrhage, and vascular events (venous thromboembolism, stroke, heart failure, and myocardial infarction).

Secondary polycythemia results from an abnormal increase in erythropoietin production (e.g., because of hypoxia that occurs with chronic lung disease or prolonged living in altitudes greater than 10,000 ft) or with other conditions, such as apnea, renal disorders (e.g., renal cell carcinoma), and liver disorders. *Polycythemia vera* (PV) is a primary disorder arising from a chromosomal mutation (a JAK2 mutation*) most often affecting men of Jewish descent, with onset in late midlife. PV results in increased RBC mass, leukocytosis, and thrombocytosis. Because of increased viscosity and decreased microcirculation, mortality is high if the condition is left untreated. In addition, there is potential for this disorder to evolve into other hematopoietic disorders, such as myelofibrosis and acute leukemia.

HEALTH CARE SETTING

Primary care; acute care for complications

---

*The JAK2 is a point mutation change that causes continuous activation of intracellular pathways responsible for erythropoiesis independent of erythropoietin stimulus (Randolf, 2012).

ASSESSMENT

Signs and symptoms: Fatigue, muscle pain, headache, dizziness, tinnitus, paresthesias, visual disturbances, dyspnea, thrombophlebitis, joint pain, painful pruritus, night sweats, chest pain, abdominal discomfort, dull foot pain at night, and a feeling of "fullness," especially in the head.

Physical assessment: Hypertension, engorgement of retinal blood veins, crackles (rales), weight loss, cyanosis, changes in mentation or mood (delirium, psychotic depression, mania), ruddy complexion (especially palmar aspects of hands and plantar surfaces of feet), splenomegaly, hepatomegaly, gastrointestinal (GI) disturbances (ulcers, GI bleed), nosebleeds.

DIAGNOSTIC TESTS

Complete blood count: Increased RBC mass (8-12 million/mm³), Hgb (more than 18.5 g/dL in women and 16.5 g/dL in men), hematocrit ([Hct] more than 48% in women and 52% in men), and leukocytes (more than 10,000/mcl); and overproduction of thrombocytes (more than 400,000/mcl) are diagnostic of polycythemia.

Platelet count: Elevated as a result of increased production.

Bone marrow aspiration: Reveals RBC proliferation, and 95% of patients demonstrate a JAK2 mutation.

Uric acid levels: May be increased because of increased nucleoprotein, an end product of RBC breakdown.

Erythropoietin levels: Elevated in secondary polycythemia and decreased in polycythemia vera.

O₂ saturation: Normal (greater than 92%).

Nursing Diagnosis:

Acute Pain

related to headache, angina, pruritus, and abdominal and joint discomfort occurring with altered circulation caused by blood hyperviscosity

Desired Outcomes: Within 1 hr of intervention, the patient's subjective perception of discomfort decreases, as documented by a pain scale. Objective indicators, such as grimacing, are absent or diminished. The patient states that lifestyle behaviors are not compromised because of discomfort.

ASSESSMENT/INTERVENTIONS	RATIONALES
Assess for the presence of headache, angina, abdominal pain, and joint pain. Devise a pain scale with the patient, rating discomfort from 0 (no pain) to 10 (worst pain).	The patient provides a personal baseline report, enabling the nurse to more effectively monitor subsequent increases and decreases in pain. Use of a pain intensity scale allows more accurate documentation of discomfort and subsequent relief obtained after analgesia has been administered.
Monitor for complaints of calf pain and tenderness.	These are indicators of peripheral thrombosis, which can lead to pulmonary embolus or stroke and therefore should be reported promptly for immediate intervention.
In the presence of joint or skin discomfort, rest the joint and elevate the extremity. Use gentle range-of-motion (ROM) exercises as tolerated. Caution patients to avoid crossing legs and wearing restrictive clothing. Apply cool compresses or ice.	Elevation may help increase circulation and prevent pooling of hyperviscous blood in the joints. ROM helps improve circulation. Ice is used (short term) to decrease severe joint pain. **Note:** In the presence of pruritus, skin may become painful and swollen, exacerbated by heat or exposure to water. Topical antihistamines or lotions generally are not helpful.
Administer analgesics as prescribed.	Analgesics reduce pain.
Avoid analgesics containing aspirin or nonsteroidal antiinflammatory drugs unless prescribed by the health care provider.	These medications may exacerbate bleeding associated with thrombocytosis (high number of ineffective platelets) but may be helpful in alleviating microvascular symptoms.
Instruct the patient to request analgesia before pain becomes too intense.	Pain is easier to control before it becomes severe. Prolonged stimulation of pain receptors results in increased sensitivity to painful stimuli and will increase the amount of medication required to relieve pain.
Teach measures that reduce pruritus, such as avoiding hot baths and taking medications as prescribed.	Hot baths exacerbate pruritus. Medications that may be prescribed include paroxetine, antihistamines, and steroids. In PV, there is potentially an increased number of mast cells in the skin and elevated histamine levels. Paroxetine (a selective serotonin reuptake inhibitor and antidepressant) potentially works by its vasomotor effects. Antihistamines and steroids reduce the inflammatory manifestations of the vascular congestion.
Encourage use of nonpharmacologic pain control, such as relaxation and distraction.	These are pain measures that potentiate analgesics and do not have side effects.

For more information, see "Pain," p. 39.

Nursing Diagnoses:

Ineffective Peripheral Tissue Perfusion
Risk for Decreased Cardiac Tissue Perfusion
Risk for Ineffective Cerebral Tissue Perfusion
Risk for Ineffective Renal Perfusion

related to blood hyperviscosity

Desired Outcome: The patient has adequate renal, peripheral, cardiac, and cerebral perfusion as evidenced by urinary output 30 mL/hr or more; peripheral pulses 2+ or more on a scale of 0-4+; distal extremity warmth; adequate (baseline) muscle strength; no mental status changes; and orientation to person, place, and time.

ASSESSMENT/INTERVENTIONS	RATIONALES
Assess intake and output; report significant findings.	Urine output less than 30 mL/hr in the presence of adequate intake can signal renal congestion and decreased perfusion.
Assess circulation by palpating peripheral pulses; assess distal extremities.	Pulse amplitude 2+ or less on a scale of 0-4+ and coolness in distal extremities can signal disruption of peripheral tissue perfusion secondary to hyperviscosity of the blood.

ASSESSMENT/INTERVENTIONS	RATIONALES
[!] Assess for muscle weakness and decreases in sensation and level of consciousness (LOC).	These are indicators of thrombosis. Any new signs or symptoms could indicate a medical emergency.
If these indicators are present, assist with ambulation or initiate fall prevention measures, depending on degree of deficit.	These measures reduce risk of further thrombosis as well as protect patients from injury caused by declining neurologic status.
In the absence of signs of cardiac and renal failure, provide prescribed intravenous (IV) hydration and encourage fluid intake to decrease viscosity.	Inadequate hydration can increase blood viscosity and contribute adversely to polycythemia.
Perform or coordinate phlebotomy as prescribed.	Phlebotomy to maintain a hematocrit of less than 42% in women and 45% in men has been shown to improve survival.
Encourage the patient to change position every hour when in bed or to exercise and ambulate to tolerance.	These measures promote circulation and reduce the risk of thrombosis.
Instruct the patient to avoid tight or restrictive clothing, and teach signs and symptoms of venous thromboembolism.	Tight clothing could impede blood flow/circulation, increasing the risk of thromboses.
Administer antiplatelet and myelosuppressive agents, as prescribed.	Anticoagulants (low-dose aspirin or anagrelide) and/or chemotherapy agents are given to inhibit bone marrow function and reduce overproduction of blood cells and potential for thrombosis. For example, low-dose aspirin may be used alone with phlebotomy initially. More aggressive treatment with hydroxyurea (preferred), busulfan, imatinib mesylate (Gleevec), or alpha interferon may be given to those refractory to the initial therapy. Ruxolitinib (a JAK1 and JAK2 inhibitor) may be used for patients who progress to myelofibrosis.
Monitor blood counts.	Because these agents can affect bone marrow function and place the patient at risk for myelosuppression, blood counts should be monitored.
If the patient smokes, encourage enrollment in a smoking cessation program.	Smoking significantly increases the potential of a thromboembolic event.

Nursing Diagnosis:

Imbalanced Nutrition: Less Than Body Requirements

related to anorexia due to feelings of fullness occurring with organ system congestion

Desired Outcome: By at least 24 hr before hospital discharge, the patient exhibits adequate nutrition as evidenced by maintenance of or return to baseline body weight or a 1- to 2-lb weight gain.

ASSESSMENT/INTERVENTIONS	RATIONALES
Assess fluid and nutrition balance by weighing the patient daily.	This will help identify trend of the patient's nutritional status.
Assess fluid volume intake; encourage intake if indicated.	These measures will maximize hydration and vascular blood flow.
Encourage the patient to eat small, frequent meals. Document intake.	Smaller, more frequent meals usually are better tolerated than larger, less frequent meals.
Request that significant others bring in the patient's favorite foods if they are unavailable in the hospital.	This promotes the likelihood the patient will eat.
Advise the patient to avoid spicy foods and to eat mild foods.	Mild foods are better tolerated.
Teach the patient to avoid intake of iron and citrus with meals.	These restrictions help minimize abnormal RBC proliferation and iron overload. Citrus increases absorption of iron.

continued

ASSESSMENT/INTERVENTIONS	RATIONALES
As indicated, obtain dietary consultation.	Such a referral will enable more detailed instruction/discussion about foods to eat and those to avoid.
Teach the patient or significant other how to record and maintain fluid and food intake diary.	This will help them monitor trends in food intake and ensure monitoring of hydration status.

Nursing Diagnoses:

Risk for Ineffective Cerebral Tissue Perfusion
Risk for Decreased Cardiac Tissue Perfusion

related to hypovolemia occurring with phlebotomy

Desired Outcome: The patient has adequate cerebral and cardiopulmonary perfusion as evidenced by no mental status changes; orientation to person, place, and time; heart rate (HR) 100 bpm or less; blood pressure (BP) 90/60 mm Hg or greater (or within the patient's baseline range); absence of chest pain; and respiratory rate (RR) 20 breaths/min or less.

ASSESSMENT/INTERVENTIONS	RATIONALES
Before the procedure, review the patient's Hgb, Hct, and platelet counts.	This is to assess the appropriateness of therapy and goal of treatment.
During the procedure assess for tachycardia, hypotension, chest pain, or dizziness; notify the patient's health care provider of significant findings.	These are signs of ineffective perfusion as a result of phlebotomy. A large-bore needle and a vacuum bottle are used. Blood is withdrawn from the vein to decrease blood volume (and decrease Hct to 45%). Usually 500 mL is removed over a period of 15-30 min every 2-4 days until Hct is 42%-47%. For the older adult, 250-300 mL is removed.
During the phlebotomy procedure, keep the patient recumbent.	This position helps prevent dizziness or hypotension as a result of phlebotomy.
After the procedure, assist the patient into a sitting position for 5-10 min before ambulation and assess for headache and weakness.	This will help prevent orthostatic hypotension. For more information about orthostatic hypotension, see "Prolonged Bedrest" for **Risk for Ineffective Cerebral Tissue Perfusion**, p. 67.
Teach the patient about the potential for orthostatic hypotension and need for caution when standing for at least 2-3 days after phlebotomy.	This information will help protect against injury caused by falling as a result of orthostatic hypotension.
Provide IV hydration as prescribed.	Adequate hydration improves blood flow to the tissues.
Explain that vigorous exercise should be avoided within 24 hr after phlebotomy and that adequate hydration should be maintained.	Vigorous exercise and lack of hydration could cause further fluid loss, hypotension, and red cell vascular congestion, whereas maximizing fluids improves blood flow.

PATIENT-FAMILY TEACHING AND DISCHARGE PLANNING

When providing patient-family teaching, focus on sensory information, avoid giving excessive information, and initiate a visiting nurse referral for necessary follow-up teaching. Include verbal and written information about the following:

✓ Need for continued medical follow-up, including potential for phlebotomy.
✓ Medications, including drug name, purpose, dosage, schedule, precautions, and potential side effects. Also discuss drug-drug, herb-drug, and food-drug interactions.

✓ Importance of augmenting fluid intake (e.g., greater than 2.5 L/day) to decrease blood viscosity and of avoiding smoking; provide smoking cessation information as appropriate.
✓ Signs and symptoms that necessitate medical attention: angina, muscle weakness, numbness and tingling of extremities, decreased tolerance to activity, mental status changes, joint pain, and bleeding.
✓ Nutrition: Importance of maintaining a balanced diet to increase resistance to infection, and limiting dietary or supplemental intake of iron to help minimize abnormal RBC proliferation and iron overload.

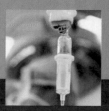

Thrombocytopenia 65

OVERVIEW/PATHOPHYSIOLOGY

Thrombocytopenia is a relatively common coagulation disorder that results from a decreased number of platelets. It can be congenital or acquired, and it is classified according to cause. Causes include deficient production of thrombocytes, as occurs with bone marrow disease (e.g., leukemia, aplastic anemia) or accelerated platelet destruction occurring from loss or increased use, as in hemolytic anemia, thrombotic thrombocytopenic purpura (TTP), idiopathic (immune) thrombocytopenic purpura (ITP), disseminated intravascular coagulation (DIC), or damage by prosthetic heart valves, as well as hypersplenism and hypothermia. Potential triggers include an autoimmune disorder, severe vascular injury, and spleen malfunction. In addition, thrombocytopenia can occur as a side effect of certain medications, such as chemotherapy. Regardless of cause or trigger, the disorder affects coagulation and hemostasis. With chemical-induced thrombocytopenia, prognosis is good after withdrawal of the offending drug. Prognosis for other types depends on the form of thrombocytopenia and the individual's baseline health status and response to treatment.

> **Note:** *Thrombocytopenia may be the first sign of systemic lupus erythematosus (SLE) or infection.*

TTP is characterized by thrombocytopenia, hemolytic anemia, neurologic abnormalities, fever (in the absence of infection), and renal abnormalities, although all features may not be present. TTP is often associated with hemolytic-uremic syndrome (HUS) and thus referred to as TTP-HUS. It is often caused by a deficiency of a plasma enzyme (ADAMTS13), which is responsible for regulating von Willebrand factor (vWF) and platelet adhesion. Without the enzyme, large vWFs attach to activated platelets, thereby promoting platelet aggregation and loss of circulating platelets. This syndrome may be triggered by certain medications (e.g., cyclosporine, clopidogrel), infections (shigella), pregnancy, or autoimmune disorders, such as SLE. Another potential cause is complement dysregulation, triggering excess clotting of platelets. Thus, this disorder is associated with both clotting and bleeding.

ITP is caused by proteins on the platelet cell membrane that stimulate production of antiplatelet immunoglobulin G (IgG) antibodies. These platelets travel to the spleen, where they are recognized as foreign and destroyed by macrophages. Additionally, platelet production from megakaryocytes is impaired. This immune reaction may be caused by medications (e.g., phenytoin, vancomycin) or even food and beverages (e.g., walnuts and quinine in tonic water). The acute form is most often seen in children (2-6 yr of age) and may be related to a previous viral infection. The chronic form is seen more often in adults (18-50 yr of age) and may be of unknown origin.

Heparin-induced thrombocytopenia (HIT) is a disorder in which heparin triggers an antibody response. Another name is *heparin-induced thrombocytopenia and thrombosis syndrome, or HITTS).* The heparin-antibody complexes bind to platelet surfaces, causing activated platelets to aggregate, leading to further thrombosis and, because of increased utilization, thrombocytopenia. Because the platelets are activated (although low in number), HIT is also associated with both arterial and venous thrombosis rather than bleeding.

HEALTH CARE SETTING

Primary care; hospitalization for complications

ASSESSMENT

Chronic indicators: Long history of mild bleeding or hemorrhagic episodes from the mouth, nose, gastrointestinal (GI) tract, or genitourinary (GU) tract. Increased bruising (ecchymosis) and petechiae also have been noted.

Acute indicators: Fever, splenomegaly, acute and severe bleeding episodes, weakness, lethargy, malaise, hemorrhage into mucous membranes, gum bleeding, and GU or GI bleeding. Prolonged bleeding can lead to a shock state with tachycardia, shortness of breath, and decreased level of consciousness (LOC). Optic fundal hemorrhage decreases vision and may preclude potentially fatal intracranial hemorrhage.

> **Note:** *With TTP and HIT, the individual may exhibit signs associated with platelet thrombus formation (such as skin necrosis) and ischemic organ failure (decreased renal function or neurologic changes).*

History of: Recent infection, myeloproliferative disease, or aplastic anemia; recent vaccination; binge alcohol consumption; positive family history of thrombocytopenia; or use of chlorothiazide, digoxin, quinidine, rifampin, sulfisoxazole, clopidogrel, phenytoin, chemotherapy, or heparin.

DIAGNOSTIC TESTS

Platelet count: Can vary from only slightly decreased to nearly absent. Less than 100,000/mm³ is significantly decreased; less than 20,000/mm³ results in a serious risk of hemorrhage.

Peripheral blood smear: May reveal megathrombocytes (large platelets), which are present during premature destruction of platelets, as well as reticulocytosis and fragmented red cells.

Lactate dehydrogenase: May be elevated.

Bilirubin: Increased.

Complete blood count: Low hemoglobin (Hgb) and hematocrit (Hct) levels because of blood loss or aggregates with clotting; white blood cell (WBC) count usually within normal range.

Coagulation studies:
Bleeding time: Increased because of decreased platelets.
Partial thromboplastin time: May be increased or normal.
Prothrombin time: May be increased or normal.
International normalized ratio: Increased.
International sensitivity index: Increased.

Bone marrow aspiration: Reveals increased number of megakaryocytes (platelet precursors) in the presence of ITP and HIT but may be decreased in other causes of thrombocytopenia.

Antibody screen: May be positive because of the presence of IgG platelet antibodies, positive HIT or drug-dependent antibodies, and ADAMTS13 deficiency.

Nursing Diagnosis:

Risk for Bleeding

related to decreased platelet count

Desired Outcome: The patient is free of the signs of bleeding as evidenced by secretions and excretions negative for blood, blood pressure (BP) 90/60 mm Hg or greater or within the patient's baseline range, heart rate (HR) 100 bpm or less, respiratory rate (RR) 12-20 breaths/min with normal depth and pattern (eupnea), and absence of bruising or active bleeding.

ASSESSMENT/INTERVENTIONS	RATIONALES
Assess for hematuria, melena, epistaxis, hematemesis, hemoptysis, menorrhagia, bleeding gums, petechiae, or severe ecchymosis.	These are signs of bleeding that could occur as a result of thrombocytopenia.
Teach the patient to be alert to and report these indicators promptly as well as any headache or changes in vision.	Prompt patient-reported outcomes may improve treatment decisions and control of the disorder.
Monitor platelet count daily and coagulation studies at least weekly or as prescribed.	Optimal range is 150,000-400,000/mm³. Less than 100,000/mm³ is significantly decreased; less than 20,000/mm³ results in a serious risk of hemorrhage.
Ensure that there is a current type and crossmatch in the blood bank for red blood cells (RBCs).	RBC transfusions would be necessary to help maintain intravascular volume in the event acute bleeding occurs.
Prevent or promptly control symptoms that can trigger bleeding, such as retching, vomiting, coughing, and straining with bowel movements.	Straining and similar actions increase intracranial pressure and can result in intracranial hemorrhage.
When possible, avoid venipuncture. If performed, apply pressure on site for 5-10 min or until bleeding stops. Do not give intramuscular (IM) injections. If injections are necessary, use the subcutaneous route with a small-gauge needle.	The patient is at risk for prolonged bleeding because of the decreased platelet count.
Advise the patient to avoid straining at stool and other strenuous activities.	Straining increases intracranial pressure and can result in intracranial hemorrhage.
Obtain prescription for stool softeners, if indicated. Teach the anticonstipation routine as described in "Prolonged Bedrest" for **Constipation,** p. 68.	These measures help prevent constipation, thereby minimizing need to strain at stool and risk for bleeding.
Teach the patient to use an electric razor and soft-bristle toothbrush.	These items minimize risk of injury and hence bleeding.

ASSESSMENT/INTERVENTIONS	RATIONALES
[!] Teach about the association of alcohol consumption, smoking, and use of aspirin or nonsteroidal antiinflammatory drugs (NSAIDs) with increased risk of bleeding.	Alcohol may suppress bone marrow production of blood cells, smoking affects circulation, and aspirin and NSAIDs reduce platelet adhesion.
As prescribed, administer treatments described in the rationale column. Monitor the patient appropriately, and provide the patient and family education regarding these treatments.	*Corticosteroids* enhance vascular integrity and diminish platelet destruction. *Intravenous immunoglobulin (IV IgG)* increases platelet count by impeding the antibody production that destroys platelets. *IV anti-D immune globulin* increases platelet count by impeding antibodies that destroy platelets because the antibodies are bound to red cells versus the platelets *Rituximab* increases platelet count by its immunosuppressive properties in ITP. *Thrombopoietin receptor agonists* (e.g., Romiplostim, Eltrombopag) may be indicated for ITP for patients who fail other therapies. *Eculizumab* may be prescribed for complement-associated TTP-HUS syndrome by inhibiting complement.
Administer platelets as prescribed.	Platelet transfusion is used if platelet destruction or deficient formation is the primary cause of the disorder or if risk of increased microthrombi and organ ischemia is not of primary concern. It provides only temporary relief because the half-life of platelets is only 3-4 days and may be even shorter with ITP (i.e., minutes to hours). Platelet transfusions may be avoided in patients with TTP or active HIT because they may increase thrombosis (the primary problem) except in life-threatening or organ-threatening hemorrhage. If used, HLA-matched or cross-matched platelets may improve clinical response.
[!] Double-check blood product and type with a colleague, and monitor for and report signs of transfusion reaction, including chills, back pain, dyspnea, hives, and wheezing.	These precautions help ensure that the patient receives the correct blood product and type, which otherwise could result in transfusion reaction.
[!] Make sure the patient has been informed of risks and benefits of all blood product transfusions by the health care provider and that the patient signs consent to the transfusion.	Although risk of life-threatening reactions and infections is low, patients must be informed as to the risks and benefits by the health care provider according to the Paul Gann Act.
[!] Ensure that if thrombocytopenia was caused by a medication, the medication is noted in the patient's chart as an allergen.	Removal of the offending agent (e.g., medication-induced TTP) is the first step in resolving the disorder.
[!] Monitor for infection and bleeding postoperatively after splenectomy.	Splenectomy may be indicated for ITP that is not responsive to medical therapies, such as steroids, IV IgG, and others. Surgical procedures may pose risk of infection and bleeding.

Nursing Diagnoses:

Ineffective Peripheral Tissue Perfusion (or risk for same)
Risk for Ineffective Cerebral Tissue Perfusion
Risk for Ineffective Renal Perfusion

related to interrupted blood flow occurring with the thrombotic component in TTP and HIT, which results in sensitization and clumping of platelets in the blood vessels

Desired Outcome: The patient's perfusion is adequate as evidenced by no mental status changes; orientation to person, place, and time; normoreactive pupillary responses; absence of headaches, dizziness, and visual disturbances; peripheral pulses greater than 2+ on a 0-4+ scale; and urine output 30 mL/hr or more.

ASSESSMENT/INTERVENTIONS	RATIONALES
Assess for changes in mental status, LOC, and pupillary response. Monitor for headaches, dizziness, or visual disturbances.	These changes and findings are indicators of ineffective cerebral tissue perfusion and may indicate a medical emergency.
Palpate peripheral pulses on all extremities. Compare distal extremities for color, warmth, and character of pulses.	Pulse amplitude 2+ or less on a 0-4+ scale is a signal of ineffective peripheral tissue perfusion (thrombosis), as are differences in color, warmth, and pulse character when comparing one extremity to the other.
Assess urine output.	Adequate renal perfusion is reflected by urine output 30 mL/hr or more for 2 consecutive hours. Amounts less than that may signal decreased renal perfusion as a result of thrombosis.
Monitor fluid intake.	The patient should be well hydrated (2-3 L/day) to increase perfusion to the small vessels.
Coordinate care for plasma exchange, which may entail physician placement of a large-bore apheresis catheter.	Plasma exchange may be performed in TTP and HIT to remove large platelet complexes from the patient's plasma and replace normal plasma.

Nursing Diagnosis:

Acute Pain

related to joint discomfort occurring with hemorrhagic episodes or blood extravasation into the tissues

Desired Outcomes: Within 1 hr of intervention, the patient's subjective perception of discomfort decreases, as documented by pain scale. Objective indicators, such as grimacing, are absent or diminished.

ASSESSMENT/INTERVENTIONS	RATIONALES
Assess for fatigue, malaise, and joint pain. Devise a pain scale with the patient, rating discomfort on a scale of 0 (no pain) to 10 (worst pain).	This assessment will help determine the degree and type of discomfort. The pain scale also will help assess degree of relief obtained after treatment/intervention.
Maintain a calm, quiet environment. Facilitate coordination of care providers, allowing time for periods of undisturbed rest.	These measures promote rest, which will help decrease discomfort and fatigue.
Elevate the patient's legs. Support legs with pillows.	These measures help minimize joint discomfort in the lower extremities.
Avoid gatching the bed at the knee. Choose chairs with or provide padding on seats.	These measures help prevent occlusion of popliteal vessels.
Use a bed cradle; provide socks, as needed, for warmth.	A bed cradle will decrease pressure on tissues of the lower extremities. Decreased circulation results in extremity coolness.
Administer analgesics as prescribed. Reassess pain and document relief obtained, using the pain scale.	Analgesics reduce pain. The pain scale will help assess the degree of relief obtained after treatment/intervention.
Avoid use of aspirin and NSAIDs.	These agents are contraindicated because of their antiplatelet action, which would increase risk of bleeding.
Instruct the patient to request analgesic before pain becomes severe.	Pain is more readily controlled when it is treated before it gets severe. Prolonged stimulation of pain receptors results in increased sensitivity to painful stimuli and will increase the amount of drug required to relieve pain.

See "Pain," p. 39, for more information.

ADDITIONAL NURSING DIAGNOSES/PROBLEMS:

"Perioperative Care" for **Risk for Bleeding/Risk for Shock** *related to* invasive procedure   p. 55

✓ PATIENT-FAMILY TEACHING AND DISCHARGE PLANNING

When providing patient-family teaching, focus on sensory information, avoid giving excessive information, and initiate a visiting nurse referral for necessary follow-up teaching. Include verbal and written information about the following:

✓ Importance of preventing trauma, which can cause bleeding.

✓ Seeking medical attention for any signs of bleeding, infection, or clotting. Review signs and symptoms of common infections, such as upper respiratory, urinary tract, and wound infections. Signs and symptoms of common infections are described in "Care of the Renal Transplant Recipient," **Risk for Infection,** p. 220. Also teach the patient to assess for hematuria, melena, hematemesis, hemoptysis, menometrorrhagia, oozing from mucous membranes, and petechiae.

✓ Importance of regular medical follow-up for laboratory studies.

✓ If the patient is discharged taking corticosteroids, an explanation of side effects of steroids, including weight gain, headache, capillary fragility, hypertension, moon facies, thinning of arms and legs, mood changes, acne, buffalo hump, edema formation, risk of GI hemorrhage, delayed wound healing, and increased appetite. Review need to take medication with food, immediately take missed doses, and not precipitously discontinue medication.

✓ Other medications, including drug name, dosage, purpose, schedule, precautions, and potential side effects. Also discuss drug-drug, herb-drug, and food-drug interactions.

✓ Importance of obtaining a medical alert bracelet and identification card outlining diagnosis and emergency treatment. Contact MedicAlert Foundation at *www.medicalert.org* or MedicAlert Foundation (Canada) at *www.medicalert.ca.*

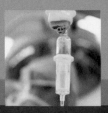

Amputation 66

OVERVIEW/PATHOPHYSIOLOGY

Amputation, the removal of part or all of a limb through bone, is now less commonly performed as an orthopedic surgical intervention than it was before advances in antibiotic therapy, treatment for musculoskeletal neoplasms, and microsurgery/limb salvage techniques. Lower extremity amputation may still be the treatment of choice for complications of diabetes mellitus (DM) such as peripheral arterial disease (PAD), for severe trauma, or for osteomyelitis or other infections that are refractory to antibiotic treatment. Persons with PAD account for approximately 80% of lower extremity amputations in the Western world. Amputation may be necessary on rare occasions because of tumors or due to congenital limb deficiencies in infants and children.

While the majority of lower extremity amputations are performed due to disease, most upper extremity amputations are the result of trauma. Amputation and prosthesis use may offer the patient improved functional ability.

HEALTH CARE SETTING

Critical care unit, acute care surgical unit, orthopedic rehabilitation unit

ASSESSMENT

Chronic disease: Patients with advanced PAD often complain of extremity pain in a definable muscle group (usually calf muscles) precipitated by exercise and promptly relieved by rest. This pain is distinguished from that of diabetic neuropathy, which is distributed along dermatomes rather than confined to a specific muscle group; neuropathy is also constant and unrelated to exercise. The affected limb is often a dark red color (rubor) when it is dependent; atrophy of skin and subcutaneous tissue may be apparent. Amputation also may be needed because of metabolic disorders (e.g., osteosarcoma of Paget's disease) or massive muscle necrosis that results from an acute thromboembolic event or untreated compartment syndrome. Amputation in the event of a bone or soft tissue tumor is much less common than in the past because of the advent of sophisticated limb salvage procedures.

Trauma: A mangled extremity is common with high-energy injuries. The patient may have multiple injuries, and surgical priority must be given to those injuries that may be life threatening. Trauma may result in a complete amputation, a near or partial amputation, or a segmental amputation of an extremity.

DIAGNOSTIC TESTS

Ankle-arm (ankle-brachial) index: The most widely used noninvasive test for evaluating PAD. Blood pressure is measured at the ankle and in the arm while the patient is at rest. For an ambulatory patient, measurements can then be repeated at both sites after the patient has walked 5 min on a treadmill. Ankle-brachial index (ABI) is calculated by dividing the highest blood pressure at the ankle by the highest recorded pressure in either arm. A normal resting ABI of 1.0-1.4 indicates the pressure in the ankle is equal to or greater than the pressure in the arm, suggesting no significant narrowing or blockage of blood flow. A decrease in the ABI (0.9 or lower) is a sensitive indicator that significant PAD is present.

Doppler ultrasound: Evaluates blood flow to the extremities. It can reliably distinguish exercise-related effects from severe ischemia.

Transcutaneous O_2 pressure: Measured after oxygen sensors are applied to the skin. By determining oxygen tension (desired value is 30-50 mm Hg), the provider can identify areas of lesser perfusion in the affected extremity. This test offers the most accurate assessment of blood supply and the best prediction of residual limb healing potential.

Angiography: Confirms circulatory impairment to determine appropriate level for amputation. This invasive study involves radiographic imaging after injection of a contrast dye into a blood vessel. It is most useful if the patient is a candidate for angioplasty or arterial reconstruction.

Xenon-133: A radioactive isotope injected intradermally at the midpoint of the intended incision for amputation. Skin clearance of this agent reflects skin blood flow as a measure of the appropriate level of amputation.

Nursing Diagnoses:

Acute Pain
Chronic Pain

related to phantom limb sensation

Desired Outcome: Within 1 hr of intervention, the patient's subjective perception of pain decreases as documented by pain intensity rating scale.

ASSESSMENT/INTERVENTIONS	RATIONALES
Assess the patient's pain using an appropriate pain intensity rating scale, such as the visual analog scale (VAS), Wong Baker FACES Pain Rating Scale, Faces Pain Scale—Revised, or FLACC (face, legs, activity, crying, consolability) scale.	The patient provides a personal baseline report, enabling the nurse to more effectively assess subsequent increases and decreases in pain. For the patient who is too young or unable to comprehend the quantitative scales, the nurse will use the FLACC scale based on observations.
Administer simple (nonopioid) analgesics (i.e., nonsteroidal antiinflammatory drugs, acetaminophen), opioid analgesics, and adjuncts as prescribed and reassess their effectiveness in approximately 1 hr using the pain intensity rating scale. Document preintervention and postintervention pain scores.	Although opioids provide effective treatment of incisional pain, they may be ineffective for phantom limb sensation because they do not alter response of afferent nerves to noxious stimuli. Higher opioid doses are often required to treat phantom limb sensation. Anticonvulsants such as gabapentin, pregabalin, and topiramate may be effective for neuropathic pain, and the muscle relaxer baclofen may be used to control spasms and cramps in the phantom limb. Tricyclic antidepressants (e.g., amitriptyline) not only offer analgesia but also may be used to elevate mood. A lidocaine patch also may be helpful when applied near the surgical wound. Beta-blockers such as propranolol have been used as adjuncts, but their efficacy is unclear.
Ensure adequate pain management before elective amputation surgery.	This measure decreases the likelihood that phantom limb sensation will develop. Patients with unrelieved preoperative pain are more likely to experience phantom limb sensation.
Explain that continued sensations often arise postoperatively from the amputated part and may be painful, irritating, or simply disconcerting. Instruct the patient to report any of these sensations if experienced.	This information prepares patients for the potential experience of phantom limb sensation.
Teach use of counterirritation to manage painful sensations.	Counterirritation is based on the gate control theory of pain. It may manage painful sensations by providing a new stimulus to compete with the patient's pain. The simplest form of counterirritation involves systematic rubbing of the painful part.
Apply and maintain an elastic dressing over the residual limb.	Use of an elastic dressing will decrease swelling and thus pain. Its use also facilitates measurement and use of a prosthetic.
As indicated, use transcutaneous electrical nerve stimulation (TENS) on the contralateral limb.	TENS may provide effective short-term management of phantom limb sensation. Use on the residual limb has been associated with exacerbation of pain and should be avoided.
Consider pain management interventions such as distraction, guided imagery, relaxation, and biofeedback.	These nonpharmacologic methods augment pharmacologic pain relief.
Instruct the patient to begin to massage the residual limb 3 wk postoperatively.	Massage will desensitize the area in preparation for the prosthesis. Early prosthesis use may reduce incidence of phantom limb sensation. After surgical wound healing is complete, vigorous stimulation of the end of the residual limb may be prescribed. This can be accomplished by hitting the end of the limb with a rolled towel.
Encourage the patient to consider use of sympathetic blocking agents, acupuncture, ultrasound, and injection with local anesthetics if standard treatment is ineffective.	Additional modalities may be used to decrease phantom limb sensation.

continued

ASSESSMENT/INTERVENTIONS	RATIONALES
Refer the patient to a pain clinic.	Pain clinics enable a comprehensive interdisciplinary program to manage chronic phantom limb sensation.
Explore the possible impact of phantom limb pain on the patient's ability to function on the job or in interpersonal relationships.	Attempts to cope with chronic pain can cause fatigue and deplete the patient's resources, leaving little energy for work and relationships.
For more information, including use of patient-controlled analgesia, see "Pain," p. 39.	

Nursing Diagnosis:

Risk for Disuse Syndrome

related to severe pain and immobility occurring with lower extremity amputation

Desired Outcomes: Within 24 hr of instruction, the patient verbalizes understanding of the prescribed exercise regimen and performs exercises independently. The patient is free of symptoms of contracture as evidenced by optimal range of motion (ROM) of joints and maintenance of muscle mass.

ASSESSMENT/INTERVENTIONS	RATIONALES
Assess ROM of the affected extremity and the patient's ability to perform prescribed exercises.	Accurate assessment ensures creation of an individualized exercise program that will enable appropriate progression of the patient's activity.
Collaborate with the patient to establish a goal for pain management, using both pharmacologic and nonpharmacologic measures.	Effective pain management promotes early movement and ambulation, which in turn aid in prevention of flexion contractures. An early return to activity also prevents loss of muscle strength and increases local circulation to improve wound healing.
If prescribed, elevate the affected extremity for the first 24 hr postoperatively.	During the first 24 hr after surgery, elevation decreases swelling and thus aids in pain management and mobility. Elevation is discontinued after 24 hr to prevent hip flexion contracture.
Assist in performance of ROM exercises daily for mobility of proximal joints.	Performance of ROM exercises contributes to optimal joint function and decreases the risk for development of flexion contractures.
Perform extremity elevation and ROM exercises *only* if prescribed by the health care provider.	A residual limb with deficient vascular supply must not be elevated in order to avoid further compromise of circulation.
On the second postoperative day, ensure the patient keeps the residual lower limb flat when at rest.	This position will decrease risk for hip flexion contracture. Other strategies to prevent contracture include assisting the patient to lie prone for 1 hr qid.
Teach prescribed exercises that increase strength of muscle extensors.	Prescribed exercises may include the following: - Above-knee amputation (AKA): The patient attempts to straighten the hip from a flexed position against resistance or perform gluteal-setting exercises. - Below-knee amputation (BKA): The patient attempts to straighten the knee against resistance or perform quadriceps exercises. The patient also should perform exercises for AKA.

Nursing Diagnoses:

Disturbed Body Image
Ineffective Role Performance

related to traumatic loss of limb

Desired Outcome: Within 72 hr after surgery, the patient begins to show adaptation to loss of the limb and demonstrates interest in resuming role-related responsibilities.

ASSESSMENT/INTERVENTIONS	RATIONALES
Assess the patient's current perception and acceptance of the amputation and residual limb.	The patient's current response to the residual limb will guide the nurse's interventions.
Assist the patient with adapting to loss of the limb while maintaining a sense of what is perceived as the normal self.	Strategies Include introducing the patient to others who have successfully adapted to a similar amputation (e.g., via local or national support, such as Amputees in Motion). Teaching aids such as books, pamphlets, audiovisuals, and videotapes can be used to demonstrate how others have adapted to amputation.
Encourage the patient to look at and touch the residual limb, and verbalize feelings about the amputation. Provide privacy for the patient and significant others to express feelings regarding the amputation.	The patient may have a stereotyped image of disability and unattractiveness following amputation. These emotions may be suppressed during rehabilitation but reemerge later. Addressing stereotypical thinking early in recovery and actively involving the patient in education will help provide a sense of participation and control. All caregivers must show an accepting attitude and encourage significant others to accept the patient's new appearance.
Discuss ways the patient may alter task performance to continue to function in vocational and interpersonal roles.	Assistive devices may be needed for continued functioning in the current vocational role. If the patient's health precludes continued performance in the current vocational role, referral and counseling for retraining may be needed.
Encourage use of a prosthesis (if prescribed) as soon as possible after surgery.	Whether the amputation is the result of trauma, chronic illness, or cancer, the patient is likely to experience a period of grieving. Disbelief and anger often mark the initial response. The patient may believe attainment of independence and future goals is impossible. Early use of a prosthesis helps patients promptly return to mobility and resume typical activities.
For patients who continue to have difficulty adapting to the amputation, provide a referral to a mental health professional such as an advanced practice psychiatric nurse or a psychologist.	Trained professionals can help explore the impact of amputation on the patient's life and review strategies for adaptation.

Nursing Diagnosis:

Deficient Knowledge

related to unfamiliarity with care of the residual limb and prosthesis and signs and symptoms of skin irritation or pressure necrosis

Desired Outcomes: Within 24 hr of hospital discharge, the patient verbalizes knowledge about care of the residual limb and prosthesis and correctly demonstrates how to wrap the residual limb. The patient verbalizes knowledge about indicators of pressure necrosis and irritation from the shrinkage device or prosthesis.

ASSESSMENT/INTERVENTIONS	RATIONALES
Assess the patient's health literacy (language, reading, comprehension). Assess culturally specific information needs and current knowledge level.	This assessment helps ensure educational materials are selected and presented in a manner that is culturally and educationally appropriate.
Teach the Patient about the Following:	
- For the first 24 hr after surgery, elevate the residual limb as prescribed.	Elevation reduces edema and pain.
- After this period, keep the residual lower limb flat when at rest in bed.	A flat position reduces risk of hip flexion contracture after the first 24 hr after surgery.
- When seated, elevate the residual lower limb.	Elevating the residual lower limb reduces dependent edema when the patient is seated.
- Apply the prescribed shrinkage device such as an elastic wrap or sock.	A shrinkage device molds and prepares the residual limb for possible prosthesis fitting. Application of the elastic wrap is begun with a recurrent turn over the distal end of the residual limb; then diagonal circumferential turns are made, overlapping to two-thirds the width of the wrap. Wrapping in a circular pattern may compromise blood supply to the residual limb. The shrinkage device should be wrapped snugly but not too tightly to avoid impeding circulation and healing. It should remain smooth and free of wrinkles to avoid causing skin breakdown or uneven shrinkage of the residual limb.
- Ensure all tissue is contained by the elastic wrap.	The goal of wrapping is to form a cone-shaped residual limb. If any tissue is allowed to bulge, proper fitting of the prosthesis will be difficult.
- Perform rewrapping and careful inspection of the residual limb at least q4-6h or as determined by the surgeon or agency protocol. Rewrapping may need to be done more often if the elastic wrap becomes loose.	Assessment of the limb at regular intervals will detect early skin impairment and allow intervention. Rewrapping also ensures the elastic wrap remains snug enough to effectively mold the residual limb for the prosthesis.
- Use extra padding with moleskin or lamb's wool.	Extra padding prevents irritation to areas susceptible to pressure.
Teach the patient to monitor the residual limb for skin abrasions, blisters, hair follicle infection, or other impairments.	These findings indicate skin irritations or pressure necrosis caused by the shrinkage device or prosthesis.
Explain that if erythema persists after massage, the patient should notify the health care provider.	Persistent erythema may be an early sign of pressure ulcer development.
If prescribed, instruct the patient to leave any open areas on the residual limb exposed to air for 1-hr periods qid. Verify wound care preferences with the patient's surgeon.	Prolonged dressing of wounds can trap moisture that can contribute to wound maceration. Exposure to air allows the wound surface to dry naturally to facilitate healing.
Teach the daily routine of skin cleansing with antibacterial soap and water.	Soap and water have adequate antibacterial effects. Washing also helps toughen skin on the residual limb in preparation for prosthesis use. Patients should be taught to avoid applying lotions, alcohol, powder, or oils unless prescribed because they can cause excessive wound dryness.
Instruct the patient to dry the residual limb thoroughly before any shrinkage device is applied.	Retained moisture can cause skin maceration, which would contribute to fungal growth.
Instruct the patient to change the shrinkage device daily, washing it with mild soap and water and drying it thoroughly before reapplication.	Use of a soiled shrinkage device can contribute to wound infection.
Instruct the patient to begin to massage the residual limb 3 wk postoperatively.	Massage will break up adherent scar tissue and prepare the skin for the stress of prosthesis wear.
Ensure that the patient receives complete instructions in the care of the prosthesis by a nurse expert or certified prosthetist-orthotist.	Patients need to be encouraged to accept the residual limb and become adept at self-care in order to be independent as quickly as possible.

ADDITIONAL NURSING DIAGNOSES/PROBLEMS:

PATIENT-FAMILY TEACHING AND DISCHARGE PLANNING

When providing patient-family teaching, focus on sensory information, avoid giving excessive information, and make appropriate referrals (e.g., visiting or home health nurse, community health resources) for follow-up teaching. Include verbal and written information about the following:

✓ Medications and supplements, including name, dosage, purpose, schedule, precautions, and potential side effects. Also discuss drug-drug, herb-drug, and food-drug interactions.

✓ How and where to purchase necessary supplies and equipment for self-care.

✓ Care of residual limb and prosthesis.

✓ Indicators of wound infection that require medical attention such as swelling, persistent redness, purulent discharge, local warmth, systemic fever, and pain. Suggest use of a small hand mirror if needed to examine incision and residual limb.

✓ Prescribed exercise regimen, including rationale for each exercise, number of repetitions for each, and frequency of exercise periods.

✓ Ambulation with assistive devices and prosthesis on level and uneven surfaces and on stairs. The patient should demonstrate independence and achievement of physical therapy goals before hospital discharge. For the patient with upper extremity amputation, independence with performance of activities of daily living should be demonstrated before discharge.

✓ Importance of follow-up care, date of next appointment, and a telephone number to call if questions arise.

✓ Referral to visiting, public health, or home health nurses as necessary for ongoing care after hospital discharge. Also consider referral to an appropriate resource person if the patient has continued difficulty with grief or body image disturbance.

✓ Referral to community resources, including local amputation support activities, and to Amputees in Motion at *www.amputeesinmotion.org*, Amputee Coalition at *www.amputee-coalition.org*, or the Amputee Coalition of Canada at *www.amputeecoalitioncanada.org*

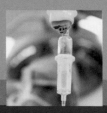

Fractures 67

OVERVIEW/PATHOPHYSIOLOGY

A fracture is a break in continuity of a bone. It occurs when stress is placed on the bone that exceeds its biologic loading capacity. Most commonly the stress is the result of trauma. Pathologic fractures can occur when the bone's decreased loading capacity cannot tolerate even normal stress, as with osteoporosis.

HEALTH CARE SETTING

Emergency care, acute care, primary care

ASSESSMENT

Physical findings: Include loss of normal bony or limb contours, edema, ecchymosis, limb shortening, decreased range of motion (ROM) of involved and adjacent joints, and false motion (occurs outside a joint). The patient may describe crepitus, but this should not be elicited by the health care provider because of risk of injury to surrounding soft tissues. Complicated or complex fractures can present with signs and symptoms of perforated internal organs, neurovascular dysfunction, joint effusion, or excessive joint laxity. Open fractures involve a break in the skin and will exhibit a wound in the area of suspected fracture; bone may be exposed in the wound.

Acute indicators: Fractures cause either insidious and progressive pain or sudden onset of severe pain. They are usually associated with trauma or physical stress, such as jogging, strenuous exercise, or a fall. In the event of pathologic fracture, the patient typically describes signs and symptoms associated with the underlying pathology.

Complications: Delayed union is failure of bone fragments to unite within the expected time frame based on factors such as the patient's age. Lack of any bony union is known as *nonunion*, which is demonstrated by nonalignment and lost function secondary to lost bony rigidity. Pseudoarthrosis is a state in which the fracture fails to heal and a false joint develops at the fracture site. Avascular necrosis occurs when the fracture interrupts blood supply to a segment of bone, causing eventual bone death. Myositis ossificans involves heterotrophic bone formation (abnormal, out of the normal area). It occurs most commonly in the arms, thighs, and hips. Complex regional pain syndrome (or reflex sympathetic dystrophy) is an incompletely understood process that results in pain out of proportion to the injury, with reduced function, joint stiffness, and trophic changes in soft tissue and skin following a traumatic event such as a fracture. Other fracture complications include altered sensation, limb length discrepancies, and chronic lymphatic or venous stasis.

> **Note:** *Any patient with a suspected fracture should be treated as though a fracture is present until diagnosis is made. Interventions should include immobilization of the affected area and careful monitoring of neurovascular function distal to the injury. Any restrictions to swelling (e.g., rings, wristwatches, bracelets) should be removed before they can contribute to neurovascular dysfunction. Ice and elevation, if tolerated and appropriate based on the type of injury, can be used to decrease swelling.*

DIAGNOSTIC TESTS

Most fractures are identified easily with standard anteroposterior (AP) and lateral x-ray examination. Occasionally special radiographic views are needed, such as the mortise view with bimalleolar ankle fractures (showing joint spaces between the fibula, tibia, and talus) or x-ray examination through the open mouth to identify fractures of the odontoid process. Magnetic resonance imaging may be useful in evaluating complicated fractures, but its ability to identify different bone densities is limited. Intraarticular fractures may be diagnosed with arthroscopy. Bone scans, computed tomography (CT) scans, tomograms, stereoscopic films, and arthrograms also can be used.

PART I: Medical-Surgical Nursing

Nursing Diagnosis:

Acute Pain

related to injury, surgical repair, and/or rehabilitation therapy

Desired Outcomes: Within 1-2 hr of intervention, the patient's subjective perception of pain decreases as indicated by a lower pain intensity rating. The patient demonstrates ability to perform activities of daily living (ADLs) with minimal complaints of discomfort.

ASSESSMENT/INTERVENTIONS	RATIONALES
Assess the patient's pain using an appropriate pain intensity rating scale, such as the visual analog scale (VAS), Wong Baker FACES Pain Rating Scale, Faces Pain Scale—Revised, or FLACC (face, legs, activity, crying, consolability) scale.	The patient provides a personal baseline report, enabling nurses to more effectively assess subsequent increases and decreases in pain. For the patient who is too young or unable to comprehend the quantitative scales, the nurse will use the FLACC scale based on observations.
If appropriate, instruct hospitalized surgical patients in the use of patient-controlled analgesia (PCA) or epidural analgesia.	Understanding principles of PCA or epidural analgesia will help patients obtain better pain management.
⚠ If PCA or epidural analgesia is used, verify with another nurse that the PCA or epidural pump contains the prescribed medication and concentration with prescribed settings for patient dosing, continuous infusion, and/or clinician-activated bolus.	Verification of the prescribed medication and pump settings is critical to the safe delivery of the analgesia.
Instruct the family/significant other that only the patient may administer a dose of analgesia from the PCA pump.	If the family administers medication via the PCA pump, the patient may experience negative effects from overmedication (e.g., excessive sedation).
Assist the patient with coordinating the time of peak effectiveness of analgesics with periods of exercise or ambulation.	Careful timing of analgesics enables patients to achieve optimal pain management before exercise or ambulation. Participation in the exercise regimen (e.g., physical therapy) contributes to expediency of recovery.
As prescribed, administer nonsteroidal antiinflammatory drugs (NSAIDs) and assess effectiveness of the patient's pain management, as well as adverse effects.	Because of the potential for excessive bleeding following NSAID administration, it is important to monitor for hemorrhage at the surgical site.
⚠ Administer anticoagulants cautiously if the patient is receiving epidural analgesia.	Anticoagulants are commonly administered following orthopedic surgery, and many are considered safe to use during epidural analgesia. However, immediate action should be taken if any signs or symptoms suggesting spinal cord compression occur. Diagnosis of epidural hematoma should be considered in the differential diagnosis if the patient using an epidural catheter develops neurovascular changes to the extremities.
Use nonpharmacologic pain management methods, such as guided imagery, relaxation, massage, distraction, biofeedback, cold therapy, and music therapy. Traditional nursing interventions such as back rubs and repositioning also should be included in the pain management plan of care.	Nonpharmacologic methods can augment pharmacologic pain management strategies. These methods may be indicated for a patient who avoids use of analgesics or experiences minimal pain management with prescribed analgesics.
⚠ If an intraarticular anesthetic or opioid was administered intraoperatively, advise the patient that lack of pain in the immediate postoperative period should *not* be mistaken for ability to move the joint excessively.	Patients with minimal postoperative pain may be tempted to increase activity, putting unnecessary stress on the fracture site. Prescribed activity and weight-bearing status must be carefully followed to avoid additional injury to the affected extremity.

Nursing Diagnosis:

Risk for Peripheral Neurovascular Dysfunction

related to interruption of capillary blood flow occurring with increased pressure within the myofascial compartment (compartment syndrome)

Desired Outcomes: The patient has adequate peripheral neurovascular function in the involved extremity as evidenced by normal muscle tone, brisk capillary refill (less than 2 sec or consistent with the contralateral extremity), normal tissue pressures (15 mm Hg or less as determined by the invasive diagnostic procedure), minimal edema or tautness, and absence of paresthesia. The patient verbalizes understanding of the importance of reporting symptoms indicative of impaired neurovascular function.

ASSESSMENT/INTERVENTIONS	RATIONALES
⚠ Assess the patient's pain at regular intervals as defined by the health care provider or agency policy, immediately informing the provider of increased pain or pain not managed by analgesia.	Increased or unrelenting pain, or pain out of proportion to the injury, is the first sign of developing compartment syndrome (pain = first "P").
⚠ Assess tissue pressures in all compartments as prescribed if an intracompartmental pressure device is available.	Continued assessment of high-risk patients (e.g., adolescents or young adults with traumatic injury; confused or developmentally disabled patients who cannot accurately report symptoms) should be done to avoid possible complications. The site of fracture or repair (e.g., high tibial osteotomy) also can increase the risk for developing compartment syndrome.
⚠ Alert the health care provider to pressures higher than 10 mm Hg.	Sustained high pressures may indicate developing compartment syndrome; if pressures exceed systolic blood pressure, perfusion to the extremity is threatened.
⚠ Assess neurovascular status at regular intervals by checking temperature (circulation), movement, and sensation in the affected extremity.	Paresthesia (second "P"), pallor (third "P"), and poikilothermia (coolness due to diminished blood flow to distal tissues) (fourth "P") are additional signs of a developing compartment syndrome. True paralysis (fifth "P") is a late sign of compartment syndrome, which indicates significant ischemia/limb impairment. **Note:** With the exception of pain and paresthesia, the so-called 5 Ps are not reliable for diagnosis, and the presence or absence of them should not affect injury management.
Apply ice and elevate the affected extremity when prescribed.	A fractured limb is typically elevated for the first 24 hr to decrease swelling. Ice is applied to cause vasoconstriction in the area of injury, which decreases edema and aids in pain management. Because edema can contribute to the development of compartment syndrome, these early interventions may be critical.
⚠ When acute compartment syndrome is suspected, avoid use of ice and elevation.	Ice and elevation may further compromise vascular supply in an extremity that is already experiencing ischemia secondary to developing compartment syndrome.
⚠ In response to changes in the neurovascular condition, contact the health care provider promptly. Adjust the constricting device as prescribed (e.g., loosen elastic wrap around a splint or bivalved cast). Wrap a dressing around a split cast.	When swelling places patients at risk for compartment syndrome, the constricting device (e.g., cast, splint, circumferential dressing) must be loosened down to skin level to prevent further swelling and compromise to the affected extremity. Wrapping a dressing around a split cast aids in continued immobilization of fracture fragments.
Teach the patient and significant others symptoms of neurovascular compromise that should be reported immediately (e.g., changes in temperature, sensation, color, or ability to move digits of the affected extremity).	Awareness of the risk of compartment syndrome will enable patients to respond more quickly to possible symptoms and reduce a delay in treatment.

Nursing Diagnosis:

Impaired Physical Mobility

related to musculoskeletal pain and unfamiliarity with use of immobilization devices

Desired Outcomes: By at least 24 hr before hospital discharge, the patient maintains appropriate body alignment with external fixation devices in place or demonstrates setup and use of a home traction device. The patient uses mobility aids safely. The patient verbalizes understanding of the use of analgesics and adjunctive methods to decrease pain.

ASSESSMENT/INTERVENTIONS	RATIONALES
Assess the patient's health literacy (language, reading, comprehension). Assess culturally specific information needs.	This assessment helps ensure that materials are selected and presented in a manner that is culturally and educationally appropriate.
Teach proper body alignment, most commonly with joints in neutral position, if an external fixation device has been applied.	Maintenance of a neutral position decreases risk of contracture formation, which would affect the patient's mobility.
If orthotic devices are used to maintain position, teach exercises and ROM to do when the device is removed.	Prolonged use of the orthotic can cause impaired joint mobility. Exercise at regular intervals will help maintain joint flexibility.
Teach the patient and significant others to perform active and/or passive ROM exercises of adjacent joints q8h as appropriate.	ROM exercises help preserve joint mobility and decrease risk of contracture formation.
When appropriate, instruct the patient and significant others in care of an extremity in traction, including signs and symptoms of complications (e.g., pressure necrosis, impaired neurovascular function, pin site infection for skeletal traction).	Knowledge will help ensure optimal healing and prompt treatment in case of complications.
Instruct the patient and significant others in care of an extremity in external fixator, performance of prescribed exercises while in the fixator, and signs and symptoms of complications (see previous intervention).	Knowledge will help ensure optimal healing and prompt treatment in case of complications.
Instruct the patient and significant others in care of the casted extremity and in signs and symptoms of complications (e.g., skin maceration, impaired neurovascular function, disuse osteoporosis).	A knowledgeable patient should be able to demonstrate cast care, describe neurovascular assessment of the distal extremity, describe assessment of evidence of pressure necrosis beneath the cast, demonstrate performance of prescribed exercises, and describe prevention of skin maceration and disuse osteoporosis to ensure optimal healing and prompt treatment in case of problems.
Instruct the patient in use of crutches, walker, cane, or other mobility aids.	Safe use enables early mobilization and decreases risk of additional injury.
Instruct the patient and significant others in use of analgesics and nonpharmacologic pain management methods.	Effective pain management will increase the patient's ability to participate in appropriate exercise and activity.

Nursing Diagnoses:

Risk for Impaired Skin Integrity
Impaired Tissue Integrity

related to irritation and pressure potentially present with an immobilization device (e.g., cast, splint)

Desired Outcomes: Within 8 hr of immobilization device application, the patient verbalizes knowledge about indicators of pressure necrosis. The patient relates absence of discomfort under the immobilization device and exhibits intact skin when the device is removed.

PART I: Medical-Surgical Nursing

ASSESSMENT/INTERVENTIONS	RATIONALES
When assisting with application of a cast or other immobilization device, ensure adequate padding is applied over bony prominences of the affected extremity.	Bony prominences are at risk for skin breakdown. Padding decreases pressure over these areas.
Handle a drying cast only with palms of the hands.	Handling a wet cast with fingers can cause indentations that create pressure points on underlying skin. Using palms of the hands ensures a smooth surface as the cast dries and decreases likelihood of underlying pressure points.
Ensure all cast surfaces are alternately exposed to air.	Exposure to air facilitates drying of the cast.
Petal edges of plaster casts with tape or moleskin if a cast liner was not applied.	Petaling prevents rough cast edges from causing skin irritation/impairment. It also prevents cast crumbs from falling into the cast and causing pressure areas with additional skin irritation/impairment.
Pad surfaces of other immobilization devices as well.	Padding decreases pressure on skin underneath the devices.
Instruct the patient never to insert anything between the immobilization device and skin.	Use of a coat hanger or stick can cause skin irritation that leads to infection. It also may cause bunching of the cotton material placed between the cast and skin, which would result in pressure points under the cast.
Advise the patient to notify the health care provider of severe itching.	The health care provider may prescribe a medication to relieve itching. Scratching the unaffected side in a similar location also may provide relief.
Teach indicators of pressure necrosis under the immobilization device, such as pain, burning sensation, foul odor from the opening, or drainage on the device.	An informed individual is more likely to report these findings quickly, which will enable prompt treatment to avoid further impairment.

Nursing Diagnosis:

Constipation

related to decreased mobility and use of opioid analgesics

Desired Outcomes: Within 8 hr of immobilization device application, the patient verbalizes understanding of strategies to maintain normal bowel elimination. The patient maintains bowel elimination in his or her normal pattern.

ASSESSMENT/INTERVENTIONS	RATIONALES
Assess the patient's usual bowel pattern and habits to ensure regular elimination.	Use of proven strategies will help patients more quickly regain their usual bowel elimination pattern.
Encourage choice of diet items that will facilitate normal bowel elimination.	High-fiber foods (e.g., bran, whole grains, nuts, raw and coarse vegetables, fruits with skins) add bulk to stool to promote bowel elimination.
If not contraindicated, encourage the patient to drink adequate fluids.	Fluid intake helps promote soft stool for easier elimination.
If the patient desires, request prescription for stool softener and/or laxative. Reassess bowel elimination for response to medication, and initiate additional treatment as needed to return normal bowel function.	Pharmacologic intervention may be needed to maintain normal bowel elimination. If a stool softener or laxative is ineffective, patients may require a rectal suppository or enema administration to assist with elimination.
Encourage mobility to the extent of the prescribed activity parameters.	Mobility promotes peristalsis and hence improves bowel elimination. The patient thus should not be left in bed or allowed to use a bedside commode if additional mobility can be tolerated.
As indicated, teach current influences on impaired bowel elimination.	Decreased mobility, use of opioid analgesics, and inconsistent food intake can adversely influence bowel elimination.

PART I: Medical-Surgical Nursing

Nursing Diagnoses:

Dressing Self-Care Deficit
Bathing Self-Care Deficit
Toileting Self-Care Deficit

related to physical limitations present with a cast, immobilizer, or orthotic devices

Desired Outcome: Within 48 hr of initiation of immobilization, the patient demonstrates optimal performance of ADLs.

ASSESSMENT/INTERVENTIONS	RATIONALES
Assess the patient's self-care limitations.	Thorough assessment enables implementation of appropriate self-care strategies.
Ensure that the patient receives the prescribed treatment for pain.	Unmanaged pain can severely limit attempts to mobilize, making performance of self-care tasks difficult or impossible.
Incorporate a structured exercise regimen that will increase strength and endurance. Direct the regimen toward development of muscle groups needed for the patient's specific activity deficit.	Patients with insufficient strength to manipulate immobilized extremities need planned exercise to assist in managing self-care while in a cast or immobilizer. Increased strength and endurance contribute to independence in self-care.
As indicated, refer the patient to occupational therapy, and use assistive devices and dressing/grooming aids as needed.	Use of appropriate assistive devices maximizes self-care ability. Sock donners, long-handled reachers and brushes, raised toilet seats, and other devices minimize stress on joints. Clothing also can be adapted for greater ease in dressing (e.g., zipper pulls, Velcro closures); adaptive clothing also accommodates a cast or external fixator.
When needed, teach significant others how to assist the patient with self-care activities.	Although independence with self-care is the goal, involvement of the significant other can minimize the need for skilled home services. A knowledgeable significant other also can reinforce professional health instructions given to the patient.
Refer to care management/social services department of the hospital.	Patients may require assistance with funding for assistive equipment or home help. Care management/social services staff also can identify community agencies that loan equipment or have other volunteer services.

Nursing Diagnosis:

Deficient Knowledge

related to unfamiliarity with function of the external fixation, performance of pin care, and signs and symptoms of pin site infection

Desired Outcomes: By at least 24 hr before hospital discharge, the patient verbalizes knowledge of the rationale for the external fixator and indicators of pin site infection. The patient or significant other demonstrates performance of pin care.

ASSESSMENT/INTERVENTIONS	RATIONALES
Assess the patient's health care literacy (language, reading, comprehension). Assess culturally specific information needs and the current knowledge level.	This assessment helps ensure educational materials are selected and presented in a manner that is culturally and educationally appropriate.

continued

ASSESSMENT/INTERVENTIONS	RATIONALES
Teach the rationale for use of the fixator with the type of fracture or injury, emphasizing patient benefits.	External fixation consists of skeletal pins that penetrate the fracture fragments and are attached to universal joints. These joints are in turn attached to rods, which provide stabilization and form a frame around the fractured limb for immobilization. A patient who is knowledgeable about the device and its purpose is more likely to handle the device judiciously to ensure bone fragment immobilization.
Teach the patient and significant others appropriate handling and care of the external fixator.	Although some fixation devices can be used safely as a handle to lift the limb, this activity is contraindicated with other devices because it may lead to loosening of skeletal pins and loss of bone fragment immobilization. Awareness of care requirements for the patient's specific type of fixation device is critical.
Teach the patient and significant others to support the extremity with pillows, two hands, slings, and other devices as necessary.	Adequate support of the extremity prevents stress on skeletal pins. Stress on pins can contribute to loosening and loss of bone fragment immobilization.
Instruct the patient and significant others in pin care as prescribed by the health care provider.	For external fixator pins, some health care providers require daily cleansing with dilute hydrogen peroxide, chlorhexidine, or other skin preparation solution. Iodine-based mixtures may cause corrosion of some fixation devices and interfere with pin site assessment. Antibacterial ointments and small dressings also may be prescribed for pin sites.
Teach the patient and significant others to identify possible indicators of infection at pin sites, including persistent redness, swelling, drainage, increasing pain, and local warmth, and body temperature greater than 101° F (38.3° C). Instruct the patient to report abnormal findings immediately to the health care provider.	The patient and significant others must recognize signs of infection and report them to the health care provider for prompt assessment and treatment.
If an orthotic device is used, ensure the patient and significant others are aware of its purpose and able to identify areas of excessive pressure, and follow the prescribed schedule for adjunctive/ROM exercises.	Orthotics may be added to the external fixator to prevent wristdrop, footdrop, contracture, or other joint dysfunction. Devices should be kept clean and dry to decrease risk for infection at pin sites.
Advise the patient of the need for maintaining adequate fracture immobilization and scheduling follow-up care.	Failure to immobilize the fracture adequately may lead to delayed union, malunion, or nonunion. Adherence to the weight-bearing prescription for lower extremities and follow-up assessment of the device will ensure fracture immobilization is maintained.

PATIENT-FAMILY TEACHING AND DISCHARGE PLANNING

When providing patient-family teaching, focus on sensory information, avoid giving excessive information, and make appropriate referrals (e.g., visiting or home health nurse, community health resources) for follow-up teaching. Include verbal and written information about the following:

✓ Medications and supplements, including name, dosage, purpose, schedule, precautions, and potential side effects. Also discuss drug-drug, herb-drug, and food-drug interactions.

✓ Use of nonpharmacologic methods of pain management.

✓ Appropriate use of elevation and thermotherapy.

✓ Importance of performing prescribed exercises.

✓ Rationale for therapy (i.e., casting, external fixation, internal fixation).

✓ Precautions of therapy.

✓ *Casts:* Caring for the cast, monitoring neurovascular function of distal extremity, identifying evidence of pressure necrosis beneath cast, preventing skin maceration, preventing disuse osteoporosis.

✓ *Internal fixation devices:* Caring for the wound, noting signs of wound infection, following appropriate weight-bearing prescription for lower extremity fracture.

✓ *External fixator:* Demonstrating pin care, identifying evidence of pin site infection, knowing when to notify the health care provider of problems with the fixator, using prescribed orthotics, monitoring neurovascular function of the distal extremity.

✓ Use of assistive devices/ambulatory aids. Ensure the patient can perform return demonstration and is independent with devices/aids before hospital discharge.

✓ Materials necessary for wound care at home, with names of agencies that can provide additional supplies.

✓ Importance of follow-up care, date of next appointment, and telephone number to call if questions arise.

✓ For all patients who receive allograft bone for bone graft and who have questions about these grafts, resources for information include the following organizations:
- American Red Cross at *www.redcross.org*
- AlloSource at *www.allosource.org*

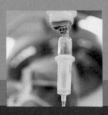

Joint Replacement Surgery 68

OVERVIEW/PATHOPHYSIOLOGY

Total hip arthroplasty

Total hip arthroplasty (THA) involves surgical resection of the hip joint and its replacement with an endoprosthesis. THA may be necessary for conditions such as osteoarthritis, rheumatoid arthritis, Legg-Calvé-Perthes disease, avascular necrosis (AVN), hip fracture, developmental hip dysplasia, and benign or malignant bone tumors. Because conservative treatments usually fail to decrease the impact of disease on the patient's functional ability, surgery becomes the next intervention. Arthroscopy, osteotomy, excision, hip resurfacing, or arthrodesis (joint fusion) may be considered before the patient and surgeon choose THA.

Historically, THA has been restricted to older patients because life of the implant has been traditionally estimated at 20 yr. However, younger patients with severe disease are now undergoing this procedure. Advanced age is not an absolute contraindication for THA because poor surgical outcomes appear to be related more to comorbidities than to aging alone. Contraindications to surgery include recent or active joint sepsis, arterial impairment or deficit to the extremity, neuropathic joint, and the individual's inability to cooperate in postoperative interventions and rehabilitation.

If the patient's condition indicates, replacement of only the femoral head can be accomplished with a bipolar or universal endoprosthesis. With THA, however, both femoral and acetabular components will be replaced. A typical prosthesis design includes a polyethylene-lined metal cup that fits over a metal femoral component. Metal-on-metal, ceramic-on-polyethylene, and ceramic-on-ceramic components are also used. The ceramic-on-ceramic components show very little wear and have minimal particle debris, thus extending the life of the hip arthroplasty. Components may be secured in place with cement (polymethylmethacrylate [PMMA]), or noncemented components with porous or roughened surfaces may be chosen to enable bony ingrowth. Because cemented components typically allow early weight bearing, they may be ideal for the patient whose activities do not place great demand on the joint but who would benefit from early mobility. The noncemented arthroplasty requires early weight-bearing restriction but accepts more strenuous activity after bony ingrowth is complete.

Early complications of infection, breakage, and loosening now occur less commonly because of improved surgical techniques and prosthetics. Infection risk has been substantially decreased with administration of prophylactic antibiotics and improved perioperative protocols. However, potential complications still include dislocation and aseptic loosening of components. The patient is also at risk for venous thromboembolism (VTE).

Total knee arthroplasty

Total knee arthroplasty (TKA) involves surgical resection of the knee joint and its replacement with an endoprosthesis. TKA may be necessary for conditions such as osteoarthritis, rheumatoid arthritis, gouty arthritis, hemophilic arthritis, osteochondritis dissecans, and severe knee trauma. Because conservative treatments have failed to decrease the impact of disease on functional ability in most patients, surgery is the next intervention. Arthroscopy, osteotomy, unicompartmental arthroplasty, arthrodesis (joint fusion), or use of a joint spacer may be considered before the patient and surgeon choose TKA.

Contraindications to surgery include recent or active sepsis in the joint, arterial impairment or deficit in the extremity, neuropathic joint, and inability of the patient to cooperate in postoperative interventions and rehabilitation. Infection in the operative joint is a possible complication, with the risk increased for patients with diabetes mellitus, immunosuppression, or significant peripheral vascular disease. Incidence of VTE ranges from 40% to 60% if prophylaxis is not initiated. Risk of dislocation is minimal, but component loosening is a long-term complication that may necessitate revision arthroplasty.

HEALTH CARE SETTING

Acute care surgical unit; rehabilitation unit

DIAGNOSTIC TESTS

Various tests are combined with patient history and physical findings to confirm presence of conditions that necessitate joint replacement. X-ray examination is commonly required, and arthroscopy may be useful in confirming extent of joint pathology and in identifying appropriate prosthesis.

Nursing Diagnosis:

Risk for Peripheral Neurovascular Dysfunction

related to interrupted arterial blood flow occurring with compression from the abduction wedge after THA and edema or use of a bulky postoperative dressing after TKA

Desired Outcomes: The patient maintains adequate peripheral neurovascular function distal to the operative site as evidenced by warmth, normal color, and ability to dorsiflex/plantar flex the foot and feel sensations with testing of the area enervated by peroneal and tibial nerves and L4-L5 nerve roots. The patient verbalizes understanding of the potential peripheral neurovascular complications and importance of promptly reporting signs of impairment.

ASSESSMENT/INTERVENTIONS	RATIONALES
Assess neurovascular function of the operative leg at regular intervals as prescribed by the surgeon or in accordance with hospital policy. Compare to the contralateral (nonoperative) leg and preoperative baseline assessment. Notify the health care provider of abnormal findings.	Pressure from the abductor wedge (THA) or a bulky knee dressing (TKA) can interrupt arterial blood flow and compress the peroneal and tibial nerves. These nerves provide movement and sensation to the calf and foot muscles. The peroneal nerve runs superficially by the fibular neck; it is assessed by testing sensation in the first web space between the great and second toes and by having patients dorsiflex the foot. The tibial nerve, a branch of the sciatic nerve, is assessed by testing sensation on the bottom of the foot and by having patients plantarflex the foot. Loss of sensation or movement signals impaired nerve function and must be reported promptly to the health care provider.
Apply cold therapy as prescribed at the operative site.	Swelling increases intracompartmental pressure in the lower leg, potentially interrupting arterial blood flow and compromising nerve function. Ice application is an important early intervention to decrease swelling.
Teach the potential for neurovascular impairment and importance of promptly reporting alterations in sensation, strength, movement, temperature, and color of the operative extremity.	These findings indicate impaired nerve function. Nerve damage can lead to severe disability with footdrop and paresthesias. The patient's knowledge of signs of impairment leads to prompt reporting, enabling health care providers to initiate appropriate treatment in a timely way.
Instruct the patient to perform the prescribed exercises (e.g., ankle pumps, heel slides) at regular intervals (e.g., four times an hour while awake).	Exercises stimulate circulation to the distal extremity and decrease risk for neurovascular dysfunction.

Nursing Diagnosis:

Ineffective Peripheral Tissue Perfusion (or risk for same)

related to development of VTE

Desired Outcome: The patient exhibits adequate tissue perfusion in the lower extremities as evidenced by maintenance of normal skin temperature and absence of calf pain and/or swelling.

ASSESSMENT/INTERVENTIONS	RATIONALES
Assess for and promptly report to the health care provider the patient's complaints of swelling, warmth, or pain/tenderness along the vein tracts in the lower extremities.	Close monitoring for these signs of thrombosis is imperative to ensure timely treatment. The patient's awareness of indicators also contributes to early identification and treatment of potential thrombotic complications.

continued

ASSESSMENT/INTERVENTIONS	RATIONALES
Encourage the patient to perform ankle pumps/heel slides at regular intervals.	These exercises cause calf muscle contraction. Muscle contraction increases blood return to the heart and decreases risk for thrombus development.
Maintain antiembolic stockings, intermittent pneumatic compression devices, or venous foot pump compression devices whenever the patient is in bed or chair.	These devices compress leg muscles and promote blood return to the heart, decreasing risk for thrombus development.
Remove compression devices when the patient needs to ambulate.	Attempting to ambulate without removing compression devices increases the risk of the patient falling.
Encourage the patient to perform other prescribed exercises and participate fully in the physical therapy (PT) program.	Early mobilization decreases risk of thrombus formation.
Instruct the patient regarding use of anticoagulants and other VTE prevention modalities.	Because of increased risk of VTE with joint replacement surgery, the surgeon will prescribe anticoagulant therapy. In addition, passive prevention strategies (e.g., sequential compression device) are likely to be implemented.
Administer anticoagulants as prescribed and review results of relevant blood tests (e.g., prothrombin [PT] time), ensuring that the health care provider has been informed of laboratory results.	Low–molecular-weight heparin (e.g., enoxaparin) or factor Xa inhibitor (e.g., fondaparinux) is administered by subcutaneous injection. Oral warfarin or rivaroxaban also may be used for VTE prevention. The patient should be knowledgeable about risks associated with anticoagulant use in order to report adverse effects in a timely way. Review **Risk for Bleeding** in "Pulmonary Embolus," p. 130.

Nursing Diagnosis:

Risk for Bleeding

related to joint replacement surgery

Desired Outcome: Within 24 hr of surgery, the patient is free of symptoms of excessive bleeding or hematoma formation as evidenced by maintenance of heart rate (HR), respiratory rate (RR), and blood pressure (BP) within the patient's normal range; balanced intake and output; output from wound drain 10 mL/hr or less; brisk capillary refill (less than 2 sec or consistent with preoperative assessment); peripheral pulses 2+ or more on 0-4+ scale; and warmth and normal color in the operative extremity distal to the surgical site.

ASSESSMENT/INTERVENTIONS	RATIONALES
[!] When taking vital signs (VS), assess drainage from the wound drainage system and on the surgical dressing. Promptly report to the health care provider output from the drainage system that exceeds 50 mL/hr or a dressing that is more than 50% saturated.	During wound closure, it is possible that a bleeding vessel may be overlooked or that bleeding will begin later during the patient's recovery. Careful assessment of wound drainage will detect excessive output.
Assess the patient's VS, subjective complaints, and neurovascular function. Report abnormal findings.	Patient complaints of warmth beneath the dressing, sensation of "things crawling" under the dressing, increasing pressure or pain, or coolness distal to the area of surgery can occur with hemorrhage or hematoma formation.
Reassess VS at regular intervals as determined by the surgeon's directive or agency policy for hypotension and increasing pulse rate.	These signs suggest shock or hemorrhage.
Also assess for pallor, decreased peripheral pulses, slowed capillary refill, or coolness of the distal extremity.	These signs can occur with hemorrhage or hematoma formation.
[!] If hemorrhage or hematoma formation is suspected, notify the health care provider promptly for intervention.	Interventions may include limb elevation or application of an elastic wrap or compression dressing to provide direct pressure on the site of bleeding.
[!] If the patient's VS suggest shock related to suspected hemorrhage or hematoma formation and the health care provider is unavailable, expose the surgical area by loosening the dressing.	This allows direct inspection of and pressure application to the area. Compression will usually control hemorrhage; if not, a thigh-high BP cuff over sheet wadding will serve as a tourniquet until the health care provider arrives for definitive therapy.

Nursing Diagnosis:

Impaired Physical Mobility

related to postoperative musculoskeletal pain and immobilization devices

Desired Outcomes: By at least 24 hr before hospital discharge, the patient demonstrates appropriate use of ambulatory aids. The patient verbalizes understanding of the use of analgesics and adjunctive methods to decrease pain when performing prescribed exercises or activity.

ASSESSMENT/INTERVENTIONS	RATIONALES
Assess the patient's health literacy (language, reading, comprehension). Assess culturally specific information needs and current knowledge level.	This assessment helps ensure materials are selected and presented in a manner that is culturally and educationally appropriate.
Reinforce teaching by the physical therapist on use and care of ambulatory aids such as a walker or crutches. Include use of the ambulatory aid on stairs or in other situations the patient may experience at home after discharge.	Patients need to be aware of equipment maintenance and techniques for its safe use to avoid injury.
Reinforce teaching by the physical therapist on exercises that improve muscle strength and increase joint flexibility.	Improved muscle strength and joint flexibility contribute to earlier mobilization and safe use of ambulatory aids. Exercises for both lower extremities and upper extremities should be included in the prescribed regimen.
Instruct the patient and significant others in use of analgesics and nonpharmacologic pain management methods.	Effective pain management will enable patients to become mobile more quickly, decreasing risk of complications associated with impaired physical mobility.

Nursing diagnosis (for patients undergoing the posterolateral approach to THA):

Deficient knowledge

related to unfamiliarity with appropriate activity precautions to decrease risk for dislocation of the operative hip

Desired Outcome: At least 24 hr before hospital discharge, the patient verbalizes knowledge about the potential for dislocation of the operative hip and activity precautions that decrease risk for dislocation.

> **Note:** *The following discussion relates to the posterolateral approach for THA; other approaches require different positional restrictions.*

ASSESSMENT/INTERVENTIONS	RATIONALES
Assess the patient's health literacy (language, reading, comprehension). Assess culturally specific information needs and current knowledge level.	This assessment helps ensure materials are selected and presented in a manner that is culturally and educationally appropriate.
⚠ During preoperative instruction, advise the patient of the potential for postoperative dislocation.	Risk of dislocation remains high until the periarticular tissues heal around the endoprosthesis (approximately 6 wk). If dislocation occurs once, the potential for recurrence is increased because of stretching of periarticular tissues. A confirmed dislocation is initially treated with closed reduction using conscious sedation. Recurrent dislocations may require revision arthroplasty or surgery to tighten periarticular tissues. A knowledgeable patient is more likely to understand the rationale for and adhere to activity and positional restrictions.

continued

ASSESSMENT/INTERVENTIONS	RATIONALES
Show the patient an endoprosthesis and describe how it can be dislocated when positional restrictions are not followed (i.e., flexion of the hip past 90 degrees, internal rotation, or adduction).	Actually seeing how certain positions result in dislocation will help patients understand the need for and adhere to positional restrictions.
During preoperative instruction, explain and demonstrate use of ambulatory aids and assistive devices for activities of daily living (ADLs) that enable independence without violating positional restrictions.	Preoperative introduction to ambulatory aids and ADL assistive devices enable patients to become familiar with the devices and techniques for use.
After surgery, reinforce positional restrictions and discuss activities that may violate restrictions, including pivoting on the operative leg, sitting on a toilet seat of regular height, bending over to tie shoelaces, or crossing legs.	Following a THA using the posterolateral approach, the patient may use an abduction wedge to prevent internal rotation and keep the hip from crossing the midline (i.e., maintain abducted position). Avoidance of flexion past 90 degrees also is required to decrease risk of dislocation.
Reinforce the need to get out of bed on the affected side.	Getting out of bed on the affected side decreases the risk of dislocation by keeping the patient from crossing the legs.
Advise the patient of the need for assistive devices for use at home after discharge. Refer the patient to the case manager or provide contact information for medical equipment suppliers that sell these items. Ensure the patient verbalizes understanding of the use of these devices, demonstrates positional restrictions and muscle-strengthening exercises, and can perform ADLs independently using appropriate assistive devices.	Self-care tasks such as dressing, bathing, and toileting necessitate use of assistive devices such as a long-handled reacher and sock donner. Patients with posterior precautions will need bathroom equipment such as an elevated toilet seat. Post-discharge PT generally includes a program of muscle-strengthening exercises and gait training with a walker or crutches to maximize mobility. Exercises also target the upper extremities because their weakness can make it difficult to use a walker or crutches.
Instruct the patient to report pain in the hip, buttock, or thigh, or prolonged limp after hospital discharge.	These symptoms may indicate prosthesis loosening.

Nursing diagnosis (for patients following TKA):

Deficient Knowledge

related to unfamiliarity with the continuous passive motion (CPM) machine and other prescribed exercises for the involved extremity following TKA

Desired Outcome: Within 30 min of instruction, the patient verbalizes understanding of CPM machine use and returns a demonstration of the prescribed exercises.

ASSESSMENT/INTERVENTIONS	RATIONALES
Assess the patient's health literacy (language, reading, comprehension). Assess culturally specific information needs.	This assessment helps ensure materials are selected and presented in a manner that is culturally and educationally appropriate.
Provide instructions for the muscle-strengthening and joint range-of-motion (ROM) exercise regimen. Provide written instructions that describe the exercises, listing frequency and number of repetitions for each one.	Prescribed exercises and use of CPM will facilitate return of normal joint function and reinforce gains in joint mobility. An effective method is to teach the appropriate exercise, demonstrate it, and then have patients return the demonstration.
Teach use of the CPM machine. For patients with prescribed postdischarge CPM, ensure understanding of the need to use the CPM machine for the prescribed amount of time each day.	The CPM machine supplements PT in rehabilitating the operative knee and restoring joint ROM.
Provide contact information in the event the patient has questions after hospital discharge.	The patient may need a contact with whom to discuss possible problems with the CPM machine as well as achievements with CPM therapy.

ADDITIONAL NURSING DIAGNOSES/PROBLEMS:

"Fractures" for **Acute Pain** related to injury, surgical   p. 491
  repair, and/or rehabilitation therapy

"Osteoarthritis" for **Sexual Dysfunction** related to pain,   p. 508
  decreased joint function, or body image changes
  that interfere with sexual performance

 PATIENT-FAMILY TEACHING AND DISCHARGE PLANNING

When providing patient-family teaching, focus on sensory information, avoid giving excessive information, and make appropriate referrals (e.g., visiting or home health nurse, community health resources, case manager) for follow-up teaching. Include verbal and written information about the following:

✓ Medications and supplements, including name, dosage, purpose, schedule, precautions, and potential side effects. Also discuss drug-drug, herb-drug, and food-drug interactions.

✓ Any precautions related to wound care and signs of infection (e.g., persistent redness or pain, swelling or localized warmth, fever, purulent drainage) or other complications of surgery.

✓ Need to avoid placing objects such as a pillow or towel roll under the knee for patients with TKA. Placing a towel roll under the ankle can force the knee to straighten (a desired goal) and raise the heel off the mattress to decrease pressure on the heel.

✓ Need to consult the health care provider about possible prophylactic antibiotics before any minor surgical procedure (e.g., dental surgery) in the first 2 yr after joint replacement.

✓ Activity restrictions related to surgical approach and weight-bearing restrictions related to choice of prosthesis.

✓ Use of prescribed immobilization device such as abductor wedge for patients with THA.

✓ Use of CPM machine, if prescribed for home use by patients with TKA.

✓ Frequency of exercise and rationale for exercise performance. Ensure the patient independently demonstrates each exercise.

✓ For ADL and ambulation, ensure the patient demonstrates independence in use of walker/crutches and assistive devices before hospital discharge.

✓ Assessment of neurovascular status at least four times daily, including need to immediately report to the provider symptoms such as numbness and tingling or coolness in extremity.

✓ Importance of follow-up care, date of next appointment, and a telephone number to call if questions arise.

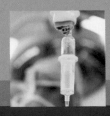

Osteoarthritis 69

OVERVIEW/PATHOPHYSIOLOGY

Osteoarthritis (OA) is the most prevalent articular disease in adults 65 yr of age and older. OA has been known by many names, including *degenerative joint disease (DJD)*, *degenerative arthritis*, or *hypertrophic arthritis*. It is no longer regarded as a wear-and-tear condition that occurs as a normal result of aging. In fact, joint changes that result from arthritis can be distinguished readily from age-related changes in articular cartilage of an asymptomatic older adult. In OA, chondrocytes within the joint fail to synthesize good-quality matrix in terms of both resistance and elasticity; this makes the cartilage more prone to deterioration. OA is recognized as a process in which all joint structures produce new tissue in response to joint injury or cartilage destruction. This chronic, progressive disease is characterized by gradual loss of articular cartilage combined with thickening of the subchondral bone and formation of bony outgrowths (osteophytes) at the joint margins. Affected individuals experience increasing pain, deformity, and loss of function. Prevalence of OA varies among different populations, but it is a universal human problem that actually may begin by 20-30 yr of age. The majority of people are affected by 40 yr of age, but few experience symptoms until after 50 or 60 yr of age. Before 50 yr of age, men are affected more often than women. After 50 yr of age, however, incidence of OA is twice as great in women as in men.

OA may be classified as either *idiopathic* or *secondary*. Idiopathic OA occurs in individuals with no history of joint injury or disease or of systemic illness that might contribute to the development of arthritis. Aging may be one influence on the deterioration of cartilage in arthritic joints, but additional evidence suggests existence of an autosomal recessive trait for gene defects that causes premature cartilage destruction. Prevalence of OA in postmenopausal women also suggests involvement of hormones in initiation of the disease. In contrast, secondary OA has an identifiable cause. Any condition or event that directly damages or overloads articular cartilage or causes joint instability can result in arthritic changes. Secondary OA typically occurs in younger individuals because of congenital processes (e.g., Legg-Calvé-Perthes disease), trauma, repetitive occupational stress, hemophilic joint hemorrhage, or infection.

OA is characterized by *site specificity*, with certain synovial joints showing higher disease prevalence. These include the weight-bearing joints (hips, knees); cervical and lumbar spine; distal interphalangeal (DIP), proximal interphalangeal (PIP), and metacarpophalangeal (MCP) joints in the hands; and metatarsophalangeal (MTP) joints in the feet (bunion deformity, or hallux valgus). The hips are most often affected in men and the hands in women, especially after menopause.

HEALTH CARE SETTING

Primary care

ASSESSMENT

Signs and symptoms: Joint pain and stiffness are the dominant symptoms and most common reason for seeking medical evaluation. However, because onset of pain is typically insidious, the patient may not be able to recall exactly when it began. The patient often describes an "aching" asymmetric pain that increases with joint use and is relieved by rest, especially in early stages of OA. Pain often is worse with using stairs, standing, and walking; less pain is experienced at night and when sitting. As the disease progresses, however, night pain or pain at rest is likely to occur. The patient also may state that pain increases with cool, damp, and rainy weather. This has been attributed to changes in intraarticular pressure associated with the fall in barometric pressure that precedes inclement weather. Joint stiffness ranges from slowness to pain with initial movement. Early morning stiffness is common but typically lasts less than 30 min. Stiffness after periods of rest or inactivity (articular gelling or gel phenomenon) is also characteristic of OA but resolves within several minutes. The patient may describe a squeaking, creaking, or grating with movement (crepitus) caused by loose cartilage particles in the joint capsule.

Physical assessment: Contralateral joints should be compared for symmetry, size, shape, color, appearance, temperature, and pain. Bony enlargement is common, and affected joints are likely to be tender to palpation. Reduced range of motion (ROM) is extremely common in osteoarthritic joints and contributes greatly to disability. Generally it is related to osteophyte formation, joint surface incongruity from severe loss of cartilage, or spasm and contracture of surrounding muscle. Locking during movement may be accentuated by mild effusion and soft tissue swelling. Large effusions are uncommon in OA and in fact would suggest other processes such as septic arthritis or gout. Crepitation during passive movement is present in more than 90% of patients with knee OA and indicates loss of cartilage integrity. Deformities may include Heberden's nodes on DIP joints and Bouchard's nodes on PIP joints of the hands. Almost 50% of patients with knee OA have a joint malalignment, typically a varus deformity due to cartilage loss in the medial compartment. Leg length discrepancy may be noted due to loss of joint space in advanced hip OA. In addition, muscular atrophy may be seen in advanced disease secondary to joint splinting for pain relief.

DIAGNOSTIC TESTS

OA almost always can be diagnosed by history and physical examination.

Laboratory tests: To rule out other arthropathic conditions (e.g., rheumatoid arthritis, septic arthritis) and to establish baselines before starting therapy.

Complete blood count (CBC): Suggested for patients who will be taking nonsteroidal antiinflammatory drugs (NSAIDs) for arthritis symptom management, with additional CBC prescribed periodically to screen for anemia caused by occult gastrointestinal (GI) bleeding.

Renal and liver function tests: For patients starting aspirin or NSAID therapy, with further testing done every 6 mo to assess for side effects such as electrolyte imbalance, hepatitis, or renal insufficiency.

Rheumatoid factor (RF), erythrocyte sedimentation rate (ESR), and C-reactive protein (CRP): None excludes a diagnosis of OA in the older patient. About 20% of healthy older adults have positive RF, and measures of inflammation tend to rise with age. Evaluation of inflammation is useful to rule out chronic conditions such as polymyalgia rheumatica. Synovial fluid analysis is another reliable method for differentiating OA from other arthritic disorders.

X-ray examination: Radiographic findings do not always correlate with severity of the patient's clinical symptoms. With disease progression, x-ray examination reveals joint space narrowing, osteophytes at joint margins, subchondral cysts, and altered shape of bone ends that suggests bone remodeling.

Magnetic resonance imaging (MRI) scan: Much more sensitive than x-ray examination in marking progression of joint destruction.

Nursing Diagnoses:

Chronic Pain
Acute Pain

related to arthritic joint changes and associated therapy

Desired Outcomes: Within 1-2 hr of intervention, the patient's perception of pain decreases as documented by a pain intensity scale. The patient demonstrates ability to perform activities of daily living (ADLs) with minimal discomfort.

ASSESSMENT/INTERVENTIONS	RATIONALES
Assess the patient's pain using an appropriate pain intensity rating scale, such as the visual analog scale (VAS), Wong Baker FACES Pain Rating Scale, Faces Pain Scale—Revised, or FLACC (face, legs, activity, crying, consolability) scale.	The patient provides a personal baseline report, enabling nurses to more effectively assess subsequent increases and decreases in pain. For the patient who is too young or unable to comprehend the quantitative scales, the nurse will use the FLACC scale based on observations.
Administer simple (nonopioid) analgesics (i.e., nonsteroidal antiinflammatory drugs [NSAIDs], acetaminophen), opioid analgesics, and adjuncts as prescribed and reassess their effectiveness in approximately 1 hr using pain intensity rating scale. Document preintervention and postintervention pain scores.	Pain management is a treatment priority for OA. Acetaminophen is recommended by the American College of Rheumatology as the initial treatment for OA pain, with doses up to 1000 mg qid for patients with normal liver function. If acetaminophen is ineffective, low-dose over-the-counter NSAIDs or salicylates are recommended for patients with normal renal function and no prior history of GI problems. Prescriptive NSAID doses are indicated if pain persists or worsens.

continued

PART I: Medical-Surgical Nursing

ASSESSMENT/INTERVENTIONS	RATIONALES
Observe for adverse effects of NSAIDs, such as GI bleeding or renal failure.	Traditional NSAIDs, such as ibuprofen or naproxen sodium, may increase risk of gastric ulceration or renal impairment because they inhibit cyclooxygenase-1 (Cox-1), which reduces prostaglandin levels in the stomach and kidneys. They also reduce renal circulation by decreasing synthesis of renal prostaglandins. The cyclooxygenase-2 selective NSAID celecoxib has shown less GI toxicity but is not without GI risk. NSAIDs can be taken with a proton pump inhibitor to minimize GI effects. An opioid analgesic can be safely added to acetaminophen or NSAID therapy if pain is unremitting.
Teach patients about the risk of cardiovascular events such as MI and stroke with high doses of NSAIDs.	Patients should know the risk of long-term NSAID use. High doses of NSAIDs are associated with increased risk of heart disease. In particular, risk of MI from NSAID use rises in proportion to the individual's underlying risk. Thus persons with a previous history of heart disease, hypertension, or hypercholesterolemia have the highest risk.
Advise the patient to coordinate time of peak effectiveness of the analgesic or NSAID with periods of exercise or other use of arthritic joints.	Careful timing of analgesics enables patients to achieve optimal pain management before exercise or ambulation. Participation in the exercise regimen helps maintain joint function.
Apply topical analgesics as prescribed.	Topical application may help with localized pain management for the OA patient. Capsaicin cream in particular has been shown to reduce knee pain significantly when used with other prescribed arthritis medications. Necessity for several applications daily often leads to poor adherence to treatment.
Use nonpharmacologic methods of pain management, such as guided imagery, relaxation, massage, distraction, biofeedback, heat or cold therapy, and music therapy. Include traditional nursing interventions such as back rubs and repositioning in the pain management plan of care.	Nonpharmacologic methods can augment pharmacologic pain management strategies. These methods may be critical for patients who avoid use of analgesics or experience minimal pain management with prescribed analgesics. Thermal therapy in particular may lessen pain and stiffness. Ice can be helpful during occasional episodes of acute inflammation, whereas heat therapy may be beneficial for stiffness. Heat therapy is delivered via numerous modalities, including hot packs, ultrasound, whirlpool, paraffin wax, and massage.
Teach the patient about the purpose and use of biologic agents.	Glucosamine sulfate and chondroitin sulfate have gained popularity because of perceived effects on cartilage regeneration. Neither supplement is directly incorporated into the extracellular matrix, so their rapid action in some patients suggests an antiinflammatory effect. Because both supplements increase the risk of bleeding, they should not be taken by patients taking prescribed anticoagulants. The dietary supplement S-adenosylmethionine (SAM-e) is believed to play a role in cell growth and repair and also may decrease arthritis pain. **Note:** Efficacy of biologic agents is not conclusively supported by scientific literature. However, anecdotal reports do indicate some patients experience positive effects. Because patients with OA continue to try these therapies, the nurse must be prepared to discuss their use.
Caution the patient to avoid joint immobilization for more than a week.	Additional stiffness and discomfort can result from prolonged joint rest.
As indicated, refer the patient to occupational therapy, and advise use of assistive devices and dressing/grooming aids as needed based on assessment of the patient's pain-related self-care limitations.	Use of appropriate assistive devices decreases pain during attempts at self-care. Sock donners, long-handled reachers and brushes, raised toilet seats, and other devices may help minimize stress on joints. Clothing also can be adapted for greater ease in dressing (e.g., zipper pulls, Velcro closures).

Nursing Diagnosis:

Impaired Physical Mobility

related to musculoskeletal impairment and need for adjustment to a new walking gait with assistive device

Desired Outcomes: Within 1 wk of instruction, the patient demonstrates adequate upper body strength for use of an assistive device. The patient demonstrates appropriate use of the assistive device on flat and uneven surfaces.

ASSESSMENT/INTERVENTIONS	RATIONALES
Before beginning gait training, assess to ensure the patient has necessary strength of the upper extremities to use the prescribed assistive device.	Many older adults have impaired upper body strength. Upper extremities must be strong enough to support body weight and allow safe use of prescribed assistive devices such as crutches or walker.
As indicated, teach armchair push-ups to attain and maintain triceps muscle strength.	Armchair push-ups target the triceps muscles, which are critically important for safe ambulation with crutches or walker. Patients should be encouraged to perform 10 repetitions several times daily if possible to improve triceps muscle strength.
Ensure height of the walker, crutches, or cane allows the patient to have approximately 15 degrees of elbow flexion when ambulating.	The assistive device must be appropriately sized to enable the patient's safe use.
Ensure crutch tops rest 1-1.5 inches (width of two fingers) below the patient's axillae.	This position avoids upper extremity paresthesia caused by pressure of the crutch tops on the brachial plexus.
Describe and demonstrate use of the prescribed assistive device, supervising the return demonstration. Ensure the patient can use the assistive device to get in and out of a motor vehicle safely.	Return demonstration and supervised practice help ensure that patients will be able to use the device safely on different surfaces and in multiple settings. Ambulation should begin in small increments on a flat surface and progress to all surfaces patients are expected to encounter.

Nursing Diagnosis:

Deficient Knowledge

related to unfamiliarity with the potential interaction between NSAIDs and herbal products

Desired Outcome: Within 1-2 hr of instruction, the patient verbalizes understanding of potential interactions between NSAIDs and herbal products that potentiate bleeding.

ASSESSMENT/INTERVENTIONS	RATIONALES
Assess the patient's health care literacy (language, reading, comprehension). Assess culturally specific information needs and current knowledge level.	This assessment helps ensure that materials are selected and presented in a manner that is culturally and educationally appropriate.
[!] Determine the patient's use of NSAIDs and herbal products that potentiate bleeding (e.g., ginkgo, ginger, turmeric, chamomile, kelp, horse chestnut, garlic, dong quai).	Herbal supplements, particularly ginger and turmeric, have been shown to reduce the pain and inflammation of arthritis. However, patients need to be aware that these herbs can potentiate bleeding.
[!] Advise the patient to discuss with the health care provider concurrent use of herbal products while taking NSAIDs for arthritis symptom management.	The provider should be aware of any products that increase the patient's bleeding risk.
Teach signs of occult bleeding such as black or tarry stools, hematuria, bleeding gums, and coughing up or vomiting blood.	A knowledgeable patient is more likely to recognize and immediately report signs of occult bleeding.

Nursing Diagnosis:

Sexual Dysfunction

related to pain, decreased joint function, or body image changes that interfere with sexual performance

Desired Outcome: Within 1 wk of intervention, the patient describes increased physical and psychologic comfort during sexual intimacy.

ASSESSMENT/INTERVENTIONS	RATIONALES
Discuss and assess possible problems with sexual performance related to decreased joint function, pain, or body image.	This discussion encourages patients to verbalize feelings related to body image changes, pain experience, and mobility that may impact interest and ability to have sexual intercourse.
Encourage the patient to use relaxation strategies (e.g., warm bath if medically permissible) to alleviate pain and stiffness before sexual intercourse.	Relaxation strategies decrease muscle tension, which contributes to joint pain, and allow increased flexibility of connective tissues that support the joints.
Encourage use of analgesics before sexual intercourse to enable easier movement.	Careful timing of analgesics enables patients to achieve optimal pain management before sexual intercourse.
Discuss other ways to preserve intimacy (e.g., caressing and holding) in a relationship if intercourse is difficult.	Exploration of additional ways to demonstrate intimacy will reinforce the patient's ability to maintain/strengthen the relationship despite effects of OA.
Instruct the patient about the disease process and alternative positions that promote comfort during sexual intercourse.	Understanding the impact of OA on mobility will allow patients to choose positions that decrease stress on joints during sexual intercourse.

ADDITIONAL NURSING DIAGNOSES/PROBLEMS:

"Rheumatoid Arthritis" for **Dressing/Bathing Self-Care Deficit** related to pain and limitations in joint range of motion   p. 518

Fatigue related to state of discomfort, effects of prolonged immobility, and psychoemotional demands of chronic illness   p. 518

✓ PATIENT-FAMILY TEACHING AND DISCHARGE PLANNING

When providing patient-family teaching, focus on sensory information, avoid giving excessive information, and initiate a visiting nurse/home health or community services referral for necessary follow-up teaching whenever possible. Include verbal and written information about the following:

✓ Medications and supplements, including name, dosage, purpose, schedule, precautions, and potential side effects. Also discuss drug-drug, herb-drug, and food-drug interactions.

✓ Importance of laboratory follow-up (e.g., blood or urine testing) for needed monitoring while the patient is taking selected medications.

✓ Proper use of heat or cold therapy, as appropriate to joint condition.

✓ Importance of joint protection, with balance of rest and activity.

✓ Use, care, and replacement of orthotics and assistive devices.

✓ Weight reduction, if indicated.

✓ Importance of follow-up care, date of next appointment, and a telephone number to call if questions arise.

✓ Referral to community resources, including local arthritis support activities, such as Arthritis Foundation at *www.arthritis.org* and The Arthritis Society at *www.arthritis.ca*

✓ Additional information on arthritis may be available through National Institute of Arthritis and Musculoskeletal and Skin Diseases (NIAMS) Information Clearinghouse at *http://www.niams.nih.gov/health_info/*

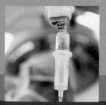

Osteoporosis 70

OVERVIEW/PATHOPHYSIOLOGY

Osteoporosis ("porous bone") is the most common metabolic bone disease. It is characterized by reduction in both bone mass and bone strength, while bone size remains constant. These changes make bone more brittle and susceptible to fractures. Osteoporosis affects 9 million people in the United States, and approximately 48 million more have low bone mass. Osteoporosis is responsible for more than 2 million fractures annually. Three types of osteoporosis have been identified: postmenopausal, senile, and secondary.

Postmenopausal osteoporosis: Affects females; clinical symptoms appear 10-15 yr after menopause as a result of lack of estrogen.

Senile osteoporosis: Affects both males and females, more commonly after 70 yr of age; related to poor nutritional status and decreased physical activity.

Secondary osteoporosis: Affects both males and females; results from another disease process (e.g., chronic kidney failure/liver disease, diabetes mellitus, rheumatoid arthritis), nutritional abnormalities (e.g., malnutrition, hypercalciuria, protein deficiency), medications and therapies (e.g., glucocorticoids, anticoagulants, anticonvulsants, cyclosporines, excessive thyroid replacement therapy, radiation therapy), and disuse (e.g., spinal cord injury/loss of biomechanical function, long-term bedrest).

HEALTH CARE SETTING

Primary care; acute care for complications. Individuals with osteoporosis are seen in all health care settings for primary diagnoses other than osteoporosis.

ASSESSMENT

Signs and symptoms: Because of the insidious onset of osteoporosis, most individuals are not diagnosed until they experience an acute fracture or receive radiographic evidence from x-ray examinations obtained for other conditions (e.g., chest x-ray examination to confirm pneumonia). Vertebral compression fractures can develop gradually, resulting in back discomfort and loss of height. Severe chronic flexion of the vertebral spine (kyphosis or "dowager's hump") may inhibit function of multiple organ systems (e.g., gastrointestinal [GI], respiratory). With severe spinal deformities, the patient often describes difficulty in obtaining clothes that fit well.

Risk factors

Unchangeable factors: Sex, age, family history, body size (small frame, slight build), ethnicity (Caucasian, Asian).

Changeable factors: Hormone levels (surgical or physiologic menopause, hypogonadism), diet (lifelong low-calcium intake, decreased protein intake, increased caffeine intake).

Lifestyle factors: Smoking, alcohol use, sedentary activity level.

Other influences: Medications, hyperthyroidism, hyperparathyroidism, multiple myeloma, transplantation, chronic diseases.

DIAGNOSTIC TESTS

Use of one or more tests is common.

Laboratory tests: Cannot accurately determine bone density or fracture risk, but serum and urinary markers of bone remodeling can help in determining disease cause. For example, urinary calcium may be elevated even if serum calcium is normal. Biochemical markers of bone resorption (e.g., osteocalcin) may be useful both for initial assessment and monitoring treatment effectiveness in confirmed disease.

Standard anteroposterior and lateral x-ray examinations of the spine: Provide a diagnosis for osteoporotic fractures or kyphosis. They have limited use in diagnosing disease before a fracture, however, because changes are not evident on plain films until at least 30% of bone mineral density has been lost.

Bone mineral density tests: Can measure the amount of bone in specific areas of the skeleton to predict risk of fracture. Dual energy x-ray absorptiometry (DEXA) is the "gold standard" for measuring bone density by testing bone mass in the spine, femoral neck, and wrist. This method is precise and economical; short procedure times mean minimal radiation exposure. Quantitative computed tomography measures bone density at sites throughout the body but is most often used in the spine. It is accurate but costly and delivers a considerable amount of radiation. In the heel, quantitative ultrasound compares favorably with density measurements obtained by DEXA. It is also an easy, low-cost, radiation-free diagnostic aid.

Bone biopsy: Useful in differential diagnosis of metabolic bone diseases such as osteoporosis and osteomalacia. It also can be useful for diagnosis in individuals with early onset of osteoporosis (age younger than 50 yr) or those with severe demineralization.

Nursing Diagnosis:

Deficient Knowledge

related to unfamiliarity with prevention of osteoporosis, its treatment, and importance of adequate dietary calcium intake/supplementation

Desired Outcome: Within 48 hr of instruction, the patient verbalizes knowledge of the disease process, possible treatments, and importance of adequate calcium intake.

ASSESSMENT/INTERVENTIONS	RATIONALES
Assess the patient's understanding of the nature of osteoporosis and the potential ineffectiveness of treatment if not initiated until symptoms appear.	Because of the insidious onset of osteoporosis, most individuals are not diagnosed until they experience an acute fracture or receive radiographic evidence from x-rays obtained for other conditions (e.g., chest x-ray to confirm pneumonia).
Include instruction on osteoporosis prevention as a routine part of health teaching for children, adolescents, and adults.	Adults need to recognize factors that increase their risk for osteoporosis (e.g., female, increasing age, small frame, Caucasian or Asian race). As children and adolescents experience bone growth, their bone quality can be improved through awareness of osteoporosis prevention strategies.
Teach the patient about proper nutrition in relation to calcium and vitamin D intake.	Appropriate nutrition is the foundation of osteoporosis prevention and treatment, and consistent calcium intake is especially important. A knowledgeable patient is more likely to adhere to prevention and treatment strategies. Vitamin D is needed for adequate intestinal absorption of calcium; see discussion of Vitamin D later in this nursing diagnosis. See **Imbalanced Nutrition: Less Than Body Requirements,** later, for more information.
Ensure that the health care provider has recommended or approves use of calcium supplements for the patient.	Although calcium is important to bone health, supplementation should be done on the advice of the health care provider. Excessive calcium intake can lead to nephrolithiasis in susceptible individuals.
Teach the patient that, although calcium supplements come in numerous forms, calcium carbonate is inexpensive and commonly available.	Calcium carbonate is best absorbed when taken with food because of its dependence on stomach acid for absorption. It contains approximately 40% calcium by weight, while calcium citrate contains approximately 21% calcium. Bone meal and dolomite should be avoided because they may contain high amounts of lead or other toxic substances.
Note: Patients taking a proton pump inhibitor (PPI) will need to take calcium citrate, an alternate form of the supplement.	Use of PPIs (e.g., esomeprazole, rabeprazole, lansoprazole) for gastric reflux or other conditions alters the acidic environment of the stomach and decreases absorption of calcium carbonate. Thus use of calcium citrate, which can be absorbed, is indicated for persons taking PPIs.
Teach the patient to recognize the amount of *elemental calcium* available in supplements and verbalize the recommended calcium dosage.	*Elemental calcium* refers to the amount of calcium in a supplement that is available for the body to absorb. Total weight in grams listed on the supplement label will reflect the weight of the calcium plus its binder (carbonate, citrate, lactate, gluconate). Adults 19-50 yr of age should take 1000 mg of calcium daily; females 51 yr and older and males 71 yr and older should take 1200 mg of calcium daily through diet and supplements. There is no added benefit in taking more calcium than is required, so supplementation is unnecessary if dietary intake is adequate.
Teach the patient not to take calcium and iron supplements at the same time.	The two elements bind with each other, and absorption of both will be impaired.
Evaluate the patient's medication profile.	Because calcium may reduce absorption of other medications, the nurse should carefully time administration of all medications to ensure maximal absorption.
Caution the patient to avoid taking more than 500-600 mg of calcium at one time and to spread doses over the entire day.	Excessive intake can lead to hypercalcemia, which may cause muscle weakness, constipation, and heart block. In addition, a dose in excess of 600 mg will not be fully absorbed.
Remind the patient to drink a full glass of water with each supplement.	Adequate hydration minimizes risk of developing renal calculi.

ASSESSMENT/INTERVENTIONS

RATIONALES

ASSESSMENT/INTERVENTIONS	RATIONALES
Remind the patient of the need for sunlight to enable vitamin D activation.	Exposure to sunlight is needed for cutaneous synthesis of vitamin D, but prolonged exposure does not necessarily increase the amount of vitamin D that is synthesized. An average of 15 minutes of exposure to the hands, face, arms, and legs typically meets the vitamin D requirement for most people.
Instruct the patient to avoid vitamin D supplementation if dietary intake is adequate.	Supplements may be needed by institutionalized persons, those living in extreme northern or southern latitudes, and people with limited sun exposure. However, excessive intake is discouraged because of risk of toxicity. Recommended amounts of vitamin D include 400 IU for neonates to age 12 months, 600 IU for persons up to age 70 yr, and 800 IU for those 70 yr or older.
⚠ If hormone replacement therapy (HRT) has been prescribed, explain its purpose, action, and precautions.	HRT is not routinely recommended for treatment of chronic disease and is prescribed only after risks and benefits have been evaluated for each patient. Women are encouraged to talk to their health care providers about personal risks and benefits. Benefits should be weighed against any risk of heart disease, stroke, and breast cancer, and health care providers should identify other prevention and treatment options when appropriate. The U.S. Food and Drug Administration also suggests using the lowest possible dose for the shortest period of time to manage symptoms of menopause.
Teach about the possible medications prescribed for treatment of osteoporosis, indications for use, possible side effects, administration time and method, and need for follow-up laboratory tests.	A knowledgeable patient is likely to adhere to the drug therapy and report necessary signs and symptoms to ensure prompt treatment of untoward side effects.
- Anabolic steroids	These medications improve bone density, but masculinizing side effects are usually prohibitive.
- Calcitonin-salmon (Miacalcin)	Calcitonin exerts a powerful inhibitory effect on osteoclasts to prevent bone resorption. It has also been used prophylactically in patients with low bone mineral density but no other symptoms of osteoporosis. It should be taken in conjunction with a high-calcium diet or with calcium supplementation and adequate amounts of vitamin D.
⚠ - Alendronate (Fosamax) - Risedronate (Actonel) - Ibandronate (Boniva) - Zoledronic acid (Reclast)	Bisphosphonates are nonhormonal oral preparations. Their highly selective inhibition of osteoclast activity is greater than that of calcitonin and accomplished without disturbing normal bone formation. Alendronate and risedronate may be taken once daily or weekly, and ibandronate requires only monthly administration. However, dosing restrictions may make adherence to the treatment regimen difficult. Zoledronic acid is given intravenously once yearly. All oral bisphosphonates must be taken with plain water on first rising, and the patient must refrain from eating or drinking for at least 30 min after taking it and remain in an upright position during this time to avoid esophageal damage. **Note:** The U.S. Food and Drug Administration issued a drug safety communication in March 2010 based on case reports of atypical subtrochanteric femur fractures in women with osteoporosis taking bisphosphonates. Review of clinical trial data did not show an increase in this risk in women using these medications. While relatively rare, cases of osteonecrosis of the jaw have been reported in persons taking oral bisphosphonates; most cases were associated with use of alendronate.
Encourage patients needing invasive dental treatment, such as tooth extractions, root canals, or dental implantations, to have dental work completed before starting treatment with a bisphosphonate.	For invasive dental treatment needed by patients already receiving a bisphosphonate, appropriate time for drug withdrawal before dental surgery has not been established. Most specialists recommend drug withdrawal 3 mo before dental surgery, but the risks and benefits of this timing are unproven because of the long half-life of bisphosphonates (Mayo Clinic, 2013).

continued

ASSESSMENT/INTERVENTIONS	RATIONALES
- Raloxifene (Evista)	In the class of medications known as selective estrogen receptor modulators (SERMs), raloxifene has had consistently positive effects on bone mineral density without stimulating the endometrium and contributing to cancer risk. Studies have documented decreased fracture risk in postmenopausal women, including those with prior osteoporotic fracture. Raloxifene can be given at any time of day without regard to meals. The patient should be taught to avoid prolonged immobility during travel because of the increased risk for venous thromboembolism.
- Teriparatide (Forteo)	Teriparatide is approved for treatment of osteoporosis in men and postmenopausal women at high risk for fracture. Teriparatide is a synthetic form of parathyroid hormone, which is the primary regulator of calcium and phosphate metabolism in bones. Daily injections of teriparatide stimulate new bone formation, leading to increased bone mineral density. **Note:** Because of increased incidence of osteosarcoma in studies of animals treated with teriparatide, the U.S. Food & Drug Administration warned against prescribing the drug for persons with increased baseline risk for osteosarcoma (e.g., persons with Paget's disease of the bone).
- Denosumab (Prolia)	Denosumab is a RANK ligand (RANKL) inhibitor/human monoclonal antibody given by injection every 6 mo to treat osteoporosis in postmenopausal women at high risk for fracture. It is also approved to treat men with high risk of fracture due to androgen deprivation therapy for prostate cancer and to increase bone mass in women receiving adjuvant aromatase inhibitor therapy for breast cancer.
Teach the importance of weight-bearing exercise and associated activity restrictions.	Weight-bearing exercise contributes to increased bone density and prevents bone loss. Individuals with established osteoporosis should avoid vigorous unsupervised exercise, and their exercise regimen should not include spinal flexion through activities such as toe touches and sit-ups. Rotational exercises such as golf and bowling may lead to vertebral injury by creating excessive compressive forces. Walking is generally considered a safe weight-bearing exercise.

Nursing Diagnosis:

Risk for Falls

related to potential for cluttered environment and other factors (see first rationale, below)

Desired Outcome: Within 24 hr of instruction, the patient describes strategies to decrease risk for fall or fracture.

ASSESSMENT/INTERVENTIONS	RATIONALES
Assess the patient's fall risk using a recognized fall risk assessment tool. Refer to the health care provider for additional evaluation of any identified deficits as necessary.	Confusion/dementia, cardiovascular disorders, decreased mobility, generalized weakness, abnormal elimination needs, impaired vision or hearing, and use of medications that affect blood pressure, balance, or level of consciousness can lead to falls and possible fracture in a patient with decreased bone density. Often the spontaneous fracture of a weakened bone causes the fall. The person with osteoporosis is also more at risk for injury (i.e., fragility fractures) if he or she falls.
Assist the patient and significant others in assessing presence of and eliminating environmental hazards that may increase risk for falls in the home.	Poor lighting, scatter rugs, electrical cords or oxygen tubing that cross floors or halls, and narrow stairs without adequate railing and lighting can increase fall risk.

ASSESSMENT/INTERVENTIONS

RATIONALES

ASSESSMENT/INTERVENTIONS	RATIONALES
Encourage the patient to avoid unnecessary inactivity because of fear of falling.	Inactivity can place an individual at greater risk for fractures by further decreasing bone density, increasing muscle atrophy, and contributing to orthostasis.
Encourage adequate intake of calcium and vitamin D, as well as appropriate use of prescribed osteoporosis medications.	Calcium and vitamin D contribute to bone health. Their adequate intake minimizes risk of injury in case a fall occurs. Other prescribed medications such as bisphosphonates or SERMs must be taken as prescribed for optimal bone health.
Instruct the patient to avoid lifting heavy objects, with weight limits stipulated by the health care provider.	Lifting puts patients with osteoporosis at risk for vertebral compression fractures. The patient needs strategies to maintain routine activities without increasing risk for vertebral injury. For example, patients interested in holding young grandchildren should be encouraged to have the child crawl, climb, or be placed in lap.
Teach exercise regimens that improve balance.	Aerobic walking and strength training via upper and lower body exercises have been shown to improve standing balance, which will help decrease risk of falls.

Nursing Diagnosis:

Imbalanced Nutrition: Less Than Body Requirements

related to inadequate intake of foods/supplements containing calcium and vitamin D

Desired Outcomes: Within 24 hr of instruction, the patient demonstrates adequate intake of calcium and vitamin D. The patient plans a 3-day menu that provides sufficient intake of both.

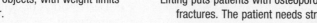

ASSESSMENT/INTERVENTIONS   RATIONALES

ASSESSMENT/INTERVENTIONS	RATIONALES
Assess the patient's knowledge of and ability to select foods high in calcium, including cheese and milk.	Food is a better source of calcium than supplements. If the patient is unable to tolerate dairy products, explore other food choices that can ensure adequate calcium intake (e.g., broccoli, sardines).
Teach the purpose and recommended daily intake for calcium and vitamin D.	Proper nutrition is the foundation of osteoporosis prevention and treatment. Consistent calcium intake alone cannot prevent or cure osteoporosis, but it is an important part of an overall prevention or treatment program.
	Adults 19-50 yr of age should take 1000 mg of calcium daily; females 51 yr and older and males 71 yr and older should take 1200 mg of calcium daily through diet and supplements. Adolescents (13-18 yr of age) need 1300 mg of calcium daily to maintain bone health. Oral calcium supplements (as calcium carbonate) may help perimenopausal women with inadequate dietary intake and may compensate for decreased intestinal absorption of calcium in postmenopausal women. Vitamin D is needed for adequate intestinal absorption and usage of calcium. Dietary sources include dairy products and vitamin-enriched cereals. Individuals who drink soy milk or another calcium-fortified liquid should be reminded to shake the container before drinking because calcium can settle to the bottom.
Provide sample menus that include adequate daily amounts of calcium and vitamin D. Guide the patient in developing a 3-day menu that includes appropriate intake of foods containing calcium and vitamin D.	Sample menus demonstrate easy ways in which adequate calcium and vitamin D can be incorporated into the daily diet.
Teach the necessity for adequate exposure to sunlight to prevent vitamin D deficiency.	Even casual sun exposure can prevent vitamin D deficiency. Individuals should be outside 15 min daily but can achieve this by walking into and out of stores during a normal routine.

continued

ASSESSMENT/INTERVENTIONS

If the patient has limited exposure to sunlight (e.g., resident of a long-term care facility), instruct the patient regarding vitamin D supplementation to ensure adequate calcium absorption.

RATIONALES

Supplementation will ensure adequate vitamin D intake. See previous discussion in **Deficient Knowledge.**

ADDITIONAL NURSING DIAGNOSES/PROBLEMS:

"Fractures" for **Constipation** related to decreased mobility, and use of opioid analgesics and calcium supplements — p. 494

"Osteoarthritis" for **Chronic Pain/Acute Pain** related to arthritic joint changes and associated therapy — p. 505

Impaired Physical Mobility related to musculoskeletal impairment and adjustment to new walking gait with an assistive device — p. 507

Sexual Dysfunction related to pain, decreased joint function, or body image changes that interfere with sexual performance — p. 508

"Rheumatoid Arthritis" for **Dressing/Bathing/Toileting Self-Care Deficit** related to pain and limitations in joint range of motion — p. 518

Disturbed Body Image related to development of joint deformities — p. 519

✓ PATIENT-FAMILY TEACHING AND DISCHARGE PLANNING

When providing patient-family teaching, focus on sensory information, avoid giving excessive information, and make appropriate referrals (e.g., visiting or home health nurse, community health resources, case manager) for follow-up teaching. Include verbal and written information about the following:

✓ Description of disease process and recommended treatment.

✓ Medications and supplements, including name, dosage, purpose, schedule, precautions, and potential side effects. Also discuss drug-drug, herb-drug, and food-drug interactions.

✓ Prescribed dietary regimen, including rationale for food choices.

✓ Prescribed exercise regimen, including need to avoid movements that twist or compress the spine (e.g., sit-ups) as well as high-impact activities.

✓ Importance of establishing fall prevention measures in the home (e.g., placing handrail in tub or shower, installing night-lights, avoiding use of throw rugs). Arrange for home visit from a nurse or physical therapist as necessary.

✓ Importance of reporting to the health care provider any indicators of pathologic fracture (i.e., deformity, pain, edema, ecchymosis, limb shortening, false motion, decreased range of motion, or crepitus). Stress need to promptly report any indicators of vertebral fractures (e.g., paresthesia, weakness, paralysis, radicular pain, or loss of bowel or bladder function) due to risk for possible spinal cord or nerve compression.

✓ Importance of follow-up care, date of next appointment, and telephone number to call if questions arise.

✓ Referral to community resources, including local osteoporosis support activities:
  • National Osteoporosis Foundation at *www.nof.org*
  • National Institute of Arthritis and Musculoskeletal and Skin Diseases (NIAMS) Information Clearinghouse, Information Specialist, at *www.niams.nih.gov*
  • Osteoporosis Canada at *www.osteoporosis.ca*

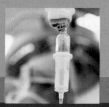

Rheumatoid Arthritis 71

OVERVIEW/PATHOPHYSIOLOGY

Rheumatoid arthritis (RA) is a chronic systemic autoimmune disease associated with severe morbidity and functional decline caused by inflammation of connective tissue, primarily in the synovial joints. Mortality rates of persons with RA are double that of the general population, particularly if the disease is not well controlled. Individuals with RA are at increased risk for cardiovascular events. Women are affected two to three times more often than men. Although no single known cause exists for RA, theory suggests that it occurs in a susceptible host who initially experiences an immune response to an antigen. Because complex genetic factors appear to be involved, the antigen is probably not the same in all patients. Autoimmunity has been suggested as a cause because of the association of RA with the occurrence of rheumatoid factor (RF), the antibody against an abnormal immunoglobulin G (IgG). Support for a genetic predisposition has come from studies of disease clusters in families, and formal genetic studies have confirmed this familial aggregation. No microorganism has been cultured from blood and synovial tissue or fluid with enough reproducibility to determine an infectious etiology for RA. In addition, no environmental factors have been identified as disease precipitators.

The immune response appears to center on synovial tissue, where disease changes are first seen. Synovitis develops when immune complexes are deposited onto the synovial membrane or superficial articular cartilage. As hypertrophied synovium invades surrounding tissues, highly vascularized fibrous exudate (pannus) forms to cover the entire articular cartilage. Pannus also scars and shortens adjacent tendons and ligaments to create the laxity, subluxation, and contractures characteristic of RA.

HEALTH CARE SETTING

Primary care; acute care for complications

ASSESSMENT

Signs and symptoms: Nonspecific symptoms such as fatigue, anorexia, weight loss, and generalized stiffness may precede onset of joint complaints. Stiffness typically becomes more localized as time progresses. Morning joint stiffness lasting at least 1 hr is common, but it may last as long as 4 hr. The patient often complains of joint pain and swelling, especially in the hands and wrists. Knees, ankles, and metatarsophalangeal joints also may be affected. The patient describes increasing difficulty with mobility and performance of activities of daily living.

Physical assessment: During early disease, examination may reveal spindle-shaped fingers, with swan-neck and boutonnière deformities becoming apparent because of flexion contractures that occur with disease progression. Ulnar deviation, a "zigzag" wrist deformity, is also likely. Metatarsal-head subluxation and hallux valgus (bunion) in the feet may lead to walking disability and pain. Affected symmetric (bilateral) joints are typically swollen, red, warm, and tender with decreased range of motion (ROM). Patients also may exhibit guarded movement and gait abnormalities due to joint changes. Subcutaneous nodules may be noted over bony prominences, extensor surfaces, or juxtaarticular areas; hoarseness may be evident if nodules have invaded the vocal chords.

DIAGNOSTIC TESTS

Diagnosis of RA is based primarily on physical findings and patient history. Radiographic studies are not usually needed to make a diagnosis. Laboratory results are helpful in confirming diagnosis and monitoring disease progression.

Rheumatoid factor: Positive in about 85% of patients. Higher titers appear to be correlated with severe and unremitting disease. However, the RF titer has little prognostic value, and serial titers have no usefulness in following disease process.

Antinuclear antibodies: Elevated titers seen in 5%-20% of patients.

Erythrocyte sedimentation rate and C-reactive protein: Elevation is a general indicator of active inflammation.

Synovial fluid analysis: Fluid is opaque and cloudy yellow, with elevated white blood cell count and polymorphonuclear leukocytes in the presence of RA. Glucose level will be lower than serum glucose.

X-ray examination of affected joints: Radiographs may be inconclusive in early disease but baseline films, especially of the hands, aid in monitoring disease progression. Presence of erosions also helps determine prognosis. With advanced disease, loss of articular cartilage leads to narrowed joint space. Subluxation and joint malalignment can be identified on x-ray film, reflecting changes noted on physical examination. Osteopenia or osteoporosis may be evident in the patient with RA who has been treated with corticosteroids.

Bone scan: Detects early synovial changes.

Arthroscopy: Reveals pale, hypertrophic synovium with destruction of cartilage and formation of fibrous scar tissue.

Nursing Diagnosis:

Deficient Knowledge

related to unfamiliarity with medications used in RA treatment

Desired Outcome: Immediately following teaching, the patient verbalizes accurate information about the prescribed RA medications.

ASSESSMENT/INTERVENTIONS	RATIONALES
Teach the patient about medications prescribed for the treatment of arthritis: indications for use, possible side effects, administration time and method, and need for follow-up laboratory tests.	Drug therapy remains the cornerstone of an interdisciplinary approach to care for patients with RA. A knowledgeable patient is likely to adhere to drug therapy and report necessary signs and symptoms to ensure prompt treatment of untoward side effects.
Disease-Modifying Antirheumatic Drugs (DMARDs)	Accurate, timely diagnosis is critical to initiation of DMARDs, which have been shown to control active synovitis and prevent joint erosions and damage. Early use is critical because they have been shown to slow the erosive course of RA and are now considered to be a first-line therapy in disease treatment. Nonsteroidal antiinflammatory drugs (NSAIDs) are often prescribed along with DMARDs to allow optimal management of pain and swelling until the slower acting disease-modifying agent begins to exert its effect.
- Methotrexate (Rheumatrex)	Most frequently prescribed by rheumatologists in the United States in doses of 7.5-25 mg weekly by mouth (PO) or intramuscular (IM).
- Other DMARDs	Include sulfasalazine (Azulfidine) (2000-3000 mg daily), hydroxychloroquine (Plaquenil) (200-400 mg daily), cyclosporine (Neoral) (1.5-2.5 mg/kg daily), cyclophosphamide (Cytoxan) (1-2 mg/kg daily), and leflunomide (Arava) (10-20 mg daily).
Biologic Response Modifiers (BRMs)	BRMs interfere with cell surface antigens of modulating cytokines to manage RA symptoms in patients with moderate to severe disease who have not responded to DMARDs. Both tumor necrosis factor (TNF) and the interleukins are cytokines considered to be markers of inflammation. BRMs are frequently given with a DMARD.
TNF Inhibitors - Adalimumab (Humira) - Certolizumab pegol (Cimzia) - Etanercept (Enbrel) - Golimumab (Simponi) - Infliximab (Remicade)	These medications block the cytokine TNF, which is involved in the inflammatory process. All TNF inhibitors are given by injection except infliximab, which is given intravenously.
Selective B Cell Inhibitors - Rituximab (Rituxan)	Two 1000-mg infusions are given 2 wk apart every 24 wk. Women of childbearing age should be reminded to use effective methods of contraception during and up to 12 mo after treatment.
Interleukin-1 Inhibitor - Anakinra (Kinaret)	A dose of 100 mg daily should be injected into the thigh, abdomen, or upper arm. The drug should be refrigerated but not frozen, and not shaken before use.
Selective Co-Stimulator Modulator - Abatacept (Orencia)	This medication can be given by infusion or injection, with dosing and time based on route of administration.

ASSESSMENT/INTERVENTIONS

RATIONALES

Interleukin-6 Inhibitor

- Tocilizumab (Actemra)

This medication is given by infusion every 4 wk.

Explain that because most BRMS are self-administered by subcutaneous injection, they may not be appropriate for all RA patients.

Self-administration by RA patients may be problematic because of muscle weakness and joint deformity. If patients do not have a family member/significant other who can be taught the injection technique, a home health care provider may need to determine the patient's ability to return to an outpatient clinic for medication administration. Infliximab is given intravenously, often in the physician's office, and offers an alternative to subcutaneous administration.

[!] Teach the patient to minimize exposure to ill individuals and immediately report personal illness to the physician.

Both DMARDs and BRMs cause immunosuppression and can increase a patient's risk for illness. Illness, particularly if resistant to conventional treatment (e.g., common cold), should be reported immediately to the health care provider for more aggressive treatment.

[!] Teach the patient that laboratory monitoring of renal and liver function is necessary with all DMARDs and BRMs.

Because the potential is great for renal and hepatic toxicity with DMARDs and BRMs, patients should be instructed to complete all follow-up laboratory tests as prescribed.

NSAIDs

A number of NSAIDs provide largely equal analgesic and antiinflammatory effects in the treatment of RA. They do not affect disease progression, and their use in alleviating RA symptoms may in fact delay initiation of DMARD therapy or referral to a rheumatologist.

[!] Teach the patient that NSAIDs are linked to increased risk for renal and gastrointestinal (GI) toxicity, and the patient should recognize signs and symptoms of internal bleeding or GI ulceration.

Patients must be able to seek prompt medical attention for any suspected bleeding or ulceration.

Corticosteroids

Injection of corticosteroids directly into affected joints can temporarily relieve the pain and inflammation of RA exacerbations. Low-dose oral prednisone may be useful in selected patients to minimize disease activity until the prescribed DMARD becomes therapeutic.

[!] Explain that caution is necessary in long-term use of oral corticosteroids.

Corticosteroids have been associated with development of avascular necrosis or osteoporosis and therefore should not be a mainstay of treatment for the patient with RA. Patients who take corticosteroids should receive additional instruction on risks associated with long-term use.

Antibiotics

Minocycline (Minocin) is the only antibiotic to be used as a DMARD in the treatment of RA. It can improve mild-to-moderate symptoms but has no disease-modifying properties. Side effects such as skin discoloration, dizziness, GI upset, and autoimmune phenomenon (including hepatitis) frequently lead to discontinuation of therapy.

Future Drug Therapies

Research on underlying causes of inflammation associated with RA may lead to development of new medications or new uses for previously marketed medications. The nurse should listen carefully to the patient's stated interest in any other pharmacologic therapies and inform the health care provider of the patient's willingness to try additional treatments.

Nursing Diagnoses:

Dressing Self-Care Deficit
Bathing Self-Care Deficit
Toileting Self-Care Deficit

related to pain and limitations in joint ROM

Desired Outcome: Within 1 wk of instruction, the patient verbalizes/exhibits increased independence in dressing/grooming.

ASSESSMENT/INTERVENTIONS	RATIONALES
Assess the impact of pain and limitations in joint ROM on performance of ADLS (e.g., dressing/bathing activities).	Recognition of the extent to which the disease has affected the patient's ability to perform ADLs independently enables the nurse and the patient to develop an individualized care/teaching plan for dressing/grooming.
Assess pain and ROM in joints used in dressing/grooming (e.g., small joints in hands; elbows, shoulders, knees).	Independence in dressing/grooming can be quickly lost as small joints become affected by the disease. Strategies for self-care must take into consideration any limitations in the small joints.
As indicated, refer the patient to an occupational therapist.	The occupational therapist is able to evaluate need for dressing/bathing/toileting aids. Sock donners, buttoners, long-handled reachers and brushes, raised toilet seats, and other devices may help minimize stress on joints. Clothing also can be adapted to promote independence in dressing (e.g., zipper pulls, elastic shoelaces, Velcro closures).
Teach the patient to coordinate the time of peak effectiveness of the prescribed analgesics and anti-inflammatory medications with periods of joint use for self-care activities.	Careful timing of analgesics enables patients to achieve optimal pain management before performing ADLs that can stress small joints.
Teach the patient about exercises that increase joint flexibility and decrease pain during joint use for self-care.	Joint flexibility is critical to a patient's ability to perform ADLs independently. Pain should be minimized to facilitate joint use as well.
Refer the patient to the Arthritis Foundation Exercise Program for local programs as well as DVDs for home use.	The Arthritis Foundation (AF) Exercise Program is available "live" in many locations, with a search function on the AF web site. The program includes ROM exercises to promote flexibility and decrease pain. AF also offers a 60-minute DVD for home use: *http://www.arthritis.org/resources/community-programs/excercise/*

Nursing Diagnosis:

Fatigue

related to state of discomfort, effects of prolonged mobility, and psychoemotional demands of chronic illness

Desired Outcome: Within 24 hr of instruction and interventions, the patient verbalizes a reduction in fatigue.

ASSESSMENT/INTERVENTIONS	RATIONALES
Assess the patient's sleep pattern and suggest strategies that facilitate adequate rest (e.g., warm bath at bedtime).	Adequate rest helps patients maintain a more normal routine and decreases risk of disease exacerbation.
Assess the patient's ability to manage pain, and encourage use of interventions to maximize quality of rest periods.	Effective use of pain management interventions enables improved quality of rest periods.

ASSESSMENT/INTERVENTIONS

Assess the patient's stress or psychoemotional distress. Suggest coping strategies or refer the patient to an appropriate clinical specialist in psychiatric nursing.

Help the patient identify the time that fatigue occurs, its relationship to necessary activities, and activities that relieve or aggravate symptoms.

Help the patient evaluate food preparation methods that may contribute to fatigue.

Encourage the patient to pace activities and allow adequate rest periods during the day.

Discuss the rationale for a stepped approach to exercise that increases endurance and strength without fatiguing the patient. Encourage the patient to set realistic exercise goals and share them with associated health care providers.

Instruct the patient in use of assistive devices.

RATIONALES

Stress and psychoemotional distress may increase fatigue and exacerbate disease symptoms. By understanding the patient's response to chronic illness, significant others may support efforts to maintain routine activities. If the patient is unable to develop and use effective coping strategies independently, referral may be warranted.

With planning, patients should be able to optimize ability to participate in routine and recreational activities. Patients also can anticipate fatigue-producing activities and plan rest periods accordingly.

For example, the patient might set the table for the next day's breakfast before going to bed at night, use convenience foods whenever possible, or prepare food while seated on a stool at the kitchen counter.

Balance of rest and activity keeps patients from becoming fatigued. Fatigue contributes to stress and possible disease exacerbations.

Endurance and strength should be increased gradually. An aggressive exercise program may cause fatigue and exacerbation of disease symptoms.

A variety of devices are available to support small joints during routine activities and to assist with ambulation, thus minimizing stress and fatigue. The patient who uses appropriate assistive devices is also generally able to continue with routine activities and avoid social isolation.

Nursing Diagnosis:

Disturbed Body Image

related to joint deformities and the effects of corticosteroid use (e.g., weight gain due to fluid retention and increased appetite)

Desired Outcome: Within 1 mo of intervention, the patient verbalizes positive adjustment to body changes.

ASSESSMENT/INTERVENTIONS

Assess the patient for negative body image.

Assess the patient for negative feelings about body image linked specifically to the use of assistive devices/mobility aids.

Provide anticipatory counseling about possible joint deformities/body image changes as the disease progresses, including ways for the patient to prepare for the reaction of others.

Encourage participation in support groups for patients with RA.

Ask the patient to complete the Baird Body Image Assessment Tool or other self-assessment survey to determine subjective response to physical changes.

RATIONALES

Manifestations of negative body image may be different in each patient. Examples may include refusal to discuss or participate in care, withdrawal from social contacts, and avoidance of intimate relationships. Early identification of a changing body image provides opportunity for overcoming isolating effects of the disease.

The nurse can help select the least obtrusive aids, which will help patients maintain a more normal body image.

Awareness of the likelihood of deformity will enable patients to develop strategies that make routine encounters and regular activities easier. Patients also can anticipate times when RA deformities may be especially apparent and respond in ways that will minimize potential embarrassment or inconvenience.

Support group members can be good role models for successful coping.

This tool encourages patients to consider the meaning and impact of any physical changes and helps the nurse suggest strategies to cope with those changes.

continued

ASSESSMENT/INTERVENTIONS

Demonstrate positive regard for the patient and acceptance of any physical changes associated with chronic illness.

RATIONALES

The nurse's consistent positive regard will help the patient avoid equating self with the disease process. It is critical that the patient recognize the disease as a separate entity rather than the defining element of his or her life.

ADDITIONAL NURSING DIAGNOSES/PROBLEMS:

"Osteoarthritis" for **Chronic Pain/Acute Pain** related to arthritic joint changes and associated therapy   p. 505

Impaired Physical Mobility related to musculoskeletal impairment and adjustment to new walking gait with an assistive device   p. 507

Deficient Knowledge (potential interaction between NSAIDs and herbal products)   p. 507

Sexual Dysfunction related to pain, decreased joint function, or body image changes that interfere with sexual performance   p. 508

✓ PATIENT-FAMILY TEACHING AND DISCHARGE PLANNING

When providing patient-family teaching, focus on sensory information, avoid giving excessive information, and make appropriate referrals (e.g., visiting or home health nurse, community health resources) for follow-up teaching. Include verbal and written information about the following:

✓ Treatment regimen, including physical therapy and exercises, systemic rest/principles of joint protection, and cryotherapy.

✓ Importance of laboratory follow-up (e.g., blood or urine testing) for needed monitoring while the patient is taking selected medications.

✓ Medications and supplements, including name, dosage, schedule, precautions, and potential side effects. Also discuss drug-drug, herb-drug, and food-drug interactions.

✓ Nutrition: Research has shown several positive connections between food or nutritional supplements (e.g., omega-3 fatty acids as in fish and fish oil) and some types of arthritis, including RA. Increased fiber intake from grains, fruits, and vegetables may also reduce inflammation. However, omega-6 fatty acids (e.g., found in some plant oils, many snack foods, margarine, egg yolks, and meats) may increase the risk of inflammation and obesity. Some specific diets that are known to have harmful side effects include those that rely on large doses of alfalfa, copper salts, or zinc, or the so-called immune power diet or the low-calorie/low-fat/low-protein diet.

✓ Patients who are taking methotrexate may experience folic acid deficiency that requires supplementation.

✓ Potential complications of disease and therapy, as well as need to recognize and seek medical attention promptly if they occur.

✓ Potential concurrent pathologic conditions, such as pericarditis and ocular lesions, and need to report them promptly to the health care provider.

✓ Use, care, and replacement of splints, orthotics, and assistive devices.

✓ Use of adjunctive aids as appropriate, including long-handled reacher, long-handled shoehorn, elastic shoe-laces, Velcro fasteners, crutches, walker, and cane.

✓ Referral to visiting/public health or home health nurses as necessary for ongoing care after discharge.

✓ Importance of follow-up care, date of next appointment, and telephone number to call if questions arise.

✓ Referral to community resources, including local arthritis support activities, and to the following:
  • Arthritis Foundation at *www.arthritis.org*
  • American Academy of Pediatrics at *www.aap.org*
  • National Institute of Arthritis and Musculoskeletal and Skin Diseases (NIAMS) Information Clearinghouse, Information Specialist, at: *www.niams.nih.gov*
  • The Arthritis Society at *www.arthritis.ca*

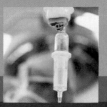

Caring for Individuals with Human Immunodeficiency Virus 72

OVERVIEW/PATHOPHYSIOLOGY

Human immunodeficiency virus (HIV) causes a life-threatening illness called *acquired immunodeficiency syndrome (AIDS)*. AIDS is characterized by disruption of cell-mediated immunity. This breakdown of the immune system is manifested by opportunistic infections such as *Pneumocystis jirovecii* pneumonia ([PCP], previously *Pneumocystis carinii* pneumonia) or tumors such as Kaposi's sarcoma (KS). According to the Centers for Disease Control and Prevention (CDC) 2012 data, there are approximately 1.1 million persons living with HIV in the United States and almost one in five are unaware of their infection.

Confirmed routes of HIV transmission include the following:

- *Blood*: Exposure to HIV-infected blood by sharing of unsterile needles or other drug paraphernalia, unsterile invasive instruments, exposure to needlesticks or sharps, transfusion with contaminated blood, mucocutaneous exposure to blood or other infected body fluids.
- *Genital secretions*: Exposure to HIV-infected genital secretions during sexual activity. Anal-receptive sex with an HIV-infected person is the greatest sexual risk for exposure to HIV, followed by vaginal sex.
- *Breast milk*: Infant exposure to HIV-infected breast milk from an HIV-infected woman.
- *Perinatal*: Fetal exposure to HIV during all stages of pregnancy with the highest rates of transmission during labor and delivery.

HIV infection has transcended all racial, social, sexual, and economic barriers, and all persons who engage in risk behaviors are at risk of transmission.

Health care workers who come into contact with infectious body fluids are also at risk. Understanding and practicing universal precautions are essential for all health care workers. Review Appendix A for a discussion of the handling of blood and body fluids for all patients. Postexposure prophylaxis is available for prevention of HIV transmission in case an occupational or high-risk nonoccupational exposure occurs but is most effective when initiated soon after exposure.

The CDC recommends all persons ages 13-64 be screened for HIV at least once in their lifetimes. Individuals with risk factors should be tested more frequently. In cases where a screening is necessary in a more time-efficient manner, HIV testing can be conducted via a rapid test, which yields results within as little as 20 minutes. Anyone with a positive HIV antibody test must be considered infectious and capable of transmitting the virus.

HIV targets CD4+ T cells, weakening the immune system. When the immune system has been significantly depleted of CD4+ T cells, the body becomes increasingly vulnerable to various infections. This phase of HIV infection is called AIDS. Thus, HIV is a chronic viral disease that covers a wide spectrum of illnesses and symptoms for a variable course of time.

Since the introduction of antiretroviral therapy (ART), there has been a dramatic reduction in HIV-related morbidity and mortality. Strict adherence to a combination of antiretroviral agents slows viral replication at different points in the life cycle of HIV. Use of antiretroviral agents reduces the amount of circulating virus (viral load). This viral load reduction has been shown to enable immune system recovery and slow progression of the disease, resulting in reduction in symptoms and opportunistic diseases; reducing risk of cardiovascular, renal, or hepatic disease; prolonging survival time; and improving quality of life. Additionally, consistent use of ART has been found to reduce the risk of HIV transmission to others (Cohen et al., 2011). Recent advances in ART have led to once-daily combinations that improve adherence and have reduced side effects. As a result ART is currently recommended for all persons living with HIV (Department of Health and Human Services Panel on Antiretroviral Guidelines for Adults and Adolescents, 2013). Plans for individuals with HIV must include discussion of adherence to medications and risk of resistance, the importance of ongoing follow-up, and prevention of HIV transmission to others through combination prevention.

HEALTH CARE SETTING

Primary care, hospice, and home care with possible acute care hospitalization resulting from complications or occurrence of opportunistic infections

ASSESSMENT

HIV risk assessment: Because of continued transmission of HIV infection and incidence of new infections regardless of race, gender, sexual preference, or age, continuous HIV risk assessment and prevention education within all clinical

PART I: Medical-Surgical Nursing

settings is essential. Health care providers have a responsibility to assess each patient's risk for HIV infection and be sensitive to issues of sexual preferences and practices, as well as cultural values, norms, and traditions. A risk assessment should be used not only for the purpose of recommending testing, but also for development of a "patient-centered" risk reduction plan.

Key components of conducting a sexual history:
- Focus on sexual "behaviors" rather than on categories or labels.
- Avoid making assumptions about individuals.
- Ask about specific sexual behavior rather than asking general questions.
  - For example, "How many sexual partners have you had?" "In the last 5 years?" "In the last month?"
  - "Do you have sex with men, women, or both?"
  - "When is the last time you had sex while under the influence of drugs or alcohol?"
- Ask nonjudgmentally about traditional and nontraditional sexual practices.
  - "What type of sexual intercourse (vaginal, anal, oral) do you have with your partner(s)?"
  - "When you have anal or oral intercourse, are you the insertive or receptive partner?"
- It is essential that clinicians provide patients with risk reduction information in a consistent and continuous process within the clinical care relationship. This intervention should include development of specific skills and ongoing monitoring of the patient's successes and continued challenges.

Key components of conducting a drug history:
- Focus on specific drug-using behaviors. For example:
  - "Do you use alcohol or tobacco?" If so, ask how much and how often.
  - "What drugs do you use?" "What drugs do you inject?"
  - "When did you last inject drugs?" "When did you last share needles?"
  - "Do you clean your works?" "How do you do this?"
- Avoid making assumptions about individuals because drug use occurs in all socioeconomic groups.
- Convey a nonjudgmental attitude.

Stages of HIV disease (for untreated individuals): The four stages of HIV infection can be categorized as acute infection, asymptomatic, symptomatic, and AIDS.

Acute or primary infection: Period of rapid viral replication during which the person may experience flulike symptoms at the time of seroconversion.

Asymptomatic stage: Immune system continues to mount a massive response to HIV, causing a drop in viral load but viral replication continues. It may last 10 yr or more, and the person may remain free of symptoms or opportunistic infections.

Early symptomatic stage: Rate of viral replication remains relatively constant; however, gradual failure of the immune system results in inability to control the virus, causing increased viral load.

Advanced stage, AIDS: The immune mechanism for virus control fails, resulting in large amounts of circulating virus and significant destruction of CD4+ T cells. Clinical manifestations include wasting and opportunistic diseases such as neoplasms and viral, bacterial, and fungal infections. Dementia also can occur, characterized by cognitive impairment and mood changes.

Physical assessment: The following indicators are commonly seen with HIV infection.

General: Fever, night sweats, weight loss.

Cutaneous: Herpes zoster or simplex lesions, seborrheic or other dermatitis, fungal infections of the skin (moniliasis, candidiasis) or nail beds (onychomycosis), KS lesions, petechiae, warts.

Head/neck: "Cotton-wool" spots visualized on funduscopic examination; oral KS; candidiasis (thrush); hairy leukoplakia; aphthous ulcers; enlarged, hard, and occasionally tender lymph nodes.

Respiratory: Tachypnea, dyspnea, diminished or adventitious breath sounds (crackles [rales], rhonchi, wheezing).

Cardiac: Tachycardia, friction rub, gallops, murmurs.

Gastrointestinal: Enlargement of liver or spleen, nausea, vomiting, diarrhea, constipation, hyperactive bowel sounds, abdominal distention.

Genital/rectal: KS lesions, herpetic lesions, candidiasis, balanitis, warts, syphilitic chancres, warts, rectal or cervical dysplasia, fistulas.

Neuromuscular: Flattened affect, apathy, withdrawal, memory deficits, headache, muscle atrophy, speech deficits, gait disorders, generalized weakness, incontinence, neuropathy.

DIAGNOSTIC TESTS

A variety of diagnostic tests are used for specific reasons in the course of HIV disease. The following tests are used to determine HIV infection. Because it can take up to 6 mo to develop enough antibodies to trigger a reactive result, the person may be infected but test negative. This is often referred to as the "window period" for HIV infection. Individuals who test negative should be retested in 3-6 mo to confirm seronegativity. The CDC currently recommends routine HIV screening for all individuals 13-64 yr old, regardless of risk factors.

Enzyme-linked immunosorbent assay (ELISA): The standard test for HIV. ELISA tests for the presence of HIV antibody. An initially reactive ELISA should be repeated on the same specimen. If reactive, a confirmatory Western blot (WB) is performed. A positive ELISA with a confirmatory WB signals infection with HIV.

Western blot: A confirmatory test used to detect immune response to the specific viral proteins of HIV. A reactive WB is defined by a specific pattern of protein bands separated by electrophoresis on a strip of nitrocellulose paper; three of the following bands must be present for reactivity: p24 (see the following), gp41, and gp210 or gp160.

p24 antigen test: Detects HIV p24 antigen in serum, plasma, and cerebrospinal fluid (CSF) of infected individuals.

Its advantage is that it may detect viral antigen (HIV p24) early in the course of infection before seroconversion.

Immunofluorescence assay: Tests for HIV antibody and is equivalent to the WB.

Rapid tests: Several relatively new Food and Drug Administration (FDA)–approved rapid antibody tests indicate presence of HIV antibodies in oral fluid, serum, and/or whole blood within approximately 20-40 min. Confirmation of positive results with a WB is imperative. This method of testing is ideal when a rapid result is critical and assists in increasing the number of persons obtaining results.

Monitoring tests

With use of ART in the clinical management of HIV disease, monitoring tests have become increasingly essential in assessing for immune reconstitution and monitoring for treatment failure or resistance.

CD4+ T cell count: A measure of the amount of CD4+ T cells per milliliter in the blood. It is a marker for the impact of HIV infection on the immune system and the individual's susceptibility to infections. With increased viral load there is a reduction in CD4+ T-cell counts because of destruction of these lymphocytes by HIV. A CD4+ T-cell count of less than 200 is diagnostic of AIDS.

Viral load testing: Only 3%-4% of the virus is located in the plasma. The remaining 90+% is located in lymphoid tissues and other blood cells. The viral load test measures the free virus in the plasma but not in these other areas. It is used to determine response of antiretroviral treatment, monitor development of drug resistance, and determine need to change antiretroviral treatment. When a patient is on ART, the viral load should be undetectable.

Viral resistance testing: Testing for viral resistance to specific antiretroviral drugs. Before initiating treatment, this test is used to determine if the virus is already resistant to a specific agent. It is also used to assess treatment failure and help determine appropriate changes in the introduction of new or alternative antiretroviral agents. The different types of resistance testing include genotypic assays, phenotypic assays, and virtual phenotype.

Nursing Diagnosis:

Noncompliance (with the antiretroviral regimen)

related to impaired judgment, socioeconomic status, antiretroviral side effects, or knowledge deficit

Desired Outcome: Following intervention, the patient exhibits improved adherence to the antiretroviral medication regimen.

ASSESSMENT/INTERVENTIONS	RATIONALES
Assess for missed doses of antiretrovirals. Note and record any missed doses.	Antiretroviral medications will help decrease the viral load and increase the CD4+ T cell count, thus decreasing risk for infection and other HIV-related complications. **Note:** Adherence is the most common issue related to individuals with HIV at the present time.
Assess for adherence to the entire antiretroviral regimen.	Antiretroviral regimens need to be taken in their entirety in order to optimize effect and decrease risk of resistance.
Assess for side effects to antiretrovirals and provide nonpharmacologic and pharmacologic interventions (as prescribed) to decrease side effects.	Side effects may be one reason for nonadherence. Interventions may help improve adherence.
Assess for the rationale behind poor adherence and help the patient develop a strategy for improving adherence.	Assessing for specific reasons behind poor adherence can assist in providing patient-specific adherence counseling.
Teach the role of antiretrovirals in improving the immune system, aiding in healing infections, preventing additional opportunistic infections and HIV-related complications, and preventing HIV transmission.	Knowledge regarding the role of antiretrovirals in improving immune system response to infections and other HIV-related complications may improve adherence.
Explain the need for almost 100% adherence in order to prevent viral resistance to antiretrovirals.	Resistance to antiretrovirals can develop with even just a few missed doses, thereby decreasing the number of treatment options and potentially increasing the pill burden.

Special Needs Care Plans

Nursing Diagnosis:

Impaired Gas Exchange

related to altered oxygen supply occurring with pulmonary infiltrates, hyperventilation, and sepsis

Desired Outcomes: After treatment/intervention, the patient has adequate gas exchange as evidenced by respiratory rate (RR) 12-20 breaths/min with normal depth and pattern (eupnea) and absence of adventitious sounds, nasal flaring, and other clinical indicators of respiratory dysfunction. By hospital discharge, the patient's oximetry demonstrates O_2 saturation greater than 92% or arterial blood gas (ABG) results as follows: PaO_2 80 mm Hg or higher; $PaCO_2$ 35-45 mm Hg; pH 7.35-7.45.

ASSESSMENT/INTERVENTIONS	RATIONALES
Assess respiratory status as often as indicated by the patient's condition. Assess rate, rhythm, quality, cough, and sputum production.	Use of accessory muscles, flaring of nares, presence of adventitious sounds, cough, changes in color or character of sputum, or cyanosis occur with respiratory dysfunction. See discussion in the next nursing diagnosis about adventitious sounds that can occur with opportunistic infections that have pulmonary signs and symptoms.
Maintain continuous or frequent monitoring of O_2 saturation via pulse oximetry. Report findings of less than 92%.	O_2 saturation 92% or less may signal the need for supplementary oxygen and should be reported to the health care provider.
Assess ABG results for changes and report abnormal findings.	Decreased $PaCO_2$ (less than 35 mm Hg) and increased pH (greater than 7.40) can occur with hyperventilation.
As prescribed, initiate or adjust oxygen therapy.	This measure helps ensure optimal oxygenation as determined by ABG values.
Administer oxygen with humidity.	Humidity alleviates convective losses of moisture and relieves mucous membrane irritation, which can predispose to coughing spells.
Instruct the patient to report changes in cough, as well as dyspnea that increases with exertion.	These indicators may be seen with opportunistic respiratory disease.
Provide chest physiotherapy as prescribed. Encourage use of incentive spirometry at frequent intervals.	These measures help loosen secretions, prevent atelectasis, and improve expectoration of secretions.
Reposition the patient q2h, and assist with ambulation and sitting up as tolerated.	Repositioning and walking help prevent stasis of lung fluids.
Assess for changes in color or character of sputum; obtain sputum for culture and sensitivity as indicated.	Changes in color and character of sputum may signal infection; a culture confirms infection type.
Group nursing activities to provide the patient with uninterrupted periods of rest, optimally 90-120 min at a time.	Rest promotes optimal chest excursion.
⚠ When administering trimethoprim + sulfamethoxazole (TMP-SMX) for PCP, monitor closely for rash, fever, or bone marrow suppression (leukopenia, neutropenia).	These symptoms, including Stevens Johnson syndrome (SJS), are side effects of TMP-SMX. SJS is a life-threatening condition with symptoms including a red or purple rash and blistering of the skin and mucous membranes. An individual with SJS should be managed in a hospital setting, and the medication should be stopped immediately.
⚠ If administering corticosteroids, be alert for additional infections or other potential side effects.	Corticosteroids may be given for PCP. Side effects of corticosteroids include masking of and increased susceptibility to infection.

Nursing Diagnosis:

Risk for Infection

related to inadequate immune system function, malnutrition, or side effects of chemotherapy

Desired Outcome: The patient is free of additional infections, as evidenced by appropriate cultures or biopsies.

ASSESSMENT/INTERVENTIONS	RATIONALES
Assess for persistent fevers, night sweats, fatigue, involuntary weight loss, persistent and dry cough, persistent diarrhea, and headache.	These are indicators of opportunistic infections that can occur as a result of breakdown of the patient's immune system.
Monitor laboratory data, especially complete blood count, differential, and cultures, to evaluate the course of infection. Be alert to abnormal results and notify the health care provider of significant findings.	Increased/positive values may signal presence/type of infection.
Assess temperature and vital signs at frequent intervals. Perform a complete physical assessment at least q8h.	These assessments identify changes from baseline assessment that signal fever or sepsis. In addition to increased temperature, other signs include diaphoresis, confusion or mental status changes, decrease in level of consciousness, increased heart rate (HR), and decreased BP secondary to the vasodilator effect of the increased body temperature.
Assess for changes in breath sounds.	Diminished or adventitious sounds may indicate opportunistic disease and/or an increasing level of pulmonary infiltrates. PCP is commonly seen in HIV disease when the immune system is extremely compromised (CD4+ T cell counts below 200). Other opportunistic infections that can manifest with pulmonary signs and symptoms include *Mycobacterium tuberculosis* (MTB) and bacterial pneumonia.
⚠ Maintain strict sterile technique for all invasive procedures.	This helps prevent introduction of new pathogens.
Assist the patient in maintaining meticulous body hygiene.	This measure helps prevent spread of organisms from body secretions into skin breaks, especially if the patient has diarrhea.
Encourage the patient to engage in frequent breathing or incentive spirometry exercises.	These exercises promote pulmonary health, which will help prevent respiratory infections.
Assess sites of invasive procedures for erythema, swelling, local warmth, tenderness, and purulent exudate.	These are signs of localized infection.
⚠ Enforce good hand hygiene practices before and after contact with the patient.	Handwashing minimizes the risk of transmitting infectious organisms from (and to) the staff and other patients.
Teach home care considerations for infection prevention after hospital discharge (see "Patient-Family Teaching and Discharge Planning").	This reinforces the importance of infection protection and promotes adherence after hospital discharge.
⚠ When providing care to patients with active tuberculosis (TB) or unknown TB status, wear respiratory protection consistent with current recommendations from the CDC and Occupational Safety and Health Administration.	This helps prevent spread of disease. See "Pulmonary Tuberculosis," p. 133, and "Infection Prevention and Control," p. 747, for more information.

Nursing Diagnosis:

Diarrhea

related to opportunistic infections; medication side effects, including chemotherapy; HIV-related gastrointestinal (GI) changes; or tube feeding/food intolerance

Desired Outcome: By the time of hospital discharge, the patient has formed stools and a bowel elimination pattern that is normal for him or her.

ASSESSMENT/INTERVENTIONS	RATIONALES
Be alert to cool and clammy skin, increased HR (greater than 100 bpm), increased RR (greater than 20 breaths/min), and decreased urinary output (less than 30 mL/hr).	These are signs of hypovolemia that could result from prolonged diarrhea.
Assess for anxiety, confusion, muscle weakness, cramps, dysrhythmias, weak pulse, and decreased BP.	These are indicators of electrolyte imbalance that could occur because of fluid loss.
Maintain accurate intake and output.	This measure monitors for changes in fluid volume status.
Assess stool for blood, fat, and undigested materials.	This may reveal presence of infection or feeding tube intolerance.
Monitor stool cultures.	Cultures identify causative organisms.
Perform hand hygiene with soap and water after handling stool.	Hand hygiene is recommended by the CDC when contact with blood or body fluids is possible. Using soap and water is the best method for infection control, particularly when spores (i.e., *C. difficile*) are found in stool cultures. In these cases, hand gels are considered ineffective.
If the patient is being given tube feedings, dilute the strength or decrease the rate of infusion to prevent "solute drag."	Solute drag (concentrated solutions that pull water into the bowel lumen) may be the cause of the diarrhea.
Encourage the patient to increase fluid intake as long as there are no fluid restrictions.	Increased hydration helps prevent dehydration.
Encourage foods high in potassium and sodium.	These foods help replace electrolyte loss.
Protect anorectal area by keeping it cleansed and using compounds such as zinc oxide or sitz baths.	This measure prevents or slows skin excoriation caused by diarrhea.
Teach the patient to avoid large amounts (greater than 300 mg/day) of caffeine.	Caffeine increases peristalsis and can promote diarrhea.

Nursing Diagnosis:

Imbalanced Nutrition: Less Than Body Requirements

related to diarrhea and nausea associated with side effects of medications, malabsorption, anorexia, dysphagia, and fatigue

Desired Outcomes: By hospital discharge, the patient has adequate nutrition as evidenced by stable weight. The patient states that nausea and other GI side effects associated with ART are controlled.

ASSESSMENT/INTERVENTIONS	RATIONALES
Assess nutritional status daily, noting weight, caloric intake, and protein values.	Progressive weight loss, wasting of muscle tissue, loss of skin tone, and decreases in total protein can adversely affect wound healing and impair the patient's ability to withstand infection.
Provide small, frequent, high-calorie, high-protein meals, allowing sufficient time for the patient to eat. Offer supplements between feedings.	Smaller, more frequent meals may be more easily tolerated. Higher calorie/protein meals will provide the adequate nutrition necessary to promote healing.
Provide supplemental vitamins and minerals as prescribed.	These supplements replace deficiencies.
Provide oral hygiene before and after meals.	Oral hygiene minimizes anorexia and helps treat stomatitis, which can occur as a side effect of chemotherapy.
If the patient feels isolated socially, encourage significant others to visit at mealtimes and bring the patient's favorite high-calorie, high-protein foods from home.	Patients likely will benefit from socialization at mealtime, which also may promote intake of these high-calorie, high-protein foods.
If the patient is nauseated, provide instructions for deep breathing and voluntary swallowing.	These measures help decrease stimulation of the vomiting center.
Administer antiemetics as prescribed.	Antiemetics help prevent or minimize nausea.

ASSESSMENT/INTERVENTIONS	RATIONALES
Encourage the patient to request medication as early as possible.	Nausea/vomiting is easier to control when it is treated before it gets too severe or is prolonged.
If the patient is dysphagic, encourage intake of fluids that are high in calories and protein; provide different flavors and textures for variation.	Fluids may be better tolerated than foods when the patient has dysphagia because they are less irritating; fluids that contain supplemental nutrients will help ensure optimal intake.
As prescribed, deliver isotonic tube feeding for patients who are unable to eat.	Isotonic fluids will help prevent diarrhea associated with hypertonic or hypotonic fluids.
Check placement of the gastric tube before each feeding.	This precaution helps prevent instillation of fluids into the respiratory tract.
Evaluate the residual feeding q4h.	This measure assesses the amount of feeding that has not been absorbed. Usually feedings are not delivered if the residual is 50-100 mL.
Keep the head of bed elevated 30 degrees while feeding, and position the patient in a right side-lying position.	This position facilitates gastric emptying and helps prevent aspiration.
Discuss potential need for total parenteral nutrition (TPN) with the health care provider.	TPN promotes caloric intake in patients whose caloric intake is insufficient.

Nursing Diagnoses:

Acute Confusion
Impaired Memory

related to altered sensory integration, reception, and transmission occurring with infection, space-occupying lesions in the central nervous system (CNS), or HIV dementia

Desired Outcomes: Following intervention, the patient verbalizes orientation to person, place, and time. Optimally, by hospital discharge, the patient correctly completes exercises in logical reasoning, memory, perception, concentration, attention, and sequencing of activities.

ASSESSMENT/INTERVENTIONS	RATIONALES
Assess for minor alterations in personality traits that cannot be attributed to other causes, such as stress or medication.	This assessment may help rule out medication side effects or opportunistic diseases.
Assess for slowing of all cognitive functioning, with problems in the areas of attention, concentration, memory, perception, logical reasoning, and sequencing of activities.	These are signs of dementia.
Encourage the patient to report persistent headaches, dizziness, or seizures.	These indicators may signal CNS involvement.
Note any cranial nerve involvement that differs from the patient's past medical history.	Most commonly the fifth (trigeminal), seventh (facial), and eighth (acoustic) nerves are involved in infectious processes of the CNS.
Assess for signs of mental aberration, blindness, aphasia, hemiparesis, or ataxia.	These indicators may signal the presence of a demyelinating disease. Blindness, for example, can occur with an opportunistic infection.
Divide activities into small, easily accomplished tasks.	Pacing activities decreases frustration and increases likelihood of completion.
Maintain a stable environment (e.g., do not change location of furniture in the room).	A stable environment helps the patient remain familiarized with the immediate surroundings.
Write notes as reminders; maintain a calendar of appointments. Provide some mechanism (e.g., pillbox) to ensure medication adherence.	Patients will require these reminders to complete tasks, take medications, and make appointments as independently as possible.
Teach the importance of reporting increasing severity of headaches, blurred vision, gait disturbances, or blackouts. Notify the health care provider of all significant findings.	These indicators identify neurologic changes that necessitate treatment intervention.

Nursing Diagnoses:

Acute Pain
Chronic Pain

related to physical and chemical factors associated with prolonged immobility, side effects of chemotherapy, neoplasms, infections, and peripheral neuropathy

Desired Outcomes: Within 1-2 hr of intervention, the patient's subjective perception of pain decreases, as documented by pain scale. Nonverbal indicators of discomfort, such as grimacing, are absent or diminished.

ASSESSMENT/INTERVENTIONS	RATIONALES
Assess and record the following: location, onset, duration, and factors that precipitate and alleviate the patient's pain. With the patient, establish a pain scale, rating pain from 0 (no pain) to 10 (worst pain).	Competent pain management requires frequent and thorough assessment of these factors. Using a pain scale provides an objective measurement that enables assessment of pain management strategies.
Administer analgesics as prescribed. Encourage the patient to request medication before the pain becomes severe.	Pain that is allowed to become severe is more difficult to control. Prolonged stimulation of pain receptors results in increased sensitivity to painful stimuli and will increase the amount of medication required to relieve pain.
Provide heat or cold applications to affected areas (e.g., apply heat to painful joints and cold packs to reduce swelling associated with infections or multiple venipunctures).	Heat and cold applications are effective nonpharmacologic measures that reduce pain, as well as augment effects of analgesics.
Encourage diversional activities (e.g., soothing music; quiet conversation; reading; slow, rhythmic breathing).	Diversion is a means of increasing pain tolerance and decreasing its intensity.
Teach techniques such as deep breathing, biofeedback, and relaxation exercises.	These techniques reduce pain intensity by decreasing skeletal muscle tension.
Discuss with the health care provider the desirability of a capped venous catheter for long-term blood withdrawal.	This measure will help reduce pain in patients in whom frequent venipunctures cause discomfort.
Administer back rubs and massage.	These measures promote relaxation and comfort.
For other interventions, see "Pain," p. 39.	

Nursing Diagnosis:

Activity Intolerance

related to generalized weakness, arthralgia, myalgia, dyspnea, fever, pain, hypoxia, and effects of chemotherapy

Desired Outcome: Before hospital discharge, the patient rates perceived exertion and/or pain on exertion at 3 or less on a 0-10 scale and exhibits tolerance to activity as evidenced by HR 20 bpm or less over resting HR, RR 20 breaths/min or less, and systolic blood pressure (SBP) 20 mm Hg or less over or under resting SBP.

ASSESSMENT/INTERVENTIONS	RATIONALES
Assess HR, RR, and BP before and immediately after activity, and ask the patient to rate his or her perceived exertion. See "Prolonged Bedrest" for **Activity Intolerance**, p. 62, for details about perceived exertion.	This assessment monitors tolerance to activity. If the patient's rate of perceived exertion (RPE) is more than 3 or he or she exhibits signs of activity intolerance, the activity should be stopped or modified.

ASSESSMENT/INTERVENTIONS

RATIONALES

ASSESSMENT/INTERVENTIONS	RATIONALES
Assess oximetry or ABG values to ensure that the patient is oxygenated adequately; adjust oxygen delivery accordingly.	Oxygen saturation 92% or less may signal the need for supplemental oxygen or an increase in oxygen delivery.
Monitor electrolyte levels.	This helps determine if muscle weakness is caused by hypokalemia.
Plan adequate (90- to 120-min) rest periods between scheduled activities. Adjust activities as appropriate.	This will help reduce the patient's energy expenditure.
As much as possible, encourage regular periods of exercise.	Exercise helps prevent cardiac intolerance to activities, which can occur quickly after periods of prolonged inactivity.
Advise the patient to keep anecdotal notes (perhaps in journal format) on exacerbation and remission of signs and symptoms.	Anecdotal notes are useful tools for self-examination as well as for reporting to the health care provider, who may use this information to alter or modify treatment or develop new strategies.

Nursing Diagnosis:

Deficient Knowledge

related to unfamiliarity with the disease process, prognosis, lifestyle changes, and treatment plan

Desired Outcome: Before hospital discharge, the patient verbalizes accurate information about the disease process, prognosis, behaviors that increase risk of transmitting the virus to others, and the treatment plan.

ASSESSMENT/INTERVENTIONS

RATIONALES

ASSESSMENT/INTERVENTIONS	RATIONALES
Assess the patient's health care literacy (language, reading, comprehension). Assess culture and culturally specific information needs.	This assessment helps ensure that information is selected and presented in a manner that is culturally and educationally appropriate.
Assess the patient's knowledge about HIV disease, including pathophysiologic changes that may occur, ways the disease is transmitted, possibility of long life expectancy with appropriate treatment, and how to prevent other infections. Correct misinformation and misconceptions as necessary.	This assessment enables formulation of an individualized teaching plan to improve the patient's health and quality of life.
Assess the patient's knowledge about ART and viral resistance. Correct misinformation and misconceptions as necessary.	This information enables nurses to formulate individualized teaching plans to improve adherence and help prevent viral resistance to ART.
Provide information about private and community agencies that are available to help with tasks such as handling legal affairs, cooking, housecleaning, and nursing care. Provide telephone numbers and addresses for HIV support groups and self-help groups.	Lack of knowledge about these services and groups may add unnecessary stress to the patient's illness.
Provide literature that explores myths and realities of the HIV disease process.	This information helps patients engage in activities that will improve, rather than harm, their health.
Teach the importance of how to inform sexual partners of the patient's HIV condition and reduce high-risk behaviors known to transmit the virus.	These measures reduce the risk of transmitting the virus to others.
Involve the significant other in the teaching and learning process.	Involving the significant other in the teaching process not only provides information to him or her but enables the significant other to reinforce teaching for the patient as well.
Provide the patient and significant other with names and addresses or phone numbers of HIV resources (see "Patient-Family Teaching and Discharge Planning").	These resources provide information about current therapies, support services, and funding for medications.

Nursing Diagnosis:

Anxiety

related to threat of death, significant life changes, and social isolation

Desired Outcome: Following intervention, the patient expresses feelings and is free of harmful anxiety as evidenced by HR 100 bpm or less, RR 20 breaths/min or less with normal depth and pattern (eupnea), and BP within the patient's normal range.

ASSESSMENT/INTERVENTIONS	RATIONALES
Assess for verbal or nonverbal expressions of anxiety, fear, or depression.	Inability to cope, apprehension, guilt for past actions, uncertainty, concerns about rejection and isolation, and suicidal ideation are likely signs of anxiety, fear, or depression.
Spend time with the patient and encourage expressions of feelings and concerns. Support effective coping patterns (e.g., by allowing the patient to cry or talk rather than denying his or her legitimate fears and concerns).	Before patients can learn effective coping strategies, they must first clarify their feelings. Verbalizing feelings in a nonthreatening, nonjudgmental environment can help patients deal with unresolved/unrecognized issues that may be contributing to the current stressor.
Provide accurate information about HIV disease, related diagnostic procedures, and emerging treatments.	Some fears and anxieties may be realistic, whereas others may necessitate clarification based on current treatment information.
If the patient hyperventilates, teach him or her to mimic your normal respiratory pattern (eupnea).	This is an effective calming technique.

Nursing Diagnosis:

Disturbed Body Image

related to biophysical changes resulting from KS lesions, chemotherapy, wasting, lipodystrophy, and lipoatrophy

Desired Outcome: Before hospital discharge, the patient expresses positive feelings about himself or herself to the family, significant other, and primary nurse.

ASSESSMENT/INTERVENTIONS	RATIONALES
Encourage the patient to express feelings, especially the way he or she views or feels about self. Provide positive feedback; help the patient focus on facts rather than myths or exaggerations.	These measures provide an environment conducive to free expression and promote understanding of health status, which may clarify misconceptions that may be contributing to the disturbed body image.
Provide a referral to a nutritionist if appropriate.	A nutrition expert will assist in establishing a healthy diet that will minimize body changes.
Provide access to clergy, psychiatric nurse, social worker, psychologist, or HIV counselor as appropriate.	The patient may require specialized counseling, especially if he or she is at risk for self-harm.
Encourage the patient to join and share feelings with an HIV support group.	Many people benefit from support groups and sharing experiences with others who are having similar experiences.
For additional information, see "Psychosocial Support" for **Disturbed Body Image,** p. 79.	

Nursing Diagnosis:

Social Isolation

related to altered state of wellness, societal rejection, loss of support system, feelings of guilt and punishment, fatigue, and changed patterns of sexual expression

Desired Outcome: Before hospital discharge, the patient communicates and interacts with others.

ASSESSMENT/INTERVENTIONS	RATIONALES
Keep the patient and significant other well informed about the patient's status and treatment plan. Provide private periods of time for the patient to communicate and interact with his or her significant other.	Information and communication help reduce a sense of isolation.
Encourage the significant other to share in the patient's care. Encourage physical closeness between them. Provide privacy as much as possible.	These actions increase the amount of time for interaction and communication with the significant other.
Involve the patient in unit or group activities as appropriate.	Such activities reduce a sense of isolation and promote socialization.
Explain the significance of transmission precautions to the patient.	Understanding the rationale for these precautions may help the patient cope with and adhere to them better and develop new approaches to life with HIV infection.
Provide a link with community support services.	This provides contact with others, psychosocial support, resources, and care.

ADDITIONAL NURSING DIAGNOSES/PROBLEMS:

"Prolonged Bedrest"	p. 61
"Psychosocial Support"	p. 72
"Psychosocial Support for the Patient's Family and Significant Other"	p. 84
"Managing Wound Care"	p. 533
"Providing Nutritional Support"	p. 539

 PATIENT-FAMILY TEACHING AND DISCHARGE PLANNING

When providing patient-family teaching, focus on sensory information, avoid giving excessive information, and initiate a visiting nurse referral for necessary follow-up teaching. Include verbal and written information about the following:

✓ Importance of reporting any new symptoms of infection or changes in neurologic status (e.g., increasing severity of headaches, blurred vision, gait disturbances, blackouts) immediately to the health care provider.

✓ Necessity of modifying high-risk sexual behaviors.

✓ Prescribed medications, including drug name, dosage, purpose, and potential side effects. Also discuss drug-drug, herb-drug, and food-drug interactions. Instruct the patient and significant other in the necessity of taking antiretroviral medications as prescribed to avoid viral resistance.

✓ Importance of the patient's adherence to ART regimens, which is critical to patients and the clinicians providing and monitoring their care. Interruptions in drug treatment can lead to development of viruses resistant to specific antiretroviral drugs, which can result in treatment failure and limiting of future treatment options. Health care provider and patient partnerships characterized by shared decision making have been identified as a key component in successful HIV treatment.

✓ Strategies for promoting HIV treatment adherence. These must be customized to meet needs of each patient. The approach must be patient centered and include ongoing education, psychosocial and community support, and resources that involve both patient-directed and provider-directed strategies.

✓ Because of decreased resistance to infection, particularly in persons with very low CD4+ T cell counts, the importance of limiting contact with individuals known to have active infections. In addition, pets may harbor various fungal, protozoal, and bacterial organisms in their excrement. Therefore, contact with birdcages, cat litter, and tropical fish tanks should be avoided.

✓ Necessity for meticulous hygiene to prevent spread of any extant or new infectious organisms. To avoid exposure to fungi, damp areas in bathrooms (e.g., shower)

should be cleaned with solutions of bleach, refrigerators should be cleaned thoroughly with soap and water, and leftover foodstuffs should be disposed of within 2-3 days.

✓ Techniques for self-assessment of early signs of infection (e.g., erythema, tenderness, local warmth, swelling, purulent exudate) in all cuts, abrasions, lesions, or open wounds.

✓ Importance of avoiding use of recreational drugs, which are believed to potentiate immunosuppressive processes, lower resistance to infection, and can be linked to transmission.

✓ Significance and importance of refraining from donating blood.

✓ Principles and importance of maintaining a balanced diet; ways to supplement diet with multivitamins and other food sources, such as high-calorie substances (e.g., Isocal, Ensure).

✓ Because of increased susceptibility to foodborne opportunistic organisms, fruits and vegetables should be washed thoroughly; meats should be cooked thoroughly at appropriate temperatures; and raw eggs, raw fish (sushi), and unpasteurized milk should be avoided.

✓ Care of the venous access device, including technique for self-administration of TPN or medications; and care of gastric tube and administration of enteral tube feedings if appropriate (see "Providing Nutritional Support").

✓ Importance of avoiding fatigue by limiting participation in social activities, getting maximum amounts of rest, and minimizing physical exertion.

✓ Importance of maintaining medical follow-up appointments.

✓ Advisability of sharing feelings with significant other or within a support group.

✓ Referral to hospice or agency that provides home help. This should occur before discharge planning begins to ensure continuity of care between hospital and home or hospice.

✓ Phone numbers to call if questions or concerns arise about hospice after discharge. Information for these patients can be obtained by contacting National Hospice Palliative Care Organization at *www.nhpco.org*

In addition, provide the following information regarding HIV resources:

✓ Public Health Service AIDS Hotline at (800) CDC-INFO or (800) 232-4636.

✓ National Sexually Transmitted Diseases Hotline/ American Social Health Association at (800) 227-8922.

✓ Local Red Cross Chapter or American Red Cross AIDS Education Office at (202) 737-8300.

✓ CDC HIV/AIDS information at *www.cdc.gov/hiv/*

✓ Association of Nurses in AIDS Care (ANAC) at *www.anacnet.org*

✓ Canadian Association of Nurses in AIDS Care (CANAC) at *www.canac.org*

✓ NIH, National Institutes of Allergy and Infectious Diseases at *www.niaid.nih.gov*

✓ DHHS HIV/AIDS Treatment Information and Clinical Trials Information at *http://aidsinfo.nih.gov*

✓ HRSA, Bureau of HIV/AIDS at *www.hab.hrsa.gov*

✓ AIDS Education and Training Centers National Resource Center at *http://aids-etc.org*

✓ National HIV/AIDS Clinician's Post-Exposure Prophylaxis Hotline (PEPline) at (800) 448-4911, *www.ucsf.edu/hivcntr*

✓ National HIV/AIDS Clinician's Consultation Center at (800) 933-3413, *www.ucsf.edu/hivcntr*

✓ Canadian AIDS Society at *www.cdnaids.ca*

✓ AIDS Foundation Canada at *www.aidsfoundation.ca*

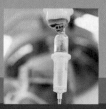

Managing Wound Care 73

A wound is a disruption of tissue integrity caused by trauma, surgery, or an underlying medical disorder. Wound management is directed at preventing infection and deterioration in wound status and promoting healing.

WOUNDS CLOSED BY PRIMARY INTENTION
OVERVIEW/PATHOPHYSIOLOGY

Clean, surgical, or traumatic wounds whose edges are closed with sutures, clips, tissue glue, or sterile tape strips are referred to as *wounds closed by primary intention*. Impairment of healing most commonly manifests as dehiscence, evisceration, or infection. Individuals at high risk for disruption of wound healing include those who are very young or very old, have diabetes mellitus, smoke cigarettes, are obese, are malnourished, or are immunosuppressed (e.g., receiving steroids or other immunosuppressive drugs, undergoing chemotherapy or radiation therapy, or have immunosuppressive disease).

HEALTH CARE SETTING

Primary care, acute care, critical care

ASSESSMENT

Normal healing: Warm, reddened, indurated, tender incision line immediately after injury. After 1 or 2 days, epithelial cells migrate across the incision line and seal the wound. Over time, a pink scar is visible. After 7-9 days, a healing ridge—a palpable accumulation of scar tissue—forms. In patients who undergo cosmetic surgery, the healing ridge is purposefully avoided to minimize scar formation. Healing is complete when structural and functional integrity is reestablished.

Impaired healing: Lack of an adequate inflammatory response manifested by absence of initial redness, warmth, and induration or inflammation that persists or occurs after the fifth postinjury day; continued drainage from the incision line 2 days after injury (when no drain is present); absence of a healing ridge by the ninth day after injury; presence of purulent exudate. Older persons may not exhibit classic signs of impaired healing but only changes in cognition or functional status that lead to search for the site of infection.

DIAGNOSTIC TESTS

Culture and sensitivity of tissue by biopsy or swab: To determine optimal antibiotic. Sample is obtained from clean tissue, not from exudate, pus, or necrotic tissue. Infection is present when there are 10^6 organisms/g or more from tissue or when there is fever and drainage.

Gram stain of drainage: Done as part of the culture procedure to identify offending organism and aid in selection of preliminary antibiotics. Data from culture confirms organisms' sensitivity to selected antibiotic or need to change antibiotic.

White blood cell (WBC) count with differential: To assess for infection.

Nursing Diagnosis:

Impaired Tissue Integrity: Wound

related to altered blood flow, metabolic disorders (e.g., diabetes mellitus [DM]), alterations in fluid volume and nutrition, and medical therapy (chemotherapy, radiation therapy, steroid or immunosuppressive drug administration)

Desired Outcome: The patient exhibits the following signs of wound healing: well-approximated wound edges, good initial postinjury inflammatory response (erythema, warmth, induration, pain), no inflammatory response past the fifth day after injury, no drainage (without drain present) 48 hr after closure, healing ridge present by postoperative day 7-9.

ASSESSMENT/INTERVENTIONS

ASSESSMENT/INTERVENTIONS	RATIONALES
Assess the wound for absence of a healing ridge, presence of drainage or purulent exudate, and delayed or prolonged inflammatory response.	These are signs of impaired healing.
Assess vital signs for elevated temperature and heart rate (HR). Document findings.	These are signs of infection, a manifestation of impaired wound healing.
Assess for hyperglycemia with serial capillary glucose measures and maintain blood glucose at the prescribed level using insulin as indicated.	Hyperglycemia increases risk for infection, thereby adversely affecting wound healing.
As indicated, assess pulse oximetry. Report O_2 saturation 92% or less, and consult the health care provider about administration of O_2.	Oxygen saturation 92% or less often signals need for supplemental oxygen to support tissue healing and prevent infection.
Assess perfusion status by checking blood pressure (BP) and HR as well as capillary refill time adjacent to the incision.	These measures determine if blood flow to the area is adequate for healing. BP and HR optimally should be within the patient's normal range; capillary refill greater than 2 sec signals inadequate tissue perfusion.
Assess hydration status by monitoring peripheral pulses, moisture of mucous membranes, skin turgor, volume and specific gravity of urine, and intake and output.	Hypovolemia adversely affects wound healing.
Assess nutritional status (see "Providing Nutritional Support" for details).	Nutrients are needed for repair.
Assess wound pain using a numeric rating scale. Treat pain with pharmacologic and nonpharmacologic interventions. Anticipate pain associated with dressing change and premedicate.	Pain causes vasoconstriction and may impair healing. See "Pain," p. 39, for details.
Follow agency policy in using sterile/clean technique when changing dressings. If a drain is present, keep it sterile, maintain its patency (e.g., empty drainage reservoir and recharge suction on closed drainage systems as needed), and handle it gently to prevent it from becoming dislodged.	Sterile technique eliminates introduction of nosocomial organisms to prevent infection. Most of the outpatient wound care is done with clean technique.
Encourage deep breathing q2h while the patient is awake. Splint the incision as needed. If indicated, provide incentive spirometry.	Deep breathing promotes oxygenation, which enhances wound healing.
Stress the importance of position changes at least q2h and activity as tolerated.	Movement, exercise, and activity promote ventilation and circulation, and hence oxygenation to the tissues.
For nonrestricted patients, ensure a fluid intake of at least 30 mL/kg body weight/day.	Adequate hydration is critical to wound healing.
Provide a diet with adequate protein, vitamin C, and calories. If the patient complains of feeling full with three meals per day, give more frequent small feedings. Encourage between-meal high-protein supplements (e.g., yogurt, milkshakes).	This diet promotes positive nitrogen balance and nutrients needed for wound healing. Smaller, more frequent meals are often more easily tolerated.
If wound care is necessary after hospital discharge, teach clean dressing change procedure to the patient and significant other. Immunosuppressed patients require sterile technique.	Clean technique is used at home because most people have antibodies to familiar organisms. Immunosuppressed patients have increased risk of Infection.

✓ **PATIENT-FAMILY TEACHING AND DISCHARGE PLANNING**

When providing patient-family teaching, focus on sensory information, avoid giving excessive information, and initiate a home health referral for necessary follow-up teaching. Include verbal and written information about the following:

✓ Local wound care, including type of equipment necessary, wound care procedure, and therapeutic and potential side effects of topical agents used. Have the patient or significant other demonstrate dressing change procedure before hospital discharge.

✓ Signs and symptoms of improvement or deterioration in wound status, including those that necessitate notification of the health care provider or clinic.

✓ Diet that promotes wound healing. Discuss importance of adequate protein and calorie intake. See "Providing Nutritional Support," p. 539. Involve dietitian, the patient, and significant other as necessary.

✓ Activities that maximize ventilatory status: a planned regimen for ambulatory patients and deep breathing and turning (at least q2h) for those on bedrest.

✓ Importance of taking pain medication, antibiotics, multivitamins, and supplements of iron and zinc as prescribed.

For all medications to be taken at home, provide the following: drug name, purpose, dosage, schedule, precautions, and potential side effects. Also discuss drug-drug, herb-drug, and food-drug interactions.

✓ Importance of follow-up care with the health care provider; confirm time and date of next appointment, if known.

✓ If needed, arrange for a visit by a home health nurse before hospital discharge.

✓ How/where to obtain wound care supplies.

SURGICAL OR TRAUMATIC WOUNDS HEALING BY SECONDARY INTENTION OVERVIEW/PATHOPHYSIOLOGY

Wounds healing by secondary intention are those with tissue loss or heavy contamination that form granulation tissue and contract in order to heal. Most often, impairment of healing is caused by contamination and inadequate blood flow, oxygenation, and nutrition. Individuals at risk for impaired healing include those who are very young or very old, have DM, smoke cigarettes, are obese, are malnourished, or are immunosuppressed (e.g., receiving steroids or other immunosuppressive drugs, undergoing chemotherapy or radiation therapy, have immunosuppressive disease).

HEALTH CARE SETTING

Acute care, critical care, primary care, long-term care, home care

ASSESSMENT

Normal healing: Initially the wound edges are inflamed, indurated, and tender. At first, granulation tissue is pink, progressing to a deeper pink and then to a beefy red; wound tissues should be moist. Epithelial cells from the tissue surrounding the wound gradually migrate across the granulation tissue. As healing occurs, the wound edges become pink, the angle between surrounding tissue and the wound becomes less acute, wound contraction occurs, and the wound gets smaller. Occasionally a wound has a tract or sinus that gradually decreases in size as healing occurs. When a drain is in place, volume, color, and odor of the drainage should be evaluated. Time frame for healing depends on wound size and location and on the patient's physical and psychologic status. Healing is complete when structure and function have been reestablished.

Impaired healing: Exudate/slough/necrotic tissue on the floor and walls of the wound. Note distribution, color, odor, volume, and adherence of the exudates/slough/dead tissue and damage to skin surrounding the wound, including disruption, discoloration, swelling, local increased warmth, and increasing pain. Older persons may not exhibit classic signs of impaired healing but only changes in cognition or functional status that lead to search for the site of infection.

DIAGNOSTIC TESTS

Culture with tissue biopsy or swab: To determine presence of infection and optimal antibiotic, if appropriate.

Gram stain: Performed as part of the culture to determine characteristics of the offending organism, if present, and aid in selection of preliminary antibiotic. Data from culture confirms organisms' sensitivity to selected antibiotic or need to change antibiotic.

Complete blood count (CBC) with WBC differential: CBC to assess hematocrit level and for presence of severe anemia (less than 25 g/dL). Increased WBC count signals infection, whereas a decrease occurs with immunosuppression. Monitor lymphocyte count (1800/mm^3 or less) as a sign of malnutrition.

X-ray examination/bone scan: To determine presence of osteomyelitis.

Nursing Diagnosis:

Impaired Tissue Integrity: Wound

related to the presence of contaminants, metabolic disorders (e.g., DM), medical therapy (e.g., chemotherapy, radiation therapy), altered perfusion, or malnutrition

Desired Outcomes: The patient's wound exhibits the following signs of healing: initially after injury, wound edges are inflamed, indurated, and tender; with epithelialization, edges become pink; granulation tissue develops over time (identified by pink tissue that becomes beefy red); and there is no odor, exudate, or necrotic tissue. The patient or significant other successfully demonstrates wound care procedure before hospital discharge, if appropriate.

ASSESSMENT/INTERVENTIONS

RATIONALES

ASSESSMENT/INTERVENTIONS	RATIONALES
Assess for the following: decreased inflammatory response in the first 5 days or inflammatory response that lasts more than 5 days; epithelialization slowed or mechanically disrupted or noncontiguous around the wound; granulation tissue remaining pale or excessively dry or moist; presence of odor, exudate, slough, and/or necrotic tissue.	These are signs of impaired healing.
Cleanse drainage or secretions from the skin surrounding the wound with a mild disinfectant (e.g., soap and water). Do not use friction with cleansing if tissue is friable.	These measures help prevent wound contamination.
Cleanse the wound with each dressing change using 100-150 mL solution (e.g., saline, water, 0.5%-1.0% acetic acid) via a 35-mL syringe with an 18-gauge angiocatheter, following infection prevention procedures outlined in agency policy (also see p. 747).	Use of an angiocatheter facilitates dislodging and removal of bacteria and loosens necrotic tissue, foreign bodies, and exudates.
When topical enzymes are prescribed, use them on necrotic tissue only and follow package directions carefully.	Enzymes remove necrotic tissue and spare healthy tissue. **Note:** Some agents, such as silver, deactivate the enzymes.
Apply prescribed dressings following meticulous infection prevention procedures (see p. 747).	Depending on the patient's individual needs, these dressings keep healthy wound tissue moist.
When prescribed, apply antimicrobial dressings for infection.	Silver dressings, honey dressings, cadexomer carbohydrate or polyethylene glycol slow-release, and polyhexamethylene biguanide (PHMB) reduce bacteria counts over a 2-4 wk period.
Insert dressing into all tracts.	This promotes gradual closure of those areas.
Ensure good hand hygiene before and after dressing changes, and dispose of contaminated dressings appropriately.	These measures prevent spread of infection to the patient and others.
When a drain is used, maintain its patency, prevent its kinking, and secure the tubing to prevent the drain from becoming dislodged.	Drains remove excess tissue fluid or purulent drainage.
Use sterile technique when caring for drains.	Organisms may move into tissue by way of the drain. Sterile technique reduces risk of contamination and ingress of organisms.
With closed drainage systems, empty the drainage reservoir and document the volume removed. Maintain suction as needed.	Suction aids in removal of excess fluid.
With negative pressure therapy, maintain pressure and change the dressing as prescribed.	This therapy reduces bacterial load and enhances blood flow to support healing.
Teach the patient or significant other the prescribed wound care procedure, if indicated.	Wound care may be required after the patient is discharged.
See discussion of diet, supplemental oxygen, insulin, hydration, and supplemental vitamins in **Impaired Tissue Integrity,** earlier, in "Wounds Closed by Primary Intention."	

✓ PATIENT-FAMILY TEACHING AND DISCHARGE PLANNING

See teaching and discharge planning interventions in "Wounds Closed by Primary Intention," earlier.

PRESSURE ULCERS
OVERVIEW/PATHOPHYSIOLOGY

Pressure ulcers result from a disruption in tissue integrity and are caused most often by excessive tissue pressure. High-risk patients include older persons and those who have decreased mobility, decreased level of consciousness (LOC), impaired sensation, debilitation, incontinence, sepsis/elevated temperature, or malnutrition.

HEALTH CARE SETTING

Primary care, acute care, critical care, long-term care, assisted care, home care

ASSESSMENT

High-risk individuals are identified on admission assessment and with daily assessments during hospitalization using a standard assessment schema. Pressure ulcer severity is categorized/staged on a scale of I to IV or classified as unstageable or having suspected deep tissue injury.

Category/Stage I: Intact skin with nonblanchable redness of a localized area, usually over a bony prominence. Discoloration of the skin, warmth, edema, hardness, or pain also may be present. Darkly pigmented skin may not have visible blanching.

Category/Stage II: Partial-thickness loss of dermis that presents as a shallow open ulcer with a red/pink bed without slough. It also may present as an intact or ruptured serum-filled or serosanguineous blister. This category does not include skin tears, tape burns, incontinence-associated dermatitis, maceration, or excoriation.

Category/Stage III: Full-thickness tissue loss. Subcutaneous fat tissue may be visible, but bone, tendon, and muscle are not exposed. Slough may be present but does not obscure the depth of tissue loss. Undermining or tunneling may be present.

Category/Stage IV: Full-thickness tissue loss with exposed bone, tendon, or muscle. Slough or eschar may be present on some parts of the wound bed. Undermining and tunneling may be present.

Unstageable: Full thickness tissue loss in which the actual depth of the ulcers is completely obscured by slough (yellow, tan, gray, green, or brown) and/or eschar (tan, brown, or black) in the wound bed.

Suspected deep tissue injury: Purple or maroon localized area of discolored intact skin or a blood-filled blister due to damage of underlying soft tissue from pressure and/or shear.

Note: *Do not downstage during pressure ulcer assessment. The ulcer is always described at its greatest depth (e.g., healing stage IV ulcer) because tissue lost in a pressure ulcer is not replaced; rather the hole is filled with scar tissue).*

See also "Surgical or Traumatic Wounds Healing by Secondary Intention," earlier, for other assessment data.

DIAGNOSTIC TESTS

See Diagnostic Tests in "Surgical or Traumatic Wounds Healing by Secondary Intention."

Nursing Diagnosis:

Impaired Tissue Integrity (or risk for same)

related to excessive tissue pressure

Desired Outcomes: The patient's tissue remains intact. The patient or significant other participates in preventive measures and verbalizes understanding of the rationale for these interventions.

ASSESSMENT/INTERVENTIONS	RATIONALES
Assess pressure ulcer risk and skin status daily, especially over bony prominences. Document findings. Use a standard risk assessment scale such as the Braden Scale (see reference section for website information).	High-risk patients include older persons and those who have decreased mobility, decreased LOC, impaired sensation, debilitation, incontinence, sepsis/elevated temperature, malnutrition, or previous pressure ulcer.
Establish and post a position-changing schedule.	This communicates established turning and position-changing schedule for the staff and the patient/family and reinforces its importance.
Assist with position changes.	Proper body alignment is provided when patients who need help receive it.
Ensure the following position changes:	
- Turn the bed-bound patient at least q1-2h and have the wheelchair-bound patient (who is able) perform push-ups in the chair q15min (and not less than q1h).	There is an inverse relationship between pressure and time in ulcer formation; therefore, heavier patients need to change position more frequently. Position changes ensure periodic relief from pressure.
- Use pillows, foam wedges, or gel pads to pad and position.	This maintains alternative positions and pads bony prominences.
- For high-risk patients and those with a history of previous pressure ulcers, provide pressure-relief measures more frequently.	Healed pressure ulcers have a lower pressure tolerance than uninjured skin.
- Use low Fowler's position and alternate the supine position with prone and 30-degree or less elevated side-lying positions.	High Fowler's position results in increased shearing when patients slide down in bed. A side-lying position at 30 degrees or less prevents high pressure on the trochanter.
For immobile patients, raise their heels off the bed surface.	This totally relieves pressure on heels.
Lift rather than drag patients during position changes and transferring; use a transfer board/draw sheet to facilitate the patient's movement.	Lifting minimizes friction and shear on tissue during activity.
Do not massage over bony prominences.	Massage can result in skin/tissue damage.

continued

ASSESSMENT/INTERVENTIONS	RATIONALES
Cleanse the skin at the time of soiling and at routine intervals. Use moisture barriers and disposable briefs as needed.	These measures minimize skin exposure to moisture and chemical irritants.
Use a mattress such as foam, low air loss, alternating air, gel, or water.	These mattresses reduce pressure on body tissues.
Encourage the patient to maintain or increase current level of activity.	Activity promotes blood flow, which helps prevent impaired skin/tissue integrity.

Nursing Diagnosis:

Impaired Tissue Integrity: Pressure Ulcer

related to altered circulation and presence of contaminants or irritants (chemical, thermal, or mechanical)

Desired Outcomes: Stages I and II show progressive healing over days to weeks; stages III and IV may require months to heal. For wounds that can be healed, expect a 30% reduction in wound size in 4 wk and complete closure in 12 wk. Following intervention and instruction, the patient or significant other verbalizes causes and preventive measures for pressure ulcers and successfully participates in the plan of care to promote healing and prevent further breakdown.

ASSESSMENT/INTERVENTIONS	RATIONALES
Assess ulcer and stage (see Assessment, earlier).	Assessment provides data on ulcer status.
Maintain a moist physiologic environment. Change dressings as needed, using meticulous infection prevention procedure (see Appendix, p. 747).	These measures promote tissue repair and minimize contaminants.
Keep the patient's skin clean with regular bathing, and be especially conscientious about washing urine and feces from the skin.	Incontinence causes chemical irritation to the skin and reduces tissue tolerance to external pressure. Soap should be used and then thoroughly rinsed from the skin.
Apply heel and elbow protection as needed.	These protectors absorb moisture and prevent shearing when the patient moves.
For patients with excessive perspiration, ensure frequent bathing and bedding changes.	Perspiration reduces tissue tolerance.
Teach the patient and significant other the importance of and measures to prevent excess pressure.	Knowledgeable individuals are more likely to adhere to prevention measures.
Provide wound care as needed (described under "Surgical or Traumatic Wounds Healing by Secondary Intention," earlier).	

ADDITIONAL NURSING DIAGNOSES/PROBLEMS:

"Surgical or Traumatic Wounds Healing by Secondary   p. 535
   Intention" for **Impaired Tissue Integrity**

✓ **PATIENT-FAMILY TEACHING AND DISCHARGE PLANNING**

When providing patient-family teaching, focus on sensory information, avoid giving excessive information, and initiate a home health referral for necessary follow-up teaching. Consider including verbal and written information about the following:

✓ Location of local medical supply stores that have pressure-reducing mattresses and wound care supplies.
✓ Planning a schedule for changing the patient's positions.

See "Wounds Closed by Primary Intention" for other teaching and discharge planning interventions.

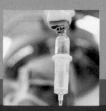

Providing Nutritional Support 74

Adequate nutrition is necessary to meet the body's demands in order to maintain normal body composition and function. A patient's nutritional status may be affected by disease or injury state (i.e., cancer or trauma), physical factors (e.g., poor dentition or mobility), social factors (e.g., isolation, lack of financial resources), or psychologic factors (e.g., mental illness). In addition, cultural beliefs (e.g., vegetarian diet) and age (e.g., older adults with cognitive impairment causing them to forget to eat) may influence overall nutrition intake.

Hospitalized patients are at high risk for developing protein-energy malnutrition. It is estimated that one third of patients arrive to the hospital malnourished. In addition, studies have shown that 40%-50% of hospitalized patients have insufficient nutrient intake while in the hospital. According to the Institute for Healthcare Improvement (ihi.org), more than 91% of patients transferred from acute care to subacute care are either malnourished or at risk of malnutrition. Malnutrition is associated with impaired wound healing, pressure ulcers, infections, and increased hospital stays and associated costs. Individuals admitted with unintentional weight loss and maintained on intravenous (IV) dextrose/electrolyte solutions alone or with poor oral intake for more than 3 consecutive days should be considered and evaluated for nutritional support.

When individuals are well nourished, there are no defined time frames during which they can be without water or food before addressing artificial replacement. The best markers to use for initiation of water and food in well-nourished people are magnitude of the injury/insult to the body and amount of time the individual will be unable to resume normal oral intake.

HEALTH CARE SETTING

Acute care

ASSESSMENT

Dietary history

A dietary history is compiled to reveal adequacy of usual and recent food intake. Based on the information obtained, the nurse may identify the need to consult with a registered dietitian for additional interventions. Be alert to excesses or deficiencies of nutrients and any special eating patterns (e.g., various types of vegetarian or prescribed diets), use of fad diets,

and excessive supplementation. The patient's perception of and actual intake may differ; therefore, include family, significant others, or caregiver when obtaining a dietary history. Include in the care plan anything that impairs adequate selection, preparation, ingestion, digestion, absorption, or excretion of nutrients as follows:

- Food allergies, food aversions, and use of nutritional supplements (prescribed or over the counter).
- Any alternative therapies such as use of herbs or other "natural" supplements.
- Any over-the-counter medications.
- Recent unplanned weight loss or gain.
- Chewing or swallowing difficulties. Include questions related to dental care, such as dentures (note presence of dentures; ask about fit of dentures or other problems), missing teeth, no teeth, and/or loose teeth.
- Nausea, vomiting, or pain with eating.
- Altered pattern of elimination (e.g., constipation, diarrhea).
- Chronic disease affecting utilization of nutrients (e.g., malabsorption, pancreatitis, diabetes mellitus).
- Surgical resection; disease of the gut or accessory organs of digestion (i.e., pancreas, liver, gallbladder).
- Currently pregnant or lactating.
- Use of medications (e.g., laxatives, antacids, antibiotics, antineoplastic drugs) or alcohol. Long-term use of drugs may affect appetite, digestion, or utilization or excretion of nutrients.

PHYSICAL ASSESSMENT

Most physical findings are not specific to a particular nutritional deficiency. Compare current assessment findings with past assessments, especially related to the following:
- Loss of muscle and adipose tissue.
  - Assess fit of clothing, rings, and watches.
  - Be aware that assessment of obese patients or individuals who have an excess of fluid accumulation due to body edema may be challenging.
  - Look for temporal wasting in individuals who have ascites or other forms of body edema.
- Work and muscle endurance.
  - Assess ability to maintain activities of daily living.
  - Query the patient regarding recent changes in mobility and/or activities.

- Muscle weakness may reflect several different deficiencies that may require additional evaluation and tests:
  - Selenium
  - Vitamin D
  - Potassium
  - Magnesium
- Changes in hair, skin, or neuromuscular function.
  - Excessive bruising or bleeding may reflect vitamin K deficiency.
  - Biotin deficiency may appear as alopecia or seborrheic dermatitis.
  - Scaly dermatitis may reflect essential fatty acid deficiency.
  - Zinc deficiency may present as sores at the edges of the mouth, facial rash, peeling of the skin on the palms of the hands and soles of the feet, and brittle nails.
  - Hypocalcemia may be accompanied by dry, scaling skin; brittle nails; and/or dry hair.

Anthropometric data

Height: Used to determine ideal weight and body mass index (BMI). If the patient's height is unavailable or impossible to measure, obtain an estimate from the family or significant other.

Weight: Used by many to determine nutritional status, but fluctuations may be a result of amputation, dehydration, diuresis, fluid retention (renal failure, edema, third spacing), fluid resuscitation, wound dressings, or clothing. (It is helpful to remember that 1 L of fluid equals approximately 2 lb or 1 kg.) More reliable information may be obtained by asking the patient to recall usual weight, weight changes (gains and losses), and the time frame in which these occurred. Unintentional loss in weight of greater than 10% over a 6-mo period is considered significant and may be associated with severe malnutrition. The greater the unintentional weight loss, the more predictive this weight loss may be of mortality.

BMI: Used to evaluate the weight of adults. One calculation and one set of standards are applicable to both men and women:

$$BMI\,(kg/m^2) = Weight/Height\,(m^2)$$

BMI values of 19-25 are appropriate for 19-34 yr olds; whereas, BMI values of 21-27 are appropriate for individuals older than 35 yr. Obesity is defined as BMI greater than 27.5, with severe or morbid obesity greater than 40. A BMI of 16-18.5 is considered mild to moderate malnutrition; whereas BMI less than 16 indicates severe malnutrition. A BMI of less than 18.5 and more than 40 is associated with increased risk of adverse clinical outcomes; referral to a clinical dietitian should be considered. Height, weight, and BMI should be documented in the medical record.

Estimating nutritional requirements

Calorie estimation: To prevent overfeeding, calculate the total calorie intake as follows:

Average nourished patient: 25 total calories per kg of body weight

Mildly stressed patient: 30 total calories per kg of body weight

Severely stressed patient: 35 total calories per kg of body weight

Morbidly obese patient: 18 total calories per kg of body weight

Protein requirements: Usually 0.8-1.5 g/kg/24 hr. (Protein will be restricted if patients have hepatic or renal failure that is not being treated with dialysis. Protein needs may be higher in patients on continuous renal replacement therapy or suffering from burns or large wounds.)

Carbohydrate (CHO) requirements: Excess amounts of CHO are not utilized or tolerated. Overfeeding of CHO may lead to hyperglycemia, increased CO_2 production, hypophosphatemia, and fluid overload in short-term use or fatty liver syndrome in long-term use. Patients with diabetes will need to be counseled regarding how to count carbohydrates for appropriate glycemic control (see "Diabetes Mellitus").

Fat requirements: Saturated fat intake should be limited, especially in patients with coronary artery disease.

Vitamin and essential trace mineral requirements: In general, follow the recommended daily allowances (RDAs) to provide minimum quantities of vitamins, minerals, and essential fatty acids. For specific patients, supplement vitamins or minerals needed in increased amounts for existing disease states (e.g., pressure ulcers/wounds: zinc, vitamins A and C; chronic alcohol ingestion: thiamine, folate, vitamin B_{12}).

Fluid requirements: Many factors affect fluid balance. Under usual circumstances an estimate of fluid needs can be made by providing 30-50 mL/kg body weight. Daily loss of water includes approximately 1400 mL in urine (60 mL/hr), 350 mL via respiration, 600 mL as evaporation through skin, and about 200 mL in feces. Fluid losses are 100-150 mL/day for each degree of temperature increase above 37° C. If loss by any of these routes is increased, fluid needs increase; if loss by any of these routes is impaired, fluid restriction may be necessary. Areas to include in the nursing assessment for fluid requirements are:
- Intake and output (I&O). Evaluate that neither one is in excess of the other and for decreases in urine output.
- Daily weights.

Note: *Rapid changes may represent problems with technique or equipment rather than actual changes in body weight. If sudden increases in weight occur, look for imbalances in I&O, occurrence of edema, and dilution of serum electrolytes.*

- Presence or absence of edema.
- Large wounds, burns, or open abdomen. Nurses should monitor the amount of exudate captured in a wound vacuum device.

- Skin turgor. This assessment may be helpful in younger patients, but is less useful in older adults due to normal changes in skin elasticity that occurs with aging.

Nutritional support modalities

Specialized nutritional support refers to provision of an artificial formulation of nutrients via oral, enteral, or parenteral route for the treatment or prevention of malnutrition. Oral supplements are the preferred route because they are less invasive, more natural, and less costly, whereas enteral nutrition is preferred over parenteral.

Types of feeding tubes

Small-bore nasal tubes: Defined as 12 French or smaller. Composition may be polyurethane, silicone, or polyvinyl chloride, and usual length is 36-55 in. It may or may not require a stylet for insertion. Location cannot be verified in the gastrointestinal (GI) tract when using auscultation after injecting an air bolus, asking the patient to speak, or submerging the tube's proximal tip into a glass of water. Standard of practice dictates that an abdominal x-ray examination is needed for confirmation of placement. The FDA has approved use of an electromagnetically guided placement device to confirm tube placement. There continues to be risk of misplacement regardless of the technique used for placement. The physician determines whether the distal tip ends in the stomach or small intestine. It also may be inserted using endoscopy- or fluoroscopy-guided placement. Because of their diameter and composition, these tubes are easily dislocated proximally in the GI tract without any resultant external signs.

Large-bore nasal tubes: Defined as larger than 12 French with composition either polyurethane or polyvinyl chloride. Usual length of the tube is 36 in. A stylet is not required for insertion. Insertion may be by a nurse. Placement is confirmed by withdrawal of gastric fluid or x-ray examination.

Gastrostomy tubes: Exit stomach directly through the abdominal wall and usually are anchored with either a balloon or disc on the inside of the stomach. Usually they are 12 French or larger. Composition may be polyurethane, silicone, or rubber and may contain multiple ports, in addition to the main lumen, for insertion of air into the balloon and delivery of medications. Initially a physician in radiology, endoscopy, or surgery performs the insertion. If not placed during surgery (i.e., open laparotomy), the common term used to describe the tube is *percutaneous endoscopically inserted gastrostomy (PEG)*. Reinsertion by a nurse is determined by agency policy. Inadvertent removal of a tube in position for less than 6 wk should be considered a medical emergency and the health care provider should be contacted immediately. To preserve the tube tract a Foley catheter may be inserted with air added to the balloon to form a bumper. An abdominal radiograph should be taken after soluble Gastrografin® has been infused into the replacement tube to ensure proper position prior to use.

Gastrostomy button: Placed into a mature gastrostomy stoma. It fits into the stoma tract flush with the outer abdominal wall. The button contains an antireflux valve to prevent leakage, but gastric samples or residuals usually cannot be obtained via the button.

Jejunostomy tubes: Placed by a physician either surgically or percutaneously (PEJ). Diameter is usually about 12-18 French. Anchoring the tube inside the jejunum presents a problem because a balloon larger than 5 mL might cause bowel obstruction. Confirmation of position requires x-ray examination with contrast. No residuals should be obtained from this tube. If the tube becomes displaced, the entry site into the jejunum will close down rapidly (approximately 20-30 min). Reinsertion by a nurse is determined by agency policy, but it is not recommended without special training.

Gastrostomy-jejunostomy tubes: Exit the stomach directly through the abdominal wall with a small-bore jejunostomy tube placed through the main lumen of the gastrostomy and the distal tip positioned in the jejunum.

Feeding sites

Stomach: Simulates normal GI functions; may be used for bolus, intermittent, or continuous feedings; indicated for patients who have intact gag or cough reflexes.

Duodenum, jejunum: Must be used for continuous feedings only to prevent dumping syndrome and diarrhea. Small-bore diameter tube is recommended.

Total parenteral nutrition

Total parenteral nutrition (TPN) provides some or all nutrients by the IV route. TPN is used to provide complete nutrition for patients who cannot receive enteral nutrition or to supplement nutritional needs of patients who are unable to absorb sufficient calories via the GI tract. TPN is more expensive than enteral nutrition and has the potential for developing severe complications more rapidly.

Parenteral solutions: IV solutions are customized combinations of dextrose (CHO), amino acids (protein), IV fat emulsions (fat), electrolytes, vitamins, and trace metals.

CHOs: Dextrose provides approximately 50%-60% of the total calories. Final compounded concentrations will range from 5% to 70%. All final mixed solutions that are more than 12.5% dextrose must be administered via a central venous catheter. (If unsure or information is unavailable on the infusion container related to infusion route, consult with a pharmacist or refer to hospital policy.) The more CHO delivered, the greater the potential for complications, which include fatty liver syndrome, increased CO_2 production, hyperglycemia, and intracellular flux of potassium, magnesium, and phosphorus.

Protein: Synthetic crystalline essential and nonessential amino acid formulations are available in concentrations of 3.5%-15%. The amount of protein delivered depends on the patient's estimated protein requirements while considering renal and hepatic function. Patients receiving dialysis have higher protein needs than a similar patient not on dialysis.

Fat: IV fat emulsion (IVFE) of 10%, 20%, or 30% is an isotonic solution providing essential fatty acids and a source of concentrated calories.

When fats are mixed in the same infusion bag with the CHO and amino acids, the solution is referred to as a *total nutrient admixture (TNA)* or *3:1 solution* (all three nutrient components in one bag). The IVFE also may be given piggyback into the amino acid/dextrose infusion to infuse over 8-12 hr. The amount of IVFE administered may be reduced or removed for patients who are septic, morbidly obese, or have hypertriglyceridemia or liver failure. IVFEs also should be held in patients with an egg allergy because long-chain triglycerides in IVFEs may originate from phospholipids in egg yolks. If a patient develops a rash during IVFE infusion, consider an allergy immediately. If the ratio of protein, CHO, and IVFE in the admixture is not stable, separation of the IV fats from the emulsion may occur, which is called "cracking" of the solution. The IV fats may float on top of the mixture much like an egg yolk floating in the solution or appear as an uneven yellow consistency. In addition, "oiling out" may occur, which looks like an oil slick or oil droplets on top of the solution. Return any solution that appears "different" to the pharmacy and do not use it.

Selection of administration site

Central venous catheter: Used for all IV solutions whose final concentration is greater than 12.5% dextrose or a solution with an osmolarity of 800 mOsm/L or greater. (If unsure or information is unavailable on the infusion container related to infusion route, consult with a pharmacist or refer to hospital policy.) Central venous catheter (CVC) use requires a large central vein with the distal tip of the catheter in the superior vena cava. The flow of blood through the large vessels rapidly dilutes hypertonic solutions and decreases the potential for thrombophlebitis.

Peripheral venous catheter: Reserved for individuals with a need for nutritional support for short-term periods, with small nutritional requirements, and for whom CVC access is unavailable. Only a low-osmolarity solution (less than 800 mOsm/L) can be used. To reduce osmolarity of the base solution, dilution of the components is usually required. The required large volume limits the type of patients in whom this admixture can be administered. (If unsure or information is unavailable on the infusion container related to infusion route, consult with a pharmacist or refer to hospital policy.)

Transitional feeding

A transition is necessary before discontinuing nutritional support. Reduce the percent of total calories supplied from enteral nutrition as oral intake increases to 60%-70% of estimated needs. Similarly, patients who have received TPN for more than 2-3 wk may have some mucosal atrophy of the bowel and will need a period of adjustment before the bowel can fully resume its usual functions of digestion and absorption. The best diet advancement includes starting with clear liquids, then advancing to a soft diet. Because these individuals have been ill, the lactase in their stomach has decreased, placing them at higher risk for lactose deficiency; therefore, they should limit or avoid a full liquid diet because of increased incidence of bloating, nausea, and diarrhea associated with lactose deficiency.

Nursing Diagnosis:

Imbalanced Nutrition: Less Than Body Requirements

related to inability to ingest, digest, or absorb carbohydrates, protein, and/or fat

Desired Outcome: The patient has adequate nutrition as evidenced by stabilization of weight at the desired level or steady weight gain of $\frac{1}{2}$-1 lb/wk; presence of wound granulation (i.e., pinkish white tissue around wound edges; wound edges approximating together), and absence of infection (see **Risk for Infection,** later).

ASSESSMENT/INTERVENTIONS	RATIONALES
For Oral Nutrition:	
Assess for nutritional deficiencies within 24 hr of admission with a nutritional screening tool; document and reassess weekly.	Hospitalized patients are at risk for developing protein-energy malnutrition. Baseline assessment enables comparison with subsequent assessments, which may reveal problems that may require interventions. Because no single sensitive and comprehensive nutritional assessment factor exists, multiple sources of information are used, including any of the following: historical data, nutritional history, anthropometric data, biochemical analysis of blood and urine, and duration of the disease process.
Assess for food allergies/intolerances and avoid these foods.	Individuals with celiac disease, for example, will have severe GI reactions (i.e., bloating, abdominal cramping, diarrhea) when exposed to even small amounts of wheat and other gluten-containing products.

ASSESSMENT/INTERVENTIONS   RATIONALES

ASSESSMENT/INTERVENTIONS	RATIONALES
Obtain weight weekly.	Stabilizing weight or a weight gain of ½-1 lb/wk is the usual goal if weight gain is desired.
Position the patient in high Fowler's position for eating.	This promotes normal position for eating and decreases risk of aspiration.
Provide small, frequent feedings of diet compatible with the disease state and the patient's ability to ingest foods.	After an illness, early satiety may be a problem. Small, frequent meals are likely to increase intake.
Respect food aversions, religious guidelines, and food preferences.	Individuals will eat more readily and frequently when consuming preferred foods that are within dietary allowances.
Provide liquid nutritional supplements as prescribed.	Supplements increase calories consumed and help meet RDAs for vitamins and minerals needed for recovery.
Serve cold or over ice.	Serving cold will help enhance palatability.
Provide psychologic support	Emotional health influences appetite.
Involve significant other in meal rituals for companionship.	Patients who eat alone tend to eat less.

For Enteral or Parenteral Nutrition in the Acute Care Setting:

Assess for nutritional deficiencies within 24 hr of admission with a nutritional screening tool; document and reassess weekly.	Hospitalized patients are at risk for developing protein-calorie malnutrition. Baseline assessment enables comparison with subsequent assessments, which may reveal problems that may require intervention. Because no single sensitive and comprehensive nutritional assessment factor exists, multiple sources of information are used, including any of the following: historical data, nutritional history, anthropometric data, biochemical analysis of blood and urine, and duration of the disease process.
Assess initial and at least weekly values of electrolytes, blood urea nitrogen (BUN), creatinine, phosphorus, and magnesium.	Values outside the normal range may signal changing metabolic status, decreased renal function, or refeeding syndrome.
[!] Assess daily if concern for refeeding syndrome exists.	Refeeding syndrome is the consequence realized after a large CHO infusion in a patient with previous inadequate food intake and may result in fluid retention, hypophosphatemia, hypokalemia, hypomagnesium, increased diarrhea, and cardiac dysrhythmias.
Assess other laboratory data initially and then at least weekly; liver function tests, including albumin, alkaline phosphatase, total bilirubin.	These laboratory values provide data about tolerance, clearance, and metabolism by organs and stabilization of the disease process.
Assess for fluid imbalance, especially fluid volume excess.	Patients may be especially susceptible to fluid excess because low protein levels in the blood cause a decrease in oncotic pressure in the vessels, resulting in fluid retention. Fluid excess may be manifested by peripheral edema, adventitious breath sounds (especially crackles), and weight gain (1 kg = 1000 mL).
Assess the patient's weight initially and daily during an acute illness, then advance to weekly.	Stabilized weight or weight gain of ½-1 lb/wk is the usual goal if weight gain is an intended goal. Weight trend also assesses fluid status and disease process.
Administer continuous enteral feedings using a pump at the prescribed rate.	A steady infusion rate decreases feelings of fullness and avoids peaks in blood glucose levels. Postoperative patients may experience gastric ileus and benefit from feeds delivered into the small bowel.
Check infused volume and rate q4h.	This helps ensure accuracy of the prescribed delivery.
Administer intermittent feeding over 30-40 min via gravity drip.	Intermittent feeding is similar to the natural pattern of eating.
Administer TPN using a volumetric pump at the prescribed rate.	There is potential for complications if dextrose or electrolytes are infused too quickly, such as hyperglycemia and hyperkalemia. An approved continuous rate for volume is better tolerated.
Check infused volume and rate q4h.	Checking volume and rate prevents volume overload and other complications that could occur when using the pump.
Ensure that the patient receives the prescribed caloric intake.	Adequate amounts of CHO, protein, and fat are necessary during the recovery phase of illness for healing and rebuilding.

Nursing Diagnosis:

Risk for Aspiration

related to GI feeding or delayed gastric emptying

Desired Outcome: The patient is free of aspiration problems as evidenced by auscultation of clear lung sounds, VS within normal limits for the patient, and no signs of respiratory distress.

ASSESSMENT/INTERVENTIONS	RATIONALES
Assess placement of the nasogastric (NG) tube. Mark the NG tube at the time of placement to determine length exiting from the body. Check this mark to determine tube migration. Secure tubing in place per agency policy.	The NG tube can easily slide out of the nose because of nasal discharge, sweat, and loosening of the tape or tube holder. The tube also may migrate beyond the pylorus over time.
Reassess tube position q4h and before each feeding.	If tube migration is suspected or the tube is reinserted, obtain x-ray to confirm placement.
Assess respiratory status q4h, including respiratory rate, effort, and adventitious breath sounds.	Lung sounds should be clear, and there should be no signs of respiratory distress before infusing a feeding.
- Regurgitation or vomiting of gastric contents	Aspiration of gastric contents is a risk factor for ventilator-associated pneumonia, which is the leading cause of hospital-associated death.
- Aspiration from the oropharynx of saliva and upper airway secretions.	Aspiration of bacteria from the oral and pharyngeal areas may cause bacterial pneumonia.
Monitor temperature q4h; report any parameters as defined by the health care provider.	Temperature outside of parameters as defined by the health care provider should be reported. An increased temperature occurs with aspiration pneumonia.
Auscultate bowel sounds q8h.	High-pitched or absent bowel sounds, abdominal distention, or nausea can occur with ileus, decreased tolerance to the feeding, and small bowel obstruction. These problems can lead to vomiting and aspiration and therefore should be reported promptly.
Depending on the patient's medical condition, raise the head of bed 30 degrees or higher or place the patient in a right side-lying position during and for 1 hr after administration of a bolus or intermittent feeding.	These positions promote gravity flow from the greater stomach curvature through the pylorus into the duodenum and decrease risk for aspiration.
Stop the tube feeding ½-1 hr before chest physical therapy or placing the patient supine.	This measure enables complete emptying of the stomach and decreases potential for aspiration.
Check residuals per agency policy.	The best practice is to hold the feeding if residuals are 200 mL from an NG or orogastric tube or 100 mL from a gastrostomy. High-volume residuals may be a sign of intolerance because of ileus or small bowel obstruction, either of which can lead to vomiting and aspiration.
Recognize that no residuals or minimal volume should be obtained from a tube placed into the small intestine.	Unlike the stomach, the small intestine does not function as a reservoir and therefore normally will not hold volume because of forward peristalsis.
Avoid use of formulas that have been tinted with coloring to assess for aspiration.	Published case reports describe fatal metabolic acidosis secondary to the excessive use of food coloring in enteral feedings. This practice has received a warning from the Food and Drug Administration and should not be used under any circumstance.

Nursing Diagnosis:

Diarrhea

related to medications, dumping syndrome, bacterial contamination, or formula intolerance

Desired Outcome: The patient has formed stools within 2-3 days of intervention.

ASSESSMENT/INTERVENTIONS	RATIONALES
Assess abdomen and GI status: bowel sounds, distention, cramping, nausea, and frequency of bowel movements.	These assessments establish a baseline and reference point from which the current trend can be compared. Hyperactive bowel sounds may occur with increased stooling, along with signs and symptoms of distention, cramping, and nausea.
Ask the patient to define diarrhea. Determine the patient's normal stool pattern.	One loose stool does not mean a patient has diarrhea. Liquid intake normally produces a pasty stool, and patients may misinterpret this as diarrhea. Enteral feedings may produce several soft-formed stools per day.
Assess hydration status by recording and evaluating I&O every shift and checking weight daily. Obtain parameter from the health care provider for notification.	An example of a parameter established by the health care provider for dehydration would be a decrease in urinary output to less than 30 mL/hr $\times$ 4 hr or increased stool output greater than a specific volume over an 8-hr period. Daily weight measurement is used to assess fluid status. For example, a loss of 1 kg/day could signal a loss of 1000 mL.
Suggest a review of medications by the pharmacy for patients with diarrhea, especially those with a history of multiple bowel surgeries, GI hypersecretion, or intestinal failure.	Pharmacists are knowledgeable about medications that cause diarrhea as well as those that are used to treat diarrhea associated with GI abnormalities. Some of these medications include prokinetic agents and stool softeners.
Contact the pharmacy about elixirs being administered. Discuss with the health care provider and pharmacist changing the form of medication or switching to another medication within the same class.	The majority of elixirs contain sorbitol, which will increase transit time in the intestines and cause diarrhea.
Consult with the health care provider regarding collection of a stool sample for bacterial culture and sensitivity, ova and parasites, or for *Clostridium difficile* toxin.	Diarrhea may be caused by bacteria or parasites. If *C. difficile* is present, the volume of the daily stool output may exceed 500 mL and will occur whether or not the individual consumes food or enteral products. This type of diarrhea is considered secretory because the fluid is secreted from the intestinal wall and can lead to imbalances in fluid status.
Do not administer an antidiarrheal medication until the stool culture is confirmed as negative.	Giving this medication when the stool culture is positive increases risk for toxic megacolon and bowel perforation.
If the patient is receiving a bolus feeding, switch to intermittent or continuous feedings.	Bolus feedings may contribute to dumping syndrome, which would result in increased diarrhea.
Follow hazard analysis and critical control point (HACCP) guidelines for handling of enteral products, feeding tube, and feeding sets. Change all equipment per agency policy.	Bacteria can grow in feeding sets and on hands of the caregiver and could cause diarrhea if allowed to be transported to the patient.
Store all products according to manufacturer's recommendations.	These products are a potential growth media for bacteria and could cause diarrhea if the product is given to the patient. All manufacturers state on their products to discard after opened for 24 hr and store in refrigerator. Unopened products should be stored at room temperature to prevent clumping of proteins in the container.
Use enteral solutions at room temperature for a maximum of 12 hr when using an open delivery system vs. 24-48 hr when using a closed system. Check with manufacturer guidelines for the specific duration of hang time.	This reduces risk of bacterial contamination. Closed systems reduce the risk of touch contamination.
Identify the tube as enteral access before attaching the closed system.	This measure reduces the risk of inadvertent infusion of enteral feeding into an IV port.

Nursing Diagnosis:

Nausea

related to underlying medical condition, too rapid infusion of enteral product, food intolerance, or medication administration

Desired Outcome: Following interventions, the patient has no nausea with food intake.

ASSESSMENT/INTERVENTIONS	RATIONALES
Assess the abdomen for distention and auscultate bowel sounds.	Absence of or high-pitched bowel sounds may signal ileus or obstruction. Decreased bowel sounds may indicate need to decrease the feeding and check stool output. Distention may appear either with ileus or with decreased motility. These signs would necessitate notifying the health care provider for intervention.
Assess for and record flatus and bowel movements.	Decreased bowel movements and flatus may indicate ileus or partial obstruction.
Assess electrolyte values, especially potassium.	Hypokalemia is associated with ileus and nausea.
Give an antiemetic as prescribed.	An antiemetic decreases/eliminates nausea.
Administer medication on an empty stomach only when indicated.	Medications such as analgesics may cause nausea if given without food.
Offer food in small portions, six times per day.	Smaller meals are better tolerated than larger meals.
Give chewing gum or hard candies prn, if permitted.	Providing some sugar to the system may stimulate the GI tract and decrease nausea.
Suggest the patient brush teeth and tongue q8h and prn.	A bad taste in the mouth may increase nausea in some individuals.
If the odor of food induces nausea, remove the food immediately.	This will help eliminate nausea caused by odor.
Reduce the rate/min of enteral formula infusion.	Nausea may be caused by an increased infusion rate, which may result in delayed gastric emptying, overdistention, or constipation.
If the patient is receiving a bolus infusion, change to intermittent or continuous.	Overdistention with a bolus infusion may cause or increase nausea, whereas a slower infusion rate with an intermittent or continuous infusion may be better tolerated.
If medically indicated, consider a bowel suppository.	This will stimulate the intestinal tract. Nausea may occur secondary to constipation or decreased motility.

Nursing Diagnosis:

Constipation

related to inadequate fluid and fiber in the diet

Desired Outcome: The patient states that he or she has had a soft bowel movement within 3-4 days of this diagnosis (or within the patient's usual pattern).

ASSESSMENT/INTERVENTIONS	RATIONALES
Assess the abdomen for distention and auscultate bowel sounds.	A distended abdomen may signal a backup of stool and gas in the colon.
If the patient is receiving a formula that contains fiber, assess intake of free water.	Fiber pulls more fluid into the intestines. When a patient is "dry" from medical therapy, there is no extra water to pull, and if no extra water is available, constipation will occur. Optimally water intake should be 1 mL/calorie of intake or 30-50 mL/kg body weight in order to compensate for losses that occur normally via respirations, urination, fever, and so on.

ASSESSMENT/INTERVENTIONS	RATIONALES
Give free water q4h or as prescribed and after each medication for enterally fed patients. Encourage adequate oral fluid intake for patients on an oral diet.	Free water helps maintain fluid balance and patency of the feeding tube, as well as promote soft stools and prevent constipation.
Discuss with the health care provider and pharmacist the possibility of a reduction in the amount of narcotics being administered.	Opioid medications are constipating. The patient may need a stool softener or motility enhancer.
Consider a stool softener, especially if the patient regularly uses a laxative at home.	If the patient is unable to increase water needs effectively, a stool softener will prevent straining and decrease risk of constipation.

Nursing Diagnosis:

Impaired Swallowing

related to decreased or absent gag reflex, facial paralysis, mechanical obstruction, fatigue, weight loss, or decreased strength or excursion of muscles involved in mastication

Desired Outcome: Before food or fluids are initiated, the patient demonstrates adequate cough and gag reflexes and the ability to ingest foods via the phases of swallowing as instructed.

ASSESSMENT/INTERVENTIONS	RATIONALES
Assess oral motor function within 24 hr of admission or on a change in a medical condition.	If the patient has adequate oral motor functioning, oral intake can be increased with dietary texture restrictions. Otherwise, texture restrictions (e.g., puree), liquid restrictions (e.g., thickened liquids), or tube feedings should be considered to prevent aspiration.
Assess cough and gag reflexes before the first feeding.	Patients who develop gastric reflux or vomit can aspirate if their cough and gag reflexes are not intact.
Offer semisolid foods and progress to thicker textures as tolerated.	If the patient is likely to have difficulty with swallowing, liquids will be the most difficult and most likely to be aspirated.
Coach the patient through the phases of ingesting food: opening the mouth, inserting food, closing the lips, chewing, transferring food from side to side in the mouth and then to the back of the oral cavity, elevating the tongue to the roof of the mouth (hard palate), and swallowing between breaths.	With illness, muscles may become weaker, and this may result in bad habits of rushing swallowing and moving food into the trachea rather than into the esophagus, where it is less likely to be aspirated.
Order extra sauces, gravies, or liquids if dryness of the oral cavity impairs swallowing ability.	This moistens each bite of food for patients in whom dryness of the oral cavity impairs swallowing ability.
If tolerated, keep the patient in high Fowler's position for ½ hr after eating.	This position minimizes risk of aspiration by promoting gravity flow through the stomach and into the duodenum.
Provide mouth care before and after meals and dietary supplements.	This measure ensures that all traces of food are removed, preventing subsequent aspiration.
Provide small, frequent meals.	Six smaller feedings per day may increase muscle strength needed for swallowing and be less likely to result in rushing, which could cause aspiration.
Provide foods at temperatures acceptable to the patient.	Foods that are too hot or too cold could rush swallowing and lead to aspiration.
As indicated, obtain services of a speech, physical, or occupational therapist.	These specialists assist in retraining or facilitating the patient's swallowing.

Nursing Diagnosis:

Risk for Infection

related to invasive procedures, nasoenteric or nasogastric tube, decreased nutritional intake, malnutrition, and suppression of the immune system

Desired Outcome: The patient is free of infection as evidenced by temperature, pulse, and respirations within the patient's normal range and absence of the following clinical signs of sepsis: erythema, swelling at the catheter insertion site, chills, fever, and glucose intolerance.

ASSESSMENT/INTERVENTIONS	RATIONALES
Assess the patient routinely for signs and symptoms of infection, including white blood cell (WBC) count with differential for values outside normal range and increased temperature.	A higher value signals infection. Infection requires extra calories. A fever increases fluid requirements.
Assess bedside glucose for values outside the normal range. If the individual is glucose intolerant, begin q4h bedside assessment and administer sliding scale insulin as prescribed by the health care provider.	Glucose intolerance is a sign of sepsis. An increase in glucose also promotes bacterial growth and increases risk of infection. Insulin is given to maintain blood glucose within normal limits.
Assess catheter insertion site q12h for erythema, swelling, or purulent discharge.	These are signs of local infection.
Change gauze dressings routinely every 48 hr or immediately if the integrity is breached. Change transparent semipermeable membrane (TSM) dressing at least every 7 days.	Gauze dressings prevent visualization of the insertion site. Blood on the gauze is considered a break in the dressing's integrity. (Infusion Nursing "The Standards of Practice" 2006 Standard S44 Dressings).
Use meticulous sterile technique when changing central line dressing, containers, or administration lines. Follow agency policy for central line dressing changes.	These measures reduce the possibility of infection.
Consult the health care provider to obtain a prescription for blood cultures at two sites as outlined by the Centers for Disease Control and Prevention (CDC) in patients with a central line who are febrile with a rising WBC count.	Two positive cultures may indicate a bloodstream infection requiring antibiotic treatment.
Restrict use of the lumen used for administration of TPN, if possible. Avoid drawing blood specimens or other fluids, pressure monitoring, or medication administration, if possible.	When TPN is being administered, most infections of catheters and blood are related to the insertion site or tubing sets.
Change all administration sets, as established by the CDC.	This is a standard infection prevention protocol.

Nursing Diagnosis:

Risk for Imbalanced Fluid Volume

related to failure of regulatory mechanisms, hyperglycemia, medications, fever, infection, fluid administration, or immobility

Desired Outcome: The patient's hydration status is adequate, as evidenced by baseline vital signs (VS), serum glucose less than 200 mg/dL, balanced I&O, 1-2 lb weight gain/wk, and serum electrolytes and WBC count within normal limits.

ASSESSMENT/INTERVENTIONS	RATIONALES
Assess rate and volume of nutritional support q4h.	This assessment helps ensure the prescribed rate and volume are delivered, thereby preventing volume overload or deficiency.
Assess the patient's weight daily initially, and advance to weekly.	Baseline will determine weight goals; subsequent assessments will determine efficacy of those goals.

ASSESSMENT/INTERVENTIONS

ASSESSMENT/INTERVENTIONS	RATIONALES
Assess I&O q8h or more frequently if medically indicated.	This measure assesses for imbalances and trends toward overhydration or dehydration.
Assess electrolytes daily, and advance to a minimum of weekly, depending on the patient's medical condition.	This assesses for hypovolemia or hypervolemia. Changes in sodium, chloride, and BUN levels may indicate changes in fluid status.
Assess for signs of circulatory overload during fluid replacement.	Signs of circulatory overload may occur during fluid replacement, including peripheral edema, bounding pulse, jugular distention, and adventitious lung sounds (especially crackles). Circulatory overload is more likely to occur in older adults or individuals with heart failure or other chronic medical conditions such as renal insufficiency in which output is decreased, even if fluids are delivered properly.

ADDITIONAL NURSING DIAGNOSES/PROBLEMS:

"Managing Wound Care" for **Impaired Tissue Integrity**　　　p. 533

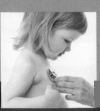

Asthma 75

OVERVIEW/PATHOPHYSIOLOGY

Asthma is a chronic, reversible (in most cases) obstructive airway disease characterized by inflammation and mucosal edema, increased sensitivity of the airways, and airway obstruction (bronchospasm and in some children, excessive, thick mucus). Increased inflammation causes increased sensitivity of the airways and is the most common feature of asthma.

The prevalence of asthma and associated morbidity rates continue to rise in children. Asthma is one of the leading causes of chronic illness in children as well as being the third leading cause of hospitalization in children under age 15 yr. An estimated 7.1 million children under age 18 yr have asthma, and 4.1 million experienced an asthma attack or episode in 2011 (American Lung Association Fact Sheet, 2012). There is an increased incidence in boys, children in poor families and/or in fair-poor health, and in African Americans (National Center for Health Statistics, National Health Interview Survey, 2013). Asthma is one of the leading causes of school absences and, in 2008, accounted for an estimated loss of 14.4 million school days in children with an asthma attack in the previous year. It is also the third leading cause of hospitalizations and resulted in 774,000 emergency room visits in 2009 of children less than 15 yr with significant direct and indirect costs totaling $56 billion. The incidence of death due to asthma has decreased, with about 3300 deaths in 2009, and is rare in children; only 157 children died from asthma that year (American Lung Association Fact Sheet, 2012).

The National Asthma Education and Prevention Program (NAEPP) published updated guidelines for diagnosis and management in 2007. The Expert Panel Report 3 (EPR-3) focuses on new guidelines for deciding treatment based on individual needs (looking at age and severity) and level of asthma control. It stresses that conditions change over time and regular monitoring is essential so that treatment can be adjusted as needed. Guidelines for children have been expanded to include 0-4 years, 5-11 years, and 12 years and older with stepwise approach for severity and control. Severity classification has been revised to include intermittent or persistent (mild, moderate, or severe). Each step includes the patient/family education, environmental control, and management of comorbidities. Assessing asthma control and adjusting therapy depend on classification of control (well controlled, not well controlled, and very poorly controlled)

(NAEPP EPR-3, 2007). National Heart, Lung, and Blood Institute (NHLBI) guidelines were revised in 2012 based on the NAEPP EPR-3 and stresses control, focusing on two areas—reducing impairment (frequency and intensity of symptoms and impairment) and reducing risk (future attacks, reduced lung growth, or side effects of medications).

HEALTH CARE SETTING

Primary care, with possible hospitalization resulting from severe acute attacks

ASSESSMENT

It is important to obtain a detailed history of current problems as well as past episodes.

Common early warning signs: Breathing changes, sneezing, moodiness, headache, itchy/watery eyes, dark circles under eyes, easy fatigue, sore throat, trouble sleeping, chest or throat itchiness, downward trend in peak flow values, cough especially at night (a common symptom of asthma), slight tightness in the chest.

Symptoms of acute episode: Coughing, shortness of breath, dyspnea, anxiety, apprehension, tightness in chest, and wheezing (primarily on expiration).

Severe asthma symptoms: Severe coughing, shortness of breath, tightness in the chest and/or wheezing, and difficulty talking, eating, or concentrating. The mucosal edema causes shortness of breath, tachypnea or bradypnea, hunched shoulders (posturing), suprasternal and intercostal retractions, cyanosis, increasing dyspnea, nasal flaring and use of accessory muscles, extreme anxiety, and apprehension.

Symptoms of severe respiratory distress and impending respiratory failure: Profuse diaphoresis, sitting upright and refusing to lie down, suddenly becoming agitated or becoming quiet when previously agitated, decrease in or absence of wheezing.

Physical assessment: Chest has hyperresonance on percussion. Breath sounds are loud and coarse, with sonorous crackles throughout the lung fields. Prolonged expiration is noted. Coarse rhonchi may be heard, as well as generalized inspiratory and expiratory wheezing. As obstruction increases, wheezing becomes more high pitched. With minimal obstruction, wheezing may be mild, heard only on end expiration with auscultation, or absent. Breath sounds and crackles may become inaudible with severe obstruction or bronchospasm.

Posturing occurs to facilitate breathing. Pulsus paradoxus (an abnormally large decrease in systolic blood pressure and pulse wave amplitude during inspiration) also may be noted because of lung hyperinflation.

Children with chronic asthma may develop a barrel chest with depressed diaphragm, elevated shoulders, and increased use of accessory muscles of respiration.

Caution: If symptoms are untreated or treated unsuccessfully, an acute asthma attack may progress to *status asthmaticus*, a severe unrelenting attack. Status asthmaticus is an acute, severe, and prolonged asthma attack in which respiratory distress continues despite vigorous therapeutic measures and may result in death.

DIAGNOSTIC TESTS

Arterial blood gas (ABG) values: Reveal status of oxygenation and acid-base balance. In severe asthma exacerbation with PaO_2 less than 60 mm Hg (on room air) and $PaCO_2$ 42 mm Hg or greater, the child may have cyanosis and may progress to respiratory failure. ABG values are not obtained often in children except in an intensive care unit and with initial assessment in order to provide atraumatic care. If possible, topical anesthetics are used to decrease pain and anxiety with blood draws.

Pulse oximetry: Noninvasive method that reveals decreased O_2 saturation (usually less than 93%-95%, depending on protocol of the facility) and helps provide atraumatic care.

Pulmonary function tests (spirometry): Provide an objective method of evaluating presence and degree of lung disease, as well as response to treatment, and usually can be performed reliably on children by 5 or 6 yr of age. These tests typically show diminished maximal breathing capacity, tidal volume, and timed vital capacity.

Chest x-ray examination: To rule out pneumonia and assess for air trapping. It is also used to evaluate possible cardiomegaly secondary to pulmonary hypertension resulting from chronic obstruction. Typical findings in a child with significant asthma symptoms are hyperinflation, atelectasis, and flattened diaphragm.

Complete blood count: May show slight elevation during acute asthma, but white blood cell elevations greater than 12,000/mm^3 or an increased percentage of band cells may indicate a respiratory infection. Eosinophils greater than 500/mm^3 tend to suggest an allergic or inflammatory disorder.

Peak expiratory flow rate: Assesses severity of asthma by measuring the maximum flow of air that can be forcefully exhaled in 1 sec using a peak flow meter (PFM). Each child's peak expiratory flow rate (PEFR) varies according to age, height, sex, and race. Once the personal best value is established, it is recommended that it be done 1-2 times/day in children with moderate-to-severe persistent asthma. The child should measure the PEFR three times with at least 30 sec between each measurement; then record the highest reading. Maintaining a diary or log book is beneficial and helps direct the plan of care. While this test is used for monitoring control, it is not used for the initial diagnosis.

Sputum: Gross examination may reveal increased viscosity or actual mucus plugs. Culture and sensitivity may reveal microorganisms if infection was the precipitating event. Cytologic examination will reveal elevated eosinophils, which is commonly associated with asthma. It is rarely done in children.

Serum theophylline level: Important baseline indicator for patients who are receiving this therapy, although it is used infrequently. NAEPP EPR-3 does not recommend oral theophylline as a long-term control medication for children 5 yr of age or less; it can be used in older children as adjunctive medication. The guidelines do not recommend it for asthma exacerbations. Current guidelines call for a serum concentration of 5-15 mcg/mL. Theophylline toxicity can occur with serum levels greater than 20 mcg/mL. Side effects include nausea, vomiting, headache, irritability, and insomnia. Early signs of toxicity are nausea, tachycardia, irritability, and seizures. Dysrhythmias occur at serum levels greater than 30 mcg/mL.

Skin testing: The 2007 revised guidelines issued by the NAEPP EPR-3 recommend consideration of subcutaneous allergen immunotherapy for patients with allergic asthma.

Nursing Diagnosis:

Ineffective Airway Clearance

related to bronchospasm, mucosal edema, and increased mucus production

Desired Outcomes: Child with a significant asthma attack: Within 48 hr of interventions/treatment, adventitious breath sounds, cough, and increased work of breathing (WOB) are decreased. Within 72 hr, the respiratory rate (RR) returns to the child's normal range, and retractions and nasal flaring disappear. *Child with a mild asthma attack:* Within 3 hr after interventions/treatment, adventitious breath sounds and cough are decreased, and retractions and nasal flaring are absent.

> **Note:** *WOB means ease or effort of breathing. Signs of increased WOB include nasal flaring, retractions, and use of accessory muscles.*

ASSESSMENT/INTERVENTIONS	RATIONALES
Assess respiratory status with the initial assessment, with each vital sign check, and prn.	After establishing the baseline, changes can be detected quickly with subsequent assessments, enabling rapid intervention.
Assess RR, heart rate (HR), O₂ saturation, and breath sounds before and several minutes after each nebulizer treatment or metered-dose inhaler (MDI) administration.	These assessments help determine the child's status and effectiveness of medication in decreasing bronchospasm or mucosal edema and enabling more effective airway clearance.
Administer nebulizer treatment or MDI, usually albuterol, as prescribed.	These therapies decrease bronchospasm or mucosal edema, thereby opening the airway and enabling more effective airway clearance.
Use a spacer or holding chamber when administering MDI.	This is the most effective method of getting the maximum amount of medication delivered to a child. A mask may be required with a spacer in children less than 5 yr of age or anyone who is unable to seal the lips effectively around the mouthpiece.
Hold the albuterol treatment if the HR is: - Greater than 180 bpm (children 2 to 3 yr) - Greater than 160 bpm (children 3 to 6 yr) - Greater than 140 bpm (children 6 to 12 yr) - Greater than 120 bpm (children older than 12 yr) Notify the health care provider as directed.	Tachycardia is a major side effect of albuterol. When it is present, the health care provider needs to assess the patient to ensure that side effects of medication do not outweigh the benefit of decreasing bronchospasm.
Position the child in high Fowler's position and encourage deep breathing.	This will ensure the child has maximum lung expansion and that medication will be dispersed more effectively, thereby improving airway clearance.
Check PEFR in children 5 yr of age and older before and after each albuterol treatment using PFM.	These assessments monitor effectiveness of the medication in decreasing bronchospasm and increasing effective airway clearance. For more information about PEFR, see the Diagnostic Tests section.
Encourage deep breathing and effective cough and expectoration q2h while awake.	This loosens and expectorates secretions (many young children cough up secretions and swallow them) and will lead to more effective airway clearance.
Teach children 7 yr old and older breathing exercises and controlled breathing.	Children younger than 7 are diaphragmatic breathers normally. Proper diaphragmatic breathing decreases WOB and improves chest wall mobility and airway clearance.
Administer other medications (inhaled, intravenous [IV], or by mouth [PO]) as prescribed (usually corticosteroids).	Corticosteroids decrease inflammation, thereby improving airway clearance. Antibiotics are given only if a bacterial infection is present.
Assess and document intake and output (I&O) q4h. Ensure that a minimum urine output (UO) of 1 mL/kg/hr is met.	Assessing I&O on a regular basis alerts one to inadequate intake or output before the child shows signs of dehydration. Dehydration thickens secretions and decreases airway clearance.
Assess hydration status q4h, including level of consciousness (LOC), anterior fontanel (if the child is younger than 2 yr old), abdominal skin turgor, and urine output.	Because of increased insensible water loss (owing to increased RR, metabolic rate, and secretions), the child may still become dehydrated *even if* receiving maintenance fluids and having appropriate I&O. Ongoing assessments detect early changes and provide more prompt resolution of the problem. Dehydration thickens secretions and decreases airway clearance. Signs of dehydration include decreasing LOC, sunken fontanel/eyes, tented abdominal skin, and decreasing urine output.
Encourage maintenance fluids, preferably orally, that are appropriate for the child's weight.	Fluids thin mucus and improve ability to expectorate it, which promotes airway clearance. Some children may need IV fluids because of increased WOB.
Provide specific guidelines for hydration (maintenance fluids).	For example, a 2-yr-old child who needs 1200 mL/day and drinks from a 4-oz "sippy" cup, needs to drink 10 "sippy" cupfuls/day. Understanding appropriate care improves adherence to the treatment regimen and decreases symptoms.
Avoid iced fluids and limit caffeinated fluids.	Iced fluids may trigger bronchospasm. Excessive intake of caffeinated fluids may increase risk of cardiovascular and central nervous system side effects of many medications.

Nursing Diagnosis:

Fatigue

related to disease state (hypoxia and increased WOB)

Desired Outcome: Within 24 hr following treatment/interventions, the child exhibits decreased fatigue as evidenced by less irritability and restlessness, improved sleeping pattern, and ability to perform usual activities.

ASSESSMENT/INTERVENTIONS	RATIONALES
Assess HR, RR, and WOB q4h or more frequently for increases from the child's normal. Report significant findings.	Recognizing and reporting changes promptly facilitates appropriate actions that resolve the problem and decrease the likelihood of fatigue.
Assess for signs of hypoxia (restlessness, fatigue, irritability, tachycardia, dyspnea, change of LOC).	Recognizing symptoms of hypoxia promptly enables timely treatment and decreases fatigue.
Provide a calm and restful environment. Ensure the child's physical comfort. Consolidate care; organize nursing care to provide periods of uninterrupted rest and sleep.	These measures promote rest and decrease stress, oxygen demand, and fatigue.
Encourage the parents' presence, especially with younger children.	The parents' presence decreases fear and anxiety, thereby decreasing O_2 consumption and fatigue.
Encourage quiet, age-appropriate play activities as the child's condition improves.	Emotional and physical comfort increases a sense of well-being, promotes rest, and decreases oxygen expenditure and fatigue.

Nursing Diagnosis:

Anxiety

related to illness, loss of control, and medical/nursing management of illness

Desired Outcome: Following interventions/treatments, the child/parents verbalize and/or exhibit decreased anxiety.

ASSESSMENT/INTERVENTIONS	RATIONALES
Assess the child's/parents' understanding of the child's anxiety.	This enables support and teaching to be more appropriate and effective.
Explain all procedures/interventions performed on the child (e.g., blood drawing, starting IVs) to the child (depending on age) and/or parents.	Knowledge often helps decrease anxiety and promotes family-centered care.
Explain the purpose of equipment used on the child (HR monitor, O_2 and pulse oximeter, blood pressure [BP] monitor). Use therapeutic play with equipment in children older than 3 yr.	Increased understanding of equipment decreases fear of pain, which in turn will decrease anxiety. For example, put a BP cuff on a doll or teddy bear or let the child put the cuff on you.
Provide a quiet room where the child can be closely observed.	Increased stimuli increase anxiety.
Encourage the parents to stay with the child if possible.	This promotes a sense of security, which will decrease the child's anxiety.
Avoid making the parents feel guilty if they are unable to stay.	Parents are already anxious about the child being ill and in a hospital.
Keep the parents informed of the child's progress, including what is being done and why.	This decreases their anxiety. The child easily perceives parental anxiety.
Talk quietly and calmly to the child in age-appropriate language. Reassure the child that you are available and will be there to help.	Establishing rapport increases trust and decreases anxiety.
Encourage transitional objects (items from the child's home such as a blanket or teddy bear).	Such items increase a feeling of security and decrease anxiety.
Facilitate coordination of care.	This avoids disturbing the child any more than necessary, which would otherwise increase the anxiety level.

Nursing Diagnosis:

Interrupted Family Processes

related to the child having a chronic illness and/or emergent hospitalization

Desired Outcome: Within 1 mo of diagnosis, the family provides a normal environment for the child and copes effectively with the symptoms, management, and effects of asthma.

ASSESSMENT/INTERVENTIONS	RATIONALES
Assess for and use every opportunity to reinforce the family's understanding of asthma and its therapies.	Accurate knowledge enables the family to cope more effectively with the child's chronic illness.
Teach the parents to have realistic expectations about the child's asthma.	Knowing what to expect enables families to cope more effectively. Expectations will vary, depending on the child's developmental age and severity of the asthma.
Encourage the parents and siblings to focus on the child as a normal child who needs some lifestyle modifications.	The child needs to be the focus, not the disease. Normalizing the environment as much as possible promotes the child as the focus.
Reinforce the importance of helping the siblings cope with/ adapt to having a sibling with a chronic illness.	This supports family-centered care and increases the likelihood of more normal family processes.
Reinforce to the parents the importance of setting consistent behavior limits and not enabling secondary gain for an asthma attack.	Discipline and guidelines are essential for all children to develop appropriate behavior.
Reinforce the need to use PFM at least 1-2 times/day and/or implement the child's asthma action plan.	Understanding the importance of monitoring the child's status enables the family to cope more effectively and incorporate monitoring into the daily routine, thereby promoting normalization and the child's optimal health status.
Teach the child/parents how to give respiratory treatments (nebulizer, MDI) correctly, using the prescribed medication and administering it with proper technique.	This information eliminates confusion about the correct administration of medications and method of delivery, thereby improving ability to cope with managing a chronic illness.
Encourage the family to contact the school (nurse, teachers, coaches) to develop a 504 plan for the child.	This promotes the family's coping while facilitating the child's improvement. A 504 plan makes accommodations in the school environment so that the child can function better and thereby learn more effectively. For example, a child who is allergic to grass will not be assigned to a classroom with windows that open near a field of grass when the grass is being mowed.
Refer the family to appropriate support groups and community agencies.	These groups/agencies help children and families function and deal with chronic illness more effectively.

Nursing Diagnosis:

Deficient Knowledge

related to unfamiliarity with the purpose, precautions, and potential side effects of prescribed medications

Desired Outcome: Following interventions/instructions, the child and/or parents verbalize accurate information about the prescribed medications.

ASSESSMENT/INTERVENTIONS	RATIONALES
Teach the Parents and Child (Depending on the Child's Age) the Following:	
Long-Term Control Medications	These are taken daily to achieve and maintain control of persistent asthma.
Corticosteroids	These are the most potent antiinflammatory medications.

ASSESSMENT/INTERVENTIONS

RATIONALES

- *Inhaled corticosteroids (ICSs), such as fluticasone (Flovent), beclomethasone (Vanceril), and flunisolide (AeroBid)*

Rinse the mouth and gargle with water after oral inhalation.	This helps prevent thrush (oral candidiasis).
Administer using a spacer or holding chamber.	These devices may enhance drug delivery and efficiency of the inhaled form and help decrease incidence of thrush.
Do not decrease dose or discontinue without consent of the health care provider.	This is a maintenance medication, and the child may have exacerbation of symptoms if it is decreased or discontinued inappropriately.

- *Oral corticosteroids, such as prednisolone and prednisone*

Monitor for and report mood changes, seizures, increased blood sugar, diarrhea, nausea, gastrointestinal (GI) bleeding (seen in emesis, stools), weight gain, and tissue swelling.	These are potential side effects; dosage may need to be changed.
Take cautiously with barbiturates, carbamazepine, phenytoin, rifampin, or isoniazid.	These medications may reduce effects of prednisone and increase risk for GI ulcer.
Observe carefully if taking salicylates, toxoids, nonsteroidal antiinflammatory drugs (NSAIDs), or diuretics that are potassium depleting.	These drugs may increase risk for GI ulcer when taken with corticosteroids.
Limit use of caffeine and alcohol.	They may increase risk for GI ulcer.
Caution: Inform all health care providers about steroid use.	It may be necessary to avoid vaccinations while taking prednisone. Live virus vaccines may increase risk of viral infection. Vaccines in general may have decreased effect.
Do not change or discontinue dose without consent of the health care provider.	Long-term steroid dosage needs to be decreased carefully in order to allow for gradual return of pituitary-adrenal axis functioning. Failure to do so can result in adrenal insufficiency.

Cromolyn

	This antiasthmatic agent prevents release of mast cells (e.g., histamine) after exposure to an allergen.
Assess for and report headache, dizziness, rash, cough, and/or nasal congestion.	These are potential side effects.
Explain that a decrease in asthma symptoms should occur after the medication has been taken for 2-4 wk on a regular basis.	Therapeutic response should occur within 2-4 wk if used on a regular basis.
Gargle or sip water to decrease throat irritation or dry mouth.	Inhaled or nebulized form of this medication may cause these symptoms.

Leukotriene Modifiers such as montelukast (Singulair)

	These antiasthmatic agents decrease inflammation and bronchoconstriction.
Assess for and report headache, changes in behavior/mood, abdominal pain, fatigue, dizziness, cough, diarrhea, laryngitis, pharyngitis, nausea, earache, sinus discomfort, and viral infections. **Note:** Side effects vary depending on age of the child..	These are potential side effects.
Use cautiously with phenobarbital and rifampin.	These medications may decrease bioavailability of Singular.
For granules: Give directly into the mouth or mixed with a small amount of cold or room temperature foods (using only applesauce, mashed carrots, rice, or ice cream). Administer within 15 min of opening the packet. Do not dissolve in liquid.	Following these guidelines ensures stability of the granules and better therapeutic response.
Check with the health care provider or pharmacist before taking any other medications.	These medications may interact with numerous other medications.

Immunomodulators such as omalizumab (Xolair®)

	These medications are used to treat moderate to severe persistent IgE-mediated allergic asthma not controlled with ICSs. This medication is administered subcutaneously. It is used only in children at least 12 yr old and in adults.

continued

ASSESSMENT/INTERVENTIONS

RATIONALES

ASSESSMENT/INTERVENTIONS	RATIONALES
Assess for and report dizziness; fatigue; pruritus; local injection site reactions (bruising and pain occur within 1 hr and may last up to 8 days); pain in joints, arms or legs; fracture; and earache.	These are potential side effects.
Assess for and report any signs of allergic reactions such as difficulty breathing, swelling of the throat or tongue, cough, chest tightness, and generalized itching to the health care provider immediately.	Anaphylaxis reactions usually occur within 2 hr but may be delayed up to 24 hr or longer. **U.S. Boxed Warning:** The patient should receive this medication only under direct medical supervision and be observed for at least 2 hr.
Do not alter medications without consulting the health care provider.	This is a maintenance medication. The child may have exacerbation of symptoms if medications are decreased or discontinued inappropriately.

Long-Acting Beta₂-Agonists (LABAs) such as salmeterol (Serevent®, Serevent Diskus®)

	LABAs relax bronchial smooth muscles to relieve bronchospasm but should only be used in patients who are not adequately controlled with long-term controller medications such as ICS or whose disease requires two maintenance therapies. **U.S. Box Warning:** LABAs increase the risk of asthma-related deaths.
Assess for and report increased blood pressure, dizziness, headache, rash, increased blood sugar, nausea, pain in joints, cough, or respiratory/sinus infections.	These are potential side effects.
Store the canister at room temperature.	Therapeutic effect may decrease when the canister is cold or hot.
Use Serevent Diskus powder up to 6 wk after removing protective foil.	Serevent powder for inhalation is stable for 6 wk after removal from the foil packet.

Methylxanthines such as theophylline (rarely used now)

	These are bronchodilators.
Assess for and report GI upset, GI reflux, diarrhea, vomiting, nausea, abdominal pain, nervousness, insomnia, agitation, dizziness, seizures, tremors, and increased pulse rate.	These are the most common side effects.
Limit caffeine (e.g., caffeinated beverages and chocolate).	Excessive intake may increase risk of cardiovascular and central nervous system side effects.
Limit intake of charcoal-broiled foods.	Excessive intake may increase elimination or decrease effectiveness of medication.
Check with the health care provider or pharmacist before taking any other medications.	Numerous medications increase or decrease theophylline level.

Quick-Relief Medications

	These agents treat acute signs and symptoms and pretreat exercise-induced asthma.
Short-acting inhaled beta₂-agonists (SABAs) such as albuterol (Proventil or Ventolin) and metaproterenol (Alupent)	SABAs are bronchodilators.
Assess for and report increased HR, palpitations, tremor, insomnia, nervousness, nausea, and headache.	These are potential side effects.
If using an MDI, use with a spacer or holding chamber.	These devices increase drug delivery and efficiency.
Limit caffeinated beverages if taking albuterol or metaproterenol.	Caffeine may increase side effects of albuterol or metaproterenol.
Check with the health care provider or pharmacist before taking other medications.	Numerous medications increase or decrease the effects/toxicity of albuterol.
Anticholinergics such as ipratropium (Atrovent®)	These bronchodilator/antiasthmatic agents should not be used for first-line therapy but rather added to SABAs (National Asthma Education and Prevention Program, NIH Guidelines, 2007); they may be used if the child cannot tolerate SABAs.
Assess for and report tachycardia, nervousness, cough, hoarseness, dry mouth, and drying of respiratory secretions.	These are potential side effects, but systemic effects are rare.

ASSESSMENT/INTERVENTIONS	RATIONALES
If using an MDI, use with a spacer or holding chamber. Shake the inhaler well before use with a spacer.	These devices increase drug delivery and efficiency. Shaking the inhaler before use ensures consistency of the dose delivered.
Oral and intravenous corticosteroids (also see under long-term control medication) such as methylprednisolone or prednisolone	These antiinflammation agents are usually given for a short time.
Assess for and report dizziness, headache, anxiety, GI discomfort, and cough.	These are potential side effects.
Give oral medication with food or milk.	Food/milk decreases GI upset.

ADDITIONAL NURSING DIAGNOSES/PROBLEMS:

"Bronchiolitis" for **Deficient Fluid Volume** p. 569

"Cystic Fibrosis" for **Impaired Gas Exchange.** p. 590
However, with asthma, be aware that oxygen saturation needs to be greater than 93%-95%, depending on agency protocol.

✓ PATIENT-FAMILY TEACHING AND DISCHARGE PLANNING

When providing patient/family teaching, focus on sensory information, avoid giving excessive information, and initiate a visiting nurse referral for necessary follow-up teaching and assessment. Stress importance of family-centered care (looking at the family as a unit that is the "constant" in the child's life and maintaining or improving the health of the family and its members in a holistic manner). Include verbal and written information about the following, ensuring that it is written at a level understandable to child/family:

✓ What is asthma? Discuss definition, signs and symptoms, and pathophysiology.

✓ Identification of specific triggers for the child that can precipitate an attack and removal of as many as possible from the environment. Asthma triggers vary for each child. Most common triggers of asthma are upper respiratory infection (URI), cigarette smoke, exercise, and weather changes. Other triggers unique to the environment are important (e.g., humid weather, frequent rainy days, local industry). Additional common triggers include pollens, dust mites, mold, cockroaches, rodents, and pet dander.

✓ Importance of personal asthma action plan with green, yellow, and red zone values specific for the child. This plan is set up by the health care provider based on the child's best score/PEFR. Zones are established similar to a stoplight. The green zone is a score 80%-100% of the child's best score and with no symptoms present. The yellow zone is a score 50%-80% of the child's best score and signals caution: the child may need extra asthma medicine. Follow guidelines in the child's personal asthma action plan. The red zone is a score that is below

50% of the child's best score and signals an emergency situation. Follow the asthma action plan and call the health care provider. A sample asthma action plan is available at *www.nationaljewish.org/healthinfo/conditions/asthma/lifestyle-management/tools/action-plan/*, *www.nhlbi.nih.gov/health/public/lung/asthma/asthma_actplan.pdf* (also includes "How to Control Things That Make Your Asthma Worse"), or the Asthma Society of Canada at *www.asthma.ca*.

✓ Correct PFM technique. Most children by 5 yr old can use PFM. Document return demonstration before discharge. The child should check this rate at least daily and more often if the rate is decreased. The child should keep a log to document PEFR.

✓ Maintaining asthma symptom diary, especially for a child with frequent symptoms.

✓ Medications, including drug name, route, purpose, type (controller: long-term management or short-acting immediate relief), dosage, precautions, and potential side effects. Also discuss drug-drug, food-drug, and herb-drug interactions.

✓ Proper technique for using MDIs with spacer (holding chamber) or spacer with a mask (usually for a child younger than 5 yr old). Document adequate return demonstration. Remind the family that over-the-counter (OTC) inhalers contain medications that can interfere with the prescribed therapy. Instruct the child/parent to contact the health care provider before trying any OTC medications. Instruct the child/parent in sequencing of inhalers; bronchodilator inhalers are used 15 min before administration of the steroid inhaler.

✓ Cleaning and care of equipment—nebulizer, MDI, or other medication delivery systems, including assessment of when the canister is low or empty.

✓ If the child is taking oral corticosteroids while at home, instructions to ensure that he or she receives the correct amount each day, especially if the medication is going to be tapered.

✓ Importance of taking medication at home and at school as directed. Medication in the original bottle/canister (with prescribing label) and written prescription from the health care provider are needed for the child to be able to take any medication at school.

✓ Importance of knowing early warning signs before an acute attack (e.g., fatigue, sneezing, sore throat, itchy/

watery eyes, headache, slight tightness in chest, drop in PFM values). These differ for each child.

✓ Signs and symptoms of increased respiratory distress in children relating to age (e.g., an infant may have increased RR when sleeping, decreased interest in eating/drinking, nasal flaring, grunting, retractions). Other signs and symptoms include difficulty speaking in sentences, inability to walk short distances, hunched posture, and PFM values in the red zone.

✓ Importance of avoiding contact with infectious individuals, especially those with respiratory infection.

✓ Recommendation that the child receive annual influenza and all age-appropriate vaccinations.

✓ Importance of follow-up care on a regular basis (not just emergency room). Confirm date and time of next appointment.

✓ Phone numbers to call should questions or concerns arise about therapy or disease.

✓ When to call the health care provider:
  • To refill medications.
  • PEFR in yellow zone 24 hr or child has an event such as coughing, wheezing, chest tightness, or shortness of breath.
  • PEFR in red zone or the child is in increased respiratory distress.
  • Immediate reliever/quick relief medication (albuterol) needed more often than q4h.
  • Reliever medication not helping.

✓ When to call emergency medical services:
  • The child is in severe respiratory distress.
  • The child is gray/blue.
  • The child is unable to answer questions or seems confused.

✓ Importance of communication with the child's school or day care regarding the child's condition, need for medication, and activity level.

✓ Legal rights of the child—Section 504 of Rehabilitation Act of 1973: Each student with a disability is entitled to accommodation needed to attend school and participate as fully as possible in school activities. This accommodation may be related to a medical condition or an education issue. More details are at *www.specialchildren.about.com/od/504s/f/504faq1.htm*

✓ Guidelines for attendance, activity level, and exercise at school/day care.

✓ Referral to community resources, such as the local and national American Lung Associations and camps for educational programs for children with asthma. Additional general information can be obtained by contacting:
  • American Lung Association at *www.lungusa.org*
  • Allergy & Asthma Network Mothers of Asthmatics (AANMA) at *www.aanma.org*
  • Asthma and Allergy Foundation of America (AAFA) at *www.aafa.org* (Asthma PACT™: Personalized Assessment and Control Tool is available at *www.asthmapact.org*)
  • Centers for Disease Control and Prevention at *www.cdc.gov/asthma*
  • Several links for children and adolescents include: The Asthma Wizard (*http://www.nationaljewish.org/healthinfo/pediatric/asthma/asthma-wizard/index.aspx*), Dusty the Asthma Goldfish and His Asthma Triggers Funbook (*http:www.epa.gov/asthma/parents.html*), and Huff & Puff: An Asthma Tale (*http://vimeopro.com/healthnutsmedia/huff-and-puff-an-asthma-tale*)
  • The Asthma Society of Canada at *www.asthma.ca*
  • Canadian Lung Association at *www.lung.ca*

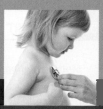
OVERVIEW/PATHOPHYSIOLOGY

Attention deficit/hyperactivity disorder (ADHD) is a neuro-developmental disorder involving developmentally inappropriate behavior. ADHD is a common chronic illness in children and the most commonly diagnosed neurobehavioral/neurobiologic disorder in children and adolescents in the United States. The statistics per the number of children affected vary depending on source and population. The American Academy of Pediatrics (AAP) in 2011 estimated that 8% of children and youth were affected. In the 2011Clinical Practice Guideline on ADHD, the AAP expanded the age range to evaluate and treat from only school age to include preschoolers and adolescents, ages 4 to 18 yr. The National Health Interview Survey conducted in 2011 noted that 8.4% of children ages 3-17 yr of age had been diagnosed with ADHD and that the average number of ambulatory care visits due to ADHD as the primary diagnosis was 9 million annually. Houck et al., in 2011 noted approximately 3%-8.7% of children and adolescents in the United States had ADHD. Although the exact etiology is unknown, it probably involves a combination of biologic, genetic, and psychologic factors. ADHD is seen more often in children who have a family member with ADHD, particularly the father, brother, or uncle. Chromosomal or genetic abnormalities such as fragile X syndrome have been seen in some children with ADHD. ADHD commonly occurs in association with emotional or behavioral (e.g., anxiety, oppositional defiant, conduct, depression disorders), developmental (e.g., language, learning or other neurodevelopmental disorders), and physical (e.g., tics, sleep apnea) conditions (AAP, 2009, 2011). ADHD is more common in males than females, and many children affected continue to demonstrate symptoms into adolescence and adulthood. There is some belief that ADHD is not "outgrown" but that people learn to compensate. The CDC's Mortality and Morbidity Weekly Report, May 2013, looked at the Mental Health Surveillance Report among U.S. children from 2005-2011 and found that children with ADHD are more likely to have higher rates of unintentional injuries, ED visits, smoking, and alcohol and illicit substance use than children without ADHD.

HEALTH CARE SETTING

Primary care

ASSESSMENT

Includes comprehensive history and physical examination with a thorough cardiovascular examination, detailed neurologic examination, family assessment, and school assessment.

Signs and symptoms: The behaviors exhibited are not unusual aspects of any child's behavior. The difference lies in the quality of motor activity and developmentally inappropriate inattention, impulsivity, and hyperactivity displayed. The symptoms vary with developmental age and may range from a few to numerous different symptoms. The core symptoms include inattention, hyperactivity, and impulsivity. Children may experience significant functional problems such as school difficulties, academic underachievement, troublesome interpersonal relationships with family members and peers, and low self-esteem.

Physical assessment: Physical examination includes vision and hearing screening, thorough cardiovascular examination, and a detailed neurologic examination that will help rule out any severe neurologic disorders.

Guidelines for the Diagnosis of ADHD (published by the American Academy of Pediatrics in October 2011)

1. Expanded the age range to include any child 4 to 18 yr of age presenting with academic or behavioral problems and symptoms of inattention, hyperactivity, or impulsivity.
2. Use of specific criteria for the diagnosis using the *Diagnostic and Statistical Manual of Mental Health Disorders*, 4th edition (DSM-IV) criteria.
3. Importance of obtaining information concerning the child's symptoms/behavior in more than one setting (especially from school). Information should be obtained primarily from parents or guardians, teachers, and mental health clinicians involved in the child's care.
4. Evaluation for coexisting conditions that may make the diagnosis more difficult or complicate treatment planning.
5. Primary care clinicians should consider this a chronic condition; thus children and youth with ADHD have special health care needs.
6. Specific guidance per treatment of preschool-aged children, school-aged children, and adolescents.
7. Primary care clinicians should titrate ADHD medications to receive maximum benefit with minimal side effects.

Multidisciplinary evaluation: Includes the primary pediatrician (and possibly a developmental pediatrician, pediatric neurologist, or pediatric psychiatrist), psychologist, pediatric/school nurse, classroom teacher, specialty teachers as appropriate, and the child's parents in order to obtain all perspectives of the child's behavior.

Detailed history: Both medical and developmental history and descriptions of the child's behavior should be obtained from as many observers as possible. Traumatic experiences and psychiatric and other disorders are ruled out, including lead poisoning, seizures, partial hearing loss, psychosis, and witnessing sexual activity and/or violence.

Psychologic testing: Valuable in determining a variety of deficits and helpful in identifying the child's intelligence and achievement levels.

Behavioral checklists and adaptive scales: Helpful in measuring social adaptive functioning in children with ADHD.

DIAGNOSTIC TESTS

ADHD is a diagnosis of exclusion. There is no definitive test for ADHD.

Nursing Diagnosis:

Ineffective Impulse Control

related to excessive environmental stimuli resulting in inability to concentrate, control impulses, and organize thoughts in a manner appropriate for age and development

Desired Outcomes: Within 1 mo of this diagnosis, the child completes activities of daily living (ADLs) and shows behavioral improvement in the school setting. Within one semester, the child shows improvement in academic activities.

ASSESSMENT/INTERVENTIONS	RATIONALES
Encourage parents/teachers to provide a structured environment and consistency.	Structure and consistency offer opportunities for children to focus on areas that need improvement.
Promote ongoing communication between parents and teachers.	Consistency among family and teachers in reinforcing same guidelines improves the child's ability to concentrate.
Encourage parents/teachers to decrease stimuli when concentration is important.	Children with ADHD are easily distracted by extraneous stimuli. Removing those stimuli should improve concentration. For example, parents/teachers should have the child do homework in a quiet area without TV or radio on or sit in a quiet section of the classroom, not near an open door or window.

Nursing Diagnosis:

Chronic Low Self-Esteem

related to negative responses and lack of approval from others regarding behavior

Desired Outcome: Within 1 mo of this diagnosis, the child achieves at least one goal, lists strengths, and elicits fewer negative responses from others.

ASSESSMENT/INTERVENTIONS	RATIONALES
Assess the child's interactions with others.	This assessment helps determine existence/degree of negative responses from other people.
Reward positive behavior and provide limit setting as needed. Avoid negative comments and giving attention for negative behavior.	Positive reinforcement is an effective way to improve behavior and self-esteem.

ASSESSMENT/INTERVENTIONS	RATIONALES
Help the child set goals that are age appropriate, realistic, and achievable. Set a timetable to achieve step-by-step progress until he or she accomplishes the overall goal.	Achieving goals increases self-esteem. If the child has difficulty completing assignments, divide the assignment into manageable tasks. For example, for an essay assignment: day 1, make outline; day 2, begin literature search; day 3, begin writing paper; day 4, finish paper and have someone review it; day 5, finalize paper.
Encourage the child to make a list of his or her strengths. Teach self-questioning techniques (e.g., What am I doing? How is that going to affect others?). Encourage positive self-talk (e.g., I did a good job with that!). Provide feedback accordingly.	These activities encourage positive self-thought and build self-esteem.

Nursing Diagnosis:

Risk for Trauma

related to increased activity level, limited judgment skills, and impulsivity

Desired Outcome: The child remains free from signs of trauma.

ASSESSMENT/INTERVENTIONS	RATIONALES
Reinforce to the parents the importance of the child using appropriate safety equipment/protective device (e.g., seat belt, bicycle helmet).	Using this equipment/device decreases likelihood of trauma.
Encourage the parents to model the use of appropriate safety equipment/protective devices.	Children are more likely to wear a seat belt or bicycle helmet if their parents wear them also.
Encourage the parents to set clear limits on where the child may ride a bike or play and to offer choices from several safe areas the child can go.	Clear, simple guidelines are easier for a child with ADHD to focus on and follow. Allowing the child some choice improves compliance, which decreases likelihood of injury.
Encourage the child's participation in active play rather than in passive activities (e.g., playing softball rather than playing video games).	Active play helps children grow physically and cognitively. It also helps the child with ADHD to redirect energy in a safe and effective manner, thus decreasing risk of injury/trauma.
Reinforce importance of the parents monitoring the child's activities frequently.	Adequate supervision decreases likelihood of injury/trauma.
Teach the parents to reinforce positive behavior with feedback and intermittent rewards.	This encourages appropriate behavior and activity, thereby decreasing risk of injury/trauma.

Nursing Diagnosis:

Deficient Knowledge

related to unfamiliarity with chronicity of ADHD and its treatment

Desired Outcome: Within 1 mo of this diagnosis, the child and/or parents verbalize accurate understanding of the chronic condition of ADHD and possible treatments.

ASSESSMENT/INTERVENTIONS	RATIONALES
Assess the parents' and child's understanding (depending on the child's age) of ADHD. As indicated, teach them about the disorder, including the fact that it is chronic.	This assessment enables development of an individualized teaching plan. Accurate knowledge about the condition facilitates understanding of the need for ongoing treatment and ways to manage it realistically.
Encourage parents/teachers to provide a calm, structured environment and consistency.	Structure and consistency offer opportunities for the child to focus on areas that need improvement.

continued

ASSESSMENT/INTERVENTIONS	RATIONALES
Promote ongoing communication between the teacher and family.	Frequent communication between the parents and teacher/school, especially when the child is first diagnosed, facilitates everyone working together to maximize the child's ability to function more appropriately.
Discuss different treatment strategies.	This information promotes understanding that no single treatment strategy is *the* answer and that there are multiple strategies that may help the child, such as medication, behavioral/psychosocial interventions (parent training and education, behavior modification, teacher training/proper classroom placement and management, counseling, psychotherapy), combined or multimodal treatment, and biofeedback.

Nursing Diagnosis:

Deficient Knowledge

related to unfamiliarity with the purpose, precautions, and potential side effects of prescribed medications

Desired Outcome: Within 1 wk of starting medication, the child and/or parents verbalize accurate information about the prescribed medications.

ASSESSMENT/INTERVENTIONS	RATIONALES
Teach the Following to the Parents/Child: **Stimulant Medications**	This is first-line treatment for children and adolescents but not for preschoolers (AAP Clinical Practice Guidelines for Treatment, 2011).
Short, intermediate, and long-acting methylphenidate (e.g., Ritalin); short, intermediate, and long-acting dextroamphetamine (e.g., Dexedrine); mixed dextroamphetamine/amphetamine salts; and dexmethylphenidate	Stimulants are given to promote attentiveness and decrease restlessness by increasing dopamine and norepinephrine levels, which leads to stimulation of the inhibitory system of the central nervous system (CNS).
- Medications can be titrated up every 3-7 days per clinician's directive until a decrease in symptoms occurs or maximum dose is reached.	A slow increase allows time to see if medication is effective. This requires close monitoring with the clinician to evaluate the child's physical condition and symptom relief. The goal is to have maximum benefit with minimal side effects.
- Assess for and report decreased appetite, weight loss, stomachache or headache, delayed sleep onset, jitteriness, increased crying or irritability, and social withdrawal.	These common side effects may require either dosage adjustment or change in schedule.
- Assess for and notify the health care provider if the child develops or has increased aggression or hostility.	These are serious side effects and will require a change in dosage or medication.
- Assess for and report tics (involuntary movements of a small group of muscles such as of the face).	Tics occur in 15%-30% of children and are usually transient. This medication is contraindicated if the child/family member has motor tics or Tourette's syndrome.
- Assess for and report the child becoming overfocused while on medication or appearing dull or overly restricted.	These changes are seen in children receiving too high a dose or who are overly sensitive. Decreasing the dose usually resolves these problems.
- Assess height, weight, and blood pressure (BP) at regular follow-up visits with the prescribing clinician.	Suppression of growth may occur with long-term use, and it can increase BP as well.
- Assess for and report decreased impulsiveness, improved social interaction, and increased academic productivity and accuracy.	This will indicate effectiveness of medication.

ASSESSMENT/INTERVENTIONS	RATIONALES
- Take the medication on an empty stomach 30-45 min before meals, if possible.	Absorption of methylphenidate is increased when taken with meals, with the exception of Concerta (this medication has the potential for GI obstruction and should not be given to children with severe GI narrowing), a long-acting form. Taking the medication at a consistent time is most important. Dosage can be adjusted to counteract effects of any decreased absorption as long as the medication is taken consistently with or without food.
- Do not crush, chew, or break sustained-release forms.	Action of the medication will change and probably not be as effective.
- Take the last daily dose several hours before bedtime.	This reduces the potential for insomnia.
- Get all prescriptions filled at the same pharmacy or give a list of all current medications to every pharmacy used.	There are many drug interactions with these medications. An informed pharmacist can identify all potential interactions among medications. For example, methylphenidate may increase serum levels of tricyclic antidepressants, phenytoin, phenobarbital, and warfarin. Monoamine oxidase inhibitors (MAOIs) or general anesthetics potentiate methylphenidate.
- Limit caffeine and decongestants.	They are stimulants and can potentiate medications the child is receiving.
- Avoid use of the above-listed CNS stimulants in patients with serious cardiac problems.	They could place the patient at increased risk for sympathomimetic effects of CNS stimulants, including sudden death in children. American Heart Association recommends that all children with ADHD being treated with stimulants have thorough cardiovascular assessments before initiation of therapy.
- Avoid use in patients with marked agitation, tension, or anxiety.	These medications may exacerbate symptoms of behavior disturbance and thought disorders.
- Prolonged use may lead to drug dependency. Abrupt withdrawal after taking high doses or after a prolonged time may cause withdrawal. Therefore patients might need to be weaned off these medications rather than abruptly stopped if possible.	**U.S. BOXED WARNING:** There is also the potential for drug dependency with these medications.
- The child should be carefully screened for any abuse history and the family should ensure the medication is secured.	**U.S. BOXED WARNING:** There is potential for abuse with these medications by the child or others.
- Avoid use of the above-listed CNS stimulants in children who have taken an MAOI within the past 14 days.	These drugs could precipitate a hypertensive crisis.
- Caution is necessary when taken by children with seizures.	These medications may lower the seizure threshold.
- Children may need a periodic drug holiday (e.g., no medication during the summer) or periodic discontinuation.	This assesses the child's requirement for medication, decreases tolerance, and limits suppression of linear growth and weight.
- The child should be reevaluated at appropriate intervals while receiving these medications.	This assesses effectiveness and if the child still needs to be on the medication at all. Some studies have shown children to have improved behavior even after going off the medication.
- Use with caution in preschool-aged children and only if behavior therapy was not effective.	Young children are more sensitive to adverse effects.
Norepinephrine Reuptake Inhibitor *atomoxetine (e.g., Straterra)*	This medication is given to improve attentiveness, enhance ability to follow through on tasks with less distraction and forgetfulness, and diminish hyperactivity. The exact mechanism of action is unknown, but it is believed to be related to the selective inhibitor of presynaptic norepinephrine transporter, resulting in norepinephrine reuptake inhibition.
- Assess for and report headache, dizziness, insomnia, upper abdominal pain, vomiting, decreased appetite, or cough.	These are the most common side effects and may require either dosage adjustment or change in schedule.
- Assess for and report chest pain or palpitations, urinary retention or difficulty voiding, appetite loss and weight loss, mood swings, or insomnia.	These are significant side effects and will require some change in either dosage or medication.

continued

ASSESSMENT/INTERVENTIONS	RATIONALES
- Assess weight on a regular basis and ensure the dose prescribed is appropriate for weight before administering.	Dose is based on weight. An accurate weight is needed to get optimal effects of the medication with minimal side effects. It is also important to note if the child is losing weight. If so, it may be necessary to interrupt therapy.
- Assess baseline heart rate (HR) and BP with dose increases and periodically while on therapy.	This medication may cause significantly increased HR, significantly increased BP, and palpitations; if so, the dose needs to be adjusted. This is especially important for a child with preexisting hypertension.
- Observe closely for and report behavioral changes, including increased aggression and hostility, which may be a precursor to emerging suicidal ideation.	**U.S. BOXED WARNING:** There is increased risk of suicidal ideation in children and adolescents with this medication for the first few months and after dose changes.
- Avoid use of atomoxetine in patients with serious cardiac problems.	This medication could put patients at increased risk for serious cardiovascular events, including sudden death in children. American Heart Association recommends that all children with ADHD who are treated with atomoxetine have a thorough cardiovascular assessment before initiation of therapy.
- Use cautiously with Albuterol or other beta$_2$-agonists, vasopressor drugs, or CYP2D6 inhibitors (e.g., paroxetine, fluoxetine, quinidine).	Beta$_2$-agonists potentiate cardiovascular effects of this medication; CYP2D6 inhibitors may increase blood levels and toxicity.
- Do not use within 2 wk of taking MAOIs.	This may precipitate a hypertensive crisis.
- Get all prescriptions filled at the same pharmacy or give a list of all current medications to every pharmacy used.	This drug interacts with many medications. An informed pharmacist can identify all potential interactions among medications.
- Assess for a decrease in ADHD symptoms within the first 4-6 wk of starting the medication.	It may take up to 4-6 wk to get the maximum response. If there is no improvement in symptoms by then, it may be necessary to get the medication dose changed or try another medication.
- Reevaluate the patient's physical condition and ADHD symptoms at appropriate intervals.	Ongoing, regular assessments will detect problems before they become severe as well as assess effectiveness and if the medication needs to be continued.

Other Approved Medications

Clonidine extended-release form only—one of two medications approved by AAP other than stimulants to treat ADHD	An alpha$_2$-adrenergic agonist, this medication regulates levels of neurotransmitters and norepinephrine. It may be effective in decreasing ADHD symptoms alone or in combination with stimulant medications.
- Avoid use of clonidine in patients with serious cardiac problems.	This medication could put the patient at increased risk for serious cardiovascular events, including sudden death in children. American Heart Association recommends that all children with ADHD who are treated with clonidine have a thorough cardiovascular assessment before initiation of therapy.
- Assess for and report dry mouth, dizziness, drowsiness, fatigue, constipation, anorexia, palpitations, and local skin reactions with patch.	These are side effects that may necessitate change in dosage.
- Assess for and report immediately: rapid heart rate or palpitations, bradycardia, edema, rapid weight gain, confusion, hallucinations.	These are serious side effects that require prompt attention.
- Do not stop the medication abruptly. It is necessary to slowly wean off the medication.	The patient will go through withdrawal symptoms.
- Watch the child closely if clonidine is given with CNS depressants.	Additive sedation would occur if given with CNS depressants, including alcohol, antihistamines, opioid analgesics, and sedative/hypnotics.
- Assess for a decrease in symptoms of ADHD, especially after 2-4 wk on the medication.	It may take this long to get maximum response from the medication. If there is no decrease in ADHD symptoms, it may be necessary to have the dose increased or the medication changed.
- Get all prescriptions filled at the same pharmacy or give a list of all current medications to every pharmacy used.	This medication interacts with many others such as cardiac, antihypertensive, tricyclic antidepressants, and psychiatric medications. An informed pharmacist can identify all potential interactions among medications.

ASSESSMENT/INTERVENTIONS	RATIONALES
Guanfacine: Extended-release form only	This medication, an alpha$_2$-adrenergic agonist, regulates levels of neurotransmitters and norepinephrine and may be effective in decreasing ADHD symptoms alone or in combination with stimulant medications. It is very similar to clonidine.
- Assess for and report immediately: bradycardia, hypotension, orthostatic hypotension, and syncope, especially during the first month of taking the medication.	These are significant side effects that may be more apparent during the first month of therapy. If severe, it may be necessary to change the dose of medication or change the medication.
- Assess for and report immediately: rash; hives; itching; difficulty breathing; tightness in the chest; swelling in the mouth, face, lips, or tongue; rapid heart rate; or palpitations.	These are significant side effects that may require immediate action.
- Assess for constipation, dizziness, drowsiness, dry mouth, or tiredness.	These are side effects that may necessitate dose change if significant. This medication causes less drowsiness than clonidine.
See "clonidine," earlier, for the last two assessments/interventions.	

Nursing Diagnosis:

Compromised Family Coping

related to need for constant and close supervision of the child, hyperactivity of the child, or the stigma associated with a child with impulsive or aggressive behavior

Desired Outcome: Within 1 wk of diagnosis, family members (including siblings depending on their developmental age) discuss the child's needs and develop a plan to provide the necessary support.

ASSESSMENT/INTERVENTIONS	RATIONALES
Assess the family's knowledge/understanding of current coping status.	This assessment will help ensure that support and assistance will be more effective.
Assist the family with problem-solving ways of managing the child's behavior and needs.	Positive reinforcement, time-out, response cost, or token rewards are examples of effective behavioral techniques for children with ADHD.
Provide handouts for caregivers explaining behavioral management techniques.	Verbal and written guidelines promote understanding. Handouts increase consistency among caregivers and improve their ability to meet the child's needs.
Enable the family (including siblings) to vent concerns and problems.	Discussing concerns increases their ability to cope with the situation.
Help identify community resources for support (e.g., many school systems have ADHD support groups, local Children and Adults with ADHD [CHADD] chapter).	Support groups often help families function and cope more effectively.
Encourage the family to advocate for their child within the school system (IEP or 504 accommodation plan as appropriate).	Many parents are unaware of the rights of disabled children. Environmental accommodation and appropriate classroom placement help children with ADHD reach their maximum potential by concentrating better, controlling impulses, and improving organizational ability. For example, for a child with ADHD, the desk may be placed in the front and on the quieter side of the classroom, and the child may be given extra time to complete tests. This involvement/support by the family increases the potential for the child to function well/succeed.

ADDITIONAL NURSING DIAGNOSES/PROBLEMS:

"Psychosocial Support for the Patient's Family and   p. 84
Significant Other," for relevant psychosocial care
plans that would help family members cope with
ADHD

✓ **PATIENT-FAMILY TEACHING AND DISCHARGE PLANNING**

The child with ADHD may have a wide variety of symptoms and treatment modalities. Providing support and information about the disease is essential because of the stigma associated with ADHD. When providing child/family teaching, focus on sensory information and avoid giving excessive information. Stress family-centered care (viewing the family as a unit that is the "constant" in the child's life and maintaining or improving the health of the family and its members). Include verbal and written information about the following (ensure that written information is at a level the reader can understand):

✓ Clarification of myths and realities concerning ADHD: The child is not "bad," "lazy," or "stupid."

✓ Safety measures relative to developmental age, impulsivity, inattentiveness, and hyperactivity.

✓ Medications, including drug name; purpose; dosage; frequency; precautions; drug-drug, food-drug, and herb-drug interactions; and potential side effects.

✓ Importance of taking medication as directed at home and school. Medication in the original pharmacy bottle and written prescription from the health care provider are needed for the child to be able to take medication at school.

✓ Importance of consistency, structure, and routine for the child with ADHD.

✓ Importance of collaboration of family, the health care provider, and school for optimal outcome.

✓ Importance of supporting siblings and including them in the "plan." Help them cope with/adapt to having a brother/sister with a chronic illness.

✓ Environmental manipulation and appropriate classroom placement, which increase the child's ability to function optimally.

✓ Suggestions regarding house rules:
  • Give clear, specific directions.
  • Use positive rewards; don't punish.
  • Implement a contingency plan.

✓ Suggestions to help children with ADHD:
  • Daily picture with schedule of activities and events.
  • Index cards with written steps or pictures.
  • Organized backpack and notebook.
  • Physical relaxation techniques.
  • Standing when needing to work at his or her desk.
  • Two chairs (can move back and forth between them).
  • Boundaries in the classroom.
  • Provide *only* needed materials.
  • Include short, fast-paced tasks.
  • Soothing music, carpet, earplugs.
  • One step at a time—the student verbalizes the step, performs the step, and then on to the next step.
  • Positive self-talk and reinforcement practices.

✓ Suggestions to facilitate communication between the family and school, including daily written communication with the teacher per behavior (gives better overall evaluation of effectiveness of medication/behavioral modification).

✓ Legal rights of the child.

✓ Individuals with Disabilities Education Act (IDEA): Requires states to identify, diagnose, educate, and provide related services for children 3-21 yr old.

✓ IEP: Multidisciplinary team designs this plan to facilitate special education and therapeutic strategies and goals for each eligible child. Parents need to be involved in this process.

✓ Section 504 of Rehabilitation Act of 1973: Each student with a disability is entitled to the accommodation needed to attend school and participate as fully as possible in school activities.

✓ Signs that indicate when to contact the health care provider:
  • Child appears very drowsy.
  • Child is unable to concentrate after being on medication several weeks.
  • Child physically harms self or others.
  • No improvement is seen in school performance over 1-2 mo.

✓ Importance of follow-up care, including the primary pediatrician and multidisciplinary team.

✓ Referral to community resources such as support groups, pediatricians who are comfortable dealing with ADHD, child psychologists, and local community services boards, including:

✓ Children and Adults with Attention-Deficit/Hyperactivity Disorder (CHADD) at *www.chadd.org*

✓ National Resource Center for ADHD (program of CHADD)—Educational/legal rights for children with ADHD in public schools at *www.help4adhd.org/en/ education/rights/wwk4* or Canadian Mental Health Association at *www.cmha.ca*

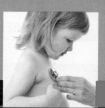

Bronchiolitis 77

OVERVIEW/PATHOPHYSIOLOGY

Bronchiolitis is an acute infection that causes inflammation and obstruction of the bronchioles, the smallest, most distal sections of the lower respiratory tract. It rarely occurs in children older than 2 yr of age and has a peak incidence between 2 and 6 mo of age. Bronchiolitis is one of the major causes of hospitalization in children younger than 1 yr. Incidence is greatest in the fall, winter, and early spring.

Acute bronchiolitis is most often a viral infection and is most often caused by the respiratory syncytial virus (RSV). Metapneumovirus, adenovirus, parainfluenza, and influenza also cause bronchiolitis. RSV is highly contagious and is transmitted by droplets and direct contact with secretions or indirectly on contaminated surfaces. Infants/children infected with RSV are usually contagious for 3 to 8 days, but some infants and immunocompromised children may be infectious for up to 4 wk (CDC, 2010). Almost 100% of young children are infected by the age of 2 yr. RSV is the leading cause of lower respiratory tract disease (e.g., bronchiolitis and pneumonia) in infants, causing more than 100,000 hospitalizations and 500 deaths annually (Crowe, March of Dimes, 2013). Most infants and young children can be cared for at home, but approximately 0.5%-2% of those infected are hospitalized (CDC, RSV, 2010).

HEALTH CARE SETTING

Primary care with possible hospitalization for respiratory distress

ASSESSMENT

Initially upper respiratory infection (URI) symptoms for 2-3 days: fever, rhinorrhea, and cough.

Acute respiratory distress: Expiratory wheezing, tachypnea with respiratory rate (RR) 60-80 breaths/min or more, nasal flaring, paroxysmal nonproductive cough, increased respiratory effort or work of breathing (WOB), cyanosis, retractions, difficulty feeding because of increased RR, irritability, lethargy.

Physical assessment: Auscultation of expiratory wheezing and crackles or rhonchi. Symptoms of dehydration may be present: decreased level of consciousness (LOC), sunken anterior fontanel (if younger than 2 yr), dry or sticky oral mucosa, decreased abdominal skin turgor, decreased urine output.

Risk factors for severe RSV bronchiolitis:

- Premature infants born at less than 35 wk gestation
- Chronic lung disease or bronchopulmonary dysplasia
- Congenital heart disease
- Low socioeconomic status
- Weight less than 5 kg or birth weight less than 1500 g
- Immunodeficiency

DIAGNOSTIC TESTS

Diagnosis should be made on the basis of history and physical examination. American Academy of Pediatrics (AAP) in Clinical Practice Guidelines for Bronchiolitis (2006) recommends not routinely prescribing laboratory and radiologic studies.

Arterial blood gases: May be done initially to determine degree of hypoxemia and acid-base imbalance in infants/children in severe distress. Topical anesthetics are used if possible to decrease pain and anxiety (atraumatic care).

Pulse oximetry: Noninvasive method of monitoring oxygen saturation. It facilitates atraumatic care of the infant.

Chest x-ray examination: Usually shows hyperinflation with mild interstitial infiltrates, but segmental atelectasis occurs infrequently.

RSV washing on nasal or nasopharyngeal secretions: To identify cause of respiratory distress; detects RSV antigen.

Nursing Diagnosis:

Ineffective Airway Clearance

related to increased mucosal edema and secretions occurring with respiratory infection

Desired Outcomes: Within 24 to 48 hr of treatment/intervention, the child exhibits decreased RR and decreased WOB. By discharge, the child is able to manage respiratory secretions as evidenced by more normal RR and minimal WOB.

ASSESSMENT/INTERVENTIONS	RATIONALES
Assess respiratory status q2h: level of consciousness (LOC), RR, breath sounds, signs of increased WOB (nasal flaring, retractions, use of accessory muscles), cough, and skin and mucous membrane color.	Early identification of changes that might indicate increasing respiratory distress (decreased LOC, increased RR, adventitious or decreasing breath sounds, increased WOB, and pallor or bluish tint) ensures prompt intervention, which results in decreased severity of respiratory symptoms.
Assess heart rate (HR), RR, O_2 saturation, and breath sounds before and after nebulizer treatment.	These assessments monitor effectiveness of treatment and for its side effects (see next rationale).
Hold the nebulizer treatment if the HR is greater than 230 bpm for a child 1 yr of age or younger or greater than 180 bpm for a child older than 1 yr. Notify the health care provider accordingly.	Tachycardia is one of the main side effects of both medications. (Side effects should not outweigh the benefit of improving airway clearance.)
Administer racemic epinephrine or albuterol with handheld nebulizer (HHN) if prescribed (not recommended to be used routinely per AAP, 2006).	These agents decrease mucosal edema, which will open the airway and decrease WOB. Racemic epinephrine is a specific type of epinephrine that is administered via nebulizer, generally for croup or bronchiolitis. Use remains controversial.
Instill saline nose drops, wait 1-2 min, and suction the nares before feedings and prn.	Instilling saline drops before suctioning is helpful if the secretions are not loose or the child sounds congested. Suctioning before feedings to clear the nares will improve intake because infants are obligate nose breathers. Suctioning too often causes nasal edema if using a bulb syringe.

Nursing Diagnosis:

Impaired Gas Exchange

related to edema of the bronchiole mucosa and the presence of increased mucus

Desired Outcomes: Immediately following treatment/intervention, the child attains O_2 saturation greater than 90% (AAP, 2006). By discharge, the child maintains O_2 saturation greater than 90% on room air (unless child was O_2 dependent before the illness).

ASSESSMENT/INTERVENTIONS	RATIONALES
Assess for signs and symptoms of hypoxia (restlessness, change in LOC, dyspnea). Remember that cyanosis is a late sign of hypoxia in children.	Ongoing observation results in early detection of problems and early intervention, thereby decreasing severity of the hypoxia if it occurs.
Assess respiratory status q2h: LOC, RR, breath sounds, signs of increased WOB (nasal flaring, retractions, use of accessory muscles), cough, and skin and mucous membrane color.	This ensures early identification of changes that might indicate increasing respiratory distress. See details in the previous nursing diagnosis.
Assess vital signs q2-4h and prn.	Hypoxia causes an increase in HR, RR, and blood pressure (BP). A drop in BP and decreasing RR may be signs of impending respiratory arrest.
Maintain continuous oximetry initially and document at least q2h if the child is receiving O_2 and/or has moderate to severe respiratory distress.	Oximetry provides continuous monitoring of O_2 saturation and alerts nurses to changes.
Spot check O_2 saturation q4-8h when the child is clinically improving (feeding well with minimal respiratory distress).	Feeding well and minimal respiratory distress are good indicators of improvement in a child, and therefore less frequent monitoring is appropriate.
Provide humidified O_2 via nasal cannula to maintain O_2 saturation greater than 90%.	Delivering oxygen increases oxygen to the tissues. Oxygen is drying to the nasal mucosa, and humidity liquefies mucus.
Report to the health care provider if O_2 saturation is 90% or less.	O_2 saturation 90% or less may indicate deteriorating condition.
Position the child for maximum ventilation (e.g., head elevated but without compression on the diaphragm).	Children are diaphragmatic breathers until 7 yr of age. Preventing compression of the diaphragm enables optimal breathing effort.

ASSESSMENT/INTERVENTIONS	RATIONALES
Use a cardiorespiratory monitor for an infant or young child at high risk for or with a history of apnea.	This monitor ensures quick detection of deterioration in status or apneic episode.
Consolidate care to provide maximum rest.	Oxygen needs decrease with decreased energy expenditure.
Provide a neutral thermal environment.	An environment in which the child does not need to use any energy to cool or warm self reduces O_2 demand.

Nursing Diagnosis:

Deficient Fluid Volume

related to increased insensible loss (owing to increased RR, fever, increased metabolic rate) and decreased intake

Desired Outcome: Within 4 to 8 hr following treatment, the child has adequate fluid volume as evidenced by alertness and responsiveness, soft anterior fontanel (in child younger than 2 yr of age), moist oral mucous membrane, elastic skin turgor, and normal urine output ([UO]; e.g., infant UO more than 2-3 mL/kg/hr, toddler and preschooler UO 2 mL/kg/hr, school-age UO 1-2 mL/kg/hr, and adolescent UO 0.5-1 mL/kg/hr).

ASSESSMENT/INTERVENTIONS	RATIONALES
Assess hydration status: LOC, anterior fontanel (in child younger than 2 yr), oral mucous membrane, abdominal skin turgor, and UO q4h.	The child may be receiving maintenance fluids but still be dehydrated because of increased insensible losses. Frequent assessment leads to early recognition of problems and quicker treatment. Deficient fluid volume may be evidenced by decreased LOC, sunken anterior fontanel, dry or sticky oral mucous membrane (if not a mouth breather), tented abdominal skin, and decreased UO.
Assess intake and output q2-4h. Weigh all diapers. Ensure minimum UO of 1 mL/kg/hr is met.	These assessments enable earlier intervention if a deficit is noted.
Assess daily weights, using the same scale at the same time of day and without any clothing (including diaper) for infants or the same clothing for a child.	Short-term weight changes are the most reliable measurement of fluid loss or gain. Consistency in the time weighed, clothing, and scale improves accuracy of weight.
Assess temperature q4h and treat per the health care provider's directive.	Increased body temperature increases insensible fluid loss.
Ensure that the child is receiving at least daily maintenance fluids based on his or her weight.	Daily maintenance fluid requirements need to be met in order for the child to have adequate hydration. The smaller the child, the greater the percentage of body weight is water. To meet minimum fluid requirements, calculate the volume needed based on the child's weight: Up to 10 kg: 100 mL/kg/24 hr = _____ 10-20 kg: 50 mL/kg/24 hr = _____ More than 20 kg: 20 mL/kg/24 hr = _____ = maintenance fluid requirement *For example, a child weighs 23 kg:* 10 kg × 100 mL/kg/24 hr = 1000 mL/24 hr 10 kg × 50 mL/kg/24 hr = 500 mL/24 hr 3 kg × 20 mL/kg/24 hr = 60 mL/24 hr 23 kg = 1560 mL/24 hr Maintenance fluid requirement for a child weighing 23 kg is 1560 mL/24 hr.
Offer a variety of liquids frequently that the child likes (e.g., frozen juices, Popsicles, Pedialyte, Rice-Lyte, breast milk, formula).	This replaces measurable and insensible fluid losses and helps liquefy secretions. A child is more likely to cooperate if offered preferred fluids.

continued

ASSESSMENT/INTERVENTIONS

Do not offer by mouth (PO) fluids if the child's RR is more than 80 breaths/min while awake.

Administer intravenous (IV) fluids as prescribed.

RATIONALES

There is increased chance of aspiration when a child is tachypneic.

The child may not be able to take adequate oral fluid because of respiratory distress. Administering IV fluids ensures that the child receives maintenance fluids.

ADDITIONAL NURSING DIAGNOSES/PROBLEMS:

"Asthma" for **Fatigue** related to hypoxia and increased WOB   p. 553

Anxiety related to illness, loss of control, and medical/nursing interventions   p. 553

✓ PATIENT-FAMILY TEACHING AND DISCHARGE PLANNING

When providing child/family teaching, focus on sensory information, avoid giving excessive information, and initiate a visiting nurse referral for necessary follow-up teaching and assessment as needed. Stress importance of family-centered care (viewing the family as a unit that is the "constant" in the child's life and maintaining or improving the health of the family and its members in a holistic manner). Include verbal and written information about the following (ensure that written information is at a level the reader can understand):

✓ Bronchiolitis: definition, signs and symptoms, basic pathophysiology, length/progression of illness, and routes of transmission.

✓ If the child is on medications, drug name, route, purpose, type, dosage, precautions, and potential side effects. Also discuss drug-drug, food-drug, and herb-drug interactions.

✓ Despite having RSV bronchiolitis, the child can develop another RSV infection.

✓ Risk factors for developing RSV infection/bronchiolitis:
  • Exposure to tobacco smoke
  • Day care attendance
  • School-age siblings
  • Crowded living conditions (two or more children in the same bedroom)
  • Multiple births and/or premature infant born at less than 35 wk gestation
  • Chronic lung disease (CLD), congenital heart disease (CHD), or immunocompromised state
  • Born within 12 weeks of RSV season (usually November-April)
  • Formula-fed (resulting in decreased maternal antibodies) rather than breastfed

✓ Guidelines for preventing RSV infection/bronchiolitis:
  • Good hand hygiene
  • Keeping anyone with a fever or cold away from the child
  • Avoiding secondhand smoke
  • Avoiding crowds/day care

✓ Importance of checking hydration status at least several times a day when the child is ill. (The younger the child is and the less he or she weighs, the greater the percentage of body weight is water. Therefore, dehydration occurs much more quickly than it would in an older child or adult.)
  • Is the child alert and interactive? The child would not be as alert and interactive as normal if dehydrated.
  • Check the anterior fontanel (soft spot) on top of the head (in children younger than 2 yr). If it is sunken, the child may be dehydrated.
  • Check inside the mouth, not the lips. If dry or sticky and the child is not a mouth breather, the child is dehydrated.
  • Pinch skin on the abdomen. If it sits up like a tent instead of falling down right away, the child is dehydrated.
  • How many wet diapers does the child normally have a day? If the number of diapers is decreased or they are not as wet as usual, the child may be dehydrated.

✓ How much should the child drink per day? Give parents information they can understand, such as an infant that weighs 9 kg needs 900 mL/day for maintenance fluids, which is 30 ounces. If the infant drinks from 4-oz bottles, he or she needs to take about eight 4-oz bottles of fluid/day to get maintenance fluids.

✓ Use of normal saline nose drops and bulb syringe to clear nares before feedings. An infant breathes primarily through the nose until 5-6 mo old, so if the nose is congested, he or she cannot breathe and therefore cannot drink or eat. Do not suction too often because it can lead to increased nasal congestion resulting from nasal edema when using a bulb syringe.

✓ Continued prophylaxis against RSV with palivizumab (Synagis) if already receiving prophylaxis or per prescription (e.g., monthly IM medication that gives passive immunity against RSV during RSV season, usually November through April). This medication is given 5 months in a row or 3 times depending on risk of severe disease per guidelines (AAP, 2009).

✓ The child may still have some signs and symptoms of RSV/bronchiolitis but may return to babysitter/day care if he or she doesn't have a fever, is eating well, has had follow-up visit to the health care provider, and is believed to be no longer contagious. Most healthy infants recover in 7 to 10 days.

✓ Importance of follow-up care; typically follow-up appointment is made within 24-48 hr after discharge.

✓ Phone number to call in case questions or concerns arise about treatment or disease after discharge.

✓ When to call the health care provider:
  • Fever increases.
  • Rate of breathing increases (more than 60 breaths/min [varies depending on age of the infant/child]).
  • Nostrils flare out with each breath when the child is resting (crying will cause this to happen when the child is not having breathing problems).
  • The chest sinks in with each breath.
  • The child looks like he or she is working harder to breathe.
  • The lips turn gray or blue (cold can make lips look very pale and almost blue).
  • The child exhibits signs of dehydration.

✓ Importance of infant/child receiving all routine childhood immunizations and rationale for giving immunizations.

✓ Importance of cardiopulmonary resuscitation (CPR) and safety training.

Refer to community resources such as local and national American Lung Associations. Additional information can be obtained by contacting:

✓ The American Lung Association at *www.lung.org/lung-disease/bronchiolitis*

✓ The Canadian Lung Association at *www.lung.ca*

✓ March of Dimes at *www.Marchofdimes.com* (type in bronchiolitis in the search box)

✓ *www.rsvprotection.com* (information about the disease, treatment, and prevention)

✓ *www.cdc.gov/rsv* (information about the disease, treatment, and prevention as well as other information about RSV)

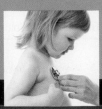

Burns 78

OVERVIEW/PATHOPHYSIOLOGY

Burn injuries represent one of the most painful and devastating traumas a person can experience. Fire and burn-related injuries are a leading cause of death from injury in children ages 1-14. Most burns in children are relatively minor and do not require hospitalization. In 2012, however, 136,453 children 19 yr and younger were seen in emergency departments for fire and burn-related injuries. In 2011, 325 children 19 yr and younger died from fires or burns, 85% of those fires were residential, and 47% of the deaths were of children 4 yr and younger. Fortunately, the death rate from burns decreased 55% from 1999 to 2011 (SAFE KIDS, 2014 Fact Sheet). Thermal burns result from contact with a thermal agent such as a flame, hot surface, or hot liquid (e.g., hair curlers/curling irons, radiators, kerosene heaters, wood burning stoves, ovens and ranges, irons, gasoline, and fireworks) and are the leading causes of fire/burn injuries in children 14 yr and younger.

The causative agent for burns varies depending on the child's developmental age. For instance, in children 4 yr and younger hospitalized with burn-related injuries, most are treated for scald burns caused by hot liquids, steam, or hot foods (e.g., coffee or soup), with the highest incidence in children younger than 2 yr. Ninety-five percent of these scald burns occur in residences and often relate to everyday activities such as bathing, cooking, and eating. Every day, 300 young children are taken to emergency departments as a result of scalds (Shriners, Scalds, May 2012). Chemical burns, another commonly seen burn in children, occur from touching or ingesting a caustic agent such as a cleaning solution and are also seen more often in younger children. The most common type of burn-related injury in older children is flame burn. In 2010, approximately 2000 children 15 yr and younger were injured and 355 were killed in fires, of which 88% were residential. Boys were at a higher risk of death from fires than girls as were African American children 4 yr and younger (USFA, August 2013). In 2013, an estimated 2960 children 15 yr and younger were treated in emergency departments for injuries involving fireworks during a 1-month special study period from June to July 2013 (CPSC, June 2014). The least common type of burn injury is electrical, usually occurring in children 12 yr and younger and often associated with household electrical or extension cords.

Another source of burn injury is child abuse. Estimates range from 1% to 35% that children admitted to burn units have an abusive burn. In the presence of unusual burns such as immersion (glove and stocking) burns, burns that spare flexor surfaces, contact burns from cigarettes or irons, and zebra burn lines from contact with a hot grate, child abuse should be suspected (Hornor, 2012).

Factors affecting severity of the burn and seriousness of the injury

1. Percentage of total body surface area (TBSA) burned: Use modified rule of nine for children (i.e., percentage of TBSA of head varies with age of child; at 1 yr old, it is 19%; at 5-9 yr old, it is 13%).
2. Burn depth:
   a. Superficial (first-degree) burn involves epidermis and heals within 5-7 days without scarring.
   b. Partial-thickness (second-degree) injury involves epidermis and varying degrees of the dermis. It may be superficial (usually healing in fewer than 21 days with variable scarring) or deep dermal (usually heals in more than 21 days if no infection occurs and with extensive scarring). The wound blanches with pressure.
   c. Full-thickness (third-degree) burn involves the epidermis and dermis and extends into the subcutaneous tissue. Nerve endings, sweat glands, and hair follicles are destroyed. It cannot reepithelialize and requires surgical excision and wound grafting. This tissue does not blanch. Frequently there are superficial and partial thickness burns to the surrounding tissue with both intact and exposed nerve endings.
   d. Fourth-degree is a full-thickness burn that involves underlying structures—muscles, fascia, and bones (Hockenberry, 2011).
3. Wound location: Certain body areas carry a higher risk of complications and require specialized care (e.g., burns of the hand and feet and across joints can interfere with growth and development because of scar formation).
4. Age of the child: For example, the very thin skin of a premature infant would take longer to heal and be damaged more easily than that of a healthy 3 yr old.
5. Causative agent.
6. Presence of respiratory involvement.
7. General health of the child.
8. Presence of concomitant injuries.

Children most at risk
- Children 4 yr and younger because of their natural curiosity and lack of awareness of danger are especially at risk for scald and contact burns and for sparkler injury.
- Children with disabilities related to developmental level or physical inability to get out of harm's way are especially at risk for scald and contact burns.
- Boys are at greater risk than girls.
- Children in homes without smoke detectors are at greatest risk for fires and fire-related death and injury.
- Children 5-14 yr old are at highest risk for fireworks-related injuries.

Differences in effects of burn injury in children
- There is a higher mortality rate in very young children who have been severely burned compared to older children and adults with comparable burns.
- Lower temperatures and shorter exposure time can cause more severe burns in children than in adults because of the child's thinner skin.
- Larger body surface area as compared with adults puts severely burned children at increased risk for fluid and heat loss.
- The greater proportion of body fluid to mass in children increases risk of dehydration and cardiovascular problems because of less effective cardiovascular response to changing intravascular volume. The younger the child, the greater the percentage of total body weight is water and the greater his or her percentage of extracellular fluid (i.e., interstitial fluid surrounds the cell; intravascular fluid is within the blood vessels or plasma; and transcellular fluid such as spinal fluid and sweat).
- Because of smaller muscle mass and less body fat than adults, children are at increased risk for protein and calorie deficiency.
- The younger the child, the less mature the immune system and the greater the risk for infection.
- Extensive burns may result in delayed growth.
- Hypertrophic scarring is increased, and scar maturation is prolonged.

HEALTH CARE SETTING

Emergency department, with possible hospitalization for significant burns; some burns are treated in primary care and others at home.

ASSESSMENT

Varies significantly depending on burn severity and seriousness of the injury.

Superficial burn (e.g., mild sunburn): Erythema, moderate discomfort/pain, blanches with pressure, good capillary refill.

Partial-thickness burn
- *Superficial:* Fluid-filled blisters, skin red to ivory with moist surfaces, considerable pain, blanches with pressure and refills.
- *Deep:* May or may not have fluid-filled blisters; blisters are often flat and dehydrated, making skin tissue-paper–like; color is mottled, waxy white, and with a dry surface. Nerve endings are intact, so pain is severe on exposure to air or water.

Full-thickness burn: Varies in color from red to tan, waxy white, brown, or black. It does not blanch with pressure. Edema is present. It has a dry, leathery appearance and lacks sensation because of destruction of nerve endings. However, because it is usually surrounded by superficial and partial-thickness burns that have intact nerve endings, adjacent areas likely will be painful.

Respiratory compromise: Upper airway edema related to injury starts within a few minutes, and the airway may occlude in minutes to a few hours, although it may be delayed up to 24-48 hr.

Respiratory distress: Abdominal breathing in a child older than 7 yr (children are primarily abdominal breathers until that age), head bobbing with respiratory effort, nasal flaring, coughing, stridor, wheezing.

Burn shock: With severe burns (greater than 15%-20% TBSA), a type of hypovolemic shock may occur with increased heart rate (HR), increased respiratory rate (RR), low blood pressure (BP), hypothermia, pallor, cyanosis, decreased level of consciousness (LOC), and poor muscle tone.

Physical assessment: In addition to signs mentioned above, the examiner may notice singed nasal hairs and nasopharynx edema. It is also important to assess for other injuries such as fractures and internal injuries.

Complications
- *Pulmonary complications are the leading cause of death in thermal trauma:* Inhalation injury, aspiration of gastric contents, bacterial pneumonia, pulmonary edema/insufficiency, and emboli. Pneumonia is the leading cause of infection and death.
- *Wound sepsis:* Disorientation is one of the first signs of overwhelming sepsis.
- *Gastrointestinal complications:* Feeding intolerance, mucosal ulceration, and bleeding, especially in the stomach and duodenum.
- *Encephalopathy:* Lethargy, withdrawal, and coma occur. Children under 10 yr of age rarely experience delirium or hallucinations; full neurologic recovery usually occurs (Hockenberry, 2011).

DIAGNOSTIC TESTS

Note: *Topical anesthetics are used with blood draws, if possible, to decrease pain and anxiety and to provide atraumatic care.*

Arterial blood gas level: To determine respiratory status/acid-base balance; variations from normal may signal respiratory compromise.

Chemistries
- *Fluid and electrolytes:* Deficits of fluid and sodium occur with burn shock.
- *Blood urea nitrogen and creatinine:* Elevations may indicate renal failure.
- *Glucose:* May be elevated in young infants. Stress may cause either hypoglycemia or pseudodiabetes, resulting in elevated glucose levels.

Nursing Diagnosis:

Deficient Fluid Volume

related to fluid shift from the intravascular to interstitial compartment, increased metabolic demands, and decreased intake

Desired Outcomes: Within 4 hr following intervention/treatment, the child has adequate fluid volume as evidenced by normal LOC for the child, soft anterior fontanel (in a child younger than 2 yr), moist oral mucous membranes, good/elastic abdominal skin turgor (on unaffected areas), and normal urine output (UO). For example, infant UO more than 2-3 mL/kg/hr, toddler and preschooler UO 2 mL/kg/hr, school-age child UO 1-2 mL/kg/hr, and adolescent UO 0.5-1 mL/kg/hr.

ASSESSMENT/INTERVENTIONS RATIONALES

ASSESSMENT/INTERVENTIONS	RATIONALES
Assess hydration status q4h: LOC, anterior fontanel (in a child younger than 2 yr), oral mucous membrane, abdominal skin turgor, and urine output. **Note:** Edema may occur around the burn or from fluid shifts.	The child may be receiving maintenance fluids but still be dehydrated due to significantly increased insensible water losses, especially in a child with burns. Frequent assessment leads to early detection of problems and quicker treatment. Signs of impaired hydration include decreasing LOC, sunken fontanel, dry and sticky oral mucous membrane, tenting of abdominal skin, and decreased UO.
Assess intake and output (I&O) q2h. Weigh all diapers, 1 mL = 1 g. Ensure minimum urine output of 1 mL/kg/hr is met	This assessment determines whether the child is receiving appropriate intake and has adequate output.
⚠ Assess vital signs (VS), capillary refill, and LOC q4h for changes related to hypovolemia.	Hypovolemia may be present because of reduced circulating blood volume that occurs with plasma loss in burns. Tachycardia, changes in tissue perfusion (e.g., capillary refill more than 2-3 sec), and alteration in LOC are early signs of hypovolemic shock. BP will be normal initially because increased systemic vascular resistance helps to maintain it. However, perfusion with a normal BP may be inadequate to meet the body's demands. Therefore, decreased BP can be a late sign of hypovolemia in children.
Assess daily weights, using the same scale at the same time of day and with the same amount of clothing (no clothes, including diaper in infants).	Short-term weight changes are the most reliable measurement of fluid loss or gain. Excessive weight gain could indicate fluid retention; weight loss could signal dehydration or excessive fluid loss. Either would interfere with wound healing. Consistency in weighing increases accuracy.
Administer intravenous (IV) fluids as prescribed.	Fluid resuscitation is required in children with burns greater than 10% TBSA. Fluids help maintain general circulation to vital organs and capillary circulation to viable skin.
⚠ Assess the IV site qh.	Peripheral IVs in children can infiltrate and cause tissue damage in a short period of time, especially in younger children. Thus, the patient would not be receiving the needed fluid systemically as well as having additional tissue damage.
Once stabilized, ensure that the child receives *at least* maintenance fluids based on his or her weight.	The smaller the child, the greater the percentage of body weight is water and the larger the percentage of extracellular fluid. Because of fluid loss from the burn injury and increased metabolic demands related to the child's age and increased catecholamine release caused by burn stress, the child probably will need more than maintenance fluids. First, use this formula to determine maintenance fluids: **Up to 10 kg: 100 mL/kg/24 hr** = _____ **10-20 kg: 50 mL/kg/24hr** = _____ **More than 20 kg: 20 mL/kg/24hr** = _____ = maintenance fluid requirement ***For example, a child weighs 33 kg:*** 10 kg × 100 mL/kg/24 hr = 1000 mL/24 hr 10 kg × 50 mL/kg/24 hr = 500 mL/24 hr 13 kg × 20 mL/kg/24 hr = 260 mL/24 hr 33 kg = 1760 mL/24 hr Maintenance fluid requirement for a child weighing 33 kg is 1760 mL/24 hr. Remember that the child probably will need *more* than maintenance fluids.
Alert the health care provider promptly to significant findings or changes.	This helps ensure timely treatment.

Nursing Diagnosis:

Acute Pain

related to thermal injuries and medical-surgical interventions

Desired Outcome: Within 30 min to 1 hr after treatment/intervention, the child's pain level is decreased (to 4 or less on the developmentally appropriate scale with 0-10 rating; FLACC [face, legs, activity, cry, consolability]; FACES; or numeric) or at a level acceptable to the child.

INTERVENTIONS	RATIONALES
Assess the child's developmental level and establish the appropriate pain scale (e.g., FLACC, Wong-Baker FACES, or numeric).	A pain scale increases the ability to accurately assess pain and the degree of relief obtained.
Assess level of pain q2-4h, as well as before and after pain medication administration (e.g., 1 hr after by mouth [PO] medications, 10-20 min after IV medications).	These assessments detect early changes in pain level and assess effectiveness of pain medications.
Provide pain medications/nonpharmacologic pain relief measures around the clock on a regular basis, not prn.	Scheduled rather than prn pain relief provides better and more reliable pain control. Prolonged stimulation of pain receptors results in increased sensitivity to painful stimuli and will increase the amount of analgesia needed to relieve pain. Pain relief measures such as distraction; relaxation; repositioning; guided imagery; cutaneous stimulation such as massage, heat, or cold; and positive self-talk increase effectiveness of medications.
Explain how patient-controlled analgesia (PCA) works and that the child cannot give self too much medication. Encourage the child/parent to use PCA when needed if it is available.	Most experts believe that when a child is capable of pushing the button on the pump, usually by 5-6 yr of age, he or she can self-administer pain medication. Some facilities allow PCA by proxy—the parent or nurse can administer the medication if the child is too ill or cannot understand the concept of pushing the button to relieve the pain.
Reassure the parent that addiction rarely occurs when medication is used to relieve pain.	Fear of addiction may decrease use of pain medication.
Premedicate the child before painful procedures. Use a topical anesthetic to decrease the trauma of blood draws/IV insertion, if possible (atraumatic care).	Pain medications given before painful procedures will help control pain. The time frame before the procedure depends on the route (e.g., 10-20 min IV and 1 hr PO).
Explain all procedures at the developmental level appropriate for the child.	Anxiety increases pain; knowing what to expect may decrease anxiety.

Nursing Diagnoses:

Impaired Skin Integrity
Impaired Tissue Integrity

related to burn injury

Desired Outcomes: The skin/graft site heals without signs of infection (e.g., drainage, erythema, edema, or pain). Superficial burns heal within 7 days without scarring; deep partial-thickness burns heal within 30 days with varying degrees of scarring.

ASSESSMENT/INTERVENTIONS	RATIONALES
Assess both the child and wound/graft/donor site(s) q4h for signs and symptoms of infection.	These assessments ensure prompt recognition of problems, more rapid treatment, and maximum healing. Infection indicators include change in LOC, hypothermia or hyperthermia, odor, drainage, increased edema, increased erythema, and increased pain.

continued

ASSESSMENT/INTERVENTIONS	RATIONALES
Assess the graft q4h for evidence of hematoma, edema, or sloughing of graft; notify the health care provider promptly if noted.	Early recognition of the problem and prompt treatment increase the chance of saving the graft.
Carefully clean the wound and tissue immediately surrounding the wound as prescribed.	Cautious cleansing is necessary to avoid damaging the epithelialization of granulating skin and decrease risk of infection. Infection would further damage the already traumatized tissue, disrupt epithelialization, and delay healing.
Provide appropriate pain control measures before removing the dressing and beginning wound care.	A relaxed, more comfortable patient facilitates careful wound cleansing.
Débride the wound as prescribed.	Débridement promotes healing by removing dead or injured tissue so that the wound has an environment conducive to healing.
Apply ointment and/or dressings as prescribed using clean/sterile technique.	These measures protect the wound, decrease risk of infection, and promote healing.
Minimize the child scratching and picking at the wound, using methods appropriate for his or her developmental age.	This promotes better wound healing and decreases scarring. Methods for developmental age include: - Young child: distraction and supervision - Older child: explanations of the importance of not scratching, picking, or hitting the wound
Perform active (or ensure passive) range-of-motion (ROM) exercises to affected joints as prescribed.	These exercises promote reabsorption of edema, prevent contracture formation, and improve healing.
Position for minimal stress/pressure on the wound/graft.	Proper positioning promotes healing and protects the wound/graft. For example, do not allow the child to lie on the wound; use a cradle to keep sheets/blankets off the graft site.
Offer high-calorie, high-protein meals and snacks, providing foods the child likes.	The child has increased metabolism and catabolism because of the burn injury and therefore needs increased calories and protein to promote positive nitrogen balance, which facilitates healing. Offering foods the child likes increases the likelihood of increased intake.
Administer vitamins and minerals (e.g., vitamins A, B, C, zinc, and iron) as prescribed.	These supplements facilitate wound healing and epithelialization.
For more detailed information, see "Managing Wound Care," p. 533.	

Nursing Diagnosis:

Risk for Infection

related to loss of skin barrier/denuded skin, increased metabolic demands, altered nutritional status, invasive procedures/lines, and the hospital environment

Desired Outcome: The child exhibits wound healing without signs of burn wound infection (e.g., odor, drainage, increased erythema or edema, increased pain) or systemic infection (e.g., pneumonia or septicemia).

> **Note:** *See assessment/interventions and rationales for* **Impaired Skin Integrity/Impaired Tissue Integrity** *plus the following:*

ASSESSMENT/INTERVENTIONS	RATIONALES
Assess VS q4h and notify the health care provider of findings indicative of infection (e.g., temperature 36° C or less or 38.5° C or greater, HR 100 bpm or greater, or RR 30 breaths/min or more, but will vary depending on age of the child).	Early signs of infection/sepsis include tachycardia, tachypnea, and fever or hypothermia. Early recognition of any abnormality enables prompt treatment and less serious infection.

ASSESSMENT/INTERVENTIONS	RATIONALES
Monitor LOC q4h.	Disorientation is one of the first signs of overwhelming sepsis/septic shock in patients with burn.
Monitor for signs of pneumonia q4h (varies depending on age of the child).	Early recognition facilitates prompt treatment and a less severe infection. - Infant: fever, restlessness, anxiety, grunting, nasal flaring, retractions, tachypnea, head bobbing. - Child and adolescent: fever, chills, cough, chest pain, restlessness, anxiety, tachypnea.
Assess IV sites (peripheral qh or central access q4h) for signs of infection (e.g., erythema, warmth, edema).	There is potential for increased rate of infection because of the child's altered immune response and because the IV site is another entry site for bacteria.
Wash your hands before and after working with a child with open wounds or if contact with blood or body fluids is possible.	Hand hygiene is the best method of preventing nosocomial infection. Hand hygiene with an alcohol-based hand sanitizer may be used before and after contact with intact skin.
Use gloves as indicated, following standard precautions.	Gloves provide an additional level of protection for the patient by reducing risk of contamination of open wounds by the bare hands of caregivers. (Wearing gloves also protects the caregiver from contact with the patient's open wounds.)
Depending on developmental age, ensure that the child turns, coughs, and deep breathes or uses incentive spirometer q2h while awake. Younger children can blow bubbles or blow on a pinwheel.	Deep breathing expands alveoli and aids in mobilizing secretions to the airways, and coughing further mobilizes and clears the secretions to help prevent pneumonia.
Position the child with the head elevated 15-30 degrees for 1-2 hr after meals.	This position decreases incidence of aspiration of gastric contents, which could lead to aspiration pneumonia.
Screen visitors for colds or other infectious illnesses before they enter the child's room.	The child has an altered immune response and is at greater risk for infection because of the following: - Open wounds or denuded skin have lost the protective skin barrier and are potential entry sites for infection. - Decreased circulation to the burned area compromises the body's ability to fight infection at the tissue level because fewer leukocytes (white blood cells, which act as scavengers and fight infection) are able to reach damaged tissue. - Mature neutrophils, the body's first line of defense against bacterial infection and severe stress, are decreased as immature neutrophils (bands) increase to digest products of the burn injury.
For more information, see Appendix A for "Infection Prevention and Control," p. 747.	

Nursing Diagnosis:

Imbalanced Nutrition: Less Than Body Requirements

related to hypermetabolic state and decreased appetite

Desired Outcome: Within 1 wk of intervention/treatment, the child exhibits adequate nutrition as evidenced by maintenance of or gaining weight.

ASSESSMENT/INTERVENTIONS	RATIONALES
Assess weight on the same scale at the same time of day with the same amount of clothing. Frequency depends on unit policy and/or prescription of the health care provider.	Consistency with weight measurements helps ensure more accurate results. Weight is a reliable indicator of nutritional status (as long as the child is not edematous).
Monitor for hypoglycemia.	Hypoglycemia can result from the stress of injury as glycogen stores in the liver are rapidly depleted.

continued

ASSESSMENT/INTERVENTIONS	RATIONALES
Monitor for hyperglycemia.	Hyperglycemia can occur because of mobilization of glucagon and decreased insulin production.
Provide high-calorie, high-protein meals and snacks, as well as foods high in vitamin C content.	Because of smaller muscle mass and less body fat than adults, children are at increased risk for protein and calorie deficiency. This diet provides positive nitrogen balance and nutrients needed for wound healing. Energy requirements increase according to size of the burn; caloric requirements may be 2 to 3 times normal because of the increased metabolic rate. High-protein meals replace protein lost by exudation.
Provide foods the child likes and encourage the child to feed self as much as possible.	These measures stimulate appetite and promote cooperation, thereby improving likelihood of increased intake.
Ensure that the child is receiving adequate nutrients. Discuss the child's needs with the health care provider.	If this cannot be accomplished orally, enteral or parenteral feedings may be necessary. Burns will not heal well without adequate nutrients.
Try to minimize anorexia in the following ways: - Offer small, frequent meals.	Anorexia occurs in many children with burn injury. - The child may eat better with 4-5 small meals/day rather than 3 large meals.
- Make mealtimes pleasant with attractive meals, companionship, and no treatments or unpleasant interruptions.	- Eating is more likely to occur in a more "homelike" environment.
Maintain a neutral thermal environment.	Caloric expenditure is minimized when the child does not need to use energy to cool or heat the body.
Ensure the child is having a normal stooling pattern. Assess for constipation or diarrhea and notify the health care provider if either occurs.	Constipation caused by decreased activity and intake could further affect intake because of discomfort and thus interfere with weight gain. Diarrhea would decrease weight as well.

Nursing Diagnosis:

Disturbed Body Image

related to the child's perception of altered appearance and mobility/skills

Desired Outcomes: The child receives emotional support from the onset of injury and discusses feelings related to the change in appearance and mobility/skills after wound healing begins. Within 48-72 hr of this diagnosis, the child relates at least one positive example of his or her appearance/abilities and expresses realistic expectations for the future, if developmentally and medically able to do this.

ASSESSMENT/INTERVENTIONS	RATIONALES
Assess support systems and coping mechanisms used in previous stressful situations.	Optimally, this assessment will mobilize previous effective strategies to assist the child in dealing with the current altered appearance and mobility/skills.
Ensure a positive attitude when caring for the child.	This shows acceptance and encourages expectation the child will get better.
Point out positive aspects of the child's appearance/abilities. Ask the child during subsequent care to give examples of positive aspects.	Positive reinforcement encourages a child to focus on positive aspects rather than on deficits.
Point out evidence of healing.	This promotes a sense of hope.
Encourage the child to provide for developmentally appropriate self-care as much as his or her condition allows.	Encouragement enables a child to focus on tasks that he or she can do and promotes a positive self-image in the process.
Give honest answers to the child and family regarding care and appearance.	Honesty facilitates building of a trusting nurse-patient/family relationship and assists in developing realistic expectations.
Arrange for continued schooling, depending on age of the child. For younger children, encourage play.	This decreases isolation and provides normalization, which may help self-image.
Promote peer contact if possible and prepare peers for the child's appearance.	These measures facilitate acceptance and support.

ASSESSMENT/INTERVENTIONS	RATIONALES
Help the child devise a plan to address and cope with the reactions of others.	This will increase a sense of control. Role playing may help the child perfect this plan.
Support appropriate adaptive behaviors.	This measure builds on strengths.
Encourage verbalization about feelings regarding appearance and changes in lifestyle.	This will help identify the child's concerns and anxieties, enabling you to provide more realistic feedback about the child's appearance if appropriate and aid in working on coping strategies.
Discuss ways the child can "cover up" disfigurement, dressings, and pressure garments.	This facilitates coping. Examples include clothing (e.g., turtleneck sweaters, larger shirt than normal), wigs, and makeup.
Facilitate transition back to day care, school, and the home environment. Encourage communication of the family and medical staff with other care providers, including school nurse and teachers.	These measures prepare other children and caregivers for the change in the child's appearance and encourage them to make the transition a positive experience.

ADDITIONAL NURSING DIAGNOSES/PROBLEMS:

"Psychosocial Support"   p. 72

"Psychosocial Support for the Patient's Family and Significant Other"   p. 84

"Managing Wound Care" for more details regarding wound treatment   p. 533

"Asthma" for **Anxiety**   p. 553

"Cystic Fibrosis" for **Impaired Gas Exchange** (for children with inhalation injury)   p. 590

✓ PATIENT-FAMILY TEACHING AND DISCHARGE PLANNING

When providing patient/family teaching, focus on sensory information, avoid giving excessive information, and initiate visiting nurse referral for necessary follow-up teaching and assessment as needed. Stress importance of family-centered care (viewing the family as a unit that is the "constant" in the child's life and maintaining or improving the health of the family and its members in a holistic manner). Include verbal and written information about the following (ensure that written information is at a level the reader can understand):

✓ Type of burn and normal healing time.
✓ Wound care as appropriate:
  • Administering oral pain medication about 1 hr before wound care if needed
  • Cleaning the wound
  • Applying ointment
  • Applying dressing
✓ Treatment of pain (e.g., administering medication on a regular basis, which gives better control and assists the healing process; use of nonpharmaceutical adjuncts such as distraction).

✓ Signs and symptoms of burn wound, graft site, or donor site infection:
  • Purulent drainage or odor
  • Increased redness or swelling
  • Temperature 101.5° F or greater or per discharge instructions
✓ Ways to prevent infection:
  • Good hand hygiene before and after caring for the wound
  • Dressing changes performed in a clean area with good light
  • Making sure the dressing stays clean and dry
✓ Methods of preventing scars and contractures:
  • Wearing pressure garments as prescribed (usually 23 hr/day)
  • Wearing splints as prescribed (over top of the pressure garment)
  • ROM exercises as prescribed and demonstrated by physical therapist (PT)
  • Child performing as many activities of daily living as possible (e.g., feeding self, combing hair, dressing self)
✓ Care of healing skin:
  • May be dry: Apply lotion (cocoa butter is most often recommended), but avoid those containing alcohol or lanolin.
  • May be itchy: Use lotion, prescribed medication (e.g., Benadryl), distraction.
  • Bathing: Use lukewarm water and be gentle!
  • Protect new skin over the burned area.
  • Wear comfortable clothing, not constrictive.
  • Try to avoid hitting or bumping the area.
  • Protect from the sun with clothing and sunscreen (SPF 15 or higher).
  • Do not stay out in cold weather; the burned area is sensitive to cold.
✓ If the child is on any medications: discuss drug name; route; purpose; type; dosage; precautions; drug-drug, food-drug, and herb-drug interactions; and potential side effects.

✓ Demonstrate drawing up and administering medication and having family member perform return demonstration.

✓ Nutritional needs (the child needs increased calories and protein to heal well):
- Make pudding with Ensure instead of milk (increases calories).
- Eat small, frequent meals or three meals with nutritious snacks between meals.
- Make mealtime a social, shared time. Turn off TV.
- Feed child when he or she is well rested.
- If receiving tube feeding: procedure for checking placement and administering feeding, checking residual, and recognizing and reporting problems.
- Vitamins that help skin heal: A and C (found in oranges, grapefruit, tomatoes, broccoli, and carrots).
- Protein, which promotes skin healing: meat, fish, eggs, peanut butter, chicken, and milk.

✓ Importance of adequate fluid intake to promote healing (the child should receive at least maintenance fluids or more per the health care provider). How much should the child drink per day? Give parents information they can understand, such as an infant that weighs 9 kg needs 900 mL/day for maintenance fluids, which is 30 oz. If the infant drinks from 4-oz bottles, he or she needs to take eight 4-oz bottles of fluid/day to get maintenance fluids. An older child weighing 40 kg would need 1900 mL/day for maintenance fluids. If this child drinks from 12-oz glasses, he or she would need at least five and a half 12-oz glasses/day. These examples are only for maintenance fluids; the child may need 1½ -2 times maintenance fluids to stay well hydrated, depending on size and stage of healing of the burn injury.

✓ Importance of checking hydration status at least several times a day while the child is still healing from the burn. The less the child weighs and the younger he or she is, the greater the percentage of body weight is water. Therefore dehydration occurs much more quickly than it would in an older child or adult. The child may still be losing fluid from the burn and using more energy to heal, therefore using more fluid.
- Is the child alert and interactive? Child would not be as alert and interactive as normal if dehydrated.
- Check soft spot on top of the head (in children younger than 2 yr). If it is sunken in, the child may be dehydrated.
- Check inside the mouth, not the lips. If dry or sticky and the child is not a mouth breather, the child is dehydrated.
- Pinch skin on the abdomen. If the skin sits up like a tent instead of falling down right away, the child is dehydrated.
- How many wet diapers does the child normally have a day or how many times does he or she normally

void? If the number of diapers is decreased, they are not as wet as usual, or the child is voiding less often, he or she may be dehydrated.

✓ Adjustment after burn injury, which is often prolonged and painful. Family and individual psychosocial support is important. Reinforce importance of helping siblings cope/adjust to having a sibling with a potentially long-term injury.

✓ Growth and development (realistic expectations of what the child should be doing at different ages and encouragement of activities that promote normal growth and development).

✓ Feelings the child may experience with reentry to school/society, which vary depending on developmental age and severity of the burn: fear, anger, guilt, depression, withdrawal, altered body image, anticipating peer response.

✓ Potential for regression. This is normal after a stressful event.

✓ Developmentally related risks for burn injuries (see introductory data).

✓ Tips for childproofing the home:
- Set water heater thermostat at 120° F or less or install antiscald devices in faucets and showerheads in buildings where one does not have access to the water tank (e.g., apartment buildings).
  - Water temperature of 120° F takes 2.5 min for full thickness burn (3rd degree).
  - Water temperature of 130° F takes 15 sec for full thickness burn.
  - Water temperature of 140° F takes 2.5 sec for full thickness burn.
- The younger the child, the thinner the skin, and the quicker the burn occurs and more deeply it penetrates.
- Never leave a young child alone, especially in the kitchen or bathroom, even to answer the telephone for a minute. Take the child with you.
- Turn pot handles toward back of the stove and use back burners when cooking.
- Cover stovetop knobs.
- Keep appliance cords out of the child's vision and reach (e.g., coffee pot), especially if the appliance contains hot food or liquid.
- Cover unused electrical outlets with appropriate outlet covers (not the ones that just plug in).
- Keep hot foods and liquids away from table and counter edges.
- Do not leave hot foods or liquids on a table with a tablecloth the child can reach.
- Never carry or hold the child and hot food and/or beverage at the same time.
- Stress the dangers of open flames; explain what "hot" means.
- Place a protective cover in front of the radiator, fireplace, or other heating element.

- Keep matches, gasoline, lighters, and all other flammable materials locked away and out of the child's reach.
- Teach children how to "*stop, drop, and roll*" if their clothes catch fire and how to crawl to safety if a fire occurs in the building they are in.
- Over 6 mo old, apply sunscreen with SPF 15 or higher when the child is exposed to sunlight.

✓ Additional tips for preventing fire-related injuries:

- Install smoke detectors in every bedroom and on each level. Test them monthly and change batteries at least yearly. Having smoke detectors cuts the risk of dying in a fire by 50%.
- Have at least two multipurpose dry chemical fire extinguishers: one in the kitchen and one in a workshop or area where potential sources of fire exist (e.g., water heater or furnace). Check monthly for signs of damage, corrosion, tampering, and leaks. Always call the fire department before using the fire extinguisher. Use the PASS method (*p*oint, *a*im at the base of the fire, *s*queeze the handle, and *s*weep from side to side).
- Set up a home emergency fire escape plan and have practice drills using the escape plan at least quarterly. Include a meeting place outside the home in your plan.

✓ First-aid emergency care for a burn injury: Put the burned area under cool running water immediately, remove clothing, cover the burned area loosely with a bandage or clean cloth, seek medical assistance.

✓ Importance of follow-up care with the health care provider, PT, and any other specialists involved.

✓ Telephone numbers to call for the health care provider, home health nurse, and PT in case any questions or concerns about treatment or injury arise after discharge.

✓ When to call the health care provider:

- If the child is not eating well or showing signs of dehydration
- If there is unmanageable behavior at home or school
- If there are any signs of infection (e.g., healing burn area or donor site looks, feels, or smells different—red, warm, swollen, very tender to the touch or there is foul-smelling drainage)
- If there is itching that is not controlled with lotion or medication
- If the healing/healed area cracks open or splits
- If contracture occurs
- If the child's temperature is higher than 101.5° F
- If the dressing change is painful despite giving pain medication as prescribed

✓ Referral to community resources, such as National SAFE KIDS Campaign, public health nurse, home health agencies, community support groups, camps for children with burns, psychologists, and financial counseling as appropriate. Additional general information can be obtained by contacting the following organizations:

- National SAFE KIDS Campaign at *www.safekids.org*
- Shriners Hospitals Burn Awareness at *www.shrinershospitals* for *children.org* and search for burns
- Alisa Ann Ruch Burn Foundation (camps in California, prevention teaching, support services) at *www.aarbf.org*
- Most burn camps are supported by local/state organizations. Search under burn camps for children for individual states. Also look at *www.kidscamps.com/special_needs/burn.html* and click on your state.
- USFA (United States Fire Association) for Kids: Interactive fire safety fun and games for kids at *www.usfa.fema.gov/kids/flash.shtm*
- USFA resources for kids, teachers, and parents/caregivers at *www.usfa.fema.gov/kids*
- Safe at Home provides safety data at *www.safeathome.ca*

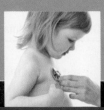

Child Abuse and Neglect 79

OVERVIEW/PATHOPHYSIOLOGY

The problem of child abuse and neglect or child maltreatment, formerly called "battered child syndrome," is now recognized as a problem of epidemic proportions to children in the United States (Hornor, 2013). A report of child abuse is made every 10 seconds. More than 4 children die every day as a result of child abuse (Child Help, 2013). In 2011 an estimated 3.4 million referrals were made to child protective services (CPS) involving an estimated 6.2 million children. About 39.2% were screened out and about 2 million reports were screened in and had a CPS response and disposition. About 27.4 referrals per 1000 children needed disposition. An estimated 681,000 children were found to be victims of child abuse or neglect with 1570 fatalities nationally, decreased from 1740 fatalities in 2009. About 80% of the fatalities were children younger than 4 yr (Administration for Children and Families [ACF] and Child Help, 2012). Many more children are left permanently disabled, and thousands of victims are overwhelmed by this trauma for the rest of their lives. The national rate of children being investigated or assessed had only slight variations over the past 5 years, but experts estimate the actual number of incidents of abuse/neglect is 3 times greater than those reported.

Child abuse and neglect occur in all cultural, ethnic, occupational, and socioeconomic groups. It is not usually a single event but rather a pattern of behavior that occurs over time. The following factors increase the likelihood of abuse or neglect occurring in families:

- **Parental characteristics:** Predisposition to maltreatment (perhaps having been victims themselves), substance abuse, lack of parenting skills, poor impulse control, and emotional immaturity.
- **Child characteristics:** Temperament, physical or cognitive disability that predisposes the child to injury, chronic illness or disability, being born to unmarried parents, or hyperactivity.
- **Environmental characteristics:** Divorce, marital problems, financial strain, poor housing, isolation from support of families or friends.
- **Societal factors:** Increased violence, children viewed as property and not valued, physical methods of punishment, lack of willingness in community to become involved in family violence issues.

The highest incidence of child abuse and neglect occurs in children younger than 5 yr, with the highest rate of victimization occurring in children from birth to 1 yr. The rate declines as children get older except for sexual abuse. In 2011, 78.5% of victims suffered neglect, 17.6% suffered physical abuse, 9.1% were sexually abused, 9.0% suffered psychologic maltreatment, and 2.2% were medically neglected, with 10.6% listed as other/unknown (e.g., abandonment, threats of harm to the child, and congenital drug/alcohol addiction). With sexual abuse, approximately 26% are 12-14 yr and 22% are 15-17 yr. Many children were victims of multiple types of maltreatment, with each type being counted individually; thus, the above categories of abuse add up to more than 100%. About 11% of victims were disabled (mental, emotional, or physical). Approximately 30% of abused and neglected children will later abuse or neglect their own children (ACF, and Child Help, 2012). The perpetrators most often are one or both of the parents, with mothers the more frequent perpetrator. Terms include:

- **Child maltreatment:** A broad term that includes intentional physical abuse or neglect, emotional abuse or neglect, and sexual abuse (younger than 18 yr) usually by an adult caregiver, most often the parent.
- **Physical abuse:** The deliberate infliction of physical injury or pain. It may result from punching, beating, kicking, biting, bruising, shaking, burning, or otherwise harming a child and can occur from overdiscipline or physical punishment.
- **Physical neglect:** Failure to provide basic necessities such as food, clothing, shelter, and a safe environment in which the child can grow and develop normally.
- **Emotional abuse:** Deliberate attempt to destroy or significantly impair self-esteem or competence by rejecting, ignoring, criticizing, isolating, or terrorizing the child. The most common form is verbal abuse or "belittling."
- **Emotional neglect:** Failure to meet the child's needs for affection, attention, and emotional support. The most common feature is absence of the normal parent-child attachment and interaction.
- **Sexual abuse:** Contacts or interactions between a child and an adult for the adult's sexual gratification, with or without physical contact. It includes pedophilia and all forms of incest and rape. It also includes fondling, oral-genital contact, all forms of intercourse, exhibitionism,

voyeurism, and involvement of children in the production of pornography. It is thought to be one of the most common but underreported crimes against children. Approximately 26% of children sexually abused are 12-14 yr, and 22% are 15-17 yr (ACF, 2012). More than 50% do not report the sexual abuse until they are adults (Jenny and Crawford-Jukubiak, 2013).

- **Medical care neglect:** Failure to provide needed treatment to infants or children who generally have life-threatening or serious medical conditions. About one third of these children are younger than 3 yr.
- **Caregiver fabricated illness (formerly Munchausen syndrome by proxy):** Abuse inflicted on a child in which a parent (usually the mother) fabricates symptoms and falsifies medical history or actually causes an illness that results in evaluation and treatment.
- **Abusive head trauma (AHT) (formerly shaken baby syndrome):** Caused by violent shaking of an infant or young child (most often younger than 1 yr with infants 1-3 mo at greatest risk) or a nonaccidental impact injury to the head, resulting in severe injury. There are high mortality rates in infant victims, estimated to exceed 20% with significant disability for nearly two thirds of the survivors. These children often have long-term consequences from their injuries including neurologic, behavioral, and cognitive (Parks et al., 2012).

HEALTH CARE SETTING

Primary care or emergency department with possible hospitalization resulting from complications. Abuse/neglect also may be found during hospitalization for other reasons.

ASSESSMENT

Note: *History is critical in making a diagnosis. Frequently in child abuse/neglect cases, the history is inconsistent with injury severity, or it changes during evaluation. It is essential that the nurse taking the history be nonjudgmental and report factual information. This is difficult to do at times, and collegial support is beneficial. History and physical examination will determine needed diagnostic tests.*

Physical abuse: Acts out violently against others; frightened of parents or caregivers; avoids changing clothes (e.g., in gym class); old, new, and multiple injuries; burn or restraint injuries; questionable bruises and welts; questionable burns (e.g., imprint or immersion); questionable fractures (e.g., spiral fracture); questionable lacerations or abrasions (e.g., human bite marks); skull fractures; or internal abdominal injuries.

Physical neglect: Consistently hungry; poor hygiene (e.g., diaper rash or lice) or inappropriate dress for weather; consistently left without supervision; abandoned; begging for or stealing food; constant fatigue and listlessness; frequently absent or tardy for school; failure to gain weight or failure to thrive (FTT); developmentally delayed; assumes adult responsibility; given inappropriate food, drink, or medication; reportedly ingests harmful substances.

Emotional abuse or neglect: Antisocial or destructive behavior; sleep disorders; habit disorders such as biting, head banging, rocking, or thumb sucking (in an older child); demanding behaviors; self-destructive, suicide attempt; overly adaptive behavior; emotional or intellectual developmental delays; speech disorders.

Sexual abuse: Recurrent abdominal pain; genital, urethral, or anal trauma; sexually transmitted diseases; recurrent urinary tract infections; enuresis (involuntary discharge of urine) or encopresis (incontinence of stool not caused by organic defect or illness); pregnancy; sleep disturbances (e.g., nightmares and night terrors); appetite disturbances (e.g., anorexia or bulimia); neurotic or conductive disorders; withdrawal, guilt, or depression; temper tantrums (in older children); aggressive behaviors; suicidal or runaway threats or behaviors; hysterical or conversion reactions; excessive masturbation; sexualized play in developmentally immature children; school problems; promiscuity; reluctance to change clothes. Many children have normal genital examinations.

Caregiver-fabricated illness: Signs and symptoms occur only when the perpetrator (usually the mother) is present. Common presenting indicators include poisoning, seizures, apnea, bleeding, vomiting, diarrhea, fever, and even cardiopulmonary arrest.

AHT: Often there are no external signs of injury other than a change in level of consciousness. The child may have history of poor feeding, vomiting, lethargy, and irritability occurring for several days or weeks. More severe shaking may cause brain damage, seizures, blindness, paralysis, and death. On ophthalmologic examination, retinal hemorrhages are seen. The anterior fontanel may be tense or full when the infant is quiet.

DIAGNOSTIC TESTS

Radiographs of injured area or skeletal survey: Certain findings on x-ray examination are strong indicators of physical abuse. These include metaphyseal "corner" or "bucket handle" fractures of long bones in infants, spiral fractures of long bones in nonambulatory infants, and multiple fractures of the ribs or long bones in varying stages of healing. These findings may help distinguish abuse from osteogenesis imperfecta (an inherited condition marked by abnormally brittle bones that are subject to fracture). A skeletal survey should be repeated in about 2 wk after the initial survey. Acute fractures may be missed initially but can be seen once periosteal new bone formation or callus formation occurs.

Computed tomography (CT) scan or magnetic resonance imaging (MRI) scan: May reveal subdural hematoma and subarachnoid hemorrhage, hallmark signs of AHT. CT scans and MRI scans may also diagnose abdominal injuries from abuse.

Ophthalmology examinations: May reveal retinal hemorrhage (usually bilateral), the hallmark sign of AHT.

Bone scans: Detect soft tissue and bone trauma, especially in locating unseen fractures or bone injuries. For example, they can define rib fractures, which are difficult to assess because of overlying structures such as the heart, lungs, and liver.

Coagulation studies: Used in children with many bruises in different stages to differentiate abuse from a medical condition such as leukemia or bleeding or clotting disorders. These studies are also used if intracranial hemorrhage is present. Use topical analgesia with blood draws to decrease anxiety and pain (atraumatic care).

Complete blood count: Helps rule out active bleeding or bleeding disorder. Provide atraumatic care.

Forensic evaluation: In sexually abused children, it may be done to identify evidence such as semen or detect sexually transmitted disease.

Nursing Diagnoses:

Risk for Trauma
Risk for Injury

related to family history of neglect or physical, emotional, or sexual abuse

Desired Outcome: Following intervention/treatment, the child exhibits no further evidence of abuse or neglect.

ASSESSMENT/INTERVENTIONS	RATIONALES
Assess the child's physical and mental status as follows: - Note bruises, scars, or other signs of abuse. - Note unusual interactions or responses of the child.	A thorough evaluation should be done on all children in all health care settings. Abuse occurs in all cultural and socioeconomic groups and may not be the admitting diagnosis.
Observe interactions between the child and family.	Signs of abuse or neglect may be detected in the way the child interacts with parents and other adults. For example, a child who is emotionally neglected may not want to be held or have eye contact with the parent or other adult.
Obtain a detailed history.	This may detect a pattern of trauma or neglect or lack of correlation between the history and severity of the trauma; or the history may change as the examination progresses.
Keep factual, detailed, objective records for documentation.	Medical records may be subpoenaed as evidence in court proceedings and therefore need to be as detailed and objective as possible. Being factual (i.e., no opinions, impressions, or interpretations) is imperative. Records should include the following: - Physical condition (e.g., "Three small, well-delineated, circular lesions, approximately 3-5 mm in diameter and 1 mm in depth, dark purple-red, noted on sole of left foot"). - Pictures, which are most beneficial in documenting injuries, need to be dated and kept in the patient's chart. - The child's behavioral response to parents, others, and environment (e.g., a child with FTT often does not verbally or physically interact with anyone). - Specific comments of the child, parents, or other family members and developmental age of the child.
Use a nonjudgmental, nonthreatening manner when interacting with the child's parents.	Frequently it is unclear who actually abused the child. The child is more likely to be helped if the parents trust the staff. If the parents feel alienated by the staff, they may deny the child access to care. Parents will be more receptive to teaching in a trusting environment.
[!] Report all cases of suspected child abuse or neglect.	All 50 states consider health care workers mandatory reporters of child abuse/neglect.
[!] Keep the child in a safe environment in the hospital (e.g., near the nurses' station).	The suspected abuser may be restricted from visiting, or only certain individuals may be approved to visit. Follow local CPS court documents for visitor information.

ASSESSMENT/INTERVENTIONS	RATIONALES
⚠ Assist in removing the child from an unsafe situation (whether verbal or physical neglect or abuse is suspected). Report any suspicious behavior to Social Services in the hospital and Child Protective Services in the community.	Nurses are mandated reporters of suspected neglect or abuse in all 50 states.
Refer families to social agencies for assistance with finances, food, clothing, and health care.	These measures help ameliorate causes of neglect.
Collaborate with the multidisciplinary health care team involved with the case.	This provides continual evaluation of progress/status of the child in the hospital, foster care, or on return to the home.
Help parents identify events that precipitate an abusive act (i.e., crying is a major trigger) and alternative ways to deal with release of anger (e.g., role playing).	This may prevent further abuse for this child or siblings.

Nursing Diagnosis:

Risk for Impaired Parenting

related to the child's, caregiver's, or situational characteristics/temperament that precipitate child abuse or neglect

Desired Outcome: Within 1 wk following interventions, the parents demonstrate more positive interactions with the child and more appropriate parenting activities and verbalize accurate understanding of normal expectations for the child.

ASSESSMENT/INTERVENTIONS	RATIONALES
⚠ Assess/identify families at risk for abuse/neglect.	Identifying at-risk families is the first step in helping prevent abuse or neglect. Such families tend to have immature, single parents; parents who were abused as children; a premature infant; a child younger than 3 yr or with a chronic illness or disability; parental substance abuse; and limited social network/support.
Assess/observe the parents' interactions with the child.	This is the best way to get a realistic view of the relationship. For example, when feeding the child, the parent may avoid making eye contact or touching the child unless absolutely necessary.
Assess the parents' strengths and weaknesses, normal coping behaviors, any cultural practices that may impact the current situation, and presence or absence of support systems.	This assessment provides the basis for developing an appropriate plan of care and making necessary referrals.
Demonstrate age-/developmentally appropriate child-rearing practices, especially communication and discipline.	Parents may care for their child in the way their parents cared for them and may not know age-/developmentally appropriate child-rearing practices.
Teach alternative methods of discipline, such as rewards, time-out, consequences, and verbal disapproval.	Parents may not know any nonviolent methods of discipline.
Provide care for the child until the parent is ready to provide care.	This allows parents time to "relax" and observe age-appropriate care.
Encourage the parents to participate in care of the child. Reinforce positive behaviors.	This helps build self-esteem and confidence in parents to improve interactions.
Focus on positive aspects of the child (e.g., "What beautiful eyes your child has" or "Tell me something your child is good at").	Parents may have a negative view of the child, and this gives them another perspective.
Teach the family what to expect in terms of growth and development for their child (physical, psychosocial, and cognitive) through role modeling and having the parents return demonstrations.	Parents will incorporate information better if not "instructed" and feeling as though they are being criticized. This increases their knowledge and reinforces accurate expectations of what is normal for their child, especially if the child has any developmental issues.
Also provide education about nutrition, care related to activities of daily living, routine well-child care, manifestations of illness, and importance of caring/loving attitude in dealing with children.	This information increases realistic expectations and chance of positive parenting.

continued

ASSESSMENT/INTERVENTIONS | RATIONALES

ASSESSMENT/INTERVENTIONS	RATIONALES
Convey a nonjudgmental attitude of genuine concern.	Such an attitude facilitates developing trust and respect and enables parents to observe and develop better methods of caring for their child.
Refer the family to appropriate social agencies to assist with financial support, adequate housing, employment, and so on.	This helps to ameliorate risk factors of abuse/neglect.
Help identify support systems for the parents such as extended family, neighbors, or support groups.	Support systems decrease family stress and hence decrease risk of abuse/neglect.

Nursing Diagnoses:

Fear
Anxiety

related to maltreatment, powerlessness, and potential loss of parents

Desired Outcome: Within 72 hr following interventions, the child verbalizes source(s) of fear/anxiety and exhibits more interactivity and sociability and less withdrawal.

ASSESSMENT/INTERVENTIONS | RATIONALES

ASSESSMENT/INTERVENTIONS	RATIONALES
Assess the child for signs or verbalization of fear/anxiety.	This enables support and reassurances that are appropriate and beneficial to the child.
Provide consistent caregivers and an age-appropriate safe environment.	These measures help relieve the child's anxiety and provide a positive role model for the family.
Reassure the child about his or her personal safety.	Verbal reassurance increases a sense of security.
Demonstrate acceptance of the child, but do not reinforce inappropriate behaviors.	Children need acceptance, as well as guidance regarding appropriate behaviors.
Support the child in talking about his or her family or stressful events.	Verbalization of fears/anxieties decreases their impact on children.
Do not ask too many questions.	This may upset the child and interfere with other professionals' interrogations.
Encourage play, especially with the family or dollhouse activity.	Play is the "work of the child" and may help reveal the types of relationships perceived by the child. This could include, for example, playing with dolls that represent father, mother, and siblings or drawing pictures of events. The child may tell the story of events with dolls. Drawings often depict fears and reactions to experiences.
Incorporate therapeutic play (for children 3 yr or older) into care activities if possible.	This helps children cope with new, frightening experiences in a nonthreatening way. For example, have the child check blood pressure on a doll before checking it on him or her.
Treat the child as you would other children, not as an "abused" victim.	This encourages the child to interact with others rather than promoting isolation.
Offer choices whenever possible regarding clothing, diet, and other activities of daily living (ADLs); recreation time; and socialization time.	Being allowed to make choices provides a sense of control and decreases a sense of powerlessness, and hence anxiety.

✓ **PATIENT-FAMILY TEACHING AND DISCHARGE PLANNING**

When providing patient-family/foster-family teaching, focus on sensory information, avoid giving excessive information, and initiate a visiting nurse referral for necessary follow-up teaching and assessment. Stress family-centered care (viewing the family as a unit that is the "constant" in the child's life and maintaining or improving the health of the family and its members in a holistic manner). Include verbal and written information about the following, ensuring that it is written at a level understandable to the child/family:

✓ Care related to any specific injury.
✓ Realistic expectations for the individual child related to:
- Growth and development (e.g., regression is normal after a child has been hospitalized or severely stressed)
- Nutrition (e.g., toddler's food jags—may only want one food for every meal for several days)

✓ Guidelines based on developmental level:
  • Safety (e.g., preschooler does not understand the danger of chasing a ball across the street)
  • Need for love and attention
✓ Methods of handling normal developmental problems that increase a parent's stress level (e.g., toddler's negativism, temper tantrums, toilet training, and need for rituals and routines).
✓ Demonstration of care related to ADLs; observe return demonstration by the parents.
✓ Importance of regular well-child visits and provision of routine well-child care.
✓ Suggestions for nonviolent, age-/developmentally appropriate methods of disciplining the child (e.g., reward, time-out, consequences, and verbal disapproval).
✓ Identification of stressful situations for the parents and ways to deal with them. For example, if an infant cries for prolonged periods, make sure that infant is clean and dry and is not uncomfortable, hungry, or ill; put the infant in a crib on his or her back and go out of the room. DO NOT SHAKE THE BABY. This can cause severe damage.
✓ Review of situations/circumstances that precipitate abuse/violence and of methods to deal with anger constructively.
✓ Importance of providing the child with positive reinforcement of appropriate behavior to build self-esteem.

✓ Teaching the child the difference between "good touch" and "bad touch."
✓ Name or place a child can go if being abused (e.g., neighborhood "safe house").
✓ Suggestions for local support systems (e.g., extended family members, church members, neighbors).
✓ Referrals to community resources, such as parenting classes, support groups, public health nurse, social worker, and financial counseling if appropriate. Additional general information/support can be obtained by contacting the following organizations:
  • Parents Anonymous, Inc., at *www.parentsanonymous.org*. This group provides support and resources for overwhelmed families/parents and caregivers.
  • National Child Abuse Hotline at (800) 4-A-CHILD (1-800-422-4453) with counselors available 24/7
  • Child Help at *www.childhelp.org* and Prevent Child Abuse America at *www.preventchildabuse.org*
  • Kids Help Phone at *www.kidshelpphone.ca*
  • National Center on Shaken Baby Syndrome at *www.dontshake.org*. This website provides family resources and support. It sponsors the Period of Purple Crying® Program: "A New Way to Understand Your Baby's Crying."
  • Caring for Kids website at *www.caringforkids.cps.ca*

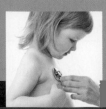

Cystic Fibrosis 80

OVERVIEW/PATHOPHYSIOLOGY

Cystic fibrosis (CF) is a chronic, progressive multisystem disease in which there is dysfunction of the exocrine (mucus-producing) glands and abnormal transport of sodium and chloride across the epithelium. This results in abnormally thick secretions, causing obstruction of the small passageways of many organs. CF is an autosomal recessive hereditary disease with more than 1940 gene mutations as of April 2011 (Nicholson, 2013). This is the reason there is such a wide variation in clinical manifestations.

In the recent past, CF was described as the most common lethal genetic illness in white children. The median life expectancy has improved dramatically from 7.5 years in 1966 (Hockenberry and Wilson, 2011) to the late 30s (CFF, 2013). The median life expectancy has increased because of specialized care, particularly through the national network of CF Foundation–accredited centers and new CF therapies that can begin with infants detected through newborn screening. Research shows that receiving CF care early in life helps children have better nutrition and better overall health than those who are diagnosed later in life (CFF, 2013).

About 30,000 people in the United States (70,000 worldwide) have CF, and more than 45% are 18 yr or older. About 1000 new cases are diagnosed each year, with over 70% diagnosed by age two. More than 10 million Americans are asymptomatic genetic carriers, which is one in every 31 Americans. CF is most often seen in Caucasians, but it can affect all races (CFF, 2013).

HEALTH CARE SETTING

Primary care, with possible hospitalization for CF exacerbation or other complications

ASSESSMENT

Initially involves overall appraisal, including monitoring general activity, physical findings, nutritional status, and chest x-ray examination.

Signs and symptoms: Vary widely, as does the severity of involvement of specific organ systems. Patients tend to have periods without acute symptoms and then periods with acute exacerbation of symptoms. The first clinical manifestation may be meconium ileus in a newborn, or the patient may not have symptoms for months or years.

Most of the usual symptoms are caused by the following:

- **Progressive chronic obstructive lung disease:** Initially wheezing and dry cough, progressing to paroxysmal cough that frequently causes posttussive emesis. Other signs include increased dyspnea, barrel chest, mild to severe clubbing of nail beds, cyanosis, and repeated pulmonary infections that cause scarring and bronchiectasis. Numerous complications such as pneumothorax and hemoptysis often occur.
- **Pancreatic enzyme deficiency** resulting from duct blockage (present in most children with CF): Stools that are frothy (bulky and large), foul smelling, fat containing (steatorrhea), and float (four Fs of CF); voracious appetite initially, progressing to loss of appetite late in the disease; weight loss, marked tissue wasting, protuberant abdomen with thin extremities, failure to thrive (FTT), anemia; and evidence of deficiency of fat-soluble vitamins (A, D, E, K). Complications include pancreatic fibrosis leading to glucose intolerance, diabetes mellitus (DM), and pancreatitis. CF-related DM (CFRD) is very common in people with CF, especially as they get older. It is found in 20% of adolescents and 40%-50% of adults (CFRD, CFF, 2013).
- **Sweat gland dysfunction** resulting in increased sodium and chloride concentrations. Infants "taste" salty and are more susceptible to dehydration.

Other GI complications: Include intestinal obstruction in infants, distal intestinal obstruction syndrome in adolescents and adults, and rectal prolapse, which occurs in children with CF usually younger than 6 yr. Many children experience transient or chronic gastroesophageal reflux (GER).

Liver complications: Biliary cirrhosis and gallbladder dysfunction.

Other: Nasal polyps and sinusitis also occur frequently in children with CF.

DIAGNOSTIC TESTS

CF has been called the "great imitator" because signs of chronic respiratory infection and FTT are symptoms of many other childhood conditions.

Newborn screening (NBS) panel: CF has been added to the panel in all 50 states as of January 1, 2010, and is done at the same time as phenylketonuria and other screening tests. The two-tiered process follows:

1. *Immunoreactive trypsinogen test (IRT)*: Enables early detection of CF and is done several days after birth. The IRT can be elevated due to prematurity or a stressful delivery or for other reasons. An elevated IRT requires a repeat test done at 2 wk of age. Some states do another IRT test, and some do an IRT-DNA screening test. If the second test is elevated/positive, referral should be made to a CF-accredited care center for further evaluation (CFF, 2013). It is confirmed by a "sweat test" or mutation analysis (i.e., genetic testing). The combination of these two tests is sensitive 90%-100% of the time.

2. *Pilocarpine iontophoresis (quantitative sweat chloride test or "sweat test")*: Production of sweat is stimulated with a special device, and the sweat is collected and measured. Diagnosis is made with sodium and chloride levels greater than 60 mEq/L (levels of 40-60 mEq/L are considered suggestive and should be repeated) and the presence of clinical symptoms or a family history of CF. Sweat test is not usually done before 4-6 wk of age because the infant has decreased sweat production until then. Infants 0-3 mo old can have a positive test at a lower level (Nicholson, 2013).
Or

3. *Polymerase chain reaction (PCR) for gene mutations (genetic testing)*: Helps determine if the child is a carrier or has CF.

Chest x-ray examination: Shows characteristic patchy atelectasis and chronic obstructive emphysema.

Pulmonary function tests (after 5-6 yr old): Assess degree of pulmonary disease and response to therapy and help distinguish between restrictive and obstructive pulmonary disease. In the presence of CF, the test will show decreased vital capacity (VC) and tidal volume, increased airway resistance, increased residual volume, and decreased forced expiratory volume in 1 sec (FEV_1) and FEV_1/VC ratio.

Pulse oximetry: Reveals decreased oxygen saturation.

Complete blood count: Increased white blood cells with increased neutrophils on differential count will be present with infection.

Sputum culture: For identification of infective organisms and sensitivity of these organisms. Many resistant organisms develop because of the frequency of respiratory infections.

DNA analysis of chorionic villi or amniotic fluid: Can establish prenatal diagnosis.

Nursing Diagnosis:

Ineffective Airway Clearance

related to thick, tenacious mucus in the airways

Desired Outcome: Immediately following treatment/interventions, the child expectorates mucus and exhibits improved airway clearance as evidenced by improved breath sounds and heart rate (HR) and a respiratory rate (RR) within the child's normal limits.

ASSESSMENT/INTERVENTIONS	RATIONALES
Assess HR, RR, and breath sounds.	This assessment establishes baseline data from which to compare later findings. With ineffective airway clearance, the child will have increased HR and RR. Breath sounds may be decreased with little air movement because of the blocked airway, or adventitious sounds may be increased because of mucus in the airway.
Assist the child with sputum expectoration (may be done by respiratory therapist):	
- Assess HR, RR, breath sounds, and O_2 saturation before nebulization and after chest physiotherapy.	Assessment before and after treatment monitors effectiveness of treatment.
- Position the child in an upright sitting position, ensuring that he or she does not slouch.	This position facilitates maximum inhalation of medication and improves effectiveness of the cough to clear secretions out of the airways.
- Administer nebulization (albuterol) as prescribed 1 hr before or 2 hr after meals.	This treatment opens bronchi and loosens secretions. It usually causes considerable coughing followed by expectoration of mucus and sometimes vomiting from excessive coughing. Scheduling in relation to meals is essential to provide maximum benefit of treatment and prevent interference with nutrient ingestion. Treatment before breakfast helps loosen secretions that built up overnight. Treatment before bedtime helps clear secretions that would otherwise provide a medium for bacterial growth.

continued

ASSESSMENT/INTERVENTIONS	RATIONALES
- Perform chest physiotherapy after nebulizer treatment. Examples follow.	This helps to loosen secretions, which will facilitate their expectoration. This treatment is performed at least 2-4 times/day for maintenance or routine daily care. The method used depends on age of the child, effectiveness of the technique, the child's/parent's ability to perform/tolerate the technique, and preference of the child/parent.
- Chest percussion and postural drainage for 20-30 min	Chest percussion loosens secretions, and postural drainage facilitates drainage of secretions so that they can be expectorated.
- Mucus clearance device (e.g., flutter valve) used for 5-15 min	This handheld pipelike device has a plastic mouthpiece on one end that the child breathes into. On the other end of the pipe a stainless steel ball rests inside a plastic circular cone. Exhaling into the device vibrates the airways, thereby loosening mucus from the airway walls and accelerating airflow, which facilitates upward movement of mucus so that it can be more readily cleared. This device is very effective and gives children control because it can be used without the assistance of others.
- Airway clearance system with high-frequency wall oscillation device, or HFCWO (e.g., the Vest) used for 30 min	This inflatable vest fits like a life jacket and is connected by tubes to a generator. The vest inflates and deflates rapidly, applying gentle pressure to the chest. It provides high-frequency chest wall oscillation to help loosen secretions and increase mucus expectoration.
- Suction as necessary.	For infants/young children or if there is a large volume of mucus, assistance may be needed to clear secretions from the airway. However, children usually cough sufficiently after nebulizer treatment and chest physiotherapy to clear secretions independently.
Ensure that the child is receiving at least maintenance fluids.	Hydration thins and loosens secretions for easier expectoration.
Administer dornase alfa (Pulmozyme) as prescribed.	This medication thins mucus, which will facilitate expectoration.

Nursing Diagnosis:

Impaired Gas Exchange

related to airway obstruction occurring with air trapping in the alveoli and airways narrowed by tenacious mucus

Desired Outcome: Within 2 hr following treatment/intervention, the child has adequate gas exchange as evidenced by O_2 saturation greater than 92% (or consistent with the child's baseline).

ASSESSMENT/INTERVENTIONS	RATIONALES
Along with vital signs, assess respiratory status q2-4h, or more frequently as indicated by the child's condition.	Increased HR and RR would occur with impaired gas exchange, as would chest retractions, increased work of breathing (WOB), nasal flaring, and use of accessory muscles of respiration. These are signs of respiratory distress necessitating prompt intervention/treatment.
Ensure continuous monitoring of pulse oximetry readings; report low value (usually 92% or lower).	Decreased O_2 saturation can indicate need for initiation of/increased O_2.
Monitor for behavioral indicators of hypoxia.	Restlessness, mood changes, and/or change in the level of consciousness are early signs of O_2 deficiency.
Be alert to changes in the child's skin color.	Cyanosis of the lips and nail beds is a late indicator of hypoxia and a signal of the need for prompt treatment/intervention.

ASSESSMENT/INTERVENTIONS	RATIONALES
Position the child in high Fowler's position and/or leaning forward.	These positions promote comfort and optimal gas exchange by enabling maximal chest expansion.
Deliver O_2 along with humidity via the most appropriate delivery system and at the rate prescribed.	The child's developmental age helps determine the most effective delivery system and flow rate (e.g., nasal cannula for infants with liter flow rate less than 4). Humidity use replaces convective losses of moisture.
Monitor the child on O_2 delivery closely.	O_2-induced CO_2 narcosis is a hazard of O_2 therapy in the child with chronic pulmonary disease. If O_2 saturation is consistently greater than 96%, for example, it is likely that the flow rate can be decreased slowly by small increments.
Encourage games or physical exercise appropriate to the child's condition (e.g., blowing bubbles or walking), but avoid overexertion.	Breathing more deeply facilitates clearing of mucus and improves oxygenation.
Provide a neutral thermal environment for the child.	This is a room temperature in which the body does not have to use as much energy to stay warm or cool off, thereby enabling the child to use energy to grow or heal. With decreased energy demands, more O_2 is available to ensure these needs are met.

Nursing Diagnosis:

Imbalanced Nutrition: Less Than Body Requirements

related to decreased appetite (advanced disease) or increased metabolic requirements because of increased WOB, infection, and/or malabsorption

Desired Outcome: By hospital discharge or within 7 days after treatment/intervention, the child/patient maintains or gains weight and does not have more than 2 or 3 stools per day.

ASSESSMENT/INTERVENTIONS	RATIONALES
Assess daily weight measurements in the hospital and teach the importance of weekly weight measurements at home.	This assesses effectiveness of nutritional interventions. If the child is losing weight, he or she may not be receiving adequate nutrients or may not be absorbing nutrients properly.
Administer pancreatic enzymes with meals and snacks per the health care provider's prescription if the child has pancreatic insufficiency (most children with CF).	Replacement of enzymes is necessary for proper digestion and absorption of nutrients. Failure to replace pancreatic enzymes would affect the child's growth and ability to fight infection.
For young children unable to swallow a capsule, mix powder, granules, or contents of the capsule with a small amount of carbohydrate food.	Protein foods break down this enzyme and can burn the mouths of infants and young children. Using the smallest amount of food possible (e.g., 1-2 tsp of applesauce) helps ensure that the child receives all the medication.
Do not administer enzymes with formula/milk in a bottle or cup.	Pancreatic enzymes curdle milk and formula. In addition, the child may not receive all the medication and may not take the milk/formula in the future if he or she associates it with medication.
Monitor and document frequency and appearance of stools.	Pancreatic enzymes are adjusted to provide normal stooling (i.e., decreased enzymes given with constipation; increased enzymes given with frequent, bulky, foul-smelling stools that float). Normal stooling indicates increased absorption of nutrients.
Provide a well-balanced, high-calorie, high-protein, medium-high–fat diet (up to 150% recommended daily allowance).	The severity of lung disease and degree of impaired intestinal absorption determine each child's needs.
Provide adequate salt, especially with fever, hot weather, or exercise.	The child/patient is at risk for electrolyte imbalance (hyponatremia) because sodium concentration in the sweat of a child with CF is 2-5 times greater than that of a child without CF.
Administer supplemental tube feedings (nasogastric tube [NGT] or gastric tube [GT]) or total parenteral nutrition (TPN) as prescribed.	Measures described in previous interventions alone are not always effective in the child exhibiting FTT. Supplemental feedings via NGT, GT, or TPN provide increased calories to treat malnutrition.

continued

ASSESSMENT/INTERVENTIONS	RATIONALES
If prescribed, administer GER medications in a timely manner.	Some reflux medications need to be given before meals or with meals to be most effective.
Position/encourage the child to maintain an upright position during and for 1 or 2 hr after eating/receiving enteral feeding.	Lying down during or right after eating increases the risk of reflux, which can increase the risk of respiratory infections.

Nursing Diagnosis:

Deficient Knowledge

related to unfamiliarity with the purpose, precautions, and potential side effects of prescribed medications

Desired Outcome: Within 1 wk of diagnosis or change in medication, the patient/parent verbalizes accurate information about the prescribed medications.

ASSESSMENT/INTERVENTIONS	RATIONALES
Teach the Following to the Patient/Parent for the Prescribed Medications: **Aerosolized Bronchodilators: Albuterol**	
	This medication helps open the bronchi for easier expectoration of mucus. The route is via nebulizer or metered-dose inhalers (MDIs).
- Be alert for and report palpitations, increased HR, chest pain, muscle tremors, dizziness, headache.	These are side effects that may indicate the need for dosage adjustment.
- Be alert for and report nervousness, central nervous system (CNS) stimulation, hyperactivity, and insomnia.	These are side effects that occur more often in younger children than in adults.
- All the above symptoms, as well as dry mouth, may occur with the MDI. Notify the prescriber if they persist.	These are additional side effects.
- Limit caffeinated beverages.	Caffeine may increase side effects such as CNS stimulation and insomnia.
- Do not take with beta-adrenergic blocking agents (e.g., propranolol), monoamine oxidase inhibitors (MAOIs), tricyclic antidepressants.	Propranolol antagonizes the action of albuterol. MAOIs potentiate sympathomimetic effects. Tricyclic antidepressants increase cardiovascular effects.
- Do not take with other sympathomimetics.	Albuterol increases cardiovascular effects.
- Rinse mouth with water following each inhalation of the MDI.	Rinsing helps moisten a dry mouth and throat.
Aerosolized Mucolytic Enzymes: Dornase Alfa (Pulmozyme)	
	This medication thins secretions and optimally decreases the number of pulmonary infections.
- Use with an appropriate nebulizer system with a compressor.	A nebulizer unit is available that is made specifically to administer this medication.
- Be alert to and report hoarseness, pharyngitis, laryngitis, rash, chest pain, and conjunctivitis.	Typically side effects are mild and subside within a few weeks.
- Do not dilute or mix with other medications in the nebulizer.	These actions may deactivate the enzyme.
- Store in the refrigerator in the foil packet and discard if unopened vials are subjected to room temperature for more than 24 hr.	Room temperature may deactivate the medication.
- Protect from strong light. Discard the solution if it is cloudy or discolored.	These are signs that the medication may be deactivated.
- Use with caution in infants and children younger than 5 yr of age.	This medication is FDA approved only for adults and children 5 yr of age and older. Some adverse side effects have been reported in children less than 5 yr of age, including cough and rhinitis.

ASSESSMENT/INTERVENTIONS	RATIONALES
Aerosolized/Oral Inhalation Antibiotics: Tobramycin (Tobi®)	
	This medication helps fight infection, which would cause an increase in symptoms. Tobi® is FDA approved for adults and children 6 yr of age and older.
- Be alert to and report hoarseness, shortness of breath, increased cough, and pharyngitis.	These are side effects.
- Store in the refrigerator. Date and time the drug when removing it from the refrigerator.	Tobi® can be used for only 28 days when stored at room temperature (no more than 77° F).
- Do not use if the medication is cloudy or contains particles.	These are signs the medication is compromised.
- Protect from intense light.	Light adversely affects Tobi®.
- Do not take with dornase alfa (Pulmozyme).	When tobramycin and Pulmozyme are mixed, a precipitate may form.
- Administer with the appropriate nebulizer system.	Medication may not be nebulized properly if it is not administered with the appropriate delivery system.
- Take the bronchodilator first, then chest physiotherapy, then other inhaled medications, and tobramycin last.	This is the most effective method of administration because when airways are clear, absorption of Tobi® is enhanced.
- Ensure that the serum aminoglycoside level is monitored for patients on high-dose aerosolized tobramycin.	This identifies patients who are significant absorbers and may be at risk for ototoxicity and nephrotoxicity.
Pancreatic Enzymes	
	These enzymes increase food and nutrient absorption.
- As prescribed, take with meals and snacks within 30 min of eating.	Taking enzymes in this manner promotes degradation and absorption of the nutrients just consumed.
- If the patient is an infant or young child, open the capsule and give it in a small amount of nonfat, nonprotein, acidic food (e.g., 1-2 tsp applesauce).	Protein/alkaline foods break down this enzyme and can burn the mouth in an infant/young child.
- Do not mix with milk or formula.	Pancreatic enzymes curdle milk or formula.
- Do not chew microspheres or microtabs; swallow capsules or tablets whole.	Chewing or mouth retention before swallowing may cause mucosal irritation and stomatitis.
- Monitor stools for frequency and appearance.	Constipation or increased stooling (more than 3 stools/day) indicates need to adjust dosage.
- Do not take if allergic to pork or if the patient has acute or chronic pancreatitis.	These are contraindications for use.
- Be alert for and report nausea, abdominal cramps, mouth irritation, sneezing, constipation, or diarrhea.	These are side effects that may indicate the need for dosage adjustment.
- Notify the prescriber if the patient is taking H2 antagonists or gastric acid pump inhibitors (e.g., ranitidine, cimetidine, omeprazole).	These agents increase the effectiveness of pancreatic enzymes; dosage adjustment may be needed.
Cystic Fibrosis Transmembrane Conductance Regulator Potentiator: Ivacaftor (Kalydeco)	
	This medication was approved in 2012 for use in children 6 yr of age or older who have the G551D mutation of CF. It is the first medication used to treat the underlying cause of CF. The route is oral.
- Be alert for and report respiratory tract infections, oropharyngeal pain, headache, stomachache, rash, diarrhea, or dizziness.	These are the most common side effects.
- Monitor liver function tests initially, then every three months for the first year, and yearly thereafter.	This medication may increase hepatic transaminases.
- Monitor for and immediately report to the health care provider abdominal pain in the right upper abdomen; yellowing of the skin or whites of the eyes; loss of appetite; nausea or vomiting; or dark, amber colored urine.	These are signs of serious adverse effects involving liver impairment.
- Monitor for low blood sugar.	This is a serious adverse effect.
- This medication interacts with numerous medications.	See a drug book for more detailed information.

continued

ASSESSMENT/INTERVENTIONS	RATIONALES
- Do not take with grapefruit or Seville oranges.	These foods/juices increase the serum concentration of this medication
- Observe for healthy weight gain.	Improved lung function and decreased sweat chloride levels help patients gain weight and are indicators of the effectiveness of this medication.
Vitamins/Minerals	They supplement the overall diet.
- Take fat-soluble vitamins in water-miscible form (i.e., mixed in a suspension that will not separate) as prescribed.	This action counteracts the malabsorption of fat-soluble vitamins (A, D, E, and K). Examples of water-miscible forms of vitamins include Aquasol A and ADEK.
- Use iron preparations as prescribed.	Malabsorption can cause iron deficiency. Review a drug handbook for more detailed information.
Antibiotics—Usually IV (e.g., Ticarcillin, Tobramycin)	These medications are used to treat infections.
- Take as prescribed, usually for at least 10 days and often for several weeks.	Children with CF have frequent respiratory infections and often develop drug resistance. Antibiotics may need to be given for an extended time.
- Monitor for side effects specific to each individual antibiotic.	Side effects vary, depending on the specific antibiotic.
Azithromycin (antibiotic)	Studies have shown an improvement in lung function, weight gain, and fewer days hospitalized for lung infections when taking this medication (CFF, 2013). Consult a drug handbook for more detailed information.
Antiinflammatory Drugs (e.g., Ibuprofen)	Studies have shown a slowed rate of pulmonary decline with better growth and fewer hospitalizations when taking an antiinflammatory drug (CFF, 2013). Consult a drug handbook for more detailed information.

ADDITIONAL NURSING DIAGNOSES/PROBLEMS:

"Psychosocial Support" for relevant nursing diagnoses that pertain to the patient's psychologic status in dealing with a chronic and potentially fatal illness — p. 72

"Psychosocial Support for the Patient's Family and Significant Other" for relevant nursing diagnoses for family members dealing with a chronic and potentially fatal illness in their loved one — p. 84

"Diabetes Mellitus" for **Risk for Infection** related to chronic disease process — p. 359

"Asthma" for **Anxiety** — p. 553

Interrupted Family Processes — p. 554

"Burns" for **Disturbed Body Image**. For patients with CF this could entail delayed puberty, copious sputum and chronic cough, inability to maintain weight, and/or possible presence of a GT — p. 578

✓ PATIENT-FAMILY TEACHING AND DISCHARGE PLANNING

When providing child-family teaching, focus on sensory data, avoid excessive information, and initiate a visiting nurse referral for necessary follow-up assessment or teaching. Stress family-centered care (viewing the family as a unit that is the "constant" in the child's life and maintaining or improving the health of the family and its members in a holistic manner). Include verbal and written information about the following and ensure that written information is at a level the reader can understand:

✓ Basic information about the disease process with emphasis on respiratory and GI components.

✓ Maintenance and exacerbation aspects of this chronic disease process.

✓ Diet, including rationale for increased calories, protein, and fat (usually two to three snacks/day).

✓ Administration of pancreatic enzymes such as Ultrase® with meals and snacks (usually a fractional dose given with snacks).

- If the patient is an infant or young child, may mix contents of capsule, granules, or powder with a small amount of applesauce or other carbohydrate food.
- Do not chew or bite capsule or enteric-coated microspheres.
- Do not administer in a bottle or cup with fluid.

✓ Need for salt replacement and free access for the child to salt, especially during hot weather, fever, diarrhea, or vomiting.

✓ GI symptoms that signal malabsorption and inadequate enzyme replacement (e.g., bloating, abdominal cramping and distention, and diarrhea).

✓ Need to monitor stools (constipation indicates too much enzyme; frequent fatty loose stools indicate insufficient enzyme).

✓ Administration of nebulizer treatment and chest physiotherapy (i.e., chest percussion and postural drainage, mucus clearance device [e.g., the FLUTTER™] or a vest airway clearance system [e.g., the Vest]). Albuterol nebulizer treatment is done first (1 hr before or 2 hr after meals), followed by chest physiotherapy and suctioning if needed. Take nebulized antibiotic and Pulmozyme after Albuterol, chest physiotherapy, and suctioning or coughing. Make sure to use the appropriate nebulizer unit with each of the above medications (they all need different nebulizer units). Stress the importance of routine pulmonary toilet because thickened mucus is an ideal medium for bacterial growth, which causes pulmonary infections.

✓ Cleaning and care of equipment (e.g., nebulizer attachments for Albuterol, Pulmozyme, and Tobi).

✓ Medications, including drug name; route; purpose; dosage; precautions; drug-drug, food-drug, and herb-drug interactions; and potential adverse effects.

✓ Importance of taking medications at home and at school as directed. Medication in the original container (with prescribing label) and written prescription from the health care provider are needed for the child to be able take medications at school.

✓ Importance of regular medical follow-up care:
- Routine immunizations plus pneumococcal polysaccharide vaccination (PPV) and yearly influenza vaccination
- Prompt attention to infection (fever, increased coughing, green sputum)
- Regular visits with the health care provider

✓ Team care approach, including pediatrician, school nurse and teachers, pulmonologist, or infectious disease physician. Ensure that a genetic referral is made.

✓ Realistic expectations for the child, especially concerning growth and development, participation in school activities and sports, and the child's participation/responsibility for self-care.

✓ Child's legal rights: Section 504 of Rehabilitation Act of 1973. Each student with a disability (physical or mental impairment) is entitled to accommodation in order to attend school and participate as fully as possible in school activities. A child with significant pulmonary involvement may need to be excused from class for 15-30 min after receiving a nebulizer treatment and chest physiotherapy because of excessive coughing and expectoration of mucus, or the class schedule might need to be rearranged to accommodate required treatment. (Day-to-Day: School and CF at www.cff.org/LivingWith CF/AtSchool/ [click on School and CF]).

✓ Telephone numbers to call in case questions or concerns arise about therapy or disease after discharge.

✓ When to call the health care provider:
- Increased respiratory effort (e.g., increased RR, nasal flaring, retractions)
- Excessive coughing and/or coughing up blood
- Color change: pallor or cyanosis (blue mucus membranes/lips/tongue or around the eyes). Stress that this is late sign of a problem.
- Temperature increase to greater than 101.5° F lasting more than a few days or a low-grade fever lasting for a week or more
- Weight loss
- Abdominal pain or distention, with or without constipation

✓ Referral to community resources such as support groups, specialists working with children affected by CF, CF care center if available, and genetic counselors.

✓ Additional information can be obtained by contacting:
- Cystic Fibrosis Foundation at www.cff.org
- STARBRIGHT Foundation at www.starbright.org: Global online community for young people dealing with chronic illness or injury
- Information for the Vest® Airway Clearance System at www.thevest.com
- CareFirst for CF (sm) at www.patientassistance.com/profile/axcanscandipharminc-96. This program helps ease the financial burden of caring for infants and children up to 2 yr of age with CF.
- Cystic Fibrosis Canada at www.cysticfibrosis.ca

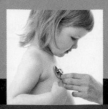

OVERVIEW/PATHOPHYSIOLOGY

Diabetes mellitus (DM) is the most common childhood endocrine disorder and one of the most costly chronic diseases of childhood. It is a disorder of carbohydrate metabolism marked by hyperglycemia and glycosuria, and it results from inadequate production or use of insulin. The major classifications seen in children are as follow:

- **Type 1 DM:** There is an absolute deficiency of insulin secretion resulting from destruction of beta cells, causing hyperglycemia and ketosis. This destruction is often an immune-mediated or related response. Previously it was called *insulin-dependent DM (IDDM)* or *juvenile-onset diabetes*. Historically, this was the primary type of diabetes seen in children and one of the most common chronic disorders of childhood. According to the CDC (National Diabetes Statistics Report, 2014), approximately 208,000 people younger than 20 have diabetes (type 1 and type 2) in the United States and they represent 0.25 of everyone in this age range. The SEARCH for Diabetes in Youth study funded by the CDC for 2008-2009 noted that about 18,436 youth were diagnosed with type 1 DM annually with the highest incidence occurring in non-Hispanic white children and adolescents (CDC, 2014). Two million adolescents between 12 and 18 yr old have prediabetes (Scott, 2013). About 75% of all newly diagnosed cases of type 1 DM occur in individuals younger than 18 yr old. These children are dependent on insulin for survival and to prevent diabetic ketoacidosis (DKA). Individuals diagnosed with type 1 DM in childhood have a high risk of early cardiovascular disease (CVD), and the American Heart Association ranks children with type 1 DM in the highest tier for risk of CVD.
- **Type 2 DM:** There is an insulin resistance with this type, so there is a relative, not absolute, insulin deficiency. Previously this was called *non–insulin-dependent DM (NIDDM)* or *adult-onset DM*. Since the 1990s, there has been an alarming epidemic of children developing type 2 DM. The National Diabetes Statistics Report for 2014 notes that more than 5000 youths younger than 20 are diagnosed with type 2 DM annually with the highest incidence from 10-19 yr (CDC, 2014). Being overweight is a strong risk factor for type 2 DM, and recent data from a 2013 evidenced-based care sheet by Schub and Caple noted that

in children 6-19 yr of age, about 16%, are overweight and 19% are obese. The prevalence of obesity (body mass index 95% or greater) has nearly tripled over the past 3 decades in the United States (American Academy of Pediatrics [AAP], Management of Type 2 Diabetes, 2013). In the past, less than 5% of children were diagnosed with type 2 DM. Now, largely due to the obesity epidemic noted above, children and adolescents make up to 45% of patients diagnosed with type 2 DM. Sedentary lifestyle is another significant risk factor. There is also an increased risk of developing type 2 DM in Black, Hispanic, Native American, and Pacific Islander populations (Schrub, 2013).

Note: *It can be difficult to distinguish between types 1 and 2 DM, especially because the prevalence of overweight in children continues to rise and autoantigen and ketones can be present in many patients with features of type 2 DM, including obesity and acanthosis nigricans (see description under Assessment) (AAP, 2013).*

- **Mature-onset diabetes of youth (MODY):** This type involves impaired insulin secretion with minimal or no defects in insulin action, usually in individuals younger than 25 yr old and symptomatic only with stress or infection. It is inherited by an autosomal dominant pattern.
- **Cystic fibrosis–related diabetes (CFRD):** This is the most common comorbidity in people with cystic fibrosis. It occurs in about 20% of adolescents with cystic fibrosis (CF), and about 40%-50% of adults with CF have CFRD. The primary cause is insulin insufficiency (Moran, 2010).
- For information on other types, see the adult Diabetes Mellitus care plan, p. 355, and "Diabetes in Pregnancy," p. 641.

HEALTH CARE SETTING

Primary care, with possible hospital admission because of complications

ASSESSMENT

Signs and symptoms: These are the same as in the adult DM care plan, except children with type 2 DM usually have hypertension, dyslipidemia, acanthosis nigricans (hypertrophy or thickening of skin with gray, brown, or black pigmentation chiefly in the axilla, other body folds, and sometimes on hands, elbows, and knees), and polycystic ovary syndrome.

Females may have vaginitis because of long-standing glycosuria. DKA also may occur in children and adolescents.

COMPLICATIONS

Potential for acute crisis: This is the same as in the adult DM care plan with the addition of idiopathic cerebral edema in resolving DKA, which occurs more often in children than in adults. To prevent the risk of this, current trends recommend cautious fluid management to replace lost fluid by replacing fluid evenly over 36-48 hr (Hockenberry, 2011). The patient may have a headache and lethargy or be asymptomatic. Symptoms can start with an abrupt change in level of consciousness (LOC); pupils dilated, fixed, or unequal; papilledema; decorticate or decerebrate posturing; and rapid progression to deep coma, respiratory arrest, or brain death (herniation of brain stem).

Long-term complications: These are the same as in adults but the micro and macro complications are very aggressive in children with type 2 DM. They occur over a much shorter time frame. With type 1 DM, retinopathy most commonly occurs after puberty and after 5-10 yr of diabetes duration but has been reported in prepubertal children who have had diabetes for only 1-2 yr.

> **Note:** *Celiac disease occurs with increased frequency in patients with type 1 DM (1%-16% of individuals compared with 0.3%-1% in the general population) per ADA's Standards of Medical Care in Diabetes (2014).*

DIAGNOSTIC TESTS

The ADA published the *Standards of Medical Care in Diabetes—2014.* This and the 2013 AAP *Clinical Practice Guideline: Management of Newly Diagnosed Type 2 Diabetes Mellitus (T2DM) in Children and Adolescents* define the following values:

A_{1C}: 6.5% or higher (test must be performed in an appropriately certified laboratory). It needs to be confirmed by repeat testing in asymptomatic children. **OR**

Fasting plasma glucose: Will reveal a value 126 mg/dL or higher. Fasting is defined as no caloric intake for at least 8 hr. This is the recommended test for children, and it should be confirmed by a second positive test on another day in an asymptomatic child. **OR**

Two-hour postprandial plasma glucose: Will reveal a value 200 mg/dL or greater during oral glucose tolerance test. It is not usually done in children. **OR**

Random/casual plasma glucose: Symptoms of diabetes (polyuria, polydipsia, polyphagia, unexplained weight loss) and a random/casual plasma glucose 200 mg/dL or greater are diagnostic of diabetes and no further testing is required.

Screening recommendations (ADA, Standards of Medical Care 2014) for type 2 DM in asymptomatic children less than 18 yr of age:
- Overweight with body mass index greater than 85th percentile for age and sex, weight for height greater than 85th percentile, or weight greater than 120% of ideal for height.
- PLUS at least two of the following risk factors:
  Family history of type 2 DM in first- or second-degree relatives.
  Belonging to certain race/ethnic groups (Native American, African American, Hispanic/Latino American, Asian/South Pacific Islanders).
  Signs of insulin resistance or conditions associated with insulin resistance such as acanthosis nigricans, hypertension, dyslipidemia, polycystic ovarian syndrome, or small-for-gestational birth weight.
  Begin screening: Age 10 yr or puberty, if puberty begins at an earlier age.
Testing should be done every 3 yr.

Fasting lipid panel, if type 2 DM suspected: Dyslipidemia is frequently seen in children in type 2 DM and also needs to be treated. Values vary depending on age of the child and if reference range is in conventional units or international units.

Basic metabolic panel (electrolytes, glucose, blood urea nitrogen, creatinine): Serum glucose will be elevated, usually greater than 250 mg/dL. Sodium and potassium may be lost because of osmotic diuresis. The higher the glucose level, the greater the dehydration and loss of electrolytes. Serum potassium may be normal on admission, but after fluid and insulin administration, rapid return of potassium to the cells decreases serum potassium, which necessitates monitoring for cardiac dysrhythmias. Blood urea nitrogen and creatinine likely will be elevated because of dehydration. Also, renal dysfunction occurs when the serum glucose level rises to greater than 600 mg/dL.

Thyroid-stimulating hormone and thyroxine: Thyroid hormone increases gluconeogenesis (synthesis of glucose from noncarbohydrate sources such as amino acids and glycerol) and peripheral use of glucose. An elevated or decreased value would impact carbohydrate metabolism and therefore plasma glucose. Normal range varies for children depending on their age and type of reference units reported. Thyroid autoantibodies occur in about 25% of children with type 1 DM at the time of diagnosis. The presence of these autoantibodies is predictive of thyroid dysfunction (Chiang: Type 1 Diabetes Through the Life Span: Position Statement, 2014).

Ketones: Elevated when insulin is not available and the body starts to break down stored fats for energy. Ketone bodies are by-products of this fat breakdown, and they accumulate in the blood and urine. Normal range for children is 0 with the qualitative test and 0.5-3 mg/dL (conventional units) or 5-30 mg/L (international units) with the quantitative test.

Additional Data:
- *Normal plasma glucose:* A value less than 100 mg/dL.
- *Impaired fasting glucose:* 100-125 mg/dL or impaired glucose tolerance if 2-hr postprandial plasma glucose is 140-199 mg/dL. Impaired fasting plasma glucose or impaired glucose tolerance should be monitored on a regular basis, but losing weight and increased activity can prevent or delay onset of DM.

Hemoglobin A₁c: Assesses control of blood glucose over the preceding 2 to 3 mo. Normal range for hemoglobin A_{1C} (HbA_{1C}) is 4%-7%. The range in children in the past varied depending on age, with higher glucose levels allowed in younger children. The ADA Type 1 Diabetes Through the Life Span position statement (2014) recommends an A_{1c} goal of less than 7.5% across all pediatric age-groups for children with Type 1 diabetes, stressing that the A_{1c} target should be individualized to achieve the best control possible while decreasing the risk of severe hyperglycemia and hypoglycemia as well as maintaining normal growth and development (Chiang, 2014).

Nursing Diagnosis:

Deficient Knowledge

related to unfamiliarity with blood glucose monitoring

Desired Outcome: Within 48 hr of this diagnosis, the child/family demonstrates and verbalizes accurate understanding of proper blood glucose monitoring and when to monitor for ketones.

ASSESSMENT/INTERVENTIONS	RATIONALES
Assess the child's/parents' knowledge base about blood glucose monitoring.	Teaching can be more effective once the receiver's knowledge/understanding has been established.
Discuss reasons for blood glucose testing.	Understanding the purpose of performing tests facilitates adherence. Reasons for blood glucose testing include: - Allows child to relate "how I feel at this time" with the actual blood glucose level. - Gives the child/family some control. - Enables understanding of the effects of food, exercise, insulin, and/or stress. - Enables adjustments in insulin or diet.
Demonstrate the correct use of a glucometer the child will use at home and the proper technique for fingerstick.	There are many different models and strips available commercially. Each system functions a little differently, and it could be overwhelming having to learn a new system at home without assistance or guidance. General guidelines include: - Use side of finger, not the tip, for fingersticks. Sides of the fingers have fewer nerve endings and hurt less. In addition, using the sides decreases loss of sense of touch in fingertips. - Clean hands with soap and warm water. Cleansing helps reduce risk of infection. Warm water facilitates circulation and hence blood flow. - Avoid regular use of alcohol to cleanse the skin. Any trace of alcohol left on the skin will interfere with the chemical reaction involved in checking blood glucose. It is okay to use occasionally (e.g., at a picnic), but the finger must be dried carefully and the first drop of blood discarded. Repeated use of alcohol also can lead to thickening of the skin, making fingerstick more difficult and painful. - Hold the hand down, not up, to facilitate blood flow.
Discuss when blood glucose testing should be done.	Knowledge and understanding facilitate adherence. - Testing normally should be done before each meal and bedtime snack. Checking blood glucose on a regular basis and documenting findings help determine if adjustments need to be made in insulin/diet/exercise/medication by assessing the pattern of blood glucose levels. - If the child is sick, blood sugar is checked q4h. Risk of hyperglycemia is increased when the child is ill (e.g., with headache, fever, sore throat) or has an infection owing to stress on the body and increased energy demands. Stress causes the adrenal glands to produce more epinephrine, norepinephrine, and cortisol. These stress hormones are "antiinsulin" in their actions, so blood glucose increases and ketones are formed by the liver, breaking down fat stores for energy. As blood glucose increases, the three *P*'s (*p*olydipsia, *p*olyuria, *p*olyphagia) occur, causing dehydration as well as nausea and vomiting owing to ketosis. Blood glucose testing will determine if changes need to be made in insulin dosage and if the health care provider should be contacted. - Blood sugar is checked with hypoglycemic or hyperglycemic symptoms to identify which event is occurring and therefore facilitate proper treatment.

ASSESSMENT/INTERVENTIONS | RATIONALES

ASSESSMENT/INTERVENTIONS	RATIONALES
Explain that if blood glucose is greater than 250 mg/dL or if the child is ill, urine should be checked for ketones with every void.	The body starts breaking down stored fats for energy because it cannot use blood glucose for energy. Ketone bodies are by-products of this fat breakdown and can lead to DKA if not controlled/treated.
Demonstrate use of a diary or log to record blood glucose levels, ketones, insulin dose, diet, exercise, and any comments.	Information in this log provides a good overview of how the child is doing and assists the health care provider in making adjustments based on the pattern seen in the log/diary.
Instruct the child/family when to call the health care provider per blood glucose levels or ketones.	Understanding when to call improves adherence and decreases complications such as DKA: - Blood glucose greater than 250 mg/dL 3 times in a row. - Blood glucose less than 70 mg/dL twice in 1 wk. - Ketones moderate or large.

Nursing Diagnosis:

Deficient Knowledge

related to unfamiliarity with causes, signs and symptoms, and treatment of hypoglycemia and hyperglycemia

Desired Outcome: Immediately following teaching, the child/family verbalizes accurate understanding of possible causes, signs and symptoms, and treatment of hypoglycemia and hyperglycemia.

ASSESSMENT/INTERVENTIONS | RATIONALES

ASSESSMENT/INTERVENTIONS	RATIONALES
Assess the child's/family's knowledge/understanding about hypoglycemia and hyperglycemia.	Teaching can be more effective when the receiver's baseline knowledge/understanding is determined.
Define hypoglycemia for the child/family.	Knowledge facilitates early recognition of the problem, enabling prompt treatment. Hypoglycemia is defined as a low blood glucose level (less than 60-70 mg/dL) that occurs rapidly with signs and symptoms noted within minutes to an hour. Hypoglycemia is a potential emergency and needs to be treated promptly.
Teach the child/family causes of hypoglycemia.	Understanding causes of hypoglycemia optimally will help them decrease occurrences. Causes include: - Too little food or not eating on time. - Increased exercise/activity with no increased intake. - Too much insulin.
Teach the child/family to recognize early and late signs and symptoms of hypoglycemia.	Signs and symptoms of hypoglycemia should prompt them to check the blood glucose level. - Early signs occurring secondary to adrenaline release are trembling, tachycardia, sweating, headache, anxiety, and hunger. - Later signs and symptoms occurring secondary to cerebral glucose deficit are dizziness, personality/mood changes, slurred speech, loss of coordination, and decreased LOC. Some children may not show early symptoms of adrenaline release or, if younger than 6 yr old, may not recognize early symptoms.
Teach the best method of assessing and treating hypoglycemia.	Some signs and symptoms of hypoglycemia and hyperglycemia are difficult to distinguish from one another, but the treatments are different. It is essential to know which reaction a child is experiencing to treat it effectively. Measures include: - Checking blood sugar to determine if the child is hypoglycemic. - In the presence of hypoglycemia, giving 15 g (range 10-20 g, depending on the child's age) of readily absorbed carbohydrates such as 4 oz orange juice, 6 oz regular soda, 4 glucose tablets, or 6 LifeSavers. If blood glucose is not increased or the child is still having signs and symptoms of hypoglycemia in 15 min, treatment is repeated. This will elevate the plasma glucose level and relieve symptoms of hypoglycemia. Understanding of the appropriate initial treatment improves ability to treat hypoglycemia successfully.

continued

ASSESSMENT/INTERVENTIONS	RATIONALES
	- In addition, if it is not time for a meal or snack within 1 hr, giving complex carbohydrates and protein such as bread or crackers with peanut butter or cheese sustains the glucose level inasmuch as readily absorbed carbohydrates (fast-acting or simple sugars) will be out of the system in 45-60 min. Complex carbohydrates (e.g., crackers) take 2-3 hr and proteins (e.g., cheese or peanut butter) 3-4 hr to be metabolized. Knowledge of the appropriate follow-up treatment and understanding necessity of this treatment improve the ability to resolve the situation successfully.
Teach strategies to prevent hypoglycemia by identifying the pattern of activity or time of day that precedes reactions.	Knowledge of these patterns enables the child/family to prevent or decrease incidence of hypoglycemia. For example, the patient/parent should record in a log/diary all unusual events or change in activity or diet to help identify patterns.
Teach care if the child is unable to eat, drink, or swallow or is unconscious.	Knowing appropriate treatment improves outcome. - Glucagon (subcutaneous or intramuscular [IM]) is administered if available to raise the blood glucose level when the child is unable to drink or eat fast-acting carbohydrate. - If glucagon is not available, the child should be positioned on his or her side and honey, corn syrup, or Cake Mate gel rubbed inside the cheek. This position prevents aspiration, especially if giving glucagon, because vomiting may occur. Fast-acting/simple sugars are absorbed through the oral mucosa without danger of aspiration.
Define hyperglycemia for the child/family.	This helps differentiate between hyperglycemia and hypoglycemia. Knowledge enables recognition and discernment of which reaction the child is experiencing. Hyperglycemia is defined as blood glucose levels higher than target range. Signs and symptoms appear within hours to several days (see signs and symptoms, below).
Teach causes of hyperglycemia.	Understanding situations that can result in hyperglycemia (e.g., increased food intake, too little insulin, decreased exercise, infection or illness, and emotional stress) can help the child/family avoid such events.
Teach signs and symptoms of hyperglycemia.	Recognition of hyperglycemia enables earlier and more effective treatment and prevents development of DKA. Signs and symptoms include the three *P*'s (*p*olydipsia, *p*olyuria, *p*olyphagia), fatigue, fruity-smelling breath, weight loss.
Teach the treatment for hyperglycemia.	Interventions prevent DKA through early treatment. These include: - If blood glucose level is greater than 250 mg/dL, urine should be checked for ketones. - If ketone results are trace to small, the child should drink extra water and be rechecked for ketones in 2 hr. - If ketone results are medium to large, the health care provider should be contacted.
Teach the child/family to call the health care provider if blood glucose is greater than 250 mg/dL three times in a row.	The provider may need to adjust insulin dosage.

Nursing Diagnosis:

Deficient Knowledge

related to unfamiliarity with meal planning and its relationship to blood glucose

Desired Outcome: Within 48 hr after teaching, the child/family demonstrates ability to perform meal planning based on blood glucose levels.

ASSESSMENT/INTERVENTIONS	RATIONALES
Assess knowledge/understanding of the child/family regarding diet and its relationship to blood glucose.	Teaching can be more effective when the receiver's baseline knowledge/understanding is determined.
Assess the child's weight on admission and daily thereafter (same time of day, same scales, same amount of clothing).	Whether the child is maintaining, losing, or gaining weight may be an indicator of the effectiveness of the diet and treatment and/or adherence to both.
Teach the action that different foods (carbohydrates, fats, proteins) have on blood glucose level.	This information facilitates understanding of the need for adhering to the prescribed diet. For example, carbohydrates raise blood sugar, and simple sugars raise blood sugar more rapidly. Fats and proteins have a less immediate effect on blood sugar level.
Involve the dietitian in developing and instructing the child/family about the prescribed meal plan. Medical nutrition therapy (MNT) is essential.	Dietitians have expertise in designing a plan appropriate for children based on age, cultural background, preferences, and caloric needs. Including these variables in the meal plan increases knowledge, understanding, and hence likelihood of adherence.
Use handouts from the dietitian and guidelines in the diabetes book used by your facility for diabetes education (see resources at the end of this care plan) to review the prescribed diet.	Written and verbal explanations increase understanding and promote adherence.
As indicated, teach carbohydrate counting.	Understanding the diet plan increases the ability to continue this regimen at home and improves adherence as well. Counting grams of carbohydrates and matching them with the amount of insulin is the diet used most often in children. A no-concentrated-sweets diet is another plan used in some facilities.
Review the child's normal schedule and set up a schedule that includes time for blood glucose tests, medication, meals, and snacks.	Having a written schedule facilitates adjustment to new routines. The meal plan is tailored to the child and his or her activity level. Ongoing assessments enable changes as necessary and/or a follow-up dietary consultation.
Identify the ideal blood glucose levels for the child.	Diet and activity levels vary more in the younger child. Generally at less than 6 yr old, a child is more likely to have hypoglycemia and less likely to recognize early signs and symptoms, so more frequent blood glucose monitoring is now recommended for all children to help maintain A_{1c} at less than 7.5%. It is strongly recommended that the range is individualized for each child to achieve the best possible goal, minimize hypoglycemia or hyperglycemia, and maintain normal growth and development. (Chiang: Type 1 Diabetes Through the Lifespan: A Position Statement of the ADA, 2014).
Instruct the family to write meal plans for several days, implementing use of prescribed foods.	This is one method of assessing and promoting the family's understanding of diet instruction.
Provide scenarios for when blood glucose is outside the normal range and have them identify ways of adjusting diet, insulin, and/or exercise to get closer to the blood glucose goal. Include how to adjust the insulin and meal plan if ill and cannot eat.	This information facilitates development of problem-solving skills within the family and assesses their understanding of the interaction among blood glucose, insulin, diet, and exercise.

ADDITIONAL NURSING DIAGNOSES/PROBLEMS:

✓ PATIENT-FAMILY TEACHING AND DISCHARGE PLANNING

Children with DM may have different classifications of DM with varying symptoms and complications. When providing patient-family teaching, focus on sensory information, avoid giving excessive information, and initiate a visiting nurse referral for necessary follow-up teaching and assessment. A part of initial assessment should include asking about existing knowledge of the disease, ability for self-care by child and/or family, and psychologic acceptance. Stress family-centered care (viewing the family as a unit that is the "constant" in the child's life and maintaining or improving the health of the family and its members). Include verbal and written information (ensuring that written material is at a level the reader can understand) about the following:

✓ DM: definition, type the child has, brief pathophysiology, characteristics of specific type.

✓ Major influences on blood sugar control: diet, exercise/activity, insulin/oral medication, stress/infection.

✓ Diet prescribed for the child (most often carbohydrate-counting or no-concentrated-sweets diet). The diet is also low in fat and high in fiber to prevent or decrease problems with blood fats, especially cholesterol and triglycerides. Provide the rationale for three meals and two to three snacks on a consistent schedule.

✓ Exercise/activity: lowers blood glucose, helps maintain normal cholesterol levels, increases circulation, and is an essential part of a child's life. If exercise is increased or has a different time frame than usual, it may be necessary to adjust the diet (add 15-30 g carbohydrates for each 45-60 min of exercise), insulin, or oral medications.

✓ Stress or illness/infection: increases blood glucose level; therefore, adjustments may be necessary in diet and/or insulin dosage.

✓ Insulin: type of insulin; characteristics of particular insulin, including onset, peak, and duration; dose prescribed; and dosing schedule.
  • Have the child/parent demonstrate drawing up each prescribed dose (e.g., lispro and NPH before breakfast, lispro before supper, and NPH at bedtime).
  • Rotation of injection sites:
    • Insulin absorption varies by site (most rapidly in the abdomen, then in the arms, in the hips, and slowest in the thighs).
    • Insulin absorption is affected by the injection site. Massage after injection, exercise of the injected limb, and body temperature increase the rate of absorption.
    • Use all spots in one site before you move on to another site or use the same site for every morning injection and the same site for every evening injection until all spots have been used (gives same absorption of insulin).
  • Have the child/parent administer insulin using proper technique.

• At least two people (one could be the child) need to know how to draw up and administer insulin.

✓ Other medications, including drug name; purpose; dosage; frequency; precautions; drug-drug, food-drug, and herb-drug interactions; and potential side effects.

✓ Honeymoon phase or period with type 1: may occur a short time after diagnosis, usually within 2 to 8 wk, and usually lasts 1-3 mo, but may last up to a year. Insulin requirement decreases. The child is *not* cured. The insulin requirement will increase again.

✓ Acute complications of DM: hypoglycemia and hyperglycemia:
  • Possible causes
  • Signs and symptoms
  • Treatment

✓ Long-term complications (avoid addressing for now if the child has just been diagnosed): microvascular, macrovascular, joint contractures.

✓ Blood glucose monitoring: See details in **Deficient Knowledge** related to blood glucose monitoring.

✓ Sick-day plan of care:
  • Always give insulin.
  • Check blood sugar at least q4h and urine ketones with each void. Document in log/diary.
  • If small amount of ketones, increase fluid intake.
  • If child does not feel like eating, give fluids with sugar such as fruit juice, regular soda, and regular Jell-O, and broth-type soups (provide some electrolytes and extra fluid) unless blood sugar is greater than 200 mg/dL. Then give diet fluids.
  • Call the health care provider or nurse educator for the following:
    ○ Nausea and vomiting
    ○ Fruity odor to breath
    ○ Deep, rapid respirations
    ○ Decreasing LOC
    ○ Moderate or high ketones in urine
    ○ Persistent hyperglycemia greater than 250 mg/dL (3 times in a row)

✓ Prevention of infection:
  • Have good body hygiene with special attention to feet.
  • Report any breaks in skin and treat promptly.
  • Wear only properly fitting shoes and do not go barefooted.
  • Get regular dental checkups.
  • Need for pneumococcal and yearly influenza vaccines.

✓ Importance of the child wearing a medical alert necklace or bracelet (depending on age) and carrying a card that states the child has diabetes, the type of diabetes, child's name, address, phone number, and the health care provider's name and number.

✓ Psychosocial adjustment:
  • Reactions of the child: shock, denial, and sadness
  • Reaction of parents: grief reaction

✓ Delegation of tasks to the child, based on age (with supervision):
- Toddler/preschooler: Chooses and cleans finger for puncture; tries to identify word or phrase to describe feeling of hypoglycemia. Help choose food; give child a choice of appropriate options.
- School-age child: Performs finger puncture and blood glucose test. Pushes plunger down on insulin syringe after needle is inserted by parent or gives own injection. Performs ketone test on urine. Recognizes need to eat on time to avoid hypoglycemia. Verbalizes the treatment for hypoglycemia.
- Older school-age child: Records blood glucose values in the log/diary. May draw up and inject insulin. Knows meal plan. Can choose correct foods for snacks.
- Adolescent: Looks for patterns in blood glucose values. Recognizes when to test for ketones. Initiates treatment for ketones (increased fluids). Can plan meals and snacks based on the dietary plan. Can choose appropriate food at a party.

✓ Coordination of care. Need to talk with school nurse and/or other adults who are in close contact with the child (e.g., teachers, scout leaders, day care provider).

✓ Legal rights of the child "Legal protections" *on ADA website*.
- Individuals with Disabilities Education Act (IDEA): Mandates federal government to provide funding to education agencies, state and local, to facilitate free and appropriate education to qualifying students with disabilities. This includes children with diabetes because diabetes can, at times, adversely affect school performance in some students. If this can be proved, the school is then required to develop an individualized education plan (IEP).
- IEP: Designed by a multidisciplinary team to facilitate special education and therapeutic strategies and goals for each child. The child does not have to be in special education classes. Parents need to be involved in this process.
- Section 504 of Rehabilitation Act of 1973: Each student with a disability is entitled to accommodation in order to attend school and participate as fully as possible in school activities. This accommodation may be related to a medical condition or an education issue. For example, the child may leave the classroom to use bathroom facilities without raising hand and will not be penalized for excessive absences from school that are caused by the diabetes. The 504 Plan may include as many accommodations as necessary for the child to function well at school. Composition of the 504 team may include teachers, school nurse, therapists (physical, occupational, or speech therapist), psychologist, and parents and child as appropriate for the child's needs. Input from the health care provider is vital.

✓ Necessity of having the health care provider's signed prescription form or individualized Diabetes Medical Management Plan (DMMP) detailing guidelines for when to check blood sugar and administer medication or treatment for diabetes-related problems, as well as medications in the original container with prescribing label intact.

✓ Goals of care for a child with diabetes:
- Focus is on a child with diabetes, *not* on the diabetic child.
- Child will have appropriate growth (height and weight).
- Child will have age-appropriate lifestyle (development).
- Child will have near normal Hemoglobin A_{1C}.
- Child will not have acute complications (hypoglycemia or hyperglycemia).
- Child will have minimal serious complications associated with long-term diabetes.
- Child will be able to perform age-appropriate self-care tasks.

✓ Importance of follow-up care and regular visits to the health care provider and any other specialists working with the child, such as dietitian, physical therapist, or endocrinologist.

✓ Telephone numbers for the family to call if any questions arise about the therapy or disease after discharge.

✓ When to call the health care provider:
- Increased blood sugar greater than 250 mg/dL 3 times in a row.
- More than two episodes of hypoglycemia per week.
- Moderate-to-large amount of ketones in urine.

✓ Diabetes camps, which are a fun way for children to learn more about their diabetes and feel less isolated. Listing is available at *www.childrenwithdiabetes.com/camps*

✓ Referrals to community resources, such as local and national chapters of the American Diabetes Association (*www.diabetes.org*) and Juvenile Diabetes Research Foundation (*www.jdrf.org*), public health nurses or home health nurse, diabetes nurse educator or endocrinologist, community teaching programs or support groups for children, diabetes camps, or other resources as necessary.

✓ See "Diabetes Mellitus," p. 363, for additional family teaching and discharge planning suggestions and resources.

✓ Additional resources include the following:
- American Association of Diabetes Educators at *www.diabeteseducator.org*
- American Diabetes Association booklet: *Be Healthy Today: Be Healthy for Life:* Information for youth and their families living with type 2 diabetes at *www.diabetes.org/living-with-diabetes/parents-and-kids/children-and-type-2*
- Blood glucose diary/logbook available at *www.rd.com/health/wellness/free-tools-for-better-blood-sugar*

and usually comes with the new meters and can be obtained from the meter manufacturer or from a local pharmacy.

- Children with Diabetes at *www.childrenwithdiabetes .com*. This is an online community for kids, families, and adults with diabetes with numerous resources: e.g., sample 504 and IEP, books/journal entries per travels of Rufus and Ruby (teddy bears with diabetes), Grandma Sandy with free games and books for young children with Type 1 DM.
- Diabetes Care at School at *www.diabetes.org/living-with-diabetes/parents-and-kids/diabetes-care-at-school*: includes DMMP under Written Care Plans and 504 Plan under Legal Protections.
- Chase HP. *Understanding Diabetes*, ed 12, 2011 ($20.00) new edition due out in 2015; *A First Book for Understanding Diabetes*, 2011 (synopsis of 12th edition with quick summary of each chapter, $12.00); *Understanding Insulin Pumps and Continuous Glucose Monitoring*, ($18.00). There is a shipping charge per book. Available at *www.ChildrensDiabetes Foundation.org* or call (800) 695-2873.
- Type One Nation (Juvenile Diabetes Research Foundation)—Social network for children over 13 yr and adults with specific groups for teens and parents of children with type 1 DM: *www.typeonenation.org*
- National Diabetes Education Program: Transitions from Pediatric to Adult Health Care—Checklist and Help planning your transition. *www.ndep.nih.gov/teens*
- *http://www.diabetes.ca/diabetes-and-you/kids-teens-diabetes/children-type-2-diabetes*

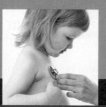

Fractures in Children 82

OVERVIEW/PATHOPHYSIOLOGY

Fractures are common childhood injuries and usually the result of trauma (falls, motor vehicle accidents, sports injuries, child abuse) or bone disease with abnormally fragile bones (osteogenesis imperfecta). Fractures usually result from increased mobility and immature understanding of potentially dangerous situations. Fractures in infancy are most often caused by trauma or child abuse.

Important variables that affect care of fractures in children as compared with adults

- Children's bones heal faster than adults'; the younger the child, the faster the bone heals.
- Children's bones are softer than adults'; rather than a complete break, they may bend, buckle, or partially break in a "greenstick" manner.
- Children's bones have a thicker periosteum and increased amount of immature bone.
- Children's bones have an open growth plate, or epiphysis. Damage to the growth plate can interrupt and alter growth.
- Children usually only complain when something is wrong. Restlessness, extended periods of crying, and calling for the parent more than usual, as well as disuse of the affected extremity, or increased use of the unaffected extremity after a fall or injury are signals that more investigation of the event is needed.

Most frequent types of fractures in children

- **Bends or plastic deformation:** A child's flexible bone can be bent 45 degrees or more before breaking and remains bent when the force is removed. Once bent, it will straighten slowly but not completely. The ossification of bones begins at birth and continues until the child is 18-21 yr old. The less ossified the bone, the more easily it bends. Thus, this type of injury occurs only in children, most often in the ulna and fibula.
- **Buckle or torus fracture:** Compression of the porous bone as a result of minimal angular trauma. It causes a bulge at the fracture site and occurs most often in young children, usually in the distal radius or ulna.
- **Greenstick:** Break occurs through the periosteum on one side of the bone but only bows or buckles the other side. It occurs most often in the forearm and is the type seen most often in children.

- **Complete fracture:** Break divides the bony fragments. It is classified by the form of the fracture line, such as spiral (from rotational force, often associated with child abuse, especially in infants), oblique, and transverse.
- **Epiphyseal growth plate fracture:** The cartilage growth plate is the weakest part of the long bones. A fracture here can be serious because it can cause growth disruption, arrest, or uneven growth. This fracture is classified by the Salter-Harris system (I-V).

Most common fracture sites in children

- Ulna, clavicle, tibia, and femur.

Most fractures are treated with closed reduction and immobilization of the affected area. Developmental age is key to the cause of injury (falls, motor vehicle accidents, sports) and type of fracture.

HEALTH CARE SETTING

Emergency department, with possible hospitalization

ASSESSMENT

The child's symptoms, trauma history (should match physical examination), and physical examination are all part of the assessment profile.

Signs and symptoms: Vary with the location, severity, and type of injury. Pain or tenderness at the site, decreased range of motion (ROM) or immobility, deformity at the fracture site, crepitus (grating sound heard on movement of the end of the broken bone), gross motion at the injured site, edema, erythema, ecchymosis, muscle spasm, and inability to bear weight may be present.

Physical assessment: Involves assessment of the location of the deformity, swelling, ecchymosis, and pain. Vital signs are checked and neurovascular assessment is performed.

DIAGNOSTIC TESTS

X-ray examination: Most effective tool for determining type and location of a fracture. Much of the skeleton of infants and young children is composed of radiolucent growth cartilage that does not appear on radiographs. Observation of gross deformity and point tenderness may be more reliable in diagnosing extremity fractures than would an x-ray. X-rays of the unaffected limb may be obtained for comparison. Radiography of the suspected limb fractures should include the joint above and below with a minimum of two views. X-rays are also taken after fracture reduction and often during the healing process to assess progress.

Computed tomography (CT) scan, magnetic resonance imaging (MRI) scan, ultrasound: May be needed to evaluate the fracture in certain circumstances.

Nursing Diagnosis:
Acute Pain
related to the fracture and other injury

Desired Outcome: Following treatment/intervention, the child's report of pain/pain level is less than 4 on a 10-point scale (e.g., FACES scale or numeric scale), or the child exhibits behavior consistent with pain less than 4 on a 10-point scale (e.g., FLACC [face, legs, activity, cry, consolability] scale).

ASSESSMENT/INTERVENTIONS	RATIONALES
Assess pain before and after analgesia administration and at least q4h using an appropriate pain scale for the child (FLACC, FACES, Oucher, Poker Chip, numeric).	This assessment helps determine the degree of pain and effectiveness of the pain medication.
Administer pain medication around the clock for the first 24-48 hr or depending on severity of the injury.	This decreases or prevents pain more effectively than when given prn. Prolonged stimulation of pain receptors results in increased sensitivity to painful stimuli and will increase the amount of medication required to relieve pain.
Administer analgesia via intravenous (IV) or by mouth (PO) route. Intramuscular (IM) route is rarely used, but if it is the only route possible, use topical anesthetic first.	These measures facilitate atraumatic care and encourage the child to give accurate pain ratings. The child may fear a "shot" and deny pain or refuse pain medication.
Position, align, and support the affected body part.	Appropriate positioning decreases tension on the affected area, thereby decreasing pain.
Use nonpharmacologic pain control measures as appropriate for the child depending on developmental age.	These are adjuncts to pain medication and include rocking, play, toys, music, distraction, relaxation techniques, humor, and massage.
Ice and elevate the extremity, especially for the first 48 hr.	These measures decrease edema, thereby decreasing pain.
Notify the health care provider if relief from pain is not obtained 15 min after IV pain medication, 30 min after IM pain medication (route rarely used), or 1 hr after PO pain medication was given and after using all the above measures.	Medication may need to be adjusted for optimal pain control. Prolonged or increasing pain also may signify a fracture complication.

Nursing Diagnoses:
Risk for Peripheral Neurovascular Dysfunction
Risk for Ineffective Peripheral Tissue Perfusion
related to edema or immobilization following fracture

Desired Outcome: The child's neurovascular checks are within normal limits within 24 hr of the fracture as evidenced by digits that are warm and sensitive to touch, brisk capillary refill (2 sec or less), peripheral pulse amplitude greater than 2+ on a 0-4+ scale, and minimal or decreased swelling in the affected limb.

ASSESSMENT/INTERVENTIONS	RATIONALES
! Assess neurovascular status (color, sensation, pulses, warmth, swelling) qh for the first 24 hr and then q2-4h. Use a measuring tape in millimeter increments to compare circumference of the area distal to the injury to that of the noninjured limb. Or, depending on size of the child, you should be able to insert one or two fingers into the cast opening.	These checks help determine the presence of peripheral neurovascular dysfunction in the injured limb, which would be evidenced by darker or lighter color than the opposite extremity, decreased sensation, decreased or absent pulse, skin cool to the touch, and increased swelling distal to the injury.
! Assess subjective and behavioral indicators of peripheral neurovascular dysfunction.	Complaints of constant or increasing pain (especially on passive movement of the digits) and numbness or tingling in the digits of the injured extremity are subjective indicators of peripheral neurovascular dysfunction. Constant crying or increasing irritability may be seen in young children.
Elevate the extremity.	Elevation helps prevent/decrease edema, thereby promoting tissue perfusion.
Apply ice during the first 48 hr.	Most swelling occurs during the first 48 hr. Ice helps decrease edema, thereby promoting tissue perfusion.
! Notify the health care provider immediately if tissue perfusion deteriorates quickly from baseline.	The child may be developing or experiencing compartment syndrome, **an emergency situation**. For details, see "Fractures" in the adult care plans for **Risk for Peripheral Neurovascular Dysfunction** related to interruption of capillary blood flow occurring with increased pressure within the myofascial compartment, p. 492.
Encourage the child to move the involved digits.	Moving toes or fingers in the affected limb improves circulation, thereby decreasing edema and increasing tissue perfusion. **Note:** Inability to move the digits is another sign of compartment syndrome.

Nursing Diagnosis:

Risk for Impaired Skin Integrity

related to presence of the immobilization device (bandages, splint, cast)

Desired Outcome: The child's skin remains intact while wearing the immobilization device.

ASSESSMENT/INTERVENTIONS	RATIONALES
Assess for erythema or irritation caused by the immobilization device q4h. - Check edges of the immobilization device above and below the fracture site. - If the edges are rough, petal moleskin to smooth the edges.	Ongoing assessment results in early detection and treatment, thereby decreasing risk of a break in skin integrity.
Assess the immobilization device by running your hand over it to feel for indentations or "hot" spots q4h.	Indentations can cause skin breakdown/pressure. Hot spots (after the cast has dried) may indicate an infection that might occur as a result of a break in skin integrity.
Feel around the edges of the immobilization device for tightness/looseness q4h.	This determines if the cast/immobilization device fits appropriately and is not too tight or loose. You should be able to insert your fingers between the cast and the child's skin after it dries. If the cast is too tight, it will cause pressure, which can result in decreased tissue perfusion and skin breakdown. If the cast is too loose, it can rub on the skin and cause skin breakdown.
Instruct the child or family not to put powder or corn starch under the cast.	These products may cake and cause skin irritation and breakdown.
Caution the child or family not to put anything inside the cast to scratch the skin.	This can cause skin breakdown or become lodged inside the cast.
Suggest that the family use cool air blown from a fan or hair dryer to relieve itching or rub the unaffected extremity.	These distraction techniques may keep the child from itching or putting things inside the cast to scratch and cause skin breakdown.
Encourage position changes q2-4h as appropriate.	This improves circulation by preventing prolonged pressure at the same area.

ADDITIONAL NURSING DIAGNOSES/PROBLEMS:

✓ PATIENT-FAMILY TEACHING AND DISCHARGE PLANNING

When providing child-family teaching, focus on sensory data, avoid giving excessive information, and initiate a visiting nurse referral for necessary follow-up teaching as needed. All information should emphasize that which is developmentally appropriate for the child. Stress family-centered care (viewing the family as a unit that is the "constant" in the child's life and maintaining or improving the health of the family and its members in a holistic manner). Include written and verbal information about the following (ensuring that information is at a level the reader can understand):

✓ Proper care of the immobilization device. See **Risk for Impaired Skin Integrity,** earlier.

✓ Medications, including drug name; purpose; dosage; frequency; precautions; drug-drug, food-drug; and herb-drug interactions; and potential adverse effects.

✓ Importance of taking medications at home and at school as directed. Medication in the original bottle (with prescribing label) and written prescription from the health care provider are needed for the child to be able to take medication at school.

✓ Legal rights of the child—Section 504 of Rehabilitation Act of 1973: Each student with a disability (whether temporary or permanent) is entitled to accommodation needed to attend school and participate as fully as possible in school activities. This accommodation may be related to a medical or an education issue. The 504 team for this child includes teachers, school nurse, possibly therapists, and parents and child, with input from the health care provider. For example, a child with a long leg cast who has to go up and down steps to change classes would need accommodation—either staying in the same room all day, leaving one class early enough to be able to get to the next class, having someone else carry his or her books, or possibly having a teacher provide lessons at home. As many accommodations can be made as necessary for the child to be able to be successful in school. More details at *www.specialchildren.about.com/od/504s/f/504faq1.htm*

✓ Adjustments needed for activities of daily living.

✓ Age-appropriate (developmental age, not just chronologic age) safety measures to help prevent further injuries:

- Childproof the home and play area (include what is appropriate for *all* children in the home).
- Avoid use of baby walkers, which are responsible for many injuries in infants.
- Proper use of protective equipment (e.g., car safety seats, bicycle helmets).
- Adaptation of a child safety restraint system to accommodate cast/immobilization device.
- Importance of supervising young children while playing.
- Not leaving a child sitting in a shopping cart because many fall out or manage to tip the cart over. Be sure the shopping cart has a safety belt and that it is secured.
- Realistic expectations for the child.

✓ When to call the health care provider:

- Child complains of pain consistently in the same spot or pain seems to be getting worse.
- Child has tingling or numbness of toes or fingers.
- Child cannot feel something touching fingers or toes.
- Red or sore areas appear around the cast edges.
- Child's fingers or toes are cold when in a warm environment.
- Child's nails stay pale when pressing on them and releasing pressure.
- Child's nails look blue even after elevating limb.
- Child's fingers or toes become very swollen several days after injury. Most swelling should occur in the first 48 hr.
- A foul smell comes from the cast.
- A "hot" spot is felt on the cast.
- Staining appears on the cast that was not there when child first came home. This could be an infected area or pressure sore.
- Child complains of constant itching that nothing helps.
- Cast is too tight or too loose.
- The cast starts to break down or fall apart or has indented areas. The cast may need to be reinforced or replaced to provide appropriate support for the injured area.
- Swelling after the first few days, pain, numbness, tingling, red marks or sores, and foul smell are serious

signs of a problem. Talk with the child's health care provider immediately. If the health care provider is unavailable, go to the nearest emergency care facility.

✓ Importance of follow-up care.

✓ Referral to community resources for assistance as needed (e.g., in providing safe home environment and transport to accommodate cast/immobilization device). Additional information can be obtained by contacting the local children's hospital, Social Services, and the following organizations:

• National SAFE KIDS Campaign at *www.safekids.org*
• Easter Seals at *www.easterseals.com*
• Parachute at *www.parachutecanada.org*

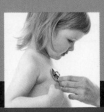

Gastroenteritis 83

OVERVIEW/PATHOPHYSIOLOGY

Gastroenteritis, one of the most common infectious diseases seen in children, is an inflammation of the stomach and intestines that accompanies numerous gastrointestinal (GI) disorders. It is one of the main causes of dehydration and can cause life-threatening complications. Acute infectious gastroenteritis is caused by a variety of bacterial, viral, and parasitic pathogens. Rotavirus infection is the most common cause of severe diarrhea in infants and young children worldwide. Before the rotavirus vaccine program started in 2006, rotavirus led to the hospitalization of 55,000 U.S. infants and children each year. Worldwide, rotavirus is estimated to cause 527,000 deaths in children annually (CDC Clinical Information Rotavirus, 2011). Because the rotavirus vaccines have been so effective against severe rotavirus disease (Cortese et al., 2013), noroviruses are the leading cause of epidemic gastroenteritis now, detected in about 50% of acute gastroenteritis (AGE) outbreaks in Europe and the United States (Hall et al., 2013). Norovirus causes 19-21 million cases of AGE, leading to 1.7-1.9 million outpatient visits and 400,000 emergency department visits, mainly in children younger than 5 yr. It is responsible for 56,000-71,000 hospitalizations and 570-800 deaths per year, most among young children and the elderly. Norovirus occurs year round but peaks in the winter. There is also 50% more norovirus illness in years when there is a new strain of the virus emerging. Norovirus outbreaks occur mainly when infected people spread the virus to others (fecal-oral route), but it is also spread by contaminated food or water or by contact with a surface the virus is on. The foods that primarily are involved in outbreaks include leafy green vegetables (e.g., lettuce), fresh fruits, and shellfish (e.g., oysters) (CDC Trends and Outbreaks, 2013).

Other common causes of infectious gastroenteritis include *Escherichia coli*, *Salmonella*, *Shigella*, and *Campylobacter* as the most common bacterial pathogens and *Giardia* and *Cryptosporidium* as the most common parasites. *Clostridium difficile* is the most common nosocomial source, and it occurs after antibiotic use.

HEALTH CARE SETTING

Primary care, with possible hospitalization depending on severity of the illness

ASSESSMENT

History is very important, as is physical examination. Signs and symptoms vary widely depending on illness severity. Age, general health, and environment are factors that predispose children to gastroenteritis.

Signs and symptoms: Children usually present with some degree of the following:
- Fever
- Vomiting
- Diarrhea: Wide range of frequency and character (e.g., watery, bloody)
- Tenesmus: Painfully urgent but ineffectual attempt to urinate or defecate
- Abdominal pain
- Dehydration: Symptoms vary depending on the degree of dehydration/water deficit (CDC MMWR, 2003).
  - Minimal (less than 3%): No physical signs and symptoms, possibly decreased urine output (UO).
  - Mild to moderate (3%-9%): May be alert, fatigued, restless, or irritable; thirsty, eager to drink; normal to increased heart rate (HR); normal to fast respiratory rate (RR); normal to decreased pulses; slightly sunken eyes; dry mucous membranes; prolonged capillary refill time; cool extremities; decreased UO.
  - Severe (greater than 9%): Apathetic, lethargic, or unconscious; minimal intake, may be unable to drink; tachycardia; weak, thready, or impalpable pulses; deep breathing; deeply sunken eyes; parched mucous membranes; prolonged or minimal capillary refill; cold, mottled, cyanotic extremities; minimal UO.
- Infants and children are at increased risk of dehydration due to many factors:
  - They have a greater percentage of body weight that is water than adults (e.g., a newborn has 75%-80% of body weight that is water, and 40% of that is extracellular; a preschooler has 60%-65% of body weight that is water, and 30% of that is extracellular).
  - Extracellular fluid is lost first with gastroenteritis.
  - The younger the child, the more quickly dehydration occurs.
  - Insensible water loss is also greater in infants and young children via the skin and GI tract because of a

proportionally greater body surface area in relation to body mass. Increased RR also increases insensible water loss as does a higher metabolic rate.

The most serious consequences of gastroenteritis are dehydration, electrolyte imbalance, and malnutrition.

DIAGNOSTIC TESTS

History is important in determining the source of gastroenteritis and if there is a need for any tests. In general, laboratory tests are not performed unless the child exhibits moderate-to-severe dehydration, appears toxic, and has abdominal pain or bloody stools.

Serum electrolytes: Determine severity of electrolyte imbalance and type of fluid replacement necessary.

Complete blood count: Hematocrit is often elevated in dehydration. The differential will determine whether viral or bacterial infection is present. In a bacterial infection, the white blood cell (WBC) count is elevated with increased polymorphonuclear leukocytes or neutrophils. In a viral infection, the WBC count is slightly elevated with increased lymphocytes.

Blood urea nitrogen: Elevated with dehydration but should return to normal with rehydration.

Blood culture: Obtained if the child is acutely ill to help determine cause of illness.

Stool specimen: Examined if diarrhea lasts more than a few days to help determine cause.

Rotazyme: Rapid test to see if rotavirus is present in stool. A positive test negates need for a stool culture.

Stool culture: Obtained if blood or mucus is present in stool, when symptoms are severe, or if there is history of travel to a developing country.

Stool for ova and parasites: May be used instead of a culture because it is less expensive and often more reliable. A specimen is obtained 3 days in a row.

Nursing Diagnosis:

Deficient Fluid Volume

related to fluid loss occurring with fever, vomiting, and diarrhea

Desired Outcome: Within 4 hr following intervention/treatment (for mild-moderate dehydration), the infant/child exhibits adequate hydration as evidenced by alertness and responsiveness, anterior fontanel soft and not sunken (in children younger than 2 yr), moist oral mucous membranes, elastic abdominal skin turgor, capillary refill less than 2 sec, and age-appropriate UO (e.g., infant 2-3 mL/kg/hr, toddler and preschooler 2 mL/kg/hr, school-age child 1-2 mL/kg/hr, and adolescent 0.5-1 mL/kg/hr).

ASSESSMENT/INTERVENTIONS	RATIONALES
Assess weight of the child on admission and daily on the same scale, at the same time of day, and wearing the same amount of clothing (infants are weighed without any clothing). Notify the health care provider if the child is losing weight.	Consistency with weight measurements helps ensure more accurate results. Weight is a useful indicator of fluid balance. Weight loss indicates the child is not receiving adequate fluid replacement and adjustments need to be made.
Assess vital signs q4h or more often if they are outside normal parameters. Report abnormalities to the health care provider.	HR is elevated and blood pressure (BP) is normal in compensated shock and low in uncompensated shock. Dehydration can quickly lead to shock in infants and young children in whom a falling BP is a *late* sign of shock.
Do not measure temperatures rectally.	Rectal temperature measurements stimulate stooling, which can lead to dehydration. Also, if the child has diarrhea, they cause further irritation to impaired skin.
Administer oral rehydration solution (ORS), for example, Pedialyte, Infalyte, Rice-Lyte, Rehydralyte.	ORS replaces fluid volume in children with minimal-to-moderate dehydration. - To make it more palatable for the child, you may add 1 tsp presweetened sugar-free Kool-Aid to chilled 1-liter bottle of ORS or try flavored brands of these solutions. - Small amounts are given frequently, especially if the child is vomiting (5 mL q5min with a gradual increase in the amount consumed). This is from the 2003 guideline issued by the CDC to improve health outcomes by replacing fluid and electrolytes, as well as glucose, with oral rehydration therapy (ORT). ORT includes rehydration with ORS and maintenance phase, including fluid and adequate dietary intake.

continued

PART II: Pediatric Nursing Care Plans

ASSESSMENT/INTERVENTIONS	RATIONALES
Do not give clear liquids such as apple juice, soda, gelatin, or sports drinks.	Liquids with a large amount of simple sugars can exacerbate osmotic effects associated with diarrhea and vomiting.
Do not give tea or soda with caffeine.	Caffeine is a mild diuretic and can increase dehydration as a result of loss of fluid and electrolytes.
Do not give chicken or beef broth.	Broths are high in salt and low in carbohydrates.
Administer and monitor nasogastric tube (NGT) fluid replacement (for mild-moderate dehydration and vomiting) or intravenous (IV) fluids as prescribed for moderate-severe dehydration and vomiting.	If the child is unable to take sufficient ORS orally, use of NGT with ORS might help initial rehydration and speed up tolerance to refeeding. IV fluid and electrolyte replacement likely will be necessary if this is not successful or if the child is severely dehydrated.
Assess hydration status q4h.	Although the child may be receiving maintenance fluids, he or she may still be dehydrated because of diarrhea, vomiting, and/or insensible water losses. A dehydrated child is likely to exhibit decreasing level of consciousness, sunken anterior fontanel (if younger than 2 yr), dry or sticky oral mucous membrane, tented abdominal skin, capillary refill greater than 2 sec, and decreasing UO.
Ensure that the child has at least minimal UO but that output is not more than intake.	This is an indicator of adequate hydration.
After the child is rehydrated, calculate maintenance fluids based on the child's current weight.	The smaller the child, the greater the percentage of body weight is water. To meet minimal fluid requirements, the necessary volume is calculated in the following way: Up to 10 kg: 100 mL/kg/24 hr = _____ 10-20 kg: 50 mL/kg/24 hr = _____ greater than 20 kg: 20 mL/kg/24 hr = _____ total amount = maintenance fluid requirement *For example, if child weighs 43 kg:* $10 \text{ kg} \times 100 \text{ mL/kg/24 hr} = 1000 \text{ mL/24 hr}$ $10 \text{ kg} \times 50 \text{ mL/kg/24 hr} = 500 \text{ mL/24 hr}$ $\underline{23 \text{ kg} \times 20 \text{ mL/kg/24 hr} = 460 \text{ mL/24 hr}}$ $43 \text{ kg} = 1960 \text{ mL/24 hr}$ Maintenance fluid requirement is 1960 mL/24 hr or 82 mL/hr.
Ensure that the child is receiving at least maintenance fluids.	This is the minimum amount of fluid needed on a daily basis to be well hydrated if there are no unusual fluid losses (e.g., fever, diarrhea, vomiting).
Administer medications as prescribed.	For example, antibiotics are given to treat the bacterial pathogen causing the diarrhea.
After the child is rehydrated, begin a regular diet as tolerated.	Enteral nutrition stimulates renewal of intestinal cells, whereas fasting increases gut atrophy and permeability, which can contribute to dehydration. A regular diet is likely to include the following factors: low in fat, avoiding high concentrations of simple sugars, and encouraging complex carbohydrates such as starches. Examples of an appropriate diet include cereals, lean meats, yogurt, and cooked vegetables.
Instruct family members in providing ORS, monitoring intake and output, and assessing for signs of dehydration.	These instructions should improve adherence and promote optimal results.

Nursing Diagnosis:

Risk for Impaired Skin Integrity

related to irritation caused by frequent stooling

Desired Outcome: The child's skin in perineal and perianal areas remains intact.

ASSESSMENT/INTERVENTIONS	RATIONALES
Assess perineal and perianal areas for signs of irritation or excoriation with every diaper change.	The earlier the problem is detected, the sooner appropriate interventions can be made to ensure the skin remains intact.
Change diapers as soon as they become wet or soiled.	This helps keep skin clean and dry.
Cleanse the buttocks gently (pat, do not rub) with water or immerse in tepid water to cleanse. Avoid using soap if possible.	Diarrheal stools are very irritating to the skin. Rubbing the skin every time the diaper is changed would irritate it further. Soap dries skin by removing normal moisturizing skin oils, thereby increasing the potential for irritation and skin breakdown.
Do not use commercial baby wipes with alcohol or perfume or baby powder on irritated or excoriated skin.	These products are painful to irritated skin. Baby powder cakes and is difficult to remove.
If not contraindicated, apply protective ointments such as Vaseline, A&D, or zinc oxide when the child is wearing a diaper.	This measure protects skin from irritation.
Leave the diaper area open to air if possible (but not in the presence of explosive diarrhea). Reapply protective ointment before putting the diaper on.	This practice facilitates drying and healing.
Instruct family members in appropriate skin care methods.	This increases the likelihood of the family using these techniques at home.

Nursing Diagnosis:

Risk for Infection

related to gastroenteritis and lack of knowledge about transmission prevention

Desired Outcome: Following intervention, family members and other children are free of indicators of gastroenteritis.

ASSESSMENT/INTERVENTIONS	RATIONALES
Implement Standard Precautions as well as appropriate Transmission-Based Precautions. For more information, see Appendix A for "Infection Prevention and Control."	Standard Precautions reduce the risk of spreading infection. These include: - Good hand hygiene: Wash hands before and after working with the child, even with appropriate gloving. - Wear gloves when changing or weighing the diaper. - Wear other personal protective equipment as designated by isolation guidelines.
Dispose of linen and other soiled items per hospital protocol.	This will prevent the spread of infection.
Apply the diaper securely.	This prevents fecal spread.
Try to keep infants and small children from placing hands or objects in contaminated areas.	Gastroenteritis is mostly spread by the fecal-oral route. Infants and young children tend to put their hands in their mouths, and if their hands get into their diaper or stool, fecal-oral spread occurs.
Teach children, as appropriate, protective measures such as washing their hands after using the toilet.	This teaching helps prevent the spread of infection.
Instruct family members and visitors in protective measures, especially handwashing and not visiting other patients.	This instruction reduces the risk of spreading infection.

Nursing Diagnosis:

Imbalanced Nutrition: Less Than Body Requirements

related to inadequate intake and fluid loss occurring with vomiting, diarrhea, and fever

Desired Outcome: Within 24-48 hr following intervention/treatment, the child maintains or gains weight and exhibits no further vomiting or diarrhea.

ASSESSMENT/INTERVENTIONS	RATIONALES
Assess weight on admission and daily (on the same scale, at the same time, with the same clothing—no diaper on infants).	These assessments measure the child's progress in attaining adequate nutrition. Consistency with weight measurements helps ensure more accurate results.
If the mother is breastfeeding, encourage her to continue along with giving ORS (if the child has mild-to-moderate dehydration) as described in **Deficient Fluid Volume,** earlier.	This practice tends to reduce the severity and duration of illness by maintaining normal intake so that the child has adequate nutrition.
Avoid the BRAT (bananas, rice, apples, and toast) diet.	These foods do not provide complete caloric and protein requirements. They provide excessive carbohydrates and, overall, are also low in electrolytes. Therefore, the child does not get needed nutrients.
Resume a regular diet when the child is rehydrated as described in **Deficient Fluid Volume,** earlier.	Enteral nutrition stimulates renewal of intestinal cells and decreases illness duration, whereas fasting increases gut atrophy and permeability.
Instruct the family in the appropriate diet as described in **Deficient Fluid Volume**, earlier.	This gains adherence to the treatment plan.
Monitor the child's response to feedings.	Monitoring helps assess feeding tolerance.
	- Some children have increased stooling with lactose-containing milk products.
	- Most children do well with lactose-containing milk products, especially if they are eating foods at the same time.
Give liquids at room temperature.	Cold liquids stimulate peristalsis and hence diarrhea.
Keep the room as odor free as possible.	Minimizing unpleasant or strong (perfume/aftershave) odors increases interest in eating and feelings of well-being.
Provide oral hygiene.	This enhances a sense of well-being and improves chances the child will eat and drink more.

ADDITIONAL NURSING DIAGNOSES/PROBLEMS:

✓ **PATIENT-FAMILY TEACHING AND DISCHARGE PLANNING**

When providing child-family teaching, focus on sensory information, avoid giving excessive information, and arrange for a visiting nurse for follow-up teaching and assessment as needed. Stress family-centered care (viewing the family as a unit that is the "constant" in the child's life and maintaining or improving the health of the family and its members in a holistic manner). Include verbal and written information about the following (ensure that written material is at a level the reader can understand):

✓ Pathophysiology of gastroenteritis.
✓ Causes of gastroenteritis: If caused by improper food storage—address proper hygiene, formula or food preparation, handling, and storage.

✓ Contagious aspect of gastroenteritis. It is important to use good handwashing technique, especially after changing a diaper. Teach children who are old enough to wash their hands after they use the toilet.

✓ Why gastroenteritis can be such a serious problem, especially for infants and young children:
  • The younger the child, the greater the percentage of body weight that is water.
    ○ Premature infant: 85%-90% of body weight is water.
    ○ Full-term infant: 75%-80% of body weight is water.
    ○ Preschooler: 60%-65% of body weight is water.
    ○ Adolescents: 50%-55% of body weight is water.
  • Therefore the younger the child, the quicker dehydration can occur (the child loses more fluid than is taken in).
  • Problems that cause or increase the severity of dehydration: fever, vomiting, diarrhea, not eating or drinking enough.

✓ Importance of checking hydration status q2-4h when the child is ill with any of the previous problems (the younger the child, the more often status is reassessed):
  • Is the child alert and interactive? The child would not be as alert and interactive as normal if dehydrated.
  • Check the soft spot on top of the head in children younger than 2 yr: if it is sunken in, the child is dehydrated.
  • No tears when crying in a child older than 6 mo old.
  • Check inside the mouth, not the lips: if dry or sticky and the child is not a mouth breather, the child is dehydrated.
  • Pinch skin on the abdomen: if the skin sits up like a tent instead of falling down right away, the child is dehydrated.
  • How many wet diapers does the child normally have per day? If the number is decreased or they are not as wet as normal, the child may be dehydrated.

✓ Feeding of child who has diarrhea:
  • If the child is breastfeeding, continue breastfeeding and supplement with ORS (e.g., Pedialyte, Infalyte, or Rehydralyte).
  • If the child is taking only formula or milk, it may not be necessary to stop that fluid as long as the child is also taking ORS.
  • 1 tsp presweetened sugar-free Kool-Aid can be added to a chilled 1-L bottle of ORS to improve taste or use flavored ORS.

✓ Change diapers frequently:
  • Clean after stool with warm water. Pat skin; do not rub.
  • Do not use soap if possible. If that is not possible, use mild, nonantiseptic soap.
  • Do not use baby wipes containing alcohol or fragrances.
  • Avoid powders and corn starch, which trap fluid and get caked in creases.
  • Leave skin open to air if irritated (but not in the presence of explosive diarrhea).
  • Put protective ointment such as Vaseline, A&D, or zinc oxide on the skin.

✓ Feeding of a child who is vomiting: Give small amounts of ORS frequently—amount varies depending on age and weight of the child.

✓ Once the child is rehydrated, begin a regular diet as tolerated.
  • Do not give BRAT (bananas, rice, apples, tea, or toast). This combination does not provide enough calories or protein.
  • Use low-fat foods (no peanut butter, potato chips, or hot dogs).
  • Give starchy foods such as cooked baby cereal, oatmeal, cream of wheat, rice, nonsugared cereals, noodles, potatoes, bread, and yogurt.
  • Give fruits (not packed in syrup), vegetables without butter, and well-cooked chicken, fish, or lean meat.
  • Avoid concentrated sweets such as candy or ice cream.
  • Most children have no problems drinking formula or milk.

✓ Call the health care provider when:
  • There are signs of dehydration.
  • There is blood or pus in the stool.
  • The child has a fever.
  • The vomiting or diarrhea lasts longer than 8-24 hr (the younger the child, the earlier the health care provider should be called).
  • Child is not drinking fluids or is less alert than usual.
  • Child has abdominal pain for 2 hr or more.
  • Child is younger than 6 mo old and is vomiting or has diarrhea.
  • Diaper area is very red or irritated and getting worse.

✓ Reinforce that the child should never receive aspirin with viral illness; acetaminophen or ibuprofen should be used for fever or discomfort.

✓ Telephone numbers to call should questions or concerns about the treatment or disease arise after discharge.

✓ Importance of follow-up care.
  • Importance of getting the rotavirus vaccine for infants less than 6 mo old.

✓ Referral to community resources as necessary.

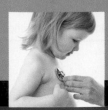

Otitis Media 84

OVERVIEW/PATHOPHYSIOLOGY

Otitis media (OM) is the most common reason for visits to the pediatrician in the first 3 yr of life, the leading cause of antibiotic use, and the most common cause of hearing loss in children. The number of clinician visits for OM decreased from 950 visits per 1000 children in 1995 to 1996 to 634 visits per 1000 children in 2005 to 2006, with a proportional decrease in antibiotic prescriptions. However, the percentage of children in visits for OM getting antibiotics remained relatively stable (from 80% to 76%). Factors that may have contributed to the decrease in visits for OM include financial issues, use of pneumococcal vaccine, increased use of influenza vaccine, and public education campaigns stressing the overuse of antibiotics (American Academy of Pediatrics [AAP], Clinical Practice Guidelines, 2013). Many factors contribute to OM development, including host (i.e., immune system or anatomic abnormality), infectious (i.e., bacterial or viral pathogen), allergic (i.e., second-hand smoke), and environmental (i.e., feeding methods and group daycare) factors. Socioeconomic factors also affect the risk of developing OM, its diagnosis, and treatment. Since the introduction of the pneumococcal conjugate vaccine, the most common bacterial pathogen for acute otitis media (AOM) is β-lactamase–producing *Haemophilus influenzae*, followed by penicillin-resistant *Streptococcus pneumoniae* (Pichichero, 2013). The AAP updated the Clinical Practice Guidelines for AOM (2013) and again recommended observation without antibiotic treatment for select, otherwise healthy children 6 mo to 12 yr of age with AOM for 48-72 hr and stressed the importance of follow-up with those children in that time frame. It was also stressed that if children treated with antibiotics did not improve or became more ill within the 48-72 hr, they needed to be reevaluated. Pain assessment and management were addressed in the new guidelines also. It noted that whether on antibiotics or not, pain would not resolve in 24 hr and, in about 30% of children younger than 2 yr, it could last 3-7 days with or without a fever. Oral pain medications such as acetaminophen and ibuprofen are very effective; topical medications have questionable benefit (AAP, 2013).

OM includes several conditions ranging from acute to chronic with or without symptoms:

- **Otitis media (OM):** inflammation of the middle ear.
- **Acute otitis media (AOM):** middle ear inflammation with symptoms of acute illness (fever, pain, irritability) and moderate to severe bulging tympanic membrane (TM) under positive pressure.
- **Otitis media with effusion (OME)** or **serous otitis media:** inflammation of the middle ear without signs and symptoms of acute infection (other than reduced hearing), TM retracted or in neutral position under negative pressure or no pressure, and fluid in the middle ear space.
- **Chronic OM with effusion:** middle ear effusion lasting more than 3 mo.

HEALTH CARE SETTING

Primary care; possible hospitalization if OM exacerbates a chronic condition or if surgical intervention is required

ASSESSMENT

Signs and symptoms: Vary depending on type of OM and age of the child.

AOM:

- *Infant or young child:* fever; possible ear drainage; crying; irritable and fussy; may tug, rub, or hold the affected ear; sleep disturbances; decreased appetite; rolling head side to side; difficult to comfort; possible difficulty hearing.
- *Older child:* fever, possible ear drainage, complaints of ear hurting, crying, irritable, lethargic, decreased appetite (chewing causes increased ear pain), possible difficulty hearing.

OME: Difficulty hearing, feeling of fullness/pressure in the ear, tinnitus or popping sounds, mild balance disturbances.

Physical assessment

AOM: Pneumatic otoscopy reveals bulging, red, immobile TM (or decreased mobility of TM). Crying, removal of cerumen and thereby irritating the auditory canal, and fever can cause redness of the TM without infection being present. Postauricular and cervical lymph nodes may be enlarged.

OME: Pneumatic otoscopy may show a slightly injected, dull gray membrane; obscured landmarks; and fluid visible behind the TM. There is also decreased mobility of the TM.

DIAGNOSTIC TESTS

Pneumatic otoscopy: A pneumatic attachment to the otoscope enables the health care provider to introduce puffs of air into the ear. The TM does not move as well with fluid behind it. This device improves diagnostic accuracy by assessing mobility of the TM, as well as visualizing it.

Tympanometry: Method of providing information about the possible presence of a middle ear effusion, including the actual pressures in the middle ear space. This is a quick and simple method of assessing TM mobility.

Acoustic reflectometry: Rapid and easy way to measure reflected sound waves from TM; the louder the sound, the greater the likelihood of middle ear effusion. Advantages over tympanometry include that it is unaffected by crying or the presence of cerumen. It is not widely used, however, as there are no specific standards established to determine results.

Tympanocentesis: "Gold standard" for diagnosis of AOM, although it is not routinely used because of cost, effort, and lack of availability. It involves removal of fluid from the middle ear to identify the bacteria causing the infection. It improves diagnostic accuracy, guides treatment by finding the causative pathogen, and avoids unnecessary medical or surgical intervention. It is especially useful in AOM unresponsive to antibiotics or recurrent AOM.

Culture and sensitivity: Not routinely done, but if drainage is present or tympanocentesis is performed, it helps guide treatment in finding the causative pathogen and antibiotics to which it is sensitive.

Nursing Diagnosis:

Acute Pain

related to increased pressure in the middle ear occurring with fluid and/or infection

Desired Outcome: The child is free from pain or has significantly decreased pain (e.g., less than 4 on a 0-10 scale: FLACC [face, legs, activity, cry, consolability], FACES, or a numeric scale [0-10]) within 1 hr after intervention/treatment.

ASSESSMENT/INTERVENTIONS	RATIONALES
Assess pain level at least q4h using developmentally appropriate pain scale for the child (FLACC, FACES, or numeric scale).	A pain scale developmentally appropriate for a child will enable accurate assessment of the pain level and help evaluate the relief obtained.
Administer antipyretics/analgesics on a regular basis, for example, acetaminophen q4-6h for a maximum of 5 doses/day and/or ibuprofen q6-8h.	This protocol provides better control of fever and pain than on a prn basis. Alternating acetaminophen and ibuprofen so that the child receives pain medication q3h gives maximum pain/fever control.
Avoid overdosage of acetaminophen.	Hepatic necrosis can occur. The child should not receive more than 4000 mg/day.
Reassess pain level and/or temperature 1 hr after administering medication.	This evaluates effectiveness of pain relief/fever control measure.
Administer antibiotics, if prescribed. Instruct parents to:	Many cases of AOM resolve in 2-3 days without antibiotics. This correlates with the 2013 Clinical Practice Guidelines from the AAP.
- Administer the correct dose of medication at the correct time.	This ensures optimal effectiveness of medication.
- Administer all doses (correct number/day and total number of doses prescribed).	The child may feel better after several days, and the parents may stop giving the medication. This may cause OM to reoccur and/or allow a more resistant bacteria to infect the child.
- Store medications appropriately.	Many antibiotics have to be refrigerated.
Use localized comfort measures based on developmental age that provide maximal comfort for the child. - Apply warm compresses to the affected ear or have the child lie on the affected ear on a heating pad on a low setting, covered with a towel to protect the child from potential burns. - Apply a wrapped ice bag over the affected ear to decrease edema and pressure.	What is comforting to an infant usually is not comforting to an adolescent. Every child has specific measures that are comforting to him or her.
Administer analgesic otic drops if prescribed.	These drops may relieve severe pain but their effectiveness is questioned in the 2013 Clinical Practice Guidelines from AAP.

continued

ASSESSMENT/INTERVENTIONS	RATIONALES
Position for comfort according to the type of OM. - AOM: Position with the affected ear in the dependent position. - OME: Elevate the head.	Positioning decreases pressure on the TM.
Teach older children to open their eustachian tube by yawning or performing Valsalva's maneuver.	This facilitates drainage of fluid from the middle ear into the pharynx and decreases pressure on the TM.

Nursing Diagnosis:

Risk for Deficient Fluid Volume

related to losses associated with fever and decreased intake

Desired Outcome: Within 24 hr of interventions, the child is alert and responsive, the anterior fontanel is soft and not sunken (in a child younger than 2 yr), the oral mucous membranes are moist, abdominal skin turgor is good, the child has age-/weight-appropriate urine output (e.g., infant 2-3 mL/kg/hr, toddler and preschool child 2 mL/kg/hr, school-age child 1-2 mL/kg/hr, and adolescent 0.5-1 mL/kg/hr), and the child receives at least maintenance-level fluids.

ASSESSMENT/INTERVENTIONS	RATIONALES
Assess hydration status q4h. Teach the parents how to do this, and explain its importance.	The younger the child is and the less he or she weighs, the greater the percentage of body weight that is water. The child can become dehydrated easily. Routinely assessing for dehydration in a child who is running a fever and/or has decreased intake facilitates rapid treatment to resolve dehydration. A child who is dehydrated may have a decreasing level of consciousness, sunken anterior fontanel (if younger than 2 yr), dry or sticky oral mucous membranes, tenting abdominal skin, and decreasing urine output.
Teach parents when to call the health care provider regarding dehydration.	This facilitates their ability to detect a problem early, thereby ensuring quicker problem resolution. Parents should call under the following conditions: - The child is not as alert as usual - The anterior fontanel is sunken - Inside of the mouth is dry or sticky if the child is not a mouth breather - Skin on the abdomen stays up like a tent when pinched - Fewer wet diapers than usual/voiding is less often than usual
Calculate maintenance fluids for the child and teach the family to provide this in terms they can understand.	Specific information enables parents to ensure that their child receives the correct fluid volume. For example, if the child weighs 15 kg, maintenance fluids are 1250 mL/day (42 oz), and if the child drinks from a 6-oz "sippy" cup (180 mL), that child needs to drink at least 7 sippy cupfuls (1260 mL) of fluid a day. Calculation for minimum daily maintenance fluids: *For the child weighing 15 kg:* Up to 10 kg: 100 mL/kg/24 hr = 10 kg × 100 mL/kg/24 hr = 1000 mL/24 hr 10 to 20 kg: 50 mL/kg/24 hr = 5 kg × 50 mL/kg/24 hr = 250 mL/24 hr 15 kg = 1250 mL/24 hr
Offer the child small amounts of fluid at a time and soft food.	Sucking on a nipple or straw or chewing can increase ear pain.

Nursing Diagnosis:

Deficient Knowledge

related to unfamiliarity with the disease process and prevention

Desired Outcome: Immediately following teaching, the parents verbalize accurate under-standing of the disease process and ways to decrease/prevent future incidents of OM.

ASSESSMENT/INTERVENTIONS	RATIONALES
Assess the parents' knowledge base/understanding of OM, its treatment, and prevention.	Identifying their knowledge/understanding facilitates more effective teaching and helps in correcting misconceptions.
Describe different types of OM and symptoms of each.	Knowledge and understanding improve adherence to the treatment plan. - AOM: infection of the middle ear; fever and pain may be treated with antibiotics. - OME: inflammation of the middle ear with fluid behind the TM without signs of acute infection; feeling of fullness in the ear; difficulty hearing; and is not treated with antibiotics.
Explain that treatment of pain is important, especially in the first few days of OM.	The child is likely to eat and drink more if comfortable, and this facilitates healing.
Instruct parents about the importance of giving the full course of antibiotics if they are prescribed and having the ear rechecked when the medication is finished.	Adequate treatment of AOM requires the full course of antibiotics; otherwise, OM can reoccur and/or allow a more resistant bacteria to infect the child. Ear rechecks assess effectiveness of treatment.
Discuss preventive feeding practices for an infant.	Feeding practices that prevent OM in infants include the following: - Feeding the infant in an upright position: facilitates drainage of the middle ear. - Not putting the infant in bed with a bottle: this increases incidence of ear infections. - Decreasing or eliminating use of a pacifier after 6 mo old: sucking on a pacifier causes bacteria to reflux back up into the ear.
Explain the importance of avoiding smoking around the child.	Passive smoking increases incidence of OM.
Encourage gentle blowing of the nose during upper respiratory infection (URI) rather than forceful nose blowing.	This decreases the risk of transferring organisms from the eustachian tube to the middle ear.
Encourage blowing activities (e.g., bubbles, pinwheels) or chewing sugarless gum during a URI.	These activities help promote equalization of pressure in the middle ear.
Explain prevention of ear pain during airplane travel.	Increased atmospheric pressure increases ear pain. - The health care provider may prescribe nasal mucosal shrinking spray if the child has URI or chronic OME to decrease pressure on the TM from edema. - The parent should offer a bottle or pacifier to the infant or give an older child gum during descent to help equalize TM pressure.
Describe potential complications of OM.	Inadequate or nonadherence to treatment may result in the following: - Hearing loss - Perforated, scarred eardrum - Mastoiditis - Cholesteatoma (a cystic mass composed of epithelial cells and cholesterol that occurs as a result of chronic OM). It may occlude the middle ear, or enzymes produced by the cyst may destroy adjacent bones, including the ossicles. - Intracranial infections such as meningitis

ADDITIONAL NURSING DIAGNOSES/PROBLEMS:

"Psychosocial Support for the Patient's Family and Significant Other" for relevant psychosocial nursing diagnoses   p. 84

"Asthma" for **Anxiety**   p. 553

✓ PATIENT-FAMILY TEACHING AND DISCHARGE PLANNING

When providing child-family teaching, focus on sensory information and avoid giving excessive information. Stress family-centered care (viewing the family as a unit that is the "constant" in the child's life and maintaining or improving the health of the family and its members in a holistic manner). Include verbal and written information about the following, ensuring that written information is at a level the reader can understand:

✓ Types of ear infections, signs and symptoms, and treatment of each type.

✓ Importance of administering antibiotics as prescribed (can develop resistant strains of bacteria otherwise).

- Return demonstration of drawing up the correct dose of medication and administering it to the child correctly.
- Use of a syringe or other calibrated device for administering medication to children.
- Administering doses at the correct time each day and for the total number of days prescribed.
- Teach the seven rights of medication administration:
  1. Right child
  2. Right medication
  3. Right dose (i.e., right concentration and right amount of medication)
  4. Right preparation
  5. Right route (e.g., ear drops or oral medication)
  6. Right time
  7. Right documentation—to help keep track of when the child received doses
- Correct storage of medication (e.g., some need to be refrigerated)

✓ Method of assessing pain in the child and importance of administering analgesic for pain on a regular basis.

✓ Treating fevers correctly:
- Discuss at what temperature an antipyretic is needed.
- Explain that fever increases ear pain.

✓ If receiving otic drops, how to administer based on the child's age:
- Child younger than 3 yr, pull earlobe down and back.
- Child older than 3 yr, pull pinna up and back.

✓ Prevention:
- Never give an infant a bottle to drink while lying down.
- Keep an infant upright during feeding.
- Breastfeed as long as possible.
- Decrease the time a pacifier is used or stop using after 6 mo (exception is when flying to prevent ear pain from atmospheric pressure changes).
- Do not smoke around the child or take him or her where smoking occurs.
- If the child has to go to day care, try to place with the least number of children possible.
- Vaccinate the child against pneumococcal and influenza infections.

✓ Signs and symptoms of dehydration:
- The child is not as alert and responsive as normal.
- Soft spot on top of the head looks sunken (for children younger than 2 yr).
- Inside of the mouth (not lips) is dry or sticky rather than moist (if the child is not a mouth breather).
- Skin on the abdomen sits up like a tent when pinched.
- Decreased number of wet diapers or same number but not as wet as normal for an infant or young child or decreased number of voids/day in an older child.

✓ Telephone number to call in case any questions arise about therapy or disease after office/emergency department visit.

✓ Importance of follow-up (e.g., many health care providers will do an ear recheck after the child finishes medication).

✓ When to call the health care provider:
- Fever or pain has not decreased after 48-72 hr while on antibiotics.
- Child is showing signs of dehydration.
- Child develops a stiff neck.
- Drainage present from the child's ear canal.

✓ If the child has had OME for more than 3 mo, he or she should have hearing evaluated.

✓ Referral to pediatric ear, nose, and throat specialist if OM or OME is chronic.

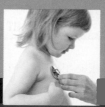

Poisoning 85

OVERVIEW/PATHOPHYSIOLOGY

Poisoning can result in death and is a leading cause of hospital visits for children. Every day in the United States, 300 children from birth to 19 yr of age are treated in emergency departments (EDs) and 2 children die due to poisoning (CDC, 2012). Poisoning may occur through ingestion, inhalation, or contact with skin or mucous membranes and is seen most often in children younger than 5 yr, with the greatest incidence in children younger than 3 yr. Curiosity and natural desire to put things in their mouths put younger children at greater risk for accidental poisoning. The 2011 Annual Report of the American Association of Poison Control Centers' (AAPCC) National Poison Data System (NPDS) showed more than 3.6 million calls were logged by the 57 poison control centers in 2011. This included calls related to human and nonhuman (animal) exposure as well as informational calls. About 2.3 million calls involved human exposure (including pharmaceuticals and nonpharmaceuticals) and 1.2 million involved informational calls. Children younger than 3 yr were involved in 36.2% of the poison exposures, while about 50% of all human exposures were in children younger than 6 yr. Despite this, only 1.7% of the fatalities in 2011 were in children younger than 6 yr. The most common poisons in children 5 yr or younger include cosmetics/personal care items such as perfume or soap (14%), analgesics such as acetaminophen or ibuprofen (9.9%), household cleaning agents such as laundry detergent or floor cleaners (9.2%), foreign bodies/toys/miscellaneous items such as the silica gel packages that remove moisture from packages and glow products (6.9%), and topical preparations such as diaper rash products and acne preparations (6.6%) (2011 AAPCC NPDS Report, 2012). According to a study in The Journal of Pediatrics in 2011, there has been a 30% increase in the visits to EDs due to medication poisoning from 2001-2008 in children 5 yr old and younger, and 95% of the time they were unsupervised ingestions (children getting the medications on their own that usually belong to a family member). The greatest cause of morbidity was with opioids, sedative-hypnotics, and cardiovascular agents. Children 13 to 24 mo are the ages most frequently seen in the ED for medication poisoning (Safe Kids, March 2013).

Inhalation of carbon monoxide is a common wintertime occurrence. Adolescents also have an increased incidence of hospitalization resulting from poisoning, but it is most often intentional and frequently involves inhaling substances (e.g., glues/adhesives, nail polish remover, paint thinner, air conditioning coolant) or ingesting alcohol or drugs (e.g., marijuana or "ecstasy"). In 2010, 89% of the deaths of children under 19 yr were the ages of 15 to 19 (Safe Kids, Fact Sheet, 2013).

About 94% of all poisoning incidents occur in the home per the 2011 Poison Control Center data. Most homes have more than 500 toxic substances in them, and one third of these are in the kitchen. The garage is also particularly dangerous for children, with gasoline and pesticides among the toxic substances housed there. Improper storage of toxic substances and caregiver distraction are major factors of poisoning in children.

Risk factors other than developmental age:
- Male children younger than 13 yr are more likely than females to be poisoned, but this is reversed in adolescents and adults.
- Children are more likely to suffer from elevated blood lead levels if they live in homes built before 1978, are low income, or live in large metropolitan areas.

HEALTH CARE SETTING

Emergency department with possible hospitalization

ASSESSMENT

Varies depending on source of the poisoning.

Gastrointestinal system: Nausea, vomiting, diarrhea, abdominal pain, anorexia.

Respiratory system: Depressed or labored respirations, unexplained cyanosis.

Circulatory system: Signs of shock, including increased, weak pulse; decreased blood pressure (BP); increased, shallow respirations; pallor; cool, clammy skin.

Central nervous system: Dizziness, overstimulation, pupillary changes, sudden loss of consciousness, behavioral changes, seizures, stupor/lethargy, coma.

Integumentary system: Skin rashes; burns to mouth, esophagus, and stomach; eye inflammation; skin irritations; stains around the mouth; oral mucous membrane lesions.

Signs, symptoms, and basic treatment specific to various poisons

Acetaminophen ingestion: Included in many over-the-counter medications, acetaminophen is the most common drug ingestion in children. Symptoms occur in stages and are dose dependent (e.g., child may not progress through all stages):

- Stage 1 (first 24 hr): malaise, nausea, vomiting, sweating, pallor, and weakness, or the child may be asymptomatic.
- Stage 2 (next 24-48 hr): decrease or disappearance of symptoms in stage 1 and right upper quadrant (RUQ) pain caused by liver damage and increase in liver enzymes.
- Stage 3 (3-7 days): jaundice, liver necrosis, and possible death from hepatic failure.
- Stage 4: occurs if the child does not die during the hepatic stage (stage 3) and involves gradual recovery.
- Treatment is with the antidote acetylcysteine (Mucomyst®).

Corrosive ingestion: Toilet and drain cleaners, bleach, ammonia, liquid dishwasher detergent, denture cleaner. Complaints of severe burning pain in the mouth, throat, and stomach; whitish burns of the mouth and pharynx with edema of the lips, tongue, and pharynx; difficulty swallowing, which leads to drooling; respiratory distress; anxiety and agitation; and shock. Treatment involves diluting the corrosive substance and avoiding emesis, which would increase damage.

Hydrocarbon ingestion: Gasoline, kerosene, paint thinner, lamp oil, turpentine, lighter fluid, some furniture polishes. Gagging, choking, coughing; nausea, vomiting; characteristic petroleum breath odor; central nervous system (CNS) depression. Respiratory symptoms of pulmonary involvement include tachypnea, cyanosis, retractions, and grunting. Treatment is symptomatic, but inducing vomiting is generally contraindicated.

Lead ingestion: Paint chips from lead-based paint, lead-contaminated dust in the home, soil contaminated with lead, lead solder used in plumbing and artwork, vinyl miniblinds, improperly glazed pottery, and traditional/folk remedies. Symptoms may be vague with insidious onset. Children absorb 50% of the lead they ingest and deposit it in their growing bones. Adults absorb only 10% of lead ingested.

- Gastrointestinal: anorexia, nausea, vomiting, and constipation.
- CNS: *low-dose exposure*—distractibility, impulsivity, hyperactivity, hearing impairment, mild intellectual deficits, loss

of recently acquired developmental skills, and loss of coordination. *High-dose exposure*—lead encephalopathy may occur 4-6 wk following the first symptoms. Mental retardation, severe ataxia, altered level of consciousness, paralysis, blindness, seizures, coma, and death all can occur.
- Cardiovascular: hypertension, bradycardia.
- Hematologic: anemia.
- Renal: glycosuria, proteinuria, possible acute or chronic renal failure, and impaired calcium function.
- Treatment depends on lead blood level.

Iron ingestion: Vitamin supplements with iron are one of most commonly ingested poisonous substances in children. Iron poisoning occurs in stages ranging from the initial stage (0.5-6 hr after ingestion) with vomiting, hematemesis, bloody stools, and abdominal pain to the hepatic injury stage (48-96 hr after the ingestion) with seizures and coma. If the child survives, pyloric or duodenal stenosis or hepatic cirrhosis may develop 2-4 wk after ingestion. Treatment may include lavage or chelation therapy.

Carbon monoxide inhalation: Improperly ventilated heaters, wood stoves, and charcoal grills; poorly ventilated automobile.
- *Low-level exposure:* headache, stomach upset, and tiredness (similar to early "flu" symptoms).
- *High-level exposure:* Within minutes, cherry red lips and cheeks, altered level of consciousness (LOC), extreme dizziness, and coma. Cherry-red skin is a late sign most commonly noted in fatalities.
- Treatment includes administration of oxygen and symptomatic treatment.

DIAGNOSTIC TESTS

History and physical examination help determine necessary tests.

Arterial blood gases: May be done if the child is hypoventilating.

Serum levels: Blood levels of acetaminophen, salicylate, lead, iron, and alcohol help determine if treatment with an antidote is necessary.

Serum carboxyhemoglobin level: To determine degree of carbon monoxide poisoning.

<u>Nursing Diagnosis:</u>

Risk for Poisoning

related to inadequate parental knowledge about poison prevention

Desired Outcomes: The child does not ingest, inhale, or touch potentially toxic substances. Immediately following teaching, the parents verbalize accurate understanding of how to childproof all areas (home, babysitter's home, grandparents' home) in which the child lives or plays.

ASSESSMENT/INTERVENTIONS

RATIONALES

ASSESSMENT/INTERVENTIONS	RATIONALES
Assess parental knowledge level/understanding of potential sources of poisoning.	Teaching can be more effective with a good baseline per the parents' knowledge/understanding.
Based on the child's developmental age, discuss ways in which the child might be exposed to poisons.	Understanding developmentally appropriate behavior enables parents to childproof the home more effectively. For example, a 1-yr-old puts everything in the mouth but is not climbing yet, so any potential poison the child could reach while crawling or standing should be secured out of his or her reach.
Going room by room, discuss areas that need to be childproofed, with special emphasis on the kitchen, storage areas, and bathroom.	Many poisonings involve household cleaners or medications. Knowledge of childproofing each area decreases risk of exposure to potentially toxic substances.
Review all materials in the home environment that could be poisonous.	Parents may not be aware of all the potentially poisonous substances in their home. Increased awareness likely will decrease the child's exposure to poisonous substances, including the following: - Household cleaners, disinfectants - Cosmetics - Insecticides - Mouthwash with alcohol in it - Alcohol (beverages or rubbing alcohol) - Liquid dishwasher detergent - Foreign bodies and toys, such as bubble-blowing solution - Arts, crafts, and office supplies, such as pen and ink - Toxic plants - Hydrocarbons - Prescription and nonprescription medications
Describe ways to childproof the home to prevent poisoning.	Guidelines enhance the parents' ability to effectively and efficiently childproof the home against poisoning. Examples include: - Put childproof locks on all kitchen, bathroom, and storage room cabinets. - Make sure all poisonous products are out of reach in locked cabinets. - Do not leave purse/briefcase sitting out that contains medication, cosmetics, or pens. - Buy medications with child-resistant caps but still store in a locked cabinet. - Do not store poisonous substances in food containers or water bottles; store them in the original containers. - Throw away all old medications and other potential poisons that are no longer being used. Dispose of poisons out of the child's reach (i.e., if poison is discarded in the kitchen trashcan and the child can reach the can, it was not disposed "out of the child's reach"). Guidelines for disposing of hazardous household waste are available from the Environmental Protection Agency at *www.epa.gov/epawaste/index.htm* and from Earth 911 at *www.earth911.org* (this website provides the closest locations for disposal of hazardous materials). - Hang or install a carbon monoxide detector on each level of the home on which bedrooms are located. - If the home was built before 1978, have it tested for lead-based paint.
Discuss these general guidelines to prevent poisoning.	
- Stay alert when using poisonous household products.	Poisoning by ingestion or inhalation can occur in a matter of seconds.
- Never refer to medicine or vitamins as "candy."	The child may think it is harmless or tastes good.
- Do not take medicine in front of young children.	Toddlers and preschoolers often imitate adult behavior.
Reinforce the importance of informing family/friends of the above guidelines.	Even with the home childproofed by the parents, visitors may bring potentially poisonous substances into the home (e.g., grandmother may visit and leave her purse containing a medicine bottle on the floor).
Encourage parents to childproof all residences/facilities visited by the child.	The child may be safe at home but not at day care or the grandparents' home.

Nursing Diagnosis:

Deficient Knowledge

related to unfamiliarity with first aid for toxic ingestion/inhalation/exposure
in accidental poisoning

Desired Outcome: Immediately following teaching, the parents verbalize accurate knowledge
of steps to take if accidental poisoning occurs.

ASSESSMENT/INTERVENTIONS	RATIONALES
Teach Parents the Following:	
Post Poison Control Center (PCC) number on all phones. Also have emergency medical services (EMS) and pediatrician's number readily available.	It is vital to call PCC for a possible ingestion of a toxic substance before administering any antidote to ensure the correct treatment is implemented. Some home treatments may interfere with effective gastric decontamination.
If syrup of ipecac is in the child's home, babysitter's home, or any other facility in which the child is cared for, it should be disposed of safely.	The current recommendation is that routine administration of ipecac be avoided in all settings. Clinical studies show that it may interfere with other methods of decontamination, there is no convincing evidence that it improves the outcome of patients that have been poisoned, and it can cause harm in some patients (Hojer et al, Clinical Toxicology 51(3), 2013).
Review the following immediate action response if a child is poisoned: - If swallowed, remove any remaining poison from the child's mouth. Call PCC immediately. - If poison is on the skin, remove contaminated clothing right away without touching the poison and rinse the child's skin with running water. Wash the skin with soap and water and rinse well. Call PCC immediately. - If poison is in the eye, flush the eye with lukewarm to cool water for a full 15 min. Call PCC immediately. - If poison is inhaled, move the child to fresh air right away. Call PCC.	Having this knowledge base enables parents to decrease absorption and provide appropriate treatment in the event of poisoning.
Discuss the following specific information parents should give to PCC: - Child's weight and age. - Time the poisoning occurred. - Amount ingested. - Name of poison, if possible. If the medicine bottle or container is available, have it on hand when speaking with PCC.	Specific information enables PCC to direct treatment more appropriately.

ADDITIONAL NURSING DIAGNOSES/PROBLEMS:

"Psychosocial Support for the Patient's Family and Significant Others" for such nursing diagnoses as **Fear**   p. 84

Compromised Family Coping for the family whose child is being seen in the emergency department or is hospitalized for a life-threatening condition   p. 86

"Bronchiolitis" for **Deficient Fluid Volume.** The child may be dehydrated related to effects of ingested substances, treatment for poisoning, or decreased fluid intake.   p. 569

 PATIENT-FAMILY TEACHING AND DISCHARGE PLANNING

When providing child-family teaching, focus on sensory information, avoid giving excessive information, and initiate a visiting nurse referral for necessary follow-up teaching or to assess safety of the home. Stress family-centered care (viewing the family as a unit that is the "constant" in the child's life and maintaining or improving the health of the family and its members). Include verbal and written information about the following (ensure that written information is at a level the reader can understand):

✓ Contributing factors to the potential for poisoning for each child in the household:
   • Developmental age of the child (e.g., cognitive, physical, and psychosocial)

- Environmental factors
- Behavioral problems
- Level of supervision

✓ Poison prevention tips:
  - Keep all poisonous products out of reach in cabinets locked with safety locks.
  - Know what household products are poisonous or potentially poisonous.
  - Be careful and alert when using poisonous household products.
  - Regularly discard old medications and other potential poisons in a safe manner.
  - Keep all products in their original containers.
  - Remember that many cosmetics and personal products may be poisonous (e.g., aftershave, cologne, hair spray, fingernail polish remover). Be sure to store them out of the child's reach and where the child cannot climb to get them.
  - Buy products with child-resistant tops.
  - Make sure that poisonous plants are not in the house or yard where the child plays.
  - Put a carbon monoxide detector on each level of the home where bedrooms are located.
  - Keep all medications (prescription and nonprescription) in labeled containers and locked in a cabinet (none in a purse or briefcase or on a counter or dresser).
  - If the child has to take prescribed medication on his or her own, leave only 1 or 2 doses accessible to the child at a time.
  - If the home was built before 1978, have it tested for lead-based paint.
  - Review sources of lead poisoning besides paint.
  - Keep alcoholic beverages out of the child's reach and locked up.

✓ Importance of having PCC, EMS, and the health care provider's phone number posted by all phones. Also have the home address and nearest intersection available in case the babysitter or other family member needs to call EMS.

✓ Necessity of close supervision of infants and young children.

✓ Anticipatory guidance for the next milestones the child will achieve and childproofing for each age, including for all children in the family (i.e., what is safe for a 6-mo-old is not safe for a 2-yr-old). Childproof all residences in which the child stays. Reassess safety/childproofing frequently.

✓ Referrals to community resources, such as local and National Safe Kids Organization, safety experts, stores with a variety of materials to help childproof a home. Additional information can be obtained by contacting the following organizations:
  - National SAFE KIDS Campaign at *www.safekids.org*
  - Parachute at *www.parachutecanada.org*
  - Nationwide Poison Control Center (PCC) at (800) 222-1222 or *www.aapcc.org*
  - The Canadian Association of Poison Control Centres provides links to Provincial Poison Control Centres, see *capcc.ca*
  - Mr. Yuk stickers and related material at *www.chp.edu/mryuk/05a_mryuk.php*
  - My Safe Home: Poison Prevention at *http://mysafehome.net/risk.php?risk=poisoning*
  - Up and Away Brochure- CDC at *www.upandaway.org*. It provides information and advice on protecting children from accidental medication overdose.
  - The Caring for Kids website at *www.caringforkids.cps.ca* provides handouts for parents on child safety and includes a home safety checklist for parents.

✓ Resources for disposal of hazardous household material:
  - EPA at *www.epa.gov/epawaste/index.htm* and Earth 911 at *www.earth911.org* (lists closest location according to zip code for disposing of hazardous material).

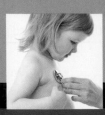

Sickle Cell Pain Crisis 86

OVERVIEW/PATHOPHYSIOLOGY

Sickle cell disease (SCD) comprises a group of hereditary blood disorders in which hemoglobin S (HbS) is the dominant hemoglobin. HbS (sickle hemoglobin) replaces normal adult hemoglobin (HbA). HbS differs from HbA in the substitution of one amino acid (valine) for another (glutamine). Under conditions of dehydration, acidosis, hypoxia, and temperature elevations, HbS changes its molecular structure and forms a crescent or sickle-shaped red blood cell (RBC). This causes the cardinal clinical features of chronic hemolytic anemia and vasoocclusion, which result from obstruction caused by the sickled RBCs and increased RBC destruction. In most instances, the sickling response is reversible with adequate hydration and oxygenation. After repeated cycles of sickling and unsickling, the RBC remains in the sickled form. The most common form of sickle cell disease is hemoglobin SS disease (HbSS), also called *sickle cell anemia* or *homozygous SCD*, in which the individual inherits a sickle cell gene from each parent.

The inheritance pattern is autosomal recessive (both parents must at least have the sickle cell trait). If both parents have the sickle cell trait, there is a 25% chance that each child will have SCD, a 25% chance that each child will have neither the trait nor the disease, and a 50% chance that each child will have the trait. Therefore, a child may be asymptomatic (except under rare circumstances) with the trait or have varying degrees of symptoms with the disease. SCD is among the most prevalent of genetic diseases in the United States and is common in individuals whose ancestors came from sub-Saharan Africa; Spanish speaking regions in the Western Hemisphere (South America, Caribbean, and Central America); Saudi Arabia; India; and Mediterranean countries such as Turkey, Greece, and Italy. It is estimated that SCD affects 90,000 to 100,000 Americans and occurs in approximately 1 in every 500 African American births and about 1 in every 36,000 Hispanic American births. About 1 in every 12 African Americans has the trait (CDC, Data and Statistics, 2011), with more than 3.5 million Americans having sickle cell trait (Platt et al., 2011). The life expectancy has increased dramatically from only 14 yr in 1973 (New York Times Health Guide, 2013) to mid 40s and 50s in 2011 due to new screening techniques, preventive treatment, ongoing education, and therapies (Platt et al., 2011).

Pain is the leading cause of emergency department visits and hospitalizations. It can occur as early as age 4-6 mo and unpredictably throughout a lifetime. There is considerable variation in the severity, frequency, and types of pain among and within affected individuals.

HEALTH CARE SETTING

Primary care with possible hospitalization for infections or pain crisis

ASSESSMENT

Signs and symptoms: Generally do not appear in infants before 4-6 mo of age because of high levels of fetal hemoglobin (HbF). Pain is the hallmark manifestation and is caused by vasoocclusion and the resulting ischemia distal to the occlusion. Pain can range from mild and transient to severe, and it can be localized or generalized, lasting from minutes to days or weeks. The acute painful episode or event is reversible and can occur in the extremities, back, chest, and abdomen. Examples include acute hand-foot syndrome (dactylitis—usually seen in children between 6 mo and 2 yr old), acute joint inflammation, acute chest syndrome (a common cause of mortality manifesting as chest pain, fever, pneumonia-like cough, anemia, abdominal pain or gallstones, and priapism). Stroke is another form of vasoocclusive event and has a high rate of recurrence. In the past, children with SCD were at more than 200 times higher risk of having a stroke than children without SCD (American Heart Association, 2010). Lehman presented research findings at the American Stroke Association meeting in February 2012 that showed a significant decrease in the risk of stroke down to only 27% higher risk in black children than in white children. It was believed that the detection of high stroke risk with transcranial Doppler ultrasound screening and chronic blood transfusions may have accounted for the significant decrease in stroke-related deaths. Children with SCD often have nonfunctional spleens due to "clogging" from the sickled RBCs, and this puts them at increased risk for sepsis. Overwhelming infection/sepsis was the leading cause of death in young children with SCD in the past, but recent studies show this changing with declining deaths in young children since the advent of universal newborn screening for SCD, daily penicillin prophylaxis for children under 5 yr with SCD, and routine pneumococcal and

Haemophilus influenzae type b vaccines for infants (Baskin et al., 2013; CDC, 2011).

Physical assessment: History and physical, including character, location, severity, and duration of pain, as well as at-home treatment. Information should be obtained about methods used in the past to treat pain crises effectively. Initial pain assessment should be done and repeated before and after analgesia.

DIAGNOSTIC TESTS

Note: *Newborn screening for sickle cell anemia is mandated in all states. Results are sent to the infant's primary care physician. If there is any HbS, a second test is done to confirm diagnosis (NHLBI, 2012).*

Hemoglobin electrophoresis, isoelectric focusing, and high-performance liquid chromatography: Enable definitive diagnosis of SCD.

Oximetry: Noninvasive method that will reveal decreased O_2 saturation if it is present.

Chest x-ray examination: Helps differentiate between acute chest syndrome and pneumonia.

Complete blood count with reticulocytes: May show increased white blood cells (WBCs) with infection. The life span of the normal RBC is decreased from 120 days to 10-14 days, so bone marrow compensates with increased production. Reticulocyte count gives an indication of RBC production by the bone marrow (reticulocytes are immature RBCs).

Blood culture: Infection may have triggered a crisis. Sepsis is a leading cause of death in children younger than 5 yr.

Basic metabolic panel: If signs and symptoms of dehydration are present, helps assess degree of dehydration and need for electrolyte replacement.

Nursing Diagnosis:

Acute Pain

related to tissue anoxia occurring with vasoocclusion

Desired Outcomes: For mild-to-moderate pain, the child states or demonstrates that pain has decreased within 1-1½ hr of receiving oral medication. For severe pain, the child states or demonstrates that pain has decreased within 24 hr of intervention/treatment. Pain is less than 4 on a 0-10-point scale such as FLACC (face, legs, activity, cry, and consolability), FACES, and numeric.

ASSESSMENT/INTERVENTIONS	RATIONALES
After establishing a pain scale appropriate for the child (FLACC, FACES, Oucher, Poker Chip, or numeric), assess pain before and after analgesic is administered (within 10-30 min after IV medication administration and within 1 hr after oral medication administration). Assess pain level q2-4h unless on continuous infusion of pain medication, in which case assess qh.	A developmentally appropriate pain scale helps monitor the degree of pain and effectiveness of the pain medication.
Assess hydration status q4h: level of consciousness (LOC), anterior fontanel if the child is younger than 2 yr, oral mucous membranes, abdominal skin turgor, and urine output.	This assessment helps detect and prevent/treat dehydration, which causes vasoocclusion/pain. A child who is dehydrated may exhibit decreased LOC, sunken anterior fontanel (if younger than 2 yr), dry or sticky oral mucous membranes if not a mouth breather, tented abdominal skin, and decreased urine output.
Plan a schedule of pain medication around the clock, not prn. (Usually patients have a continuous infusion as well as patient-controlled analgesia [PCA].)	Consistent use lowers the total amount of medication with better control. Prolonged stimulation of pain receptors results in increased sensitivity to painful stimuli and will increase the amount of analgesia required to relieve pain.
Explain how PCA works and that the child cannot give self too much medication. Encourage the child/parent to use PCA when it is needed.	Most experts believe that when a child is capable of pushing the button on the pump, usually by 5-6 yr of age, he or she can self-administer pain medication. Some facilities allow PCA by proxy: the parent or the nurse can administer the medication if the child is too ill or cannot understand the concept of pushing the button to relieve the pain.
Reassure the child/parent that addiction rarely occurs when medication is used to relieve pain.	Fear of addiction may decrease use of the PCA/request for pain medication.

continued

ASSESSMENT/INTERVENTIONS	RATIONALES
Do *not* administer meperidine (Demerol).	Demerol increases the risk of normeperidine-induced seizures, *especially* in a child with SCD.
Carefully apply warmth to the affected area.	Warmth may be soothing to the child, but it should be applied judiciously because ischemic tissue is fragile.
Do *not* apply cold compresses.	Cold promotes sickling and vasoconstriction.
Use nonpharmacologic pain control measures as appropriate for the child.	Optimally, comfort measures will distract the child from the pain and augment the effects of pharmacologic measures, but they should not be used to replace them. Examples include distraction (watching TV or playing games), deep breathing, relaxation exercises, music, touch, imagery, and massage.

Nursing Diagnoses:

Risk for Ineffective Cerebral Tissue Perfusion
Risk for Decreased Cardiac Tissue Perfusion

related to vasoocclusion and anemia

Desired Outcomes: Within 2 hr following treatment/intervention, the child's oxygen saturation is maintained at greater than 95% or at a level prescribed by the health care provider. There is no evidence of long-term complications from hypoxia.

ASSESSMENT/INTERVENTIONS	RATIONALES
Assess respiratory status and mental status q2-4h and prn.	Frequent assessment ensures early detection of changes in respiratory status. Tachypnea and increased work of breathing (WOB) are early signs of hypoxia. LOC is a good indicator of oxygen perfusion to the brain.
Monitor pulse oximetry continuously.	This is a noninvasive method of assessing oxygen saturation and noting changes promptly.
Administer oxygen as prescribed to keep oxygen saturation levels at greater than 95% or at level appropriate for each individual child.	Delivering oxygen when a child is hypoxic eases WOB. However, it does not reverse the sickling process, and long-term use can depress bone marrow activity and increase the anemia.
Elevate head of bed to a comfortable level for the child.	This facilitates chest expansion by decreasing pressure on the diaphragm.
Ensure incentive spirometry q1-2h while the child is awake.	This treatment facilitates deep breathing and decreases the incidence of acute chest syndrome.
Administer packed RBCs as prescribed.	This treatment improves tissue perfusion by correcting anemia.

Nursing Diagnosis:

Deficient Knowledge

related to unfamiliarity with the disease process of SCD, measures to avoid vasoocclusive crisis, home management to prevent severe pain crisis, and the genetics that could result in having other children with this disease

Desired Outcome: Within 48 hr following teaching, the child/family verbalizes accurate understanding of the disease process, especially a pain crisis, appropriate treatment, and the genetics of disease transmission.

ASSESSMENT/INTERVENTIONS | RATIONALES

ASSESSMENT/INTERVENTIONS	RATIONALES
Assess knowledge/understanding of SCD and its treatment.	Identifying the child's/parents' knowledge facilitates more effective teaching and helps in correcting misconceptions.
Instruct the older child/family in basic information about SCD and measures to minimize sickling.	Knowledge of the disease process promotes adherence to the plan of care, for example, taking prescribed medications such as penicillin and folic acid on a regular basis, staying up to date on immunizations, and avoiding precipitating factors (e.g., dehydration, exposure to individuals who are ill with infections, extreme temperatures, high elevations, excessive physical activity).
Encourage the child/family to obtain medical alert bracelet/necklace and inform significant health professionals/school personnel of the diagnosis.	These actions will help ensure prompt and appropriate treatment.
Explain signs of a developing pain crisis, its significance, and importance of prompt treatment. Assist parents in identifying methods of assessing pain in their child.	Knowledge about the signs of pain crisis and its significance optimally will result in prompt reporting and treatment, which may avoid a severe vasoocclusive crisis. For example, in an infant or toddler, a combination of unusual behaviors such as inconsolability, decreased appetite, unexplained crying, and rapid breathing may indicate discomfort or pain. Older children may complain of mild discomfort or aching.
Discuss the home treatment for mild/early symptoms of pain crisis.	The severity of pain crisis may be decreased by early/prompt treatment (e.g., resting, increasing fluid intake to 1-1.5× maintenance fluids, and administering pain medication).
Discuss transmission of the disease and refer for genetic counseling as indicated.	This information enables the family to make informed reproductive decisions. See discussion in the introductory data.
Encourage family members to be advocates for the child in the hospital, during appointments with the health care provider, and in day care or the school setting (e.g., individualized education plan [IEP] or 504 plan at school). Reinforce that they know the child best and understand what is normal or abnormal in relationship to the child.	Family members may be hesitant to ask questions or advocate for the child; however, they are the best resource. Encouraging advocacy increases the likelihood the child will receive the best care and facilitates optimal development.
Encourage inclusion of siblings with planning and providing care for the chronically ill child as appropriate.	Including siblings may help them cope with/adapt to having a brother/sister with a chronic illness.
Supply the family with information about support groups, local/national sickle cell organizations, and resources for additional information.	Support systems likely will improve their knowledge base about the disease process and therapeutics involved, as well as let them know they are not "alone."
Encourage the family to have the child receive follow-up visits at a sickle cell clinic on a regular basis.	Follow-up in a sickle cell clinic promotes continuity and quality of care.

Nursing Diagnosis:

Deficient Knowledge

related to unfamiliarity with precautions and side effects of prescribed medications

Desired Outcome: Within 48 hr following teaching, the child/family verbalizes accurate information about the prescribed medications, including precautions and side effects.

ASSESSMENT/INTERVENTIONS | RATIONALES

ASSESSMENT/INTERVENTIONS	RATIONALES
Morphine Sulfate	
	This medication is an opioid analgesic (administered in the hospital).
Teach the parents/child the following:	

continued

ASSESSMENT/INTERVENTIONS	RATIONALES
Assess the child for level of sedation, pain relief obtained, O_2 saturation, and respiratory and cardiac status.	This assessment helps to evaluate effectiveness of the medication and possible need to adjust dosage. Morphine can cause respiratory depression, and if it occurs, O_2 saturation would decrease along with the respiratory rate. Many hospitals have a sickle cell weaning score to facilitate adjusting the dosage appropriately.
Assess for dizziness, drowsiness, itching, nausea, vomiting, constipation, urinary retention, and low blood pressure. Explain that the parent/child should notify the staff or health care provider if any of these symptoms occur.	These side effects may indicate the need to change dosage or the medication itself or to provide additional medication, such as diphenhydramine or naloxone, via continuous IV infusion for itching or an antiemetic for nausea.
Reassure them that analgesics, including opioids, are medically indicated and that high doses may be needed to relieve pain.	There is confusion about the issues of pain control and drug dependence. Children rarely become addicted, and needless suffering may occur as a result of unnecessary fears.

⚠ Acetaminophen with Codeine

	This medication is a central analgesic/antipyretic with added opioid.
Teach the parents/child the following:	
Assess for and report palpitations, dizziness, drowsiness, itching, nausea, vomiting, cramping, low blood pressure, and constipation, as well as excessive sedation and respiratory depression.	These side effects may indicate need to adjust or change the medication.
Assess if pain has decreased within 1-1½ hr of oral administration. If the child has no relief after several doses of pain medication, the parent should notify the health care provider.	This assessment evaluates effectiveness of the medication because this is the time of peak action. If there is no relief after several doses, the health care provider may increase the dosage.
Explain that there are numerous interactions with other medications.	Administration with certain other medications may increase or decrease the effectiveness of this medication. See a drug book for more specific information.
Ensure that the child does not receive more than 4000 mg/day of acetaminophen. This includes all sources of acetaminophen. For example, it may be used for fever in addition to its use as an analgesic.	Acetaminophen may cause severe hepatotoxicity (U.S. Black Boxed Warning), potentially requiring a liver transplant or resulting in death.

Ibuprofen

	This medication augments pain control when administered with morphine or acetaminophen with codeine.
Teach the parents/child the following:	
Assess for and report dizziness, drowsiness, and heartburn.	These side effects may indicate need for the health care provider to adjust dosage or change medication.
Administer with food or milk.	This decreases gastrointestinal (GI) upset.

Folic Acid

	This medication enhances the bone marrow's ability to produce new blood cells.

⚠ Penicillin

	This is a prophylactic antibiotic. Overwhelming infection/sepsis has been the leading cause of death in young children with SCD.
Teach the parents/child the following:	
Assess for and report rash, nausea, vomiting, diarrhea, black, hairy tongue, and hypersensitivity reactions. Call 911 promptly if anaphylaxis occurs.	These side effects may indicate need for the health care provider to adjust dosage or change the medication.
Stress the importance of daily administration as prescribed at least until the child is 5-6 yr old.	This reduces morbidity risks associated with pneumococcal septicemia. It may need to be continued for a longer period if the child has experienced invasive pneumococcal infection, has not received pneumococcal immunizations, is on a hypertransfusion program, or is anatomically asplenic.

continued

ASSESSMENT/INTERVENTIONS	RATIONALES
Administer/take with water on an empty stomach 1 hr before meals or 2 hr after meals; may give with food to decrease GI upset.	Food or milk may decrease absorption.

Docusate

	This is a stool softener.
Teach the parents/child the following:	
Assess for and report rash, diarrhea, abdominal cramping, or throat irritation.	These are side effects; the health care provider may need to adjust dosage or change medication.
Administer when the child is taking analgesics.	Analgesics may cause constipation.
Monitor the stool pattern while the child is taking this medication.	It may be necessary to consider adding other medications to facilitate stool passage if docusate is not effective.
If using in liquid form, administer with a small amount of milk, fruit juice, or infant formula.	These liquids mask the bitter taste.
Ensure the child is receiving 1-1½× maintenance fluids unless pulmonary symptoms exist. For calculation of maintenance fluids, see "Bronchiolitis," p. 569, for **Deficient Fluid Volume.**	This facilitates effectiveness of the docusate and provides needed hydration for the child with sickle cell pain crisis. Increased fluids may be needed if the child is dehydrated or has insensible losses, for example, with fever.

Acetaminophen

	This is an analgesic/antipyretic.
Teach the parents/child the following:	
Administer immediately for mild complaints of pain or discomfort.	This may prevent pain crisis.
Assess for and report rash.	This side effect may indicate need for the health care provider to adjust dosage or change medication.
Ensure that child is receiving the therapeutic dose of acetaminophen.	This helps to provide effective pain relief while avoiding hepatic necrosis.
Ensure that the child does not receive more than 4000 mg/day. This includes all sources of acetaminophen. For example, it may be used for fever in addition to its use as an analgesic.	Acetaminophen may cause severe hepatotoxicity (U.S. Black Boxed Warning), potentially requiring a liver transplant or resulting in death.

Hydroxyurea

	This medication increases production of HbF, which prevents sickling of RBCs, thereby decreasing the incidence of vasoocclusive crises. Consult a drug handbook for more detailed information.

ADDITIONAL NURSING DIAGNOSES/PROBLEMS:

Constipation can occur as a result of narcotic analgesics and decreased mobility. See "Prolonged Bedrest" for **Constipation**. p. 68

"Psychosocial Support" for **Grieving/Risk for Complicated Grieving** p. 78

"Psychosocial Support for the Patient's Family and Significant Others" p. 84

"Asthma" for **Anxiety** related to illness, loss of control, and medical/nursing interventions p. 553

"Asthma" for **Interrupted Family Processes** related to having a child with a chronic illness p. 554

"Bronchiolitis" for **Deficient Fluid Volume** (however, a child with sickle cell pain crisis needs 1-1½× maintenance, unless pulmonary symptoms are present, in which case then only maintenance fluids). Increased fluids may be needed if the child is dehydrated and/or has increased insensible losses (e.g., persistent fever.) p. 569

Appendix A for "Infection Prevention and Control." Overwhelming infection/sepsis has been the leading cause of death in young children with SCD and infection risk is an ongoing concern. p. 747

✓ PATIENT-FAMILY TEACHING AND DISCHARGE PLANNING

When providing patient-family teaching, focus on sensory information. Avoid giving excessive instructions and institute a visiting nurse referral as necessary for follow-up teaching and assessment. Stress family-centered care (viewing the family as a unit that is the "constant" in the child's life and maintaining or improving the health of the family and its members). Include verbal and written information about the following (ensure written information is at a level the reader can understand):

✓ Basic pathophysiology about sickle disease and pain crisis.

✓ Cause of the pain, including precipitating factors (e.g., dehydration, infection, fever, hot or cold temperatures, high elevations, excessive physical activity) and importance of avoiding same.

✓ For boys, priapism (prolonged erection) is possible with sickle cell disease. They need to seek medical attention if erections last more than 3 hr or occur frequently.

✓ Avoiding exposure to individuals who are ill with infections (e.g., do not go in crowded areas during flu season). Overwhelming infection/sepsis is the leading cause of death in young children with sickle cell disease.

✓ Importance of maintaining adequate oral intake to prevent dehydration and thereby prevent clumping of HbS.

✓ Signs and symptoms of early pain crisis and treatment (i.e., rest, increase fluids to $1\text{-}1\text{-}1\frac{1}{2}\times$ maintenance with specific examples [e.g., a 12-kg child who drinks from a 6-oz cup needs at least $6\frac{1}{2}$ cups of fluid/day], and administer acetaminophen or ibuprofen first; if no relief, try the prescription pain medication from the health care provider).

✓ Maintaining a pain diary, which may be beneficial in finding precipitating factors and effective pain control measures. The most effective treatment in an emergency department also should be included in the event the child is seen in another hospital.

✓ Medications, including drug name; route; purpose; dosage; precautions; drug-drug, food-drug, and herb-drug interactions; and potential side effects.

✓ Importance of taking medications at home and school as directed. Medication in the original bottle (with prescribing label) and written prescription from the health care provider are needed for the child to be able to take any medication at school.

✓ Nonpharmacologic methods to relieve pain. (Stress that they are used in addition to the pain medication not in place of it):

• Psychologic strategies: distraction, imagery, education/teaching, and hypnotherapy

• Behavioral strategies: deep breathing, relaxation exercises, self-hypnosis, biofeedback, and behavior modification

• Physical strategies: careful application of heat to painful area, massage, and mild exercise, if tolerated

✓ Frequent urination, which is normal with increased fluids; enuresis may occur as a result.

✓ When to contact the health care provider:

• Temperature 101° F or higher

• Pain not relieved by prescribed pain medication (usually acetaminophen with codeine)

• The child is pale, lethargic, irritable, or dehydrated

• Vomiting and/or diarrhea lasting more than a day (time frame varies, shorter time frame for a younger child)

• Shortness of breath or other acute pulmonary symptoms

✓ Coordination of care. Parents should discuss the child's illness and needs with the school nurse and other adults who are in close contact with the child (e.g., teachers, scout leaders, day care providers).

✓ Importance of helping siblings cope with/adapt to having a brother/sister with a chronic illness and including them in planning and/or caring for the chronically ill child depending on their age and interest.

✓ Legal rights of the child:

• Individuals with Disabilities Education Act (IDEA): Mandates federal government to provide funding to education agencies for free and appropriate education to qualifying students with disabilities, including children with sickle cell disease if the disease adversely affects school performance. The school is then required to develop an IEP.

• IEP: A multidisciplinary team designs this plan to facilitate special education and therapeutic strategies and goals for each child. The child does not have to be in special education classes. Parents need to be involved in this process.

• Section 504 of Rehabilitation Act of 1973: Each student with a disability (physical or mental impairment) is entitled to accommodation to attend school and participate as fully as possible in school activities. This accommodation may be related to a medical condition or an educational issue. For example, the child may leave the classroom to use bathroom facilities without raising his or her hand and will not be penalized for excessive absences from school that are caused by sickle cell disease. The 504 Plan may include as many accommodations as necessary for the child to function well. More details at *www.specialchildren.about.com/od/504s/f/504faq1.htm*

✓ Importance of ongoing health care management with the health care provider experienced in dealing with sickle cell disease to identify and manage chronic complications:

• Receiving childhood immunizations at the appropriate age, especially pneumococcal, *Haemophilus influenzae* type b, meningococcal, and yearly flu vaccine

• Prompt attention to symptoms of infection (e.g., fever, sore throat)

- Regular visits with the health care provider, not just when ill
✓ Telephone numbers to call in case questions or concerns arise about the therapy or disease after discharge
✓ Additional general information can be obtained by contacting the following organizations:
  - The Sickle Cell Information Center at *www.scinfo.org*
  - Sickle Cell Disease Association of America at *www.sicklecelldisease.org*
  - The Sickle Cell Association of Ontario at *www.sicklecellontario.org*
  - St. Jude Children's Research Hospital. Its website has numerous downloadable handouts about sickle cell disease such as *Strokes in Children with Sickle Cell Disease* and *Hydroxyurea Treatment for Sickle Cell disease* at *www.stjude.org*. Click on patient resources,

then caregiver education resources, and then Sickle cell disease and other hematological diseases.
- Starlight-Starbright Children's Foundation at *www.starlight.org/families*. This website provides families with access to many resources.
- Starbright World®—an online social network for teens with chronic and life-threatening medical conditions at *www.starlight.org/starbright-world*.
- A fun and educational website for children with sickle cell disease is *www.sicklecellkids.org*. It needs Flash 5 to operate, but it can be downloaded from the website.
- *Hope and Destiny: The Patient and Parent's Guide to Sickle Cell Disease and Sickle Cell Trait*, revised 3rd edition by Alan Platt, James Eckman MD, and Lewis Hsu MD, published in 2011.

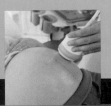

Normal Labor 87

OVERVIEW/PATHOPHYSIOLOGY

Labor and birth are natural human processes and for most women, minimal interventions are required. The philosophy that birth is a normal, natural process works best in an environment of continuous labor support, shared information and decision making, and where interventions are viewed and practiced on a continuum from noninvasive to least invasive based on the wishes of the laboring woman and at the discretion of the health care provider. Nurses working in the intrapartum setting have a broad knowledge of the physical and physiologic stresses faced by the laboring woman and provide family-centered care, supporting the labor and birthing process and the woman's wishes regarding her care. Uncomplicated labor occurs at term (completion of 38 wk gestation), with a single fetus in a vertex presentation, with labor initiated by spontaneous, effective contractions, and with birth completed within 24 hr.

Initiation of labor is a complex process involving a combination of factors that work in conjunction to stimulate myometrial activity and in turn initiate the onset of labor. These factors may include oxytocin release from the posterior pituitary, uterine distention or stretching, increasing uterine pressure due to the term fetus, increased maternal prostaglandin and fetal cortisol levels, placental aging, and changes in estrogen and progesterone ratios. The exact mechanism(s) that initiate spontaneous labor have been researched but are not completely understood.

Premonitory signs of labor such as lightening, urinary frequency, a change in vaginal discharge including bloody show, the loss of the mucus plug, and irregular contractions are often reported before true labor begins. True labor is distinguished from false labor by contractions that become progressively more frequent and regular, discomfort beginning in the back and radiating toward the abdomen causing cervical dilation, cervical effacement, and fetal descent. Duration of labor depends on fetal presentation, fetal size, position of the fetus, and a multitude of factors including pelvic structure, the woman's body mass, and birthing position. Whether the woman is a primipara (first time pregnancy past the 20th wk gestation) or multiparous (this pregnancy is past the 20th wk and the woman has already delivered an infant weighing more than 500 g) can influence how rapidly labor progresses. However, duration of labor for women, especially dilation to

6 cm, takes longer than in previous years (Zhang et al., 2010). Recognizing that labor based on current obstetrical populations is slower than in previous generations is important for avoiding early and unnecessary interventions.

Labor is divided into four stages. The first stage of labor, which is cervical dilation to 10 cm, is divided into latent (0-3 cm dilation), active (4-7 cm dilation), and transitional (8-10 cm dilation) phases. Stage two is measured from compete dilation to the birth of the baby and may have a latent or passive phase of descent and/or active open glottis pushing with contractions. Stage three is from the birth of the baby to the expulsion of the placenta. Stage four is the immediate postpartum recovery phase occurring from the delivery of the placenta and encompassing the first 2 hr postdelivery.

HEALTH CARE SETTING

Primary care and acute care in an in-patient hospital setting or free-standing birth center. Home births occur in some geographic areas.

ASSESSMENT

On the mother's arrival to the perinatal unit, the nurse obtains a thorough admission assessment. Assessment is focused on current and prior obstetric history, the patient's medical history, known allergies, and presenting labor symptoms. A review of the prenatal record is optimal and easily done with the increasing use of electronic medical records. After about 36 wk gestation most health care providers provide copies of the woman's prenatal records to the delivering hospital or birthing center so they are readily available should the woman come in to be assessed. Review of laboratory data and prenatal testing allows for a more comprehensive assessment. Risk factors for the pregnancy will be assessed and documented along with maternal preferences for childbirth, including pain control options. If the patient has had no prenatal care or no records are available, the admission assessment will include appropriate laboratory or diagnostic testing.

Signs and symptoms

Rule out labor: Women may come to the hospital to "rule out" labor, unsure if the symptoms they are experiencing indicate they are in labor. The pregnant woman is evaluated and if found to be in labor is admitted. If the woman is found not to be in labor, she is sent home with verbal and written instructions regarding the signs of true labor, when to see the health care provider, and follow-up phone numbers.

Uterine contractions: Characteristics of true labor include contractions that increase in frequency, duration, and strength over time and cause cervical dilation, effacement, and fetal descent. Typically with true labor the woman's contraction will increase with walking because this increases myometrial irritability. Uterine contractions will continue even when the woman tries to sleep or rest. In early labor the patient will be able to walk and talk through the contraction. Often the woman in early labor is encouraged to ambulate and change positions frequently rather than labor in bed, allowing gravity to facilitate labor progress.

Low back pain: Back pain that begins in the low back and radiates to the front is indicative of true labor. The woman may also report a "tightening" across the abdomen that begins in the back or back pain that does not completely go away because the fetal head is applying pressure to the maternal structures.

Bloody show: Pink or reddish-brown vaginal discharge likely will be present, resulting from cervical softening and changes due to effacement.

Mucus plug: Loss of the mucus plug will have occurred.

DIAGNOSTIC TESTS

Admission vital signs: Temperature, pulse, respirations, and blood pressure measurements are obtained. These are compared to prepregnant and prenatal records. Pain level is assessed using a valid pain tool. The woman's acceptable pain level is documented. The woman is placed in semi-Fowler's position, usually in a left tilt using a wedge or pillow under the right hip, to optimize uterine perfusion. A baseline electronic fetal heart rate monitoring strip with uterine activity of at least 20-min duration is obtained on admission. Frequency and duration of contractions are noted.

Cervical evaluation: A sterile vaginal exam is performed by the RN or health care provider to assess cervical dilation, effacement, and station of the fetal presenting part.

Sterile speculum examination: A sterile speculum is inserted into the vagina to visualize amniotic fluid leaking from the cervical os or pooling of amniotic fluid in the vagina. This fluid is tested with Nitrazine paper. If positive for amniotic fluid, the paper will turn from yellow to dark blue or green-blue, and the pH will be greater than 6.0. False-positive results may be seen in the presence of semen, blood, vaginal infections, or alkaline antiseptics. Using a cotton swab, a sample of vaginal fluid is taken from the posterior vaginal fornix (the posterior space below the cervix) and examined under the microscope for the presence of a ferning pattern that amniotic fluid makes when it dries on a slide.

PAMG-1 (AmniSure): The test detects trace amounts of a protein, PAMG-1, expressed by the cells of the decidua and found in amniotic fluid. The test is performed by swabbing a sterile polyester swab into the vaginal secretions. The swab is then rinsed with a vial of solvent for 1 min and thrown away. A test strip is dipped into the vial for 5-10 min and then read. One line indicates no rupture of membranes. Two lines is positive for rupture of membranes. No lines indicate an invalid test. The test has a 99% accuracy rate.

External uterine and fetal monitoring: Before placing the electronic fetal monitor, the RN or provider may perform Leopold's maneuvers, a systemic assessment in which the external maternal abdomen is palpated. This is intended to determine fetal presentation before placing the external fetal monitors onto the maternal abdomen. External uterine monitoring is done to evaluate fetal heart rate, variability, and periodic and episodic changes for fetal well-being. Uterine contraction presence, frequency, and duration are also monitored using a toco transducer. The RN or practitioner may also palpate the strength of uterine contraction as mild (tense fundus but easily indents to fingertip touch), moderate (firm fundus, difficult to indent with fingertip pressure), or strong (hard, firm fundus that does not indent to fingertips). The electronic fetal monitor (EFM) provides a permanent record of the fetal heart rate (FHR) and uterine contractions (UC). In the United States, the EFM may be used continuously or intermittently, or FHR may be auscultated intermittently (IA) if the patient is considered low risk. FHR will be determined, evaluated, and documented every 30 min during the first stage of labor and every 15 min during the active phase of pushing during stage two. If there are risk factors, FHR is identified, evaluated, and documented every 15 min during the first stage of labor and every 5 min during the active pushing phase of stage two (Simpson & O'Brien-Abel, 2014).

Nursing Diagnosis:

Anxiety

related to unfamiliar surroundings, processes, and procedures and hospitalization

Desired Outcome: Within 1 hr of intervention, the patient states that her anxiety has lessened or resolved, and she describes effective coping mechanisms.

ASSESSMENT/INTERVENTIONS

RATIONALES

ASSESSMENT/INTERVENTIONS	RATIONALES
On admission, provide a brief tour of the unit, familiarize the patient and family with the room and where food and supplies may be found, provide contact phone numbers and rules regarding visitation, and discuss parking and use of electronics.	Familiarity with the layout of the room and unit and knowledge of where to find important items or places such as dietary supplies, linens, pay phones, and bathrooms will increase independence and decrease anxiety. Knowing the rules for visiting, cell phone use, and taking pictures/videos, among other concerns, will help decrease anxiety.
Assess which prenatal classes, reading materials, and hospital tours the patient may have attended or participated in.	Assessment of classes the patient attended and the educational needs of the patient and her family allows the nurse to teach to the patient's specific needs, thereby helping to reduce anxiety. Identifying educational gaps enables the nurse to provide materials and teach specific educational topics to women in early labor and provides distraction as well.
Engage the patient and family in discussions regarding their previous experiences being hospitalized and their expectations and methods for successful coping during stressful events in the past.	Birth is often the first time a woman is hospitalized. Assessing previous experiences and acknowledging concerns show respect and provide the nurse with helpful information. Reflecting on methods used to cope in the past during stressful situations allows the patient to call on her own strengths.
Assess for verbal and nonverbal cues regarding the patient's anxiety level.	Verbal as well as nonverbal cues can provide the nurse with insights into how the patient is coping with the hospitalization and the labor process. Examples of nonverbal cues that might indicate anxiety are not making eye contact, fidgeting, being distracted, or ignoring teaching. Anxiety decreases the patient's ability to focus and relax. Relaxation is important in labor to provide adequate oxygenation and promote optimal labor progress.
Explain the purpose of any equipment or procedure (monitoring fetal status, IV, sterile vaginal exam) to the patient along with rationales and options for care.	Explanation or demonstration of procedures or equipment and their use or purpose will provide information and decrease anxiety. Patients often are fearful or concerned that a procedure will hurt or ask, "Why is this being done?" Informed consent and explanations of treatment options are necessary to provide the opportunity for shared decision making and facilitate cooperation and trust of the patient. For example, to assess fetal well-being and contraction status, the nurse will use EFM or IA. Explanation of these methods, when and how often they will occur, and the information they provide should be shared with the patient to gain acceptance and cooperation and ease anxiety. Explanation of findings and progress is part of family-centered care and part of the shared decision-making process.
Review the stages of labor as they occur, reassuring the woman and family of normal expectations and behaviors, while providing coaching and support.	The patient may become fearful if she does not understand what is happening to her body during labor or feels something is abnormal. Explaining in lay terms the labor process, normal progress, and what to expect while providing encouragement and support enhances the patient's and family's coping skills and well-being and decreases anxiety.
Encourage doula (professional or lay-support person) support of the laboring woman when available.	The continuous support of the doula in labor has been shown to increase satisfaction with the birth experience and provide the woman with additional support that reassures her as labor progresses. Women report a greater satisfaction with their labors when they have continuous labor support (Burke, 2014).
Offer praise and encouragement to family members or other support person and offer breaks. Acknowledge that labor support can be difficult.	Teaching and supporting family members to provide relaxation techniques through demonstration and return demonstration allows the family to support the woman in labor as part of family-centered nursing care.

Nursing Diagnosis:

Deficient Knowledge

related to misinformation, late or no prenatal care, or lack of attendance of prenatal classes

Desired Outcome: Immediately following teaching, the patient verbalizes accurate knowledge of the admission procedure and expectant labor and delivery care.

ASSESSMENT/INTERVENTIONS	RATIONALES
Assess the patient's and family's understanding of the birth process and whether they attended prenatal classes.	Assessing the knowledge base and expectations of the woman and family begins a relationship based on trust. Educational assessment facilitates the nurse's teaching and helps the woman meet her individual educational needs regarding labor and birth.
Engage the patient and family in an open discussion about their birth plan if they have one, including who will attend the delivery and any wishes they may have regarding the delivery. Share the birth plan with other members of the health care team so that collaboration occurs and the patient and family feel valued and heard.	Acknowledging and assisting the woman to meet her birthing goals based on her birthing plan necessitates clear communication. Having and meeting birth plans increases the woman's sense of control and decreases anxiety. Communicating that the health and well-being of the mother and baby may necessitate adjustment of the birthing plans is important in order to gain trust and cooperation.
Assess which plans or questions the woman has regarding pain management in labor.	Acknowledging the woman's wishes for pain management is a vital part of family-centered care. Active listening to the woman shows respect. If the patient has not taken child birth classes that discussed pain and anesthesia or analgesia, the nurse should explain options for pain management, ideally in early labor when the woman is able to focus on the information and ask questions so that she can make an informed decision. Some women will want to know their options regarding pain management and will choose to wait and see how labor progresses before selecting a specific method of analgesia or anesthesia. The nurse works with the patient and family to support their goals for pain management.
Provide culturally sensitive care to the family, adapting care to their individual needs.	Culturally sensitive nursing care shows respect and acknowledges patients as individuals and the influence that culture may have on their individual coping styles. Different cultures approach labor and birth differently. For example, in some cultures the woman may labor very quietly and in others the woman may be very demonstrative. Some cultures insist on many people being present at the delivery and other cultures may not wish any men in attendance. The nurse works with the woman and family to provide safe, culturally appropriate family-centered care in an atmosphere of shared decision making.

Nursing Diagnosis:

Deficient Fluid Volume (or risk for same)

related to decreased oral intake in labor, mouth breathing, and diaphoresis

Desired outcome: The patient remains adequately hydrated throughout labor as evidenced by normal elastic skin turgor, moist mucous membranes, and urinary output measured at a minimum of 30 mL/hr.

ASSESSMENT/INTERVENTIONS	RATIONALES
Monitor hydration status (see the desired outcome), and measure urine specific gravity as needed.	Normal specific gravity range is 1.005-1.030. An excess of 1.030 indicates dehydration.
Assess her temperature q2-4h per agency policy.	An elevated temperature is associated with dehydration.

continued

ASSESSMENT/INTERVENTIONS	RATIONALES
Monitor pulse and blood pressure per agency policy.	Increased pulse and decreased blood pressure indicate dehydration.
Encourage steady, modest amounts of fluids and light snacks in early labor (e.g., fruit juice, Jello, broth, clear soups, popsicles, tea, sports drink, and clear carbonated beverages). Provide ice chips if the patient does not wish to drink fluids.	There is slowed gastric emptying in labor, so if large volumes of food or liquids are consumed, vomiting may occur, although few women choose to eat or drink large quantities once active labor begins.
Teach the patient to avoid solid foods in labor.	Solids are avoided once active labor begins due to the risk of aspiration of gastric contents if emergency anesthesia is required. Though the risk is low, solid food in labor should be provided at the discretion of the anesthesiologist and per agency policy.
Discuss IV fluids with the patient in early labor or on admission if possible to assess her preference. (An IV may or may not be part of admission protocols, depending on unit policy.)	Provide the patient with information and rationales regarding IV administration of fluids. Administration of IV fluids for hydration, commonly lactated Ringer's, is an option in labor, especially for the patient who is nauseated or not taking adequate fluids by mouth. IV hydration in labor may have the added benefit of shortening labor and is necessary for some forms of analgesia or anesthesia. Some facilities strongly suggest or require IV access in case of emergency.
Provide comfort care for the diaphoretic patient. Maintain the room at a comfortable temperature for her. Remove excess clothing or linens as needed and change her gown to keep her dry and comfortable. Provide cool washcloths or ice packs to help maintain comfort as well as hand-held or electric fans.	Labor is strenuous work and elevates the body's temperature. The woman may perspire in an attempt to cool her body.

Nursing Diagnosis:

Acute Pain

related to cervical dilation, muscle hypoxia from uterine contractions, a full bladder, or stretching of maternal tissues

Desired Outcomes: Using a pain scale, the patient states that she is coping with pain to her satisfaction using pharmacological or nonpharmacologic pain relief methods based on her preference and birth plan. Nonverbal cues, such as grimacing, are absent or declining in frequency.

ASSESSMENT/INTERVENTIONS	RATIONALES
Encourage the patient to verbalize her level of acceptable pain using a valid pain scale.	Documentation and understanding of the patient's individual acceptable pain level enables the nurse to work with the patient in providing adequate pain relief. The nurse recognizes that pain is unique for each person.
Assess for behavioral or physiologic indicators of pain at frequent intervals (e.g., q1-2h or during scheduled vital sign assessments).	Pain in labor occurs from stretching, lactic acid buildup, muscle hypoxia, and pressure on the pelvic structure and from the fetal head. Increased heart rate, respirations, and blood pressure occur in response to increased pain.
Assess for verbal and nonverbal cues indicating pain.	Examples of nonverbal cues include facial grimacing, moaning, and muscle tension in the extremities along with increased anxiety. The patient may not be aware of these cues and should be encouraged to use relaxation techniques such as breathing and visualization to decrease muscle tension and decrease the pain-fear-tension cycle.
Teach and encourage relaxation and breathing techniques.	Relaxation and breathing techniques promote adequate oxygenation to the tissues and decrease physiologic responses to pain.

ASSESSMENT/INTERVENTIONS	RATIONALES
Encourage emptying of the bladder q2h or more frequently as needed.	A full bladder can cause discomfort and impede fetal descent. Use of a bedpan or bedside commode may be necessary if the woman does not wish to ambulate or has received medications. Catheterization may be necessary with some regional anesthetics due to motor blockade.
Keep the laboring woman's environment as quiet as possible.	A quiet environment free of noise and distraction promotes rest and conserves energy.
Teach and assist with nonpharmacologic comfort measures (e.g., breathing techniques, effleurage to the abdomen, application of heat and cold, acupressure or acupuncture, continuous and firm counterpressure to the sacral area during each contraction, pelvic rocking, relaxation conditioned in response to the partner's touch, massage, music, hydrotherapy, and transcutaneous electrical nerve stimulation [TENS]).	Nonpharmacologic methods may promote relaxation, decrease muscle tension, and provide distraction from pain and give the woman a sense of control. The support person may need to vary the method, depending on the stage of labor and position of the fetus (e.g., counterpressure to the sacrum reduces pain from back labor and occiput-posterior presentations). Cutaneous methods such as therapeutic touch, massage, counterpressure, application of heat or cold, and acupressure rely on interrupting the transmission of sensation. Location, technique, and depth of massage may vary but can decrease perceptions of pain.
Use other comfort measures that incorporate the senses.	Nonpharmacologic comfort measures that incorporate the senses include stimulation of visual, olfactory, and auditory stimuli to block pain impulses. These comfort measures include use of focal points, guided imagery, music, hypnosis, and aromatherapy.
Change the woman's position frequently, at least q30min, and encourage ambulation or an upright position in labor. Explain to her that labor progresses more quickly if she remains relaxed and upright.	Frequent position changes assist in comfort and should be based on the patient's comfort level, preference, safety, and privacy. The nurse can suggest and demonstrate appropriate laboring positions that increase comfort.
Advise the laboring woman to avoid the supine position.	This position causes decreased uteroplacental blood flow and cardiac return. If the woman wishes to lie down, a side-lying or a left or right tilt to the pelvis is recommended to increase blood flow to the heart and to the uterus. **Note:** Administration of regional anesthetics may negate the use of ambulation and some positions, especially if there is motor blockade. Hands and knees position may be effective in rotation of the fetus from occiput posterior to occiput anterior and may reduce back labor. Use of this position and the upright position shortens labor for both the first and second stages of labor and is associated with decreased use of pain medication. Use of a birthing ball, lunging, squatting at the side of the bed, and use of the various positioning capabilities of the birthing bed to find a position of comfort should all be encouraged as long as the well-being of the mother and fetus is established. Laboring on the toilet decreases pressure of presenting parts and allows gravity to assist with dilation and descent for some women and is encouraged as long as fetal well-being is assessed.
Medicate with analgesic or anesthetics as prescribed by the health care provider or anesthetist.	The types of medications used for pain management in labor may include those that cause a sedative effect to the woman so that she may doze or sleep between contractions.
As indicated, keep the side rails up and advise the patient she will need assistance with ambulation if she is being treated with opioid-type medications.	Common medications used for pain management in labor include opioids, synthetic opioids, and opioid agonist-antagonists. These medications have differing side effects but offer some blunting or dulling of pain. Safety of the patient who has received these medications is paramount. **Note:** Medications may cause a change in the labor progress and a decrease in contractions, thus they are usually not given until labor is well established. Respiratory depression in the newborn may occur if given too close to delivery. Naloxone (Narcan) is a narcotic agonist and may be given to reverse the respiratory depressive effect to the newborn if opioids are given to the patient within 4 hr of delivery.

✓ PATIENT-FAMILY TEACHING AND DISCHARGE PLANNING

Labor and birth are a part of the normal human process. Education and teaching regarding the signs of true labor, the stages of labor, normal expectations, and labor support and pain management ideally should occur in prenatal classes or in early labor when the woman and her family are ready for this information. (For problems that can occur before or after delivery, see subsequent chapters.) Include written and verbal information about the following:

✓ Signs and symptoms of true labor.
✓ When to call the health care provider or come to the hospital.
✓ Danger signs that require prompt reporting to the health care provider.
✓ Availability and choice of pain management methods.
✓ Availability of labor support/doula services.

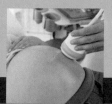

Bleeding in Pregnancy 88

OVERVIEW/PATHOPHYSIOLOGY

Hemorrhage during pregnancy continues to be a leading cause of morbidity and mortality. Although at times it may be minor, bleeding can be life threatening when profuse hemorrhage leads to maternal hypovolemia, anemia, and complications such as infection. Major causes of hemorrhage during pregnancy include *ectopic pregnancy* (implantation outside of the uterus), *threatened spontaneous abortion* (confirmed pregnancy with vaginal bleeding), *inevitable spontaneous abortion* (ruptured membranes with progressive cervical dilation before 20 wk gestation), *complete spontaneous abortion* (bleeding and cramping until passage of the whole conceptus (before 20 wk gestation), *incomplete abortion* (bleeding and cramping with retention of some of the conceptus), *missed abortion* (fetus has died but is retained with the placenta in the uterus), *septic abortion* (from infection), *gestational trophoblastic disease* ([GTD]; and includes hydatidiform mole [molar pregnancy]), *cervical insufficiency* (painless dilation of the cervix in the absence of contractions), *placenta previa* (abnormally implanted placenta that partially or completely covers the cervix), *placental abruption* (premature separation from the uterine wall of a normally implanted placenta), and *uterine rupture*.

HEALTH CARE SETTING

Primary care or acute care when bleeding persists or surgical intervention is necessary

ASSESSMENT

In early pregnancy, assessments begin with confirmation of pregnancy, determination of gestational age, and correlation of gestational age with fundal height. The amount and characteristics of bleeding as well as its origin, the severity of pain, and other accompanying signs determine priorities in physical assessment. *In late pregnancy*, medical and nursing assessments are often simultaneous. Bleeding can range from light pink spotting to dark brown (old blood). It may be like a heavy menses (up to 1000 mL of blood flows through the placenta). Bleeding can progress rapidly to massive hemorrhage with significant morbidity or mortality for the mother and fetus. When bleeding is associated with a complication of pregnancy, the priorities focus on:

Amount of and characteristics of the bleeding: Vaginal bleeding can occur at any time during pregnancy. Is the blood viscous, thin, and watery; does it contain clots; is it light pink or bright red or deep red or brown? Is there other tissue, odor, or continuous or recurrent bleeding? A pad count is conducted to maintain an accurate measurement of blood loss.

Pain: Was the onset sudden or gradual? Is it localized or generalized, intermittent or continuous, sharp, dull, aching, radiating, or changing? What is its relationship to the uterus or to activities? Pain may be the only sign of an ectopic pregnancy if bleeding is concealed within the abdomen. The abdomen may be tender and exceptionally hard (boardlike) as occurs with abruption, and bleeding may be concealed or apparent as the uterine cavity fills with blood.

Cardiovascular and respiratory status: Assess for hypertension or hypotension, tachycardia, tachypnea, shortness of breath, postural hypotension, dizziness, lightheadedness, or syncope.

Uterine contractions: Assess for frequency, duration and intensity, resting tone, rupture of membranes, and uterine irritability.

Condition of the fetus: Assess for decreased or absent fetal activity relative to gestational age. After 20 wk gestation, monitor fetal heart rate (FHR) and assess baseline variability, FHR accelerations, FHR decelerations, and FHR changes associated with uterine contractions. Note changes in status from the previous fetal monitor tracings and report to the provider. FHR is assessed as follows: Category 1 is normal, well oxygenated. Category 2 is indeterminate and needs further observation. Category 3 is abnormal and requires action.

Accompanying signs: Assess for additional signs of shock with massive blood loss, including cool, pale skin and mucous membranes; oliguria; and altered consciousness. Vaginal discharge before a bleeding episode may range from thin to thick and may be white, yellow, or green. Fever and malodorous vaginal discharge are indications of infection. Assess the woman's anxiety state, as well as her family's emotional response to the bleeding episode.

Obstetric history: A thorough history includes total number of pregnancies (gravidity), number of live births at more than 20 wk gestation (parity), and previous abortions or preterm births. Obtain any history of previous bleeding in this pregnancy and any prior pregnancy complications or testing.

DIAGNOSTIC TESTS

Obstetric ultrasound: Transabdominal, transvaginal, or translabial ultrasound locates the gestational sac as intrauterine or ectopic. Real-time ultrasound confirms cardiac activity and a viable fetus. Ultrasound identifies multiple gestation, placental position, number of umbilical vessels, presence of subchorionic hemorrhage (bleeding beneath the outer membrane), and abruption. Ultrasound allows differential diagnosis between the two types of gestational trophoblastic disease (GTD).

Speculum examination: A careful speculum vaginal examination safely visualizes the cervix during and after vaginal bleeding, when a sterile-gloved vaginal exam is contraindicated. The examiner can observe dilation and effacement, presence of tissue in the cervix or vaginal vault, polyps, cervical friability, lacerations, or other lesions. Cultures may be obtained. Rupture of membranes can be evaluated using Nitrazine paper or a specimen for microscopic evaluation of ferning (the fern leaf pattern seen with a microscope when amniotic fluid dries).

Qualitative and quantitative pregnancy tests: Urine or serum pregnancy tests measure the presence of human chorionic gonadotropin (hCG). The presence of hCG in serum or urine can confirm a pregnancy. Positive results are possible after implantation is complete, 8-10 days after conception, which may occur before or after a missed period. Because the serum concentration of hCG doubles every 1-2 days, serial testing can indicate gestational age. Declining numbers generally indicate spontaneous abortion or ectopic pregnancy.

Complete blood count (CBC): Reflects the amount of blood lost, especially by falling levels of hemoglobin (Hgb) and hematocrit (Hct). One pint of blood loss equals approximately 1½-g drop in Hgb and 1%-3% decrease in Hct. Likewise these factors will rise with each unit of blood replaced. A rising WBC count may signal infection. Falling platelets indicate an increasing risk of disseminated intravascular coagulation (DIC). (See "Disseminated Intravascular Coagulation," p. 471.)

Blood Rh factor and antibody screen: Maternal blood group (ABO) and Rh factor (positive or negative) are determined when medical prenatal care is initiated. An antibody screen (indirect Coombs test) is done to determine whether the Rh-negative woman is sensitized to the Rh antigen. Rh immune globulin (RhoGAM or HypRho-D) is administered within 72 hr after a spontaneous or induced abortion, ectopic pregnancy, or GTD pregnancy; after an external version attempt; after birth with or without a placenta previa or abruptio placenta; at any gestational age; and after maternal abdominal trauma.

Kleihauer-Betke test: Checks for the presence of fetal erythrocytes in maternal blood. Fetal-maternal bleeding occurs 3-5 times more often in pregnancy when the mother experiences abdominal trauma.

Uterine and FHR monitoring: Before gestational viability, uterine activity monitoring alone may be done to demonstrate contraction presence and pattern. In the second and third trimesters, FHR monitoring reveals fetal well-being or fetal response to blood loss, labor, or induction procedures.

Continuous FHR monitoring is used to identify signs of a compromised fetus. Fetal oxygenation may be compromised with a disrupted placental surface area for gas exchange, maternal hypotension, and uterine irritability. The Category 2 or Category 3 FHR pattern seen with bleeding may include loss of baseline variability, tachycardia or bradycardia, late decelerations in labor, prolonged decelerations, progressively severe variable decelerations, and a sinusoidal pattern. With acute abruptio placenta, there is rapid FHR deceleration indicating imminent fetal demise.

Twenty-minute nonstress test: Beginning at 27-32 wk gestation, this test can demonstrate reactive FHR activity, which indicates adequate fetal oxygenation and an intact central nervous system. Measurement standards differ for the fetus between 32 wk gestation and term from the fetus under 32 wk gestation because the latter's central nervous system is less mature.

Nursing Diagnoses:

Risk for Bleeding

related to pregnancy-related conditions (spontaneous abortion [threatened, inevitable, incomplete, complete, or missed], ectopic pregnancy, placenta previa, or abruptio placenta)

Risk for Shock

related to hypovolemia

Desired Outcome: Within 2-3 hr of appropriate intervention, the patient returns to a functional level of blood volume/body fluids as measured by return to urinary output greater than 30 mL/hr with urine specific gravity less than 1.030, normotensive blood pressure (BP) (90-130/60-80 mm Hg), heart rate (HR) 60-100 bpm, respiratory rate (RR) 12-20 unlabored breaths/min, capillary refill 2 sec or less, absence of signs of shock (e.g., alert without anxiety, skin warm and pink, bowel sounds active × 4), and a reactive FHR.

ASSESSMENT/INTERVENTIONS	RATIONALES
Assess the amount and begin measurement of continuing blood loss, including characteristics and the source/site of blood. As indicated, weigh saturated linen or peripads and keep a pad count.	Hemorrhage from spontaneous abortion, placenta previa, or abruptio placenta have different characteristics (see Assessment data, earlier). One gram of weight per scale represents 1 mL blood lost.
Assess accompanying signs and symptoms with blood loss (i.e., pain, fever, malodorous vaginal discharge), and their duration and association with behaviors (intercourse, activity).	Uterine cramping with hemorrhage may indicate one of the spontaneous abortions. Deep abdominal pain may signal ectopic pregnancy (with or without bleeding). Painless vaginal bleeding in the third trimester may indicate placenta previa. A boardlike, painful abdomen may indicate abruption (with or without dark red bleeding). Malodorous vaginal discharge may indicate chorioamnionitis (bacteria-caused inflammation of placental membranes).
! Assess maternal vital signs (VS) for signs of shock (hypotension, decreased pulse pressure, tachycardia, delayed capillary refill, cool clammy or mottled skin, and change in mentation and functional ability). Begin assessments q5-15min and decrease in frequency as her condition improves per agency protocol/health care provider directive.	In a pregnant woman, signs of shock manifest after 25%-30% blood loss. Assessment findings reveal cardiovascular status, degree of hemorrhage, and the results of continuous therapeutic adjustments related to fluid replacement needs.
! Start and maintain an intravenous (IV) site as soon as possible if one is not in place already. Use a large-bore needle.	Veins collapse with advancing hemorrhage. Venous access is necessary for administration of IV fluids. A large size needle is necessary for blood transfusions.
! Collect a blood specimen for blood type, Rh and antibody screen, CBC, and type and crossmatch per agency protocol and health care provider directives.	This action anticipates the need for fluid replacement therapy as soon as it is available.
! Administer and carefully monitor fluid replacement by crystalloid solutions in conjunction with plasma expanders or blood products (e.g., cryoprecipitate, plasma, packed red blood cells). Monitor for signs of fluid overload (e.g., dyspnea, lung crackles, or cough).	Regardless of the protocol followed, constant adjustments in fluid resuscitation and replacement are necessary during the first 24 hr. Too rapid correction of fluid deficit causes fluid overload, edema, and pulmonary congestion.
Insert indwelling catheter and measure urine output hourly.	Urine output returns with recovery from hemorrhagic shock. Its measurement determines replacement adequacy and the patient's changing needs.
Monitor laboratory reports: CBC, clotting factors, blood group and Rh, activated partial thromboplastin time (APTT), prothrombin time (PT), and hCG levels.	Hgb and Hct will be lower in the pregnant patient due to hemodilution, and their values will guide fluid replacement. Replacement with packed RBCs raises Hgb 1 g/dL and Hct approximately 3%. Platelet transfusions increase platelets by 5000/mm³. Fresh frozen plasma (FFP) raises each clotting factor by 2%-3%. Maintenance of Hct at 30% or greater supports oxygenation and nutrient transport. Platelet levels identify if thrombocytopenia is present. Platelet values, APTT, PT, and clotting factor values may signal complications (e.g., DIC); hCG levels reveal gestational age/complications (GTD, ectopic pregnancy).
Administer O₂ by snug face mask at 8-10 L/min.	Administering oxygen increases oxygen tension in the circulating blood volume and oxygen delivery to the end organs and fetus. A snug face mask more effectively delivers the higher Liters/min flow rate.
Position the patient for optimal perfusion, e.g., avoid supine position or use a hip wedge. Use the side-lying position when possible. Change position q30min while the patient is awake. Include semi-Fowler's position as well, but avoid Trendelenburg position.	These positions ensure adequate circulation to the mother and fetus. When in the supine position a hip wedge prevents compression to the descending aorta or inferior vena cava by the gravid uterus. Semi-Fowler's position may enable the fetus to act as a tampon in the third trimester, thereby minimizing bleeding. Trendelenburg position could interfere with adequate maternal respirations.
! Avoid vaginal or rectal examinations.	These exams may increase hemorrhage, especially with partial or complete placenta previa.
Save expelled conceptus (placenta, membranes, embryo, or fetus).	Anything remaining in the uterus contributes to continued bleeding. The health care provider will evaluate if the complete or only partial conceptus was passed. Histology studies may be necessary to determine cause.

continued

ASSESSMENT/INTERVENTIONS	RATIONALES
Ensure meticulous reporting and documentation.	Detailed and accurate communication ensures coordination of diagnosis, changing condition, and therapeutic interventions and maximizes effectiveness of the entire health care team.
Also see "Perioperative Care," p. 45.	Dilation and curettage is necessary for a missed or incomplete abortion; laparotomy may be necessary with ectopic pregnancy; cesarean delivery may be necessary for third trimester bleeding.

Nursing Diagnosis:

Impaired Gas Exchange (or risk for same)

related to diminished maternal circulation to the utero-placental unit

Desired Outcomes: Adequate oxygenation/perfusion to the fetus is demonstrated by fetal activity and FHR accelerations. After the age of viability, FHR maintains reassuring (Category 1) characteristic patterns (i.e., moderate variability, FHR at 110-160 bpm, accelerations, and no late decelerations in labor).

ASSESSMENT/INTERVENTIONS	RATIONALES
Monitor for fetal distress by repeated nonstress test (NST) as indicated or maintain continuous FHR monitoring at or after 20 wk gestation.	In the first half of pregnancy, no FHR determination is made. Thereafter FHR and fetal activity reflect fetal oxygenation status. A reactive FHR tracing (an increase of 15 bpm lasting 15 sec occurring twice in the 20-min tracing) indicates fetal well-being. Nonreactive FHR indicates hypoxia. Initially fetal response to hypoxia is increased movements and tachycardia. Bradycardia and decreased movements occur with continued/deepening hypoxia. Consideration of preterm behavior and response during the NST is crucial. Before 32 wk some practitioners consider the NST reactive with an increase in HR of 10 bpm that lasts 10 sec, occurring twice in the 20-min period.
Administer O$_2$ by snug face mask at 8-10 L/min.	Oxygen administration increases oxygen tension in the circulating blood volume and oxygen delivery to the fetus. A snug face mask enhances oxygen delivery to the fetus as well as to the mother.
Position the patient for optimal perfusion. For example, if unable to avoid the supine position use a hip wedge. Encourage a side-lying position. Include semi-Fowler's position, as well, but avoid Trendelenburg position. Ensure position change q30min while the patient is awake.	These positions ensure adequate circulation to the mother and fetus. In the supine position, a hip wedge prevents compression to the descending aorta or inferior vena cava by the gravid uterus. Semi-Fowler's position may enable the fetus to act as a tampon in third trimester, thereby minimizing bleeding. The Trendelenburg position may interfere with adequate maternal respirations.
At or after 20 wk gestation, assist with amniocentesis and interventions to delay delivery, or facilitate vaginal delivery or cesarean delivery as determined by the health care provider.	Hemorrhage may stop once the placenta (or total conceptus) is removed. After assessment of fetal lung maturity, the health care provider will determine the path for the best outcome.
When the fetus is at 20 wk or later gestation, call the neonatal resuscitation team before delivery.	This helps to prepare the team for delivery of a compromised newborn. Before 20 wk, the fetus is unable to sustain life after delivery. Twenty weeks or 500 g is used because dating can be off by a few wk unless the date of conception is medically confirmed. To err on the side of caution, a resuscitation team would be called until weight and age can be determined.

Nursing Diagnosis:

Acute Pain

related to uterine contractions, distention of the lower uterine segment, cervical changes, pressure on adjacent tissues, or tissue trauma (ectopic pregnancy or abruptio placenta)

Desired Outcomes: Within 1 hr of intervention the patient's subjective perception of pain is at an acceptable level, as evidenced by a report of no more than 2-3 on a 0-10 scale; objective measures such as grimacing are diminished or absent. The patient verbalizes understanding of her medications and the nonpharmacologic interventions used.

ASSESSMENT/INTERVENTIONS	RATIONALES
Assess duration and type of pain, characteristics (intensity, quality, onset, alleviating or aggravating factors), severity by a standard pain scale, and location.	Characteristics and location of pain indicate cause. Uterine contractions and cramping pain occur with spontaneous abortion (SAB) or GTD. Ectopic pregnancy may yield dull aching or severe pain (with ruptured fallopian tube). Abruptio placenta (concealed) may cause severe abdominal pain.
Assess and systematically monitor the patient for a verbal report and behavioral signs of pain q2h.	Changes in pain indicate improvement in the patient's condition or development of complications. Behavioral and physiologic responses clarify the presence of pain when the patient is unable to self-report pain.
Position for comfort and physiologic response; promote position changes q30min while the patient is awake.	Positioning in labor affects anatomic and physiologic responses (i.e., alters cardiac output, enhances or reduces effectiveness of uterine contractions, synchronizes abdominal muscle work, and reduces pressure on the preterm fetal head). Frequent position changes increase comfort and circulation and relieve fatigue.
Teach and assist with appropriate nonpharmacologic methods of pain relief (e.g., breathing and relaxation techniques, application of heat or cold, hydrotherapy, acupressure, effleurage to the abdomen or continuous and firm sacral pressure during each contraction, relaxation conditioned in response to the partner's touch, massage, and music).	Nonpharmacologic methods reduce stress, relieve body tension by promoting relaxation, often increase endorphin levels, and have fewer side effects than medications. Sacral pressure relieves strain put on the sacroiliac joint from the fetal head in the occiput posterior position.
Medicate with analgesics or anesthetics as prescribed by the health care provider or anesthetist using the seven rights of medication administration.	The goal of medication administration is to adequately relieve pain without causing maternal or fetal risk. Seven rights of administration means right drug, right dose, right preparation, right route, right time, right patient, and right documentation.

For other assessments, interventions, and rationales, see "Pain," p. 39.

Nursing Diagnoses:

Anxiety
Fear

related to threat of change in health or death (perceived or actual) to the unborn child or self and/or unknown invasive treatment and its outcome

Desired Outcome: Following intervention(s), the patient and family state that their anxieties and fears have lessened or resolved.

ASSESSMENT/INTERVENTIONS	RATIONALES
Assess and acknowledge fears or anxieties.	This will help identify causes of anxiety/fear and focus on what the potential loss of this pregnancy means to the patient and her family.
Encourage verbalization of fears.	Discussion of fears makes them more concrete and strengthens coping ability.

continued

ASSESSMENT/INTERVENTIONS	RATIONALES
Provide support with attentive and active listening.	Restating what you have heard them say empowers the patient and family with self-understanding and a sense of control and fosters decision making.
Provide verbal and written sources of information throughout care.	Honest and individualized information develops a knowledge base and helps eliminate fears and anxieties. However, the amount of information and their anxieties may interfere with assimilation. Written information enables later review of information.
Discuss the meaning of symptoms and medical interventions ahead of time (if possible).	Knowledge reduces fear and body tension and fosters participation in decision making when possible.
For other assessments, interventions, and rationales see these nursing diagnoses in "Psychosocial Support," pp. 73 and 75.	

Nursing Diagnoses:

Grieving
Risk for Complicated Grieving

related to anticipated or actual loss of the unborn child

Desired Outcome: Within 24 hr after guidance and support are given by the health care team, the patient, her partner, and family begin expressing their grief or anger, acknowledge that grieving takes a long time with no specific time frames, and begin working with other support persons in or out of the family.

ASSESSMENT/INTERVENTIONS	RATIONALES
Assess the patient's, partner's, and family's coping methods, strengths, and support system(s).	Early, individualized, and continued support help prevent delayed or complicated grief reactions.
Encourage verbalizing feelings and concerns regarding potential or actual loss of the unborn child.	The grief and feelings of pregnancy loss are complex and unique for each woman, partner, and family member. The ability to communicate fears and express feelings are important elements of sharing grief.
Per agency protocol, refer to a social worker, chaplain, and/or grief counselor as needed.	The multidisciplinary team supports the needs of both intuitive and instrumental styles of coping. They assist with decisions and provide support related to pregnancy loss, both in hospital and after discharge.
Encourage continuation with support system(s) after hospital discharge.	Grief and recovery after losing the pregnancy or child continue for a long time—through as much as a year of bereavement or more and with shadow grief episodes appearing later.
Explain that everyone grieves differently. Provide space for and communicate support.	Coping styles vary with individuals and can differ between women and men.
Grieve with the patient, partner, and family if this is helpful.	People with intuitive styles of coping (i.e., insightful without consciously reasoning) prefer care that emphasizes emotional and psychologic support.
For other assessments, interventions, and rationales, see "Psychosocial Support" for **Grieving/Risk for Complicated Grieving**, p. 78.	

Nursing Diagnosis:

Deficient Knowledge

related to unfamiliarity with the effects of bleeding on the pregnancy, fetus, and self; the treatment regimen; and medications

Desired Outcome: Following instruction, the patient and her family members begin to verbalize understanding of the patient's changing condition, diagnostic and therapeutic procedures, signs and symptoms of developing complications, and plans for follow-up care, and return demonstrations of prescribed procedures.

ASSESSMENT/INTERVENTIONS	RATIONALES
Assess understanding of the hemorrhagic condition, treatments, and possible outcomes.	This assessment enables clarification of information and correction of misunderstanding.
Ascertain religious practices or preferences.	For example, religious faith may prohibit use of blood products and indicate need for alternative treatment.
Explain the diagnosis to the patient, her partner, and family; reinforce information provided by other health care providers. Explain the changing maternal and fetal condition, treatment regimen, tests, and medications.	These explanations not only provide accurate information but also reduce stress by eliminating confusion.
Speak calmly and clearly in words appropriate to the patient's, partner's, and family's understanding.	In an already emotionally charged situation the nurse's voice can either increase or reduce anxiety.
Anticipate concerns, encourage questions, and include the patient, partner, and family in decision making as much as possible during hospitalization and follow-up care after discharge.	Evidence-based nursing practice stresses the importance of patient and family preferences in decision making. For example, with ectopic pregnancy, fertility may be reduced; with GTD, hCG levels need to be monitored; if the client has experienced a repeated spontaneous abortion (SAB), a cervical cerclage may be helpful.
For other assessments, interventions, and rationales, see this nursing diagnosis in "Psychosocial Support," p. 82.	

ADDITIONAL NURSING DIAGNOSES/PROBLEMS:

✓ **PATIENT-FAMILY TEACHING AND DISCHARGE PLANNING**

Include verbal and written information about the following:
- ✓ Importance of reporting vaginal bleeding to the health care provider in a timely manner
- ✓ Importance of reporting signs of a complication or worsening condition
- ✓ Necessity of adhering to prescribed medications, treatment regimen, and scheduled appointments
- ✓ Medications, including purpose; name; dose; frequency; precautions; and potential side effects or interactions with drugs, foods, and herbs
- ✓ Measures that help constipation (resulting from bedrest, medications, pregnancy)
- ✓ How to evaluate fetal movements and contractions (when appropriate)
- ✓ Balanced diet high in iron; hydration with 8-10 (8-oz) glasses of fluid daily (water is best; avoid caffeinated and sugary drinks)
- ✓ Adherence to restrictions on intercourse
- ✓ Referral to The American Congress of Obstetricians and Gynecologists, which has an extensive collection of patient education materials available at *www.acog.org/Resources_And_Publications/Patient_Education_FAQs_List*
- ✓ Referral to local or national support organizations:
  - Sidelines is a national organization providing support for women and families experiencing a complicated pregnancy at *www.sidelines.org*
  - March of Dimes: *www.marchofdimes.com*
  - Caring Bridge: *www.caringbridge.org*
  - The Society of Obstetricians and Gynecologists of Canada at *http://sogc.org* (requires subscription)

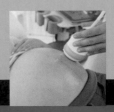

OVERVIEW/PATHOPHYSIOLOGY

According to the National Diabetes Data Group Classification, there are four types of diabetes (ADA, 2008). They are type 1 diabetes mellitus (DM), called *insulin-dependent diabetes*; type 2 DM, called *insulin-resistant diabetes*; *diabetes dependent* on other specific conditions such as infection or drug induced; and *gestational diabetes mellitus (GDM)*. GDM is defined as carbohydrate intolerance that is first recognized during pregnancy (Gilbert, 2011). There is a 50% risk of GDM turning to chronic DM within 5 yr after diagnosis if no lifestyle changes are made. Diabetes poses significant risks to maternal/fetal morbidity and mortality. Incidence of diabetes in pregnancy has increased because more women are delaying pregnancy until relatively late into their reproductive years. Currently the incidence is 4%-14% with GDM accounting for almost 90% (Gilbert, 2011).

HEALTH CARE SETTING

Primary care (outpatient obstetric clinic, high-risk perinatal clinic); or acute care (inpatient). Hospitalization is sought when starting or adjusting insulin, if an infection develops, or during the third trimester when diabetes has been poorly controlled and closer maternal and fetal surveillance is indicated.

ASSESSMENT

At the first prenatal visit all women are screened for clinical risk factors when obtaining a history. If risk factors are identified such as previous history of GDM, known impaired glucose metabolism, previous macrosomic baby (greater than 4000 g), and obesity (BMI greater than 30), early screening is recommended. An early screen that is negative is repeated for these high-risk women at 24-28 wk. Between 24 and 28 wk gestation, it is recommended that *all pregnant women* be screened for GDM. A two-step screening process is currently supported by ACOG. The approach begins with administration of 50 g of oral glucose solution with a 1-hr serum glucose measurement as the initial screening. Screening is recommended even for patients with low risk factors (age younger than 25 yr, not a member of an ethnic group at risk for developing type 2 DM, BMI less than 25, no previous history of abnormal glucose tolerance, no previous history of adverse obstetric outcomes that are usually associated with GDM, and no known diabetes in a first-degree relative [mother, father, siblings]).

Type 1 DM: Increased risk of abnormal embryogenesis (growth, differentiation, and organization of fetal cellular components), spontaneous abortion, sacral agenesis or caudal regression syndrome (absence or deformity of the sacrum), pyelonephritis, preterm labor/birth, polyhydramnios (abnormally high level of amniotic fluid), preeclampsia, ketoacidosis, cesarean section, fetal hypoxia, stillbirth, fetal macrosomia (birth weight 4000 g or more) or intrauterine growth restriction, birth trauma (e.g., shoulder dystocia because of macrosomia), congenital anomalies (ventral septal defect, transposition of the great vessels, anencephaly (absence of neural tissue in the cranium), open spina bifida (a defect in the closure of the neural tube), holoprosencephaly (absence of midline cerebral structures because of the incomplete division of the forebrain), respiratory distress syndrome (RDS), and neonatal hypoglycemia.

Type 2 DM/GDM: Increased risk of macrosomia or intrauterine growth restriction (depending on extent of the maternal illness and glycemic control), pregnancy-induced hypertension (preeclampsia), ketoacidosis, cesarean section, hypoxia, RDS, stillbirth, birth trauma, and neonatal hypoglycemia.

Note: *During pregnancy the classic symptoms of diabetes (polydipsia, polyphagia, and polyuria) cannot be used as diagnostic tools because they are normal changes of pregnancy.*

Renal-urinary: Glucosuria is not a reliable sign of diabetes during pregnancy because of a lowered renal threshold that occurs at that time. If glucose (+1 or higher) appears consistently (2 times or more) in the urine, however, the patient needs to be evaluated for GDM.

Neurologic: Frequent headaches, fatigue, and drowsiness may be present as a result of maternal insulin resistance. Retinopathy is commonly seen in women with type 1 DM (preexisting disease) caused by abnormal vasculature, capillary rupture, or hemorrhage within the retina. An ophthalmic examination during the pregnancy is recommended.

Cardiovascular: In patients with long-term diabetes, deterioration of glomerular function can lead to hypertension and superimposed preeclampsia. These women can also develop arteriosclerosis.

Other symptoms: Pregnant women with diabetes are at an increased risk of developing preeclampsia. See additional symptoms in "Preeclampsia," p. 674.

Complications—fetal
- Miscarriage/fetal death
- Embryonic growth delay
- Congenital malformations, especially cardiac and skeletal
- Hypertrophic and congestive cardiomyopathy
- Fetal macrosomia (gigantism)
- Hypoglycemia
- RDS
- Hyperbilirubinemia
- Hypocalcemia
- Intrauterine growth restriction

Risk factors: BMI above 30 kg/m^2, family history of DM, previous history of GDM, previous macrosomic infant, previous unexplained stillbirth, polyhydramnios (past or present), excessive weight gain, history of congenital anomalies in offspring, chronic hypertension, recurrent infections including vaginal monilial, recurrent glucosuria, age older than 30 yr, and family origin with high prevalence of diabetes (African American, Hispanic, Native American, South Asian [India, Pakistan, Bangladesh], Black Caribbean, Middle Eastern, and South Pacific Islanders).

DIAGNOSTIC TESTS

1-hr glucose screening: Performed between wk 24 and 28 of the pregnancy or earlier if the patient is identified as high risk. If results are negative in an earlier test, the test is repeated between 24 and 28 wk in the pregnancy if the patient meets risk factors (discussed earlier). This test requires the patient to drink a 50-g glucose load, followed in 1 hr by venous plasma measurement. Traditionally a value of 140 mg/dL or greater was considered abnormal and indicated need for the 3-hr 100-g oral glucose tolerance test. There is evidence that a 130 mg/dL cutoff level identifies 10% more women at risk for GDM. A single set of cutoff criteria is suggested. When a 1-hr value is 190 mg/dL or greater, a fasting glucose should be done before proceeding to the 3-hr test. If the fasting value is 95 mg/dL or greater, the patient is treated for GDM.

3-hr glucose tolerance test: After fasting for 8-12 hr and abstaining from smoking, a fasting blood sugar (FBS) is drawn, after which the patient drinks a 100-g glucose load followed by serum venous plasma measurements at 1, 2, and 3 hr. Two of the four values need to be abnormal to make the diagnosis of GDM.

Note: *Screening guidelines differ for diagnosing GDM, depending on medical facility preference. The American College of Obstetrics and Gynecology (ACOG) recommends the 3-hr oral glucose tolerance test (OGTT) for women who test positive with a 1-hr, 50-g OGTT. If two or more blood glucose levels are elevated, the diagnosis is established for GDM.*

Fasting: greater than 95 mg/dL

1-hr: greater than 180 mg/dL

2-hr: greater than 155 mg/dL

3-hr: greater than 140 mg/dL

Note: *The International Association of Diabetes and Pregnancy Study Group recommend using a single 2-hr, 75-g OGTT to screen for gestational diabetes. The American Diabetes Association has endorsed this criterion.*

Fasting: 92 mg/dL or higher

2-hr: 153 mg/dL or higher

Glycosylated hemoglobin (Hemoglobin A$_{1c}$): Reflects the average blood sugar levels for the 2- to 3-mo period before the test. Values may be increased in iron-deficient anemia and decreased in pregnancy. Levels less than 6% are desired in pregnancy. Recent studies have raised questions about the reliability of Hemoglobin A$_{1C}$ results in the second and third trimesters of pregnancy; therefore, it is no longer recommended as a routine assessment of glycemic control in those trimesters.

Home glucose monitoring: The patient at home performs glucose monitoring (obtaining whole blood from a fingerstick) at given intervals prescribed by the health care provider. Taking into account the risk of hypoglycemia, target values during pregnancy are FBS less than 95 mg/dL and 2-hr postprandial (pp) 120 mg/dL or less. Patients with poor glucose control will have FBS well above 90-95 mg/dL and 2-hr pp well above 120 mg/dL. Careful regulation of maternal glucose levels during pregnancy leads to decreased maternal/fetal compromise and better outcomes.

Renal function studies: Normally during pregnancy creatinine clearance is increased, but it is decreased in GDM because of deterioration in glomerular function. A 24-hr urinalysis for protein is recommended early in the pregnancy that can be used as a comparison later if renal function worsens.

Obstetric ultrasound: May be done at 2- to 4-wk intervals to monitor fetal growth, placental function, amniotic fluid levels, and fetal position and check for the presence of polyhydramnios (excess amniotic fluid). If the primary Hemoglobin A$_{1C}$ is elevated, a fetal echocardiogram may be done between 20 and 22 wk gestation. Ultrasounds also assess fetal anomalies for women with pregestational diabetes.

Antepartum fetal monitoring: Patients with GDM whose blood glucose levels are well controlled by diet are at low risk for fetal complications. Antepartum fetal heart rate testing is limited unless they have hypertension, history of prior stillbirth, or current fetal macrosomia. Any of these conditions would necessitate weekly to twice weekly testing starting at 32 wk (or sooner if necessary) to monitor fetal well-being. Ultrasound monitoring of fetal growth is recommended in the last few weeks of pregnancy because of the risk for macrosomia.

Nursing Diagnosis:

Risk for Unstable Glucose Level

related to fluctuations occurring during pregnancy

Desired Outcome: Euglycemia is maintained as evidenced by daily maternal records and prenatal testing results.

ASSESSMENT/INTERVENTIONS	RATIONALES
PRENATAL: Assess the patient's Hemoglobin A$_{1C}$ and blood glucose by the method and timing prescribed by the health care provider.	Hemoglobin A$_{1C}$ testing is recommended for patients with pregestational DM. Hemoglobin A$_{1C}$ levels above 6% are associated with a higher rate of congenital anomalies. Recent studies raise questions about its reliability in the second and third trimesters. Target daily glycemic controls in pregnancy by fingerstick are FBS of 95 mg/dL or less and 2-hr pp levels of 120 mg/dL or less.
Assess the patient's urine by dipstick for glucose and ketones, and review maternal monitoring charts as prescribed by the health care provider.	The renal threshold for glycosuria is lower in pregnancy. Glycosuria predisposes the patient to urinary tract infections.
Assess daily diet compliance according to the American Diabetic Association (ADA) diet prescribed by the dietitian.	GDM may be controlled by diet alone.
Explain to the patient with GDM and her family that insulin administration may be necessary as pregnancy progresses.	The body's insulin requirements double or quadruple by the third trimester. If diet repeatedly fails to keep fasting glucose at 95 mg/dL or less, insulin therapy is recommended.
Assess the patient's self-administration of human insulin according to the regimen prescribed by the health care provider.	Many pregnant women with diabetes want to administer their own insulin dose. Professional assessment identifies whether the patient's technique is safe or needs refinement by education.
Assess fundal height and compare to the previous level and gestational week as prescribed by the health care provider.	If euglycemia is not maintained throughout the pregnancy, the fetus is at risk for macrosomia or intrauterine growth restriction (IUGR).
Coordinate referrals after hospital discharge as prescribed, for example, to a perinatologist, endocrinologist, diabetic nurse, dietitian, and medical social worker (MSW).	Coordination of referrals fosters continuity of care and timely communication among many health care providers.
INTRAPARTUM: Assess and document blood glucose levels hourly by fingerstick and as prescribed after insulin administration.	Maintenance of euglycemia (75-126 mg/dL [4.0-7.0 mmol/L]) in labor reduces the risk for neonatal hypoglycemia, which is especially critical during the first hour of birth when the newborn is no longer experiencing the same glucose level as the mother.
If blood glucose rises to 126 mg/dL (7 mmol/L) or higher, begin insulin infusion by a secondary intravenous line at 2 units/hr in 0.9% normal saline as prescribed by the health care provider.	Blood glucose requirements vary in labor (e.g., food intake is reduced), and oxytocin acts like insulin and drives glucose into the body cells. Normoglycemia in Intensive Care Evaluation (NICE) guidelines for labor (2014) recommend that blood glucose remain between 75 and 126 mg/dL (4.0-7.0 mmol/L) by glucometer.
POSTPARTUM: Assess fasting blood glucose levels as prescribed. Encourage the patient to maintain a balanced diet, and have a snack available during breastfeeding bouts.	After the placenta is expelled, human placental lactogen (hPL) decreases and the insulin resistance during pregnancy resolves quickly. Insulin needs in the pregestational patient with diabetes are markedly reduced, often below prepregnant needs for 24 hr. The patient with GDM returns to nonpregnant carbohydrate metabolism.
Encourage breastfeeding.	Breastfeeding decreases blood glucose levels, while insulin needs are considerably decreased postpartum. Monitoring of blood glucose levels will continue because levels may fluctuate. Because hypoglycemia can occur, regular snacks are encouraged.

Nursing Diagnosis:

Deficient Knowledge

related to unfamiliarity with the effects of diabetes on self, the pregnancy, and the fetus

Desired Outcome: Immediately following teaching, the patient verbalizes accurate knowledge about the effects of diabetes on self, the pregnancy, and fetus and adheres to the treatment accordingly.

ASSESSMENT/INTERVENTIONS	RATIONALES
Explain to the patient and significant others how diabetes affects pregnancy and pregnancy affects diabetes for the mother, fetus, and newborn.	An informed patient is more likely to adhere to the therapeutic plan, which will change frequently as pregnancy advances (e.g., frequent blood sugar checks, frequent clinic visits, insulin injections, dietary monitoring, and fetal surveillance tests) and understand possible problems encountered with pregestational DM and GDM.
Encourage adherence to prenatal appointments, daily glucose testing, dietary regimen, and exercise program.	Frequent prenatal visits enable timely modification in the therapeutic regimen to promote optimal pregnancy outcomes (e.g., vaginal delivery without complications, newborn's growth average for gestational age [AGA] without hypoglycemia, nonworsening DM in postpartum patients with pregestational diabetes, and return to normal FBS for patients with GDM).
Encourage patients with pregestational diabetes to develop an individualized plan with their health care provider to maintain good glycemic control before becoming pregnant.	For the woman with pregestational diabetes, euglycemia at conception is associated with fewer congenital malformations in the newborn. Any reduction in Hemoglobin A_{1c} levels toward the nonpregnant value of 6.1 reduces the risk of congenital malformations.
Inform all patients with diabetes about a probable increased need for insulin to maintain euglycemia during the pregnancy.	The body's insulin requirements increase as the pregnancy advances. For the patient with pregestational diabetes taking oral glycemic agents or the patient with GDM, insulin therapy should be considered when nutritional therapy fails to keep FBG at or less than 95 mg/dL.
For patients with GDM, arrange for one-on-one teaching with a diabetes educator for the following: how to check blood sugars with a glucometer, how to document blood sugars, and the importance of exercise during pregnancy.	A one-on-one session with a diabetes educator experienced with GDM provides an opportunity for questions/interactions and greater patient comprehension.
Teach the patient and her significant others the signs and symptoms of hypoglycemia, hyperglycemia, diabetic ketoacidosis, and insulin shock. For more information, see "Diabetes Mellitus," p. 355, and "Diabetic Ketoacidosis," p. 365.	A knowledgeable patient likely will report these symptoms promptly. Although hPL causes tissue resistance (prolonging hyperglycemia after meals), during periods of fasting, blood glucose levels fall precipitously. Target blood sugar levels during pregnancy are lower to protect the fetus. Therefore, the patient is more likely to experience swings between hyperglycemia and hypoglycemia.
Develop a sick-day plan with the patient.	This information will help the patient maintain adequate glycemic control. For example, the patient should do the following: - Check blood sugar and urine for ketones q2-4h during illness. - Maintain normal insulin schedule. - Maintain normal meals when possible. Drink plenty of water and/or calorie-free liquids if unable to maintain solid foods. Consume a minimum of 150 g of carbohydrates per day, taken in small amounts over 24 hr. - Call the provider if temperature is 101°F (38.3°C) or greater, ketone level is moderate to high, or if vomiting and unable to keep anything down. - The patient may need to be hospitalized for intravenous (IV) fluids and regulation of blood sugar. - In diabetes associated with pregnancy, early detection of ketones is critical to fetal mortality because ketoacidosis is a significant factor that contributes to intrauterine death.

continued

ASSESSMENT/INTERVENTIONS	RATIONALES
Encourage the patient to maintain or initiate an exercise program.	Exercise improves both cardiopulmonary fitness and glucose metabolism.
Suggest that she have hard candy on hand when exercising.	Because moderate exercise increases glucose utilization, hypoglycemia can develop while exercising.
Teach daily fetal movement counts.	Fetal movement counts are a good first-line indicator of fetal well-being and are performed as follows, beginning at 28 wk gestation: The patient lies on her side and counts "distinct fetal movements" (hiccups do not count) daily; 10 movements within a 2-hr period is reassuring. After 10 movements are noted, the count is discontinued. Fewer than 10 movements indicates need for fetal nonstress testing.

Nursing Diagnosis:

Imbalanced Nutrition: Less Than Body Requirements/ More Than Body Requirements

related to inability to follow prescribed dietary regimen for effective glycemic control

Desired Outcome: The patient follows the prescribed dietary regimen.

ASSESSMENT/INTERVENTIONS	RATIONALES
Assess the patient's cultural habits surrounding diet (foods she can and cannot eat, who shops, who cooks) and exercise patterns.	Working within cultural habits aids in dietary adherence. For example, there may be high carbohydrate consumption, depending on her cultural group: rice for Asian women; tortillas and rice for Hispanic women; and breads and pasta for non-Hispanic white women.
Arrange for a meeting with a dietitian who specializes in diabetes in pregnancy.	A dietitian is trained to answer questions regarding specific foods and meal plans that are appropriate for glycemic control and can act as a resource person for the patient. Nutritional interventions should achieve normal glucose levels and avoid ketosis while maintaining appropriate nutrition and weight gain in pregnancy.
Encourage the patient to keep a daily dietary and exercise log.	A log provides a quick reference to compare blood sugars and foods eaten as well as the amount of exercise achieved on a given day. Exercise increases glucose utilization.
Praise the patient when blood sugars are within normal limits.	Good glycemic control reduces incidence of maternal and fetal morbidity and mortality.
Inform the patient of the risks to self and fetus associated with poor glycemic control related to dietary nonadherence.	Knowledge aids in adherence to the treatment plan. Dietary nonadherence can result in miscarriage, fetal anomalies, fetal macrosomia and increased risk of shoulder dystocia with a vaginal delivery, and increased potential for cesarean delivery.
Teach the patient with insulin-dependent diabetes that she may need to test blood glucose levels at bedtime and during the night.	During periods of fasting, hypoglycemia can develop more quickly when the woman is pregnant. Maternal blood glucose crosses the placental membrane and is taken into fetal circulation.
Teach the patient with type 1 DM to monitor urine with ketone testing strips and to test for ketonuria or ketonemia if becoming hyperglycemic or unwell.	Ketones are weak acids produced when blood sugar is poorly controlled and the body burns fat instead of sugar for energy. Moderate to large (2-4+) ketones may signal ketoacidosis, which necessitates immediate evaluation. If untreated, prolonged ketoacidosis can result in fetal brain damage.
Develop a "sick-day plan" with the patient.	See discussion in **Deficient Knowledge** related to the effects of diabetes on self, pregnancy, and fetus, earlier.

Nursing Diagnosis:

Fear

related to effects of GDM on self, pregnancy, and fetus; potential complications; and insulin injections

Desired Outcomes: Immediately following interventions, the patient and significant other express fears and concerns. Within 24 hr of interventions, the patient reports feeling greater psychologic comfort, understanding of the effects of diabetes on the pregnancy, and confidence in administering insulin if needed.

ASSESSMENT/INTERVENTIONS	RATIONALES
Assess for and encourage and support the patient and significant other in verbalizing their fears and concerns.	This validates their fears/concerns and enables development of an individualized care plan.
Acknowledge the patient's fears.	Acknowledging feelings in an empathetic manner encourages communication, which optimally will reduce fear. For example, "I understand that giving yourself injections frightens you, but it is necessary to control your blood sugar."
When appropriate and if available, involve Social Services in patient management. Provide a list of support groups available for patients with GDM.	Social Services can provide individual counseling and information on referrals, support groups, and Internet chat groups for patients with GDM. Some support groups are listed at the end of this care plan.
Encourage the patient to ask questions and become as knowledgeable as possible about her condition and treatment.	Increasing knowledge levels about appropriate dietary intake and blood sugar control reduces/eliminates fear of the unknown and affords a sense of control.
Teach the patient appropriate techniques for checking blood sugar, documenting results, and drawing up, injecting, and storing insulin (see "Diabetes Mellitus," p. 355).	This teaching provides an opportunity to assess and validate the patient's knowledge and fears. Knowledge likely will help decrease fear of self-administration of insulin and aid in compliance with treatments.

Nursing Diagnosis:

Anxiety

related to actual or perceived threat to self or fetus because of the effects diabetes may have on the pregnancy

Desired Outcome: Within 1-2 hr of intervention, the patient states that her anxiety has lessened or resolved, and she describes appropriate coping mechanisms in managing the anxiety.

ASSESSMENT/INTERVENTIONS	RATIONALES
Engage in honest communication with the patient; provide empathetic understanding. Listen closely.	This establishes an atmosphere that enables free expression.
Assess for verbal and nonverbal cues about the patient's anxiety level.	These cues aid in providing appropriate assistance and support. Levels of anxiety include: - *Mild:* restlessness, irritability, increased questions, focusing on the environment. - *Moderate:* inattentiveness, expressions of concern, narrowed perceptions, insomnia, increased heart rate. - *Severe:* expression of feelings of doom, rapid speech, tremors, poor eye contact. Patients may be preoccupied with the past or unable to understand the present and may have tachycardia, nausea, and hyperventilation. - *Panic:* inability to concentrate or communicate, distortion of reality, increased motor activity, vomiting, tachypnea.

continued

ASSESSMENT/INTERVENTIONS	RATIONALES
Explain that patients with poor glycemic control or who need to initiate first-time insulin use usually are admitted to the hospital for teaching and monitoring.	This offers the potential of a supportive environment that decreases anxiety and increases patient confidence.
Encourage the patient to communicate the cause of anxiety, for example, dietary changes, failure to maintain adequate glycemic control, checking blood sugars, insulin injections.	This information helps determine the patient's knowledge of diabetes in pregnancy and ways in which patient teaching can alleviate anxiety.
Provide reassurance and a safe, quiet environment for relaxation.	An anxious person has difficulty learning.
Assess at each appointment if the patient has enough supplies to maintain self-care.	Having adequate supplies (e.g., glucometer, test strips, lancets, record book, insulin, syringes, alcohol wipes, sharps disposal box) on hand may increase adherence to therapy and decrease anxiety.
Encourage the patient to attend diabetes classes and support groups for patients with diabetes.	Talking with others who had or are experiencing diabetes in pregnancy aids in establishing outside support resources. Some support groups are listed at the end of this care plan.
Inform the patient with GDM that although she has diabetes associated with the pregnancy, her efforts to return to an appropriate weight for height and body build (with a healthy diet and physical activity) can delay or prevent lifelong diabetes.	Having this information may alleviate anxiety and increase adherence to the therapeutic plan. Obesity is strongly associated with development of type 2 DM.
However, advise her that if she has other risk factors such as a first-line relative with a history of type 1 or type 2 DM, obesity, and a diet high in carbohydrates and fats, these factors can increase the risk for developing chronic DM during the next 10-15 yr.	This information identifies some factors over which she has control, which optimally will decrease anxiety and encourage weight loss, dietary control, and exercise postpartum to prevent future development of chronic DM.

Nursing Diagnosis:

Deficient Knowledge

related to unfamiliarity with benefits and potential side effects of prescribed medications used to treat GDM

Desired Outcome: Immediately following teaching, the patient and significant other verbalize accurate understanding of the risks and benefits of medications used during the pregnancy to treat diabetes.

ASSESSMENT/INTERVENTIONS	RATIONALES
Teach the following about the patient's prescribed medications:	A knowledgeable patient is more likely to adhere to the therapy, identify and report side effects, and recognize and report precautions that might preclude use of the prescribed drug.
Sulfonylureas: Second-Generation	These agents lower blood glucose by stimulating release of insulin from the pancreas.
Glucophage (Metformin) **Glyburide (Micronase, DiaBeta, Euglucon)**	Metformin is currently the preferred oral glycemic agent. Patients on all other glycemic agents are encouraged to switch, although glyburide has been shown to be safe and effective in GDM. There is concern for teratogenicity with other oral agents. Most patients with type 2 DM who have been managed on oral agents are changed to insulin during the pregnancy. Administration: PO.
Teach the patient to be alert for and report shakiness, sweating, nervousness, headache, and blood sugar level less than 60 mg/dL.	These are signs of hypoglycemia.

ASSESSMENT/INTERVENTIONS	RATIONALES
Teach the patient to be alert for and report blurred vision.	This is a side effect caused by fluctuation in blood glucose levels.
Stress the importance of monitoring blood glucose levels as directed.	This helps detect hypoglycemia or hyperglycemia promptly. The usual routine in pregnancy is to monitor blood glucose fasting (first thing in the morning before breakfast or taking medications), 2 hr after eating, at bedtime, and when glucose levels have been low or high. Poor glycemic control when taking the oral agent necessitates initiation of insulin.
Teach the patient to be alert for and report nausea, epigastric fullness, and heartburn.	These are adverse reactions. If these reactions occur consistently, the patient may require dose adjustment or be started on insulin—whichever maintains glycemic control.
⚠ Caution patients taking nonsteroidal antiinflammatory drugs (NSAIDs) and beta-adrenergic blocking agents to notify the health care provider before taking sulfonylureas.	The hypoglycemic reaction may be potentiated by these medications.
Insulin	Insulin is the gold standard for glycemic control. It is more protective for perinatal mortality than the oral hypoglycemic agents.
Regular Humalog and Lispro (Rapid Acting), NPH (Intermediate Acting)	These are parenteral blood glucose–lowering agents that regulate glucose metabolism. Lispro has a more rapid onset of action than regular insulin and does not cross the placenta. Administration: subcutaneous or by insulin pump. Some patients may be started on subcutaneous insulin as an outpatient. This choice is individualized based on patient adherence and comprehension of insulin therapy (drawing up insulin, injecting accurately, and timing doses). Inpatient setting is required for initial teaching for how to use the pump, including monitoring of glucose levels and making necessary insulin dose adjustments.
Teach the patient to be alert for and report shakiness, sweating, nervousness, headache, and low blood sugar levels.	These are signs of hypoglycemia, a potential side effect. Some patients may be symptomatic between 60 and 70 mg/dL and others not until 50-60 mg/dL (or lower).
Teach the patient to be alert for and report blurred vision.	This is a side effect secondary to fluctuations in blood glucose levels.
Stress the importance of monitoring blood glucose levels as directed.	This aids in prompt identification of hypoglycemic reactions.
⚠ Caution patients taking NSAIDs, salicylates, and beta-adrenergic blocking agents to notify their health care provider.	Insulin requirements may be decreased when also taking drugs with hypoglycemic activity. Beta-blockers may mask the symptoms of hypoglycemia and alter glucose metabolism.
Caution patients taking terbutaline to notify their health care providers.	Terbutaline is used to decrease uterine myometrial activity (contractions). Beta-sympathomimetics, such as terbutaline can cause hyperglycemia, and their use is not usually recommended for patients with diabetes.

ADDITIONAL NURSING DIAGNOSES/PROBLEMS:

"Psychosocial Support" for relevant nursing diagnoses such as **Ineffective Coping**   p. 75

"Psychosocial Support for the Patient's Family and Significant Other" for such nursing diagnoses as **Compromised Family Coping**   p. 86

"Diabetes Mellitus"   p. 355

"Diabetic Ketoacidosis"   p. 365

✓ PATIENT-FAMILY TEACHING AND DISCHARGE PLANNING

Patients with GDM require close monitoring for maternal and fetal well-being. Education is the key to making the pregnancy a success. When providing patient-family teaching, avoid giving excessive information. Part of the initial assessment should include asking about existing knowledge of the disease, ability for self-management, and psychologic acceptance. Include written and verbal information about the following:

✓ Recommended glucose levels in pregnancy: Fasting, 60-90 mg/dL; before lunch, dinner, or bedtime snack, 60-105 mg/dL; 2-hr pp, 120 mg/dL or less.

✓ Reminder that stress from illness or infection can increase insulin requirements.

✓ Recognizing warning signs of both hyperglycemia and simple and advanced hypoglycemia and insulin shock, treatment, and factors that contribute to both conditions.

- *Hyperglycemia:* Possible causes include not enough insulin or increased insulin resistance (as seen with advancing gestational age), too much food, stress of illness, emotional stress, and decreased exercise. Patients should call the health care provider for treatment, which may include increasing insulin dose and/or self-administering an insulin bolus.

- *Hypoglycemia:* Possible causes are too much insulin, too little food, not eating on time, vomiting, and too much exercise. (See next three items for treatment options.)
  - Review "Diabetes Mellitus," p. 355, for further information.
  - Foods to treat hypoglycemia such as 4-oz orange juice, 4-oz milk, 4-oz cola drink (not diet cola), 3-4 pieces of hard candy, 3-4 sugar cubes, 2-3 glucose tablets.
  - How and when to take glucose tablets. The patient should keep glucose tablets with her when away from home and available food sources. Instruct the patient to use glucose tablets if becoming shaky, nauseated, nervous, headachy, drowsy, and diaphoretic and blood sugar is 60 mg/dL or less.

✓ When to call for emergency services. With advanced hypoglycemia (blood sugar 20-50 mg/dL) the patient may not be the person calling in an emergency situation; this information needs to be communicated to the significant other and family members as well.

✓ Importance of carrying an identification card or wearing a bracelet or necklace that identifies the patient as having diabetes in case of emergency. For patients with GDM, the necklace or bracelet may be obtained at a local pharmacy. If the patient has preexisting diabetes, the above information may be obtained by contacting the following organization: MedicAlert Foundation, 323 Colorado Avenue, Turlock, CA 96382, (209) 668-3333.

✓ Importance of adherence to the prescribed health care plan and ready access to hospital and family/social support.

✓ Parameters and guidelines for blood sugar levels as recommended by the health care provider.

✓ Nutritional regimen as recommended by the health care provider. Adequate nutrition and controlled calories are essential to maintaining normoglycemia and appropriate fetal growth.

✓ Medications, including drug name, purpose, dosage, frequency, precautions, administration, and potential side effects. Also discuss potential drug-drug, food-drug, and herb-drug interactions.

✓ How to monitor urine for ketones.

✓ Fetal movement counts (gestational age appropriate).

✓ Referrals to local and national support organizations, including:

- American Diabetes Association (ADA) at *www.diabetes.org*
- The Canadian Diabetes Association at *www.diabetes.ca*
- Sidelines, a national support organization for women and their families experiencing complicated pregnancies, at *www.sidelines.org*
- Joslin Diabetes Center at *www.joslin.harvard.edu*

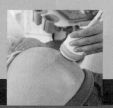

OVERVIEW/PATHOPHYSIOLOGY

Nausea and vomiting are common symptoms of unknown cause in the first trimester of pregnancy. Although mildly or moderately distressing, they do not cause metabolic imbalance. Hyperemesis gravidarum is a rare condition of excessive vomiting in pregnancy that causes weight loss of 5% or more from prepregnancy weight, dehydration, electrolyte imbalance, acidosis from starvation, and alkalosis from loss of hydrochloric acid. This condition usually begins during the first trimester, after which vomiting becomes intractable and may last throughout the entire pregnancy. The cause is unknown, but theories include rising estrogen and human chorionic gonadotropin (hCG) levels, displacement of the gastrointestinal (GI) tract, decreased motility caused by an increase in progesterone, decrease in motilin levels, *Helicobacter pylori (H. pylori)* infection, and psychogenic factors. Affected women may face multiple disruptions of work, family, and social responsibilities because of the debilitating nature of the condition and repeated hospitalization. Goals of treatment include control of nausea and vomiting, correction of dehydration, restoration of electrolyte balance, and maintenance of adequate nutrition to optimize maternal and fetal/newborn outcomes.

HEALTH CARE SETTING

Patients are often treated on an outpatient basis with oral medications, home intravenous (IV) infusion therapy to replace fluids and electrolytes, or total parenteral nutrition. Approximately 1%-5% of women who develop hyperemesis gravidarum require multiple hospitalizations.

ASSESSMENT

The first priority of care is to determine severity of the nausea and vomiting problem in patients who can no longer retain solids or liquids as well as the degree of dehydration and weight loss. Laboratory studies are prescribed to identify electrolyte imbalances. Patients may exhibit a low-grade fever, increased pulse rate, decreased blood pressure, weakness, dry skin, cracked lips, and poor skin turgor. Patients may appear extremely fatigued and listless with a possible loss of 5%-10% of total body weight, be constipated as a result of dehydration, and have a markedly decreased urinary output with ketonemia (presence of ketones in the blood). Women with diabetes who have hyperemesis need to be monitored closely to maintain glycemic control and avoid ketoacidosis. See "Diabetes in Pregnancy," p. 648.

Gastrointestinal: GI motility is reduced because of increased progesterone and decreased motilin levels. "Normal" nausea and vomiting of pregnancy usually has an onset between 4 and 6 wk, peaks at about the 12th wk, and resolves between 16 to 20 wk. Hyperemesis usually begins in the first trimester but may extend throughout the entire pregnancy.

Fluid and electrolyte imbalance: With the inability to maintain adequate fluids for hydration and solids for fuel and nutrients, the body experiences an imbalance of the elements necessary for health maintenance, which can lead to maternal ketosis.

Cardiopulmonary: The patient may experience one or all of the following: tachycardia, hypotension, postural changes, and tachypnea.

Renal: Possible presence of oliguria and ketonuria.

Complications—fetal: With prolonged dehydration and maternal weight loss, fetal intrauterine growth restriction (IUGR), prematurity, low birth weight, and lower Apgar scores may be seen.

Physical assessment: The pregnant patient with hyperemesis looks debilitated and is ill. She is extremely fatigued and pale. A thorough systems assessment is needed to rule out other causes of severe nausea and vomiting, such as gastroenteritis, cholecystitis, pyelonephritis, GI ulcers, or a molar pregnancy (intrauterine benign or neoplastic mass of grapelike vesicles of trophoblastic cells—the embryonic cells that form the chorion).

Risk factors: Previous history of hyperemesis, molar pregnancy, multiple gestation, emotional/psychologic stress, gastroesophageal reflux, primigravida, uncontrolled thyroid disease, increased body weight/obesity.

DIAGNOSTIC TESTS

Urine chemistry: The most important initial laboratory test is urine dipstick measurement of ketonuria (or a specimen may be sent for microscopic urinalysis). Ketones are present with cellular starvation and dehydration from prolonged vomiting.

Complete blood count (CBC): With dehydration, there likely will be evidence of hemoconcentration (i.e., elevated red blood cell and hematocrit levels).

Serum chemistry: Azotemia (increased blood urea nitrogen [BUN]) is seen with salt and water depletion. Serum creatinine will be elevated because of changes in renal function caused by dehydration. Hyponatremia and hypokalemia also may be present because of fluid loss.

Liver enzymes: Slight elevations of aspartate aminotransferase and alanine aminotransferase reverse with IV fluid hydration, adequate nutrition, and cessation of vomiting.

Obstetric ultrasound: Ultrasound is used to evaluate a normal intrauterine pregnancy versus a molar pregnancy, presence of multiple gestation, fetal growth for IUGR, and amniotic fluid volume/amniotic fluid index (AFI).

Results for CBC, electrolyte panel, laboratory tests for liver enzymes and bilirubin levels, and kidney function: Help to rule out the presence of underlying diseases previously listed.

Nursing Diagnoses:

Deficient Fluid Volume
Risk for Electrolyte Imbalance

related to excessive gastric losses and reduced intravascular and intercellular fluid occurring with nausea and vomiting

Desired Outcome: Within 24 hr after initiation of treatment, the patient begins to show signs of adequate hydration, as evidenced by decreased emesis, balanced intake and output, and improvement in acid-base balance and electrolyte status.

ASSESSMENT/INTERVENTIONS	RATIONALES
Assess characteristics of the patient's nausea/vomiting: frequency, duration, and severity; amount and color of vomitus; accompanying symptoms (abdominal pain, diarrhea, dyspepsia [a vague feeling of discomfort or bloating after eating]); and precipitating factors. Reassess q8h or as indicated.	This comprehensive initial assessment provides a basis for nursing interventions/teaching and a subsequent comparison for changes.
Assess for signs of dehydration: dry mucous membranes, poor skin turgor, decreased blood pressure (BP), increased pulse, possible low-grade fever, and increases in urine specific gravity, BUN, and hematocrit.	With fluid losses, blood and urine become concentrated, circulating blood volume decreases, BP may decrease, and the heart rate increases to compensate.
Assess for signs of electrolyte imbalance q8h (muscle weakness, cramps, irritability, irregular heartbeats), and monitor results of the prescribed laboratory studies.	Potassium and magnesium are lost with prolonged vomiting. Muscles, including the myocardium, are weakened by the loss of these electrolytes. Severe potassium loss impacts the kidneys' ability to concentrate urine.
Initiate and monitor IV hydration, including electrolyte replacement, while keeping the patient NPO (nothing by mouth) for 48 hr, as prescribed by the health care provider.	This approach aids in resting GI motility, resolving dehydration, and improving electrolyte balance caused by intractable vomiting.
Administer parenteral nutrition as prescribed by the health care provider. Secure the assistance of the hyperalimentation team to manage the patient's nutrition.	Total nutritional needs can be met with parenteral nutrition, thereby helping ensure adequate fetal growth and preventing maternal malnutrition.
Encourage the patient to take approximately 100 mL (e.g., in 1-oz portions qh) of liquid between each meal and avoid fluids with meals.	This measure prevents dehydration between meals and over-distension of the stomach during meals, allowing more space for caloric foods, and may prevent nausea.

Nursing Diagnosis:

Imbalanced Nutrition: Less Than Body Requirements

related to inability to ingest, digest, and absorb sufficient nutrients and calories because of prolonged vomiting.

Desired Outcome: Within 1 wk of diagnosis, the patient increases her nutritional intake and demonstrates improvement in her acid-base balance, electrolytes, and nutritional status.

ASSESSMENT/INTERVENTIONS	RATIONALES
Assess weight at admission (or initial encounter), and document daily morning weight on the same scale. Compare with prepregnant weight, and monitor continued weight loss or gain.	Weight changes indicate progress with treatment and resolution of the condition or severity of losses and risk of maternal and fetal malnutrition.

ASSESSMENT/INTERVENTIONS	RATIONALES
Assess for signs of starvation q8h (e.g., jaundice, bleeding from mucous membranes, and ketonuria).	Insufficient nutrition may cause hypothrombinemia, depleted vitamin C and B complexes, and ketosis.
Initiate and titrate enteral (nasogastric) feeding or hyperalimentation (parenteral nutrition by intravascular therapy) as prescribed by the health care provider and agency protocols.	These are effective methods with which to administer nutrients and hydration when oral ingestion of food and fluids is not possible.
Start the patient on oral intake when acute nausea resolves, beginning as prescribed with clear liquids (broth and bland juices) and advancing to solid foods as tolerated.	Because an individual tolerates liquids and foods differently, it is important to gradually test which food(s) and pattern of eating is better tolerated.
Suggest alternative dietary patterns (e.g., frequent small and dry meals, six or more per day, followed by clear liquids).	Small, frequent, dry meals may reduce nausea and vomiting from a distended stomach.
Suggest eating meals with the highest protein/calorie intake when the nausea is the least problematic, possibly within 30 min to 1 hr after taking medication for nausea and vomiting.	When the meal providing the most nutrition is consumed at the time the patient is most likely to retain it, the patient may be able to absorb higher protein and nutrient levels necessary for pregnancy.
Suggest high-protein supplemental beverages.	Liquids may be easier to tolerate than solid foods.
As indicated, suggest that the patient avoid food odors and foods that are greasy, highly spiced, rich, or overly sweet.	These measures prevent stimulating the gag reflex or increasing acid reflux. However, because some individuals prefer salty and spicy foods, the patient should try anything that is appealing and that she believes she will be able to keep down.
Encourage the patient to stay upright for 2 hr after eating.	This prevents esophageal spasms that can be caused by reflux of acid and food into the esophagus. Gravity aids in facilitating movement of food through the esophagus to the stomach and into the small intestine.
Administer prescribed therapies for nausea, e.g., ginger or ginger syrup; antiemetic medications such as pyridoxine (vitamin B₆), metoclopramide (Reglan), or promethazine (Phenergan).	These therapies are known to decrease nausea and may enable the patient to ingest and retain fluid and food nutrients, vitamins, proteins, carbohydrates, and fats from oral intake.
Refer for acupuncture as prescribed by the health care provider to stimulate the median nerve at the PC6 point, or encourage the patient to wear an acupressure wristband.	Acupuncture at this site acts on the GI system. Many women report less nausea and vomiting with the wristband.

Nursing Diagnosis:
Anxiety
related to actual or perceived threat to self and fetus because of inadequate nutritional status and increasing debilitation from prolonged vomiting

Desired Outcome: Within 1-2 hr of intervention, the patient verbalizes her anxieties, assesses her support system(s), and uses appropriate coping mechanisms for management of self and family needs.

ASSESSMENT/INTERVENTIONS	RATIONALES
Establish a therapeutic relationship with honest nurse-patient communication, unconditional positive regard, active listening, and empathetic understanding.	Fostering a trusting relationship promotes the patient's ability to assess her feelings, discuss her situation, and freely express her needs and concerns.
Encourage the patient to develop self-awareness and communicate cause(s) of her anxiety.	Self-awareness and the ability to communicate anxiety and characteristics of her situation aid in developing a care plan specific to her needs, such as whether home or hospital treatment will be more helpful. Examples of causes that may be contributing to the patient's anxiety include weight loss, frustration with constant nausea and vomiting, ambivalence about the pregnancy, fear for the well-being of the preborn baby, lack of support from significant other and family, inability to care for self or others, and loss of income if unable to work.

continued

ASSESSMENT/INTERVENTIONS	RATIONALES
Assist with making arrangements for entering the hospital, if prescribed by the health care provider, or arrange for assistance of the medical social worker (MSW) as soon as possible after admission, per hospital protocol.	Patients with severe nausea and vomiting who demonstrate changes in laboratory values and weight loss should be admitted to the hospital for hydration, nutritional supplementation, medications, and monitoring of weight loss or gain. This assistance will provide a supportive environment that decreases anxiety and increases the patient's comfort.
Be alert for verbal and nonverbal cues about the patient's anxiety level.	These cues aid in providing appropriate assistance and support. Levels of anxiety include: - *Mild:* restlessness, irritability, increased questions, focusing on the environment. - *Moderate:* inattentiveness, expressions of concern, narrowed perceptions, insomnia, increased heart rate. - *Severe:* expression of feelings of doom, rapid speech, tremors, and poor eye contact. The patient may be preoccupied with the past or unable to understand the present and may have tachycardia, increased nausea and vomiting, and hyperventilation. - *Panic:* inability to concentrate or communicate, distortion of reality, increased motor activity, increased vomiting and tachypnea.
Refer to Social Services when available to assist with psychosocial needs and discharge planning.	Social Services provides counseling, support, and resources for written material. Other options include Internet chat groups, which enable communication with others who are experiencing similar circumstances, as well as other resources within the community.
In collaboration with the health care provider, refer to a psychologist as needed.	A psychologist enables evaluation for possible psychologic factors that may be contributing to the anxiety and hyperemesis. Supportive counseling or intervention may be beneficial in identifying the cause.
Involve assistance from the hospital chaplain or the patient's personal spiritual/religious advisor if the patient desires.	Pastoral care and sharing of concerns with a trusted spiritual advisor may decrease anxiety and provide continuity of support after hospital discharge.
Assist the patient to have undisturbed sleep, and provide a quiet, restful environment free of odors that cause discomfort.	Rest enhances coping mechanisms by decreasing physical and psychologic stress. The nurse can coordinate treatment interventions and visitation around the patient's need for rest.

Nursing Diagnosis:

Ineffective Coping

related to loss of control over changing health status, changing role with her family's needs, and maintenance of adequate nutritional intake

Desired Outcome: Within the 24-hr period after diagnosis is made, the patient verbalizes her concerns, fears, strengths, and weaknesses and identifies personal coping mechanisms and support systems.

ASSESSMENT/INTERVENTIONS	RATIONALES
Establish honest and empathetic communication with the patient.	Empathy and honesty promote effective communication. For example, "Please tell me what I can do to help you through this stressful time in your pregnancy."
Assess the patient's stressors and perceptions and ability to understand her current health status.	Evaluation of the factors that stress the patient as well as her perceptions and comprehension level enable mutual development of an individualized care plan.
Identify the patient's support systems. If possible, assess their interactions with the patient and assist with development of a family plan to adapt to daily living changes.	Involvement of the family unit enables identification of strengths and weaknesses and aids in planning the patient's care, thereby reducing stress and promoting effective coping.

ASSESSMENT/INTERVENTIONS	RATIONALES
Discuss the patient's cultural beliefs that impact her present situation, decision-making abilities, and previous methods of coping with life problems.	Cultural beliefs positively or negatively impact her ability to handle her condition. Maximizing her participation in planning and home management increases successful planning. Previous styles and successes with problems in the past may empower the patient and be reliable predictors of how she will cope with current problems.
Enlist assistance from MSW, dietitian, and spiritual support individuals as indicated.	The MSW can follow the patient after hospital discharge, knows community resources, and is trained to assist with financial and psychosocial needs. The dietitian develops parenteral and oral diet plans to enhance the patient's ability to ingest, digest, and absorb fuels and nutrients. Spiritual support, related to the patient's spiritual/religious preferences, assists with finding meaning and hopefulness in a debilitating situation.
Teach the patient how to effectively use her time when she feels well (e.g., performing activities of daily living or doing errands).	This information will give some sense of control over her situation while also promoting involvement with her larger life and family.

Nursing Diagnosis:

Deficient Knowledge

related to unfamiliarity with the effects hyperemesis has on self, the pregnancy, her fetus, and family; the treatment; and expected outcomes of care

Desired Outcome: Immediately following teaching, the patient, family, and significant others verbalize accurate knowledge about hyperemesis, its treatment, and the expected outcome.

ASSESSMENT/INTERVENTIONS	RATIONALES
Assess the patient's and family's knowledge and past experiences with hyperemesis. As indicated, explain the effect hyperemesis has on the patient and the fetus.	Hyperemesis causes decreased maternal-fetal placental transfer of nutrients and IUGR. Information motivates adherence to treatments and enables understanding of possible consequences from nonadherence.
Explain the various treatment options, as described in earlier nursing diagnoses.	Treatments may include intravenous (IV) hydration, medications (IV, intramuscular [IM], by mouth [PO]), total parenteral nutrition, home care, and hospitalization. Explanation of treatment options helps the patient and health care provider decide on a care plan that is most beneficial to the patient and fetus.
Teach signs and symptoms that may indicate worsening hyperemesis and dehydration (e.g., inability to keep solids or liquids down for the previous 12 hr, dizziness, extreme fatigue, poor skin turgor, caramel-colored urine, and weight loss).	A knowledgeable patient likely will report symptoms promptly. Early evaluation and treatment may decrease severity of the condition.
Explain expected outcomes that adequate fluid and nutritional intake will have on fetal development (i.e., it will increase maternal fetal placental transfer of nutrients and optimize intrauterine fetal growth).	This information reinforces need for the patient's adherence to possible hospitalization or home infusion, IV fluids, or parenteral nutrition.
Encourage the patient to avoid brushing her teeth within 1-2 hr after meals or on arising in the morning.	This action may stimulate the gag reflex and aggravate vomiting in women who are pregnant.
Encourage good daily oral hygiene after vomiting bouts.	This prevents dental decay that may accompany contact with the acids present in emesis and for some may help decrease nausea. For example, the patient may use mouthwash and brush and floss teeth when she feels the least nauseated.

Nursing Diagnosis:

Deficient Knowledge

related to unfamiliarity with the purpose, potential side effects, and safety of prescribed medications and nonprescribed devices used during hyperemesis gravidarum

Desired Outcome: Immediately following teaching, the patient verbalizes accurate understanding of the risks, benefits, and precautions of medications used during pregnancy in the treatment of hyperemesis.

ASSESSMENT/INTERVENTIONS	RATIONALES
Teach the following about the patient's prescribed medications:	A knowledgeable patient is more likely to adhere to the therapy, identify and report significant side effects, and recognize and report precautions that might preclude use of the prescribed medication.
Metoclopramide Hydrochloride (Reglan)	This is an antiemetic that works on the chemoreceptor trigger zone in the brain to decrease nausea and vomiting. It helps move food through the GI tract, counteracting the effects of progesterone produced at higher levels in pregnancy. Reglan may be given inpatient or outpatient. Administration: PO/IM/IV.
Caution the patient to be alert for and report twitching of the eyelids or muscles surrounding the eyes, hands, or legs.	These are extrapyramidal reactions seen with high IV doses.
Caution the patient to be alert for and report involuntary repetitious movements of the muscles of the face, limbs, and trunk.	This is a sign of tardive dyskinesia (a syndrome of potentially irreversible involuntary repetitious movements) and a serious side effect seen with long-term use.
Teach the patient to be alert for and report drowsiness, agitation, seizures, hallucinations, lactation, constipation, and diarrhea.	These are common side effects.
Explain that caution is necessary in patients with seizure disorders.	This medication may lower the seizure threshold.
Explain that caution is necessary in patients taking this medication with sedatives, narcotics, and tranquilizers.	Additive sedative effects may occur.
Pantoprazole (Protonix)	Antiulcer/proton pump inhibitor. Administration: PO/IV.
Teach the patient to be alert for and report diarrhea, stomach pain, loss of appetite, headache, heartburn, muscle pain, skin rash, and drowsiness.	These are possible side effects. Patients should avoid activities that require alertness until the medication's effect on the central nervous system (CNS) is known.
Caution the patient to be alert for and report weakness, sore throat, fever, sores on mouth, unusual bruising, cloudy or bloody urine, difficult or painful urination.	These are rare but serious side effects that necessitate discontinuance of the medication.
Explain that caution is necessary in patients taking anticoagulants.	This medication increases their anticoagulant effect.
Promethazine (Phenergan)	Antiemetic/antihistamine/tranquilizer. Administration: PO/IV/IM/rectal.
Teach the patient to be alert for and report sedation, blurred vision, fatigue, ringing in the ears, nervousness, insomnia, and tremors.	These are common side effects. Patients should avoid activities that require alertness until the medication's effect on the CNS is known.
Explain that precautions are needed for patients taking other CNS depressants such as opioids.	Medication interactions can occur, necessitating a lower dose of opioids.
Caution the patient to be alert for and report involuntary movements and decreased BP.	Extrapyramidal reactions (involuntary movements) and hypotension are seen with rapid IV administration.

ASSESSMENT/INTERVENTIONS	RATIONALES
Teach the patient to be alert for and report dry mouth and blurred vision.	These are anticholinergic side effects.
Explain that caution is necessary in patients taking monoamine oxidase (MAO) inhibitors.	Medication interactions can occur, causing increased incidence of extrapyramidal reactions.

[!] Prochlorperazine (Compazine)

Antiemetic.
Administration: PO/IM/IV/rectal.

Teach the patient to be alert for and report blurred vision, fatigue, ringing in the ears, nervousness, insomnia, and tremors.	These are common CNS side effects. Patients should avoid activities that require alertness until the medication's effect on the CNS is known.
Explain that precautions are needed for patients taking other CNS depressants such as narcotics.	Medication interactions can occur, necessitating decreasing the opioid dose by half.
Caution the patient to be alert for and report involuntary movements and decreased BP.	Extrapyramidal reactions and hypotension are seen with IV administration.
Teach the patient to be alert for and report heart palpitations, seizures, dry mouth, constipation, and urinary retention.	These are less common side effects.

[!] Ondansetron (Zofran)

Antiemetic.
Administration: PO/IM/IV.

Teach the patient to be alert for and report pain, redness, and burning at the site of injection.	These signs can occur as a local reaction with IM injection or IV infiltration.
Teach the patient to be alert for and report headache, fever, constipation, and diarrhea.	These are common side effects.
Caution the patient to be alert for and report involuntary movements.	Extrapyramidal reactions are rare CNS side effects.
Caution the patient to be alert for and report rapid heart rate, dizziness, feeling faint, and chest pain.	These are cardiac side effects.
Explain that caution is necessary in patients with liver disease.	Liver clearance of this medication is reduced in patients with hepatic impairment.

Doxylamine (Unisom Nighttime Sleep Aid)

Antihistamine. It may be used as an antiemetic with mild symptoms of nausea and vomiting caused by pregnancy. It is often used in combination with pyridoxine (vitamin B_6).
Administration: PO.

Teach the patient that sedation can occur.	This is a common side effect. The patient needs to avoid activities that require alertness until the medication's effect on the CNS is known.

Pyridoxine (Vitamin B_6)

It may be used as an antiemetic for mild symptoms of nausea and vomiting in pregnancy. It is often used in combination with doxylamine (Unisom).
Administration: PO.

Caution the patient to be alert for and report nausea, headache, and numbness or tingling in hands or feet.	These are rare but serious side effects and necessitate discontinuance of the medication.

Diphenhydramine (Benadryl)

This antihistamine can be used as an antiemetic, reducing nausea and vomiting in mild cases. It also may be given in combination with droperidol (Inapsine).
Administration: PO, IV

Teach the patient of the potential for mild drowsiness and dry mouth.	These are common side effects.

continued

PART III: Maternity Nursing Care Plans

ASSESSMENT/INTERVENTIONS	RATIONALES
Droperidol (Inapsine)	Antidopaminergic, sedative. Administration: IM, IV
Teach the patient of the potential for sedation.	This is a common side effect. The patient needs to avoid activities that require alertness until the medication's effect on the CNS is known.
Caution the patient to be alert for and report involuntary movements.	These extrapyramidal symptoms are rare but have been reported.
Explain that caution is necessary when standing or changing position.	Hypotension may occur.
Motion Sickness Band	This motion sickness device is worn on both wrists, applying gentle pressure to acupressure points on the wrists. It is available without a prescription and comes in various brands; some are battery operated.

ADDITIONAL NURSING DIAGNOSES/PROBLEMS:

✓ PATIENT-FAMILY TEACHING AND DISCHARGE PLANNING

Include verbal and written information about the following:
- ✓ Possible causes and effect hyperemesis has on the pregnancy and fetus.
- ✓ Signs and symptoms the patient should report to her health care provider.
- ✓ Treatment interventions and medications for hyperemesis gravidarum.
- ✓ Importance of attaining as much rest as possible.
- ✓ Nutritional options that would be most beneficial to the patient.
- ✓ Importance of eating small, frequent meals during the day.
- ✓ Importance and timing of oral hydration.
- ✓ Importance of avoiding lying down or reclining for 2 hr after eating.
- ✓ If parenteral nutrition is needed, the importance of maintaining insertion site and reporting any signs of site infection and pump malfunction.
- ✓ Importance of frequent clinic visits if being monitored on an outpatient basis and the date and time of the next clinic visit.
- ✓ Importance of informing the health care provider of any physical and emotional changes that may exacerbate the hyperemesis.
- ✓ Medications, including drug name, purpose, dosage, frequency, precautions, and potential side effects. Also explain relevant food-drug and herb-drug interactions.
- ✓ Importance of monitoring fetal well-being with ultrasound and nonstress test (NST).
- ✓ Referral to local and national support organizations, including Sidelines, a national support organization for women and their families experiencing complicated pregnancies, at *www.sidelines.org*.
- ✓ Patient education materials may be found at:
  - The American Congress of Obstetricians and Gynecologists has an extensive collection of patient education materials available at *www.acog.org/Resources_And_Publications/Patient_Education_FAQs_List*
  - The Society of Obstetricians and Gynecologists of Canada at *http://sogc.org* (requires subscription)

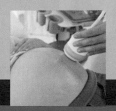

Postpartum Wound Infection 91

OVERVIEW/PATHOPHYSIOLOGY

Wound infection is one of the postpartum (puerperal) infections that can develop after childbirth. Puerperal infection is a leading cause of maternal death worldwide. In the United States the infection rate for patients with a cesarean delivery is approximately 10%-15%, whereas it is approximately 2% for patients who give birth vaginally. Prophylactic antibiotic therapy is common for women undergoing cesarean section or having a vaginal delivery who experience a fourth-degree laceration. Wound infections after childbirth can develop anywhere there is a break in the skin or mucous membranes to provide a portal of entry for bacteria. Wound infections are classified as early onset (within 48 hr) or late onset (after the first 48 hr) and develop from endogenous or exogenous bacteria. When identified early, most postpartum wound infections can be successfully treated with antibiotic therapy. Late-onset wounds may require incision and drainage, wound débridement, and multiple antibiotic therapy. Wound cultures may be necessary to identify the causative organism. When there is little to no improvement in wound site infection with first-choice antibiotics, methicillin-resistant *Staphylococcus aureus* (MRSA) infection must be considered and treated appropriately and aggressively.

The definition for puerperal infection centers on fever. A diagnosis is established with a fever of 38°C (100.4°F) or higher in 2 of the first 10 days postpartum, not including the first 24 hr (when dehydration and the exertion of labor can contribute to a low-grade fever).

The following are other types of postpartum infections:

Endometritis: An infection of the endometrium is the most common postpartum infection. It usually starts at the open site of placental attachment. It can spread easily through the interconnected genital tract or to a wound.

Urinary tract infection ([UTI] or cystitis): Bladder infections readily respond to antibiotics when identified early. Postpartum women with diabetes, women who have been catheterized, and women with lacerations extending into the urethral meatus are most at risk for UTI.

Mastitis: Infections of the breast usually involve one breast, manifest about 2 wk after delivery, and are usually preventable with good hand hygiene, frequent feedings with adequate transfer of milk, and daily variation of the newborn's feeding positions at the breast. If left untreated, mastitis may become an abscess.

Septic pelvic thrombophlebitis: Patients generally do not appear ill and may have minimal to no pain. A patient who persistently has a fever and does not respond to multiple antibiotic therapies may have this condition. Treatment includes both anticoagulant and antibiotic therapy.

HEALTH CARE SETTING

Primary care (outpatient clinic), acute care (hospital), or home care; rehospitalization is common.

ASSESSMENT

Assessments of the wound and other systemic signs of infection are necessary for all postpartum patients. Assess the postcesarean patient and those with other risk factors more frequently to monitor and report early signs of infection. The defining characteristics of wound infection are fever, pain or tenderness, edema, redness (erythema) surrounding the wound, induration (hardened tissue under the skin), purulent drainage, and separation of wound edges or wound dehiscence.

Cardiopulmonary: Tachycardia, hypotension, tachypnea, or syncope may be seen in the acutely ill patient when sepsis is present.

Fever: The temperature pattern may vary with the type of infection. It may be 101°F (38.3°C) or higher, with or without spiking episodes. With mild infection the patient may remain afebrile. Headache and overall "body aches" may accompany fever.

Chills: The patient may feel she cannot get warm even in the presence of an elevated temperature. Body shakes may accompany the chills. An overall flulike feeling may be present.

Malaise: A feeling of generalized uneasiness, discomfort, and fatigue may be present.

Pain: Pain may be present with light or deep external palpation of the abdomen or wound site, or with bimanual palpation of the uterus. Cervical motion tenderness on bimanual exam may be present with a uterine infection. With an episiotomy infection, pain may be localized (throbbing, aching, or sharp) and deep tissue in nature. The patient may describe a sensation of vaginal pressure or "fullness."

Vaginal discharge: With an episiotomy infection, discharge may be purulent. It may be foul smelling if endometritis coexists with the infected episiotomy.

Abdominal surgical incision: The area around the incision is often erythematous and warm to the touch, and it may become edematous. If the tissue is very congested (indurated), it may have a "woody" appearance and feel hard to palpation. If the wound is not already open and draining bloody, serosanguineous, or purulent discharge, it may be probed with a cotton-tipped applicator to promote drainage. Dehiscence may or may not occur.

Episiotomy or perineal laceration: A thorough wound assessment may be guided by the acronym "REEDA" to monitor localized redness (erythema), edema, ecchymosis (bruising), drainage (exudates), and approximation of skin edges. Dehiscence of the episiotomy may or may not occur. Any episiotomy or laceration, whether infected or not, interrupts tissue integrity and can lead to stress incontinence, pelvic floor prolapse, anal incontinence, and pelvic floor muscle dysfunction.

Complications—neonatal: If the maternal infection is caused by an antepartum uterine infection (chorioamnionitis), the neonate is at increased risk for infection or sepsis and generally would be admitted to the intensive care nursery (ICN) for close and careful monitoring. Group B streptococcus is the leading cause of newborn sepsis. When an infection appears in the newborn, it usually manifests as pneumonia and/or meningitis within the first 24 hr of life. The presentation is fulminant and the neonate deteriorates rapidly. Untreated, the infant mortality rate is high. A late-onset GBS infection typically presents as meningitis after 7-10 days. Mortality rate is low; however, survivors have significant neurologic sequelae.

Physical assessment: Not every patient with a wound infection looks or feels acutely ill. Some mild infections, such as cellulitis, respond well to early oral antibiotic therapy. Others will require double or triple intravenous (IV) antibiotic therapy administration, wound débridement, or daily wound packing that allows the open incision to heal from the inside out via secondary intention (tissue granulation). In some instances, as in the case when there is a large blood clot behind the incision, reopening of the complete incision may

be necessary. This condition requires use of a wound vacuum device or secondary surgical closure using retention sutures and extended hospitalization.

Early assessment and treatment are critical in reducing maternal morbidity/mortality. Sepsis is rare but can occur.

Risk factors: Risk factors associated with postpartum infections include obesity, hemorrhage, anemia, history of chorioamnionitis, prolonged rupture of membranes, multiple vaginal examinations, corticosteroid therapy, advanced age, malnutrition, immunosuppression, type 1 diabetes, low socioeconomic status, malnutrition, positive group B streptococci culture, prolonged preoperative hospitalization, long labor, hemorrhage (loss of leukocytes), duration of the surgery (cesarean delivery or postpartum tubal ligation), razor shaving the operative site, use of electrosurgical knife, use of open drains (e.g., Jackson Pratt, Penrose), closure technique (suture vs. staples), and emergency surgery (e.g., for fetal distress).

DIAGNOSTIC TESTS

Complete blood count with differential: Leukocytes (white blood cells) will be elevated in the presence of infection. The differential lists the five types of leukocytes, which all perform a special function. The type of leukocyte elevation will depend on the type of infection present (e.g., monocytes = severe infection by phagocytosis; lymphocytes = viral infections).

Blood cultures: During acute febrile illness, blood cultures identify the source of bacteria causing the infection, and sensitivity analysis determines the most effective antibiotic therapy.

Gram stain and culture of foul-smelling lochia: Helps to identify *Clostridia*, anaerobes, and *Chlamydia* and indicates sensitivity analysis for the most effective antibiotic to use.

Urinalysis for microscopy: Detects presence of UTI, which may be seen postoperatively after removal of an indwelling urinary catheter.

Pelvic ultrasound: Detects and locates possible abscesses and hematomas.

Computed tomography (CT) scan and magnetic resonance imaging (MRI) scan: In patients who do not respond to antibiotic therapy and have a negative ultrasound examination, these studies can detect obscure pelvic abscesses and pelvic thrombi.

Nursing Diagnoses:

Impaired Skin Integrity
Impaired Tissue Integrity

related to wound infection and/or dehiscence

Desired Outcome: After initiation of therapy, the patient describes sensations and characteristics of the infected wound that necessitate nursing intervention and measures she can take to improve wound condition, and she begins to regain integrity in skin and underlying tissue without evidence of complications.

ASSESSMENT/INTERVENTIONS	RATIONALES
Assess pain q2h after vaginal and cesarean childbirth, and provide pain relief with analgesics, warm compresses, or sitz baths for episiotomy incisions, as prescribed by the health care provider.	Pain relief encourages patient movement. Both increased movement and heat increase circulation to promote wound healing.
[!] Assess the cesarean surgical site, episiotomy, or other wounds q4h for REEDA (see description under "Assessment," earlier).	Early identification of infection and prompt reporting of the need for medical intervention reduces maternal morbidity, the possibility of rehospitalization, and the length of treatment. - *Cesarean surgical site:* redness surrounding incision, abdomen warm to touch, drainage from incision, wound dehiscence (incision partially or fully open), and evisceration (protrusion of an organ, usually bowel, through open surgical wound). - *Episiotomy:* extreme pain in any position but especially sitting, foul-smelling vaginal odor in the absence of abdominal tenderness, drainage of pus, or dehiscence of sutures. The patient may use a mirror for self-examination or ask a family member to examine her perineum.
Assess temperature, pulse, respirations, and pain characteristics q2-4h.	This assessment aids in early identification of a developing postpartum infection. A temperature increase of 38°C (100.4°F) or higher in 2 of the first 10 days postpartum indicates infection. Pulse rises with fever and increases more with sepsis. Tachypnea may develop with sepsis.
Demonstrate and have the patient, family, or significant other return demonstrations of their ability to practice scrupulous hand hygiene, cleansing of the wound area, and aseptic techniques to care for the wound, such as wearing gloves (nonsterile acceptable) after thorough hand washing, disposing of soiled dressings in plastic bags, maintaining a clean field for irrigation and packing, using alternatives to tapes for holding dressings in place, applying a new dressing as prescribed, and maintaining a clean and dry wound environment after discharge to home with outpatient care.	Hand hygiene and regular changes of dressings, including frequent changing of peripads, remove bacteria and thereby reduce incidence of contamination. Tape can cause skin reactions and break down sensitive tissue. Maintaining a clean and dry wound provides an optimal environment to assist the body's natural healing processes. See Appendix A for "Infection Prevention and Control," p. 747, for more information.
As prescribed by the health care provider at hospital discharge, provide a referral to community health nursing for supervision of progressive wound changes, monitoring the patient's care, or providing daily dressing changes if wound care is complex.	Professional referral decreases stress on the patient and family, reinforces newly learned skills, improves knowledge, and assists with unforeseen problems during the transition to home care (e.g., adaptation to the home environment, conflict with work commitments, or uneasiness in self-management of a surgical wound). Home care also enables the patient to be home, which decreases medical costs.
Encourage the patient to eat a well-balanced diet that includes protein, carbohydrates, fruits, vegetables, and adequate fluid intake.	An adequate diet provides nutrients, especially vitamin C, and a positive nitrogen state, which promote wound healing. Adequate hydration also promotes wound healing.
Encourage the patient to report changes that indicate complications and to keep all medical appointments.	Good communication likely will promote early identification of complications. Adherence to appointments enables timely evaluation of the wound's healing process and initiation of care in response to complications.
Provide abdominal support or a binder after a cesarean delivery or bilateral tubal ligation.	A binder provides support and decreases stretching/tension on muscles or the surrounding tissue of the wound to promote healing. This is especially important with patients who are obese.

Nursing Diagnosis:

Deficient Knowledge

related to unfamiliarity with the therapeutic medication regimen and potential side effects of the prescribed medications used for treating wound infections

Desired Outcome: Immediately following teaching, the patient and significant others verbalize accurate understanding of the risks and benefits of medications used in treating postpartum wound infections.

ASSESSMENT/INTERVENTIONS	RATIONALES
Teach the following about the patient's prescribed medications:	A knowledgeable patient is more likely to adhere to the therapy, identify and report side effects, and recognize and report precautions that might preclude use of the prescribed medication.
Antimicrobials	These agents may be used as a perioperative prophylaxis, treating potential wound cellulitis/infection.
Cephalosporins Cefazolin (Ancef, Kefzol), cefoxitin (Mefoxin), cefotetan (Cefotan), cefoperazone (Cefobid), cephalexin (Keflex)	Administration: IV, by mouth (PO), intramuscular (IM).
Teach patients who are breastfeeding that this drug will be present in low concentrations in breast milk.	Patients can breastfeed without it causing a problem to the infant.
Explain that caution is necessary for patients with sensitivity to penicillins.	Cross-sensitivity with penicillins is possible. Serious and possible fatal reactions can occur.
Teach the importance of following the complete course for all prescribed medications and taking them on time.	These measures reduce risk of reinfection, prevent development of antibiotic resistance, and maintain a constant level of medication in the bloodstream.
Teach the patient to be alert for and report diarrhea, nausea, vomiting, stomach cramps, and anorexia.	These are possible side effects.
Caution the patient to be alert for and report excessive and explosive diarrhea.	*Clostridium difficile* infection is a potentially serious side effect in which the normal flora of the bowel are reduced by antibiotic therapy and the anaerobic organism *C. difficile* multiplies and produces its toxins, causing severe diarrhea. This problem necessitates discontinuation of the antibiotic and laboratory evaluation of a stool sample.
Caution the patient to be alert for a rash and pruritus.	These may be signs of an allergic reaction.
Penicillins Penicillin, amoxicillin, amoxicillin/clavulanate potassium (Augmentin), ampicillin-sulbactam (Unasyn)	Administration: IV/IM/PO. Breastfeeding: okay with amoxicillin.
Caution the patient that this medication is not to be used if allergic to penicillins.	Serious and possible fatal reactions can occur.
Caution use in patients with sensitivity to cephalosporins.	Possible cross-sensitivity can lead to serious and sometimes fatal reactions.
Advise the patient to follow the complete course for all prescribed medications and take them on time.	These measures reduce risk of reinfection, prevent development of antibiotic resistance, and maintain a constant level of medication in the bloodstream.
Teach the patient to be alert for and report nausea, indigestion, and vomiting.	These are possible side effects.
Teach the patient to monitor for and report itching, rash, and shortness of breath.	These indicators may signal an allergic reaction.
Caution the patient to be alert for and report excessive and explosive diarrhea.	See discussion of *C. difficile,* earlier.
Aminoglycosides Gentamicin (Garamycin)	Gentamicin is not administered during pregnancy because it crosses the placenta and can cause total irreversible bilateral congenital deafness. Gentamycin is given postpartum. Administration: IM/IV. Breastfeeding: May continue.
Teach the patient to be alert for and report lethargy, confusion, respiratory depression, visual disturbances, depression, weight loss, hypotension or hypertension, decreased appetite, rash, itching, headache, nausea, vomiting, and hearing loss.	These are potential adverse and allergic reactions.

ASSESSMENT/INTERVENTIONS | RATIONALES

ASSESSMENT/INTERVENTIONS	RATIONALES
Caution the patient to be alert for and report excessive and explosive diarrhea.	See discussion of *C. difficile,* earlier.
Caution use in patients with neuromuscular disorders and in patients with impaired renal function.	This medication may lead to neurotoxicity and nephrotoxicity.

Other Antibiotics
! *Clindamycin (Cleocin)*

	Administration: IV/IM/PO. Breastfeeding may continue.
Teach the patient to monitor for and report itching and rash.	These signs can occur with allergic reactions.
Teach the patient to be alert for and report diarrhea, nausea, vomiting, stomach cramps, and anorexia.	These are possible adverse reactions.
Advise the patient to follow the complete course for all prescribed medications and take them on time.	These measures reduce risk of reinfection, prevent development of antibiotic resistance, and maintain a constant level of medication in the bloodstream.
Caution the patient to be alert for and report excessive and explosive diarrhea.	See discussion of *C. difficile,* earlier.
Caution use in patients with a history of colitis.	This drug may exacerbate the colitis.
Teach the patient to be alert for and report redness, swelling, and pain at IV insertion site.	Thrombophlebitis can occur after IV infusion of clindamycin.
Caution use in patients with renal disease.	The injectable drug is potentially nephrotoxic.

! *Linezolid (Zyvox)*

	This antibiotic is used to treat complicated skin and skin structure infections caused by MRSA. Administration: IV/PO.
Caution use in patients with hypertension.	This drug may increase preexisting hypertension.
Teach patients who are breastfeeding that caution should be used when taking this medication.	It is unknown whether linezolid is excreted in breast milk.
Teach the patient to be alert for and report diarrhea, headache, nausea, vomiting, insomnia, constipation, rash, dizziness, and fever.	These are possible side effects.
Caution patients taking selective serotonin reuptake inhibitors (SSRIs) to be alert for and report cognitive dysfunction, hyperpyrexia, hyperreflexia, and incoordination.	Serotonin syndrome can be associated with the coadministration of Zyvox and SSRIs.
Teach the patient to be alert for and immediately report visual blurring, changes in color vision, or loss of vision.	Peripheral and optic neuropathy may be associated with the drug when it is used beyond the recommended treatment (more than 28 days).
Teach the patient to be alert for and immediately report repeated episodes of nausea and vomiting.	Lactic acidosis is a possible side effect.
Teach the patient to be alert for and report excessive and explosive diarrhea.	See discussion of *C. difficile,* earlier.
Teach patients to avoid ingesting excessive amounts of foods or beverages with high tyramine content while taking this drug.	Foods with greater than 100 mg of tyramine (e.g., red wine, aged cheese) may enhance the pressor response of this drug and increase blood pressure (BP).
Teach the patient to avoid medications containing pseudoephedrine HCL or phenylpropanolamine HCL.	Zyvox enhances the increases in systolic BP caused by pseudoephedrine HCL or phenylpropanolamine HCL.

Analgesics
! **Morphine Sulfate**

	This opiate analgesic (opioid) is used in the treatment of moderate-to-severe pain. Administration: IV/IM/PO.

continued

ASSESSMENT/INTERVENTIONS	RATIONALES
Encourage breastfeeding before taking the analgesic.	Breastfeeding generally is accepted as safe. Taking the medication after breastfeeding reduces the possibility of medication influence on the infant.
Teach the patient to be alert for and report itching and rash.	These are possible allergic reactions.
Teach the patient to be alert for and report weakness, headache, restlessness, agitation, hallucinations, and disorientation.	These are possible adverse reactions.
Teach the patient to be alert for and report shortness of breath.	This is a possible adverse reaction that may indicate overdose.
Caution the patient to arise slowly from a supine position or have assistance with ambulating after receiving this medication.	Morphine is a central nervous system (CNS) depressant. It may impair mental and/or physical abilities and cause hypotension.
Caution the patient to avoid activities that require alertness until the drug's effect on the CNS is known.	Drowsiness is a common side effect.
Caution use with other CNS depressants.	Morphine can potentiate CNS effects of these drugs.
Caution use in patients with seizure disorder.	Seizures may result from high doses.
Caution use in patients with renal/hepatic insufficiency.	Morphine's active metabolite may accumulate and potentiate the sedative effects.

⚠ Oxycodone with Acetaminophen (Percocet) and Hydrocodone with Acetaminophen (Vicodin)

	These are opioid analgesics used to treat moderate to moderately severe pain.
	Administration: PO.
Encourage the patient to breastfeed before taking the medication and to follow carefully the prescribed dose regimen.	Both analgesics are commonly used in postpartum women. Breastfeeding just before taking the medication and adhering to the prescribed therapy reduces any threat to the newborn.
Teach the patient to be alert for and report itching, rash, nausea, and vomiting.	These are signs of a possible allergic reaction.
Teach the patient to be alert for and report dizziness and headache.	These are common adverse reactions.
Teach the patient to be alert for and report shortness of breath.	This adverse reaction may indicate overdose.
Caution the patient to arise slowly from a supine position or have assistance with ambulating after taking this medication.	These drugs are CNS depressants. They may impair mental and/or physical abilities and cause hypotension.
Caution the patient to avoid activities that require alertness until the drug's effect on the CNS is known.	Drowsiness is a common side effect.

Anticoagulant
⚠ Heparin

	Heparin inhibits the reaction that leads to formation of fibrin clots and clotting of blood. It is used in treating septic pelvic thrombophlebitis.
	Administration: subcutaneous/IV. IM not recommended.
Teach the patient to be alert for and report increase in vaginal bleeding (saturating one regular-size sanitary pad/hr and/or passing golf-ball–sized clots).	Hemorrhage can occur at any site in patients receiving heparin.
Caution the patient about using aspirin or aspirin-containing products and nonsteroidal antiinflammatory drugs (NSAIDs; e.g., ibuprofen) or NSAID-containing products while taking heparin.	Aspirin and NSAIDs are platelet aggregation (clotting) inhibitors that can lead to increased bleeding.
Inform the patient that bleeding and bruising at the site of injection is not unusual.	Heparin can lead to bleeding and bruising. The tendency for bleeding at the injection site will necessitate prolonged compression over the site.
Teach the patient to be alert for and report redness, pain, swelling, and firmness at the injection site.	These are signs of local irritation that may indicate injection site cellulitis.
Advise the patient to take a calcium supplement while receiving heparin.	Heparin affects bone density and may lead to osteoporosis.

Nursing Diagnosis:

Deficient Knowledge

related to unfamiliarity with the effects of postpartum wound infection on the self and neonate and the importance of following the treatment course

Desired Outcome: Immediately following teaching, the patient and/or significant other verbalize accurate knowledge about the effects of postpartum wound infections and the associated treatment on the patient and neonate.

ASSESSMENT/INTERVENTIONS	RATIONALES
Teach the patient, significant other, and family about the effects postpartum wound infection may have on the mother and newborn and the likely treatments for the infection.	Information helps patients adhere to treatments, report symptoms in a timely manner, and understand consequences of nonadherence. Effects an infection may have on the mother include pain, fever, chills, wound dehiscence, sepsis, and increased morbidity/mortality. For the neonate, effects include fever, possible rapid deterioration, and increased morbidity/mortality. Rehospitalization or illness may interrupt breastfeeding and attachment. Likely treatments include IV antibiotics and fluids, wound packing, secondary wound closure, and possible lengthy hospitalization or home treatments.
Teach signs and symptoms of worsening wound infection and its complications that should be reported after hospital discharge.	This teaching intervention enables the patient/family to recognize and report such signs as increasing fever; foul-smelling vaginal discharge; failure of lochia to progress from rubra to serosa to alba and its timely completion; spreading abdominal cellulites; severe pain; vaginal bleeding; wound drainage; seroma; hematoma; dehiscence; necrotizing fasciitis; and signs of disseminated intravascular coagulation (see "Disseminated Intravascular Coagulation," p. 471). Early evaluation and treatment result in decreased maternal morbidity.
Explain treatment options such as daily wound packing or secondary wound closure and IV or PO antibiotics used to treat the infection and decrease risk for further infection.	After hospital treatment of acute infection with IV antibiotics, treating the patient at home is preferred. If a secondary wound closure is done, it requires readmittance to the hospital (or an extended stay if the infection occurs before hospital discharge). Daily wound care consists of inspection, irrigation, débridement, packing, and dressing applications. (See "Managing Wound Care," p. 533, for more information.)
Explain to the patient and her partner that intercourse is not recommended during the process of wound healing, especially in the presence of wound dehiscence.	Usually intercourse is not recommended until 6 wk postpartum. This time frame allows the placental attachment site to heal, cervical closure, lochia (vaginal discharge) to stop, and incisions to heal without risk of introducing bacteria.

Nursing Diagnosis:

Interrupted Family Processes

related to a shift in health status of the family member, the need to provide an optimal environment for wound healing while providing for newborn care and feeding, or family roles shift

Desired Outcome: Within 2-4 hr of this nursing diagnosis, the patient and family begin to express their feelings and identify ways to modify their daily living patterns to meet physical, psychosocial, and spiritual needs of the patient and newborn.

ASSESSMENT/INTERVENTIONS	RATIONALES
Assess the patient's and family's acceptance and confidence in caring for the wound on an outpatient basis, clarifying their perceptions about the patient's current health status and daily needs.	This assessment evaluates their comfort level with providing home wound care and enables mutual development of an individualized plan for the patient to take control of her own care.
Review attachment documentation immediately after birth and observe variations in the patient's/family's attitudes and behaviors with their newborn over the course of the hospital stay. Provide family-centered care (FCC) in the hospital.	Appropriate support and interventions depend on accurate assessment of attitudes and behaviors to distinguish what is related to the complication versus psychologic causes, cultural practices, or interrupted attachment. FCC prevents needless separation of the mother and newborn.
Assess for signs of complications with parenting (e.g., being unable to take on the role of daily infant care and feeding; lack of interest in caring for and feeding the newborn; lack of consistent and ongoing support from family members, friends, church group support, and neighbors; reference to self or newborn as ugly or problematic; difficulty with sleep; and loss of appetite).	Parents usually attach without ambivalence to their newborn, want to parent their newborn, and have the energy and motivation to do so, but they also may need to develop infant care and decision-making skills as new parents and learn to balance individual needs with infant needs on a daily basis. A maternal infection complicates this process.
Establish empathetic communication and encourage open expression of feelings and thoughts by the patient, family, and significant others involved with the patient, newborn, and family after hospital discharge.	Honesty and empathy promote effective therapeutic communication and support. For example, "I know this is difficult to deal with while also caring for a newborn. Let's talk about it. I want to be of support to you in this unexpected transition."
Help the patient and family identify and develop a daily pattern to meet individual needs, incorporate the newborn into the family, continue with lactation preferences (pumping, breastfeeding, or bottle feeding), promote wound healing, support maternal rest, and have an effective support system.	The healthy family pulls together in a crisis. Adaptation is most effective when the support system is consistent, flexible, and related to individual needs. The patient may need assistance with personal care, newborn care/feeding, parenting her other children, and homemaking tasks in order to modify her daily living so that wound healing can occur.
Arrange community referrals (e.g., visiting nurse service, lactation consultant, or postpartum doula support as appropriate).	Support in the home environment is likely to promote healthier adaptation and strengthen the family system.
Affirm that lifestyle adjustments are for a limited time (e.g., increased rest, dressing changes, frequent clinic visits, taking medications, interrupted maternal role fulfillment).	This information may promote family decision-making, facilitate acceptance of outside support and assistance, and reinforce patience with the healing process of an infected wound.
Explain diagnostic tests and medical interventions (e.g., blood work to monitor for further infection, ultrasound to check for abscess), and procedures (e.g., wound packing, secondary wound closure).	Anticipating needs of the patient and family and explaining what to expect strengthen their coping mechanisms.

ADDITIONAL NURSING DIAGNOSES/PROBLEMS:

PATIENT-FAMILY TEACHING AND DISCHARGE PLANNING

Wound infections place a great deal of strain on the patient and family dynamics. A proactive approach to anticipating patient and family needs for education and support will decrease their level of anxiety and optimize outcomes. Referral to a wound care specialist may be necessary at any time during the assessment/healing process. Include verbal and written information about the following:

✓ Signs and symptoms of wound infection.

✓ Wound care (cleansing, packing, and dressing); instructions will vary depending on facility and provider preference. Check with the health care provider for specific instructions. Also see care plans in "Managing Wound Care," p. 533.

✓ Importance and timing of good hand hygiene.

✓ Where to obtain dressing materials for home care (prescriptions for supplies that may be acquired via a pharmacy or medical supply store).

✓ Importance of adequate rest, nutrition, and oral hydration for effective wound healing.

✓ Importance of compliance with the prescribed health care regimen and ready access to hospital and family/social support.

✓ Medications, including drug name, purpose, dosage, frequency, precautions, potential drug reactions, and side effects. Also discuss potential drug-drug, food-drug, and herb-drug interactions.

✓ Referral to local and national support organizations, including lactation consultants and Sidelines, a national support organization for women and their families experiencing complicated pregnancies, at *www.sidelines.org*

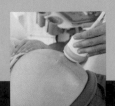

Preeclampsia 92

OVERVIEW/PATHOPHYSIOLOGY

Hypertensive disorders of pregnancy are one of the most frequently reported medical complications of pregnancy and are steadily increasing in incidence. The American College of Obstetrics and Gynecology (ACOG) lists four categories of hypertension: chronic hypertension, gestational hypertension, preeclampsia, and chronic hypertension with superimposed preeclampsia.

Preeclampsia/eclampsia: Occurs after 20 wk gestation. Blood pressure (BP) is elevated (more than 140 mm Hg systolic, more than 90 mm Hg diastolic) and accompanied by significant proteinuria (see Assessment, below). Preeclampsia may be mild, moderate, or severe in presentation and can progress to eclampsia or HELLP syndrome.

- *HELLP syndrome* is a laboratory diagnosis for a severe variant of preeclampsia associated with high maternal and fetal morbidity. "H" stands for hemolysis of red blood cells; "EL" stands for elevated liver enzymes; and "LP" stands for low platelets.
- *Eclampsia:* When severe preeclampsia has progressed to generalized seizures, it is called eclampsia. Seizures may occur during the antepartum, intrapartum, or postpartum period. Coma often follows a seizure.

Gestational hypertension: BP elevation after 20 wk gestation occurs without proteinuria. It may be transient or chronic and resolves before 12 wk postpartum. Despite the hypertension, good pregnancy outcomes are expected.

Chronic hypertension: BP elevation occurring prior to pregnancy. Chronic hypertension is defined by ACOG as systolic BP 140 mm Hg or greater, diastolic blood pressure 90 mm Hg or greater, or both, documented on two occasions more than 6 hr apart. Chronic hypertension is more prevalent with increasing late childbearing and rising rates of obesity.

Chronic hypertension with superimposed preeclampsia: A common complication for a chronic hypertensive woman, superimposed preeclampsia occurs in 25% of these pregnancies. Preconception screening and lifestyle changes are encouraged to attain a normotensive state prepregnancy.

Although the cause of preeclampsia remains unknown, the resulting generalized vasoconstriction, vasospasms, and endothelial cell damage result in decreased circulation and oxygenation for all organ systems, including the gravid uterus and fetus, and result in redistribution of intravascular fluid (edema). Serious and life-long complications can develop in any affected organ system, including the brain, kidney, liver, and uteroplacental unit. Often the presenting signs are the classic signs of hypertension accompanied by proteinuria. As this multisystem disorder progresses from mild to severe preeclampsia, varied clinical manifestations demonstrate the more severe effects on each organ system. The only known cure is delivery of the newborn and removal of the placenta.

HEALTH CARE SETTING

Primary care and acute care antepartum and intrapartum hospital units. Home care is possible for mild preeclampsia.

ASSESSMENT

Signs and symptoms: The focus of this nursing care plan is preeclampsia.

Additional reportable signs include decreased fetal movement (fetal compromise), spontaneous bruising, prolonged bleeding, and epistaxis (thrombocytopenia).

Risk factors: Nulliparity (status of a woman who has not carried the pregnancy and given birth after 20 wk gestation), African American race, history of preeclampsia, renal disease, diabetes mellitus, hypothyroidism, age younger than 20 yr or older than 40 yr, family history of preeclampsia (mother/sister), chronic hypertension, thrombophilias (antiphospholipid syndrome, proteins C and S, antithrombin deficiency, factor V Leiden), multifetal pregnancy, oocyte donation or donor insemination, urinary tract infections, obesity, gestational trophoblastic disease (molar pregnancy) (Levine et al., 2009; Rath & Fischer, 2009), and male partner whose previous partner had preeclampsia (*www.acog.org*, 2002).

DIAGNOSTIC TESTS

Complete blood count (CBC): May be within normal limits. Changes reflect hemodynamic changes. Hct rises with hemoconcentration. Platelets drop (thrombocytopenia) with hemoconcentration and with HELLP syndrome. Hemoglobin (Hgb) falls with hemolysis.

Renal function studies: Proteinuria 0.3 g or more in a 24-hr urine specimen is diagnostic for preeclampsia. With kidney involvement, blood tests may show rising serum creatinine, uric acid, and blood urea nitrogen (BUN). Elevated creatinine clearance in a 24-hr urine collection indicates reduced renal function.

Mild Preeclampsia

- BP elevated × 2, 6 hr apart on bedrest: systolic blood pressure (SBP) 140-160 mm Hg or 30 mm Hg over baseline; diastolic blood pressure (DBP) 90-110 mm Hg or 15 mm Hg over baseline (DBP 90 mm Hg or higher in second trimester)
- Mean arterial pressure (MAP) 105 mm Hg or higher or increased by 20 mm Hg from baseline
- Proteinuria: 0.3-4.0 g in 24-hr collection; 2+ or 3+ on random dipstick (without urinary tract infection)
- Reflexia: 2+ or less (normal response)
- Headache: Absent or transient
- No vision changes
- No epigastric pain
- Normal urine output
- Laboratory studies: Platelets normal, hematocrit (Hct) decreased, liver enzymes begin to rise
- Weight gain: More than 1.5 kg (3.3 lb)/month or more than 0.5 kg (1.1 lb/week) in third trimester. Edema is not considered diagnostic but should not remain after 8-12 hr bedrest.
- Placenta: Decreased placental perfusion
- Risk of oligohydramnios
- Early placental aging not apparent yet

Severe Preeclampsia

- BP elevated × 2, 6 hr apart on bedrest: SBP greater than 160 mm Hg; DBP greater than 110 mm Hg
- MAP higher than 105 mm Hg
- Proteinuria: More than 5 g/L in a 24-hr collection; 2+, 3+ or more by dipstick
- Increased sodium retention
- Hyperreflexia: 3+ or more; clonus
- Headache: Continuous or severe, affective changes, nausea/vomiting
- Vision: Blurred, scotoma, diplopia, photophobia, retinal detachment (spontaneously reattaches later)
- Epigastric pain: Present (impending convulsion)
- Oliguria: Urine output less than 20 mL/hr
- Laboratory studies: Liver enzymes (alanine aminotransferase [ALT], aspartate aminotransferase [AST], and lactate dehydrogenase [LDH]) will be elevated. Increased Hct indicates hemoconcentration. Elevated serum creatinine signals renal compromise. When these values are accompanied by thrombocytopenia, it is crucial to monitor for HELLP syndrome.
- Edema: Generalized, dyspnea, rales/crackles (pulmonary edema)
- Placenta: Markedly reduced perfusion results in intrauterine growth restriction (IUGR)
- Risk of abruptio placenta
- Labor: Late decelerations
- Placental evaluation after birth: Intervillous thrombosis, ischemic necrosis (white spots), smaller than expected for gestational age

Liver function tests: ALT, AST, and LDH rise with severe preeclampsia and rise even further with HELLP syndrome.

Coagulation studies: Platelet count decreases in severe pre-eclampsia and HELLP syndrome. Intrinsic or extrinsic factors may induce clot formation and deplete clotting factors, leading to hemorrhage.

Obstetric ultrasound: Serial ultrasounds are commonly used to estimate fetal growth and amniotic fluid index (AFI).

Daily fetal activity monitoring, nonstress testing (NST), and biophysical profile (BPP): These tests assess uteroplacental perfusion.

Nursing Diagnoses:

Decreased Cardiac Output
Risk for Ineffective Renal Tissue Perfusion

related to hypertension, generalized vasospasms, vascular wall damage, and hypovolemia with decreasing venous return

Desired Outcome: Within 24 hr after interventions, the patient begins to return to normotensive BP and pulse for pregnancy and participates in her health care regimen.

ASSESSMENT/INTERVENTIONS	RATIONALES
Assess and document BP and pulse q1-4h as indicated.	Hypertension results from biochemical changes that cause vasoconstriction and vasospasm. Rising BP values indicate progression of preeclampsia.

continued

ASSESSMENT/INTERVENTIONS	RATIONALES
Measure urine volume and proteinuria qh or per protocol. Maintain strict intake and output.	As preeclampsia becomes severe, glomerular endothelial damage allows protein molecules to pass into the urine. Hypovolemia and damage to blood vessel walls decrease circulation to the kidneys.
For patients with worsening preeclampsia, explain the importance of bedrest with bathroom privileges and frequent use of left lateral position.	Bedrest and left lateral positioning facilitate venous return to the heart, which lowers BP and increases perfusion of the kidneys and uteroplacental unit.
Administer prescribed antihypertensive medication (i.e., hydralazine [Apresoline], labetalol HCl [Normodyne], or methyldopa [Aldomet]).	Antihypertensives lower BP via vasodilation and decreasing systemic vascular resistance.
Prepare for cesarean delivery if indicated by the severity of preeclampsia and as determined by the health care provider.	Delivery (of placenta) is the definitive way to halt the progression of preeclampsia. Cesarean is selected when induction and vaginal delivery are ruled out.

Nursing Diagnosis:

Risk for Imbalanced Fluid Volume

related to vasospasm, endothelial cell damage, and fluid shifts from intravascular to extravascular spaces

Desired Outcome: Signs and symptoms of imbalanced fluid volume diminish within 8-12 hr, as evidenced by decreased BP, normal rate and quality of pulse, unlabored respirations, urine output greater than 30 mL/hr without proteinuria, normal pregnancy weight gain, absence of pitting edema, and Hct within normal limits.

ASSESSMENT/INTERVENTIONS	RATIONALES
Assess BP; heart rate, rhythm, and quality; respiratory rate (RR); and lung sounds q1-4h.	Increasing hypertension occurs with worsening vasoconstriction and increasing peripheral vascular resistance. Pulse increases and quality changes occur to compensate for hypovolemia. Pulmonary edema causes dyspnea.
Assess presence, degree, and location of edema q1-8h. Weigh the patient daily. Report significant findings.	Edema develops as fluid shifts from the vascular to the extravascular spaces. Weight gain is an indicator of fluid retention.
Assess deep tendon reflexes (DTRs) and for the presence of clonus q1-4h.	Increasing hyperreflexia signals a worsening condition. DTRs correspond to the peripheral neurologic condition. Clonus relates to central neurologic irritability. For more details about DTRs and clonus, see **Risk for Injury: Maternal**, later.
Assess for headaches: presence, location, and severity q1-4h.	Headaches increase in intensity and frequency with advancing brain edema.
Assess for mental changes, irritability, and level of consciousness q1-4h.	Changes in mentation indicate a worsening condition with increased central nervous system (CNS) edema.
Monitor fluid intake and urine output q1-4h. If indicated, limit fluid intake to 2000-3000 mL/day (PO and IV).	Fluid retention could lead to pulmonary edema when severe. Oliguria signals renal system compromise.
Collect a 24-hr urine specimen to measure proteinuria and creatinine if prescribed by the health care provider. Measure proteinuria with a dipstick every void.	As preeclampsia becomes severe, glomerular endothelial damage allows protein molecules and creatinine to pass into the urine.
Monitor for hemodynamic changes via the following laboratory values:	Hemodynamic changes result from increasingly severe preeclampsia.
- Hct	Hct rises with hemoconcentration.
- Hgb	Hgb falls as red blood cells (RBCs) are damaged in turbulent blood flow (vasospasms).
- Platelets	Platelet decrease indicates HELLP syndrome.
- Liver enzymes	Liver function enzymes rise with increased liver compromise.
- Serum creatinine and uric acid	Serum creatinine and uric acid increase with reduced glomerular filtration and indicate nephron function.

Nursing Diagnosis:

Impaired Gas Exchange (to the fetus)

related to progressive vasospasms of the uterine spiral arteries and reduced blood flow to the placenta

Desired Outcome: Within 8-12 hr of interventions, fetal status stabilizes and improves as evidenced by improved fetal activity, reassuring NST, and fetus tolerating labor and vaginal delivery.

ASSESSMENT/INTERVENTIONS	RATIONALES
Measure fundal height.	Monitoring progressive fetal growth identifies the potential development of intrauterine growth retardation (IUGR), which results from maternal vasospasm, vasoconstriction, and hypovolemia and will affect uteroplacental blood flow and oxygenation.
Monitor ultrasound (US) and AFI results after 28 wk gestation.	Serial US monitors for the potential development of IUGR. AFI measurement identifies oligohydramnios. Maternal vasospasms and vasoconstriction decrease uteroplacental perfusion, causing fetal hypoxia, and can result in IUGR and oligohydramnios.
Teach the mother assessment of fetal activity by performing and recording daily fetal movement counts per agency/hospital protocol.	Decreased fetal movements may indicate fetal hypoxia.
Assess fetal heart rate (FHR) patterns by continuous FHR monitoring or twice-a-day NST.	These procedures monitor for uteroplacental insufficiency and fetal hypoxia. Reactive NST: 2 FHR accelerations in a 20-min period are indicative of adequate oxygenation and an intact fetal CNS.
[!] Assess for signs of abruptio placenta: uterine hypertonus; dark, nonclotting vaginal bleeding; abdominal pain; uterine tenderness; and fetal distress signs.	Abruptio placenta may occur spontaneously with hypertension.
[!] Assess fetal response to medication: misoprostol (Cytotec), dinoprostone (Cervidil insert or Prepidil Gel), oxytocin induction, and magnesium sulfate.	Some cervical ripening agents (misoprostol) or oxytocin may cause uterine hyperstimulation resulting in fetal hypoxia with nonreassuring (Category 2, Category 3) FHR pattern. Magnesium sulfate may cause hypermagnesemia In the newborn (depression of respiratory and neurologic systems).

Nursing Diagnosis:

Risk for Injury: Maternal

related to abnormal blood profile; effects of vasoconstriction, vasospasm, endothelial cell damage, and tissue hypoxia in every organ system; and/or development of complications (disseminated intravascular coagulation [DIC])

Desired Outcomes: The patient remains free of injury from the effects of preeclampsia on the maternal cardiovascular, hematologic, renal, neurologic, respiratory, and hepatic systems as evidenced by a return to normotensive BP, MAP below 105 mm Hg, negative or trace proteinuria, normal urine output, reflexes of 2+, and clear vision. The patient has normal hematology values within 12-24 hr after expulsion of an intact placenta.

ASSESSMENT/INTERVENTIONS	RATIONALES
[!] Assess symptoms along with maternal reports of worsening disease: changes in CNS signs, visual changes, pain (degree, type, and location), urinary output and proteinuria, and weight gain. In addition, assess FHR pattern, maternal vital signs, and effects of medications q1-4h. Document and communicate results as indicated.	Symptoms from organ system damage with progressive vasoconstriction, vasospasms, and endothelial cell damage reflect the severity of preeclampsia. Epigastric pain is considered a late sign and is associated with impending convulsion. Twitching of facial muscles often precedes a grand mal seizure. Confusion, combative behavior, or coma often follows a seizure.

continued

ASSESSMENT/INTERVENTIONS	RATIONALES
Maintain a therapeutic environment: quiet, darkened room; limited visitors; and left lateral positioning. Initiate seizure precautions.	A therapeutic environment reduces stimuli that may heighten seizure activity.
Teach the patient the importance of eating a balanced pregnancy diet at least TID with adequate protein, calcium, zinc, magnesium, sodium, folate, vitamins C and E, and roughage. Explain that her food should contain no added salt, and she should drink 8-10 (8-oz) glasses of water/day.	Diet influences disease progression. Protein replaces protein lost in the urine. Adequate dietary antioxidants may facilitate prostacyclin/thromboxane balance, leading to vasodilation and lower BP. Roughage and fluids may prevent constipation.
Administer intravenous (IV) magnesium sulfate as prescribed with before and after assessments of DTR/clonus, BP, respirations, urine output, FHR, medication effects, and signs of magnesium toxicity.	Magnesium sulfate depresses the CNS and relaxes smooth muscle, thereby dropping BP into normal range and slowing respirations. If respirations fall to less than 12/min, this is a sign of too much magnesium. In fact, the cascade into respiratory arrest followed by cardiac arrest can be quite rapid (1 hr to a few hours); whereas DTRs become hyperreactive along with signs of clonus (rapidly alternating contractions and relaxations of a skeletal muscle) before a seizure, and depressed DTRs can occur with too much medication (see next rationale). Because magnesium sulfate is excreted via the kidneys, urinary output of at least 30 mL/hr is a sign that the kidneys are functioning adequately. A reactive (Category 1) fetal heart rate is reassuring of fetal well-being.
As prescribed, administer IV magnesium sulfate as an IV piggyback (IVPB) by infusion pump.	The IV route most accurately controls dosage and intervention responses if toxicity develops.
Follow agency protocols to ensure safe medication administration.	Overdose and overhydration are best prevented with an infusion pump.
Assess therapeutic blood levels of magnesium periodically per the health care provider directive during pregnancy, labor, and postpartum.	A loading dose of 4-6 g over 20 min, followed by 2 g/hr as a maintenance dose provides a therapeutic plasma level of 4-8 mg/dL (4-7 mEq/L) without toxicity. At 8-12 mg/dL (8-10 mEq/L) DTRs become absent, at 14 mg/dL (13-15 mEq/L) respiratory arrest occurs, at 30 mg/dL (more than 20-25 mEq/L) cardiac arrest occurs.
[!] Keep an ampule of calcium gluconate at the bedside. Administer 1 g (10 mL of a 10% solution) over a period of 3 min as prescribed and if symptoms indicate.	Calcium gluconate is the antidote administered to counteract adverse toxic effects from magnesium.
[!] Assess renal function q2h or as often as prescribed by the health care provider: i.e., strict hourly intake and output (I&O), proteinuria assessment, and periodic serum magnesium assessments.	Magnesium is excreted via the kidneys. Oliguria indicates renal compromise (if fluid intake is adequate). Serum toxic levels develop quickly with renal failure.
[!] Obtain baseline parameters (FHR pattern, maternal VS, uterine activity) prior to administration of oxytocin or cervical ripening agent.	Baseline findings within normal limits (WNL) rule out maternal or fetal contraindications. Infusion pump and IVPB administration of oxytocin decrease risk of fluid overload and allow rapid response to complications. Follow agency protocols for the safe administration of these medications.
[!] Administer the following cautiously and as prescribed: cervical ripening agents, i.e., misoprostol (Cytotec) or dinoprostone (Cervidil insert or Prepidil Gel), and oxytocin for labor induction.	Hyperstimulation of the uterus from ripening agents or oxytocin can cause rupture of the uterus.
[!] Perform invasive procedures as minimally as possible.	Invasive procedures (e.g., vaginal examination, internal maternal or fetal monitoring, intravenous therapy, catheterization, anesthesia [epidural or spinal], or cesarean birth) may cause infection as external microscopic organisms are moved internally.
[!] Maintain a safe environment with padded bedside rails, oxygen via face mask, connected and working suctioning equipment, and maternal and fetal assessment equipment.	Preparation before a seizure occurs enables immediate response by the health care team.
[!] Assess for complications: blood oozing at the IV site, epistaxis, and petechiae.	These are early signs of DIC. Vascular endothelial damage from preeclampsia can activate the intrinsic coagulation pathway and result in DIC.

Nursing Diagnosis:

Risk for Injury: Fetal

related to the progressively severe effects of vasospasm and decreased circulation to the uteroplacental unit leading to intrauterine growth restriction and decreased fetal oxygenation (may require preterm delivery of the newborn and the placenta)

Desired Outcome: Daily and timely interventions limit the progression of preeclampsia (see previous nursing diagnoses for optimal signs) and promote delivery of a healthy newborn as close as possible to term.

ASSESSMENT/INTERVENTIONS	RATIONALES
! Assess carefully for side effects when administering the following medications to prevent eclampsia in pregnancy and labor: magnesium sulfate, labetalol (Trandate), and hydralazine (Apresoline).	Tetanic contractions in an eclamptic convulsion block oxygen delivery to the fetus. Newborn hypermagnesemia (depression of the neurologic and respiratory systems) may follow maternal magnesium sulfate therapy (see discussion, earlier). Good maternal renal functioning is needed for elimination of labetalol. Hydralazine (Apresoline) overdose can lead to abruptio placenta.
! Administer prescribed oxytocin safely via IVPB with infusion pump and following the agency/health care provider protocol for increasing and decreasing the dosage.	Uterine hyperstimulation with oxytocin causes fetal hypoxia, rapid labor and delivery, and may cause CNS injury in the preterm newborn. Higher oxytocin dosages are often needed for a woman on magnesium sulfate during labor. Follow agency protocols for the safe administration of this medication.
Confer with the health care provider regarding results of the test for fetal lung maturity if a preterm birth is planned.	Respiratory distress syndrome (RDS) develops in the preterm born before lung surfactant is mature (evidenced by two parts lecithin per one part sphingomyelin [L/S ratio]). RDS is a leading cause of infant mortality. In the United States approximately 24,000 preterm infants are born each year, and mortality rate for RDS related to prematurity still remains at 10% regardless of advances in treatment (Smith & Carey, 2014).
Administer maternal corticosteroid therapy (betamethasone 12 mg intramuscular [IM] × 2 doses 24 hr apart or dexamethasone 6 mg IM × 4 doses 12 hr apart).	Corticosteroids stimulate fetal lung maturity by inducing release of lung surfactants.
Administer NST q4h or as prescribed in pregnancy and perform FHR and uterine monitoring in labor, with documentation q½-1 h or per agency protocol.	Adverse effects of severe preeclampsia, magnesium, cervical ripening agents, and oxytocin may cause fetal distress as reflected by non-reassuring (Category 2 or Category 3) FHR patterns.
! Arrange for neonatologist and resuscitation team to be present at the delivery for newborn care with delivery of an infant of a preeclamptic mother, whether preterm or term delivery.	Their presence is vital during preeclampsia and after an eclamptic seizure. Disease progression, gestational age limitations, and medications may lead to asphyxia and other severe complications in the newborn.

Nursing Diagnosis:

Deficient Knowledge

related to unfamiliarity with the effects of preeclampsia on the mother, fetus, and delivery; effects of treatments and medications; and the potential impact of medications and treatment regimen on daily family life

Desired Outcome: Immediately after teaching, the patient and her significant others begin to participate in her therapeutic regimen by accurately monitoring and reporting weight, BP, urine protein, edema, fetal activity, signs of improving or worsening preeclampsia, and side effects or effectiveness of medications.

ASSESSMENT/INTERVENTIONS	RATIONALES
Assess the woman's ability to assume self-care responsibilities, report symptoms, the impact of language on communication, and her support systems, culture and beliefs about illness, and the home environment.	Physical, psychosocial, and environmental factors determine whether home care is a viable option in mild preeclampsia. Some patients and families need more educational and medical intervention than others.
Develop an educational plan that uses several modes of instruction tailored to the patient's and family's information needs and cognitive ability.	Comprehension improves when education is given at an individual's level of understanding. Using verbal, auditory, and kinesthetic modes enhances learning and retention.
Inform the patient and her family about the effects of preeclampsia on pregnancy, delivery, and maternal and fetal well-being.	An informed patient and family are more likely to adhere to the prescribed therapy and participate in the therapeutic regimen.
As indicated, teach self-assessment and reporting of clinical signs: how to take and record her own BP, measure urine protein, maintain a daily weight record, assess edema, count and report fetal activity, and report signs of worsening preeclampsia.	Self-care instruction provides closer surveillance of changing preeclampsia, improves responses by health care providers, and may prevent worsening of preeclampsia.
Teach self-care with a balanced pregnancy diet (adequate protein, calcium, zinc, magnesium, sodium, folate, vitamins C and E, and roughage); adequate fluids as prescribed; preference for left side-lying positions; sufficient rest and relaxation; understanding treatments and medications; and the impact of the above on maternal and fetal well-being.	A nutritious diet and adequate fluids influence disease progression. Rest and relaxation promote diuresis. Antihypertensive medications (hydralazine [Apresoline] and labetalol HCl [Normodyne or Trandate]) are preferred in a hypertensive crisis. Patients with chronic hypertension prior to preeclampsia may be on labetalol HCl (beta-blocker), methyldopa (Aldomet), or nifedipine (Procardia).
Teach the patient to distinguish between magnesium sulfate side effects and toxicity.	The most common side effects of magnesium sulfate therapy include lethargy, weakness, sweating and flushing, nausea and vomiting, headaches, and slurred speech. Signs of developing toxicity include loss of DTRs, oliguria, respiratory depression (RR of less than 12/min), respiratory arrest, and cardiac arrest.
Support the family in assisting with the patient's responsibilities, helping manage the preeclampsia regimen, and providing emotional support.	Family involvement promotes the patient's self-efficacy with participation in the regimen and her sense of control, enhances her coping skills, and reduces anxiety and fears.

Nursing Diagnosis:

Caregiver Role Strain

related to care the significant other, family member, or support person needs to provide not only to the patient but also possibly to other children in order for the patient to remain compliant and thereby prolong the gestational period

Desired Outcome: Within 24 hr of this diagnosis, the caregiver verbalizes concerns/frustrations about caregiving responsibilities, identifies at least one other support person, and recognizes at least one change that would make his or her job easier.

ASSESSMENT/INTERVENTIONS	RATIONALES
Assess and encourage the caregiver to relate feelings and concerns regarding added responsibilities. Help the caregiver clarify responsibilities with the patient and other family members.	This validates the caregiver's concerns and helps him or her understand if expectations are realistic.
Encourage the caregiver to identify activities that would benefit from outside assistance.	This confirms the caregiver's need to seek help and facilitates that help.
Involve Social Services in support of the caregiver establishing a plan for time-outs or for referrals to community support groups.	This also confirms the need to seek help and provides the caregiver with coping mechanisms. During times of stress, caregivers may know they need help but may not know where to find it.

Nursing Diagnosis:

Risk for Disturbed Maternal/Fetal Dyad

related to interruption of bonding and attachment processes during separation from preterm or compromised newborn

Desired Outcome: Within 24 hr of receiving encouragement, information, and support from the health care team, the parents verbalize concerns and begin parenting of their newborn.

ASSESSMENT/INTERVENTIONS	RATIONALES
Assess parental perception of their situation, individual concerns, and strengths.	Identifying perceptions, verbalizing concerns, and identification of strengths (sensitivity to newborn cues, understanding of preterm abilities, provision of reciprocal relationship) enable effective and realistic planning.
Establish a trusting and nurturing nurse, patient, and family relationship.	The quality of the nurse-patient relationship is key to successful transitioning and parenting a preterm or compromised newborn. Nurturing the parents nurtures development of the parent-infant relationships.
Encourage the parents and family to verbalize fears and concerns.	Parents and family are already grieving real and potential losses (e.g., possible newborn death, inability to deliver at term or deliver a healthy newborn, idealized dreams of parenting the newborn, and seeing the newborn attached to tubes and ventilators). Verbalizing fears and concerns provides validation of their concerns and enables reassessment.
Prior to labor, provide anticipatory guidance for the realities of a possible preterm birth, a preterm infant, and separation from the newborn in the newborn intensive care unit (NICU).	Time to process, rehearse, and develop understanding empowers parents and fosters self-efficacy.
Encourage and assist parents to attach and interact with their newborn in the NICU.	Parents may have to resolve the realities of the NICU, along with the newborn's preterm appearance and capacity, and learn new ways to interact in an NICU setting. The newborn could have tubes inserted, be attached to a heart rate monitor and pulse oximeter, and be in an Isolette. Over time parents can learn to do some daily care (e.g., take axillary temperatures, change diapers, bathe very delicate skin, and learn preterm cues that signal fatigue and other issues).
Encourage the mother to breastfeed or provide breast milk for her baby.	Breastfeeding enhances maternal sensitivity to her newborn. Support and assistance by the hospital staff significantly influences success with breastfeeding and development of maternal role attainment. Establishing an early pumping regimen can be beneficial in creating an adequate milk supply for the baby in NICU or who is premature and unable to latch.
Support and praise the parents' behaviors that foster secure rather than avoidant or ambivalent attachment.	The parents' support, consistency, warmth, and sensitivity in responding to their baby facilitate secure attachment.
If the mother is too ill to be with her newborn, arrange for the father, family, and others to visit, keep her informed of the baby's condition, and bring her photos or other mementos.	These actions encourage development of mother-infant attachment. They may decrease her fears as well.
Refer the parents to a perinatal social worker and offer referrals to ongoing support groups as appropriate.	Professional support may facilitate parental adaptation and foster self-efficacy.

ADDITIONAL NURSING DIAGNOSES/PROBLEMS:

✓ PATIENT-FAMILY TEACHING AND DISCHARGE PLANNING

Preeclampsia is a progressive disease in which monitoring for maternal and fetal changes is of critical importance. Include verbal and written information about the following:

- ✓ Signs and symptoms of worsening preeclampsia (headache, increased edema, oliguria, right upper quadrant [RUQ] pain, decreased fetal movement, nausea, and vomiting) and importance of contacting the health care provider promptly should they occur.
- ✓ Seizure precautions.

- ✓ Medications, including drug name, purpose, dosage, frequency, precautions, potential drug reactions, and side effects. Also discuss potential drug-drug, food-drug, and herb-drug interactions.
- ✓ Importance of adherence to the prescribed health care regimen and ready access to hospital and family/social support.
- ✓ Parameters and guidelines for home bedrest.
- ✓ Measures that help with side effects of prolonged bedrest such as constipation, muscle pain, back pain, and muscle weakness.
- ✓ Fetal movement counts.
- ✓ The American Congress of Obstetricians and Gynecologists has an extensive collection of patient education materials available at *www.acog.org/ Resources_And_Publications/Patient_Education_FAQs _List*
- ✓ Referrals to national and local support agencies, including:
  - Sidelines, a national support organization for women and their families experiencing complicated pregnancies at *www.sidelines.org*
  - March of Dimes at *www.marchofdimes.com*
  - The Society of Obstetricians and Gynecologists of Canada at *http://sogc.org* (requires subscription)

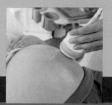

OVERVIEW/PATHOPHYSIOLOGY

Preterm labor (PTL) is the onset of contractions that effect cervical change, either dilation or effacement, after 20 wk gestation and before the 37th wk of gestation. Birth before completion of the 37th wk is considered preterm. Most preterm births (PTB) occur between 34 and 36 wk. *Late-preterm infant birth (LPI)* is the term given to infants born between $34^{0/7}$ wk and $36^{6/7}$ wk. All pregnant women are considered at risk for PTL, although approximately 12% of all pregnancies end in PTL (Hamilton et al., 2011).

It is not known what causes PTL; however, it is associated with infections such as chorioamnionitis, periodontitis, and vaginal bacteriosis. Because the mechanisms that initiate term labor are multifactorial and not completely understood, exactly what causes PTL continues to be researched. Some risk factors for PTL have been identified. See table, below, for details. The end results of PTL are increased uterine irritability, decreased placental functioning, increased prostaglandin synthesis, cervical changes, and the risk for PTB. Prematurity is the second leading cause of infant mortality in the United States after congenital anomalies. Many preterm infants who survive have long-term neurologic and/or physical impairments.

HEALTH CARE SETTING

Some patients may be managed via primary care on an out-patient basis with frequent clinic evaluation or in a high-risk perinatal clinic. Others may receive acute care in an inpatient antepartum setting.

ASSESSMENT

Symptoms of PTL may range from subtle to obvious. Many symptoms do not cause pain. PTL does not present in the same way as labor at term. All pregnant women should be taught the symptoms of PTL during early prenatal visits and then be reassessed at each prenatal visit. The mother may feel that the baby is "balling up" in her abdomen and describe a "heavy" feeling in the perineum or pelvic pressure.

Contractions/uterine tightening: As the pregnancy progresses, so does the frequency of uterine activity. Uterine tightening/contractions begin in the first trimester as the uterus enlarges and continue throughout the pregnancy. These contractions are called *Braxton-Hicks*. They occur at irregular intervals, usually are painless, and do not change the cervix. PTL may feel like light menstrual-like cramping or strong, palpable contractions. PTL is diagnosed when uterine contractions are persistent and accompanied by cervical change, either dilation or effacement.

Backache: This is a very common complaint in pregnancy. Any woman with a history of preterm labor/delivery who complains of new-onset backache needs to be evaluated for cervical changes, especially if she describes the backache as low and lumbar/sacral in location, deep tissue in nature, or a dull aching sensation that radiates around the hips to the lower abdomen/pelvic area and down the thighs.

Pelvic pressure: The woman may state that she feels the "baby has dropped." Pelvic pressure may be described as a constant or intermittent "heaviness" or a sensation of "fullness in the pelvis."

Abdominal cramping: Gastrointestinal (GI) symptoms such as increased flatus or diarrhea may be present. The abdomen may be tender to palpate, as is seen with chorioamnionitis (inflammatory reaction in the amniotic membranes caused by bacteria or virus).

Vaginal discharge: An increase in vaginal discharge is normal during pregnancy. It can be clear, thick, or thin and "milky white" or light yellow. It may become watery, as with preterm premature ruptured membranes (PPROM), or bloody, as with placental abruption or when the cervix dilates and its surface vessels break. Vaginal itching or burning or a foul odor may indicate an infection. Vaginal bleeding may range from light pink spotting to bright red bleeding.

Fever: Temperature may range from 98.6° F (37° C) to 101° F (38.3° C) or higher if an infection is present.

General complaints: Other symptoms may include a feeling of unease and body aches. The woman may state, "I just feel different."

Physical assessment: Even with vague symptoms, cervical changes may be taking place. Therefore, it is important not to underestimate reported symptoms. Early evaluation and treatment are critical in attempting to stop PTL and preventing fetal morbidity and mortality.

Complications—fetal
- Preterm delivery
- Respiratory distress syndrome (RDS)
- Patent ductus arteriosus (PDA—an abnormal opening between the pulmonary artery and aorta)

Medical Risks

Three groups of women are at greatest risk of PTL and PTB:

- Women who have had a previous preterm birth
- Women who are pregnant with twins, triplets, or more
- Women with certain uterine or cervical abnormalities

If a woman has any of these three risk factors, it is especially important for her to know the signs and symptoms of PTL and what to do if they occur.

Certain medical conditions during pregnancy may increase the likelihood that a woman will have PTL. These conditions include:

- Urinary tract infections, vaginal infections, sexually transmitted infections, and possibly other infections
- Diabetes
- High blood pressure
- Clotting disorders (thrombophilia)
- Bleeding from the vagina
- Certain birth defects in the baby
- Being pregnant with a single fetus after in vitro fertilization (IVF)
- Being underweight before pregnancy
- Obesity
- One or more midtrimester pregnancy losses
- Polyhydramnios
- Placenta abruption; placenta previa

Lifestyle and Environmental Risks

Some studies have found that certain lifestyle factors may put a woman at greater risk of PTL. These factors include:

- Late or no prenatal care
- Grand multiparity
- Smoking
- Drinking alcohol
- Using illegal drugs
- Exposure to the medication diethylstilbestrol (DES)
- Domestic violence, including physical, sexual, or emotional abuse
- Lack of social support
- Stress
- Working the night shift
- Long working hours with long periods of standing

- Short time period between pregnancies (less than 6-9 mo between birth and the beginning of the next pregnancy)

http://www.marchofdimes.com/21191_5804.asp
Retrieved from March of Dimes on August 30, 2013

- Intraventricular hemorrhage (IVH)
- Sepsis
- Necrotizing enterocolitis (ischemic, inflammatory bowel disorder that can lead to perforation and peritonitis)
- Hyperbilirubinemia
- Hypoglycemia
- Impaired/immature immunologic system
- Neonatal death

DIAGNOSTIC TESTS

There are several biochemical markers and assessments that assist in the diagnosis of PTL.

Cervical evaluation: Sterile speculum cervical exams provide information about cervical effacement, cervical dilation, and whether amniotic fluid is leaking or abnormal secretions are present in the vagina. Cervical or vaginal secretions can be collected for a ferning test (rupture of membranes) or fetal fibronectin (fFn) test, or cultures may be obtained to diagnose an infection.

Transvaginal ultrasonography: May be used to measure cervical length when cervical effacement is less than 80% and to evaluate funneling of the internal cervical os as well as effacement and dilation of the cervix. The shorter the cervix,

the greater the risk of PTL. The shortest acceptable length is 30 mm. Less than 25 mm is considered a shortened cervix and is associated with PTL (Romero et al., 2012).

Fetal fibronectin (fFn): Fetal fibronectins are glycoproteins present in the cervical and vaginal secretions early in pregnancy. After 22 wk gestation, they are not detectable in vaginal secretions. Their presence returns within 2 wk of delivery, whether it is preterm or term. Therefore negative fFn results between 24 and 35 wk gestation are strongly associated with not going into labor for the next 1-2 wk. The negative predictive power of fFn is used to avoid further and unnecessary interventions for the woman at risk for PTL. A positive fFn finding is less predictive of labor because false positives occur with recent sexual intercourse, vaginal bleeding, amniotic fluid, or recent cervical examinations. The health care provider gathers the sample for testing before doing a vaginal examination for cervical changes because the lubricant used for manual vaginal exams may interfere with test results.

Uterine contraction evaluation: A diagnosis of preterm labor is made when the cervix is more than 2 cm dilated and the patient presents with regular contractions. Other criteria include a cervical examination showing more than or equal to 80% effaced or a change in cervical dilation with regular contractions. The focus of care is on stopping PTL if the intervention can begin before the woman has reached 3-cm cervical dilation. If PTL cannot be stopped, management is focused on maternal safety and reduction of the preterm infant's risk for respiratory distress syndrome.

PPROM: Preterm premature rupture of membranes precedes PTL in 25% of preterm births. See discussion, p. 693.

Urinalysis for microscopy: Urinary tract infections (UTIs) are associated with PTL. A clean-catch urine specimen should be obtained when attempting to rule out PTL, even when the patient is asymptomatic. When a UTI is present, antibiotic therapy will be initiated.

Nursing Diagnosis:

Anxiety

related to perceived or actual threats to self and well-being of the fetus and inadequate time to prepare for labor/delivery

Desired Outcomes: Immediately after intervention, the patient describes the symptoms of anxiety she is feeling. Within 1-2 hr of intervention, the patient reports that the detrimental anxiety reactions are lessened.

ASSESSMENT/INTERVENTIONS	RATIONALES
Assess maternal level of understanding, language, and ability to communicate her feelings and concerns, cultural-bound anxiety, and the impact of fatigue.	Assessment provides information about the woman's and family's emotional needs, communication needs, and cognitive level. When interventions are provided at the appropriate level and understood, behavioral changes take place. Anxiety can be culture-related and is manifested differently from culture to culture.
Assess maternal vital signs (VS) q2-4h and fetal heart rate (FHR) patterns per agency protocol.	Maternal temperature and pulse rise if an infection is present. Physiologic stress reaction also increases pulse and respirations. Muscle tension and vasoconstriction may cause uteroplacental insufficiency and reduce oxygenation to the fetus as evidenced by nonreassuring (Category 2 or Category 3) FHR patterns.
Help the patient anticipate and problem solve her needs related to procedures, procedural side effects, how they affect her and her unborn baby, her changing labor status, the fetal condition, and hoped-for outcomes.	Anxiety is reduced with clarification of needs, medical interventions, procedures, and anticipated medications.
Encourage questions and verbalization of concerns. Answer honestly, while maintaining an optimistic attitude.	When concerns are verbalized and clarified, the nurse can give realistic feedback and provide appropriate emotional support.
Assess and guide the patient to develop a personal support system and use community resources while in the hospital in anticipation of her return home to self-care and outpatient monitoring.	Refer to interventions and rationales for support under **Ineffective Coping**, later.
Encourage self-nurturing with rest, assistance with relaxation techniques, prayer or meditation as related to the woman's faith, and by administration of sedatives if prescribed when other measures are insufficient.	When the usual quiescence of the uterus is interrupted by the threat of preterm delivery, the mother and family can become severely stressed. Rest, meditation, prayer, and focused relaxation improve physiologic, psychologic, and spiritual well-being.

Nursing Diagnosis:

Activity Intolerance

related to the need for rest to prevent the effects of activity on advancing PTL

Desired Outcomes: Within 1-2 hr after interventions, the patient describes her at-home situation, mobilizes appropriate support for home care (or family while in the hospital), and verbalizes plans to reduce her activity level as prescribed.

ASSESSMENT/INTERVENTIONS	RATIONALES
Assess readiness of the patient, her partner, and family to learn from within their cultural context. Assess ability of the family unit to assume care responsibilities in preparation for the patient's discharge to home care.	Changes in family functioning and behavior occur when education is given at the appropriate level of understanding. Barriers to effective functioning may include anemia, physical weakness, impaired mental functioning relative to the prescribed medications, familial conflicts, and uncontrollable outside stressors.
Explain ways to maintain muscle strength with prescribed activity reduction or possible bedrest, the reasons for bedrest or activity reduction, and the frequent use of left lateral positioning.	Physical deconditioning develops quickly with bedrest and may take weeks to reverse (muscle atrophy, cardiovascular changes, maternal weight loss). Understanding the value of reducing fetal pressure on the cervix and increasing uterine perfusion promotes adherence to left lateral positioning. There is no current evidence that supports *strict* bedrest as beneficial or identifies the level of reduced activity that is beneficial for the mother or baby. A thorough explanation of activity limits and positioning encourages compliance through improved understanding.
Provide comfort measures (back rubs, frequent position changes while awake, reduced noise and stimuli in the room) and uninterrupted periods of rest/sleep.	These interventions decrease muscle tension and fatigue while promoting relaxation and a sense of well-being.
Assist with the development of plans for adjustments in family functioning and mobilizing a support team, which may include personal and community resources.	Being able to rely on a team of support for the care of other children and accomplishing family needs reduces physical tension and mental anxiety.
Assist with diversional activity plans (e.g., at home get dressed daily and rest on the couch; learn sedentary hobbies [knitting etc.]; read; watch television; use a laptop computer, smart phone, or other method to communicate with friends and access support and information; listen to books on tape; and plan appropriate friend/family visits [at home or in hospital]).	Making plans for acceptable diversional activities decreases anxiety and a sense of isolation.

Nursing Diagnosis:

Risk for Injury: Maternal and Fetus

related to toxic side effects of tocolytics

Desired Outcome: After 1-4 hr of tocolytic therapy, uterine contractions begin to decrease without manifestation of toxic side effects in the mother or the fetus.

ASSESSMENT/INTERVENTIONS	RATIONALES
Assess VS (especially blood pressure [BP], heart rate [HR], respiratory rate [RR]) and cardiac rhythm. Auscultate lung sounds. Note reports of dyspnea or chest tightness.	Many adverse side effects of tocolytic medications alter these physiologic parameters.
Before beginning tocolytic therapy, hydrate with a bolus if intravenous (IV) fluids are prescribed.	Hydration reduces risk of hypotension and promotes renal clearance. It also may decrease uterine contractions.

ASSESSMENT/INTERVENTIONS	RATIONALES
⚠ Administer tocolytic medications (magnesium sulfate, terbutaline) per agency policy. Use an infusion pump if IV magnesium sulfate is being administered.	IV administration via infusion pump takes effect quickly and can be discontinued quickly if adverse reactions occur. Commonly used in the United States as tocolytics, magnesium sulfate and terbutaline are not FDA approved for this purpose and are used off label to inhibit the contractions of PTL. However, they should not be used for more than 5-7 days.
⚠ Assess for side effects of tocolytics.	
- Terbutaline: Monitor serum potassium level before administration and periodically afterward, along with glucose level. Teach the patient to report and assess for tachycardia (maternal or fetal), heart palpitations, shortness of breath, headache, weakness, and nausea.	As a beta-adrenergic agonist (betamimetic or beta-sympathomimetic), terbutaline relaxes smooth muscles, thus inhibiting uterine contractions while causing bronchial dilation and accelerating the heart rate. A HR greater than 120 bpm is associated with decreased cardiac output and may necessitate discontinuance of the medication. An overdose may cause cardiac arrest. Common adverse metabolic side effects with this medication are hyperglycemia and hypokalemia. Terbutaline is recommended for use for 48-72 hr and only in an inpatient setting. The neonate needs to be closely monitored for hypoglycemia after birth until feeding is well established.
- Magnesium sulfate: Assess serum magnesium levels as prescribed during therapy. Assess for and report depressed deep tendon reflexes (DTRs), significant changes in VS from baseline, including decreased BP, reduced respirations (less than 14/min), drowsiness, oxygen saturation less than 95%, changes in level of consciousness, hot flashes, blurred vision, slurred speech, reduced FHR variability, and serum hypocalcemia.	As a central nervous system (CNS) depressant, magnesium sulfate relaxes smooth muscles, thereby decreasing uterine contraction frequency/intensity and relaxing blood vessel walls. An overdose may cause respiratory paralysis and cardiac arrest.
Keep calcium gluconate on hand.	Normal magnesium levels are 1.5-2.5 mEq/L or 1.7-2.4 mg/dL. *Therapeutic* levels are 4-7 mEq/L or 5-8.4 mg/dL. Magnesium sulfate affects the actions/concentrations of K^+ and Ca^{2+}, and therefore calcium gluconate is used as an antidote.
⚠ Administer nifedipine as prescribed. Assess for hypotension, dizziness, weakness, fatigue, facial flushing, nausea, proteinuria, and peripheral edema (fluid retention).	As a calcium channel blocker, nifedipine relaxes smooth muscles, thereby decreasing amplitude and frequency of uterine activity and contractility of the cardiac muscle and dilating blood vessel walls. An overdose may cause heart failure.
⚠ Administer indomethacin as prescribed. Assess for side effects, e.g., headache, nausea, dizziness, hypertension, and peripheral edema.	As a prostaglandin inhibitor, indomethacin plays a role in decreasing uterine contractions of labor. When given after 32 wk gestation, it has been associated with premature closure of patent ductus arteriosus in the fetus and persistent pulmonary hypertension in newborns. After 48 hr, amniotic fluid index (AFI) measured by ultrasound, perinatology consult, and weekly fetal echocardiography may be prescribed.
Administer betamethasone or dexamethasone as prescribed by the health care provider.	These corticosteroids reduce the effects of respiratory distress syndrome (RDS), intraventricular hemorrhage (IVH), and necrotizing enterocolitis in the preterm neonate when delivery is anticipated to be less than 34 wk and after the gestation of viability. They also accelerate maturation of the CNS and fetal organs, including cardiovascular.
Assess intake and output (I&O) q1-8h as prescribed.	Assessing I&O promotes interventions for adequate hydration while reducing the risk of fluid overload. Pulmonary edema is a risk with tocolytic medications. Magnesium sulfate is excreted through the kidneys, and therefore urinary output of at least 30 mL/hr is a sign the kidneys are functioning properly.

<u>Nursing Diagnoses:</u>

Constipation
Dysfunctional Gastrointestinal Motility

related to decreased peristalsis occurring with immobility, stress, lack of exercise, and prolonged bedrest

Desired Outcome: The patient has normal bowel movements and minimal discomfort from gas and hard stooling within 2-3 days of interventions, thereby reducing the risk of preterm contractions.

ASSESSMENT/INTERVENTIONS	RATIONALES
Assess the patient's normal bowel status and whether she requires laxatives or stool softeners on a routine basis.	This assessment identifies if constipation is playing a role in PTL. Constipation is a normal symptom of pregnancy because the descending colon vies for space with the uterus as it enlarges and because progesterone, one of the hormones produced in pregnancy, decreases gastric motility. However, in a patient prone to PTL who is on bedrest, constipation can be exacerbated because of the decrease in peristalsis associated with inactivity.
Explain the effects of constipation in a patient prone to PTL.	Constipation or gastric irritability can increase uterine irritability in the form of contractions. This would increase risk of PTL.
Encourage intake of at least 8-10 glasses of water/day and increasing dietary fiber or adding a fiber laxative or stool softener to her daily regimen.	These measures provide bulk and aid in keeping the stool soft to promote evacuation.

<u>Nursing Diagnosis:</u>

Deficient Knowledge

related to unfamiliarity with the effects of PTL on self and the fetus

Desired Outcome: The patient, her partner, and her family verbalize accurate knowledge about the effects of PTL on the patient, her pregnancy, and her fetus.

ASSESSMENT/INTERVENTIONS	RATIONALES
Assess the patient, her partner, and her family regarding attitudes about the patient's care (allowed self-care and care contributed by the family). Encourage self-efficacy for learning about her condition and the necessary care for herself and the fetus.	When patients and significant others believe they cannot contribute to the patient's well-being, research identifies that they may become ambivalent, passive, and be "problem takers" rather than proactive in the care and reporting of problems.
Discuss with the patient and her family the signs of PTL, its treatment, and its effects on delivery and on the newborn. Develop an assessment and reporting plan with her.	Adequate information helps to identify problems early and promote adherence to the therapeutic regimen. The effects PTL and delivery have on the newborn can be life threatening (i.e., RDS, hypoglycemia, IVH, sepsis, necrotizing enterocolitis, and neonatal death).
Actively use written material in the discussion.	Written materials reinforce learning and retention.
Explain the importance of access to a specialized facility and the possible need to transport the pregnant woman (if she lives in a rural area) to a distant hospital.	Delivering a preterm infant at a tertiary or secondary hospital facility with perinatal and neonatal specialists and a neonatal intensive care unit (NICU) provides the greatest opportunity for infant survival.
Teach signs and symptoms of PTL to *all* pregnant women.	An informed patient likely will report these symptoms promptly. See introductory information for detailed signs and symptoms of PTL. Barring the presence of chorioamnionitis, the earlier PTL is diagnosed, the better the chance for prolonging the pregnancy and decreasing fetal morbidity and mortality.

ASSESSMENT/INTERVENTIONS	RATIONALES
Question the patient at each prenatal visit, starting at the beginning of the second trimester, if she is experiencing any signs or symptoms of PTL/contractions.	Early recognition of PTL (see signs and symptoms in the introductory data) may lead to prolonging the gestational period and decreasing fetal morbidity and mortality.
Encourage the patient to report even vague or subtle symptoms no matter the time of day or night. Provide written instructions and telephone numbers to call should concerns or changes arise.	Uterine contractions may be painless. Fewer than 50% of patients in PTL are aware of their contractions, and many do not realize that PTL can be serious. Women who present with PTL account for approximately 12% of PTB (ACOG, 2012), and PTB accounts for almost 70% of all neonatal mortality not caused by congenital anomalies (ACOG, 2012).
Teach daily fetal movement counts.	Fetal movement counts done twice a day are a good first-line indicator of fetal well-being and are performed as follows: beginning at 28 wk gestation: The patient lies on her side and counts "distinct fetal movements" (hiccups do not count); 10 movements within a 2-hr period are considered reassuring. After 10 movements are discerned, the count is discontinued. Fewer than 10 movements in a 2-hr period signals need for fetal nonstress testing.
Teach the patient how to palpate contractions.	Timely reporting of preterm contractions to her health care provider can play a significant role in affecting outcome. Palpation and awareness of contractions enable the patient to be an active participant in her health care.
	To palpate contractions, the patient lies comfortably on her side. She spreads her fingers apart and places one hand on the left side and the other on the right side of her abdomen. She will palpate the abdomen using her fingertips. When the uterus is relaxed, the abdomen should feel soft. She should palpate contractions for 1 hr.
	In the presence of a contraction, the uterus should feel hard, tight, or firm under her fingertips. She then times the duration of the contraction from the beginning of one contraction to the end of that contraction. Frequency of contractions is measured from the beginning of one contraction to the beginning of the next contraction. Contractions will vary in frequency and duration. The patient should record whether contractions are palpated only or also experienced as a specific sensation. If the patient experiences more than 4 contractions/hr, she needs to call her primary provider. Contractions may be mild to severe in intensity and difficult for a gravida I (first pregnancy) mother to discern as PTL.
Instruct the patient to drink at least 10 8-oz glasses of water per day, tapering her intake during the last few hr before sleep.	The uterus is a muscle and will respond to dehydration by cramping/contracting. Adequate oral hydration is a preventive measure for PTL.
Teach the patient and her partner the effect that sexual foreplay or intercourse may have on PTL. Advise the patient to avoid all forms of sexual stimulation.	This information promotes patient/partner understanding and adherence. Sexual intercourse may increase uterine contractions and promote cervical change. Increased uterine activity also may be caused by breast stimulation, female orgasm, and prostaglandin in male ejaculate.

Nursing Diagnosis:

Ineffective Coping

related to adjustment in lifestyle to provide an optimal environment for the fetus or lack of support from family, friends, and community

Desired Outcome: Within the 24-hr period after intervention, the patient verbalizes feelings and identifies strengths and coping behaviors that provide the best pregnancy outcome for herself and her fetus.

ASSESSMENT/INTERVENTIONS	RATIONALES
Assess the patient's perceptions and ability to understand her current health status regarding PTL.	Evaluation of the patient's perceptions and comprehension enables development of an individualized care plan.
Provide referral sources for support groups, written material, Internet chat groups, or home help if the patient is on home bedrest or hospitalization. Involve Social Services as needed.	Communicating with or learning about others who have experienced similar circumstances may aid in the development of positive coping mechanisms.
Help the patient identify or develop a support system.	Having a support system will aid in the patient's overall care and reduction of stress to promote positive coping behaviors.
Arrange community referrals as appropriate or at the request of the patient.	Support in the home environment promotes healthier adaptations and may avert crises.
Offer realistic hope for continuing the pregnancy to a safe gestation. Help the patient and family develop realistic expectations for the future if a preterm delivery occurs and to identify support persons or systems that will help them plan for the future.	These measures foster realistic expectations about a preterm neonate's health status (in the absence of congenital anomalies) and promote adaptation to possible changes in family dynamics.
Advise the patient and family that hospitalization and medical interventions in preventing a preterm birth may not always be effective or wise.	Medications, bedrest, and hydration are not always successful in stopping PTL. In some instances an early delivery may be in the best interest of the mother, fetus, or both, as would be the case in the presence of infection, nonreassuring (Category 2, Category 3) fetal heart rate tracings, severe oligohydramnios (abnormally low amount of amniotic fluid), anhydramnios (no amniotic fluid), and congenital anomalies.
Affirm that lifestyle adjustment (e.g., no work, bedrest, no intercourse) is for a limited time.	This information facilitates acceptance of outside support and assistance and reinforces knowledge that routine or increased activity with PTL may increase risk of cervical change and possible preterm delivery.

Nursing Diagnosis:

Caregiver Role Strain

related to the care the significant other, family member, or support person needs to provide not only to the patient but also possibly to other family members in order for the patient to remain compliant and prolong the gestational period

Desired Outcome: Within 24 hr from this diagnosis, the caregiver verbalizes concerns/frustrations about caregiving responsibilities, identifies at least one other support person, and recognizes at least one change that would make his or her job easier.

ASSESSMENT/INTERVENTIONS	RATIONALES
Encourage the caregiver and the patient to relate their feelings and concerns regarding their roles and to problem solve together.	This validates concerns and helps them understand if expectations are realistic. Mutual participation in planning fosters self-efficacy for both.
Acknowledge the caregiver's role in the patient's care; identify and praise strengths.	This reinforces positive ways of dealing with the current health crisis and promotes a sense of involvement and appreciation.
Involve Social Services in support of the caregiver in helping establish a plan for time-outs.	Social Services can provide the caregiver with a weekly viable goal and coping mechanisms and validate the need to seek help.
Provide the patient and caregiver with status reports on effectiveness of the patient's bedrest, decreased activity, stopping work, or inability to participate in routine household activities.	Reassuring the patient and caregiver that the support and assistance are positively affecting the patient's health likely will promote more of the same.
Affirm that this situation is for a limited time.	This information facilitates the patient's and caregiver's acceptance in receiving and giving support and assistance.
Encourage diversional activities (e.g., time alone away from home or hospital and other children) and interactions with support persons or systems outside the family.	Promoting respite enhances coping and helps family members remain focused and supportive of the patient. For example, "I know this must be a difficult time and you want to stay with your wife, but I will call you if any changes occur."

Nursing Diagnosis:

Interrupted Breastfeeding

related to break in continuity of the normal process resulting from a premature and/or ill infant

Desired Outcome: The patient produces breast milk using a breast pump or makes an informed decision regarding which method of feeding most benefits the infant's needs and her own emotional/physical state of well-being.

ASSESSMENT/INTERVENTIONS	RATIONALES
When possible, encourage the mother to visit the baby in NICU as soon as possible after the delivery. Provide the mother with written information on care, including breastfeeding support provided in the NICU.	These measures promote the bonding process, encourage communication with the baby's care providers, and provide an opportunity to have questions answered. Breastfeeding support enables the new mother to reach her goals to provide milk for her baby.
Encourage the mother to breastfeed or express milk for later feeding of the infant.	In the preterm infant, it is not always possible or recommended to feed at the breast. However, supporting the mother's efforts to provide breast milk by teaching manual hand expression and pumping facilitates lactogenesis and promotes psychologic benefits for the mother by involving her in the infant's daily care and reinforcing the importance her breast milk has to the health of her infant.
Explain benefits of breast milk for the preterm infant.	For the preterm infant, breast milk decreases incidences of infectious complications and metabolic disturbances. Maternal antibodies in breast milk also promote immunologic health because the preterm infant's immune system is immature. Breast milk also helps establish nonpathogenic bacterial flora in the newborn intestinal tract and stimulates passage of stool.
If the mother chooses to breastfeed by expressing milk for later infant feeding, assist her with breast pump operation and arrange for acquisition of an electric breast pump for home use as needed.	A breast pump aids in producing/sustaining breast milk for later infant feeding.
As indicated, teach manual expression, storage, and transport of milk.	These measures aid in the success of producing milk and the safety of its storage.
Encourage the mother to verbalize her feelings and concerns and to clarify her questions.	Verbalizing feelings and concerns makes them more concrete and manageable. Clarification of questions enables development of self-efficacy. Tension can interfere with establishing an adequate milk supply.
Reassure the patient that breastfeeding can be successful even with initial separation after birth. Teach her the physical process of how lactation occurs after birth.	This information helps decrease her anxiety about "not having enough milk" and helps her understand the importance of breast stimulation via actual breastfeeding or pumping. Delivery of the placenta causes a decrease in progesterone and an increase in prolactin, the hormone that stimulates lactogenesis (milk production). Prolactin is released from the anterior pituitary gland during breastfeeding or with nipple stimulation as with breast pumping and manual hand expression. Prolactin levels increase with each breastfeeding session and in turn stimulate milk production. Oxytocin is released from the posterior pituitary gland at the same time and causes the milk ejection reflex, or milk "let down." During the course of breastfeeding, these hormones are released and regulated on a supply and demand basis. Encouragement of a regular pumping and manual hand-expression regimen (8 times in 24 hr) promotes the best milk supply.
Provide support to the mother through referral to a lactation consultant (IBCLC) available within the hospital or as outside consultants.	Lactation consultants teach the mother how to use a breast pump or, in actual infant breastfeeding, how to position the infant for comfort and ease of nursing, how to use nipple shields and other lactation support as needed, and how to manage engorgement, inverted or flat nipples, milk supply problems, plugged ducts, sore nipples, and infant sucking problems.

continued

ASSESSMENT/INTERVENTIONS

Teach the importance of adequate oral hydration (10-12 glasses of fluids per day), nutrition (balanced diet with about 300-500 calories more than a nonpregnant diet), and rest.

RATIONALES

Adequate maternal caloric intake, oral hydration, and rest help meet the periods of increased demand for breast milk during the infant's growth spurts and maintain a consistent supply of breast milk.

ADDITIONAL NURSING DIAGNOSES/PROBLEMS:

"Psychosocial Support" for relevant nursing diagnoses such as:

Disturbed Sleep Pattern	p. 73
Anxiety	p. 73
Fear	p. 75
Spiritual Distress	p. 77
Grieving/Risk for Complicated Grieving	p. 78
Disturbed Body Image	p. 79
Social Isolation	p. 81

"Psychosocial Support for the Patient's Family and Significant Other" for such nursing diagnoses as:

Interrupted Family Process	p. 85
Compromised Family Coping	p. 86

 PATIENT-FAMILY TEACHING AND DISCHARGE PLANNING

Preterm labor and birth can have lifelong effects on the child and family. Early diagnosis and treatment are imperative. Education about signs and symptoms of PTL should be a part of every woman's prenatal care. Include verbal and written information about the following:

✓ Potential risk factors for PTL that may be present early in prenatal care.
✓ Signs and symptoms of PTL.
✓ Palpation of contractions.
✓ Promptly reporting any signs of UTI.
✓ Importance of adequate oral hydration during the pregnancy.
✓ Importance of compliance with routine prenatal care.
✓ Medications, including drug name, purpose, dosage, frequency, precautions, potential drug reactions, and potential side effects. Also discuss potential drug-drug, food-drug, and herb-drug interactions.
✓ Measures that help with constipation, which occurs frequently in pregnancy and can be exacerbated with bedrest.
✓ Measures for coping with muscle pain, back pain, and muscle weakness that can be present with prolonged bedrest.
✓ Fetal movement counts.
✓ Referral to local and national support organizations, including:
  • Sidelines, a national support organization for women and their families experiencing complicated pregnancies, at *www.sidelines.org*
  • The March of Dimes at *www.marchofdimes.com*
  • La Leche League at *www.lalecheleague.org*
  • The American Congress of Obstetricians and Gynecologists has an extensive collection of patient education materials available at *www.acog .org/Resources_And_Publications/Patient_Education_ FAQs_List*
  • The Society of Obstetricians and Gynecologists of Canada at *http://sogc.org* (requires subscription)

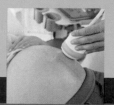

Preterm Premature Rupture of Membranes 94

PATHOPHYSIOLOGY

When membranes rupture before the onset of labor it is called *premature rupture of membranes (PROM)*. Preterm premature rupture of membranes (PPROM) is the leakage of amniotic fluid before term (38-41 wk gestation). From early in pregnancy, the slightly alkaline (pH 7.0-7.5) amniotic fluid is produced within the amniotic sac. As pregnancy advances, fetal urine significantly contributes to the volume. Fetal breathing and swallowing reabsorb the amniotic fluid, which is formed, absorbed, and replaced within a 4-hr period. Amniotic fluid volume at term is approximately 500-1000 mL. It provides an environment that protects the fetus from trauma and injury, provides even distribution of temperature, contains an antibacterial substance, and enables the fetus to move and develop without pressure. Amniotic fluid levels are a good indicator of kidney function and lung maturity. Although the cause of PPROM is unknown, it is considered the cause of one-third of the preterm births before 36 wk gestation (Jorgensen, 2008). Risk for a preterm birth is high when PPROM occurs. The majority of patients with PPROM deliver from within 24 hr to 2 wk of onset.

HEALTH CARE SETTING

The woman may be evaluated in the health care provider's office or clinic. She is managed by obstetricians or perinatologists as an outpatient or inpatient, depending on the week of gestation. Hospital sites may vary depending on gestational age and level of care needed for a high-risk pregnancy and neonate. Before 23 wk gestation, PPROM management is planned around the risks for infection and fetal-developmental anomalies. Parents are included in decision making.

ASSESSMENT

Patients may have difficulty determining the presence of ruptured membranes because symptoms are not always obvious, and leaking amniotic fluid can be confused with leaking urine. Consider carefully any complaint of watery vaginal discharge or sudden gush of fluid. Assess the timing and occurrence of the initial loss of fluid. On some occasions, leakage of amniotic fluid may stop, or it may resume without signs of infection.

Vaginal discharge: Patients may experience a "sudden gush" or sensation that something "popped" followed by a constant slow leakage of clear, watery fluid from the vagina and may state that the amount being leaked requires use of a sanitary pad. The fluid may be blood-tinged or meconium-stained. The amount, color, and odor of the fluid should be evaluated. Vaginal bleeding may accompany PPROM and range from light pink spotting to bleeding as with a heavy menses.

Backache: May or may not be present with PPROM. In the presence of infection, there may be low lumbar/sacral pain that is deep tissue in nature or a dull, aching sensation that may radiate around the hips to the lower abdomen/pelvic area. If abruptio placenta is present with PPROM, the back pain may be mild or severe.

Abdominal pain/cramping or uterine cramping contractions: There may be a feeling of pelvic pressure or fullness, menstrual-like cramping, or contractions. Aching thighs may accompany uterine cramping. In the presence of infection, the patient may complain of abdominal/uterine tenderness or pain. If abruptio placenta accompanies PPROM, the pain may be mild or severe.

Fever: May occur in the presence of an infection and temperature may be 101° F (38.3° C) or higher.

Complications—fetal: Risks to the fetus depend on gestational age at the time of PPROM, the severity of PPROM (the amount of amniotic fluid remaining), and the presence of infection.

- Prematurity
- Fetal infections/sepsis
- Hypoxia and asphyxia caused by umbilical cord compression/prolapse
- Fetal deformities with PPROM at an early gestational age (i.e., pulmonary hypoplasia, facial anomalies, limb position defects)
- Amniotic band syndrome (an abnormal condition characterized by development of fibrous bands within the uterus that entangle the fetus, leading to deformities in fetal structure and function)
- Abruptio placenta
- Fetal death

Physical assessment: In most cases, the cause of PPROM is unknown and there is no forewarning. Therefore, it is important to evaluate changes in vaginal discharge. A timely diagnosis of PPROM is critical to optimize outcomes.

Risk factors: Maternal infections precede PPROM 30%-40% of the time. Urinary tract infections (UTI); genital tract infections such as *Chlamydia trachomatis*, gonorrhea, bacterial vaginosis, or trichomoniasis; chorioamnionitis (intraamniotic infection); and group B streptococcus are contributing factors to PPROM. Other risk factors include low socioeconomic status, smoking, multiple gestation, incompetent cervix (painless cervical dilation before term without contractions), previous history of PPROM, diethylstilbestrol (DES) exposure, amniocentesis, chorionic villi sampling (CVS), coitus, poor nutrition, bleeding in pregnancy, polyhydramnios (excess of amniotic fluid), cervical cerclage (a suture used for holding the cervix closed during a pregnancy), previous cervical laceration or surgery, placental abruption (abnormal separation of the placenta from the wall of the uterus before delivery), history of midtrimester pregnancy loss, cocaine use, hypertension, diabetes, and Ehlers-Danlos syndrome (a group of inherited connective tissue diseases).

DIAGNOSTIC TESTS

Sterile speculum examination: A sterile speculum is inserted into the vagina to visualize amniotic fluid leaking from the cervical os or pooling of amniotic fluid in the vagina. This fluid is tested with Nitrazine paper. If positive for amniotic fluid, the paper will turn from yellow to dark blue or green-blue, and the pH will be greater than 6.0. False-positive results may be seen in the presence of semen, blood, vaginal infections, or alkaline antiseptics. Using a cotton swab, a sample of vaginal fluid is taken from the posterior vaginal fornix (the posterior space below the cervix) and examined under the microscope for the presence of a ferning pattern that amniotic fluid makes when it dries on a slide. A digital examination of the cervix is not recommended in a patient with suspected PPROM who is not in labor. Some agencies use an immunoassay test PAMG-1 (AmniSure) to confirm rupture of membranes. The test detects trace amounts of a protein, PAMG-1, expressed by the cells of the decidua and found in amniotic fluid. The test is performed by swabbing a sterile polyester swab into the vaginal secretions. The swab is then rinsed with a vial of solvent for 1 min and thrown away. A test strip is dipped into the vial for 5-10 min and then read.

One line indicates no rupture of membranes. Two lines is positive for rupture of membranes. No lines indicate an invalid test. The test has a 99% accuracy rate.

External uterine and fetal monitoring: External uterine monitoring is done to evaluate fetal well-being and uterine contraction presence, frequency, and duration. Category 1 fetal heart rate (FHR) pattern is a sign that the fetus is well oxygenated. Category 2 is indeterminate and needs further observation, and Category 3 is abnormal and requires action. Category 2 or Category 3 FHR patterns (decreased variability, moderate-to-severe variable decelerations, and late decelerations) suggest fetal compromise, which can be caused by umbilical cord compression, cord prolapse, or infection that may accompany PPROM.

Obstetric ultrasound: Abdominal ultrasound is used to confirm gestational age, calculate amniotic fluid index (AFI) and biophysical profile (BPP), rule out multiple gestation, and determine placental location and fetal presentation. A normal value for the AFI is between 10 and 20 mL of amniotic fluid. A normal rating on the BPP is 6-8 out of 10.

Amniocentesis: Transabdominal aspiration of amniotic fluid to test for fetal lung maturity and the presence of chorioamnionitis.

Intrauterine dye test: Done only if other tests are inconclusive in determining PPROM or to document that the membranes have sealed over. Resealing is rare, but it can occur. Under ultrasound guidance a diluted solution of indigo carmine dye is inserted with a spinal needle transabdominally into the uterus. The patient is observed for passage of blue fluid from the vagina, which would indicate rupture of membranes.

Blood Rh factor and antibody screen: This test should be a part of the routine prenatal screening. In patients with no prenatal care who have PPROM, this laboratory test is performed on admittance to determine need for administration of Rh-immune globulin to an Rh-negative mother if her newborn is Rh positive.

Nursing Diagnosis:

Risk for Infection

related to bacterial spread (often from ascending movement of vaginal bacteria)

Desired Outcome: The amniotic fluid is clear without offensive odor; maternal temperature remains less than 99.5° F.

ASSESSMENT/INTERVENTIONS	RATIONALES
Assist the health care provider with sterile speculum examination, collection of amniotic fluid, Nitrazine paper test, PAMG-1 immunoassay test, and observation of ferning by microscope.	These assessments can confirm the diagnosis of PPROM.
Assist with collecting specimens from amniocentesis or vaginal secretions for laboratory culture.	Group B streptococcus, *Chlamydia trachomatis,* gonorrhea, bacterial vaginosis, or trichomoniasis organisms are common causes of maternal vaginal tract infections and chorioamnionitis.

ASSESSMENT/INTERVENTIONS	RATIONALES
[!] After PPROM has been confirmed, begin maternal assessments: monitor maternal vital signs q4h; palpate the uterus for tenderness; and observe vaginal secretions for color, amount, and odor q8h.	Fever, uterine tenderness, and changes in vaginal discharge characteristics are signs of infection. Prompt notification of these signs to the health care provider may decrease the risk of further compromise to the fetus or mother.
[!] Apply an external fetal heart rate (FHR) monitor and perform a nonstress test (NST) q8h.	A reactive NST reflects adequate fetal oxygenation status. Category 2 or Category 3 FHR patterns (decreased variability, variable decelerations, or late decelerations) are associated with fetal compromise and indicate a need for further testing or action. Fetal tachycardia is a sign of infection, as is decreased variability.
Arrange for other tests of fetal well-being (e.g., BPP, amniocentesis for lecithin to sphingomyelin [L/S] ratio, and phosphatidyl glycerol [PG] and ultrasound for AFI).	BPP assesses deviations in growth and development and assesses for subclinical infection. L/S ratio and PG identify lung maturity/readiness for neonatal breathing. AFI measurement, a part of the BPP, identifies oligohydramnios by measuring amniotic fluid volumes and helps the health care provider make decisions for the optimal time of delivery.
Collect serial maternal specimens of blood for complete blood count (CBC) and urine for urinalysis as prescribed by the health care provider (e.g., daily).	White blood cell differential rises with infection. Bacteria are present in the urine if a urinary tract infection (UTI) develops.
Administer antibiotics as prescribed by the health care provider.	Prophylactic antibiotics prevent or reduce the effects of maternal-fetal infections and may reduce morbidity and prolong the pregnancy.
Instruct and assist the patient with good hygiene: frequent hand hygiene, daily showering, wiping the perineum from front to back, and changing the peripad q2h (if a pad is worn).	These practices prevent the spread of microorganisms from the environment to the genital area. A moist, warm peripad fosters bacterial growth.

Nursing Diagnosis:

Deficient Knowledge

related to unfamiliarity with the signs and symptoms of PPROM, its effects on the pregnancy and fetus, and guidelines to follow for an optimal outcome

Desired Outcome: Immediately following teaching, the patient and significant other verbalize accurate knowledge about the effects of PPROM on the patient and fetus, as well as its signs and symptoms, prescribed medications, and treatment guidelines for an optimal outcome.

ASSESSMENT/INTERVENTIONS	RATIONALES
Teach the patient and family or significant other signs and symptoms of PPROM and chorioamnionitis (intraamniotic infection), which may be present after PPROM.	A knowledgeable patient likely will report symptoms promptly and understand consequences of nonadherence. PPROM plays a major factor in the morbidity and mortality of the neonate, depending on gestational age. See introductory information for signs and symptoms of PPROM. Indicators of chorioamnionitis include abdominal pain, uterine tenderness, fever, chills, foul vaginal odor, and contractions.
Inform the patient and significant other about the effects PPROM can have on the patient and fetus.	Information facilitates adherence to the treatment regimen. Amniotic fluid is critical to fetal development. See Assessment, earlier, for fetal and newborn risks. PPROM also increases maternal risks: chorioamnionitis (see above symptoms), abruptio placenta (premature separation of the placenta), and a postpartum risk of endometritis (inflammation of the endometrial lining of the uterus). Maternal death from sepsis is rare, but it can occur.

continued

ASSESSMENT/INTERVENTIONS	RATIONALES
Discuss risks/benefits of conservative management (delaying delivery and monitoring the pregnant woman for signs of infection and the fetus for signs of distress) vs. active delivery with anticipated extrauterine support for a preterm infant, in spite of the risk for respiratory distress syndrome (RDS), infection, and neonatal death.	When there are no signs of maternal infection or cervical change and the intrauterine environment is safe for both the mother and fetus, conservative management may buy time for fetal lung maturation. In the presence of a uterine infection, however, delivery is advised. Treating the mother postpartum and the fetus in an extrauterine environment improves maternal/fetal well-being.
Teach daily fetal movement counts.	Beginning at 28 wk gestation, fetal movement is assessed as an indicator of fetal well-being. One of several methods is performed as follows: The patient lies on her side and counts "distinct fetal movement" (hiccups do not count) daily; 10 movements within a 2-hr period is reassuring. After 10 movements, the count is discontinued. Fewer than 10 movements indicates need for fetal NST.
Teach palpation of contractions, which may accompany PPROM (gestation appropriate).	A knowledgeable patient likely will report an increase in contractions promptly: for a singleton pregnancy, 4 contractions/hr or more; for a multiple pregnancy, 6 contractions/hr or more. Palpation and awareness of contractions enable the patient to be an active participant in her health care. Timely reporting of contractions can play a significant role in optimal maternal-fetal outcome. Although contraction frequency alone is insufficient in diagnosing preterm labor, it can serve as a helpful guideline.
	The patient lies comfortably on her side. She will spread her fingers apart and place one hand on the left side and the other on the right side of the abdomen. Palpation is done with the fingertips of both hands. When the uterus is relaxed, the abdomen should feel soft. When a contraction occurs, the uterus will feel hard, tight, or firm under the fingertips. She will time the duration from the beginning of one contraction to the end of the contraction. Duration of the contraction may or may not be an indication of contraction intensity. It is believed that the longer the contraction in true labor, the more effective it is in progressing dilation and effacement. She will also note the frequency of contractions—the time from the beginning of one contraction to the beginning of the next contraction.
Teach the patient to report signs of infection (elevated fever, chills, body aches), decrease in fetal movement (gestation appropriate), and elevated maternal blood glucose levels in patients with diabetes.	After prolonged rupture of membranes an intraamniotic infection often develops. These are common signs of an intraamniotic infection.
For patients on antibiotic therapy, caution about the importance of following the complete course and taking them on time.	These measures prevent development of antibiotic resistance and maintain a constant level of medication in the bloodstream.
⚠ Teach the patient on antibiotic therapy to be alert for and report excessive and explosive diarrhea.	*Clostridium difficile* is a potentially serious side effect in which the normal flora of the bowel are reduced by antibiotic therapy and the anaerobic organism *C. difficile* multiplies and produces its toxins, causing severe diarrhea. This problem necessitates discontinuation of the antibiotic and laboratory evaluation of a stool sample.
Explain the purpose of the antenatal glucocorticoids betamethasone or dexamethasone if these medications are prescribed.	Antenatal glucocorticoids accelerate the development of fetal lungs and help reduce effects of RDS, intraventricular hemorrhage, and necrotizing enterocolitis in the neonate when delivery is anticipated to be preterm and after 20 wk gestation. They also accelerate maturation of other organs (e.g., the central nervous system [CNS] and the cardiovascular system). - Betamethasone: two doses of 12 mg given IM 24 hr apart. - Dexamethasone: four doses of 6 mg given IM 12 hr apart. - Maximum benefit is 48 hr after administration.
⚠ Teach the patient to observe for side effects of corticosteroid therapy and to promptly report her observations.	Possible side effects of corticosteroid medication include reduced maternal-fetal resistance to infection, impaired glucose tolerance (people with borderline gestational diabetes may develop true gestational diabetes), and suppression of maternal or neonatal adrenal function. Usually a rise in blood glucose is seen for approximately 48-96 hr after administration, and it may necessitate intravenous (IV) insulin.

ASSESSMENT/INTERVENTIONS	RATIONALES
Explain the purpose of Rh-immune globulin (human) RhoGAM if it is prescribed.	This agent prevents the formation of antibodies to the Rh-positive antigen in the mother's blood and prevents hemolytic disease in a future Rh-positive fetus/newborn as long as the mother has not already been sensitized by the presence of Rh-positive blood. Administration: Intramuscular (IM) only to nonsensitized Rh-negative women after bleeding any time during the pregnancy, after spontaneous abortion, or after delivery. Recommended administration is within 72 hr after the bleeding episode or delivery.
Advise the patient that she may note discomfort at the site of injection.	This is a common side effect.

Nursing Diagnosis:

Ineffective Coping

related to health crisis, sense of vulnerability, inadequate support systems, and needed adjustment in lifestyle to provide an optimal environment for the fetus and prolong the gestational period

Desired Outcome: Within 24 hr of this diagnosis, the patient verbalizes feelings, identifies strengths, exhibits positive coping behaviors, and modifies her lifestyle to provide the best pregnancy outcome for her fetus.

ASSESSMENT/INTERVENTIONS	RATIONALES
Assess the patient's perceptions and ability to understand the current health status of herself and fetus.	Evaluation of the patient's comprehension enables development of an individualized care plan.
Help the patient identify previous stressors and methods of coping with stressful situations in life.	Recalling previous situations when she was able to handle the problem may strengthen effective coping now with current problems.
Provide the patient with resources for support groups, written information, Internet chat groups, or home helpers.	Talking with others who have experienced similar circumstances may aid in the development of coping mechanisms. A home helper, for example, likely will decrease pressure on the patient and thereby promote coping abilities.
Assist and affirm the patient's efforts to set realistic goals for lifestyle adjustments and for her support systems.	Participation in decision making, use of realistic personal and professional resources, and evaluation of potential effects or problems enable a more successful adaptation and facilitate effective coping.
Assess and acknowledge the influence of the patient's cultural beliefs, norms, and values regarding coping during pregnancy.	This shows respect for the patient's coping style and a willingness to integrate her beliefs and practices into health care prescriptions. You might ask, "Could you tell me how you and your family are coping with this pregnancy?" Different cultures perceive pregnancy in various ways. For example, some patients come from countries in which maternal and fetal mortality rate is high and daily survival is the major focus. Their method of coping may be emotional detachment from the fetus. The current pregnancy may not seem as important as the children and family that are already at home and need care. In the Hmong culture, for example, women and their families do not appear to bond with their infant after birth. Many believe to do so would be prideful and welcome evil spirits who would take the infant away (infant death).
Involve assistance of Social Services when available.	Social Services provides counseling and makes recommendations for referrals. Both home management and hospital management may require outside assistance to care for family members or pets at home.

continued

ASSESSMENT/INTERVENTIONS	RATIONALES
Provide the patient and family with information regarding the effectiveness of hospitalization bedrest vs. home bedrest.	This information helps the patient and her health care provider decide the best method of management. Before viability (20 wk), when the fetus is incapable of surviving outside the uterus, home management with bedrest in the absence of signs of maternal and fetal infection may be assumed. Patients on bedrest at home must be able to remain in bed in alternating side-lying positions (occasionally sitting up propped with pillows) and avoid doing housework, laundry, cooking, or shopping. The side-lying position improves uteroplacental blood flow and oxygenation, which in turn improves the chance of reaccumulation of amniotic fluid. After 20 wk gestation, hospitalization is usually recommended to monitor signs of infection or fetal compromise. Providers inform, educate, and involve parents in the decision-making process after increasing their knowledge level.
Encourage the patient and family to verbalize their concerns in a supportive environment.	This will help alleviate stress, anxiety, and misconceptions. See **Anxiety,** p. 685.

Nursing Diagnosis:

Deficient Knowledge

related to unfamiliarity with deconditioning, muscle weakness, back pain, and decreased circulation that can occur with prescribed bedrest

Desired Outcome: Within 24 hr of this diagnosis, the patient verbalizes understanding of and demonstrates measures to reduce or relieve back pain and improve circulation.

ASSESSMENT/INTERVENTIONS	RATIONALES
Teach the patient to recognize signs and symptoms of back pain related to bedrest vs. back pain associated with contraction activity.	A knowledgeable patient optimally will discern the different causes of back pain and report these symptoms accordingly. Back pain related to bedrest is usually thoracic to lumbar and superficial and will be improved by position change or massage to promote circulation. Back pain related to contraction activity is usually lumbar/sacral and deep tissue, and it may radiate to the hips and low abdominal/pelvic area. Position change and massage may decrease intensity.
Teach the patient the probable causes of muscle pain, weakness, and back pain.	This information aids in patient understanding and optimally in adherence to therapeutic management. For example, probable causes include lack of use of certain muscles, delay in change of positioning, increasing weight of the uterus, and dehydration, which can lead to the buildup of lactic acid in the muscles and cause pain.
Teach the patient leg exercises for the period in which she is on bedrest.	Leg exercises promote peripheral tissue perfusion and decrease risk of deep vein thrombosis (DVT) and muscle wasting. Calf-pumping (ankle dorsiflexion–plantar flexion) and ankle-circling exercises are examples of leg exercises. The patient should repeat each movement 10 times, performing each exercise hourly during extended periods of immobility, provided the patient is free of symptoms of DVT. Passive and active range-of-motion (ROM) exercises are other options.
Encourage the patient to change positions frequently in bed, from alternating side-lying positions to sitting propped up with pillows. Teach use of pillows between the knees to prevent pressure on the back.	Changing position at frequent intervals (e.g., q2h) promotes circulation and decreases pressure and hence discomfort on tissues, joints, and muscles. Pillows provide support and decrease strain on muscles and promote comfort.

ASSESSMENT/INTERVENTIONS	RATIONALES
⚠ Caution the patient to *avoid* the supine position.	The supine position places pressure on the aorta by the enlarging fetus. This could result in a vasovagal response, which would decrease maternal blood pressure and cause diaphoresis, nausea, dizziness, and decreased uteroplacental perfusion.
Provide the patient with a referral for physical or massage therapy for back pain related to prolonged bedrest.	Professional interventions likely will aid in promoting circulation and patient comfort.

Nursing Diagnosis:

Grieving

related to the potential fetal loss that could occur with PPROM

Desired Outcome: The patient and significant other verbalize their feelings and identify and use support systems to aid them in the grief process within 24 hr of this diagnosis.

ASSESSMENT/INTERVENTIONS	RATIONALES
Encourage the patient and significant other to verbalize their feelings and concerns regarding the potential for loss of their baby.	This measure validates concerns and conveys the message that grief is a normal and expected reaction to the potential loss of a baby.
Assess and accept the patient's behavioral response.	Disbelief, denial, guilt, anger, and depression are normal reactions to grief.
Teach the patient the stages of grief and explain that there is no specific time frame in which to go through the process.	This information enables the patient to understand where she or her family members may be in the grief process. Stages include (1) shock and numbness; (2) denial and searching-yearning; (3) anger, guilt, and sense of failure; (4) depression and disorganization; and (5) resolution.
Clarify misconceptions about the potential risk for fetal loss with PPROM.	This allows the patient and significant other to process the information regarding PPROM appropriately while not providing false hope. The gestational age at which PPROM occurs plays a significant role in the outcome. The earlier the gestational age at delivery, the higher the risk of fetal loss. A gestational age of 25 wk is considered viable, but with each passing day and week, there is better opportunity for fetal survival and decreased morbidity barring preexisting fetal complications such as cardiac, respiratory, and CNS problems.
If available, involve Social Services when a loss is perceived or present.	Social Services provides resources and referrals for individual counseling and support groups for bereaved parents and grandparents, which may help the participants feel less isolated. Social Services also can guide the family through the disposition of the infant should the death occur.
If a loss occurs, provide the patient and family with support if they decide to see and hold the baby and place appropriate items in a memory/keepsake box.	These measures assist with the grieving process by enabling parents/grandparents to spend time with and affirm their baby. Such items as footprints and a lock of hair may be tucked away and not looked at right away, but it may help to know they are there.

ADDITIONAL NURSING DIAGNOSES/PROBLEMS:

"Prolonged Bedrest" for such nursing diagnoses as **Constipation** — p. 68

"Psychosocial Support" for such nursing diagnoses as:

Disturbed Sleep Pattern — p. 73

Anxiety — p. 73

Fear — p. 75

Ineffective Coping — p. 75

Spiritual Distress — p. 77

Grieving/Risk for Complicated Grieving — p. 78

Social Isolation — p. 81

"Psychosocial Support for the Patient's Family and Significant Other" for such nursing diagnoses as:

Interrupted Family Processes — p. 85

Compromised Family Coping — p. 86

✓ PATIENT-FAMILY TEACHING AND DISCHARGE PLANNING

PPROM is potentially life threatening to the fetus, depending on gestational age at the time of occurrence. When reviewing the symptoms of PPROM and the importance of the patient adhering to the therapeutic regimen with the hope of decreasing fetal morbidity and mortality, include verbal and written information about the following:

✓ Signs and symptoms of ruptured membranes, a developing infection, and the importance of contacting the health care provider in a timely manner.

✓ Signs and symptoms of preterm labor (see p. 683) because it may precede or follow PPROM.
✓ Palpation of contractions and uterine tenderness.
✓ Importance of adherence to prenatal care.
✓ Importance of a well-balanced prenatal diet.
✓ Potential risk factors for PPROM that may be present early in the pregnancy.
✓ Measures for muscle pain, back pain, and muscle weakness that can be present with prolonged bedrest with bathroom privileges. See **Deficient Knowledge,** earlier.
✓ Measures that help with constipation, which occurs frequently in pregnancy and can be exacerbated with bedrest.
✓ How to read a thermometer accurately.
✓ How to avoid intercourse but maintain intimacy with her husband or partner.
✓ Availability of Social Services and spiritual care.
✓ Medications, including drug name, purpose, dosage, frequency, precautions, and potential side effects. Also discuss potential drug-drug, food-drug, and herb-drug interactions.
✓ Fetal movement counts.
✓ The American Congress of Obstetricians and Gynecologists has an extensive collection of patient education materials available at *www.acog.org/Resources_And_Publications/Patient_Education_FAQs_List*
✓ Referral to local and national support organizations, including:
  • Sidelines, a national support organization for women and their families experiencing complicated pregnancies, at *www.sidelines.org*
  • March of Dimes, at *www.marchofdimes.com*
  • The Society of Obstetricians and Gynecologists of Canada at *http://sogc.org* (requires subscription)

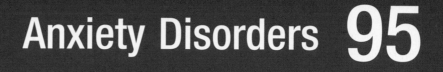

Anxiety Disorders 95

OVERVIEW/PATHOPHYSIOLOGY

Anxiety is a diffuse response to a vague threat, as opposed to fear, which is an acute response to a clear-cut external threat. Anxiety often precedes significant changes, for example, beginning new employment. When it is prolonged or excessive, crippling physical and psychologic symptoms may develop. The anxiety disorders are a group of conditions characterized by anxiety symptoms and behavioral efforts to avoid these symptoms. They are the most common psychiatric disorders in the United States, affecting more than 40 million people or about 18.1% of American adults aged 18 and older. Comorbidity with depression is common. Acute anxiety creates physical sensations of arousal (fight or flight), an emotional state of panic, decreased cognitive problem-solving ability, and altered spiritual state with hopelessness and/or helplessness. Anxiety is considered abnormal when reasons for it are not evident or when manifestations are excessive in intensity and duration. Psychologic *stress* refers to the response of an individual appraising the environment and concluding that it exceeds his or her resources and jeopardizes well-being. Some stressors are universal, whereas others are person specific because of highly individual interpretations of events.

Anxiety is always part of the stress response and has four levels, ranging from mild to panic. Normally, a person experiencing mild-to-moderate anxiety uses voluntary behaviors called *coping skills*, that is, distraction, deliberate avoidance, and information seeking. Another common response is use of unconscious defense mechanisms, including repression, suppression, projection, introjection, reaction formation, undoing, displacement, denial, and regression. If stress continues at an unbearable level or if the individual lacks sufficient biologic mechanisms for coping, an anxiety disorder may develop. There are eight major categories.

Generalized anxiety disorder: Characterized by excessive, uncontrollable worrying over a period of at least 6 months. Symptoms include motor tension (trembling; shakiness; muscle tension, aches, soreness; easy fatigue), autonomic hyperactivity (shortness of breath, palpitations, sweating, dry mouth, dizziness, nausea, diarrhea, frequent urination), and scanning behavior (feeling on edge, having an exaggerated startle response, difficulty concentrating, sleep disturbance, irritability).

Panic disorder: Characterized by a specific period of intense fear or discomfort with at least four of the following symptoms: palpitations or pounding heart, sweating, trembling or shaking, sensations of smothering or difficulty breathing, feeling of choking, chest pain, nausea, feeling dizzy or faint, feeling of unreality or losing control, numbness, and chills or flushes.

Phobias: Characterized by a persistent and severe fear of a clearly identifiable object or situation despite awareness that the fear is unreasonable. There are two types, specific and social. Specific phobias are subdivided into five types: animals, natural environment (e.g., lightning), blood-injection-injury type, situational (e.g., flying), and other (situations that could lead to choking or contracting an illness). Social phobia relates to profound fear of social or performance situations in which embarrassment could occur.

Agoraphobia is characterized by feelings of intense fear of being alone in open or public places where escape might be difficult. Individuals with agoraphobia become immobilized with anxiety and may find it impossible to leave their homes.

Acute stress disorder: Like posttraumatic stress disorder (PTSD), the problem begins with exposure to a traumatic event, with a response of intense fear, helplessness, or horror. In addition, the person shows dissociative symptoms, that is, subjective sense of numbing, feeling "in a daze," depersonalization, or amnesia and clearly tries to avoid stimuli that arouse recollection of the trauma. But just like PTSD, the victim reexperiences the trauma and shows functional impairment in social, occupational, and problem-solving skills. The key difference is that this syndrome occurs within 4 wk of the traumatic event and only lasts 2 days to 4 wk.

Anxiety disorder caused by a general medical condition: May be characterized by severe anxiety, panic attacks, or obsessions or compulsions, but the cause is clearly related to a medical problem, excluding delirium. History, physical examination, and laboratory findings support a specific diagnosis, for example, hypoglycemia, pheochromocytoma, or thyroid disease.

Anxiety disorder not otherwise specified: Describes individuals with significant anxiety or phobic avoidance but not enough symptoms to meet the criteria for a particular anxiety or adjustment disorder diagnosis. The patient may show a mixed anxiety-depressive picture or demonstrate social phobic symptoms related to having another medical problem, for example, Parkinson's disease, or present with insufficient data to rule out a general medical condition or substance abuse.

HEALTH CARE SETTING

Depends on the type of anxiety disorder. Primary (outpatient) care is likely for most categories, and possibly emergency department care for panic disorders. If the patient has developed agoraphobia, psychiatric home care may be the best care option. Some patients may be hospitalized for physiologic problems or to treat psychiatric needs.

ASSESSMENT

Physical indicators: Dry mouth, elevated vital signs, diarrhea, increased urination, nausea, diaphoresis, hyperventilation, fatigue, insomnia, sexual dysfunction, irritability, tenseness.

Emotional indicators: Fear, sense of impending doom, helplessness, insecurity, low self-confidence, anger, guilt.

Cognitive indicators: Mild anxiety produces increased awareness and problem-solving skills. Higher levels produce narrowed perceptual field; missed details; diminished problem-solving skills; and catastrophic, dichotomous thoughts resulting in deteriorated logical thinking.

Social indicators: Occupational, social, and familial role, e.g., marital and parental functioning may be adversely affected by anxiety and therefore should be assessed.

Spiritual indicators: Hopelessness/helplessness, feeling of being cut off from God, and anger at God for allowing anxiety may be experienced.

Suicidality: Suicide assessment is critical with anxious patients, especially those with panic disorder. For patients suffering dual diagnoses of depression and substance abuse or other anxiety disorders, risk of self-injury is even greater. Suicidal assessment includes questions to determine presence of suicidal ideation, intent, presence, and lethality of any plan. Essential questions to ask include:

- Have you thought of hurting yourself?
- Are you presently thinking about hurting yourself?
- If you have been thinking about suicide, do you have a plan?
- What is the plan?
- Have you thought about what life would be like for others if you were no longer a part of it?

A previous history of suicide attempts combined with depression places the patient at higher risk in the present. A patient whose depression is lifting is at higher risk for suicide than a severely depressed individual. The improvement may result in an increase in energy. This increased energy is not enough to make the patient feel well or hopeful, but it is enough to carry out a suicidal plan.

DIAGNOSTIC TESTS

There is no specific diagnostic test for anxiety disorders. The diagnosis of anxiety is made through history, interview of the patient and family, and observation of verbal and nonverbal behaviors. A number of effective scales are available to quantify the degree of anxiety, such as the Hamilton Rating Scale for Anxiety, Panic Attack Cognitions Questionnaire, State-Trait Anxiety Inventory, Sheehan Patient Rated Anxiety Inventory, and the Beck Anxiety Inventory.

Nursing Diagnosis:

Deficient Knowledge

related to unfamiliarity with the causes, signs and symptoms, and treatment of anxiety or specific anxiety disorder

Desired Outcome: By discharge (if inpatient) or after 2 wk of outpatient treatment, the patient and/or significant other verbalize accurate information about at least two of the possible causes of anxiety, four of the signs and symptoms of the specific anxiety disorder, and the available treatment options.

ASSESSMENT/INTERVENTIONS	RATIONALES
Assess the patient's understanding of anxiety, its signs and symptoms, and its treatment.	This assessment helps the nurse reinforce, as needed, information about anxiety and correct any misunderstanding. Many people lack understanding about the physiologic basis for anxiety and that feeling a little worry is different from the overwhelming anxiety experienced by those who have an anxiety disorder.
Inform the patient and significant other that anxiety disorders are physiologic disorders caused by the interplay of many factors, such as stress, imbalance in brain chemistry, psychodynamic factors, faulty learning, and genetics.	Many people who suffer from anxiety disorders accept that they are just "nervous worriers" and lack the knowledge that anxiety disorders represent a complex interplay of treatable biologic, genetic, and environmental factors.

ASSESSMENT/INTERVENTIONS	RATIONALES
Inform the patient and significant other about the holistic nature of anxiety, which produces physical, emotional, cognitive, social, and spiritual symptoms.	Many people believe that anxiety equates with nervousness and fail to recognize the many other signs and symptoms that make this a holistic disorder.
Inform the patient and significant other that anxiety disorders are treatable.	Medications are usually indicated for the treatment of these disorders and may include antidepressants and anxiolytics or a combination of medications. In addition, other interventions are useful, including dietary interventions (e.g., elimination of caffeinated products), and behavioral therapy, which may include breathing control, exercise, relaxation techniques, and psychological interventions (i.e., distraction, positive self-talk, psychoeducation, exposure therapy, systematic desensitization, implosive therapy, social interventions, cognitive therapy, and stress and time management interventions). For more information about medications, see **Deficient Knowledge** *related to* unfamiliarity with prescribed medications, their purpose, and their potential side effects, later.

Nursing Diagnosis:

Anxiety (Recurring Panic Attacks)

related to lack of knowledge regarding cause and treatment

Desired Outcome: Within 48 hr of treatment/intervention the patient verbalizes methods for dealing with panic attacks and the understanding that panic attacks are not life threatening and that they are time limited and demonstrates this knowledge accordingly.

ASSESSMENT/INTERVENTIONS	RATIONALES
Assess the patient's current understanding of the nature and cause of and treatments for panic disorders as well as current coping strategies employed by the patient.	Most patients who experience panic attacks have experienced several attacks before obtaining an accurate diagnosis. Patients sometimes adopt unhealthy coping strategies, such as restricting their movement (i.e., avoiding bridges if they have experienced a panic attack on a bridge or avoiding shopping in stores if this is where a panic attack occurred). It is important to provide information that the patient can understand and use to make appropriate lifestyle changes.
Administer medication as prescribed for panic attacks.	Panic attacks are neurobiologic events that respond to medications. See **Deficient Knowledge** *related to* unfamiliarity with prescribed medications, their purpose, and their potential side effects, later.
Teach the patient to reduce or eliminate dietary substances that may promote anxiety and panic, such as caffeine, food coloring, and monosodium glutamate (MSG).	Caffeine increases feelings of anxiety. However, caffeine withdrawal symptoms also can stimulate panic. Therefore, the plan should include focus on reducing consumption first, followed by elimination from the diet. Some individuals are sensitive to food colorings and MSG. This sensitivity is experienced as increased anxiety.
Teach relaxation techniques; assist with practicing imagery, deep breathing, progressive relaxation, and use of relaxation tapes.	Relaxation is effective in reducing anxiety. The patient's ability to master relaxation techniques provides a sense of control and enhances self-care ability.
Stay with the patient during panic attacks. Use short, simple directions. Encourage the patient to use relaxation, remind the patient that the attack is time limited, and reduce environmental stimulation. **Remain calm**.	During a panic attack, the ability to refocus is limited. The patient needs reassurance that he or she is not dying and that this will pass. Therefore, it is important that the nurse remain calm and not respond to the patient's anxiety with anxiety.
Teach the patient to self-administer anxiolytic medication when the first signs and symptoms of a panic attack start and initiate coping strategies to ward off the most severe symptoms.	This information empowers the patient by providing a strategy to deal with panic attacks. As patients become aware of early signs of oncoming panic, taking the prescribed anxiolytics and initiating relaxation and cognitive strategies to reduce the magnitude of the event will increase a sense of mastery over panic anxiety.

Nursing Diagnosis:

Social Isolation

related to agoraphobia

Desired Outcome: By discharge (if inpatient) or after 4 wk of outpatient treatment, the patient demonstrates behavior consistent with increased social interaction.

ASSESSMENT/INTERVENTIONS	RATIONALES
Assess the degree of social isolation experienced by the patient in response to agoraphobia.	It is critical to know how isolated the patient has become secondary to agoraphobia. If the patient no longer leaves her or his home and has no contact with anyone except those who either live in the home or those who come to visit, the social phobia is very severe and will require more intense work to overcome it, including home visits.
Assist the patient in a graded exposure plan to gradually increase independent functions and interactions with others.	Gradual exposure is effective in treating agoraphobia.
Assist the patient with practicing relaxation techniques.	Relaxation helps mitigate impending panic attacks.
Discuss alternatives for social interaction.	Patients may need assistance with developing activity plans. Appropriate alternatives for social interaction may be volunteer work in small groups and taking a friend to a social event to increase comfort.

Nursing Diagnosis:

Ineffective Coping

related to perceived inadequate level of control or support/resources in dealing with situational crises

Desired Outcome: Within 24-48 hr of intervention/treatment, the patient begins to identify ineffective coping behaviors and consequences, expresses feelings appropriately, identifies options, uses resources effectively, and uses effective problem-solving techniques.

ASSESSMENT/INTERVENTIONS	RATIONALES
Assess the patient's previous methods of coping with life problems.	How individuals have handled problems in the past is a reliable predictor of how current problems will be handled.
Determine use of substances (alcohol, other drugs, smoking and eating patterns).	The patient may have used substances as coping mechanisms to control anxiety. This pattern can interfere with the ability to deal with the current situation.
Provide information regarding different ways to deal with situations that promote anxious feelings, for example, identification and appropriate expression of feelings and problem-solving skills.	This information provides patients with an opportunity to learn new coping skills.
Role-play and rehearse new skills.	Role-playing promotes skill acquisition in a nonthreatening environment.
Encourage and support patients in evaluating their lifestyle and identifying activities and stresses of family, work, and social situations.	These measures enable patients to examine areas of life that may contribute to anxiety and make decisions about how to engender changes gradually without adding undue anxiety.
Assist with identifying some short- and long-term goals focused on making life changes and decreasing anxiety.	Goals help provide direction in making necessary changes.
Teach the patient how to break responsibilities into manageable units.	Small steps enhance success and avoid the anxiety that comes from facing a huge task and feeling overwhelmed.
Suggest incorporating stress management techniques (e.g., relaxation) into a normal day.	This encourages the patient to take care of self, take control, and decrease stress.

ASSESSMENT/INTERVENTIONS	RATIONALES
Teach the importance of balance in life.	A life out of balance adds tremendously to stress and anxiety. Changes such as getting adequate sleep, nutrition, exercise, quiet time, work time, family time, and spiritual time enhance quality of life, decrease anxiety, and increase a sense of power and control.
Refer to outside resources, including support groups, psychotherapy, religious resources, and community recreation resources.	Many people benefit from the support of other people and resources to help keep life in balance and monitor stress level.

Nursing Diagnosis:

Compromised Family Coping

related to family disorganization and role changes

Desired Outcome: Within 24 hr of this diagnosis, family members begin to identify resources within themselves to deal with the situation; interact appropriately with the patient, providing support and assistance as needed; recognize own needs for support; seek assistance; and use resources effectively.

ASSESSMENT/INTERVENTIONS	RATIONALES
Assess the level of information available to and understood by the family.	Lack of understanding about the patient's anxiety disorder can lead to unhealthy interaction patterns and contribute to anxiety felt by family members.
Identify role of the patient and current family roles, and discuss how illness has changed the family organization.	Patients' disabilities (e.g., resulting in inability to go to work or maintain the household) interfere with their usual role in the family structure and can substantially contribute to family stress and disorganization.
Help the family identify other factors besides the patient's illness that affect their ability to provide support to one another.	This takes the focus off of the patient as "the problem" and helps family members examine each of their individual responsibilities and behaviors.
Discuss the psychoneurologic basis of anxiety to reduce stigmatizing the patient with having an anxiety disorder.	This helps the family understand and accept behaviors that may be very difficult and reduces labeling the patient as weak or "crazy," which can aggravate the stigma of having an anxiety disorder.
Help the family to be supportive of the patient but to recognize to whom the disorder belongs and who is responsible for resolution of the disorder.	This recognition promotes self-responsibility. The individual with the disorder can seek support and ask for help, but it is not the responsibility of the family to seek treatment.
Teach the family constructive problem-solving skills.	These skills help the family learn new ways to deal with conflicts and reduce anxiety-provoking situations.
Refer the family to appropriate community resources.	The family may need additional assistance (e.g., from counselors, psychotherapy, Social Services, financial advisors, and spiritual advisor) to work through family issues and remain intact.

Nursing Diagnosis:

Deficient Knowledge

related to unfamiliarity with the prescribed medications, their purpose, and their potential side effects

Desired Outcome: By discharge (if inpatient) or after 4 wk of outpatient treatment, the patient verbalizes accurate information about the prescribed medications and their side effects.

ASSESSMENT/INTERVENTIONS	RATIONALES
Assess the patient's knowledge about the prescribed medications and her or his understanding of the importance of taking medications as prescribed.	This assessment helps the nurse to reinforce, as needed, information about the medications and correct any misunderstanding.
Teach the physiologic action of anxiolytics and/or antidepressants and how they alleviate symptoms of the patient's anxiety disorder.	Anxiety disorders are neurobiologic occurrences that respond to both anxiolytics and antidepressants. Many people who suffer from anxiety are fearful of taking medications because they fear drug dependence and view taking it as a sign of weakness.
Explain the importance of taking antidepressant medications as prescribed.	These medications require certain blood levels to be therapeutic; therefore, patients need to take them daily at the dose and time interval prescribed.
Teach the side effect profile and its management of the patient's prescribed medications that follow:	The anxiolytic medications, as well as each class of antidepressants, carry specific side-effect profiles. Knowledge about expected side effects, ways to manage these side effects, and how long these side effects last is important for ensuring therapy adherence.
⚠ **Tricyclic antidepressants:** amitriptyline (Elavil), desipramine (Norpramin), doxepin (Sinequan), imipramine (Tofranil), nortriptyline (Pamelor), protriptyline (Vivactil), and trimipramine (Surmontil)	Imipramine and desipramine are very effective in anxiety disorders due to their sedating properties to promote sleep restoration.
For patients taking tricyclic antidepressants, teach the following:	
- Drink at least 8 glasses of water a day and add high-fiber foods to the diet.	Water and high-fiber foods combat constipation, a potential anticholinergic effect.
- Rise from a sitting position slowly. Discuss risks of falling related to dizziness associated with hypotension.	Orthostatic hypotension is a potential side effect.
- Suck on sugar-free candy or mints or use sugar-free chewing gum.	These products combat dry mouth, a potential anticholinergic effect.
- Establish a sleep routine and regular exercise.	Regular sleep and exercise combat feelings of fatigue associated with these medications.
- Limit intake of refined sugars and carbohydrates.	Weight gain is a common occurrence with these medications, and eating sugar and carbohydrates can cause added weight gain and carbohydrate cravings.
- Caution is needed for patients with epilepsy or other seizure disorder.	Tricyclic antidepressants lower the seizure threshold.
- Be alert for and report signs of cardiac toxicity. Explain that patients older than 40 yr need an electrocardiogram evaluation before treatment and periodically thereafter.	These medications may decrease the vagal influence on the heart secondary to muscarinic blockade and by acting directly on the bundle of His to slow conduction. Both effects increase risk of dysrhythmias.
- Discuss possible drug interactions.	The combination of tricyclics with monoamine oxidase (MAO) inhibitors can cause severe hypertension. The combination of tricyclics with central nervous system (CNS) depressants, such as alcohol, antihistamines, opioids, and barbiturates, can cause severe CNS depression. Because of the anticholinergic effects of tricyclics, any other anticholinergic drug, including over-the-counter antihistamines and sleeping aids, should be avoided.
⚠ **Selective Serotonin Reuptake Inhibitors (SSRIs):** fluoxetine (Prozac), fluvoxamine maleate (Luvox), sertraline (Zoloft), paroxetine (Paxil), citalopram (Celexa), and escitalopram (Lexapro)	SSRIs are helpful not only for patients with depression and obsessive-compulsive symptoms but for patients with panic and anxiety disorders as well.
Teach the patient that the following can occur: nausea, headache, nervousness, insomnia, anxiety, agitation, sexual dysfunction, dizziness, fatigue, rash, diarrhea, excessive sweating, and anorexia with weight loss.	These are reported side effects. Because these medications can increase anxiety, it is recommended that treatment be started at very low doses and increased gradually.
Discuss possible drug interactions.	Interaction with MAO inhibitors can cause serotonin syndrome, a potentially life-threatening event. Symptoms include anxiety, diaphoresis, rigidity, hyperthermia, autonomic hyperactivity, and coma. Because of this possibility, MAO inhibitors should be withdrawn at least 14 days before starting an SSRI, and when an SSRI is discontinued, at least 5 wk should elapse before an MAO inhibitor is given.

ASSESSMENT/INTERVENTIONS

RATIONALES

ASSESSMENT/INTERVENTIONS	RATIONALES
Other Antidepressant Medications: bupropion (Wellbutrin); mirtazapine (Remeron); nefazodone (Serzone); trazodone (Desyrel); duloxetine (Cymbalta); venlafaxine (Effexor); and desvenlafaxine (PRISTIQ)	Antidepressants are frequently prescribed for treatment of anxiety disorders because of their effectiveness and low side effect profile.
Remind the patient to take the medication as prescribed daily and not to abruptly discontinue the medication. Explain that a gradual tapering is necessary when being taken off the medication.	Effexor in particular, when abruptly withdrawn, causes an uncomfortable discontinuation syndrome including dizziness, nausea, blurred vision, headache, and general malaise. Patients must be monitored carefully during the tapering period to avoid serious withdrawal symptoms.
Benzodiazepines: diazepam (Valium), chlordiazepoxide (Librium), clorazepate (Tranxene), lorazepam (Ativan), oxazepam (Serax), alprazolam (Xanax), halazepam (Paxipam), and clonazepam (Klonopin)	These benzodiazepines are used for generalized anxiety disorder. Alprazolam also can be used for panic disorder.
Teach the patient the following about benzodiazepines:	
- Drowsiness, impairment of intellectual function, impairment of memory, ataxia, and reduced motor coordination can occur.	These are common side effects that subside as tolerance to the drug develops.
- For patients who use these medications for sleep, there may be daytime fatigue, drowsiness, and cognitive impairments that can continue while awake.	These are common side effects that subside as tolerance to the medication develops.
- A gradual tapering is necessary when being taken off the medication.	Abrupt discontinuation of the benzodiazepines can result in a recurrence of target symptoms such as anxiety. Gradual tapering is also necessary to prevent occurrence of seizures.
- Nausea, vomiting, impaired appetite, dry mouth, and constipation may occur.	These are gastrointestinal (GI) symptoms associated with this medication.
- Take the medication with food.	Taking the medication with food may ease GI distress.
- Report worsening of depression symptoms.	This effect may occur in patients who are both depressed and anxious.
- Older adults should take the smallest possible therapeutic dose.	Older adults taking this drug are at increased risk for incontinence, memory disturbances, dizziness, and falls.
- Pregnant women and nursing mothers should avoid using benzodiazepines.	Benzodiazepines are excreted in breast milk of nursing mothers. They also cross the placenta and are associated with increased risk of certain birth defects.
- Decrease or stop smoking altogether.	Nicotine decreases effectiveness of benzodiazepines.
Nonbenzodiazepines: buspirone	Buspirone is indicated in treatment of generalized anxiety disorder. It does not increase depression, so it is a good choice when anxiety and depression coexist. It is not effective in treating other anxiety disorders.
Teach patients taking buspirone the following:	
- Be alert for dizziness, drowsiness, nausea, excitement, and headache.	These are common side effects.
- Take buspirone on a continual dosing schedule bid or tid.	Buspirone has a short half-life.
- Caution should be used with patients on digoxin.	In vitro, buspirone may displace less firmly protein-bound medications such as digoxin. However, the clinical significance of this property is unknown.
- This medication can cause liver and kidney toxicity. Patients with kidney or liver impairment must be monitored for this adverse effect.	Buspirone is metabolized in the liver and excreted predominantly by the kidneys.
Noradrenergic Medications: clonidine (Catapres), propranolol (Inderal), and pregabalin (Lyrica)	These medications are used for off-label treatment of anxiety. Propranolol is used in the treatment of performance anxiety found in some forms of social phobia and in panic disorder. Clonidine is used to block physiologic symptoms of opioid withdrawal. Pregabalin, an anticonvulsant medication, is showing positive results in the treatment of anxiety disorders.

ADDITIONAL NURSING DIAGNOSES/PROBLEMS:

"Major Depression" for:

Hopelessness   p. 727

Risk for Suicide   p. 727

Self-Esteem: Chronic Low   p. 729

✓ PATIENT-FAMILY TEACHING AND DISCHARGE PLANNING

The patient with an anxiety disorder experiences a wide variety of symptoms that affect ability to learn and retain information. Teaching must be geared to a time when medication has begun to calm the person and improve abilities to concentrate and learn. Verbal teaching should be simple and supplemented with written materials to which the patient and family can refer at a later time. Demonstrate and practice with the patient self-calming strategies, e.g., relaxation techniques, deep breathing, and "5 senses" exercise, and teach the patient to practice daily even when not anxious. Ensure that follow-up treatment is scheduled and that patient and family understand the need to take medication as prescribed. Psychiatric home care might be a valuable part of the discharge planning to facilitate compliance with the discharge plan. In addition, provide verbal and written information about the following issues:

✓ Medications, including drug name; purpose; dosage; frequency; precautions; drug-drug, food-drug, and herb-drug interactions; and potential side effects.

✓ Thought-stopping techniques to deal with negativism.
✓ Reducing catastrophic, dichotomous thinking to promote realistic appraisal of anxiety-provoking event.
✓ Importance of maintaining a healthy lifestyle—balanced diet, minimal to no caffeine, decrease or stop smoking, exercise, and regular adequate sleep patterns—for remaining in remission.
✓ Importance of continuing medication use long after symptoms have gone.
✓ Importance of social support and strategies to obtain it.
✓ Importance of using constructive coping skills to deal with stress.
✓ Importance of using relaxation techniques to minimize stress.
✓ Importance of maintaining or achieving spiritual well-being.
✓ Importance of follow-up care, including day treatment programs, appointments with psychiatrist and therapists, and vocational rehabilitation program if indicated.
✓ Referrals to community resources for support and education. Additional information can be obtained by contacting the following organizations:
  • Anxiety Disorders Association of America (ADAA) at *www.adaa.org*
  • The Anxiety Disorders Association of Canada at *www.anxietycanada.ca*
  • National Alliance for the Mentally Ill (NAMI) for information on all of the anxiety disorders.
  • National Institute of Mental Health (NIMH) for information on anxiety disorders at *www.nimh.nih.gov*
  • The Canadian Mental Health Association at *www.cmha.ca*

Bipolar Disorder (Manic Component) 96

OVERVIEW/PATHOPHYSIOLOGY

Bipolar disorder is a mood disorder characterized by episodes of major depression and mania or hypomania. (For the purpose of this chapter we will focus on the assessment and treatment of mania; see the care plan on "Major Depression," p. 725, for specifics regarding depression.) *Mania* is characterized by a period in which there is a dramatic change in mood; the individual is either elated and expansive or irritable. For the diagnosis to be made, this change in mood must last 1 wk (or any duration if hospitalization is required). At least three other symptoms from the following list must be present: inflated self-esteem or grandiosity; decreased need for sleep; pressured speech; flight of ideas; distractibility; increased involvement in goal-directed activities or psychomotor agitation; and overinvolvement in pleasurable activities with potentially damaging consequences. Examples of this behavior include hypersexuality, impulsive spending, and other reckless and dangerous behaviors.

Hypomania is characterized by at least 4 days of abnormally and persistently elevated, expansive, or irritable mood accompanied by at least three additional symptoms seen in a manic episode.

About 25% of the first episodes of bipolar disorder occur before age 20. In women, hormonal factors may account for a greater rate of rapid cycling (meaning highs and lows in a short period), but in general, women and men are equally affected with this disorder. There is no difference in prevalence rates by race or ethnicity. Bipolar disorder is a chronic, relapsing, and episodic disease. In individuals 40 yr of age or older who experience a first episode of mania, it is most likely related to medical conditions such as substance abuse or a cerebrovascular disorder. About 50% of bipolar patients have concurrent substance abuse disorders. Cigarette smoking is significantly more prevalent among individuals with bipolar disorder than among those without the disorder. Theories that explain causation of bipolar disorder include disorders in brain function or structure and genetic factors. Sleep deprivation may trigger manic/hypomanic episodes.

HEALTH CARE SETTING

Most patients may be treated outpatient except those who are at high risk for suicide, represent a danger to others, or are experiencing a psychotic mania. Acute care (inpatient psychiatric unit) stays are brief and focus on restabilization. Patients with bipolar disorder require long-term medication management; intensive psychosocial support to function within the community; and possibly individual, group, and family therapy.

ASSESSMENT

Similar to depression, the assessment of mania involves much more than an assessment of mood. This is a holistic disorder that results in changes in self-attitude (feelings of self-worth), as well as vital sense (sense of physical well-being) and spiritual sense. Depression diminishes self-worth, self-attitude, and vital sense, whereas mania may increase these perceptions.

Feelings, attitudes, and knowledge: During manic episodes, patients express inflated views of themselves. Many manic patients state that they enjoyed being high and because of this refused medications. After the mania has subsided, the patient is confronted with the consequences of behaviors and actions engaged in while manic. Being faced with the reality of those behaviors and their consequences produces negative feelings expressed as shame, humiliation, denial, anger, fear of experiencing a relapse, fear of passing the disorder onto children, and fear of cycling into an episode of depression.

Elevated mood or irritability: Patients may be excessively cheerful and unusually elated or display irritability over the smallest matters. This irritability increases when others attempt to reason with them. A manic person may display a haughty or superior attitude toward others. He or she may display overt anger, particularly if his or her requests or behaviors are curtailed.

Increased self-attitude: Patients may express and act in unusually optimistic fashion, engaging in behaviors that reflect poor judgment, and may act in inappropriate, dangerous, or indiscreet ways. For example, a normally conservative person may engage in sexual indiscretions or speak in overly critical or judgmental terms, often at inappropriate times and about sensitive subjects.

Increased vital sense: The person with mania has increased energy and may appear tireless in the face of physical and mental efforts that would greatly tax unaffected individuals. He or she may feel completely refreshed after only a few minutes or hours of sleep.

Spiritual issues: Bipolar disorder mania carries with it many negative experiences—such as marital and family problems, divorce, legal difficulties, financial ruin, and unemployment—that contribute to the downward spiral of self-appraisals. Spirituality is an important, though often a neglected, aspect of assessment, especially during the acute episode. Bipolar disorder can lead to a crisis in faith, in self, others, life, and ultimately God. This loss of faith and hope contributes significantly to the risk of suicide.

Additional sign: Manic individuals may experience a voracious appetite or may be too busy to eat.

Suicidality: Suicide assessment is critical with manic patients. The presence of psychotic thinking, hyperactivity, impulsiveness, and possible substance abuse increases suicide risk significantly. It is important to ask questions to determine the presence of suicidal ideation and the lethality of any plan. Essential questions to ask include:

- Have you thought of hurting yourself?
- Are you presently thinking about hurting yourself?

- If you have been thinking about suicide, do you have a plan? What is the plan?
- Have you thought about what life would be like if you were no longer a part of it?

A previous history of suicide attempts places the patient at high risk for attempting suicide.

DIAGNOSTIC TESTS

There are no diagnostic tests to diagnose bipolar disorder mania. Diagnosis is made through history, interview of the patient and family, and observation of verbal and nonverbal behaviors. To be diagnosed with bipolar disorder, the individual must meet the criteria spelled out in the Diagnostic and Statistical Manual of Mental Disorders (DSM). The Young Mania Rating Scale (YMRS) is an effective instrument to quantify the degree of mania.

Nursing Diagnosis:

Risk for Other-Directed Violence

related to impulsivity/agitation occurring with manic excitement

Desired Outcome: By the time of discharge from an inpatient psychiatric unit, the patient demonstrates increased self-control and decreased hyperactivity.

ASSESSMENT/INTERVENTIONS	RATIONALES
Continually assess the patient's response to frustrations or difficult situations.	This enables early intervention and helps patients manage situations independently, if possible.
Continually assess to ensure that the patient's environment is safe. Remove objects that could be dangerous and rearrange the room to decrease environmental risks to prevent accidental/purposeful injury to self or others.	Hyperactive behavior and grandiose thinking can lead to destructive actions with possible harm to self or others.
Decrease environmental stimuli, assign a private room (if possible), avoid exposure to situations of predictable high stimulation, and remove the patient from the area if he or she becomes agitated.	Patients may be unable to focus attention on relevant stimuli and will be reacting/responding to all environmental stimuli.
Intervene at the earliest signs of agitation. Use direct verbal interventions prompting appropriate behavior, redirect or remove the patient from the difficult situation, establish voluntary time-out or move to a quiet room, use physical control (e.g., hold the patient). Offer PRN medications.	Early intervention assists patients in regaining control, defuses a difficult situation, prevents violence, and enables treatment to continue in the least-restrictive manner. **Note:** Physical hold/restraints are used only as a last resort.
Until the patient is calm, avoid analyzing or problem solving regarding prevention of violence or collecting information about precipitating events or provoking stimuli.	Any questioning will only add to agitation. Analyze and problem solve when the patient is calm.
Communicate the rationale for taking action using a concrete, direct, and simple approach.	People are unable to process complicated communication when they are agitated or upset.
When the patient is ready to leave the quiet area or time-out location, allow gradual reentry to the area of greater stimulation.	The patient has diminished tolerance for environmental stimuli; gradual reentry fosters coping skills.
Do not argue with the patient if he or she verbalizes put-downs or unrealistic or grandiose ideas.	Arguing only increases agitation and reinforces undesirable behavior.
Ignore and minimize attention given to bizarre dress or use of profanity, while placing clear limits on destructive behavior.	This avoids reinforcing negative behavior while providing controls for potentially dangerous behavior.

ASSESSMENT/INTERVENTIONS	RATIONALES
Avoid unnecessary delay of gratification when the patient makes a request. If refusal is necessary, make sure the rationale is given in nonjudgmental and concrete manner.	Patients in a hyperactive state do not tolerate waiting or delays, which add to frustration or agitation level. Any unnecessary delays could trigger aggressive behavior.
Offer alternatives when available.	This uses the patient's distractibility to decrease the frustration of having a request refused. For example, "I don't have any soda. Would you like a glass of juice?"
When the patient is less agitated and labile, provide information about alternative problem-solving strategies.	When calm, patients are able to hear and retain information.
When the patient is calm, help to examine the antecedents/precipitants to agitation.	This promotes early recognition of the developing problem, enabling patients to plan for alternative responses and intervene in a timely fashion.
Collaborate with the patient to identify alternative behaviors that are acceptable to both the patient and staff. Role-play how to use these behaviors if appropriate.	Patients are more apt to follow through if the alternatives are mutually agreed on. This practice enables patients to "try on" new behaviors while calm and ready to learn.
Give positive reinforcement when the patient attempts to deal with difficult situations without violence.	Praise increases patients' sense of success and increases likelihood that desired behaviors will be repeated.
Administer the following medications as prescribed:	
Antimanic medications: lithium carbonate (Lithobid, Eskalith), divalproex sodium (Depakote), valproic acid (Depakene), valproate (Depacon), carbamazepine (Tegretol), topiramate (Topamax), oxcarbazepine (Trileptal), tiagabine (Gabitril), and lamotrigine (Lamictal).	Lithium is the drug of choice for mania and is indicated for alleviation of hyperactive symptoms. Some patients do not respond to or are intolerant of lithium and may need alternative medications, which may include divalproex, carbamazepine, topiramate, valproic acid, valproate, tiagabine, or lamotrigine.
Atypical antipsychotics with mood-stabilizing effects: olanzapine (Zyprexa), quetiapine (Seroquel), aripiprazole (Abilify), clozapine (Clozaril), paliperidone (Invega), risperidone (Risperdal Consta, M-tabs), ziprasidone (Geodon)	Atypicals have been found to be helpful as adjuncts to mood stabilizers. Olanzapine is well-tolerated and is also helpful in treating the anxiety symptoms in bipolar depression. Each of the atypical antipsychotics is effective in managing mania.
Provide restraint or seclusion per agency policy.	These measures may be necessary for brief periods to protect the patient, staff, and others.
Prepare the patient for electroconvulsive therapy (ECT) if indicated.	In a severely manic episode, ECT may be recommended. ECT is one of the most effective treatment options and is especially useful for individuals who are in need of a rapid treatment response, cannot take or are refusing medications, or do not respond to other treatment modalities.

Nursing Diagnosis:

Deficient Knowledge

related to unfamiliarity with causes, signs and symptoms, and treatment of bipolar disorder mania

Desired Outcome: Within 24 hr of teaching, the patient and/or significant other verbalize accurate information about at least two possible causes of bipolar disorder, four signs and symptoms of the disorder, and available treatment options.

ASSESSMENT/INTERVENTIONS	RATIONALES
Assess level of knowledge of the patient and significant other(s) regarding the causes of bipolar disorder, signs and symptoms of the disorder, and the available treatment options.	Initially it is difficult to diagnose bipolar disorder. Patients as well as their significant other(s) may have faulty perceptions about it. Unless corrected, these faulty perceptions may interfere with treatment adherence on the part of the patient and weaken support for treatment adherence from the significant other(s).

continued

ASSESSMENT/INTERVENTIONS	RATIONALES
Inform the patient and significant other that bipolar disorder is a physiologic disorder caused by the interplay of many factors, such as imbalance in brain function and structure, psychodynamic factors, and genetics.	Providing education about the physical basis for the disorder increases understanding and acceptance and decreases blaming behavior.
Inform the patient and significant other that there are treatments available for bipolar disorder.	Medications are essential to stabilize and maintain mood. However, they are not enough. Comprehensive treatment involves intensive outpatient programs, frequent office visits, crisis telephone calls, family involvement, and psychosocial interventions including psychoeducation, suicide prevention, psychotherapy for depression, and limit setting in mania and hypomania. Management of bipolar disorder is a lifelong commitment.

Nursing Diagnosis:

Imbalanced Nutrition: Less Than Body Requirements

related to inadequate intake in relation to metabolic expenditures

Desired Outcome: Immediately following interventions, the patient displays increased attention to eating behaviors.

ASSESSMENT/INTERVENTIONS	RATIONALES
Establish a baseline regarding nutritional and fluid intake, as well as activity level.	This assessment is necessary to quantify deficits, needs, and progress toward goals.
Weigh the patient daily.	This is another form of quantification that provides information about therapeutic needs and effectiveness of interventions.
Serve meals in a setting with minimal distractions.	This encourages patients to focus on eating and prevents other distractions from interfering with food intake.
Stay with the patient during mealtime, even if this means walking with the patient.	This provides support and encouragement for patients to take in adequate nutrition and does not set the unrealistic expectation that patients must sit during mealtime.
Provide finger foods, snacks, and juices.	Patients will most likely eat small frequent meals on the move and this allows a reasonable accommodation for this behavior.
Enable the patient to choose food when he or she is able to make choices.	Encouraging choices before patients are ready may add to confusion. However, if patients are able to handle choices, this increases a sense of control.
Refer to a dietitian as indicated.	It may be useful to involve an expert in determining patients' nutritional needs and the most appropriate options for meeting these needs.
Administer vitamins and mineral supplements as prescribed.	Supplements correct dietary deficiencies and improve nutritional status.

Nursing Diagnosis:

Dressing/Bathing Self-Care Deficit

related to impulsivity and lack of concern

Desired Outcome: Immediately following interventions, the patient performs self-care activities within his or her level of ability.

ASSESSMENT/INTERVENTIONS	RATIONALES
Assess the patient's current level of functioning; reevaluate daily.	Patients' abilities for self-care may change daily. This information is needed to plan or modify care.
Provide physical assistance, supervision, simple directions, reminders, encouragement, and support as needed.	This helps patients focus on the task. Providing only required assistance fosters independence.
If possible, use the patient's clothing and toiletries.	Patients may have been disorganized entering the hospital or hospitalized as an emergency measure, so their own belongings were left at home. Having personal clothing and supplies supports autonomy and self-esteem.
As appropriate, limit choices regarding clothing.	During periods of extreme hyperactivity and distractibility, patients may be unable to make appropriate choices or to care for personal belongings.
As the patient's condition improves, set goals to establish minimum standards for self-care (e.g., taking a bath every other day).	Setting goals promotes the idea that patients are responsible for themselves and enhances a sense of self-worth.

Nursing Diagnosis:

Deficient Knowledge

related to unfamiliarity with medication use, including purpose and potential side effects of prescribed medications

Desired Outcome: Immediately following teaching interventions, the patient verbalizes accurate information about the prescribed medications.

ASSESSMENT/INTERVENTIONS	RATIONALES
It is vital that the nurse assess the patient's level of knowledge regarding the prescribed medications.	Education should be directed to assessed deficits in knowledge regarding the expected benefits of taking the prescribed drug, potential side effects, and how to deal with them. Knowledge increases adherence to taking the prescribed medications.
In simple terms teach the physiologic action of mood stabilizers.	Patients may have little or no understating regarding the purpose and actions of these medications.
Teach the importance of taking the medication as prescribed and the need for follow-up blood tests to monitor medication serum level.	The medication requires certain blood levels to be therapeutic, and therefore patients need to take it at the dose and time interval prescribed. The scheduled serum evaluations ensure that the medication level remains within therapeutic range.
Antimanic medications for adults: lithium carbonate (Lithobid, Eskalith, Duralith) or lithium citrate (Cibalith)	Lithium provides mood stability and prevents dangerous highs and despairing lows experienced in bipolar disorder.
Teach the patient the following:	
- How to monitor for swelling of feet or hands, fine hand tremor, mild diarrhea, muscle weakness, fatigue, memory and concentration difficulties, metallic taste, nausea or abdominal discomfort, polydipsia, polyuria.	These are common side effects.
- The importance of monitoring intake and output, sodium intake, and weight and how to elevate legs when sitting or lying down.	These are interventions for the prevention of edema of the feet and hands.
- The importance of notifying the health care provider if urinary output decreases.	This may be a sign of increasing serum level of lithium.
- When to notify the prescriber if tremors interfere with work.	A medication that interferes with work may result in compliance issues. Smaller, more frequent doses may help. In addition, tremors worsen when patients are anxious.
- The need to take lithium with meals, replace fluids lost secondary to diarrhea, and notify the prescriber if diarrhea becomes severe.	Some people can have nausea from lithium. At higher doses, loose stools or even diarrhea are frequently noted. The prescriber may need to change the medication.

continued

ASSESSMENT/INTERVENTIONS	RATIONALES
! Caution the patient that if any of the following symptoms occur while taking lithium—muscle weakness, fatigue, memory problems, or concentration difficulties—the patient should avoid driving or operating hazardous equipment during this period, use reminders and cues for memory deficits, and notify the prescriber if these symptoms become severe.	These are interventions to prevent harm to self and others. The prescriber may change to another medication.
Encourage the patient to use sugarless candies or throat lozenges and engage in frequent oral hygiene.	These are interventions for metallic taste and the dry mouth that can be associated with some medications.
Explain that drinking large amounts of fluids is a normal mechanism for coping with the side effect of increased urine.	This information provides reassurance for polydipsia.
! Explain in simple terms the importance of having laboratory work done as prescribed as well as being alert to signs and symptoms of lithium toxicity.	This helps ensure that the serum lithium level is maintained between 0.6 and 1.2 mEq/L. Mild toxic lithium effects, including impaired concentration, lethargy, tremor, slurred speech, and nausea, may be seen at plasma levels of 1.0 to 1.5 mEq/L. Moderate toxic lithium effects, including confusion, disorientation, drowsiness, unsteady gait, dysarthria, and muscle fasciculations, may be seen at plasma levels of 1.6 to 2.5 mEq/L. Severe toxic lithium effects, including impaired consciousness with progression to coma, delirium, ataxia, impaired renal function, and convulsions, may be seen at plasma levels greater than 2.5 mEq/L. Laboratories have established critically high lithium values that are used for clinician notification. Usually, these concentrations are greater than 2.0 mEq/L, although some facilities may consider lithium concentrations greater than 1.5 mEq/L as their critically high lithium level (Lum, 2007). Usually, once stabilization is achieved, laboratory work is done q1-2 wk during the first 2 mo and q3-6 mo during long-term maintenance.
! Caution the patient to avoid alcohol or other central nervous system (CNS) depressant medications.	These substances may increase serum lithium level. Risk of injury may increase due to the combination secondary to sedation and/or dizziness.
! Advise the patient to notify the prescriber if pregnant or planning to become pregnant and to avoid breastfeeding while taking this medication.	Safe use during pregnancy and breastfeeding has not been established.
! Advise the patient to notify the prescriber before taking any other prescription or over-the-counter (OTC) medication.	Many other medications interact with lithium to either increase or decrease the serum level. For example, when combined with lithium, NSAIDs can increase lithium levels in the blood, resulting in an increased risk for serious adverse effects.
Caution the patient not to discontinue this medication abruptly.	This could lead to exacerbation of manic symptoms.
Antiseizure medications with mood-stabilizing effects: divalproex sodium or valproic acid (Depakote or Depakene), carbamazepine (Tegretol), topiramate (Topamax), lamotrigine (Lamictal), oxcarbazepine (Trileptal), and tiagabine (Gabitril).	These medications are generally used when lithium does not work or when side effects from lithium are intolerable to the patient.
Atypical antipsychotics with mood-stabilizing effects: olanzapine (Zyprexa), quetiapine (Seroquel), aripiprazole (Abilify), clozapine (Clozaril), paliperidone (Invega), risperidone (Risperdal Consta, M-tabs), ziprasidone (Geodon)	Olanzapine is often better tolerated than lithium. Quetiapine is also effective in treating the anxiety symptoms in bipolar depression. Each of the atypical antipsychotics is effective in managing mania.
Teach the patient to be alert for anorexia, nausea, vomiting, drowsiness (most common), and tremor.	These are common side effects.

ADDITIONAL NURSING DIAGNOSES/PROBLEMS:

"Major Depression" for:

Hopelessness	p. 727
Risk for Suicide	p. 727
Self-Esteem: Chronic Low	p. 729

✓ PATIENT-FAMILY TEACHING AND DISCHARGE PLANNING

The patient with a bipolar disorder mania experiences a wide variety of symptoms that affect the ability to learn and retain information. Patient teaching must be geared to a time when medication has begun to decrease hyperactive symptoms and improve abilities to concentrate and learn; otherwise, it is a wasted effort. Verbal teaching should be simple and supplemented with reading materials the patient and/or significant other and family can refer to at a later time. Ensure that follow-up treatment is scheduled and that the patient and/or significant other and family understand the need to get prescriptions filled and the importance of taking the medication as prescribed. Consider whether or not the patient has transportation available to get to follow-up treatment. Psychiatric home care might be a valuable part of the discharge planning to facilitate adherence to the discharge plan. In addition, provide the patient and/or significant other/family with verbal and written information about the following issues:

- ✓ Medications, including drug name; purpose; dosage; frequency; precautions; drug-drug, food-drug, and herb-drug interactions; and potential side effects.
- ✓ Importance of laboratory follow-up tests for serum lithium levels.
- ✓ Importance of maintaining a healthy lifestyle—balanced diet, minimal to no caffeine or alcohol, exercise, and regular adequate sleep patterns—to ensure remaining in remission.
- ✓ Importance of continuing medication use for life.
- ✓ Importance of social support and strategies for obtaining it.
- ✓ Importance of using community follow-up resources; for example, psychiatrist, psychiatric nurse, intensive outpatient, support groups, family counseling.
- ✓ Importance of maintaining or achieving spiritual well-being.
- ✓ Referrals to community resources for support and education. Additional information can be obtained by contacting the following organizations:
  - Depression and Related Affective Disorders Association (DRADA) at *www.drada.org*. This nonprofit organization is composed of individuals with mood disorders, family members, and mental health professionals. It offers information, education, referral, and support services to people nationwide. DRADA sponsors a nationally renowned training program for group leaders.
  - Depression Awareness, Recognition, and Treatment Program (D/ART), 5600 Fishers Lane, Suite 10-85, Rockville, MD 20857, (301) 443-4140, Fax: (301) 443-4045. D/ART is a national self-help clearinghouse. It provides a list of resources throughout the United States that can help in networking and providing consultative assistance.
  - Depression and Bipolar Support Alliance (DBSA) at *www.dbsalliance.org*. The DBSA provides education as well as support to individuals and families affected by depression and bipolar illnesses.
  - NAMI is the National Alliance on Mental Illness, the nation's largest grassroots mental health organization dedicated to building better lives for the millions of Americans affected by mental illness. NAMI advocates for access to services, treatment, support services, and research. They are steadfast in their commitment to raise awareness and building a community of hope for all of those in need (*www.nami.org*).
  - The Mood Disorders Society of Canada provides links to support groups as well as patient education materials (*www.mooddisorderscanada.ca*).
  - The Canadian Mental Health Society's website (*www.cmha.ca*) provides patient education information and allows the user to search for patient support services available in the patient's community.

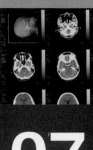

Dementia—Alzheimer's Type 97

OVERVIEW/PATHOPHYSIOLOGY

Dementia is a chronic cognitive disorder that is part of a category of psychiatric disorders classified as *Neurocognitive Disorders* in the 5th edition of the *Diagnostic and Statistical Manual of Mental Disorders* (*DSM-5*; American Psychiatric Association, 2013). Delirium is characterized by an acute change in cognition and consciousness that occurs over a short period of time. Dementia is characterized by multiple cognitive deficits that include impairment in memory. The dementias are also classified according to etiology: dementia of the Alzheimer's type; vascular dementia; Lewy body disease; frontotemporal degeneration; and neurocognitive disorder due to other general medical conditions, such as human immunodeficiency virus (HIV) disease, head trauma, Parkinson's disease, Huntington's disease, Pick's disease, and Creutzfeldt-Jakob disease; substance-induced persisting dementia; dementia due to multiple etiologies; and dementia not otherwise specified.

The most common form is Alzheimer's disease (AD), a primary dementia accounting for approximately 60%-80% of dementia cases (Alzheimer's Association, 2012), and it is the focus of this care plan. Although AD is age related, it does not represent the normal process of aging. It occurs with distinctive brain lesions without any certain physiologic basis. The brain lesions are neurofibrillary tangles and neuritic plaques that take up space in the brain, replacing normal tissue in the cell body of the neuron. There are multiple theories to explain the occurrence of AD, including genetic transmission, a decrease in acetylcholine, beta-amyloid activity, impact of a head injury, mini strokes, lack of estrogen, immunologic factors, effects of a slow-acting virus, and environmental factors.

AD affects more than 5.1 million Americans, making it the most common neuropsychiatric illness in older adults. Its diagnosis covers deficits in memory, problem solving, attention, and cognition. The actual course of the disorder follows a predictable pattern of early, middle, and late stages of progression, each displaying characteristic behaviors and requiring a different focus of treatment. The early stage is frequently referred to as the *amnestic stage*, the middle stage as the *dementia stage*, and the late stage as the *vegetative stage*. As the disease progresses, patients lose control over their bladder and bowel functions and develop apraxia (incoordination of movements), and later they lose control over speech and swallowing. Seizures and psychotic symptoms are common in late stages. Death inevitably occurs as a result of neurologic complications imposed by the brain lesions.

AD represents the clinical prototype for chronic cognitive disorders. The care required by the Alzheimer's patient, especially in the middle and late stages of the disorder, is essentially the same care required by all dementia patients regardless of type. The cognitive symptoms of dementia involve serious memory impairment, as well as significant alterations in language and perceptual acuity and abilities to abstract, problem solve, and make appropriate judgments. Patients ultimately experience loss of all memory (amnesia), agnosia (inability to recognize objects, people, places), and aphasia (loss of meaningful verbal communication). Noncognitive behavioral symptoms can be just as profound. These include significant personality changes, purposeless movements, agitation and aggression, overreaction to situations, irritable and repetitive behavior, and emotional disinhibition.

HEALTH CARE SETTING

In the early stage of AD, care takes place in the home and primary care setting. By the end of the early stage of the disease, additional services such as home care and use of adult day care are needed to safely maintain the patient at home. At the end of the early stage and moving into the middle stage, the decision regarding where to place the patient begins. The patient is generally moved into residential care in the middle stage, and during the late stage, care is frequently provided in a skilled nursing facility and sometimes a specialized, locked dementia unit for safety.

ASSESSMENT

Psychiatric assessment

Involves assessment of primary and secondary psychiatric manifestations of AD and differential diagnosis from psychosis, depression, anxiety, and phobias.

Family history: Dementing illness, psychiatric disease, neurologic disease, substance-use disorders.

Social history: Education, past level of functioning per occupational history, close relationships and children, current living situation, and history and present substance use.

Medical history: All past and present medical illnesses, especially cardiovascular; past surgeries; past trauma especially to the head; allergies; and medications.

Psychiatric history: Psychotic illness; depressive illness; other psychiatric illnesses; psychiatric symptoms, especially mood lability and psychotic symptoms; past and current treatments; hospitalizations; suicidal ideation; and violence or aggression.

Present illness: Length of cognitive loss and degree of memory loss:

- Is short-term memory loss so significant that the patient is no longer able to remember and perform activities of daily living (ADLs)?
- Other presenting problems, physical symptoms and injuries, functional deficits, psychiatric symptoms.
- Personality changes, including low tolerance for normal frustrations, oversensitivity to remarks of others, lack of initiative, decreased attention span, diminished emotional presence, emotional lability, restlessness.
- Difficulty with word finding and comprehension; thought blocking.

Mental status examination: Appearance, behavior, speech, mood, hallucinations, delusions, paranoid ideation, anxiety, phobias, cognition, insight and judgment, behavioral disturbances such as agitation, combativeness, screaming, catastrophic reactions.

Physical assessment

Psychomotor functioning: Difficulty carrying out new or complex motor tasks is apparent in the early stages; difficulty carrying out activities such as dressing, eating, and walking becomes apparent in the middle stages. Unsteadiness of gait coupled with confusion pose a significant risk for falls during the middle stages. In addition, marked psychomotor agitation is common. Restlessness, agitation, and aimless pacing replace normal motion.

Nutrition and elimination: Eating difficulties may present in the early stages. The patient may forget that he or she has just eaten, exhibit lax table manners, fail to know it is mealtime without prompting, experience changes in taste and appetite, express denial of hunger or need to eat, and experience weight loss. As the disease progresses, the patient does not respond to the need for elimination, which necessitates the caregiver to plan regular bathroom breaks. Constipation and incontinence of urine and feces become problems. Additionally, patients may forget to swallow food, which increases risk for choking and/or aspiration.

Activity and rest: Fatigue increases severity of symptoms, especially as evening approaches. Patients may reverse days and nights, with wakefulness and aimless wandering at night indicative of disturbance of sleep rhythms. Patients may be content to sit and watch others. The main activity may be hoarding inanimate objects, hiding articles, wandering, or engaging in repetitive motions.

Hygiene: As the disease progresses, so does dependence on the caregiver to meet basic hygiene needs. Appearance may be disheveled, and patients may have body odor. Clothing may be inappropriate for the situation or weather conditions. Patients may forget to go to the bathroom and the steps involved in toileting.

Social assessment: Patients may ignore rules of social conduct and exhibit inappropriate behavior and disinhibition. Speech may be fragmented; family roles may be altered/reversed as patients become more dependent.

Spiritual assessment

An assessment of the patient's faith tradition, practices, level of commitment, and connection to a faith community is critical. In the early stage of AD, the patient may have full awareness of the journey that lies ahead, and spirituality may offer support and comfort in ways that nothing else can. As the disease progresses and deficits become greater, it is difficult to assess the patient's spiritual needs. However, because long-term memory remains intact long after the short-term memory is gone, patients may still be comforted by spiritual traditions such as worship services, prayers, and hymns that are a vivid part of his or her history. Moreover, care of the Alzheimer's patient is so demanding that spiritual needs of the caregiver must be assessed and support provided. A faith community may provide invaluable assistance in the actual care of the patient, providing the caregiver with respite and help with day-to-day activities.

DIAGNOSTIC TESTS

Obtaining an accurate differential diagnosis of dementia is essential. AD is basically a rule-out disorder; that is, the diagnosis is made after family history, laboratory tests, and brain imaging eliminate other disorders with similar cognitive deficits. Sources of information needed to make a differential diagnosis of dementia include a full neurologic assessment, laboratory tests to rule out metabolic factors, and family history of the patient's past behavior and symptom progression. Mini-Cog (or other cognitive screening) and functional assessment of ADLs provide necessary information. A computed tomography (CT) scan identifies structural deficits. Brain imaging with positron emission tomography (PET) provides the clinician with information about changes in the metabolic activity and neurochemical characteristics associated with dementia. Typically, testing of patients in the early stage of AD reveals a normal electroencephalogram, CT scan, and magnetic resonance imaging (MRI) study, and generally laboratory tests are within normal range. A comprehensive psychiatric assessment provides additional information. Use of the Functional Assessment Staging Tool (FAST) allows for staging the disease, recognizing cognitive and functional abilities and deficits of each stage of AD, and enables planning for the appropriate adjustments to care.

Nursing Diagnosis:

Deficient Knowledge

related to unfamiliarity with the disease progression and care of the dementia patient

Desired Outcome: By the time the diagnosis of AD is confirmed, significant other/family relay accurate information and expectations about the course of the disease and the role they will play in the care of their loved one.

ASSESSMENT/INTERVENTIONS	RATIONALES
Assess the significant other's/family's understanding about the disease process and expected care that will be needed for their loved one.	This assessment enables the nurse to reinforce, as needed, information about AD and correct any misunderstandings.
Provide information about the staging of the disease and changes to expect in their loved one.	The family plays an integral role in the care of their loved one. Initially, they are the informants, providing information that facilitates diagnosis; they move into role of advocate, then primary caregivers, and finally the patient supporter. Staging is discussed in the introductory data.
Provide written information regarding educational resources, such as *The Thirty-Six Hour Day* (2012) by Mace and Rabins and identification of appropriate support groups.	The cited book presents a compilation of family experiences with the disorder at different stages. Although there are other helpful books, this one remains the definitive resource for family caregivers. Support groups for family members offer an ongoing, practical socioeducational source, even in the early stage. They provide a safe place to explore issues such as whether or not the patient should stop driving; whether other people should be told about the diagnosis; whether the patient should wear an ID bracelet or carry a card indicating a dementia diagnosis; what the healthy spouse should do to handle the sexual desires of the affected spouse when the unaffected spouse no longer feels as though he or she has an adult relationship.
Coach the family to recall past memories in talking with their loved one.	Families feel more comfortable and are more likely to continue to interact with the patient if they know that reduced animation in the patient's face is part of the disease. Conversation may have noticeable pauses with less spontaneous speech; conversations should be short and simple. Reassuring the patient decreases overconcern about minor matters; touch continues to be important; and sharing important memories from the past helps maintain links to the patient even if the response is minimal.
Teach about safety issues.	Safety issues become the responsibility of the caregiver early in the disorder. The patient with Alzheimer's needs room to pace and may fail to notice scatter rugs, spills on the floor, and changes in floor elevations, which increase the risk for falls. Other safety concerns deal with wandering, unsteady gait, forgetting the stove is turned on, and using toxic substances inappropriately.
Provide information about legal matters.	Decisions about durable and health care power of attorney need to be decided in the early stage of the disease, when the patient is still competent. Legal counsel may be desirable for decisions regarding financial matters.
Provide information about health care resources.	The job of the family caregiver is overwhelming. Family members need to consider use of adult day care centers and varieties of respite care, even in the early stage of the illness. Use of home health services also may be of valuable assistance.
Teach strategies to deal with behavioral issues such as wandering, rummaging, incontinence, difficulty following directions, and profound memory loss.	The more knowledge the family has regarding strategies to deal with these various behaviors, the better they will be able to care for the patient.

Nursing Diagnosis:

Risk for Trauma

related to impaired judgment and inability to recognize danger in the environment

Desired Outcome: The patient remains free of signs and symptoms of trauma/injury.

ASSESSMENT/INTERVENTIONS	RATIONALES
[!] Assess the degree of impairment in the patient's abilities. Assist the caregiver to identify risks and potential hazards that may cause harm in the patient's environment and the necessary interventions that must be made to ensure safety.	Patients with impulsive behavior are at increased risk for harm because they are less able to control their own behaviors. Patients may have visual/perceptual deficits that increase risk of falls. Caregivers need heightened awareness of potential risks in the environment and need to take appropriate action.
[!] Eliminate or minimize identified environmental risks.	Because a person with a cognitive deficit is unable to take responsibility for basic safety needs, the caregiver must eliminate as many risks as possible: take knobs off of stove, remove scatter rugs, place a safety gate at the top and bottom of stairs, and make sure doors to the outside are locked.
Routinely monitor the patient's behavior. Initiate interventions to prevent negative behaviors from escalating.	Close observation of the patient's behavior allows early identification of problematic behaviors (e.g., increasing agitation) and enables early intervention.
Use distraction or redirection of the patient's attention when agitated or dangerous behavior such as climbing out of bed occurs.	Using the patient's distractibility avoids confrontation or behavioral escalation and helps maintain safety.
[!] Ensure that the patient wears an ID bracelet providing name, phone number, and diagnosis. Do not allow the patient to have access to stairways or exits.	Because of memory deficits and confusion, these patients may not be able to provide this basic identifying information. The ID bracelet facilitates the patient's safe return.
Ensure that doors to the outside are locked. Make sure there is supervision and/or activities if the patient is regularly awake at night.	Taking appropriate preventive measures facilitates safety without constant supervision. Activities keep the patient occupied and limit wandering.
Ensure that the patient is dressed appropriately for weather/physical environment and individual need.	Patients with cognitive disorders many times experience seasonal disorientation. In addition, AD affects the hypothalamic gland, making the person feel cold. The patient is not able to make appropriate choices regarding dress.
Inspect the patient's skin during care activities.	Identification of rashes, lacerations, and areas of ecchymosis enables necessary treatment and signals need for closer monitoring and protective interventions.
Attend to nonverbal expressions of physiologic discomfort.	The patient may lack the ability to express needs clearly but may give clues to a problem by grimacing, sweating, doubling over, or panting.
[!] Monitor for medication side effects; signs of overmedication, for example, gastrointestinal (GI) upset; extrapyramidal symptoms; and orthostatic hypotension.	Drugs easily build up to toxic levels in older adults, and the patient may not be able to report any signs or symptoms that would indicate drug toxicity.

Nursing Diagnoses:

Chronic Confusion
Impaired Environmental Interpretation Syndrome

related to physiologic changes/dementia occurring with the progressive course of AD

Desired Outcome: The patient remains calm and displays fewer undesirable behaviors.

ASSESSMENT/INTERVENTIONS	RATIONALES
Assess the degree of confusion experienced by the patient with AD and how much short-term memory the patient still retains.	In the middle stage of AD individuals have only about 5 min of short-term memory and no longer can learn. This fact carries with it significant environmental safety issues that must be confronted. For instance, a person could exit from the home or facility where he/she resides and may become lost.
Provide a predictable environment with orientation cues.	A calm environment with scheduled activities, adequate lighting, low noise level, calendars, clocks, and frequent verbal orientation helps maintain the patient's sense of calm and security.
Always address the patient by name.	Patients may respond to their own name long after they no longer recognize their significant others. Names are an integral part of self-identity; using the person's name is a part of reality orientation.
Communicate with the patient using a low voice, slow speech, and eye contact.	Deliberate communication techniques such as these increase the patient's attention and chance for comprehension. Calm begets calm.
Break directions into a simple step-by-step process, giving one direction at a time and using simple and clear words.	As the disease progresses, the patient's ability to comprehend complex directions and interactions diminishes greatly. Direct simplicity is the key to effective communication.
Encourage the patient's response, allow pauses in interaction, and use open-ended comments and phrases.	These interventions invite a verbal response.
Listen carefully to the content of the patient's speech even if it is incomprehensible.	The patient may be having difficulty processing and decoding messages. However, listeners need to continue to show interest and encouragement to keep communication going.
Offer interpretations regarding the patient's statements, meanings, and words. If the patient struggles to find a word, supply the word if possible.	Assisting patients in processing words promotes continuing communication efforts and decreases frustration.
Avoid negative comments, taking argumentative stands, confrontations, and criticism.	These aggressive responses only serve to increase frustration, agitation, and inappropriate behaviors. Cognitively impaired patients have no internal controls over their thinking and communications.
Listen carefully to the patient's stories.	As memory continues to fail, patients are unable to reenter the reality of their caregivers. To argue or reason with the patient only causes more anxiety. It is more important to provide an emotional connection with the patient than to correct the details of his or her stories.
Monitor for hallucinations. Observe the patient for verbal and nonverbal cues of responding to hallucinations. Validate the presence of the patient's hallucinatory experiences.	Validating that the patient is hearing voices allows some discussion of fears associated with the experience and permits assurance that the experience is part of the illness.
Allow the patient to hoard safe objects within reason.	This provides patients with a sense of security.
Provide musical stimulation using selections that would have been popular during the patient's adolescent and early adult years.	Music is a powerful intervention. People who no longer can speak can many times sing. Music can calm an agitated mood and encourage socialization and movement.
Provide useful and productive outlets for the patient to engage in repetitive activities, for example, folding and unfolding laundry, collecting junk mail, dusting, and sweeping floors.	This measure acknowledges that repetitive activities are a normal expression of illness but channels these activities in a way that increases the patient's self-esteem and may decrease restlessness.
Ensure that the environment is quiet, calm, and visually nondistracting.	These qualities help to avoid visual/auditory overload.
Provide touch to the patient in a caring way.	Touch enhances perception of self and body boundaries, as well as communicates caring.
Use reminiscence therapy with props such as photo albums, old music, historic events, and mementos. Encourage the patient to talk about memories and feelings attached to these items.	This measure aids in preservation of self by recalling past accomplishments and events, increases the patient's sense of security, and encourages sharing that keeps the patient linked to others socially.
Encourage intellectual activity such as word games, discussion of current events, and story telling.	This provides patients with normalcy and connection to others and the world and stimulates remaining cognitive abilities.
Suggest that the caregiver accompany the patient on short outings in the car, taking walks, and going shopping.	This decreases sense of isolation, increases physical stamina, and provides sensory pleasure.

Nursing Diagnosis:

Grieving

related to awareness on the part of the patient and significant other/family that something is seriously wrong as changes in memory and behaviors are increasingly evident

Desired Outcome: The patient and family discuss loss and participate in planning for the future.

ASSESSMENT/INTERVENTIONS	RATIONALES
Assess for and encourage the patient and family to discuss feelings associated with anticipated losses.	This conveys the message that grief is a normal and expected reaction to the diagnosis of AD, with which progression and decline are certain.
Acknowledge expressions of anger and statements of despair and hopelessness, such as, "I and my family would be better off if I were dead."	Feelings of anger may be the patient's way of dealing with underlying feelings of despair. Despairing and hopeless statements may be indicative of suicidal ideation. These should be explored and appropriate action taken to protect the patient from self-directed violence (see **Risk for Suicide,** p. 727, in "Major Depression").
Provide honest answers and do not give false reassurances or gloomy predictions.	Honesty promotes a trusting relationship and open communication. False reassurances or predictions of gloom are not helpful.
Discuss with the patient and significant other/family ways they can plan for the future. Recognize and respect generational and cultural differences.	Participation in problem solving increases a sense of control. Effective communication, respect, and compassion are strengthening (Donald W. Reynolds Foundation, 2013).
Emphasize that this is a disease in which research is active and ongoing, as well as the possibility the disease will progress slowly.	Real hope may exist for the future.
Assist the patient, significant other, and family to identify strengths they see in themselves, each other, and in available support systems.	This emphasizes that there are supports and resources to help work through grief.
Encourage the family to participate in a support group for caregivers of Alzheimer's patients.	Support groups not only provide valuable information but also communicate to caregivers that they are not alone as they struggle to manage the illness.

Nursing Diagnosis:

Risk for Caregiver Role Strain

related to severity of the patient's illness, duration of care required, and complexity and number of care-giving tasks required

Desired Outcome: The caregiver exhibits behaviors consistent with a healthy lifestyle.

ASSESSMENT/INTERVENTIONS	RATIONALES
Assess the caregiver's physical/emotional/spiritual condition and the care-giving demands that are present.	This assessment helps to determine individual care needs of the caregiver.
Determine the caregiver's level of responsibility, involvement in, and anticipated duration of care involved.	This helps the caregiver realistically assess what is involved in a commitment to providing care.
Identify strengths of the caregiver and the patient.	This identifies positive aspects of each so that they may be incorporated into daily activities.
Encourage the caregiver to discuss personal perspectives and views about the situation.	This allows venting of concerns and provides opportunities for validation and acceptance of the caregiver's issues.

continued

ASSESSMENT/INTERVENTIONS	RATIONALES
Explore available supports and resources. Facilitate decision-making regarding the least restrictive, safe living environments.	This enables evaluation of adequacy of current resources. For example, "What is currently used? Is it effective? What else is needed?" This allows patients to maintain a level of personal independence (Donald W. Reynolds Foundation, 2013).
Encourage and offer to facilitate family conferences to develop a plan for family involvement in care activities.	The more people involved in care, the less risk that one person will become overwhelmed.
Identify additional resources, including financial, legal, and respite care.	These issues of concern can add to the burden of caregiving if not resolved.
Identify equipment needs/resources and other environmental adaptations.	Appropriate equipment and environmental modifications promote patient safety and ease the care burden on the primary caregiver. An Occupational Therapy consult may be helpful.
Teach caregiver/family techniques and strategies to deal with acting out and disoriented behaviors, as well as incontinence and other physical challenges.	This increases a sense of control and competency of the caregiver and family.
Teach the caregiver the importance of continuing own activities.	Risk of caregiver burden, burnout, and stress is greatly diminished if the caregiver takes time for self, for example, continuing a hobby, pursuing social activities, and taking care of personal needs.
Encourage and help the caregiver/family to plan for changes that may be necessary, such as home care services, use of adult day care, and eventual placement in a long-term facility.	Planning is essential for these eventualities. As the disease progresses, the burden of care outstrips the resources of the caregiver.

Nursing Diagnosis:

Deficient Knowledge

related to unfamiliarity with the rationale, potential side effects, and interventions for side effects of the prescribed medications

Desired Outcome: Immediately following teaching, the caregiver and/or family verbalize accurate information about the rationale for use of certain medications, their common side effects, and methods for dealing with those side effects.

ASSESSMENT/INTERVENTIONS	RATIONALES
In the early stages of AD for the patient, as well as ongoing for the caregivers and/or family, assess their knowledge level regarding the use of cholinesterase inhibitors and/or memantine as part of the treatment plan for AD.	As the disease progresses and the patient's memory continues to deteriorate, the caregiver's and/or family's role in administering and monitoring the effects of the prescribed medications becomes increasingly important.
Describe the physiologic action of **cholinesterase inhibitors** and how they improve cognition.	There are four cholinesterase inhibitors. Tacrine (Cognex) was the first to be developed and is no longer prescribed. The three others in this category, including donepezil (Aricept), rivastigmine tartrate (Exelon), and galantine (Razadyne, formerly Reminyl) do not cure AD. Instead, they slow cognitive decline by slowing the breakdown of acetylcholine released by intact cholinergic neurons.
Describe the physiologic action of **memantine** and the rationale for including it in the medication regimen along with a cholinesterase inhibitor.	Memantine (Namenda) is an NMDA receptor antagonist that targets glutamate, the main excitatory neurotransmitter, and blocks the glutamate from attaching to nerve cells. Specifically, memantine targets the N-methyl-D-aspartate receptors, another chemical and structural system involved in memory. Researchers believe that too much stimulation of nerve cells by glutamate may be responsible for the degeneration of nerves that occurs in some neurologic disorders such as AD. It is the first medication to be developed that targets symptoms during the moderate to severe stages of AD. It is taken in conjunction with a cholinesterase inhibitor.

ASSESSMENT/INTERVENTIONS

ASSESSMENT/INTERVENTIONS	RATIONALES
Advise the patient, caregiver, and family that these medications ideally will return the patient's function to the level that was present 6-12 mo before the medication was started.	This is a significant improvement and may delay nursing home placement for as much as a year.
Teach the side effect profile of the specific prescribed medication and methods for dealing with those effects as follows:	Knowledge about expected side effects and adverse effects is important for promoting adherence to the therapeutic regimen.
- Be alert for headache, fatigue, dizziness, confusion, nausea, vomiting, diarrhea, upset stomach, poor appetite, abdominal pain, rhinitis, and skin rash.	These are common side effects, which, if severe, should be reported to the prescriber for possible decrease in dosage or gradual discontinuation.
- Take the medication exactly as prescribed around the clock and on an empty stomach.	This helps ensure medication effectiveness.
- However, if GI upset occurs, administer with meals.	A full stomach may decrease gastric upset.
- Maintain appointments for regular blood work and medical follow-up while adjusting to the medication.	This is especially important if the patient has preexisting medical conditions, such as renal, liver, or cardiac disease, because these medications may affect these organs.
- Caution is necessary for patients with renal and hepatic disease, seizures, sick sinus syndrome, and GI bleeding.	These medications can worsen these conditions.
- Avoid concomitant use with nonsteroidal antiinflammatory drugs. Explore any herbs or supplements taken in conjunction with prescriptions.	Concomitant use may increase effects and risk of toxicity. Potential drug-herb interactions should be examined.
See care plans for "Anxiety Disorders," p. 705, "Major Depression," p. 730, and "Schizophrenia," p. 735, for a review of antidepressants, anxiolytics, and antipsychotic medications.	Patients with AD may also suffer from depression, anxiety, and psychosis at a clinically significant severity. If depression or anxiety symptoms are severe, psychotropic medications may be indicated and can significantly decrease distress.

ADDITIONAL NURSING DIAGNOSES/PROBLEMS:

✓ PATIENT-FAMILY TEACHING AND DISCHARGE PLANNING

The patient with dementia—Alzheimer's type—progresses through predictable stages, each with characteristic symptoms and behaviors that directly affect the ability to effectively process and use new information. As the disease progresses, the patient requires increasing amounts of physical care, and the caregiver/family require information and support. Dementia is a family disease.

As soon as the diagnosis is made, education and support of the family begins. They need information on the nature and expected progress of the disease and use of memory triggers; establishment of a schedule for basic activities, such as bathing, toileting, meals, and naps; monitoring for intake and output, weight, and skin status; recognition of nonverbal indications of needs and problems; use of redirection and distraction to reduce difficult behaviors; identification of new symptoms or changes; physical and mental activities; necessary environmental modifications, safety measures, and legal issues; sources of information and support; and community resources for caregiving assistance and respite.

Teaching must be geared to a time when medication has begun to lift mood and clear thinking processes; otherwise, it is a wasted effort. Verbal teaching should be simple and supplemented with reading materials the patient and family can refer to at a later time. Ensure that follow-up treatment is scheduled and that the patient and/or significant other and family understand the need to get prescriptions filled and to consistently take medication as prescribed. Consider whether or not the patient has transportation available to get to follow-up treatment. Psychiatric home care might be a valuable part of the discharge planning to facilitate compliance with the discharge plan and for caregiver support. In addition, provide the patient and/or significant other and family with verbal and written information about the following issues:

✓ Nature and expected course of AD.
✓ Medications, including drug name; purpose; dosage; frequency; precautions; drug-drug, food-drug, and herb-drug interactions; and potential side effects.

✓ Strategies to deal with difficult behaviors.
✓ Strategies to maintain patient safety.
✓ Importance of self-care for the caregiver.
✓ Importance of using all available supports to aid in caregiving.
✓ Importance of caregiver and family engaging in honest expression of feelings and confronting negative emotions.
✓ Importance of caregiver using relaxation techniques to minimize stress.
✓ Importance of maintaining or achieving spiritual well-being for the patient and caregiver.
✓ Referrals to community resources for support and education. Additional information can be obtained by contacting the following organizations:

- Alzheimer's Association at *www.alz.org*. It provides a 24-hour hotline, free publications, and information for local chapters. *Worship Services for People with Alzheimer's Disease and Their Families: A Handbook* is also available through this organization.
- American Association of Retired Persons (AARP) at *www.aarp.org*. This is an advocacy group for elderly; it also provides (for a reasonable fee) training materials associated with reminiscence therapy.
- National Institute on Aging (NIA) at *www.nia.nih.gov*. Alzheimer's Disease Education and Reference Center (ADEAR) is available through NIA, which provides electronic newsletters and evidence-based resources.
- The Alzheimer Society of Canada at *www.alzheimer.ca*

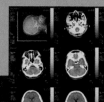

Major Depression 98

OVERVIEW/PATHOPHYSIOLOGY

Major depression is one of the mood disorders, a category of disorders characterized by profound sadness or apathy, irritability, or elation. These disorders rank among the most serious and poorly diagnosed and treated of the health problems in the United States. Major depression is defined as an illness characterized by either depression or the loss of interest in nearly all activities. The symptoms must be present for at least 2 wk. At least four other symptoms must be present from the following list: changes in appetite or weight, sleep, and psychomotor activity; feelings of worthlessness and guilt; difficulty concentrating or making decisions; and recurrent thoughts of death or suicidal ideation, plans, or attempts.

Major depression affects emotional, cognitive, behavioral, and spiritual dimensions. Depression may range from mild-to-moderate states to severe states with or without psychotic features. Major depression can begin at any age, although it usually begins in the mid-20s and 30s. The risk factors for depression include prior history of depression, family history of depression, prior suicide attempts, female gender, age of onset younger than 40 yr, postpartum period, medical comorbidity, lack of social support, stressful life events, personal history of sexual abuse, and current substance abuse. There are many theories to explain causation of depression. Research supports influence of the following factors: sleep disturbance; effects of pharmacologic substances, including many of the antihypertensive, steroidal, cardiovascular, and antipsychotic medications; neuronal factors that involve injury or malfunction of the brain, such as stroke, Parkinson's disease, and deficiencies in neurotransmitters; thyroid dysfunction; genetic factors; and psychodynamic factors.

HEALTH CARE SETTING

Primary care provider, psychiatrist, psychologist, or psychiatric nurse practitioner with occasional brief acute care hospitalization in a psychiatric unit for severe depression, especially if there is a serious suicide threat.

ASSESSMENT

The assessment of major depression involves much more than an assessment of mood. It is a disorder that results in changes in the following:

Feelings, attitudes, and knowledge: Sadness, lack of joy and happiness about anything, shame, humiliation, fear of stigma if others find out about depression, denial, anger, fear of experiencing a relapse, and fear of passing the disorder on to children.

Signs of low mood: Withdrawal from activities that once provided pleasure, as well as from social interactions; negativism and unhappiness expressed in persistent sadness or frequent crying.

Signs of lowered self-worth: Self-deprecating, guilty, or self-blaming comments are common; hopelessness.

Signs of decreased physical well-being: A depressed person may neglect personal appearance or let assignments, tasks, and projects slide. Decreased energy is common, with the depressed person complaining of fatigue and inanition (exhaustion; lack of vigor or enthusiasm). A decreased ability to concentrate makes problem solving difficult. Decision making also may be difficult.

Spiritual issues: Depression carries with it many negative experiences, such as marital and family problems, divorce, and unemployment, which contribute to the downward spiral of self-appraisals. Depression can lead to a crisis in faith in self, others, life, and ultimately God. This loss of faith and hope contributes significantly to the risk of suicide.

Additional signs: Some depressed individuals experience decreased appetite leading to weight loss. Others experience an increase in appetite and weight gain. A change in sleep pattern is characteristic of depression, with difficulty falling asleep, middle of the night awakening, and/or awakening in the early morning hours being common. Others may experience a need for excessive sleep and have difficulty awakening. A decline in sexual interest and activity is characteristic of depressed individuals.

Suicidality: Suicide assessment is critical with depressed patients and includes questions to determine the presence of suicidal ideation and the lethality of any plan. Essential questions to ask include:

- Have you thought of hurting yourself?
- Are you presently thinking about hurting yourself?
- If you have been thinking about suicide, do you have a plan?
- What is the plan?
- Have you thought about what life would be like for others, if you were no longer a part of it?

A previous history of suicide attempts combined with depression places the patient at higher risk in the present for attempting suicide. A patient whose depression is lifting is at higher risk for suicide than a severely depressed individual, because increased energy usually is manifested before improved mood. This increased energy is not enough to make the patient feel good or hopeful, but it is enough to carry out a suicidal plan.

DIAGNOSTIC TESTS

The diagnosis of depression is made through history, interview of the patient and family, and observation of verbal and nonverbal behaviors. Laboratory tests that can rule out a medical basis for depression symptoms include thyroid and liver function tests. A number of effective scales are available to quantify the degree of depression, such as the Zung Self-Rating Depression Scale, the Beck Depression Inventory, the Hamilton Depression Scale, and the Geriatric Depression Scale. The SAD PERSONS scale for suicide assessment is also useful and easy to use.

Nursing Diagnosis:

Deficient Knowledge

related to unfamiliarity with the causes, signs and symptoms, and treatment of depression

Desired Outcome: By discharge (if inpatient) or after 4 wk of outpatient treatment, the patient and significant other verbalize accurate information about at least two of the possible causes of depression, four of the signs and symptoms of depression, and use of medications, psychotherapy, and/or electroconvulsive therapy (ECT) as treatment.

ASSESSMENT/INTERVENTIONS	RATIONALES
Assess the patient's and significant other's knowledge about depression and its causes.	Depression is a physiologic disorder caused by the interplay of many factors such as stress, loss, imbalance in brain chemistry, and genetics. Many people believe that depression is caused by character weakness. This belief contributes to the stigma experienced by the person suffering with depression and interferes with seeking treatment.
Inform the patient and significant other about the major symptoms of depression.	Many people believe depression equates with sadness and fail to recognize the many other signs and symptoms that make this a holistic disorder. These include sadness and loss of interest in normal activities, plus at least four of the following: changes in appetite or weight, sleep, interest in sex, or psychomotor activity; feelings of worthlessness and guilt; difficulty concentrating or making decisions; recurrent thoughts of death or suicidal ideation, plans, or attempts. If the depressed individual displays sadness through irritability, the conclusion that depression is present may be missed and, consequently, necessary treatment may be delayed or avoided entirely.
Explain that depression is treatable.	Medications are usually indicated for treatment. They do not solve the stressors or problems that may have precipitated or resulted from the depression, but they provide the energy to deal with these issues. A combination of antidepressants and psychotherapy generally helps to relieve the symptoms of depression in weeks. Psychotherapy alone may be indicated for mild depression related to situational causes.
Explain about the use of ECT if this is appropriate.	ECT may be used to treat patients who do not respond to antidepressant medications after several trials and psychotherapy. It is generally well tolerated and is given as a series of treatments, usually between 6 and 12 on a 3×/week basis under brief anesthesia. The patient and significant other/family may fear ECT due to misinformation in media portrayals; thus if it is recommended, it provides an opportunity for education that presents ECT as a positive treatment alternative.

Nursing Diagnosis:

Hopelessness

related to losses, stressors, and the burdensome symptoms of depression

Desired Outcome: By discharge (if inpatient) or by the end of 4 wk of outpatient treatment, the patient verbalizes feelings and acceptance of life situations over which he or she has no control, demonstrates independent problem-solving techniques to take control over life, and does not demonstrate or verbalize suicidality.

ASSESSMENT/INTERVENTIONS	RATIONALES
Assess individual signs of hopelessness.	This helps focus attention on areas of individual need. These signs may include decreased physical activity, social withdrawal, and comments made by patients that indicate hopelessness and despair.
Assess unhealthy behaviors used to cope with feelings.	The patient may have tried to overcome feelings of hopelessness with harmful and ineffective behaviors (e.g., withdrawal, substance abuse, avoidance). Recognizing these behaviors provides an opportunity for change.
Encourage the patient to identify and verbalize feelings and perceptions.	The process of identifying feelings that underlie and drive behaviors enables patients to begin taking control of their lives.
Express hope to the patient with realistic comments about the patient's strengths and resources.	Patients may feel hopeless, but it is helpful to hear positive expressions from others.
Help the patient identify areas of life that are under his or her control.	A patient's emotional state may interfere with problem solving. Assistance may be required to identify areas that are under his or her control and to have clarity about options for taking control.
Encourage the patient to assume responsibility for self-care, for example, setting realistic goals, scheduling activities, and making independent decisions.	Helping patients set realistic goals increases feelings of control and provides satisfaction when goals are achieved, thereby decreasing feelings of hopelessness.
Help the patient identify areas of life situations that are not within his or her ability to control. Discuss feelings associated with this lack of control.	The patient needs to recognize and resolve feelings associated with inability to control certain life situations before acceptance can be achieved and hopefulness becomes possible.
Encourage the patient to examine spiritual supports that may provide hope.	Many people find that spiritual beliefs and practices are a great source of hope.
Conduct a suicide assessment to determine the level of suicide risk.	High risk will necessitate hospitalization.
Teach the patient about crisis intervention services such as suicide hotlines and other resources.	It is vital to provide patients with resources for support and safety when thoughts and feelings about suicide become difficult to manage.
Administer antidepressant medication or teach the importance of taking medication as prescribed (see **Deficient Knowledge** *related to* unfamiliarity with medication use in depression, including potential side effects), later.	Suicidal thinking is a symptom of depression that is ameliorated through appropriate medication.

For additional interventions, see **Risk for Suicide,** which follows.

Nursing Diagnosis:

Risk for Suicide

related to depressed mood and feelings of hopelessness

Desired Outcome: By discharge (if inpatient) or by the end of 4 wk (if outpatient), the patient expresses and demonstrates that he or she is free of suicidal thinking.

ASSESSMENT/INTERVENTIONS	RATIONALES
Complete an initial suicide assessment (see specific questions under "Assessment"). Consider using a standardized assessment tool such as SAD PERSONS suicide risk assessment scale.	The degree of hopelessness expressed by the patient is important in assessing risk for suicide. The more the patient has thought out the plan, the greater the risk. Risk for suicide is increased if the patient has a history of a previous attempt or there is family history of suicide and depression. Patients who display impulsive behaviors are more likely to attempt suicide without giving clues. Patients who are experiencing psychotic thinking, especially when there are "voices" that encourage self-harm, are at great risk. Use of alcohol/substance abuse in the presence of any of the above risk factors increases the overall risk for a suicide attempt. A high risk for suicide should prompt hospitalization.
Reassess for suicidality, especially during times of change.	Changes such as the patient's mood improving, medication regimen being altered, discharge planning being initiated, and increasing withdrawal are all signals to reassess suicidality. Suicide risk is greatest in the first few weeks after treatment is begun. The patient may be feeling a little better but not well enough to feel hopeful and may have regained enough energy to actually act on suicidal thoughts.
Administer antidepressant medication or instruct the patient regarding the importance of taking medication as prescribed.	Suicidal thinking is a symptom of depression, which is ameliorated through appropriate medication.
Teach the significant other safety precautions and to be alert for changes in the patient's behavior and/or verbalization that would indicate an increase in suicidal thinking.	Using available support provides a safety net for the patient and communicates that he or she is not alone but that others are concerned and involved in care.
If the patient is hospitalized, implement the following:	
- Monitor at least q15min for moderate risk, preferably staggering monitoring times so that the patient does not take advantage of a guaranteed window of time to engage in suicidal behavior. Provide constant one-on-one observation for serious risk. Place the patient in a room close to the nurses' station. Do not assign to a single room. Accompany the patient to all off-unit activities or restrict him or her to the unit. Ask the patient to remain in view of the staff at all times.	Providing close observation may prevent suicidal attempts.
- Remove items such as belts, scarves, razor blades, shoelaces, scissors—anything that could be used for self-harm. Check all items brought into the unit by patients. Instruct family members to avoid bringing into the unit any hazardous items.	This provides environmental safety and removes potential suicide weapons.
- Provide supervision when the patient is in the bathroom—the door must remain open with a staff member outside.	It is important to remove all opportunities to engage in self-harmful behaviors.
- Perform a mouth check to make sure the patient swallows medications that are administered.	This prevents saving up medications to overdose or discarding and not taking.
- Ensure that nursing rounds are made at frequent but irregular intervals, especially at times that are predictably busy for the staff such as a change of shift.	It is important that staff surveillance not be predictable; otherwise, patients would be able to identify a possible suicide time. In addition, it is essential to maintain awareness of the patient's location at all times.
- Routinely check the environment for hazards and ensure environmental safety.	Minimizing opportunities for self-harm (e.g., keeping doors, windows, and access to stairways and the roof locked and monitoring cleaning, chemical, and repair supplies) is an ongoing concern requiring constant vigilance.
- Initiate a safety plan with the patient.	Involving the patient in creating a safety plan advances trust between the patient and nurse while promoting self-care and monitoring. The safety plan may include a set of actions the patient agrees to initiate when suicidal feelings increase, e.g., approaching the nurse for one-on-one interactions, requesting a prn medication to reduce anxiety, and creating a list of friends or support persons the patient can call.

Nursing Diagnosis:

Grieving

related to actual, perceived, or anticipated loss

Desired Outcome: By discharge (if inpatient) or by the end of 4 wk of outpatient treatment, the patient demonstrates progress in dealing with stages of grief at his or her own pace, participates in work/self-care activities at his or her own pace, and verbalizes a sense of progress toward resolution of grief and hope for the future.

ASSESSMENT/INTERVENTIONS	RATIONALES
Assess losses that have occurred in the patient's life. Discuss the meaning these losses have had for the patient.	Many people deny the importance/impact of a loss. They fail to recognize, acknowledge, or talk about their pain and act as if everything is fine. This has a cumulative effect on the individual. Denial requires physical and psychic energy. When individuals become clinically depressed, they likely do so in a physically and emotionally depleted state.
Discuss cultural practices and religious beliefs and ways in which the patient has dealt with past losses.	Cultural practices and religious beliefs influence how people express and accept the grieving process.
Encourage the patient to identify and verbalize feelings and examine the relationship between feelings and the event/stressor.	Verbalizing feelings in a nonthreatening environment can help patients deal with unrecognized/unresolved issues that may be contributing to depression. It also helps patients connect the response (feeling) to the stressor or precipitating event.
Discuss healthy ways to identify and cope with underlying feelings of hurt, rejection, and anger.	This helps expand the patient's repertoire of coping strategies.
If indicated, tell stories of how others have coped with similar situations.	This not only provides possible solutions but also suggests that the problem is manageable.
Teach the normal stages of grief and acknowledge the reality of associated feelings, such as guilt, anger, and powerlessness.	This information helps the patient realize the normalcy of feelings and may alleviate some of the guilt generated by these feelings.
Help the patient name the problem, identify the need to address the problem differently, and fully describe all aspects of the problem.	Before patients can agree to change, they need clarity about what the problem is.
Help the patient identify and recognize early signs of depression and plan ways to alleviate these signs. Assist with formulating a plan that recognizes the need for outside support if symptoms continue and/or worsen.	This actively involves the patient and conveys the message that the patient is not powerless but rather that options are available.

Nursing Diagnosis:

Chronic Low Self-Esteem

related to repeated negative reinforcement of self-appraisal, which is symptomatic of depression

Desired Outcome: By discharge (if inpatient) or after 4 wk of outpatient treatment, the patient demonstrates behaviors consistent with increased self-esteem.

ASSESSMENT/INTERVENTIONS	RATIONALES
Assess the patient's level of self-esteem.	It is essential to identify the manifestations of low self-esteem, including neglect of personal hygiene and dress, withdrawal from social activities, and self-deprecatory comments, any of which signals a negative thought pattern.
Encourage the patient to engage in self-care grooming activities.	Attending to grooming is often an initial step in feeling better about oneself.

continued

ASSESSMENT/INTERVENTIONS	RATIONALES
Provide positive reinforcement for all observable accomplishments.	Patients with low self-esteem do not benefit from flattery or insincere praise. Honest, positive feedback enhances self-esteem.
Encourage the patient to participate in simple recreational activities or art projects, proceeding to more complex activities in a group setting.	Initially patients may be too overwhelmed to engage in activities that involve more than one person.
If the patient persists in negativism about self, place a limit on the length of time you will listen to negativity.	Time limits allow patients a safe time and place to vent negative feelings and demonstrate thought stopping, the conscious interruption of negative thoughts. For example, agree to 10 min of negativity followed by 10 min of positive comments.
Teach thought-stopping techniques and positive reframing.	Many depressed people engage in self-critical thinking and need to be taught to consciously stop that type of thinking and substitute positive thinking in its place.
Explore the patient's personal strengths and suggest making a list to use as a reminder when negative thoughts return.	Having a written list to review can help patients during difficult times.

Nursing Diagnosis:

Deficient Knowledge

related to unfamiliarity with medication use in depression, including potential side effects

Desired Outcome: By discharge (if inpatient) or after 4 wk of outpatient treatment, the patient verbalizes accurate information about the prescribed medications and their potential side effects.

ASSESSMENT/INTERVENTIONS	RATIONALES
Assess the patient's knowledge level regarding the use of medication to improve depressive symptoms.	It is essential to ascertain what patients know and do not know about the medications prescribed to treat their depression. Frequently patients hold faulty and inaccurate views about medications, which interfere with adherence to a prescribed medication regimen.
Teach the physiologic action of the prescribed antidepressant and how it alleviates symptoms of depression.	Many depressed patients resist taking medications because they fear becoming "addicted"; however, antidepressants are not addictive drugs. Providing the patient with information about the medication's physiologic action helps with adherence.
Caution about the importance of taking the medication at the prescribed dose and time interval.	Some medications require certain blood levels to be therapeutic; therefore, patients need to take them at the dose and time prescribed.
Teach the side-effect profile of the specific prescribed medication, including interventions to combat these effects, for the following:	Each class of antidepressants carries with it a specific side-effect profile. Knowledge about expected side effects, ways to manage these side effects, and the length of time these side effects last is important in ensuring adherence.
Tricyclic antidepressants: amitriptyline (Elavil), desipramine (Norpramin), doxepin (Sinequan), imipramine (Tofranil), nortriptyline (Pamelor), protriptyline (Vivactil), and trimipramine (Surmontil). For more information, see this nursing diagnosis in "Anxiety Disorders," p. 705.	These older antidepressant medications are effective in decreasing signs and symptoms of depression but can produce some troublesome anticholinergic side effects, including urinary hesitancy or retention, dry mouth, blurred vision, fatigue, weight gain, and orthostatic changes, some of which are transient in nature. Additionally, they can cause cardiac QT prolongation (heart block); therefore, ECGs must be monitored intermittently.
Selective Serotonin Reuptake Inhibitors (SSRIs): fluoxetine (Prozac), fluvoxamine maleate (Luvox), sertraline HCl (Zoloft), paroxetine (Paxil), citalopram (Celexa), and escitalopram (Lexapro). For more information, see this nursing diagnosis in "Anxiety Disorders," p. 705.	SSRIs are as effective as tricyclic antidepressants but have a better safety profile and are generally better tolerated. These agents enhance serotonergic function by inhibiting serotonin uptake, which increases bioavailability, thus promoting an antidepressant effect.

ASSESSMENT/INTERVENTIONS	RATIONALES
Dual-mechanism agents: venlafaxine (Effexor), nefazodone HCl (Serzone), mirtazapine (Remeron), duloxetine (Cymbalta), and desvenlafaxine (PRISTIQ).	These medications inhibit both norepinephrine and serotonin uptake and are used when tricyclics and SSRIs fail to improve symptoms.
- Teach the importance of frequent blood pressure (BP) measurements for patients taking venlafaxine. For more information, see this nursing diagnosis in "Anxiety Disorders," p. 705.	At doses greater than 200 mg/day, venlafaxine causes an increase in BP.
Selective Norepinephrine Reuptake Inhibitor: reboxetine (Vestra)	This medication blocks reuptake of norepinephrine.
Norepinephrine-Dopamine Reuptake Inhibitor: bupropion (Wellbutrin)	This medication blocks reuptake of both norepinephrine and dopamine.
- Teach the patient to be alert for anticholinergic side effects, decreased libido, and the potential for drug interactions.	These are common side effects.
- Be aware of the risk for seizures.	Risk increases with bupropion although seizures have been reported with reboxetine use as well.
Miscellaneous antidepressants: trazodone (Desyrel), amoxapine (Asendin), and maprotiline (Ludiomil)	
Teach the patient the following:	
- Watch for anticholinergic effects (except trazodone) such as urinary hesitancy or retention, dry mouth, blurred vision, sedation, hypotension, and risks of falling related to dizziness associated with hypotension.	These are common side effects and can be managed by encouraging patients to drink sufficient water and avoid exertion in high temperatures and activities that require mental alertness while adjusting to the medication.
- Be aware of the risk for seizures.	Risk is moderate with trazodone and increases with amoxapine and maprotiline.
- Be aware of the risk of cardiac toxicity. Patients older than 40 yr need an ECG evaluation before treatment and periodically thereafter.	Risk is minimal with amoxapine and trazodone. There is significant risk with maprotiline.
MAO inhibitors: isocarboxazid (Marplan), phenelzine (Nardil), tranylcypromine (Parnate), selegiline transdermal	MAO inhibitors are used when patients have not responded to other antidepressants. When MAO activity is reduced in the CNS, there is increased dopamine, serotonin, norepinephrine, and epinephrine at the receptor sites, thereby promoting an antidepressant effect.
- Teach the patient to be alert to the potential for mild sedation and hypotension.	These are common side effects.
- Teach the patient about MAO inhibitor restrictions.	MAO inhibitors combined with dietary tyramine can cause a life-threatening hypertensive crisis. Dietary restrictions include avocados; fermented bean curd; fermented soybean; soybean paste; figs; bananas; fermented, smoked, or aged meats; liver; bologna, pepperoni, and salami; dried, cured, fermented, or smoked fish; practically all cheeses; yeast extract; some imported beers; Chianti wine; protein dietary supplements; soups that contain protein extract; shrimp paste; and soy sauce. Large amounts of chocolate, fava beans, ginseng, and caffeine may also cause a reaction. The transdermal form of the MAO inhibitor selegiline does not require dietary restrictions.
- Teach the patient to watch for possible drug interactions and the need to avoid all prescription and over-the-counter drugs unless they have been specifically approved by the provider.	MAO inhibitors can interact with many medications to cause potentially serious results. Use of ephedrine or amphetamines can lead to hypertensive crisis. The interaction of tricyclic antidepressants with MAO inhibitors can cause severe hypertension. Selective serotonin reuptake inhibitors (SSRIs) should not be used with MAO inhibitors because together they can cause serotonin syndrome, a potentially life-threatening event. Symptoms include anxiety, diaphoresis, rigidity, hyperthermia, autonomic hyperactivity, and coma. Because of this possibility, MAO inhibitors should be withdrawn at least 14 days before starting an SSRI, and when an SSRI is discontinued, at least 5 wk should elapse before an MAO inhibitor is given. Antihypertensive drugs combined with MAO inhibitors may result in excessive lowering of blood pressure. MAO inhibitors with meperidine (Demerol) can cause hyperpyrexia (excessive elevation of temperature).

ADDITIONAL NURSING DIAGNOSES/PROBLEMS:

"Anxiety" for Social Isolation	p. 704
"Bipolar Disorder" for:	
Imbalanced Nutrition: Less Than Body Requirements	p. 712
Dressing/Bathing Self-Care Deficit	p. 712
"Substance-Related and Addictive Disorders" for Dysfunctional Family Processes	p. 741

✓ PATIENT-FAMILY TEACHING AND DISCHARGE PLANNING

Patients with major depression experience a wide variety of symptoms that affect their ability to learn and retain information. Teaching must be geared to a time when medication has begun to lift their mood and clear thinking processes; otherwise, it is a wasted effort. Verbal teaching should be simple and supplemented with reading materials the patient and/or significant other and family can refer to at a later time. Ensure that follow-up treatment is scheduled and that the patient and/or significant other and family understand the need to get prescriptions filled and the importance of taking medication as prescribed. Consider whether or not the patient has transportation available to get to follow-up treatment. Psychiatric home care might be a valuable part of the discharge planning to facilitate adherence to the discharge plan. In addition, provide the patient and/or significant other/family verbal and written information about the following issues:

- ✓ Remission/exacerbation aspects of depression.
- ✓ Medications, including drug name; purpose; dosage; frequency; precautions; drug-drug, food-drug, and herb-drug interactions; and potential side effects.
- ✓ Thought-stopping techniques for dealing with negativism.

- ✓ Importance of maintaining a healthy lifestyle—balanced diet, exercise, and regular adequate sleep patterns—to facilitate remaining in remission.
- ✓ Importance of continuing medication use long after depressive symptoms have gone.
- ✓ Importance of social support and strategies for obtaining it.
- ✓ Importance of using constructive coping skills to deal with stress.
- ✓ Importance of honest expression of feelings and confronting of negative emotions.
- ✓ Importance of using relaxation techniques to minimize stress.
- ✓ Importance of maintaining or achieving spiritual well-being.
- ✓ Importance of follow-up care, including day treatment programs, appointments with psychiatrist and therapists, and vocational rehabilitation program if indicated.
- ✓ Referrals to community resources for support and education. Additional information can be obtained by contacting the following organizations:
  - Depression and Related Affective Disorders Association (DRADA) at *www.drada.org.* This nonprofit organization is composed of individuals with mood disorders, family members, and mental health professionals. It offers information, education, referral, and support services to people nationwide. DRADA sponsors a nationally renowned training program for group leaders.
  - Depression Awareness, Recognition, and Treatment Program (D/ART) at (301) 443-4140. D/ART is a national self-help clearinghouse. It provides a list of resources throughout the United States that can help in networking and providing consultative assistance.
  - Depression and Bipolar Support Alliance (DBSA) at *www.dbsalliance.org.* The DBSA provides education as well as support to individuals and families impacted by depression and bipolar illnesses.
  - The Canadian Mental Health Association at *www .cmha.ca*

Schizophrenia 99

OVERVIEW/PATHOPHYSIOLOGY

Schizophrenia is a neurobiologic disorder of the brain categorized as a thought disorder with disturbances in thinking, feeling, perceiving, and relating to others and the environment. Schizophrenia is a mixture of both positive and negative symptoms that are present for a significant part of a 1-mo period but with continuous signs of disturbances persisting for at least 6 mo. It is characterized by delusions, hallucinations, disorganized speech and behavior, and other symptoms that cause social or occupational dysfunction.

Schizophrenia is considered one of the most disabling of the major mental disorders, with an estimated 2.4 million or about 1.1 percent of Americans afflicted. It can occur at any age, but it tends to first develop (or at least become evident) between adolescence and young adulthood. Risk factors include maternal starvation and infections during fetal development, complications during childbirth, childbirth that occurs in late winter or early spring, and living in an urban environment. Theories of causation include genetics, autoimmune factors, neuroanatomic changes, the dopamine hypothesis (people with schizophrenia appear to have excessive dopamine levels), and psychologic factors. There are several subtypes of schizophrenia, including paranoid, disorganized, catatonic, undifferentiated, and residual.

HEALTH CARE SETTING

Most patients with schizophrenia receive treatment across a variety of settings, including inpatient and partial hospitalization (day treatment), psychiatric home care, and crisis stabilization units. Community services include assertive community treatment, outpatient therapy, case management, and psychosocial rehabilitation.

ASSESSMENT

Schizophrenia affects many aspects of a person's being. How the individual looks, feels, thinks, interacts with others, and moves in the world are all drastically affected by this disorder. A thorough assessment focuses not only on the bizarre behaviors characteristic of the disease but on the whole person—his or her physical, emotional, social, and spiritual dimensions.

Biologic: A thorough history and physical are essential to rule out a medical illness or substance abuse that could cause the psychiatric symptoms. It is essential to screen for comorbid treatable medical illnesses. People with schizophrenia have a higher mortality rate from physical illness and often have smoking-related illnesses such as emphysema and other pulmonary and cardiac disorders. The patient may appear awkward and uncoordinated, with poor motor skills and abnormalities in eye tracking.

Psychologic: Many patients report prodromal symptoms of tension and nervousness, lack of interest in eating, difficulty concentrating, difficulty in making choices, disturbed sleep, decreased enjoyment and loss of interest, poor hygiene, restlessness, forgetfulness, depression, social withdrawal from friends, feeling that others are laughing at them, feeling bad for no reason, thinking about religion more, hearing voices or seeing things, and feeling too excited. These symptoms are often ignored and may result in treatment delays.

Appearance: Patients may appear in bizarre and eccentric dress, be disheveled, and have poor hygiene.

Objective behaviors: Patients may display stereotypy (idiosyncratic, repetitive, purposeless movements), echopraxia (involuntary imitation of another's movements), and waxy flexibility (posture held in odd or unusual fixed position for extended periods). Patients may display altered mood states ranging from heightened emotional activity to severely limited emotional responses. Affect, the outward expression of mood, may be described as flat, blunted, or full range, or it may be described as inappropriate. Other common emotional symptoms include affective lability, ambivalence, and apathy.

Delusions: Delusions are beliefs that are held despite clear contradictory evidence. Sometimes they are plausible; at other times the delusions expressed are bizarre, implausible, and not derived from ordinary life experiences. Delusions of persecution are the most common type. Delusions of grandeur are also commonly expressed. Ideas of reference are delusional ideas in which patients believe actions of others are directed toward them. Two other forms of delusional thinking include thought broadcasting—the belief that one's thoughts can be heard by others—and thought insertion—the belief that thoughts of others can be inserted into one's mind. It is important to assess content of the delusion; the degree of conviction with which the delusion is held; how extensively other aspects of the patient's life are incorporated into the delusion; the degree of internal consistency, organization, and logic evidenced in the delusion; and the impact exerted on the patient's life by this delusion.

Hallucinations: A hallucination is an alteration in sensory perception. Although hallucinations can be experienced in all sensory modalities, auditory hallucinations are the most common in schizophrenia. Patients may not spontaneously share their hallucinations, and in order to assess for them, nurses may need to rely on observations of the patient's behavior, including pauses in a conversation during which the patient seems to be preoccupied or appears to be listening to someone other than the interviewer, looking toward the perceived source of a voice, or responding to the voices in some manner.

Disorganized communication: Both speech content and patterns are important to assess. Abrupt shifts in conversational focus are typical of disorganized communication and are referred to as *loose association*. The most severe shifts may occur after only one or two words, referred to as *word salad*—a jumble of unrelated words. A less severe shift may occur after one or two phrases, referred to as *flight of ideas*. The least severe shift in the focus occurs when a new topic is repeatedly suggested and pursued from the current topic, referred to as *tangentiality*. In addition to abrupt shifts from one topic to another, the person with schizophrenia experiences thought blocking, in which thoughts and psychic activity unexpectedly cease. Language may be difficult to understand and may begin to serve as a tool of self-expression rather than a tool of communication. Sometimes the person creates completely new words, referred to as *neologisms*.

Cognitive impairments: Although cognitive impairments vary widely from patient to patient, several problems are consistent across most patients; these include hypervigilance (increased and sustained attention to external stimuli over an extended time), a diminished ability to distinguish relevant from irrelevant stimuli, familiar cues going unrecognized or being improperly interpreted, and diminished information processing leading to inappropriate or illogical conclusions from available observations and information.

- *Memory and orientation:* Individuals with schizophrenia display impairments in memory and abstract thinking. Although orientation to time, place, and person remains relatively intact unless the person is preoccupied with delusions and hallucinations, all aspects of memory are affected in schizophrenia. Patients may experience a diminished ability to recall within seconds newly learned information. Both short- and long-term memories are often affected.
- *Insight and judgment:* Insight and judgment depend on cognitive functions that are frequently impaired in people with schizophrenia.

Social issues: As the disorder progresses, individuals become increasingly socially isolated. People with schizophrenia have difficulty connecting with others on a one-to-one basis. Emotional blunting, inability to form emotional attachments, problems with face and affect recognition, inability to recall past interactions, problems making decisions or using appropriate judgment in difficult situations, and poverty of speech and language all serve to separate and isolate the individual.

Spiritual issues: Persons with schizophrenia may experience delusions and hallucinations with religious content, and some health care providers tend to dismiss religious verbalizations as psychotic expressions. However, the contrary is true. Religion and spirituality can be a source of comfort to patients dealing with a terrible disease. It is important to assess religious commitment, religious practices, and spiritual issues such as the meaning of the illness to the individual, the role of God, and sources of hope and support.

Suicidality: Suicide assessment is critical in schizophrenia. The presence of psychotic thinking and command hallucinations, coupled with possible substance abuse, increases the suicide risk significantly. It is important to ask questions to determine the presence of suicidal ideation and the lethality of any plan. Essential questions to ask include:

- Have you thought of hurting/killing yourself?
- Are you presently thinking about hurting/killing yourself?
- If you have been thinking about suicide, do you have a plan? What is the plan?
- Have you thought about what the life of others would be like if you were no longer a part of it?
- Consider using the SAD PERSONS suicide assessment tool to quantify the risk of suicide.

DIAGNOSTIC TESTS

There are no specific tests to diagnose schizophrenia. Diagnosis is made using the diagnostic criteria put forth in *The Diagnostic and Statistical Manual-5* (American Psychiatric Association, 2013). Diagnosis is made through history, interview of the patient and family, and observation of verbal and nonverbal behaviors. There are several reliable rating scales that are useful in the assessment of schizophrenia. These include the Scale for the Assessment of Negative Symptoms (SANS), Scale for the Assessment of Positive Symptoms (SAPS), Positive and Negative Syndrome Scale (PANSS), and the Brief Psychiatric Rating Scale (BPRS).

The Abnormal Involuntary Movement Scale (AIMS), and Simpson-Angus Rating Scale are tools used to evaluate movement abnormalities related to medications. These tools are beneficial in assessing severity of extrapyramidal symptoms or tardive dyskinesia.

Nursing Diagnosis:

Deficient Knowledge

related to unfamiliarity with the causes, signs and symptoms, and treatment of schizophrenia

Desired Outcome: Before discharge from the care facility or after 4 wk of outpatient treatment, the patient and/or significant other verbalize accurate information about at least two of the possible causes of schizophrenia, four of the signs and symptoms of the disorder, and the available treatment options.

ASSESSMENT/INTERVENTIONS	RATIONALES
Assess the patient's and significant other's understanding of schizophrenia.	Schizophrenia is a physiologic disorder caused by the interplay of many factors such as stress, genetics, infectious-autoimmune factors, neuroanatomic changes, the dopamine hypothesis, and psychologic factors. Providing education about the physical basis for the disorder increases understanding and acceptance and decreases blaming behavior.
Explain that there are treatments available for schizophrenia.	Medications are essential to stabilize and maintain patients with schizophrenia. They decrease psychotic thinking, hallucinations, and delusions. Some, but not all, drugs target negative symptoms. However, medications are not enough. Comprehensive treatment involves inpatient and partial hospitalization, day treatment, psychiatric home care, and crisis stabilization. Community services include assertive community treatment, outpatient therapy, case management, and psychosocial rehabilitation.

Nursing Diagnosis:

Deficient Knowledge

related to unfamiliarity with the medications used in schizophrenia, including their purpose and potential side effects

Desired Outcome: Before discharge from the care facility or after 4 wk of outpatient treatment, the patient verbalizes accurate information about the prescribed medications.

ASSESSMENT/INTERVENTIONS	RATIONALES
Assess the patient's knowledge about the physiologic action of antipsychotic medications.	Education should be directed to assess deficits in knowledge regarding the expected benefits of taking the prescribed drug, potential side effects, and how to deal with them. Knowledge increases adherence to taking the prescribed medications.
Teach the following side-effect profiles of the specific prescribed medication, as well as interventions to mitigate the effects.	A knowledgeable patient is likely to report adverse symptoms and know how to intervene properly for others, which optimally will promote adherence.
Typical (1st-generation) antipsychotic agents: chlorpromazine (Thorazine), thioridazine (Mellaril), mesoridazine (Serentil), loxapine (Loxitane), perphenazine (Trilafon), trifluoperazine (Stelazine), thiothixene (Navane), fluphenazine (Prolixin), haloperidol (Haldol), and pimozide (Orap)	Typical antipsychotics block all dopamine receptors in the central nervous system (CNS) and can produce serious movement disorders, referred to as *extrapyramidal side effects (EPS).*
Explain that sedation, orthostatic hypotension, and anticholinergic effects can occur.	These are common side effects of traditional antipsychotic agents.

continued

PART IV: Psychiatric Nursing Care Plans

ASSESSMENT/INTERVENTIONS	RATIONALES
Teach the patient to be alert for EPS, including acute dystonia (impaired muscle tone), parkinsonism, akathisia (restlessness, agitation), and tardive dyskinesia (involuntary movements of the face, trunk, and limbs) using the AIMS.	These are adverse effects of traditional antipsychotic drugs, with tardive dyskinesia being the most serious. Use of AIMS enables objective quantification of changes in movements and permits early intervention before the appearance of tardive dyskinesia. AIMS shall be assessed at least once every 6 months or more frequently as necessary by symptom assessment or as determined by the prescribing practitioner.
Explain the potential for neuroleptic malignant syndrome (NMS).	This is an idiosyncratic hypersensitivity to antipsychotics that is believed to affect the body's thermoregulatory mechanism. It is a rare but serious reaction that carries with it a 4% risk of mortality. Symptoms include high fever, sweating, unstable blood pressure, stupor, muscular rigidity, and autonomic dysfunction. Early identification of and treatment for individuals with neuroleptic malignant syndrome improve outcome.
Caution the patient that there is a risk for seizures.	Antipsychotics can reduce the seizure threshold and should be used with caution for patients with epilepsy or other seizure disorder.
Teach the importance of avoiding all products with anticholinergic actions, including antihistamines and specific over-the-counter sleeping aids.	Products with anticholinergic properties intensify the anticholinergic responses to antipsychotic drugs, including dry mouth, constipation, blurred vision, urinary hesitancy, and tachycardia.
Explain the importance of avoiding alcohol and other medications with CNS-depressant actions, for example, antihistamines, opioids, and barbiturates.	Antipsychotics can intensify CNS depression caused by alcohol and other medications.
For patients taking Thorazine, Mellaril, Prolixin, Trilafon, or Stelazine, teach the importance of avoiding excessive exposure to sunlight, using sunscreen, and wearing protective clothing.	These medications belong to the phenothiazine class, which causes sensitization of the skin to ultraviolet light, thus increasing the chance of severe sunburn.
Teach the patient that sexual dysfunction is a possible side effect and should be reported to the prescriber rather than stop the medication.	It is important that the patient not discontinue the medication abruptly, but rather report it so that the prescriber can intervene accordingly.
Atypical (2nd-generation) antipsychotic agents: clozapine (Clozaril), risperidone (Risperdal Consta, M-tabs), olanzapine (Zyprexa), quetiapine (Seroquel), ziprasidone (Geodon), aripiprazole (Abilify), lurasidone (Latuda), asenapine (Saphris), iloperidone (Fanapt), and Paliperidone (Invega)	Atypical antipsychotics are more selective in blocking specific dopamine receptors. Because of this, they have less risk of EPS.
Explain that patients taking clozapine should be watchful for drowsiness and sedation, hypersalivation, tachycardia, constipation, and postural hypotension.	These are common side effects.
Explain that patients taking clozapine need weekly hematologic monitoring for the first 6 mo of treatment, and after 6 mo, monitoring is monthly. Advise the patient that clozapine will not be dispensed if a blood test is not done.	Agranulocytosis occurs in 1%-2% of patients, with an overall risk of death of about 1 in 5000. Agranulocytosis usually occurs in the first 6 mo.
Caution that patients taking clozapine, especially those with seizure disorder, are at risk for seizures.	Generalized tonic-clonic seizures occur in 3% of patients, and the risk is dose related, with higher incidence in patients receiving doses greater than 600 mg. Patients who have experienced a seizure should be warned not to drive a car or participate in other potentially hazardous activities while on this medication.
Explain that patients taking clozapine should avoid medications that can suppress bone marrow function, such as carbamazepine (Tegretol) and many cancer drugs. Cimetidine and erythromycin increase levels of clozapine, leading to toxicity. Smoking, Tegretol, and phenytoin can decrease levels of clozapine, diminishing its efficacy.	These are drug-to-drug interactions that can occur when they are combined with clozapine.
Advise patients taking risperidone that there is a risk for insomnia, agitation, anxiety, constipation, nausea, dyspepsia, vomiting, dizziness, and sedation.	These are common side effects.

ASSESSMENT/INTERVENTIONS

ASSESSMENT/INTERVENTIONS	RATIONALES
Advise patients taking risperidone to be watchful for EPS.	This is an adverse effect that is dose related (reported in doses greater than 10 mg/day).
Explain that patients taking olanzapine should be watchful for headache, insomnia, constipation, weight gain, akathisia, and tremor.	These are common side effects.
Explain that patients taking quetiapine should be watchful for headache, somnolence, constipation, and weight gain.	These are common side effects.
Caution patients taking ziprasidone (Geodon) who have a history of cardiac disease, low electrolyte levels, or family history of QT prolongation that they are at risk for electrocardiogram changes, specifically QT prolongation.	This is a common side effect.

ADDITIONAL NURSING DIAGNOSES/PROBLEMS:

✓ PATIENT-FAMILY TEACHING AND DISCHARGE PLANNING

Patients with schizophrenia experience a wide variety of symptoms that affect their ability to learn and retain information. Teaching must be geared to a time when medication has begun to decrease the psychotic symptoms, thoughts are more organized, and communication is more effective. Verbal teaching should be simple and supplemented with reading materials that the patient and/or significant other and family can refer to at a later time.

Most patients with schizophrenia experience memory deficits, so retention of new information does not come easily. Repetition and attention to clarity and simplicity of teaching approaches and materials facilitate learning. Ensure that follow-up treatment is scheduled and that the patient and/or significant other and family understand the need to get prescriptions filled and to take medications as prescribed. Consider whether or not the patient has transportation available to get to follow-up treatment. Psychiatric home care might be a valuable part of the discharge planning to facilitate adherence to the discharge plan. In addition, provide the patient and/or significant other/family with verbal and written information about the following issues:

✓ Medications, including drug name; purpose; dosage; frequency; precautions; drug-drug, food-drug, and herb-drug interactions; and potential side effects.

✓ Importance of laboratory follow-up tests if the patient is taking Clozaril.

✓ Importance of maintaining a healthy lifestyle—balanced diet, minimal to no caffeine or alcohol, exercise, limit the amount of smoking, and regular adequate sleep patterns—to facilitate remaining in remission.

✓ Importance of continuing medication use, probably for a lifetime.

✓ Importance of social support and strategies to obtain it.

✓ Importance of using community resources, for example, psychiatrist, psychiatric nurse, intensive outpatient support groups, family counseling, psychosocial programs including club houses, and other patient-run support groups.

✓ Importance of following up with medical care, as well as psychiatric care.

✓ Importance of maintaining or achieving spiritual well-being.

✓ Referrals to community resources for support and education. Additional information can be obtained by contacting the following organizations:

• Johnson & Johnson Patient Assistance Foundation, Inc. (JJPAF) provides access to medicines for uninsured individuals who lack the financial resources to pay for them (1-800-652-6227).

• Lilly Cares Patient Assistance Program, at Eli Lilly and Company, Lilly Corporate Center, Indianapolis, IN 46285, (800) 545-9962. This program was designed to assist providers, patients, and the patient caregivers through reimbursement support and temporary provision of Zyprexa and other drugs at no charge to eligible patients.

• National Alliance for the Mentally Ill (NAMI) at *www.nami.org*. Contact NAMI chapter in local state for information and schedule or contact national office of NAMI. The NAMI Family to Family Education Program is a 12-session comprehensive course for families of people with serious mental illnesses.

- Mental Illness Education Project, Inc., at *www.miepvideos.org*, has a videotape for families and mental health professionals entitled, "Families Coping with Mental Illness."
- MedicAlert Foundation at *www.medicalert.org* provides a simple tool to ensure that people with schizophrenia receive proper care in an emergency department or to help family members find a loved one who has stopped taking medication and is experiencing behavioral problems in public. MedicAlert has a program for people who cannot afford the membership fees.

- National Institute of Mental Health (NIMH) Public Inquiries at *www.nimh.nih.gov* has a booklet prepared by the Schizophrenia Research Branch titled, "Schizophrenia: Questions and Answers" (DHHS Publication No. ADM 90-1457).
- National Alliance for Research on Schizophrenia and Depression (NARSAD) at *www.narsad.org*
- Schizophrenia Society of Canada at *www.schizophrenia.ca*
- American Psychiatric Association: Healthy Minds TV—Living with Schizophrenia, at *http://www.psychiatry.org/mental-health/more-topics/healthy-minds-tv*

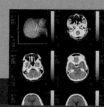

Substance-Related and Addictive Disorders 100

OVERVIEW/PATHOPHYSIOLOGY

Substance use disorders are a major health issue in the United States. The connection between substance use and social and health problems is well documented and includes such issues as an increase in illegal and violent activities associated with the sale and distribution of illegal drugs, major health problems including the spread of human immunodeficiency virus (HIV) and other communicable diseases among intravenous (IV) drug users, developmental issues of "crack babies" born to addicted mothers, fetal alcohol syndrome babies, low-birth-weight babies, and domestic violence and child abuse and neglect. Deaths caused by motor vehicular accidents are directly linked to alcohol consumption. In addition, there are a full range of medical complications that are a direct result of alcohol use disorders, including cardiovascular, respiratory, hematologic, nervous, digestive, endocrine, metabolic, skin, musculoskeletal, and genitourinary problems, as well as nutritional deficiencies.

According to the *Diagnostic and Statistical Manual of Mental Disorders-5* (*DSM-5*; American Psychiatric Association [APA], 2013), the essential feature of a substance use disorder is a cluster of cognitive, behavioral, social, and physiologic symptoms indicating that the individual continues using a substance despite significant substance-related problems and dangers. There is an underlying change in brain circuits that may persist beyond detoxification. The distinction between substance abuse and substance dependence made in DSM-IV-TR has moved toward a DSM-5 diagnosis for each substance based on a continuum from mild to severe: mild (2-3 symptoms), moderate (4-5 symptoms), and severe (6 or more symptoms). Each substance the person uses will receive its own diagnosis in relation to its severity on this spectrum, e.g., Alcohol Use Disorder—Severe; Stimulant Use Disorder—Moderate.

Identifying the specific drug(s) used is essential for individualized treatment of toxicity and withdrawal. However, it is the outcome of psychoactive drug use, shared in common by all drug classifications, that is most likely to account for the problems associated with the disorder. These properties include acute and chronic structural and functional changes in the brain associated with drug intake; variable effects on the person taking the drugs; tolerance and reinforcing properties that are unique characteristics of most psychoactive substances and are not found in other pharmacologic classifications; and the treatment concepts of recovery and relapse prevention after cessation of drug intake.

HEALTH CARE SETTINGS

Treatment of substance use disorders occurs over the full range of the health care continuum. Acute detoxification usually takes place in an acute care/hospital facility. However, long-term care takes place in various community settings: outpatient or partial hospitalization therapy, vocational supports, family therapy, residential programs, and employee assistance programs. Treatment adjuncts include support group programming such as Alcoholics Anonymous (AA) and Narcotics Anonymous (NA).

ASSESSMENT (ALCOHOL USE DISORDER)

Assessment focuses on alcohol use disorder (or alcoholism) as a prototype for the category of *Substance Use Disorders* because it constitutes the most frequently used and misused psychoactive substance in the United States.

Major symptoms supportive of a diagnosis of alcohol use disorder:

- Withdrawal symptoms
- Tolerance, as evidenced by needing more alcohol to get the same effect or consuming the same amount with less effect.
- Indiscriminate or regular drinking (or cravings) despite social or medical contraindications.
- Significant interference with psychosocial functioning in family and job relationships.
- Drinking in hazardous situations or arrests for driving while under the influence of alcohol.

Assessment interview: This should include family history, history of drug use, and a description of behavior patterns described above. It is important to ask about preexisting mental disorders, metabolic conditions, cardiac and gas exchange problems, prescribed medications, and head injuries, all of which have symptoms that sometimes mimic acute intoxication or withdrawal symptoms.

Psychologic symptoms, behavior patterns, and defense mechanisms: The patient uses *denial* to insist that she or he does not have a problem despite concrete evidence to the contrary. *Rationalization* appears in the form of self-imposed rules that explain the person's drinking habits as legitimate. Statements may be made such as, "I only drink on weekends" or "I limit myself to a beer, none of the hard stuff for me." *Projection* is evidenced in the blaming of external forces for stimulating the need to drink, for example, a nagging spouse or a stressful job. *Blackouts* occur when there is a neuronal irritability that erases the memory of behaviors while under the influence.

Physical indicators/examination:

- **Activity/rest:** Difficulty sleeping, not feeling well rested.
- **Cardiovascular:** Peripheral pulses weak, irregular, or rapid; hypertension common in early withdrawal stage from alcohol but may become labile and progress to hypotension as withdrawal progresses; tachycardia common in early withdrawal; dysrhythmias may be identified; other abnormalities depending on underlying heart disease/concurrent drug use.
- **Elimination:** Diarrhea, varied bowel sounds resulting from gastric complications such as gastric hemorrhage or distention.
- **Nutrition and fluid intake:** Nausea, vomiting, and food intolerance; difficulty chewing and swallowing food; muscle wasting; dry, dull hair; swollen salivary glands, inflamed buccal cavity, capillary fragility (malnutrition); possible generalized tissue edema resulting from protein deficiency; gastric distention, ascites, liver enlargement (seen in cirrhosis with long-term use).
- **Pain/discomfort:** Possible constant upper abdominal pain and tenderness radiating to the back (pancreatic inflammation).
- **Respiratory:** History of smoking; recurrent/chronic respiratory problems; tachypnea (with hyperactive state of alcohol withdrawal); diminished breath sounds.
- **Neurosensory:** Internal shakes or tremors, headache, dizziness, blurred vision, blackouts.
- **Psychiatric:** Possible dual diagnoses of mental illness, for example, schizophrenia, bipolar disorder, and major depressive disorder.
- **Level of consciousness/orientation:** Confusion, stupor, hyperactivity, distorted thought processes, slurred/incoherent speech.
- **Affect/mood/behavior:** May be fearful, anxious, easily startled, inappropriate, irritable, labile, physically/verbally abusive, depressed, or paranoid.

Withdrawal assessment: Monitor the patient q4-6h with Clinical Institute Withdrawal Assessment—Alcohol, Revised (CIWA-Ar) until the score is less than 10 for 24 hr, when medication for withdrawal is usually no longer necessary.

- **Early symptoms (6-12 hr after alcohol use cessation):** temperature, pulse, respirations (TPR) and systolic blood pressure (SBP) elevated; palpitations; slight diaphoresis; oriented × 3; mild anxiety and restlessness; restless sleep; tremulousness; decreased appetite; nausea.
- **12-24 hr after alcohol use cessation:** increased diaphoresis; intermittent confusion; transient visual and auditory hallucinations, primarily at night; increased anxiety and motor restlessness; insomnia; nightmares; nausea, vomiting, anorexia.
- **24-48 hr after alcohol use cessation:** additional symptoms may include generalized tonic-clonic seizures.
- **Later (48-72 hr after alcohol use cessation):** severe additional symptoms. Pulse 120-140 bpm; increased temperature; increased diastolic blood pressure (DBP) and SBP; marked diaphoresis; marked disorientation and confusion; frightening visual, auditory, and tactile hallucinations (predominantly visual); illusions (misinterpretation of objects); delusions; delirium tremens; disturbances in consciousness; agitation, panic states; inability to sleep; gross uncontrollable tremors, convulsions; inability to ingest any oral fluids or foods.

Safety assessment: History of recurrent accidents, such as falls, fractures, lacerations, burns, bruises, blackouts, or automobile accidents.

Suicidal assessment: Alcoholic suicide attempts may be as much as 30% higher than the national average, and impulsivity is increased during intoxication.

Social assessment: Dysfunctional family system; problems in current relationships; frequent sick days off work/school; history of arrests because of fighting with others or driving while intoxicated, disorderly conduct, or automobile accidents.

Spiritual assessment: It is important to assess for spiritual beliefs, practices, faith traditions, and commitment to those traditions. Many alcoholics and others addicted to substances find recovery through the spiritual program models of AA and NA. Additionally, spiritual beliefs may provide the anchor that prevents an addicted individual from considering suicide.

DIAGNOSTIC TESTS

Blood alcohol and drug levels can be obtained. However, diagnosis of *Alcohol Use Disorder* is generally made through interview history and physical and psychiatric examinations. The diagnosis is made by confirmation of the presence of the four major symptoms of alcoholism listed above. Two of the most common assessment screening tools used to establish problem severity are the Michigan Alcohol Screening Test (MAST) and the CAGE-AID questionnaires.

Nursing Diagnosis:

Risk for Trauma

related to altered cognitive function occurring with alcohol withdrawal

Desired Outcome: The patient does not exhibit evidence of physical trauma caused by alcohol withdrawal.

ASSESSMENT/INTERVENTIONS — RATIONALES

ASSESSMENT/INTERVENTIONS	RATIONALES
⚠ Assess the stage of alcohol withdrawal and severity of symptoms. Monitor vital signs, gait and motor coordination, presence and severity of tremors, mental status, and electrolyte status.	The greater the severity of symptoms, the more likely the patient will experience increasing disorientation, confusion, and restlessness. As the withdrawal progresses, the risk for a fall or injury increases significantly.
⚠ Monitor for seizure activity; institute seizure precautions: bed in lowest position with side rails padded.	Withdrawal seizures usually occur within 24-48 hr following the last alcoholic drink.
Keep communication simple.	As withdrawal progresses, the patient's ability to comprehend complex directions and interactions diminishes greatly. Simplicity is the key to effective communication.
Continue to orient the patient to surroundings and call light or communication system.	As the blood alcohol level drops, disorientation increases and can last several days.
Maintain a calm, quiet environment.	Controlling the amount of external stimulation and keeping it at a minimal level promotes calm in the patient.
⚠ Administer IV/PO fluids with caution as indicated.	Careful fluid replacement corrects dehydration and facilitates renal clearance of toxins. Excessive alcohol use damages the cardiac muscle and/or conduction system. Overhydration poses significant risk to cardiac functioning.
⚠ Administer medications as prescribed and be alert for side effects:	
- Benzodiazepines: lorazepam (Ativan), diazepam (Valium), or chlordiazepoxide (Librium)	These medications are commonly used to control neuronal activity as alcohol is detoxified from the body. Either IV or PO route is preferred. These agents produce muscle relaxation, which is effective in controlling the "shakes," trembling, and ataxic movements, as well as preventing seizures. They are usually initiated at a high dose and tapered and discontinued within 96 hr. They must be used cautiously in patients with hepatic disease because the liver metabolizes them.
- Benzodiazepine: oxazepam (Serax)	This may be the medication of choice for patients with liver disease. Although it does not produce quite the dramatic effects of controlling withdrawal symptoms, it has a shorter half-life, so it is safer in the presence of hepatic disease.
- Phenobarbital or carbamazepine	This medication is highly effective in suppressing withdrawal symptoms and is an effective anticonvulsant. Use must be monitored to prevent exacerbation of respiratory depression.
- Haloperidol or olanzapine	Antipsychotic medications may be used with delirium tremens, specifically for symptoms of psychosis or severe agitation.

Nursing Diagnosis:

Dysfunctional Family Processes

related to long-term pattern of the patient's alcoholism

Desired Outcome: Before the patient is discharged from the care facility or after 4 wk if the patient is outpatient, family members verbalize the dysfunctional behavioral dynamics present within the family system, the difference between caring and enabling, and the available services and treatment options that would help the family.

ASSESSMENT/INTERVENTIONS — RATIONALES

ASSESSMENT/INTERVENTIONS	RATIONALES
Assess for and provide family members with an opportunity to discuss their experiences of living with the disabling effects of alcoholism.	This validates their experience and encourages open discussions of the problem.
Educate family members about the effects of alcoholism on the family system.	This information enables recognition that the dynamics in their family, although dysfunctional, is a predictable response to having a family member addicted to alcohol. It also encourages engagement in a realistic appraisal of the family's dynamics.

continued

ASSESSMENT/INTERVENTIONS	RATIONALES
Provide family members with a list of services and treatment options available.	This validates that the dysfunction within the family is serious and requires and normalizes support of professionals to correct the patterns.
Define the term *enabling* for family members. Encourage each of them to identify at least one time when he or she enabled the patient. Offer family members alternative choices to enabling behaviors. Have them practice what they will do and say when a situation arises.	It is important to reframe helping behavior as enabling behavior in order for family members to recognize the pattern. It is also important for them to realize that changing these patterns requires practice and feedback. During times of anxiety, it is normal to fall back on previous patterns of behaving.
If in a relationship, encourage the couple to consider couples therapy to begin to discuss regrets and resentments that have occurred as a result of alcoholism.	After many years of denial, it is important to begin to talk about feelings that have been buried. This process should be undertaken with a professional who can act as a mediator and teach the couple how to communicate without blaming, a common dynamic in a marriage affected by alcoholism.
Explain how roles have changed within the family as a result of alcoholism.	Teaching may have to be repeated frequently based on the family's readiness to learn. Alcoholism produces dramatic role shifts that families are unaware of when they are in the midst of problems such as codependence. Presenting this emotionally charged information in a concrete, didactic manner increases their ability to hear.
Encourage family members to tell one another their needs and that caring about them is different from enabling.	Social and emotional isolation and denial of needs are common in alcoholic families. Enabling behaviors are frequently intended to be caring.
Encourage the family to attend Al-Anon meetings.	Significant change will require long-term commitment and support.

Nursing Diagnosis:

Ineffective Denial

related to lack of control of alcoholism resulting in minimization of its symptoms and effects

Desired Outcome: Before discharge from the care facility or after 4 wk if outpatient, the patient acknowledges that his or her drinking is out of control and his or her life has become unmanageable.

ASSESSMENT/INTERVENTIONS	RATIONALES
Assess the patient's level of denial vs. acceptance that his/her alcohol use is a major problem and responsible for disruption in every area of his or her life.	Denial interferes with the patient's ability to participate in treatment.
Encourage the patient to self-admit to an alcoholism treatment program.	Self-admittance is preferred because the element of denial has been addressed to a certain degree.
Assure the patient that alcoholism is a physiologic, chronic illness and not a moral problem.	This demonstrates a nonjudgmental attitude; it is easier to accept treatment for an illness than it is for what may be perceived as a moral weakness or flaw.
Encourage the patient to compile a written list of the deleterious consequences of excessive alcohol use experienced over the time he or she has been drinking. Ask the patient to show the list to another nurse, peer, or member of AA (if the patient is participating in AA programming).	These interventions help break through the process of denial.
Ask the patient to compile a list of situations that influenced excessive drinking and discuss ways to respond that do not involve drinking.	To help avoid relapse, it is important to know which situations triggered excessive drinking in the past.

Nursing Diagnosis:

Imbalanced Nutrition: Less Than Body Requirements

related to poor dietary intake

Desired Outcome: Within 1 wk of this diagnosis, the patient verbalizes accurate understanding of the effects of alcohol and reduced dietary intake on nutritional status and demonstrates nutritional intake adequate for his or her needs.

ASSESSMENT/INTERVENTIONS	RATIONALES
Assess for abdominal distention, tenderness, and the presence and quality of bowel sounds.	Excessive alcohol intake may irritate gastric mucosa and result in epigastric pain and hyperactive bowel sounds. Other, more serious gastrointestinal (GI) effects may occur secondary to hepatitis and cirrhosis.
Note the presence of nausea/vomiting and diarrhea.	These signs are frequently among the first indicators of alcohol withdrawal and may interfere with establishing adequate nutritional intake.
Assess the patient's ability to feed self.	A number of factors, including tremors, mental status changes, and hallucinations, may interfere with independent feeding and signal the need for assistance.
Refer to a dietitian as indicated.	Expert advice may be necessary to coordinate the patient's nutritional regimen.
Provide small, easily digested, and frequent feedings/snacks as desired; increase as tolerated.	Small feedings may enhance intake and toleration of nutrients by limiting gastric distress. As appetite and ability to tolerate food increase, adjustments are made to the diet to ensure that adequate calories and nutrition are supplied for tissue repair and healing and restoration of energy and vitality.
Review liver function tests.	Liver function status influences the choice of diet and need for/effectiveness of supplemental therapy.
Provide a diet high in protein with about 50% of the calories supplied by carbohydrates.	This diet provides for energy needs and tissue healing while stabilizing blood sugar levels.
Administer medications as prescribed:	
- Antacids, antiemetics, and antidiarrheals	These medications reduce gastric irritation.
- Thiamine and vitamins	All substance users should receive thiamine and vitamins because most have these deficiencies.
Keep the patient nothing by mouth (NPO) if indicated.	It may be necessary to reduce gastric/pancreatic stimulation in the presence of GI bleeding or excessive vomiting.

Nursing Diagnosis:

Deficient Knowledge

related to unfamiliarity with the prescribed medications, rationale for use, and potential side effects

Desired Outcome: The patient verbalizes accurate information about the prescribed medication, including rationale for use and common side effects.

ASSESSMENT/INTERVENTIONS	RATIONALES
Assess the patient's level of knowledge of the medications used in treatment.	Knowledge increases adherence to a prescribed medication regimen. In addition, because some of the medications used to treat alcoholism carry significant and dangerous risks, the patient must be informed regarding these risks.
Teach the patient about the medications that are sometimes used as adjuncts to alcohol use disorders treatment:	

continued

ASSESSMENT/INTERVENTIONS	RATIONALES

Disulfiram (Antabuse)

	This agonist medication is used as a deterrent to impulsive drinking.
Teach the risks of drinking while taking Antabuse.	Response of taking alcohol while on Antabuse includes the following: severe nausea, vomiting, hypotension, headache, cardiovascular collapse, heart palpitations, seizures, or death.
Inform the patient both verbally and in writing of the serious side effects that occur while taking Antabuse when ingesting alcohol or other substances containing alcohol such as cough syrups or cold remedies.	Potential side effects are so serious that informed consent is essential.

Reinforce the following:

- Do not take any form of alcohol (beer, wine, liquor, vinegars, cough medicines, sauces, aftershave lotions, liniments, or cologne).	Doing so may cause a severe, even life-threatening reaction.
- Take the medication daily (at bedtime if it produces fatigue or dizziness). Crush or mix the tablet with liquid if necessary.	
- Wear or carry medical identification with you at all times.	This alerts any medical emergency personnel that the patient is taking Antabuse.
- Keep appointments for follow-up laboratory tests.	Disulfiram may worsen coexisting conditions such as diabetes mellitus, hypothyroidism, chronic and acute nephritis, and hepatic disease. It also increases prothrombin time. When these conditions exist, blood sugar monitoring, kidney and liver function tests, thyroid tests, and prothrombin times need scheduled follow-up evaluations.
- The metallic aftertaste is temporary and will disappear after the medication is discontinued. - Avoid drinking for 14 days after discontinuing disulfiram (Antabuse).	It takes up to 2 weeks for Antabuse to be totally metabolized by the body. Drinking before the drug is fully metabolized can lead to unpleasant symptoms such as nausea, vomiting, and sweating.
- Avoid driving or performing tasks that require alertness.	Drowsiness, fatigue, or blurred vision may occur.

Naltrexone (Re-Via); Long-Acting Injectable Formulation (Vivitrol)

	This is a narcotic antagonist originally used as a treatment for heroin abuse but has now been approved for treatment of alcoholism. The drug reduces the cravings for alcohol and works best when accompanied by psychosocial treatment.
Teach the patient about adverse effects: difficulty sleeping, anxiety, nervousness, headache, low energy, abdominal pain, cramps, nausea, vomiting, delayed ejaculations, decreased potency, skin rash, chills, increased thirst, and joint and muscle pain.	These common adverse effects should be reported to the prescriber.

Reinforce the following:

- This medication will make it easier not to drink and it blocks the effects of narcotics.	
- Wear a medical identification tag. Notify other health professionals that you are taking this medication.	This alerts emergency medical personnel that the patient is taking this medication.
- Avoid use of heroin or other opiate drugs.	Small doses may have no effect, but large doses can cause death, serious injury, or coma.
- Report any signs and symptoms of adverse effects.	
- Keep appointments for follow-up blood tests and treatment program.	

Ondansetron (Zofran)

	Zofran is a serotonin receptor antagonist and is useful in reducing alcohol consumption and craving in patients with early onset alcohol use disorders.

ASSESSMENT/INTERVENTIONS	RATIONALES
Nalmefene (Revex)	
	Revex is an opioid antagonist that is similar in structure to naltrexone and is used often in emergency department treatment. It is less toxic to the liver and effective in preventing relapse to heavy drinking. It has few side effects.
Acamprosate (Campral)	
	Campral is a synthetic compound that is associated with increased abstinence through decreased alcohol craving.
Medications being Investigated for Treatment of Alcoholism **Topiramate (Topamax)**	
	Topiramate is an antiseizure agent that also helps control impulsivity and has shown some evidence of decreasing days and amounts of drinking.
Baclofen (Lioresal)	
	Baclofen is a muscle relaxant and antispasmodic agent and has shown some benefit in helping patients maintain abstinence, particularly in those with alcoholic cirrhosis.

ADDITIONAL NURSING DIAGNOSES/PROBLEMS:

 PATIENT-FAMILY TEACHING AND DISCHARGE PLANNING

The patient with a substance use disorder suffers from a problem that can and will affect every area of his/her life. To remain free of the use of substances, the patient will likely benefit from lifelong adjunctive treatment support through AA or NA. The patient and family need to recognize that substance use disorders are family problems necessitating professional counseling and that alcoholism is a relentlessly progressive disease with profound medical, psychologic, social, and spiritual implications. Provide the patient and family with verbal and written information about the following issues:

✓ Nature and expected course of alcoholism/alcohol use disorder/substance use disorder.

✓ Medications, including drug name; purpose; dosage; frequency; precautions; drug-drug, food-drug, and herb-drug interactions; and potential side effects.

✓ Withdrawal process—what to expect.

✓ Nutrition issues.

✓ Emergency measures.

✓ Importance of social support and strategies to obtain it; importance of changing social support if that support promotes drug use.

✓ Importance of using relaxation techniques to minimize stress.

✓ Importance of maintaining or achieving spiritual well-being.

✓ Importance of lifestyle issues such as benefits of exercise.

✓ Importance of group support for continued adjunctive treatment through AA or NA.

✓ Additional information can be obtained by contacting the following organizations:
  • National Clearinghouse for Alcohol and Drug Information (NCADI) at *http://www.dhs.state.il.us/page .aspx?item=4843*

- National Institute on Alcohol Abuse and Alcoholism (NIAAA) at *www.niaaa.nih.gov*
- National Institute on Drug Abuse (NIDA) at *www.nida.nih.gov*
- Online Alcoholics Anonymous (AA) Recovery Resources at *www.recovery.org/aa* or at *www.aacanada.com*

- Research Institute on Addictions at *www.ria.buffalo.edu*
- The Centre for Addiction and Mental Health at *www.camh.ca*

Appendix A
Infection Prevention and Control

SYSTEMS OF TRANSMISSION PRECAUTIONS

Many different systems of transmission precautions have been used in health care facilities over the years and are commonly called *isolation precautions*. The 1996 Standard Precautions system synthesized the major features of *universal precautions and body substance isolation* and applied them to (1) blood; (2) all body fluids, secretions, and excretions, except sweat, regardless of whether they contain visible blood; (3) nonintact skin; and (4) mucous membranes. In addition, standard precautions were designed to reduce risks of transmission of microorganisms from both recognized and unrecognized sources of infectious agents. Standard precautions include the use of personal protection equipment (PPE) (e.g., gloves, gowns, and masks) and hand hygiene to interrupt transmission of organisms among and between patients and health care workers.

These recommendations are updated periodically, with the most recent revisions occurring in 2007 by the Centers for Disease Control and Prevention (CDC), intended to reflect evidence-based practices and current knowledge (Siegel, Rhinehart, Jackson, and Chiarello, 2007). The 2007 guidelines continue these same principles of standard precautions and apply them to a broader range of situations and care settings. Additionally, specific recommendations for multidrug-resistant organisms (MDROs) were published in December of 2006 by the CDC.

The 2007 guideline contains two tiers of precautions (Table A-1): (1) *standard precautions*, which are designed for the care of all patients in any health care setting, regardless of diagnosis or presumed infection status, and (2) *transmission-based precautions*, which are used for patients known to be or suspected of being infected or colonized with epidemiologically important pathogens that can be transmitted by airborne transmission, droplet transmission, or by contact transmission. Another type of transmission-based precaution has also been added, the protective environment, which is specifically for patients receiving hematopoietic stem cell transplantation (HSCT) and are at particular risk for infections with airborne fungi. Guidelines are updated regularly and can be accessed through the CDC web site.

The CDC offers hospitals and other types of health care settings the option of modifying the recommendations according to their needs and circumstances and as directed by federal, state, or local regulations. For example, the Occupational Safety and Health Administration (OSHA) Bloodborne Pathogens Standard (1991; revised 2001) is still operable, and all facilities are required to comply with its provisions. The CDC's 2007 standard precautions incorporate all requirements of the OSHA bloodborne pathogens standard. See Table A-2 for a discussion of pathogen transmission types.

TRANSMISSION PRECAUTIONS FOR PATIENTS WITH SUSPECTED OR DEMONSTRATED AIRBORNE INFECTIONS

Airborne infection isolation precautions are for persons diagnosed with or suspected of having microorganisms that can be transmitted to others via the airborne route. Examples of airborne infections include pulmonary or laryngeal tuberculosis (TB), measles (rubeola), varicella (chickenpox), and smallpox. These guidelines focus on early identification and treatment of persons with a diagnosis or suspected diagnosis of active TB as the most common airborne infection. Because infection with airborne infections can occur without face-to-face contact with an infected individual, if infection control measures are not followed, large numbers of persons can be exposed. Thus the CDC defined requirements for special ventilation and use of respiratory protection masks that provide better filtration and a tighter fit than standard surgical masks. A mask of this type is called *particulate respirator (PR)*, and the specific type of PR for TB protection is called an *N95 respirator* (CDC, 2005). The best protection for any of the vaccine-preventable infectious diseases is for all caregivers to be immunized, in which case respiratory protection masks are not necessary.

MANAGEMENT OF DEVICES AND PROCEDURES TO REDUCE RISK OF HEALTH CARE–ASSOCIATED INFECTION

Use of barriers is but one of many strategies that can reduce the risk of health care–associated infection among patients and personnel. In fact, studies from the CDC show that significant gains can be made in reducing infection risks by focusing on the management of devices and procedures commonly used in patient care. For example, many patients need intravascular devices that deliver therapeutic medications, but they are put at risk for site infections and bacteremias when these devices are used. It is well known that rotating the access site at appropriate intervals reduces these risks to the patient, while ensuring that catheters are inserted

Table A-1 Recommendations for Isolation Precautions in Health Care Settings, 2007*

Standard Precautions		Transmission-Based Precautions			Protective Environment
		Airborne Infection Isolation	Droplet	Contact	
When to use	All patients in all health care settings.	Patients with known or suspected airborne droplet nuclei	Patients with known or suspected respiratory droplets	Patients with known or suspected contact with transmitted organisms. If the patient is known or suspected to have multidrug-resistant organisms, follow specific recommendations: Management of Multi-Drug Organisms in Health Care Settings (Siegel et al., 2006).	For allogeneic hematopoietic stem cell transplantation (HSCT) patients to minimize fungal spore counts in the air.
Hand hygiene	1. When hands are visibly dirty or contaminated with proteinaceous material or visibly soiled with blood or other body fluids, wash hands with either a nonantimicrobial soap and water or an antimicrobial soap and water. 2. If hands are not visibly soiled, use an alcohol-based handrub for routinely decontaminating hands in all other clinical situations; alternatively, wash hands with an antimicrobial soap and water. 3. Decontaminate hands in the following circumstances: before having direct contact with patients; after contact with blood, body fluids or excretions, mucous membranes, nonintact skin, or wound dressings; after contact with a patient's intact skin (e.g., when taking a pulse or blood pressure or lifting a patient); if hands will be moving from a contaminated body site to a clean body site; after contact with inanimate objects in the immediate vicinity of the patient; after removing gloves.				

Gloves	Wear gloves when it can be reasonably anticipated that contact with blood or other potentially infectious materials, mucous membranes, nonintact skin, or potentially contaminated intact skin could occur. Wear gloves with fit and durability appropriate to the task; wear disposable medical examination gloves for providing direct patient care; wear disposable medical examination gloves or reusable utility gloves for cleaning the environment or medical equipment. Remove gloves after contact with patient and/or surrounding environment (including medical equipment), using proper technique to prevent hand contamination. Do NOT wear same pair of gloves for care of more than one patient. Change gloves during patient care if hands will move from a contaminated body site to a clean body site.	Wear gloves as indicated according to standard precautions and whenever touching patient's intact skin or surfaces and articles in close proximity to patient (e.g., medical equipment or bed rails), and upon entry into the room.
Mouth, nose, eye, and respiratory protection	Wear a mask and eye protection or a face shield to protect mucous membranes of eyes, nose, and mouth during procedures and patient care activities that are likely to generate splashes or sprays of blood, body fluids, secretions, and excretions. Select masks, goggles, face shields, and combinations of each according to the task performed.	Restrict susceptible health care personnel from entering rooms of patients known or suspected to have airborne infections if other immune health care personnel are available. Wear fit-tested National Institute for Occupational Safety and Health–approved N95 or higher respirator for respiratory protection when entering any space with a patient with confirmed or suspected airborne disease.	Wear a mask for close patient contact (e.g., within 6-10 ft). Use of eye protection should follow pathogen-specific recommendations in the CDC (2007) isolation guideline.	During periods of construction, to prevent inhalation of respiratory particles that could contain infectious spores, provide respiratory protection (e.g., N95 respirator) to patients who are medically fit enough to tolerate a respirator when they are required to leave the protective environment. Ensure that patients are instructed on respirator use. In the absence of construction, the CDC makes no recommendation for use of particulate respirators when leaving the protective environment.

continued

Table A-1   Recommendations for Isolation Precautions in Health Care Settings, 2007—cont'd

Standard Precautions	Transmission-Based Precautions			
	Airborne Infection Isolation	Droplet	Contact	Protective Environment
Respiratory hygiene/cough etiquette Educate staff on importance of source control measures to contain respiratory secretions and prevent droplet and fomite transmission of respiratory pathogens, especially during seasonal outbreaks of viral respiratory tract infections. Post signs in ambulatory and inpatient settings with instructions to patients and other persons to inform them to cover mouths/noses when coughing or sneezing, use and dispose of tissues, and perform hand hygiene after hands have been in contact with respiratory secretions. The health care facility should provide tissues and no-touch receptacles for disposal of used tissues as well as conveniently located dispensers of alcohol-based hand rubs, and, where sinks are available, supplies for handwashing. These are particularly important during periods of increased infections but can be instituted year round.				
Gowns Wear a gown or other personal protective equipment (PPE) attire that is appropriate to the task, to protect skin and prevent soiling of clothing during procedures and patient-care activities when contact with blood, body fluids, secretions, or excretions is anticipated. Wear a gown for direct patient contact if patient has uncontained secretions or excretions. Remove gown and other PPE attire and perform hand hygiene before leaving patient's environment.			Wear a gown whenever anticipating that clothing will have direct contact with patient or potentially contaminated environmental surfaces or items in patient's room. Don gown upon entry into the room. Remove gown and observe hand hygiene before leaving patient's environment. After gown removal, ensure that clothing and skin do not contact potentially contaminated environmental surfaces to avoid transfer of microorganisms to other patients or environmental surfaces.	

continued

Patient placement	Include the potential for transmission of infectious agents when making patient placement decisions.	Place patient in a single-patient airborne infection isolation room (AIIR) that has been constructed in accordance with current guidelines; keep AIIR door closed when not required for entry and exit. If appropriate AIIR room is not available, consult facility's infection control professional (ICP) for alternatives. Discontinue airborne precautions after signs and symptoms have resolved or according to pathogen-specific recommendations in the Centers for Disease Control and Prevention (CDC, 2007) isolation guideline.	Place patients in a single-patient room when available. If single-patient rooms are in short supply, prioritize patients who have excessive cough and sputum production for single-patient room placement because of their risk of transmission. Avoid placing patients who require droplet precautions in same room with patients who are at increased risk for infection or adverse outcomes associated with infection (e.g., immunocompromised or have anticipated prolonged length of stay). Place together (cohort) in same room patients who are infected with same organism or are suitable roommates. In other situations or care settings, consult facility's ICP for alternatives.	Place patients who may require contact precautions in a single-patient room when available. If single-patient rooms are in short supply, prioritize patients with conditions that may facilitate transmission (e.g., uncontained drainage, stool incontinence) for single-patient room placement. Place together (cohort) in same room patients who are infected or colonized with the same pathogen and are suitable roommates. Ensure patients are physically separated (i.e., more than 3 ft). Draw privacy curtain between beds to minimize direct contact. Change protective attire and perform hand hygiene between patients. For patient placement in other situations or care settings, consult facility's ICP.
Patient transport		Limit movement and transport of patients who require airborne precautions to medically necessary purposes. If transport or movement outside AIIR is necessary, instruct patient to wear a mask. Instruct patients who cannot tolerate wearing masks because of medical conditions to observe respiratory hygiene/cough etiquette procedures. Discontinue airborne precautions after signs and symptoms have resolved or according to pathogen-specific recommendations in the CDC (2007) isolation guideline.	Limit movement and transport of patient to medically necessary purposes. Instruct patient to wear a mask and follow respiratory hygiene/cough etiquette during transport. No mask is required for persons who are transporting patient. Discontinue droplet precautions after signs and symptoms have resolved or according to pathogen-specific recommendations in the CDC (2007) isolation guideline.	Limit transport and movement of patients to outside the room to medically necessary purposes. When transport is required, ensure that infected or colonized areas of the patient are contained and covered. Remove contaminated PPE and perform hand hygiene prior to transporting patient. Don clean PPE to handle patient when transport destination has been reached.

Table A-1 Recommendations for Isolation Precautions in Health Care Settings, 2007—cont'd

Standard Precautions		Transmission-Based Precautions			
		Airborne Infection Isolation	Droplet	Contact	Protective Environment
Patient care equipment	Follow established policies and procedures for containing, transporting, and handling patient care equipment that may be contaminated with blood or body fluids; always clean patient care equipment to remove organic material before disinfection and sterilization processes are used.			Manage patient care equipment according to standard precautions. Use disposable patient care items (e.g., blood pressure cuffs) whenever possible or implement patient-dedicated use of noncritical equipment to avoid sharing between patients. If use of common equipment or items is unavoidable, clean and disinfect them before use on another patient.	
Care of the environment	Follow established policies and procedures for cleaning and maintaining environmental surfaces as appropriate for level of patient contact and degree of soiling.			Ensure that rooms of patients on contact precautions are given cleaning priority and cleaned at least daily, with a focus on high-touch surfaces (e.g., bed rails, bedside commodes, faucet handles, doorknobs, carts, charts) and equipment in immediate vicinity of the patient.	
Textiles, laundry	Handle used textiles and fabrics with minimum agitation to avoid contamination of air, surfaces, and persons.				
Workers' safety	Adhere to federal and state requirements for protection of health care personnel from exposure to bloodborne pathogens.				

*Modified from Siegel et al, (2007)

Table A-2   Pathogen Transmission (Based on Siegel, Rhinehart, Jackson, and Chiarello, 2007)

Transmission Type	Mode of Transmission	Pathogen Examples
Airborne	Dissemination of airborne droplet nuclei or small particles in the respirable size range that can be dispersed over long distances by air currents and inhaled by individuals without face-to-face contact with an infectious individual	*M. tuberculosis,* measles, chickenpox, disseminated herpes zoster, smallpox
Droplet	Large particle respiratory droplets, generally but not exclusively larger than 5μ in size, generated by coughing, sneezing, or talking. Usually not transmissible over distances greater than 6-10 feet. Other modes of transmission are through suctioning, endotracheal intubation, CPR, or cough induction.	Influenza virus, *B. pertussis,* adenovirus, rhinovirus, *Mycoplasma pneumoniae,* SARS-associated coronavirus, group A streptococcus, *Neisseria meningitidis*
Contact	Direct contact: transmitted from person to person via blood or other blood-containing fluids through a cut or abrasion; transferred from skin to skin due to ungloved contact; or ungloved contact with oral fluids or membranes Indirect contact: contact with a contaminated intermediate object or person. Examples include contact with an inanimate object contaminated by unwashed health care worker's hands, contaminated thermometer or glucose-monitoring device, contaminated pediatric toys, contaminated clothing, or inadequately disinfected instruments.	MRSA, VRE, *C. difficile*
Bloodborne	Transmitted through contact with infectious blood or body fluids	HIV, Hepatitis B or C

in an upper-extremity site in adults and catheter materials are more "vein friendly," thereby reducing trauma to the vascular system. Catheters should be selected specifically for their intended purpose and duration of use and known infectious or noninfectious complications. Additionally, the insertion site should be evaluated daily to assess for tenderness or possible infection. Use of needles to deliver medications and fluids to patients through these intravascular devices can put the health care worker at risk for puncture injury. Needleless or needle-free intravenous (IV) access devices are used to access line ports so that it is not necessary to use needles once the intravascular catheter has entered the vascular system. Thus, the use of newer and safer intravascular devices and procedures can benefit both the patient and the health care worker by reducing their risk of health care–associated infection. The Guidelines for the Prevention of Intravascular Catheter Related Infections (O'Grady,

Alexander, Burns, et al, 2011) are an excellent resource for additional details.

Research studies of interventions to reduce health care–associated infection risks are published in general and specialty journals and presented at professional meetings each year. Infection control professionals (ICPs) (also called *infection preventionists*) and hospital epidemiologists use these studies to make recommendations about changes in nursing and medical practice. The Joint Commission (TJC) requires that all accredited facilities have a person qualified to provide infection surveillance, prevention, and control services. The national associations for these professionals are the Association for Professionals in Infection Control and Epidemiology, Inc. (APIC), which publishes the *American Journal of Infection Control,* and the Society for Healthcare Epidemiology of America (SHEA), which publishes the journal *Infection Control and Hospital Epidemiology.*

Appendix B

Laboratory Tests: Reference Ranges for Adult Patients

Table B-1 Complete Blood Count (CBC)

	Adult Reference Ranges* (Traditional—U.S.)	SI Adult Reference Ranges* (International System)
Hemoglobin (Hb)	Male: 14-18 g/dL	Male: 2.17-2.79 mmol/L
	Female: 12-16 g/dL	Female: 1.86-2.48 mmol/L
Hematocrit (Hct)	Male: 37%-49%	Male: 0.37-0.49 vol fraction
	Female: 36%-46%	Female: 0.36-0.46 vol fraction
Red blood cell (RBC) count	Male: $4.7\text{-}6.1 \times 10^6$/microL	Male: $4.7\text{-}6.1 \times 10^{12}$/L
	Female: $4.2\text{-}5.4 \times 10^6$/microL	Female: $4.2\text{-}5.4 \times 10^{12}$/L
RBC indices		
Mean corpuscular volume	80-100 fl	80-100 fl
Mean corpuscular hemoglobin	27-31 pg	27-31 pg
Mean corpuscular hemoglobin concentration	32-36 g/dL	320-360 g/L
White blood cell (WBC) count	4500-11,000/mm³	$4\text{-}11 \times 10^9$/L
Neutrophils	54%-75%	$2.5\text{-}7.5 \times 10^9$/L
Band neutrophils	3%-8%	0%-3%
Lymphocytes	20%-40%	$1\text{-}4 \times 10^9$/L
Monocytes	2%-8%	$0\text{-}1 \times 10^9$/L
Eosinophils	1%-4%	$0\text{-}0.7 \times 10^9$/L
Basophils	0.5%-1.0%	$0\text{-}0.3 \times 10^9$/L
Platelet count	150,000-400,000/mm³	$150\text{-}400 \times 10^9$/L

*Reference ranges may vary significantly with different laboratory methods of testing.

Table B-2   Serum, Plasma, and Whole Blood Chemistry

	Adult Reference Ranges* (Traditional—U.S.)	SI Adult Reference Ranges* (International System)
Adrenocorticotropic hormone (ACTH)	8-10 AM, less than 100 pg/mL	0-22 pmol/L
Antidiuretic hormone (ADH; vasopressin)	1-5 pg/mL	1-5 ng/L
Albumin	3.5-5.0 g/dL	35-50 g/L
Aldosterone	Male: 6-22 ng/dL	140-415 pmol/L
	Female: 4-31 ng/dL	
Alanine aminotransferase (ALT)	Male: less than 40 units/L	Male: less than 40 units/L
	Female: less than 31 units/L	Female: less than 31 units/L
Alkaline phosphatase	30-110 units/L	30-110 units/L
Ammonia	10-80 mcg/dL	6-47 micromol/L
Amylase	60-180 Somogyi units/dL	Less than 125 units/L
Aspartate aminotransferase (AST)	Male: less than 37 units/L	Male: less than 37 units/L
	Female: less than 31 units/L	Female: less than 31 units/L
Bicarbonate	22-26 mEq/L	22-26 mmol/L
Bilirubin	Total: 0.3-1.4 mg/dL	Total: 5-24 micromol/L
Blood gases, arterial		
pH	7.35-7.45	7.35-7.45
$Paco_2$	35-45 mm Hg	35-45 mm Hg
Pao_2	80-100 mm Hg	80-100 mm Hg
O_2 saturation (Sao_2)	95%-99%	95%-99%
Blood urea nitrogen (BUN)	6-20 mg/dL	2-7 mmol/L
CA-125 cancer marker	0-35 units/mL	0-35 units/mol
Calcitonin	Less than 100 pg/mL	Less than 100 ng/L
Calcium	8.5-10.5 mg/dL; 4.3-5.3 mEq/L	2.2-2.6 mmol/L
Carcinoembryonic antigen (CEA)	0-4.6 mcg/L	0-4.6 mcg/L
Chloride (Cl)	95-108 mEq/L	95-108 mmol/L
Cortisol		
8-10 AM	5-25 mcg/dL	140-690 nmol/L
4 PM-midnight	2-18 mcg/dL	55-500 nmol/L
CO_2 content (total CO_2)	22-28 mEq/L	22-28 mmol/L
C-reactive protein (CRP)	Less than 1 mg/dL	Less than 10 mg/L
Creatinine	0.6-1.5 mg/dL	53-133 micromol/L
Creatinine clearance	Male: 107-141 mL/min	Males: 1.8-2.3 mL/sec
	Female: 87-132 mL/min	Females: 1.4-2.2 mL/sec
Creatine kinase (CK)	Male: 55-170 units/L	Male: 130-150 International Units/L
	Female: 30-135 units/L	Female: 20-115 International Units/L
CK isoenzyme (MB)	5% total CK activity	Less than 5% total CK activity
D-dimer	Less than 0.5 mcg/mL	Less than 0.5 mg/L
Erythrocyte sedimentation rate (ESR)	0-10 mm/hr	
Westergren method	Male: up to 15 mm/hr	
	Female: up to 20 mm/hr	
Fibrin split products (FSPs, FDPs)	Less than 10 mcg/mL	Less than 10 mg/L
Folic acid (folate)	5-25 ng/mL	11-57 mmol/L
Follicle-stimulating hormone (FSH, follitropin)		
Adult female		Follicular: less than 16 International Units/L
	Premenopausal: 4-30 milli International Units/mL	Luteal: less than 12 units/L
	Postmenopausal: 40-250 milli International Units/mL	Postmenopausal: 23-167 units/L
Adult male	Adult male: 4-25 milli International Units/mL	Less than 18 units/L
Globulins, total	1.5-3.5 g/dL	15-35 g/L
Glucose, fasting	True glucose: 60-120 mg/dL	3.3-6.6 mmol/L
	All sugars: 80-120 mg/dL	
Glucose, random	Less than 145 mg/dL	
Glucose tolerance, oral		
Fasting	60-120 mg/dL	3.3-6.6 mmol/L
1 hr	Less than 165 mg/dL	Less than 9.2 mmol/L
2 hr	Less than 120 mg/dL	Less than 6.6 mmol/L

continued

Table B-2   Serum, Plasma, and Whole Blood Chemistry—cont'd

	Adult Reference Ranges* (Traditional—U.S.)	SI Adult Reference Ranges* (International System)
Glycosylated hemoglobin (glycohemoglobin [GHb])	4%-6.4%	0.04-0.064
Growth hormone (GH)	Less than 10 ng/mL	Less than 10 mcg/L
Homocysteine (Hcy)	4-14 micromol/L	
Insulin	Fasting: 4.24 micro units/mL	Fasting: 28-168 pmol/L
Iron	Total: 60-200 mcg/dL	11-36 micromol/L
	Male, average: 125 mcg/dL	
	Female, average: 100 mcg/dL	
	Older adult: 60-80 mcg/dL	
Total iron-binding capacity	25-420 mcg/dL	4.5-75 micromol/L
Ketone bodies	2-4 mcg/dL	Arterial: 0.30-0.80 mmol/L
Lactic acid	Arterial: 3-7 mg/dL	
	Venous: 5-20 mg/dL	Venous: 0.60-0.22 mmol/L
Lactic dehydrogenase	100-250 units/L	100-250 units/L
Lipase	0-110 units/L	0-110 units/L
Magnesium	1.3-2.1 mEq/L	0.7-1.1 mmol/L
Osmolality	280-300 mOsm/kg	280-300 mmol/Kg
Partial thromboplastin time (PTT)	25.0-35.0 sec	25.0-35.0 sec
On anticoagulant therapy	1.5-2.5 × control value	
Phosphorus	2.5-4.5 mg/dL	0.80-1.45 mmol/L
Potassium (K+)	3.5-5.0 mEq/L	3.5-5.0 mmol/L
Prolactin	Male: 0-20 ng/mL	Male: 0-20 mcg/L
	Female: 0-25 ng/mL	Female: 0-25 mcg/L
Prothrombin time (PT)	11.0-12.5 sec; INR 08.0-1.20	11.0-12.5 sec; INR: 0.80-1.2
Renin		
Normal sodium intake		
Supine	4-6 hr: 0.5-1.6 ng/mL/hr	Overnight or 6 hr: 6.4-23.8 ng/L/sec
Sitting	4 hr: 1.8-3.6 ng/mL/hr	2 hr: 9.3-43.4 ng/L/sec
Sitting		2 hr plus diuretic: 12.3-80.5 ng/L/sec
Low sodium intake		
Supine	4-6 hr: 2.2-4.4 ng/mL/hr	Overnight or 6 hr: less than 10.2 ng/L/sec
Sitting	4 hr: 4.0-8.1 ng/mL/hr	2 hr: 5.8-20.2 ng/L/sec
Reticulocyte count	0.5%-2% of total erythrocytes	0.005-0.015 (number fraction)
Reticulocyte index	1.0	1.0
Sodium (Na+)	135-145 mEq/L	134-145 mmol/L
Thyroid screen		
Free thyroxine (free T$_4$)	0.9-2.4 ng/dL	12-31 pmol/L
Free triiodothyronine	260-480 pg/dL	4.0-7.4 pmol/L
Thyroid-stimulating hormone	2-10 micro units/L	
Thyroxine-binding prealbumin	20-30 mg/dL	
Total thyroxine	4.6-10.5 mcg/dL	59-135 nmol/L
Triiodothyronine (T$_3$)	78-208 ng/dL	1.2-3.2 nmol/L
Transferrin	200-400 mg/dL	1.7-3.9 g/L
Urea clearance, serum/24 hr urine		
Maximum	64-99 mL/min	64-99 mL/min
Standard	41-65 mL/min	41-65 mL/min
Uric acid	Male: 4.0-8.5 mg/dL	Male: 0.24-0.50 mmol/L
	Female: 2.7-7.3 mg/dL	Female: 0.16-0.43 mmol/L

*Reference ranges may vary significantly with different laboratory methods of testing.

Table B-3 Urine Chemistry

	Adult Reference Ranges* (Traditional—U.S.)	SI Adult Reference Ranges* (International System)
Albumin		
Random	Negative	Negative
24 hr	10-150 mg	10-150 mg
Amylase	6.5-48.1 units/hour	6.5-48.1 units/hour
Bilirubin (random)	Negative	Negative
Calcium (Ca^{2+})		
Random	1+; less than 40 mg/dL	
24 hr	50-300 mg	1.25-7.5 mmol/L
Creatinine (24 hr)	Male: 20-26 mg/kg	Male: 177-230 micromol/kg
	Female: 14-22 mg/kg	Female: 125-195 micromol/kg
Creatine clearance	Male: 107-141 mL/min/1.73 m^2	1.5-2.2 mL/sec
	Female: 87-132 mL/min/1.73 m^2	
Glucose		
Random	Negative	Negative
24 hr	Less than 0.5 g/day	Less than 2.78 mmol/day
Ketone (random)	Negative	Negative
Microalbumin		
Random	Less than 2 mg/dL	Less than 20 mg/L
Night collection	7 ± 2 mcg/min	7 ± 2 mcg/min
24 hr	10 ± 3 mg/day	10 ± 3 mg/day
Microalbumin/creatinine ratio		
Male	Less than 2.0 mg/mmol	Less than 2.0 mg/mmol
Female	Less than 2.8 mg/mmol	Less than 2.8 mg/mmol
Osmolality		
Random	350-700 mOsm/kg H_2O	350-700 mOsm/kg H_2O
24 hr	300-900 mOsm/kg H_2O	300-900 mOsm/kg H_2O
Physiologic range	50-1400 mOsm/kg H_2O	50-1400 mOsm/kg H_2O
pH	4.6-8.0	4.6-8.0
Phosphorus (24 hr)	0.9-1.3 g	29-42 mmol/L
Protein		
Random	Negative: 2-8 mg/dL	Negative: 20-80 mg/L
24 hr	40-150 mg	40-150 mg/day
Sodium (Na+)		
Random	50-130 mEq/L	50-130 mmol/L
24 hr	40-220 mEq	40-220 mmol/day
Specific gravity		
Random	1.003-1.035	1.003-1.035
After fluid restriction	1.025-1.035	1.025-1.035
Sugar (random)	Negative	Negative
Urea clearance (24 hr)		
Maximum	64-99 mL/min	64-99 mL/min
Standard	41-65 mL/min	41-65 mL/min

*Reference ranges may vary significantly with different laboratory methods of testing.

Table B-4 Cerebrospinal Fluid (CSF)

	Adult Reference Ranges* (Traditional—U.S.)	SI Adult Reference Ranges* (International System)
Albumin	11-48 mg/dL	0.11-0.48 g/L
Blood	Not present	Not present
Cell count	0-5 mononuclear cells/microL	0-5 × 10^6 cells/L
Culture and sensitivity	No organisms present	No organisms present
Cytology	No malignant cells present	No malignant cells present
Glucose	50-75 mg/dL	2.8-4.2 mmol/L
Pressure	70-180 mm H_2O	70-180 mm H_2O
Protein	15-45 mg/dL	0.15-0.45 g/L

*Reference ranges may vary significantly with different laboratory methods of testing.

Appendix C

Laboratory Tests: Reference Ranges for Pediatric Patients

Normal Laboratory Values (Pediatric Patients)

Test/Specimen	Age/Gender/Reference	Reference Ranges	
		Conventional Units	**International Units (SI)**
Acetaminophen			
Serum or plasma	Therapeutic concentration	10-30 mcg/mL	66-200 micromol/L
	Toxic concentration	More than 200 mcg/mL	More than 1320 micromol/L
Ammonia Nitrogen			
Plasma or serum	Newborn	90-150 mcg/dL	64-107 micromol/L
	0-2 wk	79-129 mcg/dL	56-92 micromol/L
	Older than 1 mo	29-70 mcg/dL	21-50 micromol/L
	Thereafter	0-50 mcg/dL	0-35.7 micromol/L
Amylase			
Serum	1-19 yr	30-100 units/L	30-100 units/L
Antistreptolysin O Titer (ASO)			
Serum	2-4 yr	Less than 160 Todd units	Less than 160 Todd units
	School-age children	170-330 Todd units	170-330 Todd units
Base Excess			
Whole blood	Newborn	(10) − (2) mEq/L	(10) − (2) mmol/L
	Infant	(7) − (1) mEq/L	(7) − (1) mmol/L
	Child	(4) − (2) mEq/L	(4) − (2) mmol/L
	Thereafter	(−3) − (+3) mEq/L	(−3) − (+3) mmol/L
Bicarbonate (HCO_3)			
Serum	Arterial	21-28 mEq/L	21-28 mmol/L
	Venous	22-29 mEq/L	22-29 mmol/L

	Premature (mg/dL)	Full Term (mg/dL)	Premature (micromol/L)	Full Term (micromol/L)
Bilirubin, Total				
Serum Cord	Less than 2.0	Less than 2.0	Less than 34	Less than 34
0-1 d	Less than 8.0	Less than 6.0	Less than 137	Less than 103
1-2 d	Less than 12.0	Less than 8.0	Less than 205	Less than 137
2-5 d	Less than 16.0	Less than 12.0	Less than 274	Less than 205
Thereafter	Less than 20.0	Less than 10.0	Less than 340	Less than 171
Bilirubin, Direct (Conjugated)				
Serum			0.0-0.2 mg/dL	0-3.4 micromol/L
Bleeding Time				
	Blood From Skin Puncture			
Ivy	Normal		2-7 min	2-7 min
	Borderline		7-11 min	7-11 min
Simplate (G-D)			2.75-8 min	2.75-8 min

Blood volume

Whole blood	Male	52-83 mL/kg	0.052-0.083 L/kg
	Female	50-75 mL/kg	0.050-0.075 L/kg

C-Reactive Protein (CRP)

Serum	Cord	52-1330 ng/mL	52-1330 mcg/dL
	2-12 yr	67-1800 ng/mL	67-1800 mcg/dL

Calcium, Ionized

Serum, plasma, or whole blood	Cord	5.0-6.0 mg/dL	1.25-1.50 mmol/L
	Newborn, 3-24 hr	4.3-5.1 mg/dL	1.07-1.27 mmol/L
	24-48 hr	4.0-4.7 mg/dL	1.00-1.17 mmol/L
	Thereafter	4.8-4.92 mg/dL	1.2-1.23 mmol/L

Calcium, Total

Serum	Cord	9.0-11.5 mg/dL	2.25-2.88 mmol/L
	Newborn, 3-24 hr	9.0-10.6 mg/dL	2.25-2.65 mmol/L
	24-48 hr	7.0-12.0 mg/dL	1.75-3.0 mmol/L
	4-7 d	9.0-10.9 mg/dL	2.25-2.73 mmol/L
	Child	8.8-10.8 mg/dL	2.2-2.70 mmol/L
	Thereafter	8.4-10.2 mg/dL	2.1-2.55 mmol/L

Carbon Dioxide, Partial Pressure (PCO_2)

Whole blood, arterial	Newborn	27-40 mm Hg	3.6-5.3 kPa
	Infant	27-41 mm Hg	3.6-5.5 kPa
	Thereafter: Male	35-48 mm Hg	4.7-6.4 kPa
	Female	32-45 mm Hg	4.3-6.0 kPa

Carbon Dioxide, Total (tCO_2)

Serum or plasma	Cord	14-22 mEq/L	14-22 mmol/L
	Premature (1 wk)	14-27 mEq/L	14-27 mmol/L
	Newborn	13-22 mEq/L	13-22 mmol/L
	Infant, child	20-28 mEq/L	20-28 mmol/L
	Thereafter	23-30 mEq/L	23-30 mmol/L

Cerebrospinal Fluid (CSF)

Pressure		70-180 mm H_2O	70-180 mm H_2O
Volume	Child	60-100 mL	0.06-0.10 L
	Adult	100-160 mL	0.10-0.16 L

Chloride

Serum or plasma	Cord	96-104 mEq/L	96-104 mmol/L
	Newborn	97-110 mEq/L	97-110 mmol/L
	Thereafter	98-106 mEq/L	98-106 mmol/L
Sweat	Normal (homozygote)	Less than 40 mEq/L	Less than 40 mmol/L
	Marginal (e.g., asthma, Addison disease, malnutrition)	45-60 mEq/L	45-60 mmol/L
	Cystic fibrosis	More than 60 mEq/L	More than 60 mmol/L

Cholesterol, Total

	From Lipid Screening and Cardiovascular Health in Childhood	*Pediatrics* 2008;122(1): 198-208.	
Serum or plasma	Acceptable	Less than 170 mg/dL (LDL less than 110 mg/dL)	Less than 4.4 mmol/L (LDL less than 2.85 mmol/L)
	Borderline	170-199 mg/dL (LDL 110-129 mg/dL)	4.4-5.1 mmol/L (LDL 2.85-3.34 mmol/L)
	High/Elevated	More than 200 mg/dL (LDL more than 130 mg/dL)	More than 5.2 mmol/L (LDL more than 3.37 mmol/L)

Clotting Time (Lee-White)

Whole blood		5-8 min (glass tubes)	5-8 min
		5-15 min (room temp)	5-15 min
		30 min (silicone tube)	30 min

Creatine Kinase (CK, CPK)

Serum	Cord	70-380 units/L	70-380 units/L
	5-8 hr	214-1175 units/L	214-1175 units/L
	24-33 hr	130-1200 units/L	130-1200 units/L
	72-100 hr	87-725 units/L	87-725 units/L
	Adult	5-130 units/L	5-130 units/L

Creatinine

Serum	Cord	0.6-1.2 mg/dL	53-106 micromol/L
	Newborn	0.3-1.0 mg/dL	27-88 micromol/L
	Infant	0.2-0.4 mg/dL	18-35 micromol/L
	Child	0.3-0.7 mg/dL	27-62 micromol/L
	Adolescent	0.5-1.0 mg/dL	44-88 micromol/L
Urine, 24 hr	Premature	8.1-15.0 mg/kg/24 hr	72-133 micromol/kg/24 hr
	Full term	10.4-19.7 mg/kg/24 hr	92-174 micromol/kg/24 hr
	1.5-7 yr	10-15 mg/kg/24 hr	88-133 micromol/kg/24 hr
	7-15 yr	5.2-41 mg/kg/24 hr	46-362 mmol/kg/24 hr

Creatinine Clearance (Endogenous)

Serum or plasma and urine	Newborn	40-65 mL/min/1.73 m^2	40-65 mL/min/1.73 m^2
	Less than 40 yr: Male	97-137 mL/min/1.73 m^2	97-137 mL/min/1.73 m^2
	Female	88-128 mL/min/1.73 m^2	88-128 mL/min/1.73 m^2

Eosinophil Count

Whole blood, capillary blood		50-250 cells/mm^3 (microL)	$50\text{-}250 \times 10^6$ cells/L

Erythrocyte (RBC) Count

Whole blood	Cord	3.9-5.5 million/mm^3	$3.9\text{-}5.5 \times 10^{12}$ cells/L
	1-3 d	4.0-6.6 million/mm^3	$4.0\text{-}6.6 \times 10^{12}$ cells/L
	1 wk	3.9-6.3 million/mm^3	$3.9\text{-}6.3 \times 10^{12}$ cells/L
	2 wk	3.6-6.2 million/mm^3	$3.6\text{-}6.2 \times 10^{12}$ cells/L
	1 mo	3.0-5.4 million/mm^3	$3.0\text{-}5.4 \times 10^{12}$ cells/L
	2 mo	2.7-4.9 million/mm^3	$2.7\text{-}4.9 \times 10^{12}$ cells/L
	3-6 mo	3.1-4.5 million/mm^3	$3.1\text{-}4.5 \times 10^{12}$ cells/L
	0.5-2 yr	3.7-5.3 million/mm^3	$3.7\text{-}5.3 \times 10^{12}$ cells/L
	2-6 yr	3.9-5.3 million/mm^3	$3.9\text{-}5.3 \times 10^{12}$ cells/L
	6-12 yr	4.0-5.2 million/mm^3	$4.0\text{-}5.2 \times 10^{12}$ cells/L
	12-18 yr: Male	4.5-5.3 million/mm^3	$4.5\text{-}5.3 \times 10^{12}$ cells/L
	Female	4.1-5.1 million/mm^3	$4.1\text{-}5.1 \times 10^{12}$ cells/L

Erythrocyte Sedimentation Rate (ESR)

Whole blood

Westergren (modified)	Child	0-10 mm/hr	0-10 mm/hr
	Less than 50 yr: Male	0-15 mm/hr	0-15 mm/hr
	Female	0-20 mm/hr	0-20 mm/hr
Wintrobe	Child	0-13 mm/hr	0-13 mm/hr
	Adult: Male	0-9 mm/hr	0-9 mm/hr
	Female	0-20 mm/hr	0-20 mm/hr

Fibrinogen

Plasma	Newborn	125-300 mg/dL	1.25-3.00 g/L
	Thereafter	200-400 mg/dL	2.00-4.00 g/L

Galactose

Serum	Newborn	0-20 mg/dL	0-1.11 mmol/L
	Thereafter	Less than 5 mg/dL	Less than 0.28 mmol/L
Urine	Newborn	Less than or equal to 60 mg/dL	Less than or equal to 3.33 mmol/L
	Thereafter	Less than 14 mg/d	Less than 0.80 mmol/d

Glucose				
Serum	Cord	45-96 mg/dL	2.5-5.3 mmol/L	
	Newborn, 1 d	40-60 mg/dL	2.2-3.3 mmol/L	
	Newborn, more than 1 d	50-90 mg/dL	2.8-5.0 mmol/L	
	Child	60-100 mg/dL	3.3-5.5 mmol/L	
	Thereafter	70-105 mg/dL	3.9-5.8 mmol/L	

		Normal	**Diabetic**	**Normal**	**Diabetic**
Glucose Tolerance Test (GTT), Oral					
Serum					
Dosages					
Adult: 75 g	Fasting	70-105 mg/dL	More than or equal to 126 mg/dL	3.9-5.8 mmol/L	More than or equal to 7.0 mmol/L
Child: 1.75 g/kg of ideal weight	60 min	120-170 mg/dL		6.7-9.4 mmol/L	
up to maximum of 75 g	90 min	100-140 mg/dL		5.6-7.8 mmol/L	
	120 min	70-120 mg/dL		3.9-6.7 mmol/L	
		Diabetic range for all ages more than or equal to 200 mg/dL		Diabetic range for all ages more than or equal to 11 mmol/L	
Plasma	1 d	5-53 ng/mL		5-53 mcg/L	
	1 wk	5-27 ng/mL		5-27 mcg/L	
	1-12 mo	2-10 ng/mL		2-10 mcg/L	
	Fasting child/adult	Less than 0.7-6.0 ng/mL		Less than 0.7-6.0 mcg/L	
Hematocrit (HCT, Hct)					
Whole blood	1 d (capillary)	48%-69%		0.48-0.69 vol fraction	
	2 d	48%-75%		0.48-0.75 vol fraction	
	3 d	44%-72%		0.44-0.72 vol fraction	
	2 mo	28%-42%		0.28-0.42 vol fraction	
	6-12 yr	35%-45%		0.35-0.45 vol fraction	
	12-18 yr: Male	37%-49%		0.37-0.49 vol fraction	
	Female	36%-46%		0.36-0.46 vol fraction	
Hemoglobin (Hgb)					
Whole blood	1-3 d (capillary)	14.5-22.5 g/dL		2.25-3.49 mmol/L	
	2 mo	9.0-14.0 g/dL		1.40-2.17 mmol/L	
	6-12 yr	11.5-15.5 g/dL		1.78-2.40 mmol/L	
	12-18 yr: Male	13.0-16.0 g/dL		2.02-2.48 mmol/L	
	Female	12.0-16.0 g/dL		1.86-2.48 mmol/L	
Hemoglobin A (HbA)					
Whole blood		More than 95% of total		More than 0.95 fraction of Hb	
Hemoglobin A1C, HB A1C or A1c					
Serum	1-5 yr	2.1-7.7% of total Hb		0.021-0.077 fraction of total Hb	
	5-16 yr	3.0%-6.2% of total Hb		0.030-0.062 fraction of total Hb	
Hemoglobin F (HbF)					
Whole blood	1 d	63%-92% HbF		0.63-0.92 mass fraction HbF	
	5 d	65%-88% HbF		0.65-0.88 mass fraction HbF	
	3 wk	55%-85% HbF		0.55-0.85 mass fraction HbF	
	6-9 wk	31%-75% HbF		0.31-0.75 mass fraction HbF	
	3-4 mo	Less than 2%-59% HbF		Less than 0.02-0.59 mass fraction HbF	
	6 mo	Less than 2%-9% HbF		Less than 0.02-0.09 mass fraction HbF	
	Adult	Less than 2% HbF		Less than 0.02 mass fraction HbF	

Immunoglobulin A (IgA)

Serum			
	Cord	1.4-3.6 mg/dL	14-36 mg/L
	1-3 mo	1.3-53 mg/dL	13-530 mg/L
	4-6 mo	4.4-84 mg/dL	44-840 mg/L
	7-12 mo	11-106 mg/dL	110-1060 mg/L
	2-5 yr	14-159 mg/dL	140-1590 mg/L
	6-10 yr	33-236 mg/dL	330-2360 mg/L
	Adult	70-312 mg/dL	700-3120 mg/L

Immunoglobulin D (IgD)

Serum			
	Newborn	None detected	None detected
	Thereafter	0-8 mg/dL	0-80 mg/L

Immunoglobulin E (IgE)

Serum			
	Male	0-230 International Units/mL	0-230 k International Units/L
	Female	0-170 International Units/mL	0-170 k International Units/L

Immunoglobulin G (IgG)

Serum			
	Cord	636-1606 mg/dL	6.36-16.06 g/L
	1 mo	251-906 mg/dL	2.51-9.06 g/L
	2-4 mo	176-601 mg/dL	1.76-6.01 g/L
	5-12 mo	172-1069 mg/dL	1.72-10.69 g/L
	1-5 yr	345-1236 mg/dL	3.45-12.36 g/L
	6-10 yr	608-1572 mg/dL	6.08-15.72 g/L
	Adult	639-1349 mg/dL	6.39-13.49 g/L

Immunoglobulin M (IgM)

Serum			
	Cord	6.3-25 mg/dL	63-250 mg/L
	1-4 mo	17-105 mg/dL	170-1050 mg/L
	5-9 mo	33-126 mg/dL	330-1260 mg/L
	10-12 mo	41-173 mg/dL	410-1730 mg/L
	2-8 yr	43-207 mg/dL	430-2070 mg/L
	9-10 yr	52-242 mg/dL	520-2420 mg/L
	Adult	56-352 mg/dL	560-3520 mg/L

Iron

Serum			
	Newborn	100-250 mcg/dL	18-45 micromol/L
	Infant	40-100 mcg/dL	7-18 micromol/L
	Child	50-120 mcg/dL	9-22 micromol/L
	Thereafter: Male	65-170 mcg/dL	12-30 micromol/L
	Female	50-170 mcg/dL	9-30 micromol/L
	Intoxicated child	280-2550 mcg/dL	50-456 micromol/L
	Fatally poisoned child	More than 1800 mcg/dL	More than 322 micromol/L

Iron-Binding Capacity, Total (TIBC)

Serum			
	Infant	100-400 mcg/dL	18-72 micromol/L
	Thereafter	250-400 mcg/dL	45-72 micromol/L

Lead

Whole blood			
	Child	Less than 10 mcg/dL	Less than 0.48 micromol/L
	Toxic	More than or equal to 100 mcg/dL	More than or equal to 4.83 micromol/L
Urine, 24 hr		Less than 80 mcg/L	Less than 0.39 micromol/L

Leukocyte Count (WBC Count)

		$\times$ 1000 cells/mm^3 (μL)	$\times$ 10^9 cells/L
Whole blood	Birth	9.0-30.0	9.0-30.0
	24 hr	9.4-34.0	9.4-34.0
	1 mo	5.0-19.5	5.0-19.5
	1-3 yr	6.0-17.5	6.0-17.5
	4-7 yr	5.5-15.5	5.5-15.5
	8-13 yr	4.5-13.5	4.5-13.5
	Adult	4.5-11	4.5-11

CSF (cell count)		$\times$ 1000 cells/mm^3 (microL)	$\times$ 10^6 cells/L
	Premature	0-25 mononuclear	0-25
		0-10 polymorphonuclear	0-10
		0-1000 RBCs	0-1000
	Newborn	0-20 mononuclear	0-20
		0-10 polymorphonuclear	0-10
		0-800 RBCs	0-800
	Neonate	0-5 mononuclear	0-5
		0-10 polymorphonuclear	0-10
		0-50 RBCs	0-50
	Thereafter	0-5 mononuclear	0-5

Leukocyte Differential Count

Whole blood			
	Myelocytes 0%	0 cells/mm^3 (microL)	Number fraction 0
	Neutrophils—"bands" 3-5%	150-400 cells/mm^3 (microL)	Number fraction 0.03-0.05
	Neutrophils—"segs" 54%-62%	3000-5800 cells/mm^3 (microL)	Number fraction 0.54-0.62
	Lymphocytes 25%-33%	1500-3000 cells/mm^3 (microL)	Number fraction 0.25-0.33
	Monocytes 3%-7%	285-500 cells/mm^3 (microL)	Number fraction 0.03-0.07
	Eosinophils 1%-3%	50-250 cells/mm^3 (microL)	Number fraction 0.01-0.03
	Basophils 0%-0.75%	15-50 cells/mm^3 (microL)	Number fraction 0-0.0075

Lipase (serum)			
	1-18 yr	3-32 units/L	3-32 units/L

Mean Corpuscular Hemoglobin (MCH)

Whole blood			
	Birth	31-37 pg/cell	0.48-0.57 fmol/cell
	1-3 d (capillary)	31-37 pg/cell	0.48-0.57 fmol/cell
	1 wk–1 mo	28-40 pg/cell	0.43-0.62 fmol/cell
	2 mo	26-34 pg/cell	0.40-0.53 fmol/cell
	3-6 mo	25-35 pg/cell	0.39-0.54 fmol/cell
	0.5-2 yr	23-31 pg/cell	0.36-0.48 fmol/cell
	2-6 yr	24-30 pg/cell	0.37-0.47 fmol/cell
	6-12 yr	25-33 pg/cell	0.39-0.51 fmol/cell
	12-18 yr	25-35 pg/cell	0.39-0.54 fmol/cell

Mean Corpuscular Hemoglobin Concentration (MCHC)

Whole blood			
	Birth	30%-36% Hb/cell or g Hb/dL RBCs	4.65-5.58 mmol Hb/L RBCs
	1-3 d (capillary)	29%-37% Hb/cell or g Hb/dL RBCs	4.50-5.74 mmol Hb/L RBCs
	1-2 wk	28%-38% Hb/cell or g Hb/dL RBCs	4.34-5.89 mmol Hb/L RBCs
	1-2 mo	29%-37% Hb/cell or g Hb/dL RBCs	4.50-5.74 mmol Hb/L RBCs
	3 mo–2 yr	30%-36% Hb/cell or g Hb/dL RBCs	4.65-5.58 mmol Hb/L RBCs
	2-18 yr	31%-37% Hb/cell or g Hb/dL RBCs	4.81-5.74 mmol Hb/L RBCs

Mean Corpuscular Volume (MCV)

Whole blood			
	1-3 d (capillary)	95-121 microm^3	95-121 fl
	0.5-2 yr	70-86 microm^3	70-86 fl
	6-12 yr	77-95 microm^3	77-95 fl
	12-18 yr: Male	78-98 microm^3	78-98 fl
	Female	78-102 microm^3	78-102 fl

Osmolality

Serum	Child/adult	275-295 mOsm/kg H$_2$O	275-295 mOsm/kg H$_2$O
Urine, random		50-1400 mOsm/kg H$_2$O, depending on fluid intake; after 12-hr fluid restriction: More than 850 mOsm/kg H$_2$O	50-1400 mOsm/kg H$_2$O, depending on fluid intake; after 12-hr fluid restriction: More than 850 mOsm/kg H$_2$O
Urine, 24 hr		approximately equal to 300-900 mOsm/kg H$_2$O	approximately equal to 300-900 mOsm/kg H$_2$O

Oxygen, Partial Pressure (PO₂)

Whole blood, arterial	Birth	8-24 mm Hg	1.1-3.2 kPa
	5-10 min	33-75 mm Hg	4.4-10.0 kPa
	30 min	31-85 mm Hg	4.1-11.3 kPa
	Older than 1 hr	55-80 mm Hg	7.3-10.6 kPa
	1 d	54-95 mm Hg	7.2-12.6 kPa
	Thereafter (decreases with age)	83-108 mm Hg	11-14.4 kPa

Oxygen Saturation (SaO₂)

Whole blood, arterial	Newborn	85%-90%	Fraction saturated 0.85-0.90
	Thereafter	95%-99%	Fraction saturated 0.95-0.99

Partial Thromboplastin Time (PTT)

Whole blood (Na citrate)

Nonactivated		60-85 sec (Platelin)	60-85 sec
Activated		25-35 sec (differs with method)	25-35 sec
pH			H concentration
Whole blood, arterial	Premature (48 hr)	7.35-7.50	7.35-7.50
	Birth, full term	7.11-7.36	7.11-7.36
	5-10 min	7.09-7.30	7.09-7.30
	30 min	7.21-7.38	7.21-7.38
	Older than 1 hr	7.26-7.49	7.26-7.49
	1 d	7.29-7.45	7.29-7.45
	Thereafter must be corrected for body temp	7.35-7.45	7.35-7.45
Urine, random	Newborn/neonate	5-7	5-7
	Thereafter	4.5-8 (average approx. equal to 6)	4.5-8 (average approx. equal to 6)
Stool		7.0-7.5	7.0-7.5

Phenylalanine

Serum	Premature	2.0-7.5 mg/dL	120-450 micromol/L
	Newborn	1.2-3.4 mg/dL	70-210 micromol/L
	Thereafter	0.8-1.8 mg/dL	50-110 micromol/L
Urine, 24 hr	10 d–2 wk	1-2 mg/d	6-12 micromol/d
	3-12 yr	4-18 mg/d	24-110 micromol/d
	Thereafter	Trace—17 mg/d	Trace—103 micromol/d

Plasma Volume

Plasma	Male	25-43 mL/kg	0.025-0.043 L/kg
	Female	28-45 mL/kg	0.028-0.045 L/kg

Platelet count (Thrombocyte count)

Whole blood (EDTA)	Newborn (after 1 wk, same as adult)	84-478 × 10³/mm³ (microL)	84-478 × 10⁹/L
	Adult	150-400 × 10³/mm³ (microL)	150-400 × 10⁹/L

Potassium

Serum	Newborn	3.0-6.0 mEq/L	3.0-6.0 mmol/L
	Thereafter	3.5-5.0 mEq/L	3.5-5.0 mmol/L
Plasma (heparin)		3.4-4.5 mEq/L	3.4-4.5 mmol/L
Urine, 24 hr		2.5-125 mEq/d (varies with diet)	2.5-125 mmol/L

Protein

Serum, total	Premature	4.3-7.6 g/dL	43-76 g/L
	Newborn	4.6-7.4 g/dL	46-74 g/L
	1-7 yr	6.1-7.9 g/dL	61-79 g/L
	8-12 yr	6.4-8.1 g/dL	64-81 g/L
	13-19 yr	6.6-8.2 g/dL	66-82 g/L

Total

Urine, 24 hr		1-14 mg/dL	10-140 mg/L
		50-80 mg/d (at rest)	50-80 mg/d
		Less than 250 mg/d (after intense exercise)	Less than 250 mg/d (after intense exercise)
CSF		Lumbar: 8-32 mg/dL	80-320 mg/L

Prothrombin Time (PT)
One-stage (Quick)

Whole blood (Na citrate)	In general	11-15 sec (varies with type of thromboplastin)	11-15 sec
	Newborn	Prolonged by 2-3 sec	Prolonged by 2-3 sec
Two-stage modified (Ware and Seegers)			
Whole blood (Na citrate)		18-22 sec	18-22 sec

RBC Count: See Erythrocyte (RBC) Count
Red Blood Cell Volume

Whole blood	Male	20-36 mL/kg	0.020-0.036 L/kg
	Female	19-31 mL/kg	0.019-0.031 L/kg
Reticulocyte count			
Whole blood	Adult	0.5%-1.5% of erythrocytes	0.005-0.015 (number fraction)
Capillary	1 d	0.4%-6.0%	0.004-0.060 (number fraction)
	7 d	Less than 0.1%-1.3%	Less than 0.001-0.013 (number fraction)
	1-4 wk	Less than 0.1%-1.2%	Less than 0.001-0.012 (number fraction)
	5-6 wk	Less than 0.1%-2.4%	Less than 0.001-0.024 (number fraction)
	7-8 wk	0.1%-2.9%	0.001-0.029 (number fraction)
	9-10 wk	Less than 0.1%-2.6%	Less than 0.001-0.026 (number fraction)
	11-12 wk	0.1%-1.3%	0.001-0.013 (number fraction)

Salicylates

Serum, plasma	Therapeutic concentration	15-30 mg/dL	1.1-2.2 mmol/L
	Toxic concentration	More than 30 mg/dL	More than 2.2 mmol/L

Sedimentation Rate: See Erythrocyte Sedimentation Rate (ESR)
Sodium

Serum or plasma	Newborn	134-146 mEq/L	134-146 mmol/L
	Infant	139-146 mEq/L	139-146 mmol/L
	Child	138-145 mEq/L	138-145 mmol/L
	Thereafter	136-146 mEq/L	136-146 mmol/L
Urine, 24 hr		40-220 mEq/L (diet dependent)	40-220 mmol/L
Sweat	Normal	Less than 40 mEq/L	Less than 40 mmol/L
	Indeterminate	45-60 mEq/L	45-60 mmol/L
	Cystic fibrosis	More than 60 mEq/L	More than 60 mmol/L

Specific Gravity

Urine, random	Adult	1.002-1.030	1.002-1.030
	After 12-hr fluid restriction	More than 1.025	More than 1.025
Urine, 24 hr		1.015-1.025	1.015-1.025

Theophylline

Serum, plasma	Therapeutic concentration		
	Bronchodilator	10-20 mcg/mL	56-110 micromol/L
	Premature apnea	5-10 mcg/mL	28-56 micromol/L
	Toxic concentration	More than 20 mcg/mL	More than 110 micromol/L

Thrombin Time

Whole blood (Na citrate)	Control time ± 2 sec when control is 9-13 sec	Control time ± 2 sec when control is 9-13 sec

Thyroxine, Total (T_4)

Serum			
	Cord	8-13 mcg/dL	103-168 nmol/L
	Newborn	11.5-24 mcg/dL (lower in low-birth-weight infants)	148-310 nmol/L
	Neonate	9-18 mcg/dL	116-232 nmol/L
	Infant	7-15 mcg/dL	90-194 nmol/L
	1-5 yr	7.3-15 mcg/dL	94-194 nmol/L
	5-10 yr	6.4-13.3 mcg/dL	83-172 nmol/L
	Thereafter	5-12 mcg/dL	65-155 nmol/L
	Newborn screen (filter paper)	6.2-22 mcg/dL	80-284 nmol/L

		Male both (mg/dL)	Female	Male both (g/L)	Female
Triglycerides (TG)					
Serum after 12-hr fast	Cord	10-98	10-98	0.10-0.98	0.10-0.98
	0-5 yr	30-86	32-99	0.30-0.86	0.32-0.99
	6-11 yr	31-108	35-114	0.31-1.08	0.35-1.14
	12-15 yr	36-138	41-138	0.36-1.38	0.41-1.38
	16-19 yr	40-163	40-128	0.40-1.63	0.40-1.28

Triiodothyronine (T_3), Free

Serum			
	Cord	20-240 pg/dL	0.3-3.7 pmol/L
	1-3 d	200-610 pg/dL	3.1-9.4 pmol/L
	6 wk	240-560 pg/dL	3.7-8.6 pmol/L
	Adult (20-50 yr)	230-660 pg/dL	3.5-10.0 pmol/L

Triiodothyronine, Total (T_3-RIA)

Serum			
	Cord	30-70 ng/dL	0.46-1.08 nmol/L
	Newborn	72-260 ng/dL	1.16-4.00 nmol/L
	1-5 yr	100-260 ng/dL	1.54-4.00 nmol/L
	5-10 yr	90-240 ng/dL	1.39-3.70 nmol/L
	10-15 yr	80-210 ng/dL	1.23-3.23 nmol/L
	Thereafter	115-190 ng/dL	1.77-2.93 nmol/L

Urea Nitrogen

Serum or plasma			
	Cord	21-40 mg/dL	7.5-14.3 mmol/L
	Premature (1 wk)	3-25 mg/dL	1.1-9.0 mmol/L
	Newborn	3-12 mg/dL	1.1-4.3 mmol/L
	Infant/child	5-18 mg/dL	1.8-6.4 mmol/L
	Thereafter	7-18 mg/dL	2.5-6.4 mmol/L

Urine Volume

Urine, 24 hr			
	Newborn	50-300 mL/d	0.05-0.3 L/d
	Infant	350-550 mL/d	0.35-0.5 L/d
	Child	500-1000 mL/d	0.5-1 L/d
	Adolescent	700-1400 mL/d	0.7-1.4 L/d

WBC: See Leukocyte Count (WBC Count)

From Wilson D, Hockenberry MJ: Wong's clinical manual of pediatric nursing, ed 7. St. Louis, 2008, Mosby. Modified from Behrman RE, Kliegman RM, Jenson HB, editors: Nelson textbook of pediatrics, ed 17. Philadelphia, 2004, Saunders; McMillan JA, Deangelis CD, Feigin RD, et al, eds: Oski's pediatrics: principles and practice, ed 3. Philadelphia, 1999, Lippincott Williams & Wilkins; and Fischbach F: A manual of laboratory and diagnostic tests, ed 6. Philadelphia, 2000, Lippincott Williams & Wilkins.

Bibliography

Part I: Medical-Surgical Nursing
General Care Plans

Adelstein DJ, Ridge JA, Gillison ML, et al: Head and neck squamous cell cancer and the human papillomavirus: Summary of a National Cancer Institute State of the Science Meeting, November 9-10, 2008, Washington, DC, *Head Neck* 31(11):1393–1422, 2009.

Agency for Health Care Research and Quality (AHRQ): AHRQ's MCC Research Network, 2013. http://www.ahrq.gov/professionals/systems/long-term-care/resources/multichronic/index.html.

A legacy to remember. www.alegacytoremember.com.

American Cancer Society: *Breast cancer facts and figures, 2011-2013*, Atlanta, 2013a, American Cancer Society.

American Cancer Society: *Cancer facts and figures 2013*, Atlanta, 2013b, American Cancer Society.

American Cancer Society: *Colorectal cancer facts and figures 2011-2013*, Atlanta, 2013c, American Cancer Society.

American Heart Association: *2012 ACCF/AHA focused update incorporated into the ACCF/AHA 2007 guidelines for the management of patient with unstable angina/non–st elevated myocardial infarction: A report of the American College of Cardiology Foundation/American Heart Association Task Force on Practice Guidelines.* http://circ.ahajounal.org/content/127/23/e663. Retrieved July 19, 2013.

American Liver Foundation: The American Liver Foundation issues a warning on dangers of excess Acetaminophen, http://www.liverfoundation.org/about/news/33. Retrieved 2008.

American Nurses Association & American Society for Pain Management in Nursing: Pain management nursing: scope & standards of practice, www.nursesbooks.org. Retrieved 2005.

American Pain Society: *Principles of analgesic use in the treatment of acute and cancer pain*, ed 6, Glenview, IL, 2008, American Pain Society.

American Society of Anesthesiologist: *Practice guidelines for acute pain management in the perioperative setting. An updated report by the American Society of Anesthesiologist Task Force on Acute Pain Management* (Feb. 2012).

Andry JM: Dyspnea. In Esper P, Kuebler K, editors: *Palliative practices from a-z for the bedside clinician*, ed 2, Pittsburgh, PA, 2008, Oncology Nursing Society, pp 117–122.

Association of Perioperative Registered Nurses: *Perioperative Standards and Recommended Practices*, Denver, CO, 2011, AORN, Inc., p 367.

Borg GA: Psychophysical bases of perceived exertion, *Med Sci Sports Exer* 14(5):377–381, 1982.

Brunnhuber K, Nash S, Meier D, et al: *Putting evidence into practice: Palliative care*, London, 2008, BMJ Publishing Group.

Centers for Disease Control and Prevention: Occupational Exposure to Antineoplastic agents, 2013. http://www.cdc.gov/niosh/topics/antineoplastic. Retrieved August 7, 2013.

Centers for Medicare & Medicaid Innovation: Health care innovation awards, 2013. http://www.innovations.cms.gov/initiatives/Innovation-Awards/index.html.

Chaturvedi AK, Engels EA, Pfeiffer RM, et al: Human papillomavirus and rising oropharyngeal cancer incidence in the United States, *J Clin Oncol* 29(32):4294–4301, 2011.

Cherny NI, Radbruch L, Board of the European Association for Palliative Care: European Association for Palliative Care (EAPC) recommended framework for the use of sedation in palliative care, *Palliat Med* 23(7):581–593, 2009.

Close JF, Long CO: Delirium: An opportunity in palliative care, *J Hosp Palliat Nurs* 14:386–394, 2012.

Cloyes KG, Berry PH, Reblin M, et al: Exploring communication patterns among hospice nurses and family caregivers: A content analysis of in-home speech interactions, *J Hosp Palliat Nurs* 14:426–437, 2012.

D'Arcy Y: Managing end-of-life symptoms, *American Nurse Today* 7(7):22–27, 2012.

Davis MP: Pain. In Esper P, Kuebler K, editors: *Palliative practices from a-z for the bedside clinician*, ed 2, Pittsburgh, 2008, Oncology Nursing Society, pp 205–210.

de Leon-Casasola O: Implementing therapy with opioids in patients with cancer, *Oncol Nurs Forum* 35:S7–S12, 2008.

Del Ferraro C, Grant M, Koczywas M, et al: Management of anorexia-cachexia in late-stage lung cancer patients, *J Hosp Palliat Nurs* 14:397–404, 2012.

Doorenbos A, Given C, Given B, et al: Symptom experience in the last year of life among individuals with cancer, *J Pain Symptom Manage* 32(5):403–412, 2006.

Dunn GP: Surgical palliative care: Recent trends and developments, *Surg Clin North Am* 91:277–292, 2011.

Five Wishes—an advance directive document available from The Commission on Aging with Dignity. 1-888-5-WISHES or www.agingwithdignity.org.

Foley KM, Abernathy A: Management of cancer pain. In DeVita VT Jr, et al, editors: *DeVita, Hellman, and Rosenberg's Cancer: principles and practice of oncology*, ed 8, vol 2, Philadelphia, 2008, Lippincott Williams and Wilkins, pp 2757–2790.

Fournier J: End-stage disease and family education, 2013. Retrieved from: www.palliativecareeducation.org.

Global Initiative for Chronic Obstructive Lung Disease [GOLD]: *Global strategy for the diagnosis, management, and prevention of chronic obstructive pulmonary disease*, Bethesda, Maryland, 2013, U.S. Department of Health and Human Services, Public Health Services, National Institutes of Health, National Heart, Lung and Blood Institute.

Green UR, Murphy ME: Urinary elimination. In Esper P, Kuebler K, editors: *Palliative practices from a-z for the bedside clinician*, ed 2, Pittsburgh, 2008, Oncology Nursing Society, pp 251–256.

Heppner H, Cornel S, Walger P, et al: Infections in the elderly, *Crit Care Clin* 29:757–774, 2013.

Ignatavicius D, Workman ML: *Medical-surgical nursing*, ed 6, St. Louis, 2009, Saunders.

Institute for Safe Medication Practices: Safety issues with patient-controlled analgesia. Part I, How errors occur, *ISMP Medication Safety Alert* 8(14), 2003. www.ismp.org.

Institute for Safe Medication Practices: Safety issues with patient-controlled analgesia. Part II, How to prevent error, *ISMP Medication Safety Alert* 8(15), 2003. www.ismp.org.

Institute for Safe Medication Practices: Safety issues with patient-controlled analgesia. Part I, *ISMP Medication Safety Alert Nurse Advise—ERR* 3(1), 2003. www.ismp.org.

Institute for Safe Medication Practices: Safety issues with patient-controlled analgesia. Part II, *ISMP Medication Safety Alert Nurse Advise—ERR* 3(2), 2003. www.ismp.org.

Institute for Safe Medication Practices: The five rights cannot stand alone, *Nurse-Advise ERR* 2(11), 2004. http://www.ismp.org/news-letters/nursing/issues/nurse. Retrieved January 4, 2010.

Institute for Safe Medication Practices: Misprogramming PCA concentration leads to dosing errors, *ISMP Medication Safety Alert* 8(28), 2008. www.ismp.org.

Institute for Safe Medication Practices: ISMP Urges Caution with Basal Opioid Infusions 3(15), 2009. www.ismp.org.

Institute for Safe Medication Practices: Safety issues with patient-controlled analgesia. Part II, United States Department of Health and Human Services: Guide to Patient and Family Engagement in Hospital Quality and Safety, 2013. http://www.ahrq.gov/professionals/systems/hospital/engagingfamilies/patfamilyengageguide/index.html.

Institutes of Medicine (IOM): Living well with chronic disease: A Call for Public Health Action, 2012. Retrieved from: http://www.nap.edu/catalog.php?record_id=13272.

Joint Commission on Accreditation of Healthcare Organizations: *Approaches to pain management: a guide for clinical leaders*, Oakbrook Terrace, IL, 2003, Joint Commission Resources.

Joint Commission on Accreditation of Healthcare Organizations: *Universal protocol for preventing wrong site, wrong procedure, wrong person surgery*, Oakbrook Terrace, IL, 2003, TJC. www.jointcommission.org.

Kanacki LS, Roth P, Georges JM, et al: Shared presence: Caring for a dying spouse, *J Hospice Palliative Nurs* 14:414–425, 2012.

Kozlov M, Anderson MA, Sparbel KJ: Opioid-induced neurotoxicity in the hospice patient, *J Hospice Palliative Nurs* 13:341–346, 2011.

Kruse RL, LeMaster JW, Madsen RW: Fall and balance outcomes after an intervention to promote leg strength, balance, and walking in people with diabetic peripheral neuropathy: "feet first" randomized controlled trial, *Phys Ther* 90(11):1568–1579, 2010.

Kuebler K, Pompey V: Dehydration. In Esper P, Kuebler K, editors: *Palliative practices from a-z for the bedside clinician*, ed 2, Pittsburgh, 2008, Oncology Nursing Society, pp 95–98.

Kuebler K, Pompey V: Delirium. In Esper P, Kuebler K, editors: *Palliative practices from a-z for the bedside clinician*, ed 2, Pittsburgh, 2008, Oncology Nursing Society, pp 99–103.

Lewis SL, Dirksen SR, Heitkemper MM, et al: *Medical-surgical nursing: Assessment and management of clinical problems*, ed 8, St. Louis, 2011, Mosby.

Margaretta MS, Berger AM, Johnson LB: Putting evidence into practice: Evidence-based interventions for sleep-wake disturbances, *Clin J Oncol Nurs* 10(6):753–767, 2006. Retrieved from: http://ons.metapress.com/content/7l114218m6184368/fulltext.pdf.

Mayo Clinic: Magic Mouthwash: Effective for Chemotherapy Mouth Sores? 2013. http://www.mayoclinic.com/health/magic-mouthwash/AN02024.

Moore CD: Caregiver issues. In Esper P, Kuebler K, editors: *Palliative practices from a-z for the bedside clinician*, ed 2, Pittsburgh, 2008, Oncology Nursing Society, pp 55–59.

NANDA International: *Nursing diagnoses, definitions and classifications, 2012-2014*, Oxford, 2012, Wiley-Blackwell.

National Cancer Institute: Head and neck cancers, 2013. From: http://www.cancer.gov/cancertopics/factsheet/Sites-Types/head-and-neck. Retrieved October 28, 2013.

National Cancer Institute: Cancer survivorship research, 2013a. From: http://cancercontrol.cancer.gov/ocs/prevalence/index.html. Retrieved August 1, 2013.

National Cancer Institute: General information about renal cancer, 2013b. From: http://www.cancer.gov/cancertopics/pdq/treatment/renalcell/HealthProfessional. Retrieved August 4, 2013.

National Cancer Institute: Prostate-specific antigen (PSA) test, 2013c. From: http://www.cancer.gov/cancertopics/factsheet/detection/PSA. Retrieved August 3, 2013.

National Cancer Institute: SEER stat fact sheets: Testis, 2013d. From: http://seer.cancer.gov/statfacts/html/testis.html. Retrieved August 4, 2013.

National Cancer Institute: A snapshot of bladder cancer, 2013e. From: http://www.cancer.gov/researchandfunding/snapshots/bladder. Retrieved August 3, 2013.

National Cancer Institute: A snapshot of brain and central nervous system cancers, 2013f. Retrieved from: http://www.cancer.gov/researchandfunding/snapshots/brain.

National Cancer Institute: A snapshot of leukemia, 2013g. From: http://www.cancer.gov/researchandfunding/snapshots/leukemia. Retrieved August 2, 2013.

National Cancer Institute: A snapshot of lymphomas, 2013h. From: http://www.cancer.gov/researchandfunding/snapshots/lymphoma. Retrieved August 2, 2013.

National Cancer Institute: PDQ® Last Days of Life, Bethesda, Maryland, National Cancer Institute. Date last modified 06/30/2011. From: http://www.cancer.gov/cancertopics/pdq/supportivecare/lasthours/healthprofessional. Retrieved July 25, 2012.

National Consensus Project for Quality Palliative Care: *Clinical practice guidelines for quality palliative care*, ed 3, Pittsburgh, 2013, American Academy of Hospice and Palliative Medicine.

National Hospital Inpatient Quality Reporting Measures Specifications Manual, December 4, 2012.

National Lung Screening Trial Research Team: Reduced lung cancer mortality with low-dose computed tomographic screening, *New Engl J Med* 365(5):395–409, 2011.

National Quality Forum (NQF): MCC measurement framework, 2012. Retrieved from:: http://www.qualityforum.org/Projects/Multiple_Chronic_Conditions_Measurement_Framework.aspx.

Oncology Nursing Society: ONS PEP Guideline/Expert Opinion Table: Constipation, 2011. From: http://www.ons.org/Research/PEP/media/ons/docs/research/outcomes/constipation/guidelines.pdf. Retrieved August 7, 2013.

Oncology Nursing Society: ONS PEP Guidelines/Expert Opinion Table: Anxiety, 2011a. From: http://www.ons.org/Research/PEP/media/ons/docs/research/outcomes/anxiety/guidelines.pdf. Retrieved August 15, 2013.

Oncology Nursing Society: ONS PEP Guidelines/Expert Opinion Table: Fatigue, 2011b. From: http://www.ons.org/Research/PEP/media/ons/docs/research/outcomes/fatigue/guidelines.pdf. Retrieved August 14, 2013.

Oncology Nursing Society: ONS PEP Guidelines/Expert Opinion Table: Sleep/Wake Disturbances, 2011c. From: http://www.ons.org/Research/PEP/media/ons/docs/research/outcomes/sleep/quickview.pdf. Retrieved August 14, 2013.

Pasero C, McCaffery M: *Pain assessment and pharmacologic management*, St. Louis, 2011, Mosby.

Patient Safety and Quality Healthcare: ISMP: Patient-Controlled Analgesia. http://www.psqh.com/julyaugust-2013/1713-patient -controlled-analgesia.

Payne A, Savarese D: Extravasation injury from chemotherapy and other non-neoplastic vesicants, 2013. From: http://www.uptodate .com/contents/extravasation-injury-from-chemotherapy-and -other-non-neoplastic-vesicants. Retrieved August 7, 2013.

PubMed Health: Testicular cancer, from: http://www.ncbi.nlm.nih.gov/ pubmedhealth/PMH0002266/#adam_001288.disease.signs-and-tests. Retrieved August 4, 2013.

Redman B: *Advanced practice nursing ethics in chronic disease self-management*, New York, 2012, Springer.

Revier SS, Meiers SJ, Herth KA: The lived experience of hope in family caregivers caring for a terminally ill loved one, *J Hospice Palliative Nurs* 13:438–446, 2012.

Shih F, Lin H, Gau M, et al: Spiritual needs of Taiwan's older patients with terminal cancer, *Oncol Nurs Forum* 36:E31–E38, 2009.

Tanner J, Moncaster K, Woodings D: Preoperative hair removal: a systematic review, *J Perioper Pract* 17(3):118–121, 124–132, 2007.

Taylor B, Davis S: Using the extended PLISSIT model to address sexual healthcare needs, *Nurs Stand* 21(11):35–40, 2006.

The Joint Commission on Accreditation of Healthcare Organizations: *National patient safety goals*, Oakbrook Terrace, Illinois, 2013, TJC. Retrieved from: http://www.jointcommission.org/ hap_2013_npsg/.

Thomas JR, Cooney GA: Palliative care and pain: New strategies for managing opioid bowel dysfunction, *J Palliative Med* 11:S5–S6, 2008. doi: 10.1089/jpm.2008.9839.supp.

U.S. Department of Health and Human Services: Multiple chronic conditions: A strategic framework optimum health and quality of life for individuals with multiple chronic conditions, 2010. http:// www.hhs.gov/ash/initiatives/mcc/mcc_framework.pdf.

U.S. Preventative Services Task Force: Screening for cervical cancer, 2012. http://www.uspreventiveservicestaskforce.org/uspstf/uspscer .htm. Accessed August 5, 2013.

U.S. Preventive Services Task Force: Screening for testicular cancer, 2011. From: http://www.uspreventiveservicestaskforce.org/ uspstf10/testicular/testicuprs.htm. Retrieved August 4, 2013.

U.S. Preventive Services Task Force: Screening for prostate cancer: U.S. Preventive Services Task Force recommendation statement, 2012. From: http://www.uspreventiveservicestaskforce.org/ prostatecancerscreening/prostatefinalrs.htm. Retrieved August 3, 2013.

U.S. Preventive Services Task Force: Screening for breast cancer, 2013. From: http://www.uspreventiveservicestaskforce.org/uspstf/ uspsbrca.htm. Retrieved August 2, 2013.

Waszynski C: The Confusion Assessment Method (CAM). Hartford Institute for Geriatric Nursing, Issue 13, 2007.

Wierenga P, Buurman B, Parlevliet J, et al: Association between acute geriatric syndromes and medication related hospital admissions, *Drugs Aging* 29(8):691–699, 2012.

World Cancer Research Fund International: Cancer facts and figures, 2013. From: http://www.wcrf.org/cancer_statistics/cancer_facts/ index.php. Retrieved August 1, 2013.

World Health Organization: *Palliative care: what is it?* Geneva, Switzerland, 2003, World Health Organization. www.who.int/hiv/ topics/palliative/care/en/print.htm.

Yang CB, Wang YC, Gao Y, et al: Artificial gravity with ergometric exercise preserves the cardiac, but not cerebrovascular, functions during 4 days of head-down bed rest, *Cytokine* 56(3):648–655, 2011.

Zhang B, Nilsson ME, Prigerson HG: Factors important to patient's quality of life at the end of life, *Arch Int Med* 172(15):1133–1142, 2012. doi: 10.1001/archinternalmed.2012.2364.

Respiratory Care Plans

American College of Physicians, American College of Chest Physicians, American Thoracic Society, and European Respiratory Society: Diagnosis and management of stable chronic obstructive pulmonary disease: A clinical practice guideline update, 179–191, 2 August 2011. From: http://www.thoracic.org/statements/ resources/copd/179full.pdf. Retrieved July 26, 2013.

American Thoracic Society Subcommittee on Integrated Care of the COPD Patient: An Official American Thoracic Society Workshop Report: The integrated care of the COPD patient, 2012. From: http://www.thoracic.org/statements/resources/copd/integrated -care-of-copd-patient.pdf. Retrieved July 26, 2013.

American Thoracic Society: Guidelines for the management of adults with hospital-acquired, ventilator associated and health-care associated pneumonia, *Am J Resp Crit Care Med* 171(4):388–416, 2005.

Augustyn B: Ventilator-associated pneumonia: Risk factors and prevention, *Crit Care Nurse* 27(4):32–39, 2007.

British Thoracic Society Guidelines for the management of community acquired pneumonia in adults: Update 2009, *Thorax* 64(Suppl 3):S1–S55, 2009.

Burt C, Arrowsmith J: Respiratory failure, *Surgery* 27(11):475–479, 2009.

Centers for Disease Control and Prevention: Advisory Committee on Immunization Practices (ACIP). Recommended immunization schedule for adults age 19 years and older—United States, 2013, *MMWR* 62(1):9–19, 2013.

Centers for Disease Control and Prevention: Data and statistics, 2013. From: www.cdc.gov/tb/statistics/default.htm. Retrieved September 5, 2013.

Centers for Disease Control and Prevention: Guidelines for preventing the transmission of *Mycobacterium tuberculosis* in health-care settings, 2005, *MMWR* 54(RR–17):1–141, 2005.

Centers for Disease Control and Prevention: Interim-adjusted estimates of seasonal influenza vaccine effectiveness—United States, 2013, *MMWR* 62(7):119–123, 2013.

Global Initiative for Chronic Obstructive Lung Disease (GOLD): Pocket guide to COPD diagnosis, management, and prevention: A guide for healthcare professionals, 2013. From: http:// www.goldcopd.org/uploads/users/files/GOLD_Pocket_2013 _Mar27.pdf. Retrieved July 26, 2013.

Guyatt GH, Akl EA, Crowther M, et al: Executive summary: antithrombotic therapy and prevention of thrombosis, ed 9: American College of Chest Physicians evidence-based clinical practice guidelines, *Chest* 141(2, Suppl):7S–47S, 2012.

Jackson MM: Viewpoint: delayed diagnosis: the tuberculosis tragedy, *Am J Nurs* 106(4):3, 2006.

Kaynar AM, Sharma S: Respiratory failure, *Medscape* 2012. http:// emedicine.medscape.com/article/167981-overview.

King DA, Cordova F, Scarf SM: Nutritional aspects of chronic obstructive pulmonary disease, *Proc Am Thorac Soc* 5(4):519–523, 2008.

MacDuff A, Arnold A, Harvey J: Management of spontaneous pneumothorax: British Thoracic Society pleural disease guideline 2010, *Thorax* 65(Suppl 2):ii18–ii31, 2010.

NANDA International: *Nursing diagnoses, definitions and classifications, 2012-2014*, ed 9, Oxford, 2012, Wiley-Blackwell.

National Institute for Health and Care Excellence (NICE): Chronic obstructive pulmonary disease (update): NICE guideline, 2010. From: http://www.nice.org.uk/nicemedia/live/13029/49397/49397.pdf. Retrieved July 26, 2013.

National Tuberculosis Controllers Association: *Tuberculosis nursing: A comprehensive guide to patient care*, ed 2, Smyrna, Georgia, 2011, National Tuberculosis Controllers Association.

Smith SB, Geske JB, Maguire JM, et al: Early anticoagulation is associated with reduced mortality for acute pulmonary embolism, *Chest* 137(6):1382–1390, 2010.

World Health Organization: *WHO policy on TB infection control in health-care facilities, congregate settings and households*, France, 2009, WHO Press.

Cardiovascular Care Plans

AHA releases Guidelines for Hypertension Management in Adults With or At Risk of CAD, 2008. At: http://www.aafp.org/afp/2008/0715/p270.html.

American Heart Association Guidelines for Cardiopulmonary Resuscitation and Emergency Cardiovascular Care Science, 2010. Part 10: Acute Coronary Syndromes.

American Heart Association: *Women and cardiovascular diseases. Statistical fact sheet, 2012 update*, Dallas, 2012, AHA. http://www.heart.org/idc/groups/heart-public/@wcm/@sop/@smd/documents/downloadable/ucm_319576.pdf.

Buttaro T, Trybulski J, Bailey P, et al: *Primary care—A collaborative practice*, ed 4, 2013, pp 487–611.

Caboral M: Update on Cardiovascular Disease Prevention in Women, *AJN* 113:3, 2013.

Effectiveness-based guidelines for the prevention of cardiovascular disease in women—2011 update: a guideline from the American Heart Association.http://www.guideline.gov/content.aspx?id=33603.

Evaluation and Therapy for Heart Failure in the Setting of Ischemic Heart Disease, *J Cardiac Failure* 16(6):Section 13, 2010.

Fonarow GC, Albert NM, Curtis AB, et al: Improving evidence-based care for heart failure in outpatient cardiology practices: primary results of the Registry to Improve the Use of Evidence-Based Heart Failure Therapies in the Outpatient Setting (IMPROVE HF), *Circulation* 122(6):585–596, 2010. doi: 10.1161/CIRCULATIONAHA.109.934471. [Epub 2010 Jul 26].

Go AS, Mozaffarian D, Roger VL, et al: on behalf of the American Heart Association Statistics Committee and Stroke Statistics Subcommittee. Heart disease and stroke statistics—2013 update: a report from the American Heart Association, *Circulation* 127:e6–e245, 2013.

James PA, Oparil S, Carter BL, et al: 2014 Evidence-Based Guideline for the Management of High Blood Pressure in Adults. Report From the Panel Members Appointed to the Eighth Joint National Committee (JNC 8), *JAMA* 311(5):507–520, 2014. doi: 10.1001/jama.2013.284427.

Lauck S, Mackay M, Galte C, et al: A new option for the treatment of aortic stenosis: percutaneous aortic valve replacement, *Crit Care Nurse* 28:40–51, 2008.

McMillan S, Haley W, Zambroski C, et al: The COPE Intervention for caregivers of patients with heart failure: An adapted intervention, *JHPN* 15, 2013.

http://www.nhlbi.nih.gov/guidelines/hypertension
http://www.nhlbi.nih.gov/guidelines/cholesterol
http://www.heartfailureguideline.org/.

NANDA International: *Nursing Diagnoses, definitions and classifications, 2012-2014*, ed 9, Oxford, 2012, Wiley-Blackwell.

Pulmonary Arterial Hypertension; Future Directions: Report of National Heart, Lung, and Blood Institute/Office of Rare Diseases. http://www.nhlbi.nih.gov/meetings/workshops/pah-wksp.htm.

Radvany N, Seguritan V: *Abdominal aortic aneurysm, diagnosis*, 2008. emedicine.medscape.com.

Rothrock JC: *Alexander's care of the patient in surgery*, ed 15, St. Louis, 2014, Mosby.

Urden Li, Stacy K, Lough M: *Priorities in critical care nursing*, ed 5, St. Louis, 2008, Mosby.

Renal-Urinary Care Plans

American Nephrology Nurses' Association (ANNA) Transplantation Special Interest Group: ANNA transplantation fact sheet. www.annanurse.org.

Ardelt P, Woodhouse C, Riedmiller H, et al: The efferent segment in continent cutaneous urinary diversion: a comprehensive review of the literature, *BJU Internat* 109:288–297, 2012.

Beers MH, Berkow R, editors: *Merck geriatrics manual*, ed 4, Whitehouse Station, 2009, Merck Research Lab. Online edition.

Chadban S, Chan M, Fry K, et al: Nutritional management of diabetes mellitus in adult kidney transplant recipients, *Nephrology* 15:S37–S39, 2010.

Cleveland Clinic: Transplant medications, Retrieved from: www.myClevelandclinic.org/services/kidney_transplantation/hic_transplant_medications.aspx.

Craig S: Renal calculi: differential diagnoses and workup, *eMedicine* 2009. www.emedicine.medscape.com.

Danovitch GM, editor: *Handbook of kidney transplantation*, ed 5, Philadelphia, 2010, Lippincott Williams & Wilkins.

Gaston RS: Maintenance immunosuppression in the renal transplant recipient: An overview, *Am J Kidney Dis* 38(6 Suppl 6):S25–S35, 2001.

Gomez N: *ANNA nephrology nursing scope and standards of practice*, ed 7, Pitman, NJ, 2011, American Nephrology Nurses' Association.

Laederach-Hofmann K, Bunzel B: Non-compliance in organ transplant recipients: A literature review, *Gen Hosp Psychiatry* 22(6):412–424, 2000.

Levey AS, Greene T, Kusek JW, et al: A simplified equation to predict glomerular rate for serum creatinine, *J Am Soc Nephro* 11:155A, 2000.

Light TD, Light JA: Acute renal transplant rejection possibly related to herbal medications, *Am J Transplant* 3(12):1608–1609, 2003.

Luan FL, Samaniego M: Transplantation in diabetic kidney failure patients: Modalities, outcomes, and clinical management, *Sem Dialysis* 23(2):198–205, 2010.

Molzahn A, Butera E: *Contemporary nephrology nursing: principles and practice*, ed 2, Pitman, NJ, 2006, American Nephrology Nurses' Association.

NANDA International: *Nursing diagnoses, definitions and classifications, 2012-2014*, Oxford, 2012, Wiley-Blackwell.

National Kidney Foundation: Clinical practice guidelines and clinical practice recommendations for 2006 Updates: Hemodialysis adequacy, peritoneal dialysis adequacy and vascular access, *Am J Kidney Dis* 48(1 Suppl 1):S1–S322, 2006.

National Kidney Foundation: Clinical practice guidelines for chronic kidney disease: evaluation, classification and stratification, *Am J Kidney Dis* 39(Suppl 1):S1–S266, 2002.

National Kidney Foundation: Use of herbal supplements in chronic kidney disease. www.kidney.org/atoz/content/herbalsupp.cfm.

Newman DK: Using the BladderScan for bladder volume assessment. http://www.seekwellness.com/incontinence/using_the _bladderscan.htm. Accessed September 2013.

Neurologic Care Plans

Alexander S: *Care of the patient undergoing intracranial pressure monitoring/external ventricular drainage or lumbar drainage: AANN clinical practice guideline series*, Glenview, Illinois, 2012, American Association of Neuroscience Nurses.

Appleton R, Marson A: *Epilepsy: the facts*, ed 3, New York, 2009, Oxford University Press.

Bonner SM: Getting to the root of your patient's back pain, *Nursing* 39(7):36–41, 2009.

Bradley WG: *Treating the brain: what the best doctors know*, Washington DC, 2009, Dana Press.

Centers for Disease Control and Prevention: Seasonal influenza (flu) Guillain-Barré syndrome (GBS) Question & Answers Centers for Disease Control and Prevention, National Center for Immunization and Respiratory Diseases (NCIRD), August 23, 2012.

http://www.cdc.gov/flu/protect/vaccine/guillainbarre.htm. Accessed August 21, 2013.

Cram DL, Schrecter SH, Gao XK: *Understanding Parkinson's disease: a self-help guide*, ed 2, Omaha, 2009, Addicus Books.

Finlayson O, Kapral M, Hall R, et al: Canadian Stroke Network; Stroke Outcome Research Canada (SORCan) Working Group: Risk factors, inpatient care, and outcomes of pneumonia after ischemic stroke, *Neurology* 77(14):1338–1345, 2011. http://www.ncbi.nlm.nih.gov/pubmed/21940613. Accessed September 15, 2013. [Epub September 21, 2011].

Herbs at a Glance: A quick guide to herbal suppliments National Center for Complementary and Alternative Medicine (NCCAM), 9000 Rockville Pike, Bethesda, Maryland 20892. http://nccam .nih.gov/health/herbsataglance.htm. Accessed 14 Sep 2013.

Hickey JV: *The clinical practice of neurological and neurosurgical nursing*, ed 6, Philadelphia, 2009, Lippincott Williams & Wilkins.

Hreib KK: *100 questions & answers about stroke: A Lahey Clinic guide*, Boston, 2009, Jones and Barlett.

Jandial R, Aryan HE: *100 questions & answers about spine disorders*, Boston, 2009, Jones and Bartlett.

Mayo Clinic: *Mayo clinic guide to living with a spinal cord injury*, New York, 2009, Demos Medical Publishing.

Miller J, Mink J: Acute ischemic stroke, *Crit Care Nurs* 5(1):40–46, 2009.

NANDA International: *Nursing diagnoses, definitions and classifications, 2012-2014*, Oxford, 2012, Wiley-Blackwell.

Oran NT, Oran I: Carotid angioplasty and stenting in carotid artery stenosis: neuroscience nursing implications, *J Neurosci Nursing* 42(1):3–11, 2010.

Ross AP, Clesson I, Hartley G, et al: Practical approaches to spasticity management: A roundtable discussion, *Counseling Points* 5(2):2–13, 2009.

Simmons S: Guillain-Barré syndrome: A nursing nightmare that usually ends well, *Nursing* 40(1):24–29, 2010.

Taft KA: Raising awareness of hemorrhagic stroke. Nursing made incredibly easy! 7(4):42–52, 2009.

Thompson HJ, editor: *Care of the Patient with Seizure: AANN Clinical Practice guideline Series*, ed 2, Glenview, IL, 2009, American Association of Neuroscience Nurses. http://www.aann.org/pdf/ cpg/aannseizures.pdf. Accessed 13 Sep 2013.

Thompson HJ, editor: *Guide to the care of the hospitalized patient with ischemic stroke: AANN Clinical practice guideline series*, ed 2, Glenview, Illinois, 2012, American Association of Neuroscience Nurses.

Thompson HJ, editor: *Nursing management of adults with severe traumatic brain injury: AANN clinical practice guideline series*, Glenview, Illinois, 2012, American Association of Neuroscience Nurses.

Thompson HJ, Mauk K, editors: *Care of the patient with mild traumatic brain injury: AANN clinical practice guideline series*, Glenview, Illinois, 2012, American Association of Neuroscience Nurses.

Wyatt AH, Moreda MV, Olson DWM: Keeping the balance: understanding intracranial pressure, *Crit Care Nurs* 4(5):18–23, 2009.

Endocrine Care Plans

American Diabetes Association: Standards of medical care in diabetes mellitus, *Diabetes Care* 36(Suppl 1):S11–S66, 2013.

Bahn RS, Burch HB, Cooper DS, et al: ATA/AACE Guidelines. Hyperthyroidism and other causes of thyrotoxicosis: Management guidelines of the American Thyroid Association (ATA)/ American Association of Clinical Endocrinologists, *Endocrine Prac* 17(3):456–520, 2011.

Chamberlain L: Hyponatremia caused by polydipsia, *Crit Care Nurs* 32(3):e11–e20, 2012. www.ccnonline.org.

Faust AC, Attridge RL, Ryan L: How low should you go? The limbo of glycemic control in intensive care units, *Crit Care Nurs* 31(4):e9–e18, 2011. www.ccnonline.org.

Ganz F: Sleep and immune function, *Crit Care Nurse* 32(2):e19–e25, 2012. www.ccnonline.org.

Garber JR, Cobin RH, Gharrib H, et al: ATA/AACE Guidelines. Clinical practice guidelines for hypothyroidism in adults: Cosponsored by the American Association of Clinical Endocrinologists and the American Thyroid Association, *Endocrine Prac* 18(6):988–1028, 2012.

Handelmsan Y, Mechanick JI, Blonde L, et al: American Association of Clinical Endocrinologists medical guidelines for clinical practice for developing a diabetes mellitus comprehensive care plan, *Endocrine Prac* 17(Suppl 2):1–53, 2011.

Harrar S: Taking Diabetes Drugs with Nutritional Supplements, *Today's Dietitian* 13(11):32, 2011. http://www.todaysdietitian.com/ newarchives/110211p32.shtml.

Isaac S: Contrast-induced nephropathy: Nursing implications, *Crit Care Nurs* 32(3):41–48, 2012.

John CA, Day MW: Central neurogenic diabetes insipidus, syndrome of inappropriate ADH, and cerebral salt wasting syndrome in traumatic brain injury patients, *Crit Care Nurs* 32(2):e1–e7, 2012. www.ccnonline.org.

Jorgensen AL: Contrast-induced nephropathy: Pathophysiology and preventive strategies, *Crit Care Nurs* 33(1):37–46, 2013.

Khalaila R, Libersky E, Catz D, et al: Nurse Led Implementation of a Safe and Effective Intravenous Insulin Protocol in a Medical Intensive Care Unit, *Crit Care Nurs* 31(6):27–35, 2011.

Kitabchi AE, Umpierrez GE, Miles JM, et al: Hyperglycemic crises in adult patients with diabetes, *Diabetes Care* 32:1335, 2009.

NANDA International: *Nursing diagnoses, definitions and classifications, 2012-2014*, Oxford, 2012, Wiley-Blackwell.

New York Presbyterian Hospital Diabetic Ketoacidosis Guidelines. http://www.columbiaresidents.org/bb/DKA%20Protocol.pdf.

Porsche R, Brenner ZR: Amiodarone-induced thyroid dysfunction, *Crit Care Nurs* 26(3):34–41, 2006.

Robinson AG, Verbalis JG: Posterior pituitary. In Melmed S, Polonsky KS, Larsen PR, et al, editors: *Williams textbook of clinical endocrinology*, ed 12, St. Louis, 2011, Saunders, pp 291–323.

Gastrointestinal Care Plans

Atkinson J, Wolfe S, Hamborsky J, et al: Centers for disease control and prevention: *Epidemiology and prevention of vaccine-preventable diseases*, ed 11, Washington, DC, 2009, Public Health Foundations.

Benarroch-Gampel J, Boyd CA, Sheffield KM, et al: Overuse of computed tomography in patients with complicated gallstone disease, *J Am Coll Surg* 213(4):524–530, 2011.

Chapman R, Fevery J, Kalloo A, et al: Diagnosis and management of primary sclerosing cholangitis, *Hepatology* 51(2):660–678, 2010.

Colwell JC, Goldberg MT, Carmel JE: *Fecal and urinary diversions: management principles*, St. Louis, 2004, Mosby.

Crohn's and Colitis Foundation of America: The Facts on Crohn's and Colitis, Newly Diagnosed Kit, 2012.

Crohn's and Colitis Foundation of America: Anti-TNF and Immunomodulator Treatment Options program, 2013.

Crookes BA, Shackford SR, Gratton J, et al: "Never be wrong": the morbidity of negative and delayed laparotomies after blunt trauma, *J Trauma* 69(6):1386–1391, discussion 1391–1392, 2010. [Medline].

DiCiaula A, Wang D, Wang H, et al: Targets for current pharmacological therapy in cholesterol gallstone disease, *Gastroenterol Clin North Am* 39:245–264, 2010.

Dienstag JL: Acute viral hepatitis. In Longo DL, Kasper DL, Jameson JL, et al, editors: *Harrison's principles of internal medicine*, ed 18, New York, 2012, McGraw Hill.

Dienstag JL: Toxic and drug-induced hepatitis. In Longo DL, Kasper DL, Jameson JL, et al, editors: *Harrison's principles of internal medicine*, ed 18, New York, 2012, McGraw Hill.

Dienstag JL: Chronic hepatitis. In Longo DL, Kasper DL, Jameson JL, et al, editors: *Harrison's principles of internal medicine*, ed 18, New York, 2012, McGraw Hill.

Duncan CB, Riall TS: Evidence-based current surgical practice: Calculous gallbladder disease, *J Gastrointestinal Surg* 16:2011–2025, 2012.

Elfaki DA, Lindor KD: Antibiotics for the treatment of sclerosing cholangitis, *Am J Thera* 18:261–265, 2011. http://emedicine.medscape.com/article/1980980-overview/.

Emergency Nurses Association: *Sheehy's emergency nursing: Principles and practice*, ed 6, Des Peres, Illinois, 2009, ENA.

Friedman LS: Liver, biliary tract, and pancreas disorders. In Papadakis MA, McPhee SJ, editors: *Current medical diagnosis & treatment*, ed 52, New York, 2013, McGraw Hill.

Ghany MG: An update on treatment of genotype I chronic hepatitis C virus infection: 2011 practice guidelines by the American association for the study of liver diseases, *Hepatology* 54(4):1433–1444, 2011.

Goci E, Shkreli R, Haloci E, et al: Complementary and alternative medicine (CAM) for pain, herbal anti-inflammatory drugs, *Eur Sci J* 9(9):90–105, 2013.

Goldberg M, Aukett LK, Carmel J, et al: Management of the patient with a fecal diversion: best practice guidelines for clinicians, *Wound Ostomy Continence Nurs Soc* 2010.

Griffin N, Grant LA, Anderson S, et al: Small bowel MR enterography: problem solving in Crohn's disease, *Insights Imaging* 3(3):251–263, 2012.

Iacucci M, Panaccione R, Ghosh S: Advances in novel diagnostic endoscopic imaging techniques in inflammatory bowel disease, *Inflam Bowel Dis* 19(4):873–880, 2013.

Koning M, Ailabouni R, Gearry RB, et al: Use and predictors of oral complementary and alternative medicine by patients with inflammatory bowel disease: a population-based, case-control study, *Inflam Bowel Dis* 19(4):767–778, 2013.

Krawczyk M, Stokes CS, Lammert F: Genetics and treatment of bile duct stones, *Curr Opin Gastroenterol* 29:329–335, 2013.

Landy J, Al-Hassi HO, McLaughlin SD, et al: Etiology of pouchitis, *Inflam Bowel Dis* 18(6):1146–1155, 2013.

LeMone P, Burke K, Bauldoff G: *Medical-surgical nursing: critical thinking in patient care*, ed 5, Boston, 2011, Pearson.

Loomba R, Rivera M, McBurney R, et al: The natural history of acute hepatis C: clinical presentation, laboratory findings and treatment outcomes, *Aliment Pharmacol Ther* 33(5):559–565, 2011.

MacLeod R, Vella-Brincat J, Macleod AD: *The palliative care handbook: guidelines for clinical management and symptom control*, ed 6, Auckland, New Zealand, 2012, Soar Printers.

Mahid SS, Jafri NS, Brangers BC, et al: Meta-analysis of cholecystectomy in symptomatic patients with positive hepatobiliary iminodiacetic acid scan results without gallstones, *Arch Surg* 144(2):180–187, 2009.

Mayo Clinic: Appendicitis. MayoClinic.com (website), from: http://www.mayoclinic.com/health/appendicitis/DS00274. Retrieved August 17, 2013.

NANDA International: *Nursing diagnoses, definitions and classifications, 2012-2014*, Oxford, 2012, Wiley-Blackwell.

Nishijima D, Simel D, Wisner D, et al: Does this adult patient have a blunt intra-abdominal injury?, *JAMA* 307(14):1517–1527, 2012. doi: 10.1001/jama.2012.422.

Pagana KD, Pagana TJ: *Mosby's diagnostics and laboratory test reference*, ed 4, St. Louis, 2009, Mosby.

Saljoughian M: Intravenous radiocontrast media: a review of allergic reactions, *US Pharm* 37(5):HS-14–HS-16, 2012.

Sheffield KM, Ramos KE, Dijukom CD, et al: Implementation of a critical pathway for complicated gallstone disease: Translation of population-based data into clinical practice, *J Am Col Surg* 212(5):835–843, 2011.

Silen W: Acute appendicitis and peritonitis. In Longo DL, Kasper DL, Jameson JL, et al, editors: *Harrison's principles of internal medicine*, ed 18, New York, 2012, McGraw Hill.

Somers MS: *Diseases and disorders: A nursing therapeutics manual*, ed 4, Philadelphia, 2011, FA Davis.

Udeani J: Blunt abdominal trauma, 2013. http://emedicine.medscape.com/article/1980980-overview.

Vallerand AH, Sanoski CA, Deglin JH, editors: *Davis' drug guide for nurses*, ed 13, Philadelphia, 2013, FA Davis.

Wu BE, Conwell DL: Acute pancreatitis part I: Approach to early management, *Clin Gastroenterol Heoatol* 8:410, 2010.

Zheng W, Xu G, Wu G, et al: Laparoscopic exploration of common bile duct with primary closure versus t-tube drainage: a randomized clinical trial, *J Surg Res* 157:e1–e5, 2009.

Hematologic Care Plans

Antle E: Who needs therapeutic phlebotomy?, *Clin J Oncol Nurs* 14:694–696, 2010.

Arnold DM, Nazi I, Warkentin TE, et al: Approach to the diagnosis and management of drug-induced immune thrombocytopenia, *Trans Med Rev* 27:137–145, 2012.

Balducci L: Anemia, fatigue, and aging, *Transfusion Clinique et Biologique* 17:375–381, 2010.

Bross MH, Soch K, Smith-Knuppel T: Anemia of older persons, *Am Fam Phys* 82:480–487, 2010.

Diz-Kucukkaya R, Chen J, Geddis A, et al: Thrombocytopenia, Chapter 119. In Lichtman MA, Kipps TJ, Seligsohn U, et al, editors: *Williams hematology*, ed 8, New York, 2010, McGraw-Hill. http://www.accessmedicine.com. Accessed 1/9/2012.

Dressler DK: Coagulopathy in the intensive care unit, *Crit Care Nurs* 32:48–59, 2012.

Greenberg H: Polycythemia vera—An evidence-based examination from a nursing perspective, *Crit Care Nurs Q* 36:228–232, 2013.

Hunt CW: Immune thrombocytopenia purpura, *Med Surg Nurs* 19:237–239, 2010.

Imbach P, Crowther M: Thrombopoietin-receptor agonists for primary immune thrombocytopenia, *New Engl J Med* 365:734–741, 2011.

Kirsch M, Klaassen RJ, DeGeest S, et al: Understanding the importance of using patient-reported outcome measures in patients with immune thrombocytopenia, *Sem Hematol* 50(Suppl 1):539–542, 2013.

Koury MJ, Rhodes M: How to approach chronic anemia, *Am Soc Hematol Ed Prog* 12:183–190, 2012.

Kremyanskaya M, Mascarenhas J, Hoffman R: Why does my patient have erythrocytosis?, *Hematol Oncol Clin N Am* 26:267–283, 2012.

Legendre CM, Licht C, Muus P, et al: Terminal complement inhibitor eculizumab in atypical hemolytic-uremic syndrome, *N Engl J Med* 368:2169–2181, 2013.

Leung L: Clinical features, diagnosis, and treatment of disseminated intravascular coagulation in adults, 2013. www.UpToDate.com. Accessed July 31, 2013.

Lichtman MA, Kaushansky K, Kipps TJ, et al: *Williams manual of hematology*, ed 8, New York, 2011, McGraw-Hill.

Little JA, Benz EJ, Gardner LB: Anemia of chronic disease, Chapter 35. In Hoffman R, Benz EJ, Silberstein LE, et al, editors: *Hematology: Basic principles and practice*, ed 6, Philadelphia, 2013, Elsevier. http://mdconsult.com. Accessed August 1, 2013.

Levi M: Disseminated intravascular coagulation, Chapter 141. In Hoffman R, Benz EJ, Silberstein LE, et al, editors: *Hematology: Basic principles and practice*, ed 6, Philadelphia, 2013, Elsevier Chapter 35, http://www.mdconsult.com. Accessed August 1, 2013.

Levi M, Meijers JC: Which laboratory tests are most useful, *Blood Rev* 25:33–37, 2011.

NANDA International: *Nursing diagnoses, definitions and classifications, 2012-2014*, Oxford, 2012, Wiley-Blackwell.

Neunert C, Lim W, Crowther M, et al: The American Society of Hematology 2011 evidence-based practice guideline for immune thrombocytopenia, *Blood* 117:4190–4207, 2011.

Pandit TN, Sarode R: Blood component support in acquired coagulopathic conditions: Is there a method to the madness?, *Am J Hematol* 87:S56–S62, 2012.

Randolf TR: Myloproliferative neoplasms (Chapter 34). In Rodak BF, Fritsma GA, Keohane EM, editors: *Hematology: Clinical principles and applications*, St. Louis, 2012, Elsevier, pp 508–532.

Rivera JA, O'Hare AM, Harper GM: Update on the management of chronic kidney disease, *Am Fam Phys* 86:749–754, 2012.

Rodgers GM, Blinder M, Cella D, et al: Cancer—and chemotherapy-induced anemia, NCCN Clinical Practice Guidelines in Oncology version 2. 2014. Available at www.nccn.org.

Sadler J, Poncz M: Antibody-mediated thrombotic disorders: Thrombotic thrombocytopenic purpura and heparin-induced thrombocytopenia (Chapter 133). In Lichtman MA, Kipps TJ, Seligsohn U, et al, editors: *Williams hematology*, ed 8, New York, 2010, McGraw-Hill. http://www.accessmedicine.com. Accessed January 9, 2012.

Schrier SL, Camaschella C: Anemia of chronic disease (anemia of chronic inflammation), 2013. www.UpToDate.com. Accessed July 29, 2013.

Silverberg DS, Wexler D, Iaina A, et al: Anaemia management in cardio renal disease, *J Renal Care* 36(Suppl 1):86–96, 2010.

Sink BLS: Administration of blood components. In Rodak JD, Grossman BJ, Harris T, et al, editors: *Technical manual: Standards for blood banks and transfusion services*, ed 17, Bethesda, 2011, AABB., pp 617–629.

Strenger M: Update on romiplostim therapy for immune thrombocytopenic purpura, *Comm Oncol* 8:224–228, 2011.

Tefferi A: Myeloproliferative neoplasms 2012: The John M. Bennet 80th birthday anniversary lecture, *Leukemia Res* 36:1481–1489, 2012.

Tefferi A: Polycythemia vera and essential thrombocythemia: 2012 update on diagnosis, risk-stratification, *Am J Hematol* 88:507–516, 2013.

Tsai H: Untying the knot of thrombotic thrombocytopenic purpura and atypical hemolytic uremic syndrome, *Am J Med* 126:200–209, 2013.

Warkentin TE: Heparin-induced thrombocytopenia in critically ill patients, *Crit Care Clin* 27:805–823, 2011.

Winkeljohn D: Idiopathic thrombocytic purpura, *Clin J Oncol Nurs* 14:411–413, 2010.

Musculoskeletal Care Plans

Abel LE: Metabolic bone conditions. In *NAON: Core curriculum for orthopaedic nursing*, ed 7, Chicago, 2013, NAON, pp 377392.

AlloSource: Allografts, 2013. http://www.allosource.org/medical-professionals/allografts.

American Academy of Orthopaedic Surgeons (AAOS): Bone grafts in spine surgery, 2010. http://orthoinfo.aaos.org/topic.cfm?topic=a00600.

American Academy of Orthopaedic Surgeons (AAOS) and American Association of Tissue Banks (AATB): Bone and tissue transplantation, 2009. http://orthoinfo.aaos.org/topic.cfm?topic=a00115.

American College of Rheumatology: Rheumatoid arthritis, 2012. http://www.rheumatology.org/practice/clinical/patients/diseases_and_conditions/ra.pdf.

Arthritis Foundation: Arthritis Today's drug guide, 2013. http://www.arthritistoday.org/treatments/drug-guide/index.php.

Arthritis Foundation: Arthritis Today's supplement and herb guide, 2013. http://www.arthritistoday.org/treatments/supplement-guide/index.php.

Arthritis Foundation: Get the facts, 2013. http://www.arthritis.org/conditions-treatments/understanding-arthritis/.

Arthritis Foundation: Lab test guide, 2013. http://www.arthritistoday.org/tools-and-resources/tools/lab-test-guide.php.

Arthritis Foundation: Nutritional guidelines for people with rheumatoid arthritis, 2013. http://www.arthritistoday.org/about-arthritis/types-of-arthritis/rheumatoid-arthritis/daily-life/nutrition/rheumatoid-arthritis-diet-2.php.

Arthritis Foundation: Rheumatoid arthritis treatment: remission is possible, 2013. http://www.arthritistoday.org/conditions/

rheumatoid-arthritis/ra-treatment/rheumatoid-arthritis-remission
.php.

Arthritis Foundation, Association of State and Territorial Health Officials, and Centers for Disease Control and Prevention: National arthritis action plan: a public health strategy, 1999. http://www.arthritis.org/media/Delia/NAAP_full_plan.pdf.

Cash JJ, Weinblatt ME, Kavahaugh A: *Rheumatoid arthritis: early diagnosis and treatment*, ed 3, West Islip, New York, 2010, Professional Communications.

Institute of Medicine: Dietary reference intakes for calcium, phosphorus, magnesium, vitamin D, and fluoride, 1997. http://www.nap.edu/openbook.php?record_id=5776.

International Association for the Study of Pain: Faces pain scale—Revised, 2013. http://www.iasp-pain.org/Content/Navigation Menu/GeneralResourceLinks/FacesPainScaleRevised/default.htm.

Karanikolas M, Aretha D, Monantera G, et al: Optimized perioperative analgesia reduces chronic phantom limb pain intensity, prevalence, and frequency: A prospective, randomized, clinical trial, *Anesthesiology* 114:1144–1154, 2011.

Klippel JH, editor: *Primer on the rheumatic diseases*, ed 13, Atlanta, 2008, Arthritis Foundation.

Kunkler CE: Therapeutic modalities. In *NAON: Core curriculum for orthopaedic nursing*, ed 7, Chicago, 2013, NAON, pp 233–262.

NANDA International: *Nursing diagnoses, definitions and classifications, 2012-2014*, Oxford, 2012, Wiley-Blackwell.

National Osteoporosis Foundation: Exercise for strong bones. http://www.nof.org/articles/238.

National Osteoporosis Foundation: Learn about osteoporosis. http://www.nof.org/learn/basics.

National Osteoporosis Foundation: Managing and treating osteoporosis. hhttp://www.nof.org/live/treating.

National Osteoporosis Foundation: Types of osteoporosis medication. http://www.nof.org/articles/22.

Office of Dietary Supplements, National Institutes of Health: Calcium, 2013. http://ods.od.nih.gov/factsheets/Calcium -HealthProfessional/.

Office on Women's Health, U.S. Department of Health and Human Services: Menopausal hormone therapy (MHT), 2010. http://www.womenshealth.gov/menopause/symptom-relief-treatment/menopausal-hormone-therapy.cfm.

Parker R: Orthopaedic complications. In *NAON: Core curriculum for orthopaedic nursing*, ed 7, Chicago, 2013, NAON, pp 191–216.

Partners Against Pain: Wong-Baker FACES Pain Rating Scale, 2009. http://www.partnersagainstpain.com/printouts/A7012AS6.pdf.

Roberts D: Care of the patient with hip, foot and ankle problems. In Mosher CM, editor: *An introduction to orthopaedic nursing*, ed 4, Chicago, 2004, NAON, pp 67–84.

Roberts D: Nursing management: Arthritis and connective tissue disease. In Lewis SL, Dirksen SR, Heitkemper MM, et al, editors: *Medical-surgical nursing: assessment and management of clinical problems*, ed 8, St. Louis, 2011, Mosby, pp 1641–1679.

Roberts D: Arthritic and connective tissue disorders. In *NAON: Core curriculum for orthopaedic nursing*, ed 7, Chicago, 2013, NAON, pp 335–376.

Stanford Medicine 25: #18 Ankle brachial index, 2013. http://stanfordmedicine25.stanford.edu/the25/ankle.html.

Subedi B, Grossberg GT: Phantom limb pain: Mechanisms and treatment approaches, *Pain Res Treat* 2011. doi: 10.1155/2011/864605.

The Merck Manuals Online Medical Library: Acute infectious arthritis, 2013. http://www.merckmanuals.com/professional/musculoskeletal_and_connective_tissue_disorders/infections_of_joints_and_bones/acute_infectious_arthritis.html?qt=&sc=&alt=l.

The Merck Manuals Online Medical Library: Osteoporosis, 2013. http://www.merckmanuals.com/professional/musculoskeletal_and_connective_tissue_disorders/osteoporosis/osteoporosis.html?qt=&sc=&alt.

Turcotte E: Orthopaedic effects of immobility. In *NAON: Core curriculum for orthopaedic nursing*, ed 7, Chicago, 2013, NAON, pp 141–158.

U.S. Food and Drug Administration: FDA drug safety communication: Ongoing safety review of oral bisphosphonates and atypical subtrochanteric femur fractures, 2010. http://www.fda.gov/Drugs/DrugSafety/PostmarketDrugSafetyInformationforPatientsandProviders/ucm203891.htm.

U.S. Food and Drug Administration, Forteo, 2008. http://www.accessdata.fda.gov/drugsatfda_docs/label/2008/021318s015lbl.pdf.

Special Needs Care Plans

Alpers DH, Stenson WF, Taylor BE, et al, editors: *Manual of nutritional therapeutics*, ed 5, Philadelphia, 2008, Lippincott Williams & Wilkins.

Bankhead R, Boullata J, Brantley S, et al: Enteral nutrition practice recommendations, *J Parenter Enteral Nutr* 33:122–167, 2009.

Braden Scale for Predicting Pressure Sore Risk. www.bradenscale.com/braden.PDF.

Bryant RA, Nix DP: *Acute & chronic wounds: Current management concepts*, ed 4, St. Louis, 2010, Elsevier.

Centers for Disease Control and Prevention: Monitoring selected national HIV prevention and care objectives by using HIV surveillance data—United States and 6 U.S. dependent areas—2010. HIV Surveillance Supplemental Report 2012;17(No. 3, part A) http://www.cdc.gov/hiv/pdf/statistics_2010_HIV_Surveillance_Report_vol_17_no_3.pdf. Published June 2012.

Cohen MS, Chen YQ, McCauley M, et al: Prevention of HIV-1 Infection with Early Antiretroviral Therapy, *N Engl J Med* 365:493–495, 2011. doi: 10.1056/NEJMoa110524.

Franz MG, Robson MC, Steed DL, et al: Wound Healing Society. Guidelines to aid healing of acute wounds by decreasing impediments of healing, *Wound Repair Regen* 16(6):723–748, 2008.

Guo S, Dipietro LA: Factors affecting wound healing, *J Dent Res* 89(3):219–229, 2010.

Kim H, Stotts NA, Froelicher ES, et al: Why patients in critical care do not receive adequate enteral nutrition? A review of the literature, *J Crit Care* 27(6):702–713, 2012.

Kuppinger DD, Rittler P, Harti WH, et al: Use of gastric residual volume to guide enteral nutrition in critically ill patients: A brief systematic review of clinical studies, *Nutrition* 29:1075–1079, 2013.

Lim SL, Ong KCB, Chan YH, et al: Malnutrition and its impact on cost of hospitalization, length of stay, readmission and 3-year mortality, *Clin Nutrition* 31:345–350, 2012.

Marian M, McGinnis C: Overview of Enteral Nutrition. In Gottschlich MM, editor: *The A.S.P.E.N. Nutrition Support Core Curriculum: A case-based approach—the adult patient*, Silver Spring, Maryland, 2007, American Society of Parenteral and Enteral Nutrition.

McMahon MM, Nystrom E, Braunschweig C, et al: A.S.P.E.N. clinical guidelines: Nutrition support of adult patients with hyperglycemia, *J Parenter Enteral Nutr* 37(1):23–36, 2013.

NANDA International: *Nursing diagnoses, definitions and classifications, 2012-2014*, Oxford, 2012, Wiley-Blackwell.

National Pressure Ulcer Advisory Panel and European Pressure Ulcer Advisory Panel: *Prevention and treatment of pressure ulcers: Clinical practice guideline*, Washington, DC, 2009, National Pressure Ulcer Advisory Panel.

Panel on Antiretroviral Guidelines for Adults and Adolescents: *Guidelines for the use of antiretroviral agents in HIV-1-infected adults and adolescents*. Department of Health and Human Services. http://aidsinfo.nih.gov/contentfiles/lvguidelines/Adultand AdolescentGL.pdf.

Panel on Opportunistic Infections in HIV-Infected Adults and Adolescents: *Guidelines for the prevention and treatment of opportunistic infections in HIV-infected adults and adolescents: Recommendations from the Centers for Disease Control and Prevention, the National Institutes of Health, and the HIV Medicine Association of the Infectious Diseases Society of America* http://aidsinfo.nih.gov/contentfiles/lvguidelines/adult_oi.pdf.

Panel on Treatment of HIV-Infected Pregnant Women and Prevention of Perinatal Transmission: *Recommendations for use of antiretroviral drugs in pregnant HIV-1-infected women for maternal health and interventions to reduce perinatal HIV transmission in the United States.* http://aidsinfo.nih.gov/contentfiles/lvguidelines/PerinatalGL.pdf.

Rhoda KM, Porter MJ, Quintini C: Fluid and electrolyte management: Putting a plan in motion, *J Parenter Enteral Nutr* 35:675–685, 2011.

Sibbald RG, Goodman L, Woo KY, et al: Special considerations in wound bed preparation 2011: an update, *Adv Skin Wound Care* 24(9):415–436, quiz 437–438, 2011.

Swanson B: *ANAC's core curriculum for HIV/AIDS nursing*, ed 3, Sudbury, MA, 2009, Jones & Bartlett.

Tappenden KA, Quatrara B, Parkhurst ML, et al: Critical role of nutrition in improving quality of care: An interdisciplinary call to action to address adult hospital malnutrition, *Medsurg Nurs* 22(3):147–165, 2013.

Ukleja A, Sanchez-Fermin M: Gastric versus post-pyloric feeding: relationship to tolerance, pneumonia risk, and successful delivery of enteral nutrition, *Curr Gastroenterol Rep* 9:309–316, 2007.

Whitney J, Phillips L, Aslam R, et al: Guidelines for the treatment of pressure ulcers, *Wound Repair Regen* 14(6):663–679, 2006.

Windle EM, Beddow D, Hall E, et al: Implementation of an electromagnetic imaging system to facilitate nasogastric and post-pyloric feeding tube placement in patients with and without critical illness, *J Hum Nutr Diet* 23(1):61–68, 2010.

Part II: Pediatric Nursing Care Plans

Administration for Children and Families, U.S. Department of Health and Human Services: Child maltreatment 2012, Summary, December 2013 www.acf.hhs.gov/programs/research-data-technology/statistics-research/child-maltreatment. Accessed October 14, 2013, and September 29, 2014.

American Academy of Pediatrics: ADHD: Clinical practice guideline for diagnosis, evaluation, and treatment of attention-deficit/hyperactivity disorder in children and adolescents, *Pediatrics* 128(5):1007–1022, 2011.

American Academy of Pediatrics: Clinical practice guideline: Diagnosis and management of bronchiolitis, *Pediatrics* 118(4):1774–1793, 2006.

American Academy of Pediatrics: Clinical practice guideline: Diagnosis and management of acute otitis media, *Pediatrics* 131(3):e946–e999, 2013.

American Academy of Pediatrics: Clinical practice guideline: Management of newly diagnosed type 2 diabetes mellitus (T2DM) in children and adolescents, *Pediatrics* 131(2):364–382, 2013.

American Academy of Pediatrics: Policy statement—prevention of rotavirus disease: Updated guidelines for use of rotavirus vaccine, *Am Acad Pediatr* 123(5):1412–1420, 2009. http://aappolicy.aappublications.org. Accessed March 11, 2010.

American Association of Poison Control Centers: 2011 Annual report of the national poison data system, *Clin Toxicol* 50:911–1164, 2012. www.aapcc.org (click on NPDS/Poison Data, then click on Annual Reports). Accessed October 10, 2013.

American Diabetes Association: Standards of medical care in diabetes—2014, *Diabetes Care* 37(supplement1):s14–s80; 36(supplement 1):S11–S66, 2014. http://care.diabetesjournals.org/content/37/Supplement_S14.full.pdf. Accessed September 29, 2014.

American Heart Association News release: Children with sickle cell disease 221 times more likely to suffer stroke, new American Heart Association statement reveals americanheart.mediaroom.com/index.php?s=43&item=488. Accessed March 13, 2010.

American Lung Association: Asthma & children fact sheet, October 2012. www.lungusa.org/lung-disease/asthma/resources/. Accessed October 10, 2013.

Baskin MN, Goh XL, Heeney MM, et al: Bacteremia risk and outpatient management of febrile patients with sickle cell disease, *Pediatrics* 131(6):1035–1041, 2013.

Becker L, Goobie K, Thomas S: Advising families on AD/HD: a multimodal approach, *Pediatr Nurs* 35(1):47–52, 2009.

Bond GR, Woodward RW, Ho M: The growing impact of pediatric pharmaceutical poisoning, *J Pediat* 160(2):265–270.e1, 2012. www.jpeds.com/article/S0022-3476(11)00771-2/abstract. Accessed October 10, 2013.

Centers for Disease Control and Prevention: Managing acute gastroenteritis among children: Oral rehydration, maintenance, and nutritional therapy, *MMWR* 52(RR16):1–16, 2003. www.cdc.gov/mmwr/preview/mmwrhtml/rr52161a1.htm. Accessed July 14, 2006; March 3, 2010; and October 13, 2013.

Centers for Disease Control and Prevention: Mental health surveillance among children—United States 2005-2011, *MMWR* 62(2):1–35. www.cdc.gov/mmwr. Enter title of report in search box. Accessed October 16, 2013.

Centers for Disease Control and Prevention: National diabetes statistics report, 2014. www.cdc.gov/diabetes/pubs/statsreport14.htm. Accessed October 3, 2014.

Centers for Disease Control and Prevention: Clinical information: Rotavirus 2011 www.cdc.gov/rotavirus/. Accessed October 14, 2013.

Centers for Disease Control and Prevention: Data & Statistics: Sickle Cell Disease, 2011. www.cdc.gov/ncbddd/sicklecell. Accessed October 13, 2013.

Centers for Disease Control and Prevention: RSV: Infection and incidence, 2010. www.cdc.gov/rsv/about/infection.html. Accessed October 12, 2013.

Centers for Disease Control and Prevention: RSV: Transmission, 2010. www.cdc.gov/rsv/about/transmission.html. Accessed October 12, 2013.

Centers for Disease Control and Prevention: Safe kids: poisonings: the reality. www.cdc.gov/safechild. Last updated April 12, 2012. Accessed October 10, 2013.

Centers for Disease Control and Prevention: Trends and outbreaks: Norovirus 2013. www.cdc.gov/norovirus/trends-outbreaks.html. Accessed October 14, 2013.

Chase HP, Maahs DM: *Understanding diabetes*, ed 12, Denver, 2011, Barbara Davis Center for Childhood Diabetes at Denver.

Chiang J, Kirkman M, Laffel L, et al: Type 1 diabetes through the life span: A position statement of the American Diabetes Association, *Diabetes Care* 37(7):2034–2054, 2014. www.care.diabetesjournal.org/content/early/2014/06/09/dc14-1140.full.pdf. Accessed September 30, 2014.

Child Help: National child abuse statistics: Child abuse in America www.childhelp.org.pages/statistics. Accessed October 15, 2013, and September 29, 2014.

Coco A, Vernacchio L, Horst M, et al: Management of acute otitis media after publication of 2004 AAP and AAFP clinical practice guidelines, *Pediatrics* 125(2):214–220, 2010.

Consumer Product Safety Commission: 2013 Fireworks annual report, 2014. http://www.cpsc.gov//Global/Research-and-Statistics/Injury-Statistics/Fuel-Lighters-and-Fireworks/2013 FireworksReport.pdf. Accessed September 27, 2014.

Cortese MM, et al: Effectiveness of monovalent and pentavalent rotavirus vaccine, *Pediatrics* 132(1):e25–e33, 2013.

Crowe JE: March of Dimes: RSV. www.marchofdimes.com/spotlights/print/spotlight-on-james-e-crowe-md.html. Accessed October 12, 2013.

Cystic Fibrosis Foundation: About cf www.cff.org. Accessed October 9, 2013.

Cystic Fibrosis Foundation: *Managing cystic fibrosis-related diabetes (CFRD)*, ed 5, St. Louis, 2011. www.cff.org/treatments/Therapies/Nutrition/Diabetes. Accessed October 10, 2013.

D'Auria JP: All about asthma: Top resources for children, adolescents, and their families, *J Pediatric Health Care* 27(4):e39–e42, 2013.

Flaherty EG, MacMillan HL: and Committee on Child Abuse and Neglect: Clinical report: Caregiver-fabricated illness in a child: A manifestation of child maltreatment, *Pediatrics* 132(3):590–597, 2013.

Hall AJ, Lopman BA, Payne DC, et al: Norovirus disease in the United States, *Emerg Infect Dis* 19(8):1198–1205, 2013.

Hockenberry MJ, Wilson D, editors: *Wong's nursing care of infants and children*, ed 9, St. Louis, 2011, Mosby.

Hojer J, Troutman WG, Hoppu K, et al: Position paper update: Ipecac syrup for gastrointestinal decontamination, *Clin Toxicol* 51(3):134–139, 2013.

Hornor G: Child maltreatment: Screening and anticipatory guidance, *J Pediatric Health Care* 27(4):242–250, 2013.

Hornor G: Medical evaluation for child physical abuse: What the PNP needs to know, *J Pediatric Health Care* 26(3):163–170, 2012.

Jenny C, Crawford-Jukubiak JE: Clinical Report: The evaluation of children in the primary care setting when sexual abuse is suspected, *Pediatrics* 132(2):e558–e567, 2013. www.pediatrics.aapublications.org/content/early/2013/07/23/peds. Accessed October 3, 2013.

Kalydeco: Kalydeco (ivacaftor): The first and only FDA-approved medication to treat the underlying G551D-CCTR protein defect. www.kalydeco.com. Accessed October 10, 2013.

Lehman L: Sickle cell anemia stroke prevention efforts may have decreased racial disparities in childhood stroke deaths. American Stroke Association Meeting Report—Abstract 2602/MP72. 2012 http://newsroom.heart.org/news/. Enter sickle cell anemia stroke in childhood Accessed October 14, 2013.

Manworren RCB, Hyman LS: Clinical validation of FLACC: preverbal patient pain scale, *Pediatr Nurs* 29(2):140–146, 2003.

MedicineNet.com: Tobramycin inhalation solution-oral, tobi www.medicinenet.com/tobramycin_inhalation_solution-oral/page4.htm. Accessed October 10, 2013.

Moran A, Brunzell C, Cohen RC, et al: Clinical care guidelines for Cystic Fibrosis-Related Diabetes, *Diabetes Care* 33(12):2697–2708, 2010.

NANDA International: *Nursing diagnoses, definitions and classifications, 2012-2014*, Oxford, 2012, Wiley-Blackwell.

National Asthma Education and Prevention Program: Expert panel report 3 (EPR 3). Guidelines for the diagnosis and management of asthma: summary report, National Heart, Lung, and Blood Institute. NIH publication number 08-5846, 2007. www.nhlbi.nih.gov/guidelines/. Accessed January 15, 2010; October 12, 2013; and September 2014.

National Center for Health Statistics—Vital and Health Statistics Series 10, No. 258: Summary Health Statistics for U.S. Children: National Health Interview Survey, 2012, published December 2013. www.cdc.gov/nchs/nhis.htm search for Summary Health Statistics for US Children, then click on Series 10 # 258. Accessed October 10, 2013, and September 28, 2014.

National Heart, Lung, and Blood Institute: Asthma care quick reference: Diagnosing and managing asthma, published 2012 www.nhlbi.nih.gov/guidelines/asthma/asthma_quickref.htm. Accessed October 10, 2013.

National Heart, Lung, and Blood Institute, National Institute of Health: Diseases and conditions index: sickle cell anemia—How is sickle cell anemia diagnosed? www.nhlbi.nih.gov/health/dci/Diseases/Sca/SCA.html and click on Diagnosis. Updated September 28, 2012. Accessed September 28, 2014.

National Institute of Mental Health: Attention deficit hyperactivity disorder (ADHD) rev 2012. NIH Publication 12-3572 www.nimh.nih.gov/health/publications. Publications listed by topic—click on Attention Deficit Hyperactivity Disorder (ADHD) 4 items, 2nd booklet. Accessed September 28, 2014.

National Institutes of Health, National Heart Lung and Blood Institute: *The management of sickle cell disease, NIH Publication No. 02-2117*, ed 4, 2002. www.scinfo.org/health-care-providers. Accessed July 22, 2006; March 15, 2010; and September 28, 2014.

New York Times Health Guide: Sickle cell anemia: Prognosis, March 14, 2013. http://www.nytimes.com/health/guides/disease/sickle-cell-anemia/prognosis.html. Accessed October 13, 2013.

Nicholson KN: Screening for cystic fibrosis: What every NP should know, *Nurse Pract* 38(9):24–32, 2013.

Pagana KD, Pagana TJ: *Mosby's diagnostic and laboratory test reference*, ed 11, St. Louis, 2009, Mosby Elsevier.

Parks SE, Annest JL, Hill HA, et al: Pediatric abusive head trauma. National Center for Injury: Prevention & Control: Division of Violence Prevention: CDC, April 2012. www.cdc.gov/violenceprevention/pdf/pedheadtrauma-a.pdf. Accessed October 12, 2013.

Pichichero ME: Otitis media, *Pediatr Clin North Am* 60(2):391–407, 2013.

Platt AF, Eckman J, Hsu L: *Hope & destiny: The patient and parent's guide to sickle cell disease and sickle cell trait*, ed 3, Indianapolis, 2011, Hilton Publishing.

Safe Kids: Burns and fire safety fact sheet, 2014. www.safekids.org/. Then enter Burns & Fire Safety Fact Sheet in search box. Accessed September 27, 2014.

Safe Kids: Poison prevention fact sheet, 2013. www.safekids.org/our-work/research/fact-sheets/. Accessed October 10, 2013.

Safe Kids: Research report: An in-depth look at keeping young children safe around medicine, 2013. www.safekids.org. Accessed October 10, 2013.

Schrub T, Caple C, Pravikoff D: Evidence-based care sheet: Diabetes Mellitus, type 2: Prevention in children and adolescents. Cinahl

Information System (Glendale, CA.), 2013. Accessed October 16, 2013.

Scott L: Presence of Type 2 diabetes risk factors in children, *Pediatr Nurs* 39(4):190–196, 2013.

Shriners Hospitals for Children: Preventing scald injuries www.shrinershospitalsforchildren.org/en/Hospitals/BurnAwareness/ScaldInjuries.aspx. Accessed October 12, 2013.

Skidmore-Roth L: *Mosby's 2014 nursing drug reference*, ed 27, St. Louis, 2014, Elsevier.

Strayer DA, Schub T, Pravikoff D: Diabetes mellitus, type 2: prevention in children and adolescents. *CINAHL Nursing Guide*, Ipswich, MA, August 21, 2009, Cinahl Information Systems (evidence-based care sheet).

Taketoma CK, Hodding JH, Kraus DM: *Pediatric & neonatal dosage handbook*, ed 20, Hudson, OH, 2013, American Pharmaceutical Association, Lexi-Comp.

Tschudy MM, Arcara KM: *The Johns Hopkins Hospital: The Harriet Lane handbook*, ed 19, Philadelphia, 2012, Mosby.

U.S. Consumer Product Safety Commission: 2010 fireworks annual report, June 2011, www.cpsc.gov/pagesfiles/110031/2010fwreport.pdf. Accessed October 13, 13.

U.S. Fire Administration: Fire risk to children in 2010. Topical fire report series 2013;14(8) www.usfa.fema.gov/downloads/pdf/statistics/v14i8.pdf. Accessed September 27, 2014.

Wilson D, Hockenberry MJ: *Wong's clinical manual of pediatric nursing*, ed 8, St. Louis, 2012, Mosby.

Yawn B, Buchanan G, Afenyi-Annan A, et al: Management of sickle cell disease: Summary of the 2014 evidence-based report by expert panel members, *JAMA* 312(10):1033–1048, 2014.

Part III: Maternity Nursing Care Plan

American College of Obstetrics and Gynecology: *Diagnosis and management of preeclampsia and eclampsia. ACOG practice bulletin no. 33*, Washington, DC, 2002.

American College of Obstetrics and Gynecology: *Gestational diabetes, practice bulletin no. 137*, Washington DC, 2013.

American College of Obstetrics and Gynecologists: *Prediction and prevention of preterm birth. Practice bulletin no. 130*, Washington, DC, 2012.

American College of Obstetrics and Gynecologists: *Management of preterm labor. Practice bulletin no.127*, Washington, DC, 2012.

American College of Obstetricians and Gynecologists (ACOG): *Postpartum hemorrhage, ACOG practice bulletin no. 76*, Washington, DC, 2006, American College of Obstetricians and Gynecologists.

American Diabetes Association: *Diabetes in pregnancy. Management of diabetes and its complications from pre-conception to the postnatal period*, 2008, National Guidelines Clearinghouse. http://www.nationalguidelinesclearinghouse.gov. Accessed August 8, 2013.

American Diabetes Association: Position statement: Diagnosis and classification of diabetes mellitus. http://care.diabetesjournals.org/content/36/Supplement_1/S67.full. Accessed August 8, 2013.

Burke C: Pain in labor: Non pharmacologic and pharmacologic management. In Simpson K, Creehan P, editors: *Perinatal nursing*, ed 4, Philadelphia, 2014, Lippincott, Williams & Wilkins, pp 493–520.

Cashion K: Endocrine and metabolic disorders in pregnancy. In Lowdermilk DL, Perry SE, Cashion K, et al, editors: *Maternity nursing*, ed 10, St. Louis, 2012, Mosby, pp 688–690.

Craighead D: Early Term birth: Understanding the health risks to infants, *Nurs Womens Health* 16(2):136–143, 2012.

Ezzo J, Streitberger K, Sneider A: Cochrane Systematic Reviews examine P6 acupuncture-point stimulation for nausea and vomiting, *J Altern Complement Med* 12(5):489–495, 2006.

Fejzo MS, Poursharif B, Korst LM, et al: Symptoms and pregnancy outcomes associated with extreme weight loss among women with hyperemesis gravidarum, *J Womens Health* 18(12):1981–1987, 2009.

Gabel K, Weeber T: Measuring and communicating blood loss during obstetric hemorrhage, *J Obstet Gynecol Neonatal Nurs* 41(4):551–558, 2012.

Gilbert ES: *Manual of high-risk pregnancy and delivery*, ed 5, St Louis, 2011, Mosby, pp 200–242.

Hale T: *Medications & mothers milk*, ed 14, Amarillo, Texas, 2008, Hale Publishing.

Hamilton BE, Martin JA, Ventura MA: Births: Preliminary data for 2010, *DHHS CDC National Center for Health Statistics* 60(2):1–36, 2011.

Jorgensen AM: Late preterm birth: a rising trend, *Nurs Womens Health* 12(4):308–315, 2008.

Levine R, Vatten L, Horowitz G, et al: Preeclampsia, soluble FMS-like tyrosine kinase 1 and the risk of reduced thyroid function: Nested case control and population based study, *BMJ* 339:b4336, 2009.

Lo J, Mission J, Caughey A: Hypertensive disease of pregnancy and maternal mortality, *Curr Opin Obstet Gynecol* 25(2):124–132, 2013.

Lowdermilk DL: Postpartum complications. In Lowdermilk DL, Perry SE, Cashion K, et al, editors: *Maternity & women's health care*, ed 10, St. Louis, 2012, Mosby. pp 833–835.

Lyndon A, Miller S, Huwe V, et al: Blood loss: Clinical techniques for ongoing quantitative evaluation, 2010. California Maternal Quality Care Collaborative. http://www.cmqcc.org/resources/ob_hemorrhage/ob_hemorrhage_best_practice_articles_v1_4_alphabetical_order. Accessed August 10, 2013.

McCune B: Caring for the woman experiencing complications during the postpartal period. In Ward SL, Hisley M, editors: *Maternal-child nursing care: Optimizing outcomes for mothers, children, and families*, Philadelphia, 2009, Davis.

Mullin P, Ching C, Shoenberg F, et al: Risk factors, treatments, and outcomes associated with prolonged hyperemesis gravidarum, *J Matern Fetal Neonat Med* 25(6):632–636, 2012.

NANDA International: *Nursing diagnoses, definitions and classifications, 2012-2014*, Oxford, 2012, Wiley-Blackwell.

National Collaborating Centre for Women's and Children's Health: *Diabetes in pregnancy. Management of diabetes and its complications from pre-conception to the postnatal period. Clinical guideline no. 63*, London, 2008, National Institute for Health and Clinical Excellence.

National Institute for Health and Clinical Excellence: *Diabetes in pregnancy overview*, London, 2014.

Rath W, Fischer T: The diagnosis and treatment of hypertensive disorders of pregnancy: new findings for antenatal and inpatient care, *Deutsches Arzteblatt Int* 106(45):733–780, 2009.

Romero R, Nicolaides K, Conde-Agudelo A, et al: Vaginal progesterone in women with an asymptomatic sonographic short cervix in the mid-trimester decrease preterm delivery and neonatal morbidity: A systematic review and metaanalysis of individual patient data, *Am J Obstet Gynecol* 206(2):124e1–124.e19, 2012. doi10.1016/ajog.2011.12.003.

Simpson KR: New evidence for reconsideration of normal labor progress, *Am J Matern Child Nurs* 37(6):408, 2012.

Simpson KR, Miller L: Assessment and optimization of uterine activity during labor, *Clin Obstet Gynecol* 54(1):40–49, 2011.

Simpson KR, O'Brien-Abel N: Labor and birth. In Simpson K, Creehan P, editors: *Perinatal nursing*, ed 4, Philadelphia, 2014, Lippincott, Williams & Watkins, pp 343–373.

Smaill FM, Gyle GM: Antibiotic prophylaxis vs. no prophylaxis for prevention of infection after cesarean section, *Cochran Review* 2010.

Smith J, Carey A: Common neonatal complications. In Simpson K, Creehan P, editors: *Perinatal nursing*, ed 4, Philadelphia, 2014, Lippincott, Williams & Wilkins, p 664.

Sosa M: Bleeding in pregnancy. In Simpson K, Creehan P, editors: *Perinatal nursing*, ed 4, Philadelphia, 2014, Lippincott, Williams & Wilkins, pp 143–160.

Tharpe N: Postpregnancy genital tract and wound infections, *J Midwifery Womens Health* 53(3):236–246, 2008.

Tipton A, Cohen S, Chelmow D: Wound infection in the obese pregnant woman, *Semin Perinatol* 35(6):345–349, 2011.

Wegrzyniac L, Repke J, Ural S: Treatment of hyperemesis gravidarum, *Rev Obstet Gynecol* 5(2):78–84, 2012.

Zhang J, Lindy H, Branch W, et al: Contemporary patterns of spontaneous labor with normal neonatal outcomes, *Obstet Gynecol* 116(6):1281–1287, 2010.

Part IV: Psychiatric Nursing Care Plans

Alcohol withdrawal syndrome, *Am Fam Physician* 69(6):1443–1450, 2004.

Alzheimer's Association: *Alzheimer's Disease Facts and Figures*, *Alzheimer's & Dementia*, vol 8, Issue 2, 2012.

American Nurses Association: *Psychiatric-mental health nursing practice: Scope and standards of practice*, Silver Spring, Maryland, 2007, ANA.

American Psychiatric Association: *Diagnostic and statistical manual of mental disorders*, ed 5, 2013. http://dx.doi.org/10.1176/appi.books.9780890425596.910646.

Anxiety Disorders Association of America: Statistics and facts about anxiety disorders, 2010. www.adaa.org/mediaroom/index.cfm.

Bayard M, Mcintyre J, Hill K, et al: Quillen College of Medicine, Johnson City, Tennessee.

Beck AT, Rector NA, Stolar N, et al: *Schizophrenia: Cognitive theory, research, and therapy*, New York, 2008, Guilford Press.

Beng-Choon H, Black DW, Andreasen NC: Schizophrenia and other psychotic disorders. In Hales RE, Yudofsky SC, editors: *Essentials of clinical psychiatry*, ed 3, Washington, DC, 2008, American Psychiatric Publishing.

Brown RL, Rounds LA: Conjoint screening questionnaires for alcohol and other drug abuse: Criterion validity in a primary care practice, *Wis Med J* 94(3):135–140, 1995.

Bulechek G, Butcher HK, Dochterman JM: *Nursing interventions classification (NIC)*, ed 6, St. Louis, 2012, Mosby.

Carson VB, Vanderhorst KJ: Becoming an Alzheimer's whisperer: Taking market share, *Caring Magazine* 28(8):36–40, 42, 2009.

Carson VB, Vanderhorst KJ: Becoming an Alzheimer's whisperer: A strategy to lovingly manage challenging behaviors, *Monroe County Women's Journal* 10, 2009.

Carson VB, Vanderhorst KJ: Communicating as an Alzheimer's whisperer, *Monroe County Women's Journal* 11, 2009.

Cruz M, Pincus HA, Welsh DE, et al: The relationship between religious involvement and clinical status of patients with bipolar disorder, *Bipolar Disord* 12:68–76, 2010.

Donald W, Reynolds Foundation: *The portal of geriatrics online education: Recommended geropsychiatric competency enhancement for entry level professional nurses. Geriatric and Palliative Medicine*, New York, 2013, Mount Sinai.

Dubovsky SL, Davies R, Dubovsky AN: Mood disorders. In Hales RE, Yudofsky SC, editors: *Essentials of clinical psychiatry*, ed 3, Washington, DC, 2010, American Psychiatric Publishing.

Heffner JL, Strawn JR, DelBello MP, et al: The co-occurrence of cigarette smoking and bipolar disorder: Phenomenology and treatment considerations, *Bipolar Disord* 13:439–453, 2011.

Kaplan BJ, Kaplan VA: *Kaplan & Sadock's concise textbook of clinical psychiatry*, ed 3, Philadelphia, 2008, Lippincott Williams & Wilkins.

Karch A: *2014 Lippincott's nursing drug guide*, Philadelphia, 2014, Lippincott, Williams & Wilkins.

Lehne RA: *Pharmacology for nursing care*, ed 7, Philadelphia, 2009, Saunders.

Lum G: Lithium self-intoxication treated with hemodialysis, *Lab Med* 38(11):667–668, 2007.

Mace N, Rabins P: *The 36-hour day: A family guide to caring for people with Alzheimer's disease, other dementias, and memory loss*, ed 5, New York, 2012, Grand Central Life and Style.

NANDA International: *Nursing diagnoses, definitions and classifications, 2012-2014*, Oxford, 2012, Wiley-Blackwell.

National Clinical Guideline Centre for Acute and Chronic Conditions: *Alcohol-use disorders. Diagnosis and clinical management of alcohol-related physical complications: Clinical guideline no. 100*, London, 2010, National Institute for Health and Clinical.

Stuart GW: *Principles and practice of psychiatric nursing*, ed 9, St. Louis, 2009, Elsevier.

Sullivan JT, Sykora K, Schneiderman J, et al: Assessment of alcohol withdrawal: The revised Clinical Institute Withdrawal Assessment for Alcohol scale (CIWA-Ar), *Br J Addict* 84:1353–1357, 1989.

Varcarolis E: *Essentials of psychiatric mental health nursing*, St. Louis, 2012, Elsevier.

Appendix A

Centers for Disease Control and Prevention: Guidelines for preventing opportunistic infections among hematopoietic stem cell transplant recipients: Recommendations of CDC, the Infectious Disease Society of America, and the American Society of Blood and Marrow Transplantation, MMWR 49(RR-10), 1–125, 2007.

Centers for Disease Control and Prevention: Guidelines for preventing the transmission of Mycobacterium tuberculosis in healthcare settings, MMWR 54(RR-17), 1–141, 2005. From http://www.cdc.gov/mmwr/preview/mmwrhtml/rr5417a1.htm. Retrieved June 13, 2014.

O'Grady NP, Alexander MA, Burns LA, et al: The guidelines for the prevention of intravascular catheter related infections. From http://www.cdc.gov/hicpac/pdf/guidelines/bsi-guidelines-2011.pdf. Retrieved June 13, 2014.

Siegel JD, Rhinehart E, Jackson M, Chiarello L and the Healthcare Infection Control Practices Advisory Committee: Management of multidrug-resistant organisms in healthcare settings. Centers for Disease Control and Prevention 2006. From http://www.cdc.gov/hicpac/pdf/MDRO/MDROGuideline2006.pdf. Retrieved June 13, 2014.

Siegel JD, Rhinehart E, Jackson M, Chiarello L, and the Healthcare Infection Control Practices Advisory Committee: Guideline for isolation precautions: Preventing transmission of infectious agents in healthcare settings. Centers for Disease Control and Prevention 2007. From http://www.cdc.gov/hicpac/pdf/isolation/Isolation2007.pdf. Retrieved June 13, 2014.

Nursing Diagnoses Index

A

Activity intolerance

anemia, acute or chronic lung changes, surgery, cancer, 18-19

decreased cardiac contractility with heart failure, 174-175

decreased RBCs in anemias of chronic disease, 469

inefficient work of breathing with COPD, 113-114

intestinal inflammatory process in Crohn's disease, 425

need for rest to prevent effects of activity on advancing PTL, 686

right and left ventricular failure with pulmonary arterial hypertension, 183-184

Activity intolerance, risk for

deconditioned status with prolonged bedrest, 61-63

with slowed metabolism and decreased cardiac output in hypothyroidism, 387

weakness

with anemia and uremia in CKD, 207-209

arthralgia, myalgia, dyspnea, fever, pain, hypoxia, and effects of chemotherapy in HIV/AIDS, 528-529

bedrest following cardiac surgery, 150

with tissue ischemia post-MI, 155-156

Acute confusion

age-related, altered sensory/perceptual reception, brain oxygenation, 90-92

altered sensory integration, reception, and transmission, space-occupying lesions in CNS, or HIV dementia, 527

cerebral retention of water in hypothyroidism, 389

dehydration or cerebral edema associated with DKA, 369

irrigation fluid with BPH; cerebral hypoxia with sepsis, 198-199

Acute confusion, risk for

neurosensory changes occurring with cerebral accumulation of ammonia or GI bleeding in cirrhosis, 418-419

neurosensory changes with ARF, 192-194

normal process of death and dying and its effects on the body, 108-110

Acute pain

angina, 154-155

arthritic joint changes and associated therapy in osteoarthritis, 505-506

bladder spasms

with BPH, 201

with urinary tract obstruction, 240

blood hyperviscosity in polycythemia, 475-476

Cervical dilation, contractions, full bladder, muscle stretching for a woman in labor, 638

disease process

injury, surgical procedure, 39-44

surgical intervention, or treatment effects for cancer, 5

fracture and other injury, 606

headache

occurring with TBI, 346

photophobia, neck stiffness with bacterial meningitis, 264

Headache, angina, pruritus, abdominal/joint discomfort with polycythemia, 475

impaired pleural integrity, chest tube, surgery, 125

increased pressure in the middle ear occurring with fluid and/or infection, otitis media, 617-618

inflammatory process

in appendicitis, 407

fever, and tissue damage in peritonitis, 456

of pancreas, 443-444

injury, surgical repair, and/or rehabilitation therapy for fractures, 491

intestinal inflammatory process

in Crohn's disease, 424

in ulcerative colitis, 462-463

irritation, trauma or surgical incision, or manipulation of organs during surgery, 399

joint discomfort with hemorrhagic episodes or blood extravasation into the tissues in thrombocytopenia, 482

muscle tenderness, hypersensitivity to touch in Guillain-Barré syndrome, 272-273

obstructive or inflammatory process in cholelithiasis, cholecystitis, and cholangitis, 410-411

phantom limb sensation, 485-486

prolonged immobility, chemotherapy, neoplasms, infections, and peripheral neuropathy in HIV/AIDS, 528

spasms, headache, photophobia with neurologic dysfunction, 256

subtotal thyroidectomy surgical procedure, 382-383

thermal injuries and medical-surgical interventions, 575

thrombus formation with VTE, 187

tissue anoxia with vasoocclusion in sickle cell pain crisis, 627-628

unfamiliarity with pain control measures in intervertebral disk disease, 276-278

ureteral calculus or surgical procedure to remove it, 225

uterine contractions, distention of lower uterine segment, cervical changes, pressure on adjacent tissues, or tissue trauma, 645

Adult failure to thrive

loss of independence or functional abilities, depression, malnutrition, chronic disease, 101-102

normal process of death and dying and its effects on the body, 108-110

Adverse reaction to iodinated contrast media, risk for

Administration during CT scan procedure, 407

Allergy response, risk for

Immunomodulator and biologic/anti-TNF medications in Crohn's disease, 425

Peristomal hypersensitivity (contact dermatitis) with fecal diversion, 430

Anticipatory grieving, risk for

potential fetal loss that could occur with PPROM, 699

Anxiety

actual or perceived threat to self or fetus in diabetes in pregnancy, 653-654

illness, loss of control, and medical/nursing management of illness, asthma, 553

Index

Page numbers followed by "f" indicate figures, "t" indicate tables, and "b" indicate boxes.

Index